Designing functional foods

Related titles:

Understanding and controlling the microstructure of complex foods
(ISBN 978-1-84569-151-6)
Awareness of the interrelationship between the nanoscopic, microscopic and macroscopic features of foods and their bulk physiochemical properties, sensory attributes and healthfulness is increasing. It is now widely recognised that creation of novel foods or improvement of existing products depends largely on a better understanding of this complex interrelationship. This important collection presents current understanding of significant aspects of food structure and methods for its control. The main structural elements in foods, their interactions and newer analytical techniques for structure assessment are reviewed. Subsequent chapters then discuss the use of structural design principles in product development and structural issues in particular foods, such as ice cream and chocolate.

Delivery and controlled release of bioactives in foods and nutraceuticals
(ISBN 978-1-84569-145-5)
Active ingredients in foods must remain fully functional for as long as necessary and be transported and discharged appropriately to have the desired nutritional effect. Controlled release and delivery systems are used to achieve these aims. Edited by a leading expert in the field, this collection discusses materials and techniques for the controlled release and delivery of nutraceuticals. Opening chapters review factors affecting nutrient bioavailability and methods to test delivery system efficacy. Part II addresses materials used and specific techniques, such as nanoemulsions. The final chapters focus on the delivery of particular nutraceuticals, such as vitamins and probiotics.

Food, diet and obesity
(ISBN 978-1-85573-958-1)
Obesity is a global epidemic, with significant numbers of adults and children overweight or obese in many developed and developing countries. As a result, there is an unprecedented level of interest and research in the complex interactions between our genetic susceptibility, diet and lifestyle in determining individual risk of obesity. With its distinguished editor and international team of contributors, this collection sums up the key themes in weight control research, focusing on their implications and applications for food product development and consumers.

Designing functional foods

Measuring and controlling food structure breakdown and nutrient absorption

Edited by
D. Julian McClements and Eric A. Decker

CRC Press
Boca Raton Boston New York Washington, DC

WOODHEAD PUBLISHING LIMITED
Oxford Cambridge New Delhi

Published by Woodhead Publishing Limited, Abington Hall, Granta Park,
Great Abington, Cambridge CB21 6AH, UK
www.woodheadpublishing.com

Woodhead Publishing India Private Limited, G-2, Vardaan House, 7/28 Ansari Road,
Daryaganj New Delhi – 110002, India

Published in North America by CRC Press LLC, 6000 Broken Sound Parkway, NW,
Suite 300, Boca Raton, FL 33487, USA

First published 2009, Woodhead Publishing Limited and CRC Press LLC

British Library Cataloguing in Publication Data
A catalogue record for this book is available from the British Library.

Library of Congress Cataloging in Publication Data
A catalog record for this book is available from the Library of Congress.

Woodhead Publishing ISBN 978-1-84569-432-6 (book)
Woodhead Publishing ISBN 978-1-84569-660-3 (e-book)
CRC Press ISBN 978-1-4200-9485-5
CRC Press order number: WP9485

The publishers' policy is to use permanent paper from mills that operate a sustainable forestry policy, and which has been manufactured from pulp which is processed using acid-free and elemental chlorine-free practices. Furthermore, the publishers ensure that the text paper and cover board used have met acceptable environmental accreditation standards.

Typeset by SNP Best-set Typesetter Ltd., Hong Kong
Printed by TJ International Limited, Padstow, Cornwall, UK

Contents

Contributor contact details

(* = main contact)

Chapter 1

Dr A. van der Bilt
Dept. of Oral-Maxillofacial Surgery
Prosthodontics and Special
Dental Care
Faculty of Medicine
University Medical Center Utrecht
Str 4.115
Universiteitsweg 100
3584 CG Utrecht
The Netherlands

E-mail: a.vanderbilt@umcutrecht.nl

Chapter 2

H. J. Flint*, S. H. Duncan and
P. Louis
Microbial Ecology Group
Rowett Institute of Nutrition
and Health
University of Aberdeen
Greenburn Road
Bucksburn
Aberdeen
AB21 9SB
UK

E-mail: h.flint@rowett.ac.uk

Chapter 3

Professor D. Lairon
INSERM, 476; INRA, 1260
Université de la Méditerranée
Nutriments Lipidiques et
Prévention des Maladies
Métabolique
Faculté de médecine
27 Bd Jean Moulin
13385 Marseille cedex 05
France

E-mail: Denis.Lairon@medecine.
univ-mrs.fr

Chapter 4

C. M. Lo and P. Tso*, PhD
Department of Pathology &
Laboratory Medicine
University of Cincinnati Medical
Center
2120 E. Galbraith Road, Bldg. A
Cincinnati, OH 45237
USA

E-mail: tsopp@email.uc.edu

Chapter 5

A. C. Ouwehand*, K. Tiihonen, H. Mäkeläinen and N. Rautonen
Health & Nutrition
Danisco
02460 Kantvik
Finland

E-mail: cultures@danisco.com; Arthur.ouwehand@danisco.com

O. Hasselwander
Technology & Business Development
Danisco
Redhill
RH1 6YS
UK

G. Sworn
Innovation & Technology Development
Danisco
75017 Paris
France

Chapter 6

P. J. Moughan
Riddet Institute
Massey University
Palmerston North
New Zealand

E-mail: p.j.moughan@massey.ac.nz

Chapter 7

Dr M. J. Amiot-Carlin
INRA
UMR1260
Nutriments Lipidiques et Prévention des Maladies Métabolique
INSERM
U476
Université Aix-Marseille
Faculté de Médecine
IPHM-IFR 125
Marseille
F-13385
France

E-mail: Marie-Jo.Amiot-Carlin@medecine.univ-mrs.fr

Chapter 8

Professor Dr F. A. Tomás-Barberán*, Dr A. Gil-Izquierdo and Dr D. A. Moreno
Research Group on Quality, Safety and Bioactivity of Plant-based Foods
Food Science and Technology Department
CEBAS-CSIC
PO Box 164
Campus Universitario de Espinardo
E-30100 Espinardo
Murcia
Spain

E-mail: fatomas@cebas.csic.es

Chapter 9

S. Lahtinen, N. Rautonen and A. Ouwehand*
Danisco Finland H&N
Sokeritehtaantie 20
02460 Kantvik
Finland

E-mail: cultures@danisco.com; Arthur.ouwehand@danisco.com

A. Henrikson
Danisco Singapore
61 Science Park Road
Singapore 117525

P. Steele
Danisco USA
3329 Agriculture Drive
Madison
WI 53716
USA

Chapter 10

Dr I. A. M. Appelqvist
CSIRO
11 Julius Avenue
Riverside Corporate Park
North Ryde
NSW 2113
Australia

E-mail: Ingrid.Appelqvist@csiro.au

Chapter 11

A. J. Taylor
Division of Food Sciences
University of Nottingham
Sutton Bonington Campus
Loughborough
LE12 5RD
UK

E-mail: andy.taylor@nottingham.ac.uk

Chapter 12

K. Venema*, R. Havenaar and M. Minekus
TNO Quality of Life
Dept. BioSciences
PO Box 360
3700 AJ Zeist
The Netherlands

E-mail: koen.venema@tno.nl

Chapter 13

R. Glahn
USDA-ARS
Courtesy Associate Professor of Food Science and Division of Nutrition
Robert W. Holley Center for Agriculture and Health
Cornell University
Tower Road
Ithaca
NY 14853
USA

E-mail: rpg3@cornell.edu

Chapter 14

Professor R. Spiller* and Dr L. Marciani
Nottingham Digestive Diseases Centre Biomedical Research Unit
C Floor South Block
Nottingham University Hospitals
Queen's Medical Centre Campus
University of Nottingham
Nottingham
NG7 2UH
UK

E-mail: Robin.Spiller@nottingham.ac.uk; Luca.Marciani@nottingham.ac.uk

Professor P. Gowland
Sir Peter Mansfield Magnetic Resonance Centre
School of Physics and Astronomy
University of Nottingham
Nottingham
NG7 2RD
UK

E-mail: Penny.Gowland@nottingham.ac.uk

Chapter 15

H. Xiao
Department of Food Science
University of Massachusetts
100 Holdsworth Way
Amherst
MA 01003
USA

E-mail: hangxiao@foodsci.umass.edu

Chapter 16

S. A. Abrams
United States Department of Agriculture/Agricultural Research Service
Children's Nutrition Research Center
Department of Pediatrics
Sections of Nutrition and Neonatology
Baylor College of Medicine and Texas Children's Hospital
Houston
TX 77030
USA

E-mail: sabrams@bcm.edu

Chapter 17

Dr S. Bayarri and Professor Dr E. Costell*
Instituto de Agroquímica y Tecnología de Alimentos. CSIC
PO Box 73
46100 Burjassot
Valencia
Spain

E-mail: ecostell@iata.csic.es

Chapter 18

G. J. van den Oever, J. Busch, E. van der Linden, G. Smit and N. J. Zuidam*
Unilever Research and Development
Olivier van Noortlaan 120
PO Box 114
3130 AC Vlaardingen
The Netherlands

E-mail: klaas-jan.zuidam@unilever.com

Chapter 19

G. A. van Aken*, E. H. A. de Hoog
TI Food and Nutrition
Nieuwe Kanaal 9A
PO Box 557
6700 AN Wageningen
The Netherlands

G. A. van Aken and
Els H. A. de Hoog
NIZO Food Research
Kernhemseweg 2
PO Box 20
6710 BA Ede
The Netherlands

E-mail: george.van.aken@nizo.nl

M. H. Vingerhoeds
TI Food and Nutrition

and

Wageningen University and
Research Centre
Centre for Innovative Consumer
Studies
Bornsesteeg 59
PO Box 17
6700 AA Wageningen
The Netherlands

Chapter 20

D. J. McClements and E. A. Decker
Department of Food Science
University of Massachusetts
Amherst
MA 01003
USA

E-mail: mcclements@foodsci.
umass.edu; edecker@foodsci.
umass.edu

Chapter 21

G. Zhang
Jiangnan University
Wuxi
China

Z. Ao
Mead Johnson Nutrition
2400 W. Lloyd Expressway
Evansville
IN 47721
USA

B. R. Hamaker*
Whistler Center for Carbohydrate
Research
Purdue University
West Lafayette
IN 47907
USA

E-mail: hamakerb@purdue.edu

Chapter 22

Professor L. Chen
Department of Agricultural
Food and Nutritional Science
Agriculture/Forestry Center
University of Alberta
Edmonton
AB
Canada
T6G 2P5

E-mail: lingyun.chen@ualberta.ca

Chapter 23

Dr T. J. Foster*
Division of Food Sciences
School of Biosciences
University of Nottingham
Sutton Bonington Campus
Loughborough
Leicestershire
LE12 5RD
UK

E-mail: tim.foster@nottingham.ac.uk

Professor I. T. Norton
Department of Chemical Engineering
University of Birmingham
Edgbaston
Birmingham
B15 2TT
UK

E-mail: nortonit@bham.ac.uk

Chapter 24

R. M. A. J. Ruijschop, MSc*, K. M. M. Burseg, PhD, T. T. Lambers, PhD, and J. Overduin, PhD
NIZO Food Research
Kernhemseweg 2
PO Box 20
6710 BA Ede
The Netherlands

E-mail: Rianne.Ruijschop@nizo.nl

Chapter 25

G. S. M. J. E. Duchateau* and W. Klaffke
Unilever Research and Development
Olivier van Noortlaan 120
PO Box 114
3130 AC Vlaardingen
The Netherlands

E-mail: guus.duchateau@unilever.com

Chapter 26

I. Amar-Yuli, A. Aserin and Professor N. Garti*
Casali Institute of Applied Chemistry
The Institute of Chemistry
Givat Ram Campus
The Hebrew University of Jerusalem
Jerusalem 91904
Israel

E-mail: garti@vms.huji.ac.il

Preface

During the past decade or so there has been an increasing awareness by the food industry that the composition and structural organization of the components within a food matrix can strongly increase or decrease the bioavailability and/or bioactivity of any nutritional components that it contains. In principle, the digestion, absorption and biological activity of functional food components can therefore be controlled by altering the nature of the food matrix. Consequently, there has been an increasing emphasis on studying the complex relationship between the composition and structure of food matrices on the one hand, and the bioactivity of specific food components on the other. Ultimately, the knowledge gained from these studies will facilitate the rational design and fabrication of foods known to enhance, reduce or control the biological activity of specific food components. Hence, the bioactivity of potentially beneficial food components could be increased, whereas that of potentially detrimental food components could be decreased. This is a particularly exciting field of research because it brings together scientists from a wide range of different disciplines, including food chemistry, microbiology, physics, engineering, physiology, nutrition, medicine, physics and sensory science. In addition, the results of this research could lead to the availability of a diverse range of high-quality and economic foods that have beneficial effects on the health and wellbeing of the general population.

This book provides a comprehensive overview of some of the most important current areas of research on the rational design of functional foods. The first section contains chapters that review the physiology of the mouth and gut, as well as the digestion and adsorption of major functional food components (lipids, carbohydrates, fibers, proteins, peptides, vitamins, minerals, probiotics, nutraceuticals, etc.). The second section contains chapters on the various research methods that are needed to study the digestion, absorption and bioactivity of food components. This section includes reviews of methods for measuring the behavior of foods in the mouth, the release of flavors from foods, and the simulation of the behavior of foods and their digestion products as they pass through the gastrointestinal tract using *in vitro* physicochemical, cell culture and animal models. Part III focuses on the implications of understanding the impact of food composition and structure on the bioactivity of food components for the rational design of functional foods. It includes sections on designing food structure so as to: reduce fat content; to improve flavor; to control the bioavailability and bioactivity of specific food components (lipids, carbohydrates, proteins, nutraceuticals); and to induce satiety. We hope that this book will stimulate further research in this growing area, and that it will provide the food industry with valuable information that will lead to the production of novel, high-quality functional foods.

Finally, we must thank all of the authors of the various chapters for taking valuable time out of their busy schedules to contribute to this project. We also thank all of the excellent editorial staff at Woodhead Publishing for their invaluable support in selecting, contacting and following up authors for their chapters. Without their help this book would not have been possible. Finally, we would like to thank our families, friends and colleagues for all their help and support throughout the process of editing the book.

D. Julian McClements
Eric A. Decker
University of Massachusetts

Part I

Digestion and absorption of food components

1

Oral physiology, mastication and food perception

A. van der Bilt, University Medical Center Utrecht, The Netherlands

Abstract: During chewing, food is reduced in size, while saliva moistens the food and binds the masticated food into a bolus that can be easily swallowed. Characteristics of the oral system, such as bite force, number of teeth and salivary flow, will influence the masticatory process. Properties of the food, such as hardness, moisture and fat content, will also have an influence on chewing. Numerous receptors in the mouth and nose respond to the ingested food and monitor the changes during chewing. This leads to perception of taste, odour and texture of the food. An overview of the neuromuscular control of chewing and swallowing is presented. Finally, the influence of age on oral physiology, food perception and nutrient intake is discussed.

Key words: oral physiology, mastication, food perception, neuromuscular control of chewing and swallowing, nutrient intake.

1.1 Introduction

Chewing is the first step in the process of digestion and is meant to prepare the food for swallowing and further processing in the digestive system. In the mouth, the food is subjected to several mechanical and chemical processes. Taste and texture of the food are perceived and have their influence on the chewing process. The water in the saliva moistens the food particles, whereas the salivary mucins bind masticated food into a coherent and slippery bolus that can be easily swallowed.

In Section 1.2 oral factors determining the chewing result are introduced. The teeth are important in the masticatory system. They form the occlusal area where the food particles are fragmented. This fragmentation depends on the total occlusal area and thus on the number of teeth. Another important factor in mastication is the bite force. The bite force depends on muscle volume and jaw muscle activity. Furthermore, the production of sufficient saliva is indispensable for good chewing.

Section 1.3 deals with the influence of food characteristics on chewing. For instance, water and fat percentage and hardness of the food are known to influence the masticatory process. Food hardness is sensed during mastication and affects masticatory force, jaw muscle activity and movements of the lower jaw.

Food perception is discussed in Section 1.4. Numerous receptors in the oral cavity and nose respond to the initially ingested food and monitor the changes during processing. This leads to central perceptions of taste, odour, and texture of the food. Most sensations associated with food texture occur only when the food is manipulated, deformed or moved across the oral receptors.

In Section 1.5 an overview of the neuromuscular control of chewing and swallowing is presented. Mastication is a complex process, involving activities of various jaw muscles and the tongue. These activities result in patterns of rhythmic jaw movements, food manipulation and the crushing of food between the teeth. The movement of the jaw, and thus the coordination between the various chewing muscles, plays an important role in the fragmentation of the food.

In Section 1.6 the influence of age on oral physiology, food perception and nutrient intake is discussed. Oral physiological parameters such as jaw muscle force, dental state, salivary flow and composition, and oral sensitivity are influenced by age. The changed oral physiology may influence perception of taste, odour and texture of the food. As a result food choice may be altered, which could lead to inadequate nutrient intake. Future trends are discussed in Section 1.7.

1.2 Food processing in the mouth

All ingested solid foods, regardless of bite size and initial texture, are processed in a stereotyped way by humans (Hiiemae *et al.*, 1978; Hiiemae, 2004; German *et al.*, 2004). After ingestion, the food is transported from the front of the mouth to the occlusal surfaces of the post-canine teeth (Stage I transport); and then the food is processed by a series of masticatory cycles needed to comminute and soften the food (food processing stage). The number of processing cycles increases as foods become more difficult to chew. When food is ready to be swallowed, it is propelled posteriorly into the oropharynx (Stage II transport). Food accumulates in the oropharynx until it is finally swallowed (Pedersen *et al.*, 2002). The initiation of swallowing, which is voluntary, has been thought to depend on separate thresholds for food particle size and for particle lubrication (Hutchings and Lillford, 1988). However, instead of this duality, it has also been suggested that swallowing is initiated when it is sensed that a batch of food particles is bound together under viscous forces so as to form a bolus (Prinz and Lucas, 1997).

1.2.1 Influence of oral physiology on chewing

Characteristics of the oral system, such as bite force, number of teeth and salivary flow rate, will influence the masticatory process, e.g. size reduction of food particles, salivation and mixing of food particles into a food bolus that can be swallowed. The number of chewing cycles needed to prepare food for swallowing (stage I transport until swallowing), defined here as swallowing threshold or moment of swallowing, is fairly constant within a subject for one type of food, whereas large variations in the number of chewing cycles until swallowing were observed among subjects (Lucas and Luke, 1986; Fontijn-Tekamp *et al.*, 2004). For instance, the number of chewing cycles needed to swallow 9.1 cm^3 of peanuts varied between 17 and 110 in a group of 87 dentate subjects (Engelen *et al.*, 2005). Furthermore, the moment of swallowing appeared to be strongly correlated among various natural foods (Fontijn-Tekamp *et al.*, 2004; Engelen *et al.*, 2005). This means that subjects who used a small number of chewing cycles for one food consistently also used small numbers for all types of food. This implies that there are 'slow' and 'fast' swallowers (subjects who swallow any food after a relative low or high number of cycles, respectively). This is partly the result of the individual's physiology, but possibly also of the social context.

Figure 1.1 illustrates the large variation in chewing behaviour among people. The jaw movement, rectified muscle activity, and muscle work (product of jaw gape and muscle activity) are shown for two healthy subjects (A and B). The subjects were instructed to chew and swallow a piece of bread (13 cm^3). Subject A chewed 8 times on the bread and then swallowed it (upper three rows), whereas the second subject chewed the bread 34 times, thus more than four times longer, before he swallowed it (lower three rows). Figure 1.1 clearly illustrates that muscle work decreases while mastication proceeds and the food bolus is softened.

1.2.2 Masticatory performance and swallowing

Masticatory performance can be determined by quantifying the degree of fragmentation of an artificial test food (Optosil, a silicon rubber) after a fixed number of chewing cycles (van der Bilt *et al.*, 1993). Subjects chew on cubes of Optosil with an edge size of 5.6 mm for 15 chewing strokes. The degree of fragmentation of the chewed food is determined by sieving the food through a stack of sieves. The amount of test food on each sieve is weighed and the median particle size of the chewed food particles is determined from the weight distribution of particle sizes. The degree of fragmentation of the chewed food is well described by the median particle size. A small median particle size after a fixed number of chewing cycles indicates

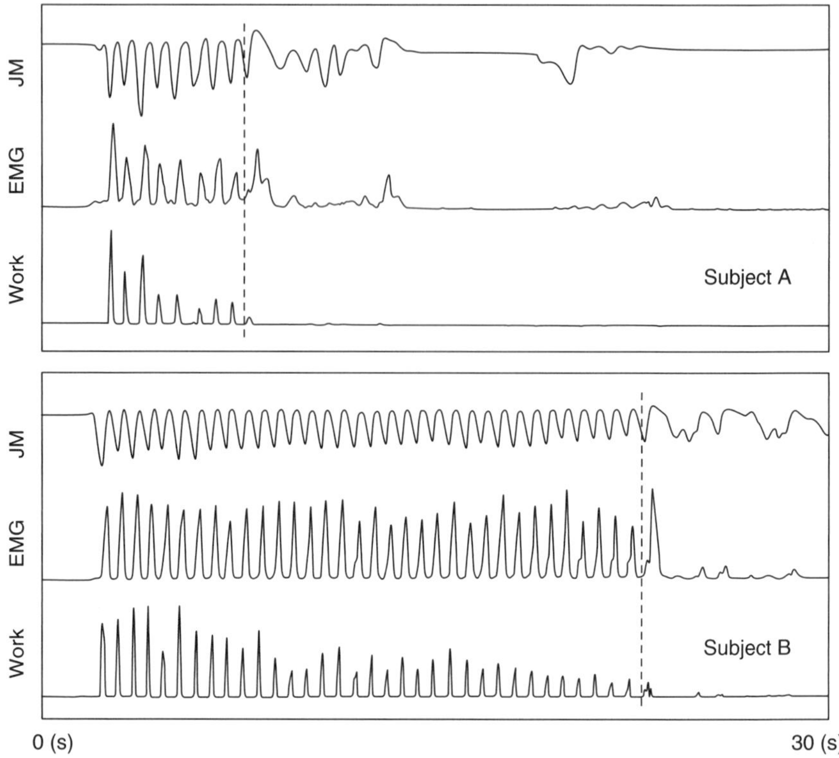

Fig. 1.1 Jaw movement (JM), rectified muscle activity (EMG) and muscle work (work) of two subjects chewing a piece of bread (13 cm^3). EMG and work bursts occur while the jaw is closing. The work bursts decline while mastication proceeds and the food bolus is softened. The dashed lines indicate the moments before the food was swallowed. Subject B chewed the bread more than four times longer than subject A.

that the food has been well fragmented and thus the masticatory performance is high. Large individual differences in masticatory performance were observed among healthy subjects (Fontijn-Tekamp *et al.*, 2004).

The number of chewing cycles needed to prepare the food for swallowing also largely varied among people. However, the moment of swallowing was shown to be only weakly correlated with the chewing performance (Fontijn-Tekamp *et al.*, 2004). Thus, a subject with a high masticatory performance does not necessarily swallow food after a smaller number of chewing strokes than a subject with a less high masticatory performance. This is illustrated in Fig. 1.2. The number of chewing cycles needed to prepare the food for swallowing is plotted as a function of the masticatory performance (median particle size after 15 chewing cycles) for 87 subjects (Fontijn-Tekamp *et al.*, 2004). Low values of the median particle size (left part of figure) indicate that the food was well fragmented and thus the masticatory performance

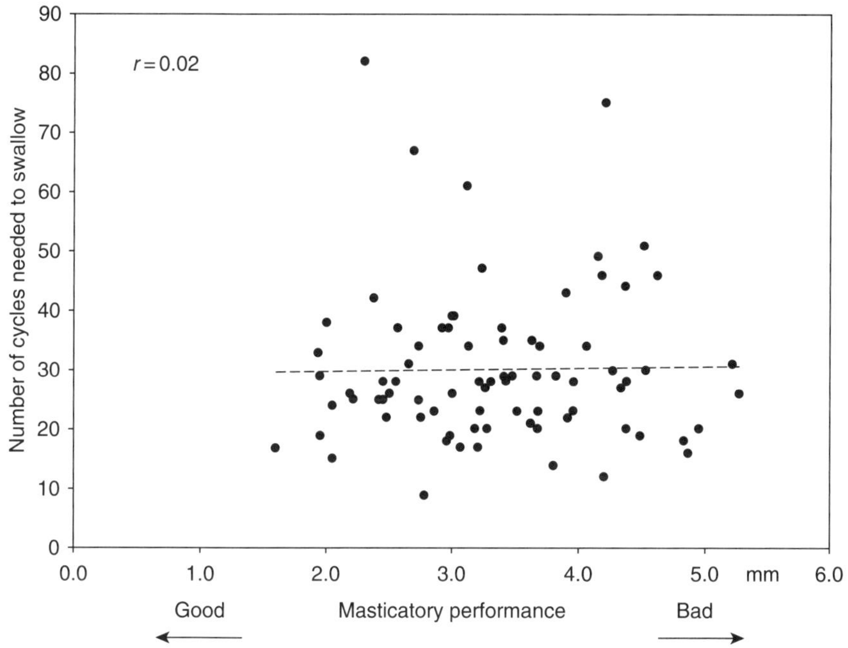

Fig. 1.2 The number of chewing strokes needed before swallowing the test food (Optocal) as a function of the median particle size obtained after 15 chewing strokes (masticatory performance). The data were obtained from 87 healthy adult subjects. Dashed line shows linear regression. A very low correlation ($r = 0.02$) was observed, which indicates that there is no relationship between the number of chewing strokes until swallowing and the masticatory performance. Reproduced from Fontijn-Tekamp *et al.* (2004).

is good, whereas large values (right part of figure) indicate that the food was not broken into small particles (bad chewing performance). As can be seen from Fig. 1.2, there is no relation between the number of chewing cycles up to swallowing and the masticatory performance. As a consequence, subjects with a high masticatory performance will, on average, swallow finer food particles (median particle size below 3 mm) than subjects with a less high performance (median particle size above 3 mm). This is illustrated in Fig. 1.3, where the median size of the swallowed food is plotted as a function of masticatory performance (Fontijn-Tekamp *et al.*, 2004). A significant correlation between the median particle size of the bolus ready for swallowing and the masticatory performance was observed ($r = 0.59$, $p < 0.001$). It could well be that this will influence the perception of the food. If so, chewers with a high performance would, on average, perceive food in a different way than subjects with a less high chewing performance.

In a study on 10 healthy subjects the food boluses ready for swallowing were analysed for six different foods, nuts and vegetables (Peyron *et al.*,

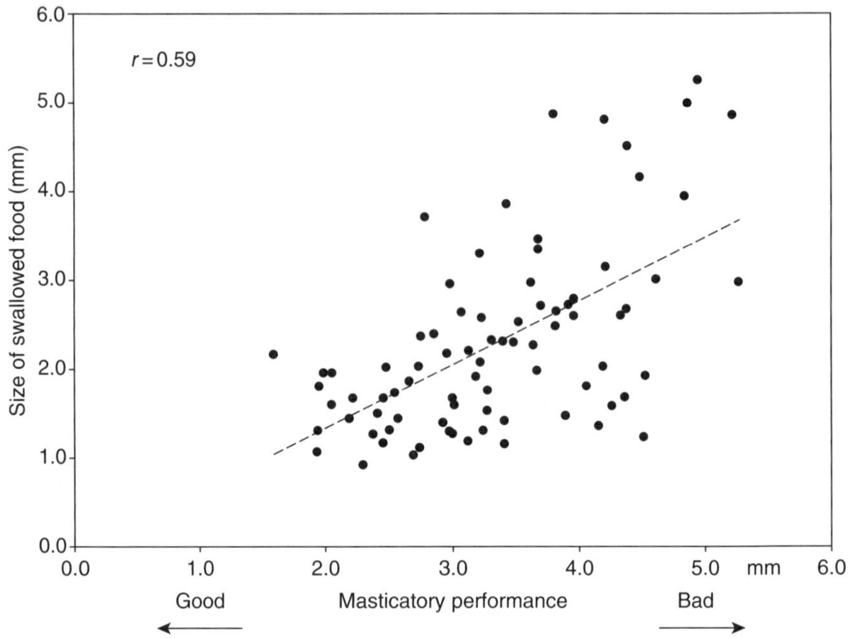

Fig. 1.3 Median particle size of the swallowed food as a function of the median particle size obtained after 15 chewing strokes (masticatory performance). The data were obtained from 87 healthy adult subjects. Dashed line shows linear regression. A significant correlation ($r = 0.59$; $p < 0.001$) was observed, which indicates that subjects with a good masticatory performance swallow finer food particles than subjects with a less good performance. Note that the median sizes of swallowed food vary from 5.23 mm (hardly fragmented particles) down to 0.92 mm (very fine grains), which indicates the large differences in chewing behaviour among the 87 healthy subjects. Reproduced from Fontijn-Tekamp *et al.* (2004).

2004b). Surprisingly, no inter-individual variability was observed in the particle distributions for the six foods. Based on this result, the authors suggested that the requirements that the food bolus must meet before it is ready to be swallowed are similar for everyone (Peyron *et al.*, 2004b). This is an unlikely assumption as it contradicts the results for the large group of subjects shown in Fig. 1.3: median particle sizes of the boluses ready for swallowing varied from 5.23 mm (hardly fragmented particles) down to 0.92 mm (very fine grains) (Fontijn-Tekamp *et al.*, 2004). The puzzling result about the absence of inter-individual variability may be caused by the relative small number of participants in that study (Peyron *et al.*, 2004b).

1.2.3 Saliva

The production of sufficient saliva is indispensable for good chewing. The water in saliva moistens the food particles, whereas the salivary mucins bind masticated food into a coherent and slippery bolus that can be easily swallowed (Pedersen *et al.*, 2002). It has been suggested that the swallowing process initiates when the cohesive forces that bind food particles together into a bolus are strongest (Prinz and Lucas, 1997). The important role of saliva for chewing and swallowing is demonstrated by the finding that the number of chewing strokes, hence time in the mouth, needed for swallowing significantly increases after experimentally induced oral dryness (Liedberg and Öwall, 1991). Additionally, significantly more saliva is required for oral manipulation of powdered crisp bread than for pieces of crisp bread (Pangborn and Lundgren, 1977) as the larger surface area of the powder requires more saliva for lubrication and cohesive binding in preparation for deglutition. In a study on rabbits, it was demonstrated that greater amounts of saliva were produced for dry food than for moist food (Anderson *et al.*, 1985). The amount of saliva also plays a role in the chewing of meat, with more saliva being incorporated into a food bolus of tough meat than into tender meat before the bolus is swallowed (Mioche *et al.*, 2003).

While saliva and chewing have been shown to be interrelated, the relationship between amount of saliva and mastication has not been studied extensively (Hector and Linden, 1999). During mastication it is likely that mechanoreceptors in the gingival tissues will be stimulated, which may result in salivary flow (Anderson *et al.*, 1996; Scott *et al.*, 1999). At chewing, forces as low as 5% of comfortable chewing forces the masticatory-salivary reflex could already be elicited (Anderson *et al.*, 1996).

Mechanically stimulated salivary flow rate can be determined in a standardized way from chewing on a piece of tasteless Parafilm. Over a period of 5 minutes, a subject expectorates saliva at 30 s intervals into a preweighed container and flow rate (ml/min) is then calculated. In a group of 266 healthy subjects salivary flow rates ranged from 0.16 to 3.8 ml/min (Engelen *et al.*, 2005). In that study it was shown that the moment of swallowing was only weakly correlated ($r = -0.13$; $p = 0.04$) with the salivary flow rate of a subject. The results of that study are shown in Fig. 1.4. Salivary flow rate explains only 2% of the variance in the swallowing threshold. This means that a subject with a relatively high salivary flow rate does not necessarily swallow food after fewer chewing cycles than a subject with less saliva. As a consequence, subjects with relative high salivary flow rates are used to swallow better moistened food than subjects with less saliva. Again, this may influence the perception of the food. However, previous work in our laboratory has shown that there was no relationship between a subject's salivary flow rate and sensory ratings (Engelen *et al.*, 2003b). Thus, a subject with a larger salivary flow rate during eating did not rate food differently from a subject with less salivary flow. An artificial increase of 0.5 ml of saliva significantly influenced the sensory ratings of semi-solids (Engelen *et al.*, 2003a). The addition of a fluid affected the mouthfeel attributes of thickness and melting of vanilla custard dessert. The facts that the perceived effect was equally strong for water as for α-amylase solution and saliva, and that a

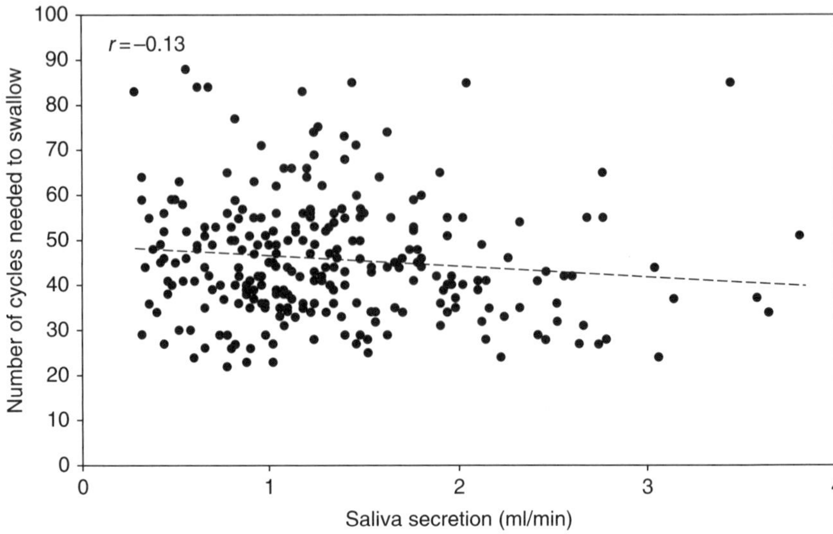

Fig. 1.4 Number of chewing strokes needed before swallowing non-buttered melba toast as a function of the salivary flow rate. The data were obtained from 266 healthy adult subjects. Dashed line shows linear regression. A small but significant correlation was observed ($r = -0.13$; $p = 0.04$; 2% explained variance only), which indicates salivary flow rate does not influence the swallowing threshold. Reproduced from Engelen *et al.* (2005).

larger fluid volume increased the effect, are evidence that the decreased sensation was mainly due to dilution.

1.3 Influence of food characteristics on chewing

Physical properties of a food can be determined from rheological measurements. An important objective method to determine properties for solid foods is a compression machine and for liquid foods a rotary viscometer. Universal testing machines can be set up to use a number of different test procedures, including deformation, puncture, extrusion, cutting-shear and crushing (Bourne, 2004). With such a machine, force–deformation curves (stress–strain curves) can be obtained. In texture profile analysis (TPA) bite-size pieces of food are compressed and decompressed two times, imitating the first two chews on a food (Bourne, 2002). This procedure allows the determination of, for example, fracturability (force at a significant break in the first bite), and hardness (maximum force of first bite) of a food sample. Solid food can also be characterized by textural parameters, such as hardness (soft, firm, hard), cohesiveness (crumbly, crunchy, brittle), viscosity (thin, viscous), springiness (plastic, elastic) and adhesiveness (sticky, gooey) (Szczesniak, 2002). Furthermore, solid food has geometrical characteristics: size, shape and orientation of particles (e.g. gritty, grainy, course, fibrous). Other characteristics of food are moisture and fat content (dry, moist, wet; oily, greasy). It should be noted that texture is a sensory attribute and therefore only people can really measure texture (Bourne, 2004). The characteristics of a food may influence the masticatory process.

1.3.1 Influence of food type on muscle activity, chewing force and jaw movement

The influence of food characteristics on the chewing process has been extensively studied. Food hardness is sensed during mastication and affects jaw muscle activity (Horio and Kawamura, 1989; Mathevon *et al.*, 1995; Agrawal *et al.*, 1998; Mioche *et al.*, 1999; Peyron *et al.*, 2002; van der Bilt *et al.*, 2007), masticatory force (Kohyama *et al.*, 2004) and jaw movements (Thexton *et al.*, 1980; Pröschel and Hofmann, 1988; Hiiemae *et al.*, 1996; Peyron *et al.*, 1997). When we chew, for instance, a crispy food, the jaw decelerates and accelerates as a result of resistance and breakage of food particles. The characteristic breakage behaviour of a food is essential for the sensory sensation.

A clear relationship between food hardness and jaw muscle activity has been reported in numerous studies. Increased jaw muscle activity and longer burst duration of the muscle activity were observed for harder foods (Plesh *et al.*, 1986; Horio and Kawamura, 1989; Agrawal *et al.*, 1998; Mioche *et al.*, 1999; Peyron *et al.*, 2002; Foster *et al.*, 2006; van der Bilt *et al.*, 2007). It was shown that the hardness of chewing gum (soft or hard gum) influenced the chewing cycle duration and the amplitude of the muscle activity. The subjects chewed slower and with more muscle activity on the hard gum (Plesh *et al.*, 1986). In another study muscle activity was measured while subjects chewed on 15 different types of food (various kinds of cheese, nuts and carrots), which largely varied in mechanical properties (Agrawal *et al.*, 1998). Young's modulus and toughness were measured for each food. Young's modulus (or elastic modulus) was determined from the slope of a force–deformation curve of the material. Toughness is the resistance to fracture of a material when stressed and was measured by a wedge test. Muscle activity needed to chew the various food types turned out to be highly significantly related to the square root of the ratio of toughness and the modulus of elasticity ($p < 0.0001$).

The influence of food characteristics on chewing was also studied using model foods (Foster *et al.*, 2006). Two model food types were used, presenting either elastic or plastic rheological properties. Each model food type consisted of four products of different hardness. The elastic model food was an edible jellied confectionery product and the plastic model food was an edible caramel confectionery product. Muscle activity was significantly affected by an increase in hardness regardless of the food type. Chewing tests were also performed with meat of two different textures: tough and dry versus tender and juicy meat (Mioche *et al.*, 2003). The mean muscle activity needed for chewing the tough meat was significantly higher than for chewing the tender meat.

Chewing force has been measured using a multiple-point sheet-type sensor (Kohyama *et al.*, 2004). The sensor was a flexible sheet, thinner than 0.1 mm, which had many pressure-sensing points (269 sensing cells) on it. Each sensing cell detects pressure in real time. With this method both chewing force and contact area between the teeth are obtained. Three silicone rubber model foods of varying hardness were used. The study clearly indicated that sample hardness modified chewing force of humans. The masticatory force during chewing samples of silicon rubber was shown to increase from 100 to 150 N, when the hardness of the samples increased by a factor of 2 (Kohyama *et al.*, 2004). Chewing force was also determined for five natural foods in the first chew (Kohyama *et al.*, 2001). Force–time curves largely varied for both foods and subjects. Various peaks occurred in the force–time curves of cracker and rice cracker, whereas only two peaks were observed for carrot. The authors suggested that the first peak corresponded to sample rupture.

Jaw movement was reported to be influenced by food hardness (Horio and Kawamura, 1989). Larger jaw opening was observed when subjects chewed on harder foods. Similar results were reported for edible model foods (Peyron *et al.*, 2002). Four gelatine-based viscoelastic foods, identical in shape but differing in hardness, were used. The amplitude of the mandibular movements increased for harder foods, especially in the first five chewing cycles.

1.3.2 Influence of food type and volume on swallowing

Food characteristics do have a large influence on the number of chewing cycles needed to prepare the food for swallowing (Hiiemae *et al.*, 1996; Mioche *et al.*, 2003; Engelen *et al.*, 2005; van der Bilt *et al.*, 2007; Jalabert-Malbos *et al.*, 2007). In a group of 87 dentate subjects the number of chewing cycles varied from on average 17 cycles for a portion of 8 cm^3 of cake up to 61 cycles for an equal portion of carrots (Engelen *et al.*, 2005). The volume of food also has a large influence on oral physiology. For larger portion sizes, subjects needed more time and chewing strokes before they swallowed the food (Lucas and Luke, 1984; Gavião *et al.*, 2004; Fontijn-Tekamp *et al.*, 2004; Blissett *et al.*, 2007). The number of chewing strokes needed to prepare the food for swallowing linearly increased as a function of the food volume ($p < 0.001$) (Fontijn-Tekamp *et al.*, 2004). Sample thickness of the food also influences chewing. The force needed to chew a piece of apple increased with sample thickness (Dan *et al.*, 2003). Food size was shown to influence jaw movement: larger food sizes led to larger jaw gapes and larger jaw velocities during chewing (van der Bilt *et al.*, 1991; Miyawaki *et al.*, 2000). These results suggest that humans chew food such that the mandibular teeth that come into contact with the food open to a height equivalent to that of the food bolus.

Dry and hard products required more chewing cycles before swallowing than moist and soft products. Evidently, more time is needed to break the food down and to add enough saliva to form a cohesive bolus suitable for swallowing (Anderson *et al.*, 1985). Thus, a dry product needs a longer time in the mouth to allow for enough secretion of saliva. Confirming this, buttering dry foods (cake, melba toast and toast) significantly reduced the number of chewing cycles of these foods (Engelen *et al.*, 2005). The reason for this is probably that butter enhances lubrication and bolus formation of dry products, decreasing the time needed in the mouth to form a coherent bolus. Similar results were observed in a study in which lubrication of the food bolus had been experimentally varied (Prinz and Lucas, 1995). In a recent study it was shown that adding small volumes of water (5 or 10 ml) to a food significantly lowered the number of chewing cycles and total muscular work until swallowing (Pereira *et al.*, 2006; van der Bilt *et al.*, 2007). Results from this study are depicted in Fig. 1.5. The average muscle activity per chewing cycle is plotted versus the number of chewing cycles for five different foods. For each food three different conditions were measured: food without additional water, and food with 5 or 10 ml additional water. The additional water reduced the number of chewing cycles until swallowing and the muscle activity for melba toast, cake, peanut and cheese, but not for carrot. The largest effects were observed for melba toast and cake, which are dry products requiring sufficient saliva to form a coherent bolus safe for swallowing. More facilitation of the chewing process was observed after adding fluid to breakfast cake for subjects with relatively low salivary flow rates. Subjects with a relatively low salivary flow rate apparently benefit more from the addition of water than subjects with a larger flow rate.

Several texture and sound attributes of melba toast, cake and peanut were also significantly affected by the additional fluids (Pereira *et al.*, 2006; Dijksterhuis *et al.*, 2007). For melba toast, cake and peanut, significant correlations between physiology parameters and several attributes for the various fluid conditions were observed. This indicates that adding a small volume of water to the food affects both the physiology (muscle activity and number of cycles) and the sensory perception of a number of texture and sound attributes.

In a recent article the particle size distributions of the food boluses suitable for deglutition and the number of chewing cycles until swallowing were determined for 10 natural foods (Jalabert-Malbos *et al.*, 2007). The number of cycles, sequence duration and particle size distributions significantly differed among subjects and foods. Large differences in average median particle size of the bolus ready to swallow were observed, ranging from 0.82 mm for peanuts (hard food) to 3.04 mm for gherkins (soft food). Foods that were rapidly swallowed were both soft and characterized by a high water content (egg white, gherkins, mushrooms and olives). The boluses obtained from these foods contained many large particles. Harder foods needed more chewing cycles before swallowing so a better particle fragmentation and bolus salivation was achieved (coconut, carrots).

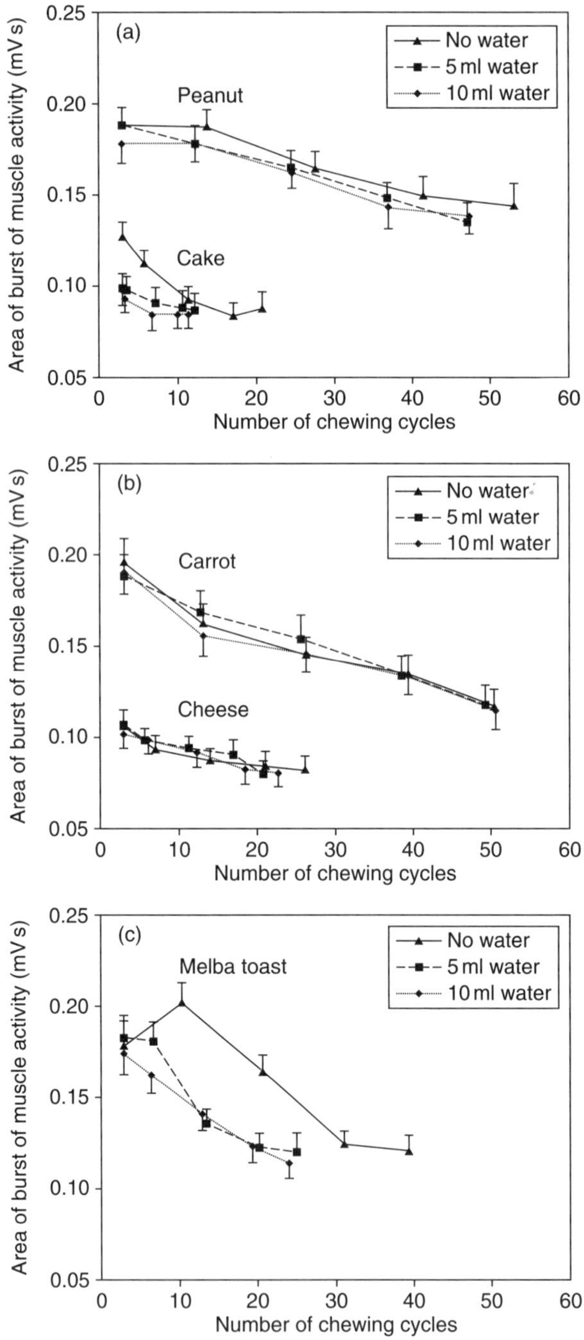

Fig. 1.5 Average muscle activity per chewing cycle in five different phases of chewing (begin, 25%, 50%, 75% and end) for various food–fluid combinations. Data points along a line represent the five phases of chewing. Five foods were chewed without added water (solid lines), with 5 ml (dashed lines) and 10 ml water (dotted lines). Reproduced from van der Bilt *et al.* (2007).

The influence of texture on the chewing process has also been studied with meat. Chewing tests were performed with meat of two different textures: tough and dry versus tender and juicy meat (Mioche *et al.*, 2003). Mechanical shear force of the meat samples was determined before chewing and after chewing, when the bolus was ready to be swallowed. Texture differences between the two types of meat remained significant even when the boluses were ready to swallow: the toughest meat gave the toughest bolus, despite being chewed with more strokes. Muscle activity was higher for the chewing of tough meat than of tender meat. The percentage of saliva incorporated into the bolus ready to swallow of the tough meat was significantly higher than the percentage of saliva in the bolus of the tender meat.

1.3.3 Muscle activity and jaw movement in various phases of chewing

During chewing, the food bolus or food particles are reduced in size, saliva is produced to moisten the food and flavours are released. As a result, jaw muscle activity and jaw amplitude decrease while mastication proceeds as the food bolus is softened (Kohyama and Mioche, 2004; van der Bilt *et al.*, 2007). The decrease in muscle activity during the chewing process is nicely illustrated in Fig. 1.5. The softening of the food is caused by structure breakdown to smaller particles (for high-moisture foods such as carrot and brittle foods such as peanut), by temperature raising (for fatty foods such as cheese) and by action of the water and α-amylase of saliva (for dry foods and foods containing starch, e.g. cake and melba toast). Adding 5 or 10 ml water to the food did have an effect on both number of cycles until swallowing as well as muscle activity for cake and melba toast (Fig. 1.5). These are dry products requiring a sufficient amount of saliva to be added to form a coherent bolus safe for swallowing. In a study on edible elastic model foods it was shown that vertical and lateral jaw amplitudes, the duration of a chewing cycle and the muscular work steadily decreased as mastication progressed (Lassauzay *et al.*, 2000). Similar results were observed for dentate subjects who chewed meat: muscle work per chewing cycle gradually decreased during the chewing process (Yven *et al.*, 2006). The change in the pattern of jaw movement during the chewing process suggests continuous sensory modulation of the motor output to the mandibular musculature (Hiiemae *et al.*, 1996). Muscle activity could thus act as a sensory clue for certain food sensory properties such as tenderness of meat (Mioche, 2004).

1.4 Oral physiology and food perception

Food undergoes many events on its way from the plate to the stomach, e.g. spooning, stirring, ingestion, mastication and swallowing. In the oral cavity, food is subjected to several mechanical and chemical processes. It is fractured by the teeth, manipulated by the tongue, diluted and broken down by saliva, heated or cooled by the ambient temperature of the mouth, formed into a bolus and finally swallowed. Numerous receptors in the oral cavity and nose respond to the initially ingested food and monitor the changes during processing. This leads to central perceptions of taste, odour, irritation and texture of the food. Most sensations associated with food texture occur only when the food is manipulated, deformed or moved across the oral receptors. In addition, people assessing the same stimulus differ in their ratings of that stimulus and their oral physiological parameters also exhibit inter-individual variations. A review on the relationship between oral physiology and texture perception, based on a PhD study in our research group, has been published recently (Engelen, 2004; Engelen and van der Bilt, 2008).

Sensation is the receptor response to bodily stimulation, whereas perception is awareness through the senses interpreted in the light of experience. The conventional categorization of the senses is touch, including temperature, in addition to taste, smell, hearing and sight. Perception can be the awareness arising through one single sense or through a combination of many. Perception of food is the result of food characteristics interacting with the processes in the mouth, as interpreted by the brain.

1.4.1 Texture

In literature, a number of definitions of texture can be found. One frequently used definition was stated by Szczesniak, who defined texture as 'the sensory manifestation of the structure of the food and the manner in which this structure reacts to the applied forces, the specific senses involved being vision, kinesthesis, and hearing' (Szczesniak, 1963a). Jowitt extended the definition of texture: 'Texture is the attribute of a substance resulting from a combination of physical properties and perceived by the senses of touch (including kinesthesis and mouthfeel), sight, and hearing. Physical properties may include size, shape, number, nature and conformation of constituent structural elements' (Jowitt, 1974). Jowitt also stated that the appreciation of texture involves the subtle interaction between both motor and sensory components of the masticatory and the central nervous system.

When asking lay people to describe food, taste and flavour are most often mentioned. However, texture of food is of great importance for the appreciation of food (Szczesniak, 1963b; Matsumoto and Matsumoto, 1977; Lucas *et al.*, 2004; Nishinari, 2004b): just think of soggy cornflakes, water-thin chocolate mousse or wilted lettuce. Conversely, very good texture, such as a soft and airy hollandaise sauce, is associated with excellent cooks. Texture is not only important for the appreciation, but also for the recognition of food. After blending food products, the lack of texture cues resulted in only 40% of the products being correctly identified from their flavour only (Schiffman, 1977). Food texture and its importance to the consumer are considerably less well understood than factors such as odour and taste (Kilcast and Eves, 1991). In contrast to odour or taste, there are no specific

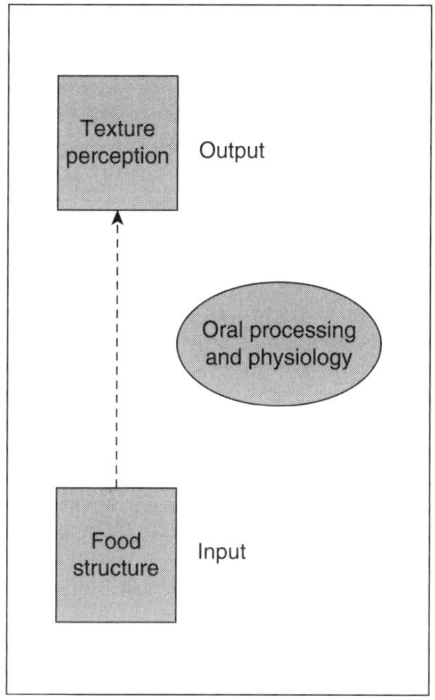

Fig. 1.6 Oral physiology as the missing link in the relationship between food structure (input) and texture perception (output). Reproduced from Engelen and van der Bilt (2008).

receptors for texture per se. Texture perception has in the past received relatively little research attention compared with odour and taste. However, this is a changing trend (Szczesniak, 1990).

1.4.2 Understanding texture

Research on food texture has focused mainly on rheological measurements, frequently correlated with sensory data of the same product (Fig. 1.6). Conventional rheological measurements, such as viscosity and puncture tests, are not based on oral systems, but have their origin in process technique and product control (Bourne, 1982). As a result, rheological measurements have often turned out not to be completely satisfactory in explaining the relationship between food structure and texture perception. This could be explained by the notion that this approach disregards the oral processing and physiology of the mouth (Bourne, 1975). Moreover, most sensations associated with food texture occur only when the food is manipulated, deformed or moved across the oral receptors. During the time in the mouth, the stimulus undergoes constant changes: it is heated or cooled; diluted and broken down by saliva; and manipulated mechanically. This makes the mouth a very challenging system to mimic *in vitro*. Recently, researchers have tried to take this into consideration by making more physiologically adapted physical measurements (Jellema *et al.*, 2005; de Wijk *et al.*, 2006a; Janssen *et al.*, 2007). It is especially important to take saliva into consideration in instrumental measurements (de Wijk *et al.*, 2006a).

Another indication that oral processes are important is that human volunteers (subjects) assessing the same stimulus do not only differ largely in their ratings of that stimulus, but the oral physiological parameters also exhibit large inter-individual variations. In this light, oral physiology, e.g. oral processes (manipulation, mixing and dilution of food in the mouth) and oral sensitivity and receptors, is possibly the 'missing link' in understanding the relationship between food structure and texture perception (Fig. 1.6). Understanding the relationship between food texture perception and food structure is of increasing importance for companies wishing to produce texturally attractive food products. The perception of texture is a complex process involving the senses of vision, hearing, somesthesis and kinesthesis. Texture perception takes place partly during the dynamic process of food breakdown in the mouth and is affected by oral processes, such as motility, saliva production and temperature (Wilkinson *et al.*, 2000).

1.4.3 Factors influencing texture

There are numerous factors, both product and subject related, that can influence texture perception (Fig. 1.7). These factors can affect texture perception directly or indirectly. Many of the factors influence each other, which makes the whole concept rather complex. This diagram is not exhaus-

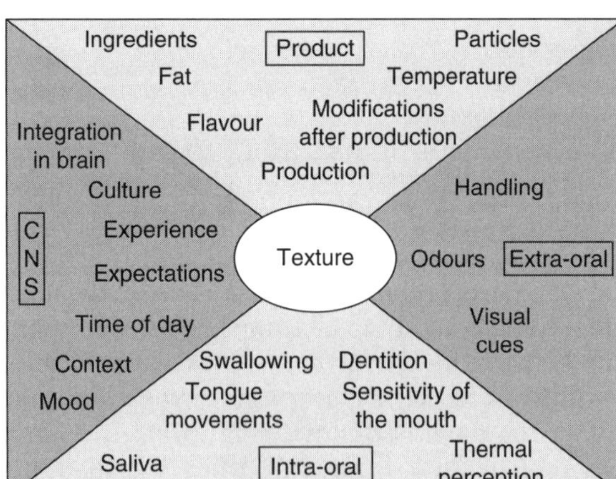

Fig. 1.7 Diagram of factors that may influence food texture. Reproduced from Engelen and van der Bilt (2008).

tive, but includes a collection of factors for food types ranging from solid to liquid.

Starting at the top left in Fig. 1.7, product ingredients are major determinants of the product structure. The ingredients include thickeners, type of starch, oil, water, etc. Moving clockwise, the level of fat is thought to influence flavour release (Barylko-Pikielna and Szczesniak, 1994; Hyvönen *et al.*, 2003), mouthfeel (de Wijk *et al.*, 2006b) and thermal perception (Engelen *et al.*, 2002). In addition, ingredients can affect the overall perception of product flavour, e.g. by having off-flavours. Product structure is of importance for how the product will be handled in the mouth. Production techniques, e.g. homogenization, baking and freezing, affect the final structure strongly. Various substances, such as particles, can be added after production, to modify the product. Temperature of the product does not only affect the structure, but can also influence the perception of food texture, flavour and irritation.

Texture is also perceived outside the mouth (extra-oral). Before the food enters the mouth, visual cues such as colour, shine, grains and heterogeneity (lumps) provide information on the texture of the food. Additional information can be obtained by handling the food, e.g. stirring, spooning and cutting. The time until swallowing was shorter and fewer chews were observed as palatability of the food increased (Bellisle *et al.*, 2000). The effects of sensory factors were most evident at the beginning of meals and decreased until the end of meals (Bellisle *et al.*, 1984).

Intra-oral factors that are subject-related can affect the food itself and how it is perceived. These are: thermal perception; sensitivity of the mouth to touch and size; dentition; swallowing; movements of the tongue in relation to the palate; and saliva amount and composition.

Finally, the central nervous system (CNS) is an important determinant in texture perception. The memory and emotional state of the person eating the food, social background, time of day and expectations could be of importance. During exposure to different foods, the perception and appreciation of food will change due to experience. In different cultures, different textures are favourable, such as stickiness and pliability in Japan (Tanaka, 1986).

A selection of factors related to oral physiology have been shown to influence texture: oral sensitivity, added particles, tongue movements, temperature and saliva (Engelen, 2004). This selection is in accordance with Szczesniak's ideas. She stressed that tactile perception, perception related to size and position of particles in the mouth and temperature are very important (Szczesniak, 2003). Texture is being looked at as a positive quality attribute, denoting freshness of produce, and excellence of food preparation and contributing to the enjoyment of eating (Szczesniak, 2002).

1.4.4 Oral physiology

The next paragraphs offer a general overview of a few aspects of physiology that could affect the perception of texture.

Receptors and sensations
Humans have four classes of receptors, each of which is sensitive primarily to one type of physical energy – chemical, mechanical, thermal and electromagnetic. In the mouth all types of receptor, except the photoreceptors sensitive to electromagnetic energy, are present. Chemical receptors include taste and odour. Thermoreceptors sense the temperature of the body and objects that we come in contact with, and nociceptors signal sensations of pain. Mechanoreceptors mediate sensations of touch and proprioception. Proprioception is the most important sense from inside our bodies. It is the sense of what the muscle itself is doing: sense organs in the tendons signal how hard the muscles are pulling, and sense organs within the muscles signal how much and how fast the muscles are being stretched (Brooks, 1986). All these types of receptors contribute to the total sensation and perception of food that we ingest. However, in the sensation and perception of oral texture, the tactile stimuli are probably the most prominent clues to texture.

The somatic sensory system
The mouth is a very sensitive organ. The oral cavity is one of the regions of the body most densely innervated with nerve fibres and receptors (Mountcastle, 1974) and is exquisitely sensitive to tactile stimulation (Ringel and Ewanowski, 1965; Van Boven and Johnson, 1994). This means that thresholds for somethetic stimuli are lower and discrimination is better than on most other skin areas of the body. Thresholds for detection of touch are lowest on the tip of the tongue and hard palate (Ringel and Ewanowski, 1965; Henkin and Banks, 1967). Somesthetic receptors are found in all regions of the oral cavity, including the lips, tongue, teeth and mucosa. The somatic sensory system transmits information about four modalities: touch, temperature, pain and proprioception. The receptors for each modality are specialized structures, allowing them to sense specific types of stimuli. Cutaneous receptors can be subdivided according to the type of stimulus to which they respond.

The major types of receptors include mechanoreceptors responding to tactile stimuli, thermoreceptors, responding to cold and warm stimuli, and nociceptors, responding to pain. Mechanoreceptors respond to tactile stimuli, such as pressure or tapping. In the mouth and lip, three different types of mechanoreceptors have been described: slowly adapting type I and II (SA I and SA II) and rapidly adapting type I (RA I) (Johansson *et al.*, 1988; Trulsson, 1993; Trulsson and Essick, 1997). These are associated with a particular type of tactile perception: pressure, stretch of skin, and taps on skin, respectively. Thermal sensations result from differences between temperature of the air or of objects contacting the body and the normal skin temperature. There are two types of thermoreceptors in the skin, responding to specific temperatures and changes in temperature: cold (range: 20–40 °C) and warm (range: 30–48 °C) receptors (Goldstein, 1996). Pain is mediated by specialized free nerve endings, called nociceptors. The sensation of pain serves an important protective function: it warns of injury that should be avoided or treated. The nerve endings respond to stimuli that may produce tissue damage, such as intense pressure, extreme temperature or burning chemicals (Gardner *et al.*, 2000).

1.4.5 Saliva

Saliva is always present in the mouth, where it serves many functions. The amount and composition of saliva, however, varies with the state (sleep/awake; relaxed/stressed) of the individual (Nieuw Amerongen, 1994). During eating, the amount of saliva increases and the degree depends on the type of stimulation. Saliva consists of 99% water, and in the remaining 1% there is a multitude of other components, such as ions, enzymes and other proteins (Schneyer *et al.*, 1972). Thus, tastants are dissolved in saliva, and are therefore more easily transported to the taste buds, enabling us to taste the food (Guinard *et al.*, 1997; Ruth and Roozen, 2000). Between meals, saliva wets and protects the mucosa and the teeth, and it also has antibacterial and anti-inflammatory properties (Lindberg, 1973; Adams, 1975; Gibbons, 1979; Tabak *et al.*, 1982).

Saliva is expected to be involved in our perception of the taste, flavour and texture of foods. The effects of saliva on food leading to changes in perception are plentiful. Mixing saliva with food can have a diluting effect (Christensen, 1985) and plays a role by initial breakdown of food (Engelen *et al.*, 2003a), by effecting flavour release (Guinard *et al.*, 1997; Ruth and Roozen, 2000), transport of taste compounds to the taste buds (Ruth and Roozen, 2000), precipitation of proteins by tannins, e.g. resulting in a sensation of astringency (Green, 1993), and acting as a buffering system (Larsen *et al.*, 1999), affecting the degree to which we perceive sourness (Christensen *et al.*, 1987). Saliva is also important for lubrication. It has been shown that whole mouth saliva reduced the in-mouth coefficient of friction significantly, facilitating manipulation of food in the oral cavity and swallowing (Ranc *et al.*, 2006). The large salivary proteins are believed to influence lubrication (Nieuw Amerongen, 1994) and hence perhaps the perception of attributes such as smoothness and astringency (Kallithraka *et al.*, 2001). Salivary flow rate has an influence on the chewing process (Gavião *et al.*, 2004; Engelen *et al.*, 2005). The food is mixed, diluted and broken down by saliva, which changes the texture of the food (Mioche *et al.*, 2003; Pereira *et al.*, 2006; van der Bilt *et al.*, 2007). Mixing the food with saliva, including breakdown and dilution, is considered to be of large importance for semi-solids as these products are masticated without chewing. Saliva volume and composition were demonstrated to influence flavour and texture sensations in custard and mayonnaise (Engelen *et al.*, 2003b, 2007). These examples indicate the value of saliva for the appreciation and acceptance of food.

1.5 Neuromuscular control of chewing and swallowing

The movement of the jaw, and thus the neuromuscular control of chewing, plays an important role in the comminution of the food. Chewing requires muscle activity to make the movements of the jaw and to exert forces in order to cut or grind the food. A relatively low level of muscle activity is observed in the surface electromyography of the closing muscles of subjects making pseudo-chewing movements without food. Surface electromyography (EMG) is obtained from electrodes placed on the belly of the muscle. The electrodes record the electrical potentials generated by the motor units of the muscles. More muscle activity is generated if the closing movement is counteracted by food resistance (van der Glas *et al.*, 1987; Thexton, 1992). Apparently, a small part of the muscle activity observed during chewing is needed just for the basic rhythmic movements of the jaw, and additional muscle activity is required to overcome the resistance of the food. The total amount of EMG activity has been shown to depend on the texture of food: more EMG activity is observed for harder foods (Mathevon *et al.*, 1995; Agrawal *et al.*, 1998; Mioche *et al.*, 1999; Peyron *et al.*, 2002; van der Bilt *et al.*, 2007).

1.5.1 Central pattern generator

The brain stem has been shown to be an essential part of the central nervous system that is necessary for mastication, because decerebrate animals and animals without a cerebellum or spinal cord can still chew (Dellow and Lund, 1971; Lund, 1976, 1991; Nozaki *et al.*, 1986; Goldberg and Chandler, 1990). The basic rhythmic activity of the jaw-opening and jaw-closing muscles is probably evoked by a central pattern generator located in the brain stem (Thexton, 1992). Cortically evoked rhythmic trigeminal activity remained present in animals after elimination of sensory feedback from peripheral receptors (Dellow and Lund, 1971; Goodwin and Luschei, 1974). This shows that neither muscle spindle afferents nor periodontal afferents are essential to the basic rhythmic activity patterns of mastication. Cortical stimulation of the anaesthetized rabbit induced rhythmical mandibular movements in the awake animal (Morimoto *et al.*, 1989). The central pattern generator may be switched on by activity of higher centers or by intra-oral stimuli (Thexton, 1973; Lund, 1976).

1.5.2 Peripheral feedback

Comparison of the movements and the activity patterns in the motor nerves evoked by cortical stimulation of the paralysed animal with those of natural chewing before paralysis has demonstrated the important role of sensory feedback in mastication (Lund, 1991). During cortical stimulation, the central pattern generator produces stereotyped open–close cycles, whereas during natural chewing the movement trajectories of the consecutive chewing cycles vary considerably (Lund, 1991). Moreover, the activity of the jaw-closer α-motoneurons is much smaller in fictive mastication than during natural chewing. This suggests that, to adequately fulfil the motor tasks of the mandible during chewing, the central nervous system requires information about the position and velocity of the mandible, about the forces acting on the mandible and on the teeth, and about the length and contraction velocity of the muscles involved. An increase in the amplitude and duration of the activity of the jaw-closing muscles of the rabbit was observed when cortically induced rhythmic open-close movements were obstructed by a steel ball or a foam strip between antagonistic teeth (Lavigne *et al.*, 1987; Morimoto *et al.*, 1989, 1995). This effect was reduced after elimination of feedback from the periodontal pressoreceptors by deafferentation. It was concluded that periodontal pressoreceptors, and muscle spindles, provide positive feedback to the jaw-closing muscles during mastication.

1.5.3 Simulated chewing experiments

The neuromuscular control of chewing in humans has been studied in our laboratory (e.g. Ottenhoff *et al.*, 1992; van der Bilt *et al.*, 1995; Abbink *et al.*, 1997). In these studies food resistance was simulated by a computer-controlled external load, acting on the mandible in a downward direction during closing (Fig. 1.8). Sequences of cycles with a load were unexpectedly

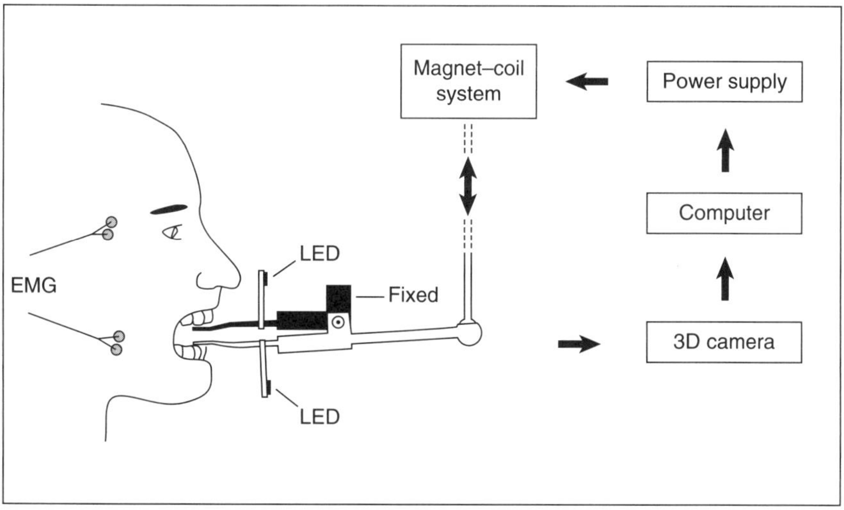

Fig. 1.8 Experimental setup for external loading of jaw muscles (LED = light-emitting diode). Reproduced from van der Bilt *et al.* (2006).

alternated with sequences of cycles without a load. Jaw movement and EMG of the masseter, temporalis and digastric muscles were recorded. It was demonstrated that the additional muscle activity, needed to counteract the external load, consists of two components: an anticipating component starting before the onset of the food-simulating load and a peripherally induced component starting after the onset of the load. The anticipating component is generated only if a counteracting load is expected. The onset of the anticipating muscle activity occurs immediately after the moment that the jaw starts closing. Peripherally induced muscle activity is generated on average 23 ms after the onset of the load. About 85% of the muscle activity needed to overcome the external load is peripherally induced, which indicates that the muscle activity is mainly of sensory origin. However, when the movement rate of chewing was doubled (fast chewing with 120 cycles per minute), the contribution of peripherally induced muscle activity decreased to only 40%. Therefore, as jaw movement speed increased, emphasis in the control of the muscle activity shifted from sensory induced (closed-loop) to feed forward (open-loop) control (Abbink *et al.*, 1999a). Muscles spindles are primarily responsible for the peripherally induced muscle activity as was demonstrated in an experiment on anaesthetized rabbits (Morimoto *et al.*, 1995).

The masticatory system is mainly closed-loop controlled. A reason for this may be the fact that the relatively large forces needed for food fragmentation must be controlled under uncertain conditions. First, no optical feedback is available in the chewing process. Furthermore, food resistance may vary largely from cycle to cycle. Thus, immediate muscle response is necessary to maintain a constant chewing rhythm. Force–velocity properties of the jaw-closing muscles play a major role if food resistance suddenly disappears (Slager *et al.*, 1997). In that case reflex activity is too slow to limit the jaw velocity at impact. The force-velocity properties of the muscles provide a quick mechanism for dealing with unexpected closing movements and so avoid damage to the dental elements.

An experiment with rhythmic arm movements, comparable to the rhythmic jaw movements described above, showed that arm and jaw muscles respond differently to loading (Abbink *et al.*, 1999b). In the arm muscles, there was little reflex activity, but a large anticipatory response. This indicates that reflexes do not play an important role in these rhythmic arm movements. This emphasizes that the mainly reflexly induced control of the jaw-closing muscles is a unique phenomenon.

1.5.4 Neuromuscular control of chewing crispy food

The crispy/crunchy nature of food products is an important sensory characteristic on which consumers base their appreciation. When we chew crispy food, the jaw decelerates and accelerates as a result of resistance and breakage of food particles. The characteristic breakage behaviour of a crispy food is essential for the sensory sensation. Our chewing muscles will generate the chewing force needed to break the food. The electrical activity of the chewing muscles will abruptly decrease when the food breaks, thus preventing too fast jaw closing and damage of the teeth. The breakage behaviour of a crispy food during chewing could be quantified by studying the neuromuscular control of the jaw movement during chewing of crispy foods. Such a study was recently performed on crispy foods (Hück *et al.*, 2005). The EMG of the jaw-closer muscles, the jaw movement and the vibrations of the skull were measured while a subject chewed Brazil nuts, carrots and biscuits. Several distinct peaks in the acceleration of the jaw and skull were detected in the first cycles while chewing on nuts and carrots (Fig. 1.9). Furthermore, unloading reflexes in the corresponding EMG signals were observed. More, but less pronounced, peaks in the acceleration of the jaw were observed when the subject chewed biscuits.

Another approach to study the chewing of crispy foods is to simulate the mechanical resistance of a crispy food (Hück *et al.*, 2005). In that way the breakage behaviour of a food during chewing can be manipulated in a reproducible way. Instead of the food resistance present while chewing on a food, an external load was generated by a magnet–coil system (Fig. 1.8). The external load thus mimics the load that would be present while chewing a crispy food. The force–deformation characteristics, as obtained from chewing a crispy food, were used to program the load for simulated chewing.

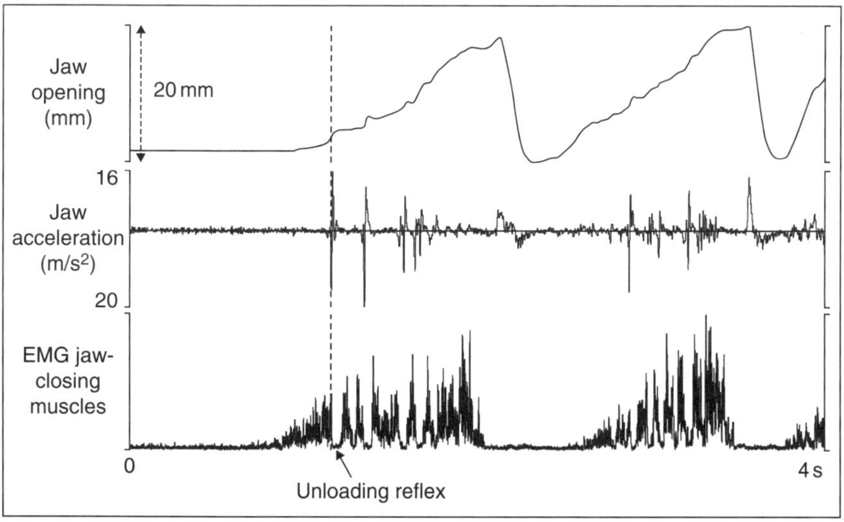

Fig. 1.9 Jaw movement, jaw acceleration and rectified jaw muscle activity of a subject who starts chewing on a Brazil nut. The dashed line indicates the first breakage of the nut. The breakage is followed by an unloading reflex in the jaw closing muscles. Reproduced from van der Bilt *et al.* (2006).

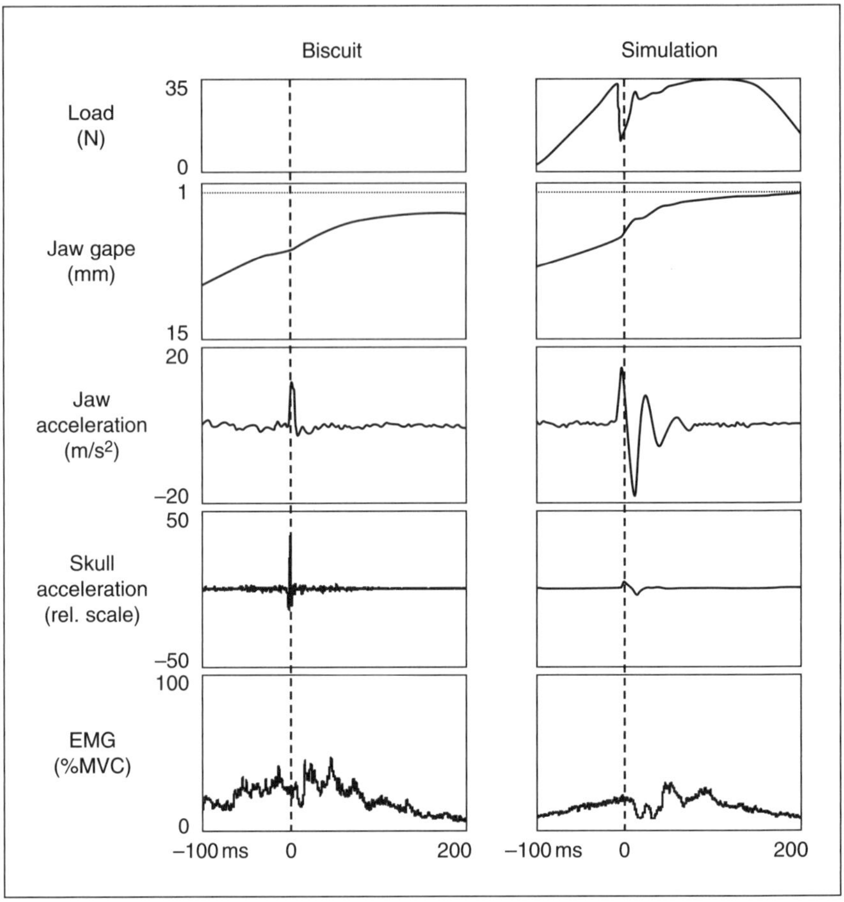

Fig. 1.10 Jaw gape, jaw acceleration, skull acceleration, and rectified muscle activity for chewing biscuit and simulated chewing (MVC, maximum voluntary contraction). Reproduced from van der Bilt *et al.* (2006).

The simulated crispy food resistance should thus show similar muscle activity and jaw movement as with the natural food. Indeed, the muscle activity evoked while chewing on a natural food was very similar to the muscle activity observed during simulated chewing with a corresponding load profile (Fig. 1.10). The skull vibrations occurred in synchronization with acceleration of the jaw, which occurs when the food breaks or after a dip in the load profile. Significant differences in texture attributes were observed for load profiles which simulate different breakage behaviour of a food. It can be concluded that simulated chewing is a promising tool for studying neuromuscular and sensory aspects of chewing crispy foods in a controlled and reproducible way.

1.6 Influence of age on oral physiology, food perception and nutrient intake

Ageing involves various changes in the oral physiology such as teeth loss, muscle fatigue, bite force reduction and decrease of tongue motor skill. Salivary flow rate and saliva composition may also change with age. A substantial number of older people have a compromised chewing performance, which may result in a diet low in fruits and vegetables. The ensuing monotonous food consumption may lead to inadequate nutrient intakes. It is commonly believed that the sense of smell decreases with age. The sense of taste, however, remains relatively robust throughout the lifespan. Texture perception appears well preserved during healthy ageing.

Elderly people may have deficiencies in masticatory performance because of deteriorated muscle strength, loss of teeth, malocclusion or periodontal disease (Fontijn-Tekamp *et al.*, 2000; Shinogaya *et al.*, 2001; Locker, 2002; Kohyama *et al.*, 2002; Mioche *et al.*, 2004; Kohyama and Mioche, 2004; Peyron *et al.*, 2004a; Ikebe *et al.*, 2005; Gotfredsen and Walls, 2007). Also salivary flow rate may decrease for the elderly, although the decrease appeared to be moderate in fit, healthy, unmedicated subjects (Heintze *et al.*, 1983; Navazesh *et al.*, 1992; Bourdiol *et al.*, 2004; Walls and Steele, 2004). However, substantial changes in salivary composition and flow rate are reported for older people as a result of diseases and conditions associated with age (Walls and Steele, 2004). The deterioration of masticatory performance and salivary flow may lead to changes in the diet, because some foods become troublesome to eat (Fontijn-Tekamp *et al.*, 1996; Hildebrandt *et al.*, 1997; Sheiham *et al.*, 2001; N'Gom and Woda, 2002; Bartali *et al.*, 2003; Roininen *et al.*, 2004; Walls and Steele, 2004; Sakurai *et al.*, 2005). The altered food choice may result in lower intakes for key nutrients as iron and fibre (Sheiham *et al.*, 2001). Quality of life could be influenced by the oral status in the elderly (Miura *et al.*, 2000; Takata *et al.*, 2006). However, in spite of their handicap, most people manage to eat successfully even though they are unable to comminute their food perfectly before swallowing. Tailored nutrition intervention aimed to increase the fruit and vegetable intake of edentulous older people can change dietary behaviour positively (Bradbury *et al.*, 2006).

In order to improve the masticatory function, missing teeth are often replaced by fixed or removable prosthodontic appliances. The provision of dental implants significantly improves oral function. After the implant treatment the patients report high levels of satisfaction regarding various aspects of their denture function and they are more satisfied than patients with similar problems who received a conventional denture without implant support (Naert *et al.*, 2004; Cune *et al.*, 2005). Improvement of the oral function after implant treatment was also demonstrated by objective methods. The maximum bite force of subjects with a mandibular denture supported by implants is 60–200% higher than that of subjects with a conventional denture (Carlsson and Lindquist, 1994; Fontijn-Tekamp *et al.*, 1998; van Kampen *et al.*, 2002). The objective masticatory performance significantly improved after implant treatment (Fontijn-Tekamp *et al.*, 2000; Bakke *et al.*, 2002; van Kampen *et al.*, 2004). The number of chewing cycles needed to halve the initial size of a test food on average decreased from 47 to 25 cycles after implant treatment (van Kampen *et al.*, 2004). Thus, after implant treatment, subjects needed only about half the number of chewing cycles as before treatment to comminute their food.

In a study on the determinants of masticatory function it was reported that age had a direct effect on bite force and on occlusal units (Hatch *et al.*, 2000). Furthermore, an indirect effect of age on bite force was reported, which was caused by a decrease in the number of occlusal units. One can only speculate why bite force decreases with age. It may be a direct effect of age on muscle strength or it may be caused by changes in food choice because of deteriorated dentition. This may lead to less trained jaw muscles. Although the correlation between age and bite force was significant, it should be realized that the effect of age on bite force was small. The correlation coefficients were between –0.22 and –0.31, which means that age explains less than 10% of the variance of bite force. In a recent study the impact of age on masticatory function was assessed (Mishellany-Dutour *et al.*, 2008). The oral function of a group of young fully dentate subjects (36.7 years) was compared with the function of aged individuals with similar dentition (68.8 years). Aged subjects used significantly more chewing strokes to reach the swallowing threshold than younger subjects and as a result they swallowed finer food particles than the young subjects.

It is well established that sensory acuity diminishes with age and that, within the chemical senses, the sense of smell is more prone to losses with age than is the sense of taste (Murphy, 1993; Mojet *et al.*, 2005). It is also widely assumed that such losses inevitably lead to less pleasure derived from eating (Mattes, 2002), and to a preference for stronger flavoured/tasting products (de Graaf *et al.*, 1996). As a consequence, age-related changes in sensory perception and preference are believed to have a major impact on appetite and food intake (Mojet *et al.*, 2005). Oral sensation, as measured with, for example, two-point discrimination, oral stereognosis, vibrotactile detection, proprioception and thermal sensistivity, was shown to remain stable with ageing, and showed only a slight decline after the age of 80 (Calhoun *et al.*, 1992; Ikebe *et al.*, 2007).

1.7 Future trends

By understanding the processes in the mouth while eating, a better understanding of the sensations and the perceptions of the food can be gained. Knowledge of physiological parameters may be of importance when performing and designing rheological/instrumental measurements for a food.

Better predictions of sensory perception of a specific food may thus be obtained. This could save time and money on time-consuming and expensive sensory panels in the earlier steps of product development and renovation. Knowing how physiological processes highlight specific flavour/texture sensations may be useful for product development or quality control where one typically wants to focus on certain sensations and ignore others. In addition, a future application could be to tailor products for personalized nutrition, individual choices or clinical nutrition based on physiological groups.

1.8 Sources of further information and advice

The following review issues/articles may be helpful in further study:

- Special issue of the *Journal of Texture Studies* on 'Mastication and food texture' (Nishinari, 2004a).
- Special issue of *Physiology and Behavior* on 'Making sense of food' (Hamer *et al.*, 2006).
- Special issue of *Archives of Oral Biology* on 'Mastication' (Türker and Cadden, 2007).
- Review article on 'Human oral function' (van der Bilt, 2002).
- Review article on 'The neurocognitive bases of human multimodal food perception: sensory integration' (Verhagen and Engelen, 2006).
- Review article on 'Oral physiology and texture perception of semisolids' (Engelen and van der Bilt, 2008).
- Review article on 'Food oral processing' (Chen, 2009).

1.9 References

ABBINK JH, VAN DER BILT A, BOSMAN F, VAN DER GLAS HW (1997), A comparison of jaw-opener and jaw-closing muscle activity in humans to overcome an external force counteracting jaw movement. *Exp Brain Res* **118**, 269–278.

ABBINK JH, VAN DER BILT A, BOSMAN F, VAN DER GLAS HW (1999a), Speed-dependent control of cyclic open-close movements of the human jaw with an external force counteracting closing. *J Dent Res* **78**, 878–886.

ABBINK JH, VAN DER BILT A, BOSMAN F, VAN DER GLAS HW, ERKELENS CJ, KLAASSEN MFH (1999b), Comparison of external-load compensation during rhythmic arm movements and rhythmic jaw movements in humans. *J Neurophysiol* **82**, 1209–1217.

ADAMS D (1975), The mucus barrier and absorption through the oral mucosa. *J Dent Res* **54**, B19–B26.

AGRAWAL KR, LUCAS PW, BRUCE IC, PRINZ JF (1998), Food properties that influence neuromuscular activity during human mastication. *J Dent Res* **77**, 1931–1938.

ANDERSON DJ, HECTOR MP, LINDEN RWA (1985), The possible relation between mastication and parotid secretion in the rabbit. *J Physiol* **364**, 19–29.

ANDERSON DJ, HECTOR MP, LINDEN RWA (1996), The effects of unilateral and bilateral chewing, empty clenching and simulated bruxism, on the masticatory-parotid salivary reflex in man. *Exp Physiol* **81**, 305–312.

BAKKE M, HOLM B, GOTFREDSEN K (2002), Masticatory function and patient satisfaction with implant-supported mandibular overdentures: a prospective 5-year study. *Int J Prosthodont* **15**, 575–581.

BARTALI B, SALVINI S, TURRINI A, LAURETANI F, RUSSO CR, CORSI AM, BANDINELLI S, D'AMICIS A, PALLI D, GURALNIK JM, FERRUCCI L (2003), Age and disability affect dietary intake. *J Nutr* **133**, 2868–2873.

BARYLKO-PIKIELNA N, SZCZESNIAK AS (1994), Taste and flavour perception in mayonnaise-type emulsion of various fat level. *Pol J Food Nutr Sci* **3**, 57–70.

BELLISLE F, LUCAS F, AMRANI R, LE MAGNEN J (1984), Deprivation, palatability and the micro-structure of meals in human subjects. *Appetite* **5**, 85–94.

BELLISLE F, GUY-GRAND B, LE MAGNEN J (2000), Chewing and swallowing as indices of the stimulation to eat during meals in humans: effects revealed by the edogram method and video recordings. *Neurosci Biobehav Rev* **24**, 223–228.

BLISSETT A, PRINZ JF, WULFERT F, TAYLOR AJ, HORT J (2007), Effect of bolus size on chewing, swallowing, oral soft tissue and tongue movement. *J Oral Rehabil* **34**, 572–582.

BOURDIOL P, MIOCHE L, MONIER S (2004), Effect of age on salivary flow obtained under feeding and non-feeding conditions. *J Oral Rehabil* **31**, 445–452.

BOURNE MC (1975), Is rheology enough for food texture measurement? *J Texture Stud* **6**, 259–262.

BOURNE MC (1982), *Food Texture and Viscosity: Concept and Measurement*. New York: Academic Press.

BOURNE MC (2002), *Food Texture and Viscosity. Concept and Measurement*, London: Academic Press.

BOURNE MC (2004), Relation between texture and mastication. *J Texture Stud* **35**, 125–143.

BRADBURY J, THOMASON JM, JEPSON NJA, WALLS AWG, ALLEN PF, MOYNIHAN PJ (2006), Nutrition counseling increases fruit and vegetable intake in the edentulous. *J Dent Res* **85**, 463–468.

BROOKS VB (1986), *The Neural Basis of Motor Control*, New York, Oxford: Oxford University Press.

CALHOUN KH, GIBSON B, HARTLEY L, MINTON J, HOKANSON JA (1992), Age-related changes in oral sensation. *Laryngoscope* **102**, 109–116.

CARLSSON GE, LINDQUIST LW (1994), Ten-year longitudinal study of masticatory function in edentulous patients treated with fixed complete dentures on osseointegrated implants. *Int J Prosthodont* **7**, 448–453.

CHEN J (2009), Food oral processing – a review. *Food Hydrocolloids* **23**, 1–25.

CHRISTENSEN CM (1985), Role of saliva in human taste perception. In: *Clinical Measurements of Taste and Smell*. Meiselman HL, Rivlin RS, editors. New York: Macmillan, pp. 414–428.

CHRISTENSEN CM, BRAND JG, MALAMUD D (1987), Salivary changes in solution pH: A source of individual differences in sour taste perception. *Physiol Behav* **40**, 221–227.

CUNE MS, VAN KAMPEN FMC, VAN DER BILT A, BOSMAN F (2005), Patient satisfaction and preference with magnet, bar-clip, and ball-socket retained mandibular implant overdentures: a cross-over clinical trial. *Int J Prosthodont* **18**, 99–105.

DAN H, WATANABE H, KOHYAMA K (2003), Effect of sample thickness on the bite force for apples. *J Texture Stud* **34**, 287–302.

DE GRAAF C, VAN STAVEREN W, BUREMA J (1996), Psychophysical and psychohedonic functions of four common food flavours in elderly subjects. *Chem Senses* **21**, 293–302.

DE WIJK RA, PRINZ JF, JANSSEN AM (2006a), Explaining perceived oral texture of starch-based custard desserts from standard and novel instrumental tests. *Food Hydrocolloids* **20**, 24–34.

DE WIJK RA, TERPSTRA MEJ, JANSSEN AM, PRINZ JF (2006b), Perceived creaminess of semi-solid foods. *Trends Food Sci Tech* **17**, 412–422.

DELLOW PG, LUND JP (1971), Evidence for central timing of rhythmical mastication. *J Physiol* **215**, 1–13.

DIJKSTERHUIS G, LUYTEN H, DE WIJK RA, MOJET J (2007), A new sensory vocabulary for crisp and crunchy dry model foods. *Food Qual Prefer* **18**, 37–50.

ENGELEN L (2004), A rough guide to texture: Oral physiology and texture perception of semi-solids. Dissertation, Utrecht University, the Netherlands.

ENGELEN L, VAN DER BILT A (2008), Oral physiology and texture perception of semi-solids. *J Texture Stud* **39**, 83–113.

ENGELEN L, DE WIJK RA, VAN DER BILT A, JANSSEN AM, BOSMAN F (2002), The effect of oral temperature on the temperature perception of liquids and semi-solids in the mouth. *Eur J Oral Sci* **110**, 412–416.

ENGELEN L, DE WIJK RA, PRINZ JF, JANSSEN AM, VAN DER BILT A, WEENEN H, BOSMAN F (2003a), A comparison of the effects of added saliva, α-amylase and water on texture perception in semisolids. *Physiol Behav* **78**, 805–811.

ENGELEN L, DE WIJK RA, PRINZ JF, VAN DER BILT A, BOSMAN F (2003b), The relation between saliva flow after different stimulations and the perception of flavor and texture attributes in custard desserts. *Physiol Behav* **78**, 165–169.

ENGELEN L, FONTIJN-TEKAMP FA, VAN DER BILT A (2005), The influence of product and oral characteristics on swallowing. *Arch Oral Biol* **50**, 739–746.

ENGELEN L, VAN DEN KEYBUS PAM, DE WIJK RA, VEERMAN ECI, VAN NIEUW AMERONGEN A, BOSMAN F, PRINZ JF, VAN DER BILT A (2007), The effect of saliva composition on texture perception of semi-solids. *Arch Oral Biol* **52**, 518–525.

FONTIJN-TEKAMP FA, VAN 'T HOF MA, SLAGTER AP, VAN WAAS MAJ (1996), The state of dentition in relation to nutrition in elderly Europeans in the SENECA study of 1993. *Eur J Clin Nutr* **50**, S117–S122.

FONTIJN-TEKAMP FA, SLAGTER AP, VAN 'T HOF MA, GEERTMAN ME, KALK W (1998), Bite forces with mandibular implant-retained overdentures. *J Dent Res* **77**, 1832–1839.

FONTIJN-TEKAMP FA, SLAGTER AP, VAN DER BILT A, VAN 'T HOF MA, WITTER DJ, KALK W, JANSEN JA (2000), Biting and chewing in overdentures, full dentures, and natural dentitions. *J Dent Res* **79**, 1519–1524.

FONTIJN-TEKAMP FA, VAN DER BILT A, ABBINK JH, BOSMAN F (2004), Swallowing threshold and masticatory performance in dentate adults. *Physiol Behav* **83**, 431–436.

FOSTER KD, WODA A, PEYRON MA (2006), Effect of texture of plastic and elastic model foods on the parameters of mastication. *J Neurophysiol* **95**, 3469–3479.

GARDNER EP, MARTIN JH, JESSELL TM (2000), The bodily senses. In: *Principles of Neural Science*. Kandel ER, Schwartz JH, Jessell TM, editors. New York: McGraw-Hill, pp. 430–450.

GAVIÃO MBD, ENGELEN L, VAN DER BILT A (2004), Chewing behavior and salivary secretion. *Eur J Oral Sci* **112**, 19–24.

GERMAN RZ, CROMPTON AW, THEXTON AJ (2004), The role of animal models in understanding feeding behavior in infants. *Int J Orofacial Myology* **30**, 20–30.

GIBBONS R (1979), On the mechanisms of bacterial attachment to teeth. In: *Saliva and Dental Caries*. Kleinberg I, Mandel ID, Ellison SA, editors. New York: Information Retrieval Inc., pp. 267–273.

GOLDBERG LJ, CHANDLER SH (1990), Central mechanisms of rhythmic trigeminal activity. In: *Neurophysiology of the Jaws and Teeth*. Taylor A, editor. Hong Kong: Macmillan Press Ltd, pp. 268–293.

GOLDSTEIN EB (1996), The somatic senses. In: *Sensation and Perception*. Pacific Grove: Brooks/Cole Publishing Company, pp. 459–487.

GOODWIN GM, LUSCHEI ES (1974), Effects of destroying spindle afferents from jaw muscles on mastication in monkeys. *J Neurophysiol* **37**, 967–981.

GOTFREDSEN K, WALLS AWG (2007), What dentition assures oral function? *Clin Oral Impl Res* **18** Suppl. 3, 34–45.
GREEN BG (1993), Oral astringency: a tactile component of flavor. *Acta-Psychol-Amst* **84**, 119–125.
GUINARD J-X, ZOUMAS-MORSE C, WALCHAK C, SIMPSON H (1997), Relation between saliva flow and flavor release from chewing gum. *Physiol Behav* **61**, 591–596.
HAMER RJ, PRINZ JF, DRANSFIELD E, WESTERTERP-PLANTENGA MS (2006), Making sense of food. *Physiol Behav* **89**, 1–3.
HATCH JP, SHINKAI RSA, SAKAI S, RUGH JD, PAUNOVICH ED (2000), Determinants of masticatory performance in dentate adults. *Arch Oral Biol* **46**, 641–648.
HECTOR MP, LINDEN RWA (1999), Reflexes of salivary secretion. In: *Neural Mechanisms of Salivary Gland Secretion*. Garrett JR, Ekström J, Anderson LC, editors. Basel: Karger, pp. 196–217.
HEINTZE U, BIRKHED D, BJÖRN H (1983), Secretion rate and buffer effect of resting and stimulated whole saliva as a function of age and sex. *Swed Dent J* **7**, 227–238.
HENKIN RI, BANKS V (1967), Tactile perception on the tongue, palate and the hand of normal man help. In: *Symposium on Oral Sensation and Perception*. Bosma JF, editor. Springfield, pp. 182–187.
HIIEMAE KM (2004), Mechanisms of food reduction, transport and deglutition: How the texture of food affects feeding behavior. *J Texture Stud* **35**, 171–200.
HIIEMAE KM, THEXTON AJ, CROMPTON AW (1978), Intra-oral food transport: the fundamental mechanism of feeding. In: *Muscle Adaptation in the Craniofacial Region*. Carlson DS, McNamara JA, editors. Ann Arbor, Michigan: University of Michigan, pp. 181–208.
HIIEMAE KM, HEATH MR, HEATH G, KAZAZOGLU E, MURRAY J, SAPPER D, HAMBLETT K (1996), Natural bites, food consistency and feeding behaviour in man. *Arch Oral Biol* **41**, 175–189.
HILDEBRANDT GH, DOMINGUEZ BL, SCHORK MA, LOESCHE WJ (1997), Functional units, chewing, swallowing, and food avoidance among the elderly. *J Prosthet Dent* **77**, 588–595.
HORIO T, KAWAMURA Y (1989), Effects of texture of food on chewing patterns in the human subjects. *J Oral Rehabil* **16**, 177–183.
HÜCK NL, ABBINK JH, VAN DER GLAS HW, VAN VLIET T, LUYTEN H, VAN DER BILT A (2005), Oral physiology of eating crispy foods. *Proceedings 6th Pangborn Sensory Science Symposium* P29 (Abstract).
HUTCHINGS JB, LILLFORD PJ (1988), The perception of food texture – the philosophy of the breakdown path. *J Texture Stud* **19**, 103–115.
HYVÖNEN L, LINNA M, TUORILA H, DIJKSTERHUIS GB (2003), Perception of melting and flavor release of ice cream containing different types and contents of fat. *J Dairy Sci* **86**, 1130–1138.
IKEBE K, NOKUBI T, MORII K, KASHIWAGI J (2005), Association of bite force with ageing and occlusal support in older adults. *J Dent* **33**, 131–137.
IKEBE K, AMEMIYA M, MORII K, MATSUDA K, FURUYA-YOSHINAKA M, NOKUBI T (2007), Comparison of oral stereognosis in relation to age and the use of complete dentures. *J Oral Rehabil* **34**, 345–350.
JALABERT-MALBOS ML, MISHELLANY-DUTOUR A, WODA A, PEYRON MA (2007), Particle size distribution in the food bolus after mastication of natural foods. *Food Qual Prefer* **18**, 803–812.
JANSSEN AM, TERPSTRA MEJ, DE WIJK RA, PRINZ JF (2007), Relations between rheological properties, saliva-induced structure breakdown and sensory texture attributes of custards. *J Texture Stud* **38**, 42–69.
JELLEMA RH, JANSSEN AM, TERPSTRA MEJ, DE WIJK RA, SMILDE AK (2005), Relating the sensory sensation 'creamy mouthfeel' in custards to rheological measurements. *J Chemometrics* **19**, 191–200.

JOHANSSON RS, TRULSSON M, OLSSON KA, WESTBERG KG (1988), Mechanoreceptor activity from the human face and oral mucosa. *Exp Brain Res* **72**, 204–208.

JOWITT R (1974), The terminology of food texture. *J Text Stud* **5**, 351–358.

KALLITHRAKA S, BAKKER J, CLIFFORD MN, VALLIS L (2001), Correlations between saliva protein composition and some T-I parameters of astringency. *Food Qual Prefer* **12**, 145–152.

KILCAST D, EVES A (1991), Integrating texture and physiology techniques. In: *Feeding and the Texture of Food*. Vincent JFV, Lillford PJ, editors. New York: Cambridge University Press, pp. 167–183.

KOHYAMA K, MIOCHE L (2004), Chewing behavior observed at different stages of mastication for six foods, studied by electromyography and jaw kinematics in young and elderly subjects. *J Texture Stud* **35**, 395–414.

KOHYAMA K, SAKAI T, AZUMA T (2001), Patterns observed in the first chew of foods with various textures. *Food Sci Technol Res* **7**, 290–296.

KOHYAMA K, MIOCHE L, MARTIN J-F (2002), Chewing patterns of various texture foods studied by electromyography in young and elderly populations. *J Texture Stud* **33**, 269–283.

KOHYAMA K, HATAKEYAMA E, SASAKI T, DAN H, AZUMA T, KARITA K (2004), Effects of sample hardness on human chewing force: a model study using silicone rubber. *Arch Oral Biol* **49**, 805–816.

LARSEN MJ, JENSEN AF, MADSEN DM, PEARCE EIF (1999), Individual variations of pH, buffer capacity, and concentrations of calcium and phosphate in unstimulated whole saliva. *Arch Oral Biol* **44**, 111–117.

LASSAUZAY C, PEYRON MA, ALBUISSON E, DRANSFIELD E, WODA A (2000), Variability of the masticatory process during chewing of elastic model foods. *Eur J Oral Sci* **108**, 484–492.

LAVIGNE G, KIM JS, VALIQUETTE C, LUND JP (1987), Evidence that periodontal pressoreceptors provide positive feedback to jaw closing muscles during mastication. *J Neurophysiol* **58**, 342–358.

LIEDBERG B, ÖWALL B (1991), Masticatory ability in experimentally induced xerostomia. *Dysphagia* **6**, 211–213.

LINDBERG AA (1973), Bacteriophage receptors. *Ann Rev Microbiol* **27**, 205–241.

LOCKER D (2002), Changes in chewing ability with ageing: a 7-year study of older adults. *J Oral Rehabil* **29**, 1021–1029.

LUCAS PW, LUKE DA (1984), Optimum mouthful for food comminution in human mastication. *Arch Oral Biol* **29**, 205–210.

LUCAS PW, LUKE DA (1986), Is food particle size a criterion for the initiation of swallowing? *J Oral Rehabil* **13**, 127–136.

LUCAS PW, PRINZ JF, AGRAWAL KR, BRUCE IC (2004), Food texture and its effect on ingestion, mastication and swallowing. *J Texture Stud* **35**, 159–170.

LUND JP (1976), Evidence for a central neural pattern generator regulating the chewing cycle. In: *Mastication*. Anderson DJ, Matthews B, editors. Bristol: John Wright and Sons, pp. 204–212.

LUND JP (1991), Mastication and its control by the brain stem. *Crit Rev Oral Biol Med* **2**, 33–64.

MATHEVON E, MIOCHE L, BROWN WE, CULIOLI J (1995), Texture analysis of beef cooked at various temperatures by mechanical measurements, sensory assessments and electromyography. *J Texture Stud* **26**, 175–192.

MATSUMOTO N, MATSUMOTO F (1977), Taste of food. Factors related to the evaluation. *Jpn J Cookery Sci* **10**, 97–101.

MATTES R (2002), The chemical senses and nutrition in aging: challenging old assumptions. *J Am Diet Assoc* **102**, 192–196.

MIOCHE L (2004), Mastication and food texture perception: variation with age. *J Texture Stud* **35**, 145–158.

MIOCHE L, BOURDIOL P, MONIER S (2003), Chewing behaviour and bolus formation during mastication of meat with different textures. *Arch Oral Biol* **48**, 193–200.

MIOCHE L, BOURDIOL P, MONIER S, MARTIN J-F, CORMIER D (2004), Changes in jaw muscles activity with age: effects on food bolus properties. *Physiol Behav* **82**, 621–627.

MIOCHE L, BOURDIOL P, MARTIN J-F, NOËL Y (1999), Variations in human masseter and temporalis muscle activity related to food texture during free and side-imposed mastication. *Arch Oral Biol* **44**, 1005–1012.

MISHELLANY-DUTOUR A, RENAUD J, PEYRON MA, RIMEK F, WODA A (2008), Is the goal of mastication reached in young dentates, aged dentates and aged denture wearers? *Brit J Nutr* **99**, 121–128.

MIURA H, MIURA K, MIZUGAI H, ARAI Y, UMENAI T, ISOGAI E (2000), Chewing ability and quality of life among the elderly residing in a rural community in Japan. *J Oral Rehabil* **27**, 731–734.

MIYAWAKI S, OHKOCHI N, KAWAKAMI T, SUGIMURA M (2000), Effect of food size on the movement of the mandibular first molars and condyles during deliberate unilateral mastication in humans. *J Dent Res* **79**, 1525–1531.

MOJET J, CHRIST-HAZELHOF E, HEIDEMA J (2005), Taste perception with age: pleasantness and its relationships with threshold sensitivity and supra-threshold intensity of five taste qualities. *Food Qual Prefer* **16**, 413–423.

MORIMOTO T, INOUE T, MASUDA Y, NAGASHIMA T (1989), Sensory components facilitating jaw-closing muscle activities in the rabbit. *Exp Brain Res* **76**, 424–440.

MORIMOTO T, NAKAMURA O, OGATA K, LIU ZJ, MATSUO R, INOUE T, MASUDA Y, SAITO O, MIZUNO J, KATO T (1995), Autoregulation of masticatory force in the anesthetized rabbit. In: *Brain and Oral Functions*. Morimoto T, Matsuya T, Takada K, editors. Amsterdam: Elsevier Science BV, pp. 115–124.

MOUNTCASTLE VB (1974), Neural mechanisms in somesthesia. In: *Medical Physiology*. Mountcastle VB, editor. St. Louis, MO: Mosby, pp. 307–347.

MURPHY C (1993), Nutrition and chemosensory perception in the elderly. *Crit Rev Food Sci Nutrition* **33**, 3–15.

NAERT I, ALSAADI G, QUIRYNEN M (2004), Prosthetic aspects and patient satisfaction with two-implant-retained mandibular overdentures: a 10-year randomized clinical study. *Int J Prosthodont* **17**, 401–410.

NAVAZESH M, MULLIGAN RA, KIPNIS V, DENNY PA, DENNY PC (1992), Comparison of whole saliva flow rates and mucin concentrations in healthy Caucasian young and aged adults. *J Dent Res* **71**, 1275–1278.

N'GOM PI, WODA A (2002), Influence of impaired mastication on nutrition. *J Prosthet Dent* **87**, 667–673.

NIEUW AMERONGEN AV (1994), *Speeksel en mondgezondheid*, Amsterdam: VU Uitgeverij.

NISHINARI K (2004a), Introduction to a special issue of JTS. *J Texture Stud* **35**, ix–xi.

NISHINARI K (2004b), Rheology, Food texture and mastication. *J Texture Stud* **35**, 113–124.

NOZAKI S, IRIKI A, NAKAMURA Y (1986), Localization of central rhythm generator involved in cortically induced rhythmical masticatory jaw-opening movement in the guinea-pig. *J Neurophysiol* **55**, 806–825.

OTTENHOFF FM, VAN DER BILT A, VAN DER GLAS HW, BOSMAN F (1992), Peripherally induced and anticipated elevator muscle activity during simulated chewing in humans. *J Neurophysiol* **67**, 75–83.

PANGBORN RM, LUNDGREN B (1977), Salivary secretion in response to mastication of crisp bread. *J Texture Stud* **8**, 463–472.

PEDERSEN AM, BARDOW A, JENSEN SB, NAUNTOFTE B (2002), Saliva and gastrointestinal functions of taste, mastication, swallowing and digestion. *Oral Dis* **8**, 117–129.

PEREIRA LJ, DE WIJK RA, GAVIÃO MBD, VAN DER BILT A (2006), Effects of added fluids on the perception of solid food. *Physiol Behav* **88**, 538–544.

PEYRON MA, MASKAWI K, WODA A, TANGUAY R, LUND JP (1997), Effects of food texture and sample thickness on mandibular movement and hardness assessment during biting in man. *J Dent Res* **76**, 789–795.

PEYRON MA, LASSAUZAY C, WODA A (2002), Effects of increased hardness on jaw movement and muscle activity during chewing of visco-elastic model foods. *Exp Brain Res* **142**, 41–51.

PEYRON MA, BLANC O, LUND JP, WODA A (2004a), Influence of age on adaptability of human mastication. *J Neurophysiol* **92**, 773–779.

PEYRON MA, MISHELLANY A, WODA A (2004b), Particle size distribution of food boluses after mastication of six natural foods. *J Dent Res* **83**, 578–582.

PLESH O, BISHOP B, MCCALL WD (1986), Effect of gum hardness on chewing pattern. *Exp Neurol* **92**, 502–512.

PRINZ JF, LUCAS PW (1997), An optimization model for mastication and swallowing in mammals. *Proc R Soc Lond B* **264**, 1715–1721.

PRINZ JF, LUCAS PW (1995), Swallow thresholds in human mastication. *Arch Oral Biol* **40**, 401–403.

PRÖSCHEL PA, HOFMANN M (1988), Frontal chewing patterns of the incisor point and their dependence on resistance of food and type of occlusion. *J Prosthet Dent* **59**, 617–624.

RANC H, ELKHYAT A, SERVAIS C, MAC-MARY S, LAUNAY B, HUMBERT P (2006), Friction coefficient and wettability of oral mucosal tissue: changes induced by a salivary layer. *Colloids Surfaces A: Physicochem Eng Aspects* **276**, 155–161.

RINGEL RL, EWANOWSKI SJ (1965), Oral perception: 1. Two-point discrimination. *J Hearing Speech Res* 8, 389–397.

ROININEN K, FILLION L, KILCAST D, LÄHTEENMÄKI L (2004), Exploring difficult textural properties of fruit and vegetables for the elderly in Finland and the United Kingdom. *Food Qual Prefer* **15**, 517–530.

RUTH SMV, ROOZEN JP (2000), Influence of mastication and saliva on aroma release in a model mouth system. *Food Chemistry* **71**, 339–345.

SAKURAI M, TADA A, SUZUKI K, YOSHINO K, SUGIHARA N, MATSUKUBO T (2005), Percentile curves for food acceptance response scores in assessing chewing functions in adults. *Bull Tokyo Dent Coll* **46**, 123–134.

SCHIFFMAN SS (1977), Food recognition by the elderly. *J Gerontology* **32**, 586–592.

SCHNEYER LH, YOUNG JA, SCHNEYER CA (1972), Salivary secretion of electrolytes. *Physiol Rev* **52**, 720–755.

SCOTT BJJ, BAJAJ J, LINDEN RWA (1999), The contribution of mechanoreceptive neurones in the gingival tissues to the masticatory-parotid salivary reflex in man. *J Oral Rehabil* **26**, 791–797.

SHEIHAM A, STEELE JG, MARCENES W, LOWE C, FINCH S, BATES CJ, PRENTICE A, WALLS AWG (2001), The relationship among dental status, nutrient intake, and nutritional status in older people. *J Dent Res* **80**, 408–413.

SHINOGAYA T, BAKKE M, THOMSEN CE, VILMANN A, SODEYAMA A, MATSUMOTO M (2001), Effects of ethnicity, gender and age on clenching force and load distribution. *Clin Oral Invest* **5**, 63–68.

SLAGER GEC, OTTEN E, VAN EIJDEN TMGJ, VAN WILLIGEN JD (1997), Mathematical model of the human jaw system simulating static biting and movements after unloading. *J Neurophysiol* **78**, 3222–3233.

SZCZESNIAK AS (1963a), Classification of textural characteristics. *J Food Sci* **28**, 385–389.

SZCZESNIAK AS (1963b), Consumer awareness of texture and other food attributes. *Food Technol* **17**, 74–77.

SZCZESNIAK AS (1990), Texture: Is it still an overlooked food attribute? *Food Technol* **44**, 86–95.

SZCZESNIAK AS (2002), Texture is a sensory property. *Food Qual Prefer* **13**, 215–225.

SZCZESNIAK AS (2003), Psychorheology and texture as factors controlling the consumer acceptance of food. *Cereal Foods World* **35**, 1201–1205.

TABAK LA, LEVINE MJ, MANDEL ID, ELLISON SA (1982), Role of salivary mucins in the protection of the oral cavity. *J Oral Pathol* **11**, 1–17.

TAKATA Y, ANSAI T, AWANO S, FUKUHARA M, SONOKI K, WAKISAKA M, FUJISAWA K, AKIFUSA S, TAKEHARA T (2006), Chewing ability and quality of life in an 80-year-old population. *J Oral Rehabil* **33**, 330–334.

TANAKA M (1986), Texture of Japanese foods. *Food Revs Intl* **2**, 247.

THEXTON AJ (1973), Some aspects of neurophysiology of dental interest. I. Theories of oral function. *J Dent* **2**, 49–54.

THEXTON AJ (1992), Mastication and swallowing: an overview. *Brit Dent J* **173**, 197–206.

THEXTON AJ, HIIEMAE KM, CROMPTON AW (1980), Food consistency and bite size as regulators of jaw movement during feeding in the cat. *J Neurophysiol* **44**, 456–474.

TRULSSON M (1993), Orofacial mechanoreception in man. Dissertation, University of Umeå, Sweden.

TRULSSON M, ESSICK GK (1997), Low-threshold mechanoreceptive afferents in the human lingual nerve. *J Neurophysiol* **77**, 737–748 (Abstract).

TÜRKER KS, CADDEN SW (2007), Preface: Special issue International Mastication Symposium Brisbane 2006. *Arch Oral Biol* **52**, 295.

VAN BOVEN RW, JOHNSON KO (1994), The limit of tactile spatial resolution in humans: grating orientation discrimination at the lip, tongue, and finger. *Neurology* **44**, 2361–2366.

VAN DER BILT A (2002), Human oral function. A review. *Braz J Oral Sci* **1**, 7–18.

VAN DER BILT A, VAN DER GLAS HW, OLTHOFF LW, BOSMAN F (1991), The effect of particle size reduction on the jaw gape in human mastication. *J Dent Res* **70**, 931–937.

VAN DER BILT A, ABBINK JH, MOWLANA F, HEATH MR (1993), A comparison between data analysis methods concerning particle size distributions obtained by mastication in man. *Arch Oral Biol* **38**, 163–167.

VAN DER BILT A, OTTENHOFF FM, VAN DER GLAS HW, BOSMAN F, ABBINK JH, WEIJNEN FG (1995), Neuromuscular control of simulated chewing in humans. In: *Brain and Oral Functions*. Morimoto T, Matsuya T, Takada K, editors. Amsterdam: Elsevier Science BV, pp. 125–140.

VAN DER BILT A, ENGELEN L, PEREIRA LJ, VAN DER GLAS HW, ABBINK JH (2006), Oral physiology and mastication. *Physiol Behav* **89**, 22–27.

VAN DER BILT A, ENGELEN L, ABBINK JH, PEREIRA LJ (2007), Effects of adding fluids to solid foods on muscle activity and number of chewing cycles. *Eur J Oral Sci* **115**, 198–205.

VAN DER GLAS HW, OLTHOFF LW, VAN DER BILT A, BOSMAN F (1987), Control of elevator muscle activity during chewing in man. *Soc Neurosci Abstr* **13**, 11.

VAN KAMPEN FMC, VAN DER BILT A, CUNE MS, BOSMAN F (2002), The influence of various attachment types in mandibular implant-retained overdentures on maximum bite force and EMG. *J Dent Res* **81**, 170–173.

VAN KAMPEN FMC, VAN DER BILT A, CUNE MS, FONTIJN-TEKAMP FA, BOSMAN F (2004), Masticatory function with implant-supported overdentures. *J Dent Res* **83**, 708–711.

VERHAGEN JV, ENGELEN L (2006), The neurocognitive bases of human multimodal food perception: sensory integration. *Neurosci Biobehav Rev* **30**, 613–650.

WALLS AWG, STEELE JG (2004), The relationship between oral health and nutrition in older people. *Mech Ageing Devel* **125**, 853–857.
WILKINSON C, DIJKSTERHUIS GB, MINEKUS M (2000), From food structure to texture. *Trends Food Sci Tech* **11**, 442–450.
YVEN C, BONNET L, CORMIER D, MONIER S, MIOCHE L (2006), Impaired mastication modifies the dynamics of bolus formation. *Eur J Oral Sci* **114**, 184–190.

2

Gut microbial ecology

H. J. Flint, S. H. Duncan and P. Louis, Rowett Institute of Nutrition and Health, UK

Abstract: Microbial colonization of the human intestine has multiple consequences. On the negative side, the gut is a source of pathogens and inflammation, and microbial activity can produce toxic metabolites. On the positive side, the gut community in healthy individuals helps to create a barrier that reduces the risk of infection by pathogens, while the major products of microbial fermentation in the colon, the short chain fatty acids, especially butyrate, play a generally beneficial role in maintaining gut health. This chapter focuses upon the influence of diet composition upon the metabolic activities and species composition of the human colonic microbiota.

Key words: colonic microbiota, functional foods, butyrate, hydrogen metabolism, pH.

2.1 Introduction

Microbial colonization of the human gastrointestinal (GI) tract has both positive and negative consequences for the host (Fig. 2.1). On the negative side, the gut is a source of pathogenic micro-organisms and potentially a major site of infection and microbially promoted inflammation. In addition, microbial metabolic activity can produce toxic and carcinogenic compounds from dietary or endogenously derived substrates. On the positive side, the resident gut community in healthy individuals helps to create a barrier that reduces the risk of proliferation and infection by pathogens. Furthermore, the major products of fermentation, the short chain fatty acids (SCFAs), are formed by the anaerobic microbial metabolism of 'low digestible' dietary carbohydrates and functional foods. These SCFAs are considered to play a generally beneficial role as energy sources for the host, and butyrate in particular exerts regulatory effects on the colonic epithelium, helping to maintain the gut mucosa in a healthy state. It has also been proposed that this microbial supply of energy might contribute to obesity, with

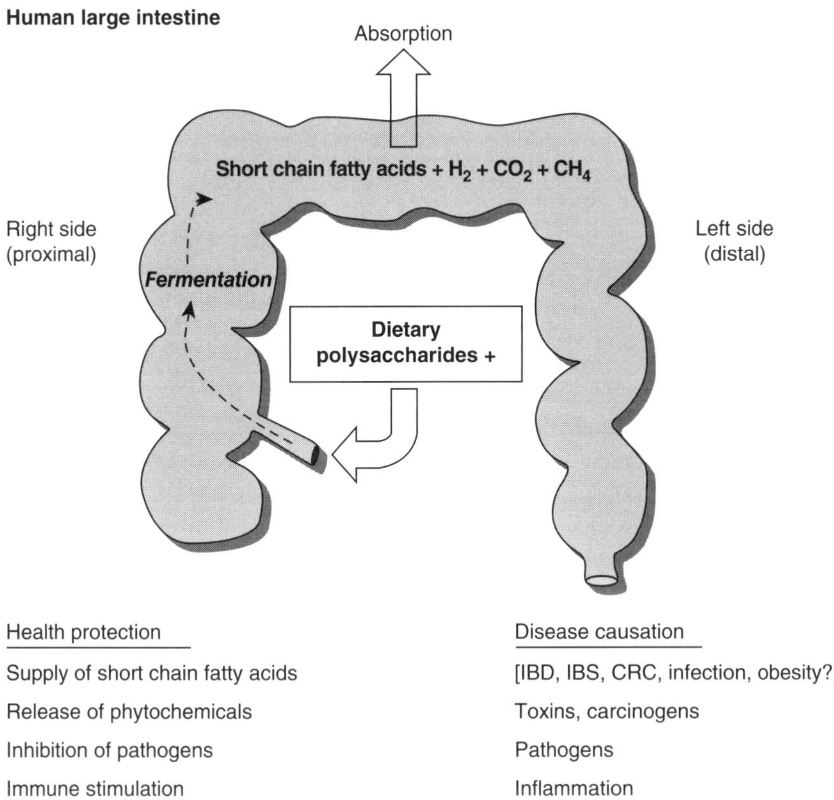

Fig. 2.1 Overview of the main activities of the gut microbiota in relation to health and disease (IBD, inflammatory bowel disease; IBS, irritable bowel syndrome; CRC, colorectal cancer).

evidence that microbial activity promotes lipogenesis in the host (Backhed *et al.*, 2004). 'Low digestible' dietary carbohydrates that reach the large intestine, however, supply considerably less energy via microbial fermentation products than the equivalent amount of absorbed glucose, and should therefore also be regarded as dietary components that make a small contribution to absorbed calories, while presumably contributing to satiety.

This chapter will review aspects of microbial diversity and metabolism in the human large intestine before moving on to consider the promise offered by recent developments in molecular methodologies for studying the gut microbiota.

2.2 Microbial community composition

2.2.1 Microbial diversity in the human large intestine

Molecular approaches based on 16S rRNA sequence analysis have provided a more complete description of the diversity of bacteria that colonize the human large intestine than was achieved previously through cultivation alone. Several hundred phylotypes or operational taxonomic units (i.e. putative species as defined by 16S rRNA sequences) can be identified within an individual faecal sample (Suau *et al.*, 1999; Hayashi *et al.*, 2002; Hold *et al.*, 2002; Eckburg *et al.*, 2005). Of these, perhaps 30% correspond to known cultured species. There are reasons to think that cultivability may be relatively high for gut bacteria, however, and it is clearly still possible to recover new species using anaerobic procedures (Flint *et al.*, 2007; Barcenilla *et al.*, 2000). Many earlier culture collections of human gut anaerobes were unfortunately lost before 16S rRNA sequencing became a standard tool in phylogeny.

Estimates of the relative abundance of major groups of gut bacteria from analysis of 16S rRNA clone libraries suggest that in healthy individuals the two dominant phyla are the Gram-negative Bacteroidetes and low % G+C Gram-positive bacteria belonging to the Firmicutes (Eckburg *et al.*, 2005). Depending in part on the primers used, however, clone libraries may underestimate the abundance of some other groups. Quantitative information from the use of group-targeted fluorescent *in situ* hybridization (FISH) probes confirms the abundance of the Bacteroidetes and of the Firmicute clostridial clusters IV and XIVa, but further demonstrates the abundance of another clostridial cluster (IX) and of the high % G+C content Gram-positive *Bifidobacterium* and *Atopobium* spp. (Franks *et al.*, 1998; Walker *et al.*, 2005). While bacterial species diversity in the human colon is high, at the phylum level the community is less diverse, with only 8 out of the 70 currently known bacterial phyla represented (Turnbaugh *et al.*, 2007).

The major Archaea found in the human gastrointestinal (GI) tract are methanogens, and appear to be dominated by *Methanobrevibacter smithii.* Eukaryotic micro-organisms are also part of the human gut community and include pathogenic protozoa such as *Entamoeba* and *Cryptosporidium*, as well as fungi, including *Candida* spp. Arguably, these are likely to show greater variability among human populations of different geographic and social origin than the bacterial flora, but their distribution and diversity has yet to receive systematic study from molecular ecologists.

2.2.2 Zonation

Distinct microbial communities are found in the oesophagus, stomach and different regions of the small intestine, reflecting the very different conditions of pH, transit and host secretions in these compartments (Bik *et al.*, 2006; Dethlefsen *et al.*, 2006; Ahmed *et al.*, 2007). The highest bacterial cell densities, exceeding 10^{11}/g, are found in the large intestine where transit is slow and a predominantly anaerobic community develops. Molecular surveys of the gut mucosa suggest that associated microbial communities do not change substantially along the length of the colon, and indeed those in the distal ileum are not very different from the colonic mucosal community (Wang *et al.*, 2005). Faecal samples are expected to reflect mainly the lumenal content of the gut, although these will include mucus and sloughed epithelial cells. Bacteria whose main site is the gut mucosa should therefore also be present in faecal samples, and comparisons suggest considerable overlap between mucosal/mucus-associated bacteria and those found in faecal samples, although there is evidence for quantitative differences in species composition (Eckburg *et al.*, 2005). Some quantitative differences in composition have also been detected between fibre-associated and planctonic bacterial communities, with a higher percentage of Bacteroidetes being found in the planctonic phase, and a higher percentage of one group of Firmicutes (cluster IV ruminococci) being found on fibre (Walker *et al.*, 2008).

2.2.3 Stability and individual variation

Evidence from denaturing gradient gel electrophoresis (DGGE) profiling suggests that the gut bacterial community monitored in faecal samples is relatively stable in healthy adult individuals over time (Zoetendal *et al.*, 1998; Franks *et al.*, 1998). On the other hand, there is evidence that sustained changes in dietary intake affect the composition of the community, as monitored using FISH probes or by 16S rRNA sequence analysis (Kruse *et al.*, 1999; Ley *et al.*, 2006; Duncan *et al.*, 2007). This suggests that the composition of the community must be subject to continual change in response to dietary intake, but also that the observed stability reflects consistent eating habits. As might be expected, serious disturbances such as antibiotic treatment or diarrhoea lead to dramatic shifts in community composition, as detected through profiling techniques (Clausen *et al.*, 1991; Frank and Pace, 2008). There are indications, again mainly from profiling methodologies, that the gut community shows a degree of resilience in returning to the pre-disturbed state following disruption (De la Cochetiere *et al.*, 2005).

Detailed analysis of 16S rRNA sequences from faecal or gut samples derived from a small number of individuals shows that, although the same phyla are typically present, there is limited overlap between the phylotypes, let alone strains, that are present in different individuals (Hold *et al.*, 2002; Eckburg *et al.*, 2005). These results agree with the findings of earlier profiling studies using DGGE (Zoetendal *et al.*, 1998). It remains possible, however, that there is significant commonality in broader functional/phylogenetic groupings. Furthermore, the likelihood of temporal changes means that we do not know with any certainty whether the dominant phylotypes are stable over time in an individual.

These important questions of stability, individual variation and resilience of human gut communities have been studied so far at a fairly superficial level, and must currently be regarded as unresolved. Major projects in the EU and USA are now under way, however, that will apply metagenome sequencing to the human gut microbiome (Turnbaugh *et al.*, 2007). The more detailed investigations triggered by these initiatives may profoundly alter our understanding of these questions.

2.2.4 Disease states

Particular components of the colonic microbiota appear to be involved in the aetiology of several gut diseases, and the exact mechanisms are under intense study. Colorectal cancer incidence in the Western world is higher than in developing countries and differences in the diet seem to be a major contributor to this difference in disease prevalence (O'Keefe, 2008). Only 15% of colorectal cancer cases are considered to be due to genetic susceptibility (Gill and Rowland, 2002). Diet can influence cancer risk directly by supplying beneficial or toxic compounds, but many dietary effects are likely to be mediated by the gut microbiota, for example by influencing inflammation status or supplying either carcinogenic or anti-carcinogenic metabolites (Huycke and Gaskins, 2004; Hope *et al.*, 2005; O'Keefe, 2008). A recent study found that the microbiota of both colorectal cancer and polyp patients were less stable and showed higher diversity for the Firmicutes, and differences were also detected in the metabolite profile of faecal waters, compared with healthy controls (Scanlan *et al.*, 2008).

Genetic susceptibility plays a role in the aetiology of inflammatory bowel disease (IBD), but there is also clear evidence that the microbiota are involved (Seksik *et al.*, 2006; Barnich and Darfeuille-Michaud, 2007; Strober *et al.*, 2007). Changes in microbiota composition in patients compared with healthy controls are currently being elucidated both in mucosal and faecal samples (Bibiloni *et al.*, 2006; Swidsinski *et al.*, 2008) and the development of more holistic approaches, such as the use of metagenomic and metabolomic analyses (Manichanh *et al.*, 2007; Marchesi *et al.*, 2007) should improve our understanding of the role the microbiota play in IBD and lead to novel therapies. Irritable bowel syndrome (IBS) is a prevalent gut disorder that encompasses several different types of symptoms, while the underlying causes seem to be complex (Foxx-Orenstein, 2006). Several studies point to an involvement of the microbiota in IBS and the effectiveness of treatments that modulate the microbiota (antibiotics, probiotics) is being investigated (King *et al.*, 1998; Quigley, 2007).

2.3 Microbial metabolism of dietary components

2.3.1 Functional groups among gut bacteria: substrate utilization

There is evidence for broad substrate-utilizing abilities in several of the predominant species of anaerobic gut bacteria. *Bacteroides thetaiotaomicron*, for example, has a very wide repertoire of genes concerned with carbohydrate utilization and is able to switch readily between host-derived and dietary carbohydrate sources of energy (Xu *et al.*, 2003; Sonnenburg *et al.*, 2005). Similarly the Firmicute species *Roseburia inulinivorans* is able to switch from utilization of dietary starch or inulin to fucose utilization (Scott *et al.*, 2006). Despite this, however, there is also evidence that many intestinal anaerobes are rather specialized in the nutritional niches that they occupy.

Much of the fermentable substrate that enters the large intestine is in the form of insoluble particles (e.g. plant fragments, starch granules). A recent study used 16S rRNA sequence analysis to show that distinct species of human faecal bacteria became closely associated with starch, wheat bran or mucin in a continuous flow fermentor model (Leitch *et al.*, 2007). Conventional cultural studies have also shown that the ability to degrade particular plant cell wall polymers is often quite restricted among human gut anaerobes (Salyers *et al.*, 1977a,b; Chassard *et al.*, 2007) (Table 2.1). Thus

Table 2.1 Utilization of dietary carbohydrate substrates and product formation by cultured bacteria from the human colon

	Bacteroidetes	Firmicutes	Actinobacteria
Substrate utilization			
Starch	*Bacteroides* spp.	*Eubacterium rectale*	*Bifidobacterium adolescentis*
		Roseburia spp. (XIVa*)	
		Ruminococcus bromii (IV)	
Xylan	*Bacteroides ovatus*	*Roseburia intestinalis* (XIVa)	
Cellulose	*Bacteroides cellulosyliticus*	*Ruminococcus* spp. (IV)	
Inulin		*Roseburia inulinivorans*	*Bifidobacterium* spp. (some strains)
		Other clostridial spp. (XIVa, IV, XVI)	
Product formation			
Propionate	*Bacteroides* spp.	*Megasphaera* spp. *Veillonella* spp. (IX)	
Butyrate		*Roseburia* spp.	
		Eubacterium rectale	
		Eubacterium hallii (XIVa)	
		Faecalibacterium prausnitzii (IV)	

* Refers to the clostridial cluster to which these species belong.

rather few strains have the ability to degrade insoluble cellulose, and only about 10% have the ability to degrade xylans. The ability to colonize and degrade a particular type of plant cell wall may therefore be restricted to the small fraction of human gut bacteria that possess suitable enzyme systems and adhesion factors (Flint *et al.*, 2008).

Resistant starch is considered to be one of the most important energy sources for microbial growth in the large intestine (Macfarlane and Gibson, 1997). Although amylase activity is likely to be widespread, occurring in many *Bacteroides* spp. and in low % G+C Gram-positives such as *Eubacterium rectale*, *Roseburia* spp. and *Ruminococcus bromii* (Ramsay *et al.*, 2006; Salyers *et al.*, 1977a,b), there are indications that a few species may dominate the breakdown of insoluble starch particles (Leitch *et al.*, 2007). Starch-utilizing bifidobacteria are readily isolated, although this characteristic is not found in all species (Macfarlane and Englyst, 1986; Belenguer *et al.*, 2006). The most abundant utilizers of inulin have yet to be fully defined (Apajalahti *et al.*, 2002) although they include some *Bifidobacterium* spp. and the low % G+C species *Roseburia inulinivorans* (Rossi *et al.*, 2005; Scott *et al.*, 2006).

There is increasing evidence for the existence of complex hierarchies involved in the utilization of polysaccharide substrates. Thus the activities of primary degraders capable of accessing and cleaving full-length polysaccharides release a variety of partial breakdown products that can be utilized by other members of the gut community (Falony *et al.*, 2006; Belenguer *et al.*, 2006). This results in a complex network of cross-feeding interactions (Flint *et al.*, 2007). One implication of this is that the chain-length of carbohydrates used as prebiotics, as observed for example with inulin/fructo-oligosaccharides (Rossi *et al.*, 2005), is likely to be critical to its effect on the gut community.

2.3.2 Key bacterial groups involved in short chain fatty acid formation

Changes in dietary intake can cause shifts in the relative rates of production of different organic acids through fermentation by the large intestinal community (Fig. 2.2). Many groups of gut bacteria are known to produce acetate, whilst bacterial groups that are involved in the formation of butyrate and propionate are more restricted. One of the major bacterial groups that generate propionate is Bacteroidetes, employing the succinate route (Table 1). Another major group of propionate-producers is likely to be clostridial cluster IX (or *Sporomusa* group) which are estimated by FISH probing to account for 7% of total human faecal bacteria (Walker *et al.*, 2005).

In general, we are much more knowledgeable about the groups of bacteria that are involved in butyrate formation. The two most abundant groups of butyrate producers are *Faecalibacterium prausnitzii* (clostridial cluster IV) and *Eubacterium rectale/Roseburia* spp. (belonging to clostridial cluster XIVa) (Barcenilla *et al.*, 2000; Aminov *et al.*, 2006; Duncan *et al.*, 2006). Both

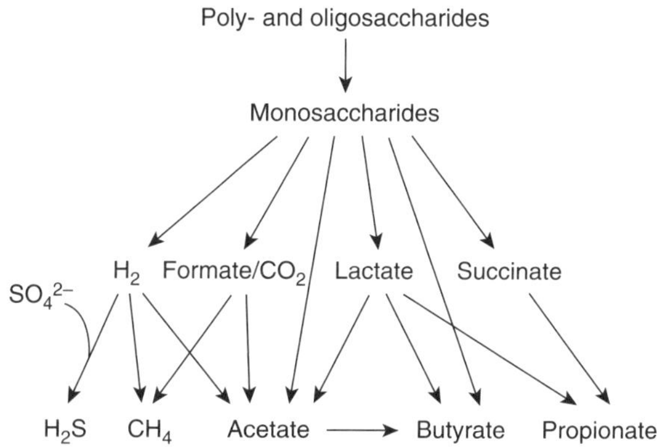

Fig. 2.2 Main microbial products formed directly from dietary carbohydrates and through microbial cross-feeding interactions in the human large intestine.

groups rely on a CoA transferase for the final step in butyrate production, and tend to be net consumers of acetate (Duncan *et al.*, 2004a; Louis *et al.*, 2004; Charrier *et al.*, 2006), whilst it seems that a minority of colonic bacteria employ the alternative butyrate kinase enzyme (Duncan *et al.*, 2002; Louis *et al.*, 2004). Populations of the *Roseburia/Eubacterium rectale* group appear to be particularly dependent on carbohydrate content of the diet (Duncan *et al.*, 2007).

Many groups of gut bacteria, including bifidobacteria, are known to produce lactate as one of several fermentation products, especially under conditions of substrate excess. The ability to utilize lactate, often considered as an intermediate product in the colon of healthy subjects, is, however, more restricted. In the human colon, recent work has shown that organisms related to *Eubacterium hallii* and *Anaerostipes caccae* have the ability to convert lactate and acetate into butyrate (Duncan *et al.*, 2004b). Efficient utilization normally means that lactate remains at low concentrations in the human colon (Belenguer *et al.*, 2007). In addition, the sulphate reducer (SRB) *Desulfovibrio piger* can convert lactate to acetate with the attendant generation of H_2S (see below). Other groups of bacteria are involved in converting lactate to propionate, including *Megasphaera elsdenii* where this conversion occurs via the acrylate pathway (Counotte *et al.*, 1981). It would appear, however, that few of these diverse lactate-utilizing bacteria are able to function when the pH falls towards 5.0 or lower, and lactate accumulates under these conditions (Belenguer *et al.*, 2007).

Stable isotopic labelling studies confirm that butyrate is a significant product from lactate in incubations with human faecal slurries (Morrison *et al.*, 2006; Bourriaud *et al.*, 2005; Belenguer *et al.*, 2007). Furthermore, populations of *E. hallii* in particular were found to increase dramatically following addition of lactate and polysaccharides to such incubations (Belenguer *et al.*, 2007).

2.3.3 The fate of hydrogen: methanogenesis, acetogenesis, sulphate reduction

Certain specialized groups of bacteria and archaea play potentially key roles in the inter-species transfer of hydrogen. Methanogenic archaea, for example, produce methane from hydrogen and CO_2, or from formate; the main species found in the human colon appears to be *Methanobrevibacter smithii* (Eckburg *et al.*, 2005). Humans can be divided into methane-producers and non-methane-producers, who possess either high ($>10^8$/ml) or low ($<10^5$/ml) methanogen populations respectively (Florin *et al.*, 2000). The underlying cause of this inter-individual variation is not entirely clear, but there is evidence for a relationship between slow gut transit and the possession of methanogens (El Oufir *et al.*, 2000). This could imply that the slow-growing methanogens can only persist under conditions of slow transit but, remarkably, there is evidence that methane itself slows gut transit (Pimentel *et al.*, 2006). Possession of methanogens may therefore have profound consequences for metabolism and microbial balance in the large intestine. For example, IBS sufferers who produce methane apparently show more severe symptoms of constipation than non-methane-producing IBS patients (Chatterjee *et al.*, 2007). Methanogenesis is more common in women than in men (Florin *et al.*, 2000), an observation that may correlate with the difference in transit time between the sexes.

Another group of hydrogen-utilizing bacteria that has a potentially important impact on health are sulphate reducers (SRBs). These bacteria, which include the Gram-negative *Desulfovibrio piger* (Fite *et al.*, 2004), can use co-substrates such as lactate in the reduction of sulphate to hydrogen sulphide. Hydrogen sulphide is toxic for colonic epithelial cells, and one of its effects is to inhibit butyrate oxidation, leading to reduced energy supply (Roediger *et al.*, 1997). A role for SRBs has been proposed in the aetiology of colitis, but clear evidence is currently lacking for an increase in SRB populations or activity in colitic patients. It has been proposed that methanogens and sulphate reducers do not occur together in high numbers as a result of competition (Gibson *et al.*, 1988), but this has not been found in all studies (Dore *et al.*, 1995; Bernalier *et al.*, 1996).

Evidence from stable isotope studies (Miller and Wolin, 1996; Wolin *et al.*, 1999) indicates substantial fixation of ^{13}C from CO_2 into acetate in faecal incubations that must be assumed to result from reductive acetogenesis. A number of species of human colonic bacteria, such as *Ruminococcus hydrogenotrophicus*, have been shown to be capable of producing acetate from CO_2, but their affinity for hydrogen is lower than that of methanogens or sulphate reducers, and they are reported to be out-competed when methanogens are present (Bernalier *et al.*, 1996). Gut pH, discussed further below, may be a critical factor in determining the outcome of competition for hydrogen. There are indications that acetogenesis may be favoured at slightly lower pH values that are suboptimal for methanogens or sulphate reducers (Macfarlane and Gibson, 1997). If so, then acetogenesis may occur mainly under mildly acidic conditions in the proximal colon where methanogens may be less able to survive (Bernalier *et al.*, 1996; Macfarlane and Gibson, 1997).

2.4 Interplay between gut transit, pH and the microbial community

Acid production resulting from fermentation by gut bacteria tends to drive down the pH of the gut lumen. This tendency is counteracted by the constant uptake of SCFAs across the gut mucosa, by the formation of ammonia, and by secretions that help to buffer the pH, especially close to the mucosal surface. A high rate of supply of fermentable substrate to the dense bacterial community of the large intestine will result in high rates of acid production, tending to increase concentrations of organic acids and reduce gut pH (Lewis and Heaton, 1997). A consequence of increased fibre intake is to increase gut transit, and this also leads to increased concentrations of fermentation acids and consequently to reduced gut pH, as SCFA production increases relative to uptake (Lewis and Heaton, 1997; El Oufir *et al.*, 2000). This effect has been demonstrated without altering diet composition, by using drugs that either increase (loperamide, codeine) or reduce (cisapride) the mean gut transit time (Stephen *et al.*, 1987; El-Oufir *et al.*, 2000).

Rapid fermentation of non-digestible substrates occurs mainly in the proximal part of the colon. Once digesta reach the distal regions, the more readily fermentable substrates such as soluble polysaccharides and oligosaccharides have been largely metabolized, leaving the more recalcitrant, slowly degradable substrates. The rate of production of fermentation acids from dietary substrates is therefore expected to be lower in the distal colon. The net consequence appears to be a pH gradient, as demonstrated by telemetry, from mildly acidic in the proximal colon to near neutral in the distal regions (Bown *et al.*, 1974; Lewis and Heaton, 1997). Diet supplementation with fermentable substrates can nevertheless have a detectable impact on faecal pH (Muir *et al.*, 2004). It is expected that colonic pH will vary significantly with time, in particular after ingesting meals containing fermentable substrates.

As discussed earlier, many species of *Bacteroides* and of Gram-positive butyrate-producers have the ability to ferment dietary polysaccharides, including starch, as energy sources and growth substrates. In a pH-controlled fermentor model of the human colonic microbial community, with starch as the main growth substrate, a one-unit change in pH was found to have a dramatic effect on the competition between these two groups of polysaccharide-utilizing bacteria. At pH 6.5, *Bacteroidetes* came to dominate the community, accounting for at least 70% of the cells detected by FISH while Gram-positive butyrate producers were almost undetectable (Walker *et al.*, 2005). At pH 5.5, however, *Bacteroidetes* accounted for only 25% of bacterial cells, while populations of the two major groups of butyrate-producers, one related to *F. prausnitzii* and the other to *Eubacterium rectale/Roseburia* spp., became significant. These population changes can be explained simply by the influence of pH on the growth of these two groups of bacteria. Representative *Bacteroidetes* isolated from human faeces grow optimally at pH 6.5 to 7.0 and show progressive growth inhibition at lower pH values (Walker *et al.*, 2005). By contrast, many of the butyrate-producers found in the human colon (notably *Eubacterium rectale*) are relatively tolerant of mildly acidic pHs in the range 5.0 to 6.0 (Walker *et al.*, 2005).

This shift in species composition is assumed to be responsible for a major shift in the proportions of SCFAs that was observed between the two pH values. At pH 5.5 butyrate was the major product, accompanied by lower concentrations of acetate and propionate. After the shift to pH 6.5, however, butyrate concentrations declined four-fold, and steady-state propionate and acetate concentrations were increased (Walker *et al.*, 2005). Interestingly, in view of the fact that butyrate producers have been shown to be net utilizers of acetate in pure culture (Barcenilla *et al.*, 2000; Duncan *et al.*, 2004a), acetate concentrations were found to decline dramatically at pH 5.5 in these mixed cultures.

One potentially fortuitous effect of this net conversion of acetate to butyrate at pH 5.5 is that it should help to stabilize the total concentration of organic acids, and therefore the pH, under *in vivo* conditions. A second is that a high proportion of the carbon from the carbohydrate substrate is directed into butyrate, which is the preferred energy source for the colonic epithelium and is rapidly taken up *in vivo* (Rizhaupt *et al.*, 1998; Pryde *et al.*, 2002). In summary, this simple experiment suggests that the delivery of sufficient fermentable carbohydrate to the large intestine may create mildly acidic conditions that have a butyrogenic effect, favouring butyrate-producing bacteria and the supply of butyrate to the colonic epithelium.

In animals it is well established that further reductions in gut pH lead to the phenomenon of lactic acidosis, with only low-pH tolerant species such as streptococci and lactobacilli able to survive at pH values of 5 or below. These species themselves produce D or L lactic acid, which tends to further reduce the external pH as a result of its low pK_a. A recent study using human faecal samples as inocula demonstrated that, although lactate concentrations were low or undetectable in incubations performed at pH 5.9 or 6.4, lactate was a major product when incubations were performed at pH 5.2 (Belenguer *et al.*, 2007). This raises the question whether lactate accumulates because its production is increased at low pH, or whether it is produced at higher pHs but is reutilized by certain members of the gut community only at near neutral pH values. Based on studies with stable isotopically labelled lactate, Belenguer *et al.* (2007) concluded that lactate was indeed produced by mixed human faecal bacteria at pH 6.5, 5.9 and 5.2. At pH 5.2, however, lactate utilization was very much reduced, resulting in its accumulation.

Mildly acidic conditions in the proximal colon resulting from the intake of non-digestible but fermentable fibre may be generally beneficial for gut health. As discussed above, these conditions are expected to favour the production of butyrate by the colonic microbial community, and there is evidence to support the view that this effect occurs *in vivo* (Folino *et al.*, 1995; De Schrijver *et al.*, 1999). In addition, prebiotic stimulation of another group of bacteria that is tolerant of low pH, the bifidobacteria, may be mediated in part by a slight reduction in the pH of the gut lumen.

More dramatic reductions in gut pH, however, have been associated with disease states, especially ulcerative colitis (Fallingborg *et al.*, 1993; Nugent, 2005). Stool samples in severe colitis show elevated lactate concentrations (Vernia *et al.*, 1988; Hove *et al.*, 1994) that are probably explained by the effect of low pH on lactate utilization by gut bacteria (Belenguer *et al.*, 2007). Reasons for the initial drop in pH are not entirely clear, but could include rapid gut transit and reduced mucosal uptake accompanying diarrhoea and mucosal damage.

2.5 Role of microbial metabolites in health and gut function

2.5.1 Short chain fatty acids

Whereas glutamine and glucose are the main fuels for small intestinal epithelial cells (Windmueller and Spaeth, 1978), colonocytes are fuelled largely by the SCFAs derived from microbial fermentation. SCFAs in fact supply approximately 10% of the host's energy (McNeil, 1984). The three major SCFAs that are detected in faecal samples are acetate, propionate and butyrate, together with smaller amounts of branched chain fatty acids that are formed mainly from protein and peptide metabolism. Total SCFA concentrations have been estimated to reach up to approximately 180 mM levels in the proximal colon and fall to as low as 20 mM in the distal colon (Macfarlane *et al.*, 1992). The molar proportions of the major SCFAs (acetate:propionate:butyrate) range from 10:2:1 to around 3:1:1 depending on diet. Approximately 95% of the major SCFAs produced by bacterial fermentation are rapidly absorbed from the colonic lumen, while lactate absorption occurs at a much slower rate (Fleming *et al.*, 1991; Ritzhaupt *et al.*, 1998; Gupta *et al.*, 2006).

SCFAs are important anions in the colonic lumen as they influence gut morphology and function, and can affect colonic mucosa blood flow, motility, mucin secretion and differentiation and proliferation of colonocytes (Scheppach, 1994). Acetate, which is the principal SCFA in the colon, may have a trophic effect on the colonic epithelium and increases mucosal blood flow. After transport across the colonic mucosa to the portal circulation, acetate passes to the liver and is recovered in peripheral blood (Scheppach *et al.*, 1991). Acetate, in particular, is involved in cholesterol synthesis (Wolever *et al.*, 1995).

Propionate is largely metabolized in the liver (Cummings *et al.*, 1987) and is gluconeogenic. In contrast to acetate, diets that promote propionate formation are considered to lower cholesterol levels. Some studies suggest that diets enriched in oats, a source of β-glucans, promote SCFA formation in the human large intestine (Drzikova *et al.*, 2005) and more recently it has been suggested that β-glucans promote butyrate formation in particular (Kanauchi *et al.*, 1999) with a concomitant decrease in acetate and plasma cholesterol levels (Queenan *et al.*, 2007).

Butyrate is the preferred energy source for the colonocytes and this preference is more pronounced in the distal than the proximal colon (Roediger, 1980). It has anti-inflammatory effects and protects against oxidative stress (Rosignoli *et al.*, 2001). It also has a wide range of effects on gene expression in host cells including induction of hyperacetylation of histones, modification of oncogene expression, alteration of DNA methylation and suppression of nuclear factor kappa B (NF-κB) activation (Hinnebusch *et al.*, 2002). The pro-apoptotic effect of butyrate on colorectal cancer cells (Avivi-Green *et al.*, 2000) may explain its cancer protective effects reported *in vivo* (McIntyre *et al.*, 1993). Butyrate up-regulates expression of the main mucin-encoding gene in human colonic epithelial cells, *muc-2* (Gaudier *et al.*, 2004) and may also contribute to maintaining the protective mucus barrier. These effects of butyrate have been extensively reviewed elsewhere (Csordas, 1996; Pryde *et al.*, 2002; Hamer *et al.*, 2008).

Low faecal butyrate has been reported in severe cases of ulcerative colitis (UC) (Vernia *et al.*, 1988) and correlates with a higher carriage of SRBs in UC compared with healthy controls (Picton *et al.*, 2007), whilst sulphide is a product that has been found to impair butyrate oxidation (Den Hond *et al.*, 1998). Butyrate concentrations may also be lower in faecal samples from polyp and cancer patients compared to healthy controls (Lambert *et al.*, 2002). In view of the role of butyrate in promoting colonic health, several trials have been conducted using butyrate enemas to alleviate bowel disease but with variable outcomes (Scheppach *et al.*, 1992). Dietary supplementation with fructooligosaccharides (FOS) and resistant starch is considered to be butyrogenic (Cummings *et al.*, 1996; Topping and Clifton, 2001; Pryde *et al.*, 2002) and represents a less invasive approach to delivery. Stimulation of butyrate formation may arise through direct utilization of these substrates by butyrate-producing bacteria, or by cross-feeding of intermediate fermentation products (Belenguer *et al.*, 2006).

Another approach that has been considered for delivery of organic acids to the colon is via their chemical linkage to dietary components. Bajka *et al.* (2006) demonstrated that feeding butyrylated starch to rats increased caecal butyrate concentrations, although it did not increase concentrations in either the proximal or distal colonic contents.

2.5.2 Other potentially significant metabolites of microbial origin

Microbial fermentation of foods that reach the colon results in the generation of a very wide range of compounds that have potential effects on colonic health and more generally on cardiovascular disease, diabetes, obesity and inflammation (Fig. 2.1). The potential impact of some of these microbially derived products has been assessed using a range of *in vitro* cytotoxicity and genotoxicity tests, but it is not easy to extrapolate these results in order to predict impacts on human health. For example, it is still not clear how much dietary protein or lipid reaches the colon. Proteolytic bacteria can give rise to ammonia, indoles and nitrosamines (Cummings and Bingham, 1987) and if the source of protein is mainly red meat then haem concentrations in the colon will also be elevated. Other fermentation products likely to have a negative impact on colonic health include phenols, cresols, fecapentanes and sulphides (Gill and Rowland, 2002). An adequate supply of non-digestible, fermentable carbohydrate in the diet may help to reduce the formation of these products by promoting microbial growth, so increasing the assimilation of amino acid nitrogen into microbial protein. Thus resistant starch may ameliorate the negative effects on gut health, such as DNA damage, induced by high-protein diets (Toden *et al.*, 2007).

Diets high in fruits and vegetables are considered to have a protective effect against disease (Riboli and Norat, 2003), and bacterial degradation of plant cell walls plays a role by releasing phenolic compounds (Russell *et al.*, 2006). These phenolic compounds have been shown to possess a wide range of effects that may include cancer prevention and anti-bacterial activity. The links between the myriad of individual metabolites of microbial origin and human health cannot be reviewed in detail here, but metabolomic approaches, which promise to yield important new insights, are considered further below.

2.6 New methods for studying the gut microbiota

Progress in techniques relevant to the dissection of complex microbial communities has never been more rapid, and the likely impact of these developments on gut microbial ecology will be considered briefly here (Table 2.2).

2.6.1 16S rRNA-based methods

The 16S rRNA gene is a good marker for the determination of the phylogenetic composition of microbial ecosystems, as it is ubiquitous and carries highly conserved and variable regions. Techniques employing the 16S rRNA gene have been developed and extensively utilized in recent years and several excellent review articles on this topic are available (Frank and Pace, 2001; Blaut *et al.*, 2002; Flint *et al.*, 2006). Therefore, we will only give a short overview of the most commonly used methodologies.

Table 2.2 Relevant techniques for studying the microbial ecology of the human large intestine

	Techniques applicable to	
	Cultured isolates	Whole community
Gene	Genomics Transcriptomics	Metagenomics Metatranscriptomics
Gene product	Proteomics	Metaproteomics
Cell	Physiology, biochemistry, metabolism	Laser-capture microdissection and genome sequencing
Community	Microbial interactions (co-cultures), metabolite fluxes	Phylogenetic composition, metabolomics, metabolite fluxes

Most techniques include a polymerase chain reaction (PCR) amplification step with either universal primers against conserved regions of the 16S rRNA gene that target the majority of known bacteria or group-specific primers for analysis of a sub-section of the microbiota. This initial PCR step may, however, introduce some bias against 16S rRNA genes that is amplified with a lower efficiency (Von Wintzingerode *et al.*, 1997). Furthermore, DNA extraction from complex samples may also lead to an under-representation of certain bacteria (Wang *et al.*, 2004).

A commonly used fingerprinting technique is DGGE or temperature gradient gel electrophoresis (TGGE). Partial 16S rRNA amplicons are resolved on a gel by either chemical or temperature-dependent denaturation dependent on their sequence composition. This method results in a banding pattern dependent on the microbiota composition and is well suited to analyse temporal changes within individuals or differences between individuals or sampling sites; however, the identity of bacteria present can be elucidated only after excision of bands and sequencing. In particular, when universal primers are used, bands often contain several different 16S rRNA amplicons, which makes the interpretation of sequencing results difficult. DGGE analysis from RNA after reverse transcription is used to preferentially detect the most active members of the gut community, and marked differences between DNA- and RNA-DGGE have been detected (Tannock *et al.*, 2004). Recently, denaturing high-performance liquid chromatography (HPLC) was applied to human gut samples as a more rapid alternative to DGGE analysis (Goldenberg *et al.*, 2007); however, it remains to be seen whether this technique has sufficient resolution to become widely applied to gut microbiology.

Some approaches rely on restriction length polymorphism (RFLP) analyses. Specific primer sets can be used to amplify DNA for a bacterial group of interest and the amplified products are then cleaved with multiple restriction endonucleases or rare site enzymes to generate banding patterns (ribotypes) (Wood *et al.*, 1998). A complex microbial community can, however, result in numerous fragments. The sensitivity of the method can be improved by using terminal fragment labelled (T)-RFLP. The advantage of this method is that digested fluorescently labelled amplicons are run on high-resolution acrylamide gels. This method can be used to track a strain of interest or to analyse complex communities (Nagashima *et al.*, 2003). Alternatively, dot blot hybridization techniques employ radioactive or fluorescently labelled oligonucleotides to target specific sequences within the 16S rRNA gene and multiple probes can be used to analyse samples.

Construction of clone libraries of amplified 16S rRNA genes and subsequent sequencing analysis results in the identification of the actual individual phylotypes present. It has led to the description of many novel 16S rRNA gene sequences and revealed that the majority of bacteria within the intestine remain uncultured (Suau *et al.*, 1999; Hold *et al.*, 2002; Eckburg *et al.*, 2005). The recently developed method of serial analysis of ribosomal sequence tags (SARST, Yu *et al.*, 2006) is based on the cloning of concatemers of single variable regions of 16S rRNA genes so that several sequence tags can be read from a single sequencing reaction. This technique has lower resolution than longer 16S rRNA gene sequences, but allows identification at the genus level.

Real-time PCR with group-specific primers allows quantification of different bacterial groups, and the number of primers targeting different members of the gut microbiota is increasing rapidly (e.g. Matsuki *et al.*, 2002; Rintillä *et al.*, 2004). However, it is important to re-validate the specificity of older primers, as our knowledge of the microbial diversity and the description of new 16S rRNA sequences are expanding rapidly. Results from real-time PCR analyses cannot be extrapolated directly to actual bacterial cell numbers, as different bacteria can carry different copy numbers of 16S rRNA genes.

A method not subjected to PCR-bias is FISH. It employs fluorescently labelled probes against regions on the 16S rRNA that are specific for certain bacterial groups. Labelled bacteria within a complex sample can directly be counted using a fluorescence microscope and related to the total bacterial population by using probes that target highly conserved regions of the 16S rRNA gene or a nucleic acid stain. The technique is quite laborious, but can be combined with fluorescence activated cell sorting (FACS) (Rigottier-Gois *et al.*, 2003).

In recent years, efforts have been made to develop array-based technologies for rapid analysis of microbial gut communities. For example, Wang *et al.* (2004) developed a microarray for the detection of 40 different bacterial species; however, the assay was qualitative rather than quantitative. A microarray consisting of 10462 oligonucleotide probes targeting different taxonomic levels (species, genus, family, class and phylum) was recently described by Palmer *et al.* (2006). A direct comparison of the results to clone library analysis performed in parallel gave similar results for both approaches both qualitatively as well as quantitatively. Thus, microarrays are a very promising tool for rapid profiling of gut communities; however, great care has to be taken when setting up microarray-based assays owing to the inherent technical challenges, such as probe specificity and hybridization bias (Wagner *et al.*, 2007).

2.6.2 Isotope-labelling technologies

A comprehensive overview of techniques utilizing stable isotopes to elucidate microbial physiology in the colon (De Graaf and Venema, 2008) and of methods employing stable and radioactive isotopes (Neufeld *et al.*, 2007) have recently been given. We will therefore give only a brief outline of these methodologies here.

Stable isotope-based methods have been used to elucidate predominant metabolic pathways of the complete microbiota. For example, Wolin *et al.* (1999) determined that the Embden–Meyerhof–Parnas pathway is the major route of glucose breakdown in faecal incubations. The contribution of acetate to butyrate formation in the presence of different carbohydrates and the fate of lactate have also been determined *in vitro* with the use of stable isotope labels (Duncan *et al.*, 2004a; Bourriaud *et al.*, 2005; Morrison *et al.*, 2006; Belenguer *et al.*, 2007). De Preter *et al.* (2004) quantified urinary breakdown products of isotopically labelled biomarkers to assess the effect of pro- and prebiotics on the colonic protein metabolism of the microbiota in human volunteers. A significant decrease of the urinary markers was found for both, the prebiotic lactulose as well as the probiotic *Lactobacillus casei* Shirota. Stable isotope labelling techniques have also been utilized to elucidate metabolic pathways in pure cultures and defined co-cultures (Duncan *et al.*, 2004a; Belenguer *et al.*, 2006).

Stable isotope probing (SIP) is used to identify microbes within the whole community that utilize certain substrates (Dumont and Murrell, 2005). Microbial communities are incubated with an isotopically labelled substrate. Community members that utilize and thus incorporate the label are identified by separation of the heavy DNA or RNA and its analysis using 16S rRNA gene-targeted or metagenomic approaches. In the field of gut microbiology, this technique has as yet only been applied *in vitro* (Egert *et al.*, 2007). While it is expected to prove extremely powerful for *in vitro* and animal model studies, its applicability to human *in vivo* studies remains uncertain, owing to the need for high levels of label reaching the colon, inaccessibility of the gut environment, and extensive cross-feeding and dilution of the label.

Exciting recent developments in the field of isotope-labelling are their combination with other techniques, such as FISH (Neufeld *et al.*, 2007), which allows one to phylogenetically identify individual cells that have incorporated the label.

2.6.3 Metagenomics

Metagenomics, i.e. the analysis of the total DNA recovered from environmental samples, enables the molecular investigation of microbial communities within an ecosystem without the need for cultivation (Riesenfeld *et al.*, 2004). Metagenomic libraries are either analysed by sequencing or by functional screening. Sequencing allows for the determination of the prevalence of the types of gene present as well as the discovery of novel sequences. Gill *et al.* (2006) sequenced approximately 78 million base pairs of DNA originating from the gut microbiota of two human volunteers. Several classes of genes, such as those involved in the metabolism of glycans and amino acids, were enriched in comparison to previously sequenced microbial genomes. However, it has to be kept in mind that the available genome sequence information does not represent a random sample of the global microbial diversity and that the amount of sequence data generated from the gut microbiome, while impressive, was nevertheless equivalent only to approximately 26 genomes (assuming an average genome size of 3 Mb). Curiously, phylogenetic analysis of the 16S rRNA gene sequences of the metagenomic library revealed that genes originating from *Bacteroidetes* were virtually absent, despite this group normally being a dominant component of the human gut microbiota (see Section 2.2.1).

A potential pitfall of metagenomic analysis exclusively based on sequencing is the accurate annotation of the vast amount of open reading frames detected, as genes exhibiting similarity can nevertheless code for proteins with different functions. Gill *et al.* (2006), for example, highlighted the prevalence of butyrate kinase genes in their metagenomic data; however, we could detect only one true match upon blast analysis.

Kurokawa *et al.* (2007) performed a metagenomic analysis of the faecal microbiota from 13 individuals, including infants. Based on the taxonomic assignment of deduced protein sequences to bacterial genera by high sequence identity of blastp hits (>90%), *Bacteroides* spp. accounted on average for approximately 16% of protein coding genes in adults and weaned children, in contrast to the results by Gill *et al.* (2006). The majority of sequences, however, could not be assigned. This will undoubtedly change with the current effort in sequencing genomes from cultured representatives of the gut microbiota. Comparing metagenomic libraries from other habitats revealed distinct patterns for the different ecosystems and between adult-type and infant-type metagenomes, and 647 orphan gene families were exclusively present in human intestinal microbiomes. Although sequence-based metagenomic analyses deliver a huge amount of information, they remain mainly descriptive and highly dependent on information gained by the analysis of bacterial isolates. Furthermore, microbial communities will consist of individual cells at different levels of metabolic activity and dead cells, which cannot be resolved with this technology, unless an initial sample fractionation (for example to separate live from dead cells) is performed. Metatranscriptomics and metaproteomics (Turnbaugh *et al.*, 2007) might provide a better tool to analyse the active component of the gut microbiota; however, the complexity of the ecosystem under study is a potential problem especially for metaproteomic analysis. Nevertheless, metagenomic sequence data are an important source of information and may also reveal insights that ultimately lead to successful culturing strategies of novel isolates.

Functional screening of metagenomic libraries is dependent on appropriate high-throughput screening assays, the expression of the genes of interest in the heterologous cloning host and the absence of gene product toxicity. The use of alternative cloning hosts will be crucial to enable the expression of genes from a wider range of original hosts. Novel screening methods that enable high-throughput and target specific functions, such as substrate-induced gene expression screening (SIGEX, Uchiyama and Watanabe, 2007), will make this approach even more powerful. Functional screens are quite widely applied in the microbial ecology of other ecosystems such as soil (Riesenfeld *et al.*, 2004) but, to date, few studies have applied them to human gut metagenomic libraries (Gloux *et al.*, 2007; Jones *et al.*, 2007).

PCR-based techniques targeting specific functional genes can also be regarded as metagenomic approaches, despite being less complex than techniques targeting the complete DNA of an environmental sample. Such approaches give phylogenetic context to specific functional groups and enable the detection of novel bacterial groups contributing to those functions. Examples include the analysis of sulphate-reducing bacteria and methanogens (Deplancke *et al.*, 2000; Denman *et al.*, 2007) and butyrate-producing bacteria (Louis and Flint, 2007).

2.6.4 Metabolomics/metabonomics

It is becoming increasingly evident that the metabolic activities of the gut microbiota and the host are intricately linked. Examples for this interplay with regard to gut function are given above; however, microbial activities may also influence wider aspects of host health, for example cardiovascular health (Ordovas and Mooser, 2006). Enterohepatic circulation enables exchange of metabolites between host and microbiota. Thus, microbial metabolites may be absorbed from the gut and further metabolized in host tissues (predominantly liver), and host metabolites can be excreted into the gut with the bile. This metabolic interplay is exemplified by the co-metabolism of bile acids (Floch, 2002) and bioactive food components such as polyphenols (Manach *et al.*, 2004; Blaut and Clavel, 2007). Modern high-throughput technologies now enable the analysis of numerous metabolites in parallel rather than focusing on specific compounds and thus allow for an integrated view of the whole system (Nicholson and Wilson, 2003; Nicholson *et al.*, 2005). This has been applied to the analysis of faeces (Jacobs *et al.*, 2008; Marchesi *et al.*, 2007) as well as other biofluids and tissues such a urine, plasma and liver (Dumas *et al.*, 2006; Martin *et al.*, 2007; Li *et al.*, 2008), facilitating the quantification of microbial metabolites outside the gut. For example, Dumas *et al.* (2006) found a correlation between low levels of plasma phosphatiylcholine and high levels of urinary methylamines, which originate from bacterial choline breakdown, in a mouse model. This indicates an involvement of the microbiota in the development of non-alcoholic fatty liver disease. Li *et al.* (2008) have correlated human microbiota composition based on DGGE patterns with urinary metabolic profiles, which indicated mainly positive links between certain bacteria and specific metabolites. These novel approaches hold great promise to improve our understanding of the complex interactions between the host and their microbiota; however, in order to exploit the full potential of the vast datasets generated, it will be of utmost importance to gain a comprehensive understanding of the functionality of the different members of the complex gut microbiota. Nevertheless, correlations found in the whole system can provide valuable hypotheses for follow-up work in more simple model systems. On the other hand, more work with model systems, e.g. gnotobiotic animals with simple microbiotas, will enable a full evaluation of the robustness of these novel techniques.

2.7 Future trends

A number of important areas have been highlighted by recent work on the human gut microbiota that require clarification. One of these is on the overall effect of different 'low-digestible' (or 'resistant' – Englyst *et al.*, 2007) carbohydrates on health and metabolism. There is evidence for example that fructo-oligosaccharides and inulin promote targeted bacterial groups, such as Bifidobacteria, but information is limited on the effects of these and other fermentable carbohydrates on other dominant groups of gut bacteria. Once this information is available, it may become apparent that any beneficial effects are attributable to changes in a variety of bacterial groups and metabolites (Flint *et al.*, 2007). Furthermore, the possibility must be entertained that some resistant carbohydrates might promote groups of bacteria that are harmful rather than beneficial. If so, we would propose that these should be termed 'dys-biotics' to distinguish them from 'pre-biotics'!

More generally, we know that increased dietary intake of resistant, fermentable carbohydrates alters the bacterial community of the gut and boosts SCFA production (Duncan *et al.*, 2007). This has generally been regarded as a net health benefit, because of the increased energy supply to the colonic mucosa, reductions in gut pH, and inhibition of pathogens (Scheppach, 1994; Topping and Clifton, 2001). Recent reports, however, suggest that SCFA promote lipogenesis (Backhed *et al.*, 2004) and also that the bacterial community in obese subjects differs from that in lean subjects, and may even be more efficient in extracting energy from the diet (Ley *et al.*, 2006; Turnbaugh *et al.*, 2006). On the other hand, another recent study on obese subjects (Duncan *et al.*, 2007) did not observe the reduction in *Bacteroides* that was reported by Ley *et al.* (2006), indicating that further work is needed on this topic.

The phylogenetic diversity and variability of the gut microbiota at the level of individual strains and species present a huge challenge. As discussed above, new molecular approaches, especially metagenomics and metabolomics, promise to produce vast datasets that will provide novel information on the abundance of gene sequences and metabolites. It seems very important, however, to balance '-omics' approaches with continued efforts to understand the functioning and interactions of major components of the gut microbiota. To this end, more studies are required on the genomics, physiology and genetics of representative cultured bacteria, together with efforts to extend the range of cultured isolates from the gut. This can greatly enhance the value of the information that will be obtained from '-omics' approaches.

2.8 Sources of further information and advice

WACKET LP (2005), Web alert: microbes in the digestive tract. *Environ Microbiol*, **7**, 602–603.

2.9 Acknowledgements

The Rowett Institute of Nutrition and Health, University of Aberdeen, receives support from the Scottish Government Rural Environment Research and Analysis Directorate.

2.10 References

AHMED S, MACFARLANE G T, FITE A, MCBAIN A J, GILBERT P and MACFARLANE, S (2007), 'Mucosa-associated bacterial diversity in relation to human terminal ileum and colonic biopsy samples', *Appl Environ Microbiol*, **73**, 7435–7442.

AMINOV R I, WALKER A W, DUNCAN S H, HARMSEN H J M, WELLING G W and FLINT H J (2006), 'Molecular diversity, cultivation, and improved detection by fluorescent *in situ* hybidization of a dominant group of human gut bacteria related to *Roseburia* spp. or *Eubacterium rectale*', *Appl Environ Microbiol*, **72**, 6371–6376.

APALAJAHTI J H, KETTUNEN H, KETTUNEN A, HOLBEN W E, NURMINEN P H, RAUTONEN N and MUTANEN M (2002), 'Culture-independent microbial community analysis reveals that inulin in the diet primarily affects previously unknown bacteria in the mouse cecum', *Appl Environ Microbiol*, **68**, 4986–4995.

AVIVI-GREEN C, POLAK-CHARCON S, MADAR Z and SCHWARTZ B (2000), 'Apoptosis cascade proteins are regulated *in vivo* by high intracolonic butyrate concentration: correlation with colorectal cancer inhibition', *Oncol Res*, **12**, 83–95.

BACKHED F, DING H, WANG T, HOOPER L V, KOH G Y, NAGY A, SEMENKOVITCH C F and GORDON J I (2004), 'The gut microbiota as an environmental factor that regulates fat storage', *Proc Natl Acad Sci*, **101**, 15718–15723.

BAJKA B H, TOPPING D L, COBIAC L and CLARKE J M (2006), 'Butyrylated starch is less susceptible to enzymic hydrolysis and increases large-bowel butyrate more than high-amylose maize starch in the rat', *Br J Nutr*, **96**, 276–282.

BARCENILLA A, PRYDE S E, MARTIN J C, DUNCAN S H, STEWART C S and FLINT H J (2000), 'Phylogenetic relationships of dominant butyrate producing bacteria from the human gut', *Appl Environ Microbiol*, **66**, 1654–1661.

BARNICH N and DARFEUILLE-MICHAUD A (2007), 'Role of bacteria in the etiopathogenesis of inflammatory bowel disease', *World J Gastroenterol*, **13**, 5571–5576.

BELENGUER A, DUNCAN S H, CALDER A G, HOLTROP G, LOUIS P, LOBLEY G E and FLINT H J (2006), 'Two routes of metabolic cross-feeding between *Bifidobacterium adolescentis* and butyrate-producing anaerobes from the human gut', *Appl Environ Microbiol*, **72**, 3593–3599.

BELENGUER A, DUNCAN S H, HOLTROP G, ANDERSON S E, LOBLEY G E and FLINT H J (2007), 'Impact of pH on lactate formation and utilization by human fecal microbial communities', *Appl Environ Microbiol*, **73**, 6526–6533.

BERNALIER A, LELAIT M, ROCHET V, GRIVET J-P, GIBSON G R and DURAND M (1996), 'Acetogenesis from H_2 and CO_2 by methane and non-methane-producing human colonic bacterial communities', *FEMS Microbiol Ecol*, **19**, 193–202.

BIBILONI R, MANGOLD M, MADSEN K L, FEDORAK R N and TANNOCK G W (2006), 'The bacteriology of biopsies differs between newly diagnosed, untreated, Crohn's disease and ulcerative colitis patients', *J Med Microbiol*, **55**, 1141–1149.

BIK E M, ECKBURG P B, GILL S R, NELSON K E, PURDOM E A, FRANCOIS F, PEREZ-PEREZ G, BLASER M J and RELMAN D A (2006), 'Molecular analysis of the bacterial microbiota in the human stomach', *Proc Natl Acad Sci USA*, **103**, 732–737.

BLAUT M and CLAVEL T (2007), 'Metabolic diversity of the intestinal microbiota: implications for health and disease', *J Nutr*, **137**, 751S–755S.

BLAUT M, COLLINS M D, WELLING G W, DORÉ J, VAN LOO J and DE VOS W (2002), 'Molecular biological methods for studying the gut microbiota: the EU human gut flora project', *Br J Nutr*, **87**, S203–S211.

BOURRIAUD C, ROBINS R J, MARTIN L, KOZLOWSKI F, TENAILLEAU E, CHERBUT C and MICHEL C (2005), 'Lactate is mainly fermented to butyrate by human intestinal microfloras but inter-individual variation is evident', *J Appl Microbiol*, **99**, 201–212.

BOWN R L, GIBSON J A, SLADEN G E, HICKS B and DAWSON A M (1974), 'Effects of lactulose and other laxatives on ileal and colonic pH as measured by radiotelemetry device', *Gut*, **15**, 999–1004.

CHARRIER C, DUNCAN G J, REID M D, RUCKLIDGE G J, HENDERSON D, YOUNG P, RUSSELL V J, AMINOV R I, FLINT H J and LOUIS P (2006), 'A novel class of CoA-transferase involved in short-chain fatty acid metabolism in butyrate-producing human colonic bacteria', *Microbiology*, **152**, 179–185.

CHASSARD C, GOUMY V, LECLERC M, DEL'HOMME C and BERNALIER-DONADILLE A (2007), 'Characterization of the xylan-degrading microbial community from human faeces', *FEMS Microbiol Ecol*, **61**, 121–131.

CHATTERJEE S, PARK S, LOW K, KONG Y and PIMENTAL M (2007), 'The degree of breath methane production in IBS correlates with the severity of constipation', *Am J Gastroenterol*, **102**, 837–841.

CLAUSEN M R, BONNEN H, TVEDE M and MORTENSEN P B (1991), 'Colonic fermentation to short chain fatty acids is decreased in antibiotic-associated diarrhoea', *Gastroenterology*, **101**, 1497–1504.

COUNOTTE G H M, PRINS R A, JANSSEN H A M and DEBIE M J A (1981), 'Role of *Megasphaera elsdenii* in the fermentation of [2-^{13}C]-lactate in the rumen of dairy cattle', *Appl Environ Microbiol*, **42**, 649–655.

CSORDAS A (1996), 'Butyrate, aspirin and colorectal cancer', *Eur J Cancer Prevent*, **5**, 221–231.

CUMMINGS J H and BINGHAM S A (1987), 'Dietary fibre, fermentation and large bowel cancer', *Cancer Surveys*, **6**, 601–621.

CUMMINGS J H, POMARE E W, BRANCH W J, NAYLOR C P E and MACFARLANE G T (1987), 'Short chain fatty acids in human large intestine, portal, hepatic and venous blood', *Gut*, **28**, 1221–1227.

CUMMINGS J H, BEATTY E R, KINGMAN S M, BINGHAM S A and ENGLYST H N (1996), 'Digestion and physiological properties of resistant starch in the human large bowel', *Br J Nutr*, **75**, 733–747.

DE GRAAF A A and VENEMA K (2008), 'Gaining insight into microbial physiology in the large intestine: a special role for stable isotopes', *Adv Microb Physiol*, **53**, 73–168.

DE LA COCHETIERE M F, DURAND T, KEPAGE P, BOUREILLE A, GALMICHE J P and DORE J (2005), 'Resilience of the dominant human fecal microbiota upon short-course antibiotic challenge', *J Clin Microbiol*, **43**, 5588–5592.

DE PRETER V, GEBOES K, VERBRUGGHE K, DE VUYST L, VANHOUTTE T, HUYS G, SWINGS J, POT B and VERBEKE K (2004), 'The *in vivo* use of the stable isotope-labelled biomarkers lactose-[^{15}N]ureide and [$^{2}H_4$]tyrosine to assess the effects of pro- and prebiotics on the intestinal flora of healthy human volunteers', *Br J Nutr*, **92**, 439–446.

DE SCHRIJVER R, VANHOOF K and VANDE GINSTE J (1999), 'Effect of enzyme resistant starch on large bowel fermentation in rats and pigs', *J Nutr*, **19**, 927–936.

DEN HOND E, HIELE M, EVENEPOEL P, PEETERS M, GHOOS Y and RUTGEERTS P (1998), '*In vivo* butyrate metabolism and colonic permeability in extensive ulcerative colitis', *Gastroenterology*, **115**, 584–590.

DENMAN S E, TOMKINS N W and MCSWEENEY C S (2007), 'Quantification and diversity analysis of ruminal methanogenic populations in response to the antimethanogenic compound bromochloromethane', *FEMS Microbiol Ecol*, **62**, 313–322.

DEPLANCKE B, HRISTOVA K R, OAKLEY H A, MCCRACKEN V J, AMINOV R, MACKIE R I and GASKINS H R (2000), 'Molecular ecological analysis of the succession and diversity of sulfate-reducing bacteria in the mouse gastrointestinal tract', *Appl Environ Microbiol*, **66**, 2166–2174.

DETHLEFSEN L M, ECKBURG P B, BIK E M and RELMAN D A (2006), 'Assembly of the human intestinal microbiota', *Trends Ecol Evol*, **21**, 517–523.

DORE J, POCHART P, BERNALIER A, GODEREL I, MORVAN B and RAMBAUD J C (1995), 'Enumeration of H_2-utilizing archaea, acetogenic and sulfate-reducing bacteria from human feces', *FEMS Microbiol Ecol*, **17**, 279–284.

DRZIKOVA B, DONGOWSKI G and GEBARDT E (2005), 'Dietary fibre-rich oat-based products affect serum lipids, microbiota, formation of short-chain fatty acids and steroids in rats', *Br J Nutr*, **94**, 1012–1025.

DUMAS M-E, BARTON R H, CLOAREC O, BLANCHER C, ROTHWELL A, FEARNSIDE J, TATOUD R, BLANC V, LINDON J C, MITCHELL S C, HOLMES E, MCCARTHY M I, SCOTT J, GAUGHIER D and NICHOLSON J K (2006), 'Metabolic profiling reveals a contribution of gut microbiota to fatty liver phenotype in insulin-resistant mice', *Proc Natl Acad Sci USA*, **103**, 12511–12516.

DUMONT M G and MURRELL J C (2005), 'Stable isotope probing – linking microbial identity to function', *Nature Rev Microbiol*, **3**, 499–504.

DUNCAN S H, BARCENILLA A, STEWART C S, PRYDE S E and FLINT H J (2002), 'Acetate utilization and butyryl coenzyme A (CoA): acetate-CoA transferase in butyrate-producing bacteria from the human large intestine', *Appl Environ Microbiol*, **68**, 5186–5190.

DUNCAN S H, HOLTROP G, LOBLEY G E, CALDER A G, STEWART C S and FLINT H J (2004a), 'Contribution of acetate to butyrate formation by human faecal bacteria', *Br J Nutr*, **91**, 915–923.

DUNCAN S H, LOUIS P and FLINT H J (2004b), 'Lactate-utilising bacteria, isolated from human faeces, that produce butyrate as a major fermentation product', *Appl Environ Microbiol*, **70**, 5810–5817.

DUNCAN S H, AMINOV R I, SCOTT K P, LOUIS P, STANTON T B and FLINT H J (2006), 'Proposal of *Roseburia faecis* (sp. nov.), *Roseburia hominis* (sp. nov.), and *Roseburia inulinivorans* (sp. nov.), based on isolates from human faeces', *Int J Syst Evol Microbiol*, **56**, 2437–2441.

DUNCAN S H, BELENGUER A, HOLTROP G, JOHNSTONE A M, FLINT H J and LOBLEY G E (2007), 'Reduced dietary intake of carbohydrate, by obese subjects, results in decreased concentrations of butyrate and butyrate-producing bacteria in feces', *Appl Environ Micobiol*, **73**, 1073–1078.

ECKBURG P B, BIK E M, BERNSTEIN C N, PURDOM E, DETHLEFSEN L, SARGENT M, GILL S R, NELSON K E and RELMAN D (2005), 'Diversity of the human intestinal microbial flora', *Science*, **308**, 1635–1638.

EGERT M, DE GRAAF A A, MAATHUIS A, DE WAARD P, PLUGGE C M, SMIDT H, DEUTZ N E, DIJKEMA C, DE VOS W M and VENEMA K (2007), 'Identification of glucose-fermenting bacteria present in an *in vitro* model of the human intestine by RNA-stable isotope probing', *FEMS Microbiol Ecol*, **60**, 126–135.

EL OUFIR L, BARRY J L, FLOURIÉ B, CHERBUT C, CLOAREC D, BORNET F and GALMICHE J P (2000), 'Relationships between transit time in man and *in vitro* fermentation of dietary fiber by fecal bacteria', *Eur J Clin Nutr*, **54**, 603–609.

ENGLYST K N, LIU S and ENGLYST H N (2007), 'Nutritional characterization and measurement of dietary carbohydrates', *Eur J Clin Nutr*, **61**, S19–S39.

FALLINBORG J, CHRISTENSEN L A, JACOBSEN B A and RASMUSSEN S N (1993), 'Very low intraluminal colonic pH in patients with ulcerative colitis', *Dig Dis Sci*, **38**, 1989–1993.

FALONY G, VIACHOU A, VERBRUGGE K and DE VUYST L (2006), 'Cross-feeding between *Bifidobacterium longum* BB536 and acetate converting, butyrate-producing colon bacteria during growth on oligofructose', *Appl Env Microbiol*, **72**, 7835–7841.

FITE A, MACFARLANE G T, CUMMINGS J H, HOPKINS M J, KONG S C, FURRIE E and MACFARLANE S (2004), 'Identification and quantitation of mucosal and faecal desulfovibrios using real time polymerase chain reaction', *Gut*, **53**, 523–529.

FLEMING S E, CHOI Y S and FITCH D M (1991), 'Absorption of short chain fatty acids from the rat caecum *in vivo*', *J Nutr*, **121**, 1787–1789.

FLINT H J, LEITCH E C M, DUNCAN S H, WALKER A W, PATTERSON A, RINCON M T, SCOTT K P and LOUIS P (2006), 'Molecular approaches to the analysis of gastrointestinal microbial ecosystems', in Perry G, *Avian Gut Function in Health and Disease*, CAB International, Wallingford, 107–123.

FLINT H J, DUNCAN S H, SCOTT K P and LOUIS P (2007), 'Interactions and competition within the microbial community of the human colon: links between diet and health', *Environ Microbiol*, **9**, 1101–1111.

FLINT H J, BAYER E A, RINCON M T, LAMED R and WHITE B A (2008), 'Polysaccharide utilization by gut bacteria: potential for new insights from genomic analysis', *Nature Rev Microbiol*, **6**, 121–131.

FLOCH M H (2002), 'Bile salts, intestinal microflora and enterohepatic circulation', *Digest Liver Dis*, **34**, S54–S57.

FLORIN T H F, ZHU G, KIRK K M and MARTIN N G (2000), 'Shared and unique environmental factors determine the ecology of methanogens in human and rats', *Am J Gastroenterol*, **95**, 2872–2879.

FOLINO M, MCINTYRE A and YOUNG G P (1995), 'Dietary-fibers differ in their effects on large-bowel epithelial proliferation and faecal fermentation-dependent events in rats', *J Nutr*, **125**, 1521–1528.

FOXX-ORENSTEIN A (2006), 'IBS – review and what's new', *Med Gen Med*, **8**, 20.

FRANK D N and PACE N R (2001), 'Molecular-phylogenetic analyses of human gastrointestinal microbiota', *Curr Opin Gastroenterol*, **17**, 52–57.

FRANK D N and PACE N R (2008), 'Gastrointestinal microbiology enters the metagenomic era', *Curr Op Gastroenterol*, **24**, 4–10.

FRANKS A H, HARMSEN H J M, RAANGS G C, JANSEN G J, SCHUT F and WELLING G W (1998), 'Variations of bacterial populations in human feces measured by fluorescent *in situ* hybridisation with group-specific 16S rRNA-targeted oligonucleotide probes', *Appl Environ Microbiol*, **64**, 3336–3345.

GAUDIER E, JARRY A, BLOTTIERE H M, DE COPPET P, BUISINE M P, AUBERT J P, LABOISSE C, CHERBUT C and HOEBLER C (2004), 'Butyrate specifically modulates MUC gene expression in intestinal epithelial cells deprived of glucose', *Am J Physiol Gastrointest Liver physiol*, **287**, G1168–G1174.

GIBSON G R, CUMMINGS J H and MACFARLANE G T (1988), 'Competition for hydrogen between sulphate-reducing bacteria and methanogenic bacteria from the human large intestine', *J Appl Bacteriol*, **65**, 241–247.

GILL C I R and ROWLAND I R (2002), 'Diet and cancer: assessing the risk', *Br J Nutr*, **88** (suppl. 1) S73–87.

GILL S R, POP M, DEBOY R T, ECKBURG P B, TURNBAUGH P J, SAMUEL B S, GORDON J I, RELMAN D A, FRASER-LIGGETT C M and NELSON K E (2006), 'Metagenomic analysis of the human distal gut microbiome', *Science*, **312**, 1355–1359.

GLOUX K, LECLERC M, ILIOZER H, L'HARIDON R, MANICHANH C, CORTHIER G, NALIN R, BLOTTIÈRE H M and DORÉ J (2007), 'Development of high-throughput phenotyping of metagenomic clones from the human gut microbiome for modulation of Eukaryotic cell growth', *Appl Environ Microbiol*, **73**, 3734–3737.

GOLDENBERG O, HERRMANN S, MARJORAM G, NOYER-WEIDNER M, HONG G, BERESWILL S and GÖBEL U B (2007), 'Molecular monitoring of the intestinal flora by denaturing high performance liquid chromatography', *J Microbiol Meth*, **68**, 94–105.

GUPTA N, MARTIN P M, PRASAD P D and GANAPATHY V (2006), 'SLC5A8 (SMCT-1)-mediated transport of butyrate forms the basis for the tumor suppressive function of the transporter', *Life Sci*, **78**, 2419–2425.

HAMER H M, JONKERS D, VENEMA K, VANHOUTVIN S, TROOST F J and BRUMMER R J (2008), 'Review article: the role of butyrate on colonic function', *Aliment Pharmacol Ther*, **27**, 104–119.

HAYASHI H, SAKAMOTO M and BENNO Y (2002), 'Phylogenetic analysis of the human gut mircobiota using 16S rDNA clone libraries and strictly anaerobic culture methods', *Microbiol Immunol*, **46**, 535–548.

HINNEBUSCH B F, MENG S F, WU J T, ARCHER S Y and HODIN R A (2002), 'The effects of short-chain fatty acids on human colon cancer cell phenotype are associated with histone hyperacetylation', *J Nutr*, **132**, 1012–1017.

HOLD G L, PRYDE S E, RUSSELL V J, FURRIE E and FLINT H J (2002), 'Assessment of microbial diversity in human colonic samples by 16S rDNA sequence analysis', *FEMS Microbiol Ecol*, **39**, 33–39.

HOPE M E, HOLD G L, KAIN R and EL-OMAR E M (2005), 'Sporadic colorectal cancer-role of the commensal microbiota', *FEMS Microbiol Lett*, **244**, 1–7.

HOVE H, NORGARD ANDERSEN I and MORTENSEN P B (1994), 'Fecal DL-lactate concentrations in 100 gastrointestinal patients', *Scand J Gastroenterol*, **29**, 255–259.

HUYCKE M M and GASKINS H R (2004), 'Commensal bacteria, redox stress, and colorectal cancer: mechanisms and models', *Exp Biol Med*, **229**, 586–597.

JACOBS D M, DELTIMPLE N, VAN VELZEN E, VAN DORSTEN F A, BINGHAM M, VAUGHAN E E and VAN DUYNHOVEN J (2008), '1H NMR metabolite profiling of feces as a tool to assess the impact of nutrition on the human microbiome', *NMR Biomed*, **21**, 615–626.

JONES B V, SUN F and MARCHESI J R (2007), 'Using skimmed milk agar to functionally screen a gut metagenomic library for proteases may lead to false positives', *Lett Appl Microbiol*, **45**, 418–420.

KANAUCHI O, FUJIYAMA Y, MITSUYAMA K, ARAKI Y, ISHII T, NAKAMURA T, HITOMI Y, AGATA K, SAIKI T, ANDOH A, TOYONAGA A and BAMBA T (1999), 'Increased growth of *Bifidobacterium* and *Eubacterium* by germinated barley foodstuff, accompanied by enhanced butyrate production in healthy volunteers', *Int J Mol Med*, **3**, 175–179.

KING T S, ELIA M and HUNTER J O (1998), 'Abnormal colonic fermentation in irritable bowel syndrome', *Lancet*, **352**, 1187–1189.

KRUSE H-P, KLEESSEN B and BLAUT M (1999), 'Effects of inulin on faecal bifidobacteria in human subjects', *Br J Nutr*, **82**, 375–382.

KUROKAWA K, ITOH T, KUWAHARA T, OSHIMA K, TOH H, TOYODA A, TAKAMI H, MORITA H, SHARMA V K, SRIVASTAVA T P, TAYLOR T D, NOGUCHI H, MORI H, OGURA Y, EHRLICH D S, ITOH K, TAKAGI T, SAKAKI Y, HAYASHI T and HATTORI M (2007), 'Comparative metagenomics revealed commonly enriched gene sets in human gut microbiomes', *DNA Res*, **14**, 169–181.

LAMBERT D W, WOOD I S, ELLIS A and SHIRAZI-BEECHEY S P (2002), 'Molecular changes in the expression of human colonic nutrient transporters during transition from normality to malignancy', *Br J Cancer*, **86**, 1262–1269.

LEITCH E C, WALKER A W, DUNCAN S H, HOLTROP G and FLINT H J (2007), 'Selective colonisation of insoluble substrates by human faecal bacteria', *Environ Microbiol*, **72**, 667–679.

LEWIS S J and HEATON K W (1997), 'Increasing butyrate concentration in the distal colon by accelerating intestinal transit', *Gut*, **41**, 245–251.

LEY R E, TURNBAUGH P J, KLEIN S and GORDON J I (2006), 'Microbial ecology – human gut microbes associated with obesity', *Nature*, **444**, 1022–1023.

LI M, WANG B, ZHANG M, RANTALAINEN M, WANG S, ZHOU H, ZHANG Y, SHEN J, PANG X, ZHANG M, WEI H, CHEN Y, LU J, SU M, QIU Y, JIA W, XIAO C, SMITH L M, YANG S, HOLMES E, TANG H, ZHAO G, NICHOLSON J K, LI L and ZHAO L (2008), 'Symbiotic gut microbes modulate human metabolic phenotypes', *Proc Natl Acad Sci USA*, **105**, 2117–2122.

LOUIS P and FLINT H J (2007), 'Development of a semiquantitative degenerate real-time PCR-based assay for estimation of numbers of butyryl-Coenzyme A (CoA) CoA transferase genes in complex bacterial samples', *Appl Environ Microbiol*, **73**, 2009–2012.

LOUIS P, DUNCAN S H, MCCRAE S, MILLAR J, JACKSON M S and FLINT H J (2004), 'Restricted distribution of the butyrate kinase pathway among butyrate-producing bacteria from the human colon', *J Bacteriol*, **186**, 2099–2106.

MACFARLANE G T and ENGLYST H N (1986), 'Starch utilization by the human large intestinal microflora', *J Appl Bacteriol*, **60**, 195–201.

MACFARLANE G T and GIBSON G R (1997), 'Carbohydrate fermentation, energy transduction and gas metabolism in the human large intestine', in ed Mackie R I and White B A, *Gastrointestinal Microbiology* Vol 1, Chapman and Hall, London 269–318.

MACFARLANE G T, GIBSON G R and CUMMINGS J H (1992), 'Comparison of fermentation reactions in different regions of the human colon', *J Appl Bacteriol*, **72**, 57–64.

MANACH C, SCALBERT A, MORAND C, REMESY C and JIMENEZ L (2004), 'Polyphenols: food sources and bioavailability', *Am J Clin Nutr*, **79**, 727–747.

MANICHANH C, RIGOTTIER-GOIS L, BONNAUD E, GLOUX K, PELLETIER E, FRANGEUL L, NALIN R, JARRIN C, CHARDON P, MARTEAU P, ROCA J and DORE J (2007), 'Reduced diversity of faecal microbiota in Crohn's disease revealed by a metagenomic approach', *Gut*, **55**, 205–211.

MARCHESI J R, HOLMES E, KHAN F, KOCHHAR S, SCANLAN P, SHANAHAN F, WILSON I D and WANG Y (2007), 'Rapid and non-invasive metabonomic characterization of inflammatory bowel disease', *J Proteome Res*, **6**, 546–551.

MARTIN F-P J, DUMAS M-E, WANG Y, LEGIDO-QUIGLEY C, YAP I K S, TANG H, ZIRAH S, MURPHY G M, CLOAREC O, LINDON J C, SPRENGER N, FAY L B, KOCHHAR S, VAN BLADEREN P and HOLMES NICHOLSON J K (2007), 'A top-down systems biology view of microbiome-mammalian metabolic interactions in a mouse model', *Mol Syst Biol*, **3**, 112.

MATSUKI T, WATANABE K, FUJIMOTO J, MIYAMOTO Y, TAKADA T, MATSUMOTO K, OYAIZU H and TANAKA R (2002), 'Development of 16S rRNA-gene-targeted group-specific primers for the detection and identification of predominant bacteria in human feces', *Appl Environ Microbiol*, **68**, 5445–5451.

MCINTYRE A, GIBSON P R and YOUNG G P (1993), 'Butyrate production from dietary fiber and protection against large bowel cancer in a rat model', *Gut*, **34**, 386–391.

MCNEIL N I (1984), 'The contribution of the large intestine to energy supplies in man', *Am J Clin Nutr*, **39**, 338–342.

MILLER T L and WOLIN M J (1996), 'Pathways of acetate, propionate and butyrate formation by the human fecal microbial flora', *Appl Environ Microbiol*, **62**, 1589–1592.

MORRISON D J, MACKAY W G, EDWARDS C A, PRESTON T, DODSON B and WEAVER L T (2006), 'Butyrate production from oligofructose fermentation by the human faecal flora: what is the contribution of extracellular acetate and lactate?' *Brit J Nutr*, **96**, 570–577.

MUIR J G, YEOW E G W, KEOGH J, PIZZEY C, BIRD A R, SHARPE K, O'DEA K and MACRAE F A (2004), 'Combining wheat bran with resistant starch has more beneficial effects on fecal indices than does wheat bran alone', *Am J Clin Nutr*, **79**, 1020–1028.

NAGASHIMA K, HISADA T, SATO M and MOCHIZUKI J (2003), 'Application of new primer-enzyme combinations to terminal restriction fragment length polymorphism profiling of bacterial populations in human feces', *Appl Environ Microbiol*, **69**, 1251–1262.

NEUFELD J D, WAGNER M and MURRELL J C (2007), 'Who eats what, where and when? Isotope-labelling experiments are coming of age', *ISME J*, **1**, 103–110.

NICHOLSON J K and WILSON I D (2003), 'Understanding "global" systems biology: metabonomics and the continuum of metabolism', *Nature Rev Drug Discov*, **2**, 668–676.

NICHOLSON J K, HOLMES E and WILSON I D (2005), 'Gut microorganisms, mammalian metabolism and personalized health care', *Nauret Rev Microbiol*, **3**, 431–438.

NUGENT A P (2005), 'Health properties of resistant starch', *Brit Nutr Foundation Bull*, **30**, 27–54.

O'KEEFE S J D (2008), 'Nutrition and colonic health: the critical role of the microbiota', *Curr Opin Gastroenterol*, **24**, 51–58.

ORDOVAS J M and MOOSER V (2006), 'Metagenomics: the role of the microbiome in cardiovascular diseases', *Curr Opin Lipidol*, **17**, 157–161.

PALMER C, BIK E M, EISEN M B, ECKBURG P B, SANA T R, WOLBER P K, RELMAN D A and BROWN P O (2006), 'Rapid quantitative profiling of complex microbial populations', *Nucl Acids Res*, **34**, e5.

PICTON R, EGGO M C, LANGMAN M J S and SINGH S (2007), 'Impaired detoxification of hydrogen sulfide in ulcerative colitis?' *Dig Dis Sci*, **52**, 373–378.

PIMENTEL M, LIN H C, ENAYATI P, VAN DEN BURG B *et al.* (2006), 'Methane, a gas produced by enteric bacteria slows intestinal transit and augments small intestinal contractile activity', *Am J Physiol*, **290**, G1089–1095.

PRYDE S E, DUNCAN S H, HOLD G L, STEWART C S and FLINT H J (2002), 'The microbiology of butyrate formation in the human colon', *FEMS Microbiol Letts*, **217**, 133–139.

QUEENAN K M, STEWART M L, SMITH K N, THOMAS W, FULCHER R G and SLAVIN J L (2007), 'Concentrated oat β-glucan, a fermentable fiber, lowers serum cholesterol in hypercholesterolemic adults in a randomized controlled trial', *Nutr J* (http:www.nutritionj.com/content/6/1/6).

QUIGLEY E M M (2007), 'Bacterial flora in irritable bowel syndrome: role in pathophysiology, implications for management', *J Dig Dis*, **8**, 2–7.

RAMSAY A G, SCOTT K P, MARTIN J C, RINCON M T and FLINT H J (2006), 'Cell associated α-amylases of butyrate-producing *Firmicute* bacteria from the human colon', *Microbiology*, **152**, 3281–3290.

RIBOLI E and NORAT T (2003), 'Epidemiologic evidence of the protective effect of fruit and vegetables on cancer risk', *Am J Clin Nutr*, **78**, 559S–569S.

RIESENFELD C S, SCHLOSS P D and HANDELSMAN J (2004), 'Metagenomics: genomic analysis of microbial communities', *Annu Rev Genet*, **28**, 525–552.

RIGOTTIER-GOIS L, LE BOURHIS A G, GRAMET G, ROCHET V and DORÉ J (2003), 'Fluorescent hybridisation combined with flow cytometry and hybridisation of total RNA to analyse the composition of microbial communities in human faeces using 16S rRNA probes', *FEMS Microbiol Ecol*, **43**, 237–245.

RINTTILÄ T, KASSINEN A, MALINEN E, KROGIUS L and PALVA A (2004), 'Development of an extensive set of 16S rDNA-targeted primers for quantification of pathogenic and indigenous bacteria in faecal samples by real-time PCR', *J Appl Microbiol*, **97**, 1166–1177.

RITZHAUPT A, ELLIS A, HOSIE K P and SHIRAZI-BEECHEY S P (1998), 'The characterisation of butyrate transport across pig and human colonic luminal membrane', *J Physiol*, **507**, 819–830.

ROEDIGER W E W (1980), 'The colonic epithelium in ulcerative colitis – an energy deficiency disease', *Lancet*, **2**, 712–715.

ROEDIGER W E W, MOORE J and BABIDGE W (1997), 'Colonic sulphide in pathogenesis and treatment of ulcerative colitis', *Dig Dis Science*, **42**, 1571–1579.

ROSIGNOLI P, FABIANI R, DE BARTOLOMEO A, SPINOZZI F, AGEA E, PELLI M A and MOROZZI G (2001), 'Protective activity of butyrate on hydrogen peroxide induce DNA damage in isolated human colonocytes and HT29 tumour cells', *Carcinogenesis*, **22**, 1675–1680.

ROSSI M, CORRADINI C, AMARETTI A, NICOLINI M, POMPEI A, ZANONI S and MATTEUZZI D (2005), 'Fermentation of fructooligosaccharides and inulin by bifidobacteria: a comparative study of pure and faecal cultures', *Appl Environ Microbiol*, **71**, 6150–6158.

RUSSELL W R, LABAT A, SCOBBIE L and DUNCAN S H (2006), 'Availability of blueberry phenolics for microbial metabolism in the colon and the potential inflammatory implications', *Mol Nut Food Res*, **51**, 726–731.

SALYERS A A, VERCELOTTI J R, WEST S E H and WILKINS T D (1977a), 'Fermentation of mucin and plant polysaccharides by strains of *Bacteroides* from the human colon', *Appl Environ Microbiol*, **33**, 319–322.

SALYERS A A, WEST S E H, VERCELLOTTI J R and WILKINS T D (1977b), 'Fermentation of mucins and plant polysaccharides by anaerobic bacteria from the human colon', *Appl Environ Microbiol*, **34**, 529–533.

SCANLAN P D, SHANAHAN F, CLUNE Y, COLLINS J K, O'SULLIVAN G C, O'RIORDAN M, HOLMES E, WANG Y and MARCHESI J R (2008), 'Culture-independent analysis of the gut microbiota in colorectal cancer and polyposis', *Env Microbiol*, **10**, 789–798.

SCHEPPACH W (1994), 'Effects of short chain fatty acids on gut morphology and function', *Gut* (Suppl 1), **35**, S35–S38.

SCHEPPACH W, POMARE E W, ELIA M and CUMMINGS J H (1991), 'The contribution of the large intestine to blood acetate in man', *Clin Sci*, **80**, 177–182.

SCHEPPACH W, SOMMER H, KIRCHNER T, PAGANELLI G M, BARTRAM P, RICHTER F, DUSEL G and KASPER H (1992), 'Effect of butyrate enemas on the colonic mucosa in distal ulcerative colitis', *Gastroenterology*, **103**, 51–56.

SCOTT K P, MARTIN, J C, CAMPBELL G, MAYER C-D and FLINT H J (2006), 'Whole-genome transcription profiling reveals genes up-regulated by growth on fucose in the human gut bacterium *Roseburia inulinivorans*', *J Bacteriol*, **188**, 4340–4349.

SEKSIK P, SOKOL H, LEPAGE P, VASQUEZ N, MANICHANH C, MANGIN I, POCHART P, DORÉ J and MARTEAU P (2006), 'Review article: the role of bacteria in onset and perpetuation of inflammatory bowel disease', *Aliment Pharmacol Ther*, **24** (Suppl 3), 11–18.

SONNENBURG E D, XU J, LEIP D D, CHEN C H, WESTOVER B P, WEATHERFORD J, BUHLER J D and GORDON J I (2005), 'Glycan foraging *in vivo* by an intestine-adapted bacterial symbiont', *Science*, **307**, 1955–1959.

STEPHEN A M, WIGGINS H S and CUMMINGS J H (1987), 'Effect of changing transit time on colonic microbial metabolism in man', *Gut*, **28**, 601–609.

STROBER W, FUSS I and MANNON P (2007), 'The fundamental basis of inflammatory bowel disease', *J Clin Invest*, **117**, 514–521.

SUAU A, BONNET R, SUTREN M, GODON J J, GIBSON G R, COLLINS M D and DORE J (1999), 'Direct analysis of genes encoding 16S rRNA from complex communities reveals many novel molecular species within the human gut', *Appl Environ Microbiol*, **65**, 4799–4807.

SWIDSINSKI A, LOENING-BAUCKE V, VANEECHOUTTE M and DOERFFEL Y (2008), 'Active Crohn's disease and ulcerative colitis can be specifically diagnosed and monitored based on the biostructure of the fecal flora', *Inflamm Bowel Dis*, **14**, 147–161.

TANNOCK G W, MUNRO K, BIBILONI R, SIMON M A, HARGREAVES P, GOPAL P, HARMSEN H and WELLING G (2004), 'Impact of consumption of oligosaccharide-containing biscuits on the fecal microbiota of humans', *Appl Environ Microbiol*, **70**, 2129–2136.

TODEN S, BIRD A R, TOPPING D L and CONLON M A (2007), 'Dose-dependent reduction of dietary protein-induced colonocyte DNA damage by resistant starch in rats correlates more highly with caecal butyrate than with other short chain fatty acids', *Cancer Biol Ther*, **6**, 253–258.

TOPPING D I and CLIFTON P M (2001), 'Short-chain fatty acids and human colonic function: roles of resistant starch and nonstarch polysaccharides', *Physiol Rev*, **81**, 1031–1064.

TURNBAUGH P J, LEY R E, MAHOWALD M A, MAGRINI V, MARDIS E R and GORDON J I (2006), 'An obesity-associated gut microbiome with increased capacity for energy harvest', *Nature*, **444**, 1027–1031.

TURNBAUGH P J, LEY R E, HAMADY M, FRASER-LIGGETT C M, KNIGHT R and GORDON J I (2007), 'The human microbiome project', *Nature*, **499**, 804–810.

UCHIYAMA T and WATANABE K (2007), 'The SIGEX scheme: high throughput screening of environmental metagenomes for the isolation of novel catabolic genes', *Biotechnol Genet Eng Rev*, **24**, 107–116.

VERNIA P, CAPRILLI R, LATELLA G, BARBETTI F, MAGLIOCCA F M and CITTADINI M (1988), 'Fecal lactate and ulcerative colitis', *Gastroenterology*, **95**, 1564–1568.

VON WINTZINGERODE F, GÖBEL U B and STACKEBRANDT E (1997), 'Determination of microbial diversity in environmental samples: pitfalls of PCR-based rRNA analysis', *FEMS Microbiol Rev*, **21**, 213–229.

WAGNER M, SMIDT H, LOY A and ZHOU J (2007), 'Unravelling microbial communities with DNA-microarrays: challenges and future directions', *Microb Ecol*, **53**, 498–506.

WALKER A W, DUNCAN S H, LEITCH E C M, CHILD M W and FLINT H J (2005), 'pH and peptide supply can radically alter bacterial populations and short chain fatty acid ratios within microbial communities from the human colon', *Appl Environ Microbiol*, **71**, 3692–3700.

WALKER A W, DUNCAN S H, HARMSEN H J M, HOLTROP G, WELLING G W and FLINT H J (2008), 'The species composition of the human intestinal microbiota differs between fibre-associated and liquid phase communities', *Environ Microbiol*, **10**, 3275–3283.

WANG M, AHRNÉ S, JEPPSSON B and MOLIN G (2005), 'Comparison of bacterial diversity along the human intestinal tract by direct cloning and sequencing of 16S rRNA genes', *FEMS Microbiol Ecol*, **54**, 219–231.

WANG R F, BEGGS M L, ERICKSON B D and CERNIGLIA C E (2004), 'DNA microarray analysis of predominant human intestinal bacteria in fecal samples', *Mol Cell Probes*, **18**, 223–234.

WINDMUELLER H G and SPAETH A E (1978), 'Identification of ketone bodies and glutamine as major respiratory fuels *in vivo* for post absorptive rat small intestine', *J Biol Chem*, **253**, 69–76.

WOLEVER T M, SPADAFORA P J, CUNNANE S C and PENCHARZ P B (1995), 'Propionate inhibits incorporation of colonic [1,2-13C] acetate into plasma lipids in humans', *Am J Clin Nutr*, **53**, 681–687.

WOLIN M J, MILLER T L, YERRY S, ZHANG Y, BANK S and WEAVER G A (1999), 'Changes of fermentation pathways of fecal microbial communities associated with a drug treatment that increases dietary starch in the human colon', *Appl Environ Microbiol*, **65**, 2807–2812.

WOOD J, SCOTT K P, AVGUSTIN G, NEWBOLD C J and FLINT H J (1998), 'Estimation of the relative abundance of different *Bacteroides* and *Prevotella* ribotypes in gut samples by restriction enzyme profiling of PCR-amplified 16S rRNA gene sequence', *Appl Environ Microbiol*, **64**, 3683–3689.

XU J, BJURSELL M K, HIMROD J, DENG S, CARMICHAEL L K, CHIANG H C, HOOPER L V and GORDON J I (2003), 'A genomic view of the human-*Bacteroides thetaiotaomicron* symbiosis', *Science*, **299**, 2074–2076.

YU Z, YU M and MORRISON M (2006), 'Improved serial analysis of V1 ribosomal sequence tags (SARST-V1) provides a rapid, comprehensive, sequence-based characterization of bacterial diversity and community composition', *Environ Microbiol*, **8**, 603–611.

ZOETENDAL E G, AKKERMANS A D L and DE VOS W M (1998), 'Temperature gradient gel electrophoresis analysis of 16S rRNA from human fecal samples reveals stable and host-specific communities of active bacteria', *Appl Environ Microbiol*, **64**, 3854–3859.

3

Digestion and absorption of lipids

D. Lairon, Université de la Méditerranée, France

Abstract: Digestion and absorption of dietary lipids is a very complex multi-step process, starting in the stomach, and ending in the small intestine. Physicochemical remodelling and lipase-catalysed hydrolysis are key events enabling efficient lipid assimilation. It results in transient marked postprandial changes in plasma lipoprotein patterns which are involved in the cardiovascular pathogenicity of fat and cholesterol. Numerous steps in this process can be modulated, thus providing a large opportunity to improve food qualities.

Key words: dietary fat, digestion, absorption, gut, health.

3.1 Introduction

Lipids are part of all human diets everywhere in the world. The quantity of fat ingested daily has markedly evolved over time, especially since the Neolithic with the development of crop and animal farming and even more markedly during the past century. Moreover, living in specific ecosystems can lead humans to adopt very specific dietary patterns with either very low-fat diets (i.e. most of Asia or Africa) or very high-fat diets (i.e. Inuits, Massai, certain segments of industrialized countries). The quality of dietary fat can also widely vary accordingly, with diets rich either in saturated fat (Northern Europe, North America), monounsaturated-rich diets (Mediterranean area), polyunsaturated fats with *n*-6 series (industrialized countries) and *n*-3 series (most coastal areas).

Overall, adult humans ingest about 20–120 g lipids daily, composed of about 97% triglycerides, a few per cent phospholipids, ≈1% cholesterol, and <1% various lipophylic moieties (phytosterols, fat-soluble vitamins, carotenoids, etc.). From an evolutionary point of view, humans needed to adapt to repeated seasonal lack of foods and famine over millions of years. To accommodate such a dramatic deficit and survive, humans as well as other non-ruminant animal species developed a highly efficient means of storing energy, i.e. in the form of lipids (adipose tissue) that have an energy efficiency among the highest of all nutrients (about 9 kcal/g). To establish such an efficient storage capacity, it was necessary to set up a high capacity for assimilation of dietary fat. Indeed, the lipid digestion and absorption process is normally extremely efficient (about 98% for fatty acids) in humans.

Nevertheless, contrary to other water-soluble nutrients (e.g. proteins, carbohydrates, minerals), all dietary lipids are insoluble in the aqueous media, where enzymes secreted by the gut are present and active. This particular condition necessitated the development of very sophisticated processes enabling an efficient and controlled uptake of dietary lipids.

It is the purpose of this chapter to describe the mechanisms of lipid digestion and uptake by the small intestine, along with the resulting post-prandial lipid occurrence in the circulation and tissues. The variability of this process can form the basis of a functional food strategy to maintain or improve human health.

3.2 Stuctural and physicochemical aspects

3.2.1 Lipids: a wide range of molecular structures

While all lipid moieties have in common an insoluble character in aqueous media, they cover a wide range of structures and thus physicochemial properties. According to Small (1986), lipids can be categorized based on their behaviour in an aqueous phase as follows (see Fig. 3.1):

- Non-polar lipids: neutral, highly hydrophobic lipids such as hydrocarbons and carotene; fully insoluble in water; do not form a stable monolayer at an air/water interface.
- Polar lipids:
  - Class I: neutral, hydrophobic lipids such as triglycerides, diglycerides, protonated fatty acids and chlolesterol; do not swell in water; can form a stable monolayer at an air–water interface or make emulsions.
  - Class II: amphipathic lipids such as phospholipids, monoglycerides and ionized fatty acids; can swell in water to make a crystalline phase or various kinds of liquid–crystalline phases; can self-assemble in water to form bilamellar vesicles and can build a stable monolayer at an air–water or oil–water interface.
  - Class III: surface active lipids such as lyso-phospholipids and bile salts; have a low monomeric solubility in water; can self-organize in a micellar form at higher concentration; do not build a stable monolayer at an air–water interface.

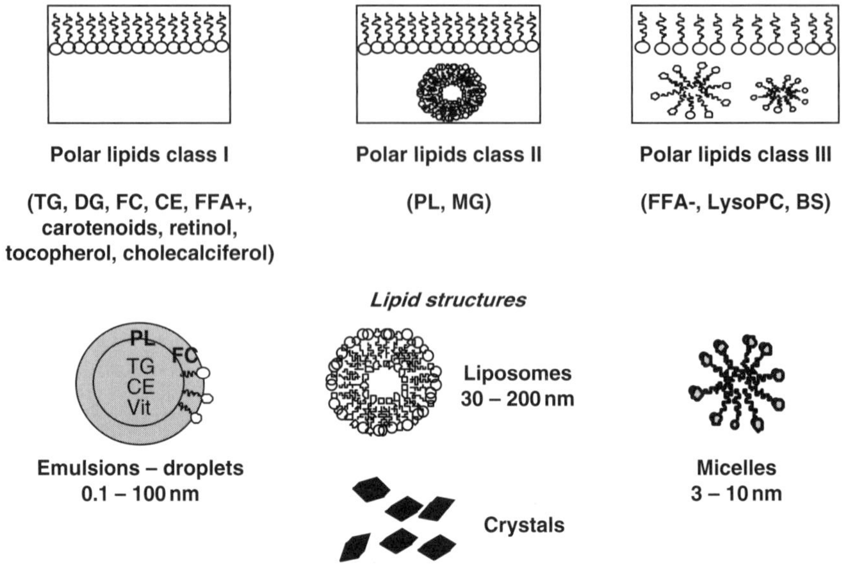

Fig. 3.1 The physicochemical properties and structures made by lipid moieties. (TG, triglycerides; DG, diglycerides; MG, monoglycerides; FFA, free fatty acids; PL, phospholipids; FC, free cholesterol; CE, cholesterol esters; BS, bile salts; LysoPC, lyso-phosphatidylcholine).

In fact, the digestion of dietary lipids involves all these kinds of lipids, organized under different forms depending on the step considered (Fig. 3.1).

3.2.2 Dietary lipids

The structure of food fat is highly variable. Triglycerides can be found as droplets or vacuoles (fatty foodstuffs), stable emulsions (milk, cream), liquids (vegetable or fish oils), solids and crystals (butter, palm oil, saturated fats at room temperature or below) or lipoproteins (egg yolk). Phospholipids comprise various moieties which are essentially present in cellular membranes of any kind of vegetal or animal tissues, or as lipoproteins (egg yolk). Cholesterol is present in all animal cell membranes, various animal fatty foodstuffs or lipoproteins (egg yolk). Phytosterols are found in cell membranes of plant origin.

3.2.3 Lipids in the gut contents

The properties of the aqueous medium found in the stomach or the small intestine are very different. Dietary lipids initially present in the stomach are mostly dietary Class I and un-ionized lipids (triglycerides, phospholipids). Given the essentially acidic nature of the stomach content (pH 1–2 at fasting up to pH 4–5 some 2–5 hours after meal intake), these lipid moieties are organized in the form of emulsions, vesicles and crystals.

In the duodenum and downward, the pH is about neutral (pH 6.5–7.0) owing to pancreatic bicarbonate secretion, allowing ionization of acid groups. In addition, several lipid moieties are provided by the bile which is concomitantly delivered from the gallbladder. Indeed, very important amounts of phospholipids (essentially phosphatidylcholines), free cholesterol and conjugated bile salts (Classes II and III) are mixed with the content delivered by the stomach through the pylorus. The bile lipids are present in the form of vesicles (phospholipids, free cholesterol), mixed micelles (phospholipids, free cholesterol, bile salts) and simple micelles and monomers (bile salts). These two events make a considerable change in the physicochemical properties of the digestive content, with a much higher total lipid concentration leading to saturation and precipitation (emulsions, crystals) and much more amphipatic lipids (vesicles, liquid–crystalline structures, micelles).

3.2.4 Lipids in the intestinal cell

After their apical uptake by the intestinal cells, the various lipid moieties are channelled through the cytosol as complexes with proteins (sterol carrier protein, SCP; fatty acid binding protein, FABP), then in the endoplasmic reticulum for *de novo* lipid synthesis (phospholipids, triglycerides, cholesterol and fat-soluble vitamins esters), packaging in triglyceride-rich vacuoles with some proteins (microsomal transfer protein, MTP; apoB-48; apoA-IV) in the Golgi apparatus and finally secretory lipoproteins (mostly chylomicrons with surface-bound apoproteins) to be delivered into the lymphatics and then the circulation. Short chain fatty acids can be channelled more simply across the enterocyte to be secreted into the portal circulation.

3.3 Lipid digestion and absorption: basics and variability

3.3.1 Lipid digestion

From the figures above, it appears clearly that digestion is a very complex process involving insoluble substrates, neutral and amphipatic lipids, and several lipases acting in the stomach (Carey *et al.*, 1983; Hamosh, 1990; Carrière *et al.*, 1993; Armand *et al.*, 1994) and the small intestine (Borgström and Hildebrand, 1975; Carey *et al.*, 1983; Verger, 1984; Armand *et al.*, 1996a; Armand, 2007; Whitcomb and Lowe, 2007). Therefore, the intestinal uptake of lipolytic products (mainly fatty acids) as well as free cholesterol and fat-soluble vitamins (see Chapter 7) is highly dependent on the efficiency of sequential actions by lipolytic enzymes on lipid substrates. The characteristic feature of these water-soluble enzymes is their specificity to act on insoluble substrates that need to provide a suitable interface in the aqueous digestive media. Emulsification is the physicochemical process by which a given amount of oil–water interface is created (Prince, 1974; Small, 1986). It depends on the concomitant availability of a mechanical energy supply to disrupt and disperse the lipid phases and surface active molecules to coat the lipid droplets formed. The concentration of the created interface (m^2/g lipid) and its qualitative properties will govern the binding of lipases onto the droplet surface and subsequently the catalytic activity of such enzymes (Sarda and Desnuelle, 1958; Armand *et al.*, 1992; Borel *et al.*, 1994b; Borgström and Hildebrand, 1975; Hamosh, 1990; Verger, 1984).

The gastric step

It has long been thought that insoluble and unemulsified fats are present in the stomach, floating as an upper layer above the aqueous phase within the content. A late gastric emptying of dietary fat has frequently been regarded as evidence of unemulsified oil in the stomach. The observations supporting this concept were made in the 1960s using very simplified lipid meals such as the 'Lund meal', essentially made of oil mixed in an aqueous phase only. In this case, triglycerides cannot be stably emulsified and dispersed, probably explaining the above observations in humans. Moreover, the most detrimental property of the stomach content in regard to emulsification of fat is its acidic pH (1 to 5) which limits ionization and therefore emulsification and can cause some emulsion breakage.

Nevertheless, it has been established that triglyceride lipolysis occurs to some extent in the stomach content in animals and humans (Hamosh, 1990; Armand *et al.*, 1994) as catalysed by gastric lipase (Armand, 2007). This suggested that dietary triglycerides need to be emulsified to some extent to be intra-gastrically hydrolysable. Our group performed a series of studies in rats and humans to test the hypothesis that dietary fats are emulsified in the stomach content, enabling their lipolysis. Fasting subjects were intragastrically intubated and received coarsely emulsified test meals (olive oil–egg yolk in water emulsions), and gastric aspirates were collected after 1, 2, 3 and 4 h (Armand *et al.*, 1994). During digestion in the stomach, unemulsified lipids (droplets above 100 µm) represented a minor fraction. A significant amount of the initial large 70–100 µm lipid droplets disappeared and fine 1–10 µm droplets were generated. The median lipid droplet diameter significantly decreased (21.9 vs 52.9 µm initially) after 1 h and kept intermediate values for longer periods of time. The emulsion surface area was 100–120 m^2/l stomach content and was basically provided by 20–40 µm droplets. Lipolysis catalysed by gastric lipase primarily occurred within the first hour of digestion at the extent of 12%. As shown *in vitro* and *in vivo*, gastric lipase preferentially splits the sn-3 ester bond in the triglyceride molecule, thus essentially generating free fatty acids, diglycerides and few

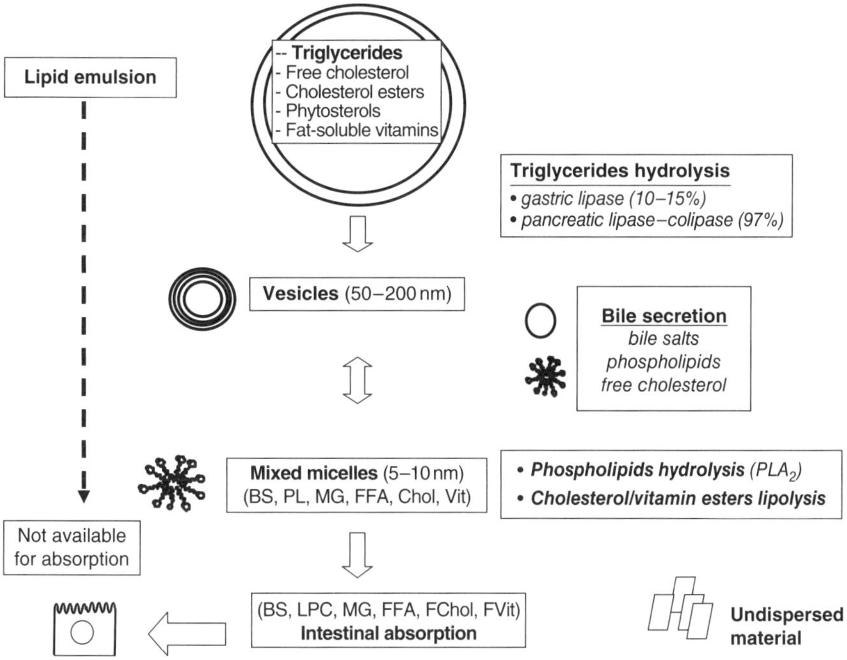

Fig. 3.2 The multi-step process of lipid digestion in the stomach and small intestine. (VitE, fat-soluble vitamin esters; FVit, free fat-soluble vitamins).

monoglycerides (Hamosh, 1990). Buds are formed at the emulsion interface (Pafumi *et al.*, 2002) and, given the acidic conditions, some precipitated materials (especially enriched in free fatty acids) accumulate. This finding demonstrated for the first time that, in the human stomach, most dietary lipids are present in the form of emulsified droplets, and that gastric lipolysis can in turn help to increase emulsification in the stomach (Fig. 3.2).

The data from these pioneering studies have been fully reproduced in another group of healthy subjects (Armand *et al.*, 1996a). In a third study we compared in humans the fate of dietary lipids emulsified in the form of a coarse (10 µm) or a fine emulsion (0.7 µm) with identical composition (Armand *et al.*, 1999). We showed that, despite an increase in droplet size in the stomach (from 0.7 up to 2.7–6.2 µm), the intubated fine emulsion retained droplets of smaller size, with the surface area of the fine emulsion being significantly higher than that of the coarse one (2.7–7.0 vs 1.3–1.8 m^2/g). At the same time, its lipolysis was significantly greater than that of the coarse emulsion (36.5% vs 15.8%) and its gastric emptying was delayed. A previous study performed in rats provided overall comparable results (Borel *et al.*, 1994a).

The rate of gastric emptying of the fine emulsions was significantly lower than that of the coarse emulsions (Borel *et al.*, 1994a; Armand *et al.*, 1999).

Some extreme conditions can be found when comparing unstable emulsions with the acidic-stable emulsions made with specific surfactants, which do not break in the stomach content and have a delayed gastric emptying (Marciani *et al.*, 2007).

Data obtained with milk fat globules are worth mentioning. Milk globule (about 4 μm diameter) lipids are mainly composed of a core of triglycerides made of noticeable proportions of short and medium chain fatty acids (about 15%) and a surrounding three-layer membrane containing various kinds of phospholipids, cholesterol and proteins. The supramolecular structure of the fat globule can be altered by several habitual processes such as milk homogenization, heat treatment, making butter or cheeses (Lopez, 2005). Gastric lipase hydrolyses 25–40% milk fat in humans, with a preferential release of short and medium chain fatty acids. The milk fat globule can be better hydrolysed in the pre-term infant stomach than dedicated formulas (Armand *et al.*, 1996b).

From these recent and replicated findings, it appeared clear that, in contrast with what was previously thought, dietary lipids can be present as an emulsion in the stomach content, they can even be further emulsified when not initially finely dispersed, and the rate of intra-gastric lipolysis is highly dependent on the size of the emulsion droplets. These new findings deserve some comments.

First, there are indeed several reasons why emulsification of dietary fat could occur to some extent in the stomach postprandially:

1. Some regular food items are already in the form of emulsions.
2. Most food products contain components with emulsifying and/or stabilizing properties.
3. The stomach may likely act as an emulsifying organ given the contractions and peristaltic waves (three cycles/min) propelling the gastric content toward the pylorus, which gathers speed as it passes through the antrum to the pylorus, thus dispersing oil droplets, as well as other solid particles.

Provided enough amphipatic moities are present, it is thus likely that the stomach provides enough mechanical energy to maintain and/or promote lipid emulsions.

Secondly, lipolysis mainly occurs within the first hour of intra-gastric digestion (Hamosh *et al.*, 1975; Armand *et al.*, 1994). From *in vitro* data (Gargouri *et al.*, 1986), it was suggested that the activity of gastric lipase on triglycerides may be inhibited by free fatty acids, especially in a protonated form and a 2–5 mmol/l concentration range. Moreover, we demonstrated that inhibition of gastric lipase is a surface-dependent phenomenon (Borel *et al.*, 1994b) and a complex multi-step process where 100–130 μmoles free fatty acid/m^2 emulsion surface area fully inhibit the enzyme activity (Pafumi *et al.*, 2002). In fact, the free fatty acid concentrations measured in the human stomach contents were almost constant over 1–4 h and in the range of 5.6–8.2 mmol/l. This means that, after 1 h digestion in the stomach, and probably less, inhibitory concentrations of free fatty acids are already produced under lipolysis. When calculated for the emulsions found in the human stomach, we found 78–180 μmoles free fatty acids/m^2 available emulsion area after 1–4 h digestion. The surface concentration reached after 1 h digestion is thus already in excess and thus the mostly protonated long chain free fatty acids released quickly and fully inhibit gastric lipolysis *in vivo*.

Third, the partial gastric fat digestion has several consequences with physiological relevance in healthy humans, such as release of readily available free fatty acids, reshaping of emulsion droplets, control of gastric emptying rate likely through the release of free fatty acids stimulating hormonal (cholecystokinine) receptors in the duodenum, stimulation of pancreatic and bile secretion through the same mechanism, and promotion of further efficient pancreatic lipase activity through changes in emulsion surface composition. Importantly, in humans with pancreatic deficiency, i.e. lacking normal bicarbonate and pancreatic lipase secretion, only gastric lipase can ensure a certain level of fat digestion.

The intestinal step

When passing from the stomach to the duodenum, two key events greatly influence the physicochemical conditions. Under some comparable hormonal stimulations, bile and pancreatic juice are concomitantly secreted and mixed in a common duodenal area. The secretion of highly concentrated bile from the gall bladder completely changes the medium properties, by providing high amounts of conjugated bile salts with detergent properties as well as phospholipids (essentially phosphatidylcholines) and free cholesterol (Small, 1986). The pancreatic secretion provides a concentrated solution of bicarbonate with a large buffer capacity that quickly raises the medium pH, as well as providing various digestive enzymes, especially pancreatic lipases and phospholipases. The stomach content will be delivered stepwise for hours through the pylorus into this new environment.

As reviewed in 1983 (Carey *et al.*, 1983), the studies on fat emulsions most frequently cited were those of Frazer *et al.* (1944) on the rat. Using a light microscope, these authors demonstrated the existence of droplets with sizes less than 0.5 μm in the duodenal content of rats fed olive oil. Later, the pioneering work done by Hoffman and Borgström (1964) and others (Mansbach *et al.*, 1975; Lindström *et al.*, 1981) on the lipid phases in the human small intestine provided some compositional data of the isolated oil phase. It was reported in the 1970s that bile lipids are part of the emulsion phase isolated during digestion in the rat upper small intestine (Nalbone *et al.*, 1974) and fat droplet–bile lipid interactions were further characterized *in vitro* (Lairon *et al.*, 1978, 1980). Later, Hernell and co-workers (Hernell *et al.*, 1990) provided detailed lipid composition on the oil phase collected from the human upper small intestine during digestion.

In order to provide lacking information on the state of emulsification of dietary lipids in the human small intestine, we performed a study in fasting subjects fitted with nasogastric and nasoduodenal tubes and receiving intragastrically a coarsely emulsified test meal (Armand *et al.*, 1996a). In the duodenum, most lipids (>90%) were present as emulsified droplets sized 1–100 μm. Large droplets and unemulsified material present in the test meal (>100 μm) disappeared, while smaller droplets (1–50 μm) were present after 1 h digestion. Thus, the median lipid droplet diameter significantly decreased in the duodenum (19.6 vs 56.5 μm in the test meal) but was overall similar to the one measured at the same 1–4 h time points in the stomach (20–46 vs 17–52 μm). The specific surface area significantly increased in the stomach (2.08 vs 0.70 m^2/g lipid in the test meal) and was comparable in the duodenum (1.6 m^2/g) and the stomach (2 m^2/g) 1 h after meal ingestion. After 2, 3 and 4 h digestion, the emulsion surface areas kept intermediate values in the duodenum contents (0.51–1.1 m^2/g). The mean concentration of emulsion surface was 78 and 70 m^2/l after 1 and 2 h in duodenum contents, respectively. Nevertheless, the extent of apparent triglyceride hydrolysis was much higher in the duodenum (42–45%) than in the stomach (6–16%), where small droplets were enriched in lipolytic products, cholesterol and phospholipids. The relative lipid composition of the various emulsion droplets was related to their size (Armand *et al.*, 1996a).

When comparing the fate of two emulsions with very different initial droplet sizes (mean diameters: 10 or 0.7 μm), we observed for a coarse and a fine emulsion that the median droplet size did not change in the duodenum compared with the stomach and that the fine emulsion still provided a significantly higher surface area than the coarse one in the duodenum (Armand *et al.*, 1999). At the same time, the apparent intra-duodenal lipolysis of the fine emulsion was noticeably greater than that of the coarse one (76 vs 46%). Comparable observations have previously been made in rats (Borel *et al.*, 1994a), showing that emulsion droplets present in the duodenum were sized 14–33 μm and that the size of the emulsion droplets in the duodenum content did not noticeably differ from those in the stomach content.

These concordant findings thus established that most dietary lipids are present in the human duodenum as emulsified droplets of 10–50 μm size and that no further marked emulsification of dietary fat occurs in the duodenum compared with the stomach. This novel view is contrary to that previously thought (in the absence of relevant data), but is supported by physicochemical considerations. Indeed, it has clearly been shown that triglyceride emulsification is very unefficiently achieved by bile salts alone, contrary to fatty acids and phospholipids (Linthorst *et al.*, 1977). While these latter are present in the duodenal medium, it is unlikely, as observed, that the intestinal peristaltism is strong enough to provide the necessary shear forces to achieve extensive lipid dispersion in the small intestine.

The intestinal lipolytic process, as illustrated in Fig. 3.2, is a very complex one as described in previous review articles (Carey *et al.*, 1983; Armand,

2007; Whitcomb and Lowe, 2007). Lipolysis is mediated by the pancreatic colipase–lipase system which adsorbs onto the emulsion interface and splits the sn-1 and sn-3 ester bonds on the triglyceride moiety, generating intermediate diglycerides and finally, fatty acids and monoglycerides. We have provided evidence that, under close to physiological conditions, bile lipids, especially phospholipid-free cholesterol complexes (mixed micelles/unilamellar vesicles), bind to water-soluble colipase–lipase complexes, forming an effecitive entity that binds to the lipid interface and directs the extent of enzyme adsorption (Lairon *et al.*, 1978, 1980). Bile salts can also exert either an inhibitory or stimulatory role in this process thanks to their detergent properties. In the absence of an efficient colipase–lipase system, triglyceride hydrolysis is impaired and lipid absorption very limited or inefficient (Verger, 1984). This intestinal step is facilitated by the previous one catalysed by gastric lipase. Indeed, fluid coming from the stomach into the duodenum provides generated tensio-active moieties such as free fatty acids, which help the emulsification process and the binding of pancreatic lipase onto the droplet surface (Bernback *et al.*, 1989; Borel *et al.*, 1994b).

Upon the lipolysis process in duodenal conditions, the excess material (lipolytic products, i.e. fatty acids and monoglycerides, and surface monolayer moieties) generated at the emulsion/water interface expands from the interface in the form of a lamellar liquid crystal phase, leading to dispersed unilamellar vesicular structures in the aqueous medium of size 20–60 nm (Hernell *et al.*, 1990). Thanks to the supramicellar bile acids concentration (5–20 mmol/l), an equilibrium is attained between vesicles (20–60 nm) and mixed micelles sized about 4 nm. This fits well with the phase behaviour and aggregation states of such lipid mixtures in an aqueous phase as modelled *in vitro* (Staggers *et al.*, 1990). A schematic representation of lipid structures present during fat digestion in the human duodenum is shown in Fig. 3.3.

During digestion in humans (Hernell *et al.*, 1990; Armand *et al.*, 1996a), the aqueous phase is thus mainly composed of bile salts (6–20 mmol/l), free fatty acids (6–20 mmol/l) and monoglycerides (3–6 mmol/l), phospholipids (1.5–4 mmol/l) and free cholesterol (0.5–1 mmol/l).

A second enzymatic step will occur, mixed micelles compounds being suitable substrates for other pancreatic enzymes. Indeed, pancreatic phospholipase A2 possesses a strict capability to efficiently hydrolyse phospholipids to lyso-phospholipids when present in the form of mixed micelles (Nalbone *et al.*, 1980). Upon digestion, about two-thirds of phospholipids are present as lyso-phospholipids. This step is critical to efficient cholesterol absorption. Other substrates are found in mixed micelles such as cholesterol esters and fat-soluble vitamin (A, E) esters. These esters will be split through the catalytic action of pancreatic carboxyl-ester lipase and/or pancreatic triglyceride lipase, enabling further absorption of these free moieties (see Chapter 7). A recent study in knockout mice has shown that both pancreatic triglyceride and carboxyl ester lipases are involved in the hydrolysis of

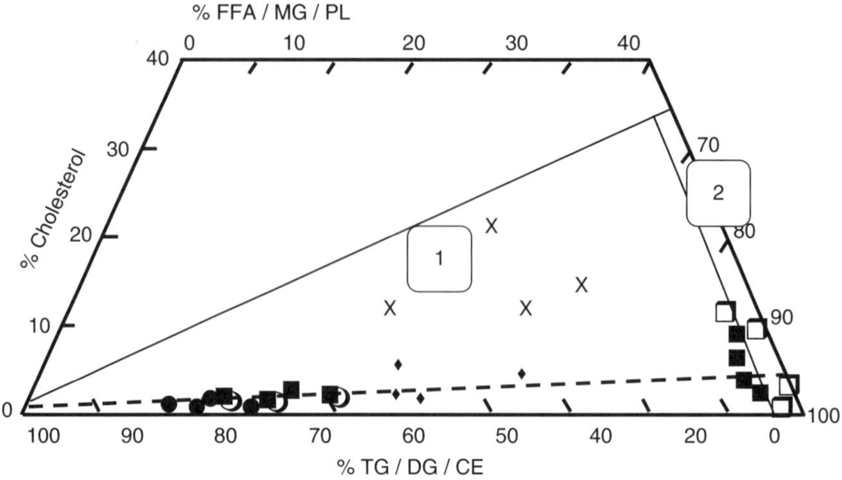

Fig. 3.3 Plots of the relative lipid compositions of emulsion droplets, intermediate fractions, pellets and aqueous phases isolated from human duodenum content during digestion (from Armand *et al.*, 1996a). Three lipid-axis with free cholesterol (CH), polar lipids (phospholipids (PL) + monoglycerides (MG) + free fatty acids (FFA)) and neutral lipids (triglycerides (TG) + diglycerides (DG) + cholesteryl esters): (1) two-phase emulsions and (2) lamellar liquid–crystalline phase essentially composed of polar lipids. The relative lipid compositions of fractions isolated after 1, 2, 3 and 4 h digestion are plotted on the diagram: emulsion droplets in the range 50–100 µm (●), 10–50 µm (○) and 1–10 µm (▲), intermediate <1 µm fraction (×), pellets (■) and aqueous micellar phase (□).

triglycerides, cholesterol esters or retinyl palmitate and synergistically enable the absorption of about half cholesterol or retinol (Gilham *et al.*, 2007). Other lipases have been found in the pancreatic juice (PLRP1 and PLRP2), whose substrates and functions are not yet clearly identified although some could be relevant to human physiology (Reboul *et al.*, 2006).

It is noteworthy that an important part of lipid moieties present in the duodenal contents are found as precipitated (pellet) material (Hernell *et al.*, 1990; Armand *et al.*, 1996a). Such precipitates are mainly composed of free fatty acids, monoglycerides, phospholipids and cholesterol in decreasing order. It is likely that these lipids are present in the form of large lamellar structures, soaps and liquid crystals in this supersaturated environment. This suggests that the overall process leading to almost complete intestinal lipid absorption is even more complex than considered, a further transfer of fatty acid and monoglyceride moieties from the insoluble material into mixed micelles in the aqueous phase being necessary. This could not be the case for free cholesterol because its intestinal absorption efficiency is only 30–80% in healthy humans (Bosner *et al.*, 1999).

The variability of lipid digestion is both linked to the nature of the lipid substrates (fatty acid composition, emulsification degree, amphipaths present, etc.) and the level of secretion of gastric and pancreatic lipases. This latter depends on many factors, including development state, level of fat content in the diet, age and pathological conditions impairing normal process such as gastric dysfunction, pancreatic insufficiency or defect in bile secretion.

3.3.2 Lipid absorption

Lipid uptake by the small intestine

The capacity of humans to take up dietary fat is extremely high, i.e. about 600 g fat can be absorbed with 95% efficiency! Conversely, our capacity to absorb cholesterol is much less, a few hundred milligrams being absorbed daily at a highly variable but limited rate (30–80%) in healthy humans (Bosner *et al.*, 1999). The uptake of digested lipid mixtures occurs at the apical side of small intestinal cells (enterocytes), mostly in the duodenum and jejunum. The apical side of enterocytes is made by a brush border membrane, offering an optimal surface area for maximum uptake.

It is thought that, given the distance (15–20 nm) between two microvilli at the cell brush border membrane, only lipid moieties in the form of mixed micelles (about 4 nm) are capable of being efficiently uptaken. This explains, at least partly, why lipid absorption is much less effective from vesicular structures with greater size (20–60 nm). Moreover, we have recently shown that the facilitated uptake of cholesterol mediated by cellular transport proteins is strictly limited to the very small cholesterol donors (Haikal *et al.*, 2008) and stimulated by a biliary protein (Jourdheuil-Rahmani *et al.*, 2002).

For a long time, a key unresolved question was: is the lipid absorption process in the small intestine passive or facilitated? Regarding fatty acids and monoglycerides, the question is still open as reviewed recently (Mansbach and Gorelick, 2007). Indeed, some data support a protein-free diffusion model where fatty acids 'flip-flop' across the brush border membrane at a non-limiting rate. In contrast, other data support a protein-mediated uptake and transport. Indeed, a number of candidate proteins have been suggested: the fatty acid transport protein 4 (FATP-4), but its role in apical uptake is controversial, the FAT/CD36 transporter whose role could be either in fatty acid uptake or detection and further intracellular signalling, and the fatty acid binding protein pm (FABP pm), a membrane protein whose inhibition reduces fatty acid uptake. It is likely that the two kinds of processes coexist but their relative importance is not yet established.

Regarding free cholesterol, impressive progress has been made during the past decade. It is now acknowledged that the intestinal absorption of cholesterol is mostly performed through transport proteins as reviewed recently (Hui *et al.*, 2007). Cholesterol apical uptake of cholesterol requires several brush border proteins such as Niemann-Pick1-like1 (NPC1-L1), the scavenger receptor B-I and possibly FAT/CD36, along with proteins located at the basal side of the enterocyte such as ATP-binding cassette half transporters (ABCG5, ABCG8). Their respective roles are not fully established but experimental data do support the concept that NPC1L1 and SR-BI can direct the apical uptake of free cholesterol, while ABCG5 and ABCG8 stimulate the release of cholesterol and phytosterols from the intestinal cell back to the lumen. This means that the overall capacity to absorb cholesterol is the result of the balance between these two antogonist processes. The new drug Ezetimide, interfering with NPC1L1 function (and possibly SR-BI and CD36), has recently been released on the market to reduce cholesterol absorption in hypercholesterolaemic humans (Miura and Saku, 2008).

The intracellular assembly, transport and secretion process

As recently reviewed (Mansbach and Gorelick, 2007), after being taken into the brush border membrane, lipid moieties must be channelled to the endoplasmic reticulum. For that, transport proteins such as FABP-1 and FABP-2 can bind fatty acids or monoglycerides, while the sterol carrier proteins (SCP1, SCP2) bind free cholesterol, whereas in the endoplasmic reticulum, numerous enzyme-catalysed reactions will take place, leading to efficient *de novo* synthesis of triglycerides, phospholipids and cholesterol esters.

The assembly of chylomicron is the next key step in the intracellular process. It involves the microsomal transfer protein (MTP) which chaperones the apoprotein apoB-48 (specific truncated form of apoB in the intestine). In the presence of lipids, apoB-48 will form dense particles with phospholipids, cholesterol and small amounts of triglycerides. At the same time, triglycerides and cholesterol esters in the smooth reticulum endothelium are carried out by MTP to build enlarged particles, which then bind the apoprotein apoA-IV. The two kinds of particles will finally merge to make pre-chylomicrons with a neutral lipid core surrounded by an amphipatic monolayer. It will then buds from the smooth endoplasmic reticulum to translocate into the Golgi complex, where apo A1 binding and protein glycosylation take place. Finally, the mature chylomicrons exit the Golgi apparatus and the transport vesicles fuse with the basal membrane to allow secretion. Chylomicrons are secreted into the lymph, which will further enter the blood circulation.

Chylomicron secretion is limited by several factors, such as the amount of biliary or dietary phospholipids, the amount of dietary fat, and the nature of dietary fatty acids, especially *n*-3 fatty acids (Lairon, 2008).

Finally, it is worth mentioning that short and, to a lesser extent, medium chain fatty acids are preferentially channelled within the enterocyte via another route, leading to their secretion at the basal membrane into the portal blood circulation as complexes with albumin. These fatty acids thus do not participate noticeably to the postprandial lipid rise observed in the peripheral circulation.

3.4 Mechanisms relating lipid absorption and health

3.4.1 Postprandial lipid metabolism and organ interplay

Most people in Western countries are used to consuming 40–120 g fat per day provided as fat-containing meals at regular 4–5 hour intervals and frequent snacks. Following consumption of a typical fat-containing meal (30–60 g fat), circulating triacylglycerols show a marked increase called postprandial lipaemia after 1 h and can remain elevated for 5–8 h. Thus, most of the state of triacylglycerol metabolism is a postprandial one in humans (Roche and Gibney, 1995; Lairon, 1996; Williams, 1997; Lopez-Miranda *et al.*, 2007).

As recently reviewed (Lopez-Miranda, *et al.*, 2007; Lairon, 2008) and illustrated in Fig. 3.4, the postprandial period is characterized by a physiological transient accumulation of triglyceride-rich lipoprotein particles in the circulation provided both by the small intestine (chylomicrons secreted specifically after lipid digestion and absorption) and by the liver (in the form of very low density lipoproteins (VLDL), as in the fasting state).

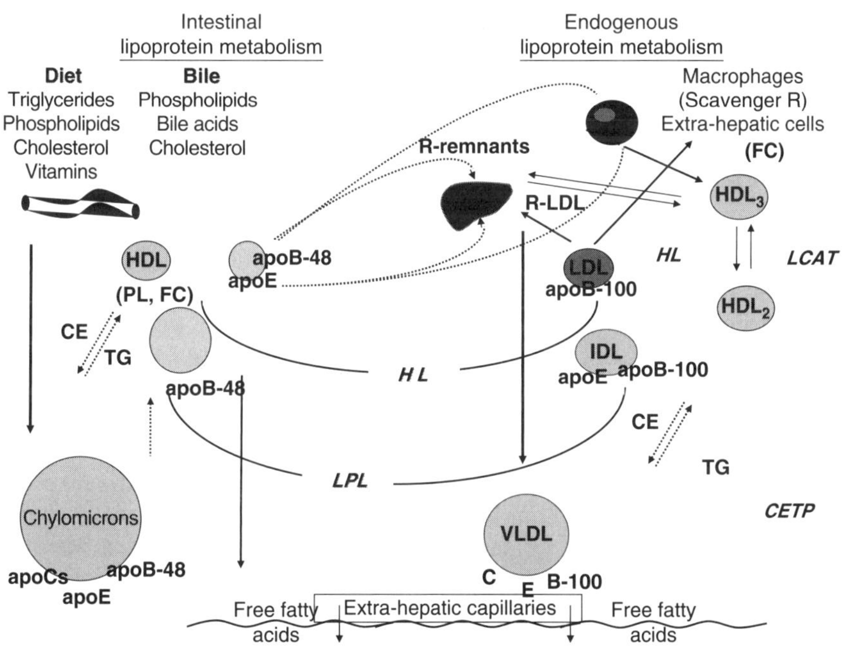

Fig. 3.4 Schematic representation of the postprandial lipid metabolism in humans. Exogenous (small intestine/chylomicrons) and endogenous (liver/very low density lipoproteins,VLDL) pathways co-exist leading to transient accumulation of triglyceride-rich lipoproteins and remnants of two origins. (IDL, intermediate density lipoprotein; LDL, low density lipoprotein; R-remnants, cellular receptor for chylomicron remmant; R-LDL, cellular receptor for LDL; apo-, apoprotein; LPL, lipoprotein lipase; HL, hepatic lipase; LCAT, lecithin cholesterol acyl-transferase; CETP, cholesterol ester transfer protein).

Through this postprandial process, adipose tissue is efficiently filled with fatty acid moieties upon chylomicron triglyceride hydrolysis catalysed by lipoprotein lipase. The resulting accumulated remnant particles in the circulation can be taken up by the liver but also by peripheral tissues including muscle and the arterial wall (atherogenic particles). It is now recognized that extended postprandial lipaemia is a characteristic metabolic abnormality of a number of lifestyle-related conditions that are associated both with increased morbidity, such as hypertriglyceridaemia, metabolic syndrome, obesity, insulin resistance, type 2 diabetes and mortality, especially from cardiovascular disease (Patsch *et al.*, 1992; Chen *et al.*, 1993; Jeppesen *et al.*, 1995; Karpe and Hamsten, 1995; Couillard *et al.*, 1998; Mekki *et al.*, 1999; Bansal *et al.*, 2007; Lopez-Miranda *et al.*, 2007; Nordestgaard *et al.*, 2007).

Through this frequent process, the organism is provided with key nutrients, such as essential or necessary fatty acids and fat-soluble micronutrients, such as vitamin A, E, D, K or carotenoids. Concomitantly, exogenous cholesterol and saturated fatty acids are provided and high amounts can have deleterious effects on lipid homeostasis (hypercholesterolaemia and elevated LDL cholesterol, insulin resistance). Exagerated lipemia is key to adipogenesis, fat storage and resulting obesity.

3.4.2 Variability in postprandial lipaemia

It is known that the capacity of individuals to regulate circulating triacylglycerol levels and clear triglyceride-rich lipoproteins can be modulated by various gene polymorphisms (Lopez-Miranda *et al.*, 2007a). Another key factor is the fact that most daily meals are mixed meals made of various foodstuffs that provide numerous macro-nutrients including lipids, digestible carbohydrates (starch, sugar, etc.), micro-nutrients (vitamins, carotenoids, phytochemicals) and indigestible carbohydrates (e.g. mostly fibres). This means that postprandial metabolism resulting from digestion and absorption of available nutrients is a highly complex process involving numerous potential interactions.

The amount of dietary triglycerides as well as the nature of the ingested fatty acids in a typical diet or in a test meal modulates the extent of chylomicron and plasma triglyceride levels postprandially (Lairon *et al.*, 2007a,b; Lopez-Miranda *et al.*, 2007; Lairon, 2008). The amount of dietary cholesterol also modulates the extent of postprandial chylomicron and plasma triglycerides. Other nutrients can alter the postprandial occurrence of chylomicrons such as proteins, alcohol, carbohydrates or fibres. For instance, addition of glucose and more markedly fructose to a fat test meal increases the accumulation of chylomicrons, as does a high-glycaemic index meal. In contrast, some sources of dietary fibres such as oat bran noticeably decrease the occurrence of chylomicron postprandially. Overall, changing the habitual dietary pattern, for instance from a Western-type diet to a Mediterranean-type one can, in turn, alter the postprandial response of the subjects

(Lairon, 2008). The last step in postprandial lipid metabolism is clearance from plasma through combined lipolysis processes and tissue uptake of chylomicron remnants. This process is influenced both by the condition of the subject and the level, size and composition of chylomicrons.

3.5 Implications for the development of functional foods and future trends

As mentioned above, the number and complexity of mechanisms involved in lipid digestion, intestinal absorption and postprandial metabolism offer a wide range of opportunities to develop new concepts aimed at modulating such processes through diet and specific foods. We will review the important and likely strategies in this area.

3.5.1 Limiting the amount of fat ingested

Obviously, this is the first direction to go from a public health point of view. Given the high habitual fat intake of about 38–40% energy in Western countries, all recommended diets are nowadays set at a lower fat level, i.e. about 30% energy, with a special emphasis on limiting saturated and *trans* fatty acids. This would help reduce energy intake (lipids: 9 kcal/g) and get a better energy balance, lower saturated/*trans* fatty acid intakes, which raise plasma and LDL cholesterol, to lower gastric and pancreatic lipase secretion, and to lower postprandial hypertriglyceridaemia, whose extent is determined by the amount of fat ingested (Dubois *et al.*, 1998; Lairon, 2008).

This opens a large window for selecting naturally low (saturated) fat foodstuffs and the important range of light foods with reduced or no fat. This raises the question of the palatability and the durability of use of such 'light' products. Regardless, having a low-fat diet nowadays is easily achievable, and more products could be developed along that line.

3.5.2 Replacing fat

A strategy developed a long time ago is the use of fat replacers and some of them have already been approved by the Food and Drug Administration in the USA. Fat replacers have diverse chemical structures, functional properties and food applications. While part of them are not lipid moieties but carbohydrate- or protein-based (Chung and Min, 2004), we will briefly focus on the lipid-based ones. Sucrose fatty acid polyesters, commonly known as Olestra (Procter & Gamble), are long chain fatty acids esterified with sucrose, which have organoleptic and thermal properties similar to fat. Conversely, it is not a suitable substrate for pancreatic lipase (and probably gastric lipase), and thus this molecule is too large to be absorbed by the small intestine and is fully excreted into the stools. Its contribution to energy is thus null. Several clinical studies have shown the beneficial effects of Olestra on weight control and cardiovascular risk (Chung and Min, 2004). It has been calculated that the intake of 2 g/day Olestra would save 6570 kcal and thus decrease body weight by 0.85 kg a year. It can be used as a baking and frying fat.

The overall safety of fat replacers has been established, but the long-term consequences should be evaluated. In the short term, they are known to lower the intestinal absorption of fat-soluble nutrients whose intakes should therefore be increased for those individuals who consume appreciable amounts of fat replacers.

3.5.3 Altering the nature of fat

Monounsaturated fatty acids and olive oil

Oleic acid (*cis* C18:9, *n*-1) is by far the predominant monounsaturated fatty acid (MUFA) and olive oil is its main source (Lopez-Miranda *et al.*, 2006). Compared with other kinds of fat-improved diets, an oleic-rich diet has a comparable cholesterol-lowering effect while maintaining the protective HDL cholesterol level and decreasing triglyceridaemia (Kris-Etherton *et al.*, 1999). While the amplitude of postprandial triglyceridaemia has not been found to be different for *n*-6 PUFA and olive oil (Mekki *et al.*, 2002), oleic acid can stimulate chylomicron secretion and clearance from the circulation (Roche *et al.*, 1998; Lopez-Miranda *et al.*, 2006). Considering the additional beneficial effects of olive oil on endothelial function, haemostasis, platelet function, and coagulation factors (Perez-Jimenez *et al.*, 2005; Lopez-Miranda *et al.*, 2006), MUFA-rich and especially olive oil-rich diets are highly recommended nowadays. This is an important feature of the Mediterranean diet acknowledged worldwide for its health-protective effects (Willett *et al.*, 1995; Giugliano and Esposito, 2008). Important improvements in food composition can be achieved by replacing part of saturated fats by MUFA-rich sources and using olive oil as the main added fat source.

n-*3 Fatty acids*

Since the pioneering studies performed in the 1970s, it is known that diets rich in *n*-3 long chain polyunsaturated fatty acids, namely EPA and DHA, are associated with a low cardiovascular risk and mortality (Dyerberg and Bang, 1982; GISSI, 1999; Albert *et al.*, 2002; Minihane and Lovegrove, 2006; Hansen and Harris, 2007). This is clearly due to a high consumption of fatty fish and seafood (Torres *et al.*, 2000), while the protective effect of the mostly vegetal *n*-3 precursor alpha linolenic acid (C 18:3, *n*-3) is probable but still debated. This protective effect could be due to the observed lowering of fasting and postprandial triglyceridaemia (Lopez-Miranda *et al.*, 2007) because *n*-3 fatty acids are a poor substrate for chylomicron or VLDL triglyceride synthesis. *n*-3 Fatty acids also reduce blood aggregation and inflammation. Increasing the intake of foods naturally rich or specifically enriched in *n*-3 fatty acids is thus highly recommended at the level of a few grams a day. The development of such enriched functional foods is an important challenge, despite the uncertain availability of these fatty acids in the near future. Improved farming systems (adding linseed kernels or oil to animal feeds, organic husbandry) are already able to increase meat or milk *n*-3 fatty acid levels.

Conjugated linoleic acids

Conjugated linoleic acids (CLAs) are a group of C18 fatty acids with consecutive double bonds, which are end products of the biohydrogenation in the rumen of ingested unsaturated fatty acids (Yacoob and Tricon, 2006). Meats and dairy products are thus the richest foodstuffs in which the *c*9, *t*11-CLA accounts for 80% of total CLA. Some supplements can be found, which contain equal amounts of *c*9, *t*11 and *t*10, *c*12-CLA. In experimental models, the *c*9, *t*11 isomer has shown anti-atherogenic effects, while the effects of the *t*10, *c*12 isomer are more controversial. Their effects on blood lipids are not yet firmly demonstrated, while the anti-inflammatory effects of the *c*9, *t*11 isomer seem established. The long-term effects of CLAs in humans have not yet been demonstrated.

Thus, there is an important challenge for the dairy industry to face in that area. Further efforts are needed to evaluate the effects of individual CLAs in humans and to improve their levels in dairy products and meats.

Short and medium chain fatty acids, structured lipids

Short (C4, C6, C8) and medium chain fatty acids (C10, C12, C14) are a natural part of milk and dairy triglycerides, being about 15% of the total fatty acids. Given their reduced hydrophobicity, these fatty acids are released faster from triglycerides upon lipase-catalysed hydrolysis than long chain ones, and are readily absorbed by the enterocyte from which they are directly secreted into the portal blood circulation as complexes with albumin, unlike long chain fatty acid moieties which are secreted after packaging through the chylomicron route. This improved capability to be handled in the gut and further used as a fuel source made them a useful source of fat for clinical purposes in situations with poor outcome (pancreatic insufficiency, cystic fibrosis, malabsorption syndromes, emergency). Their intake is as expected associated with a somewhat reduced postprandial chylomicronaemia and triglyceridaemia (Mekki *et al.*, 2002; Lopez-Miranda *et al.*, 2007).

Structured lipids are triglycerides containing both short or medium and long chain fatty acids as obtained by random *trans*-esterification. Upon lipase-catalysed hydrolysis, medium-chain fatty acids can be readily absorbed via the portal route and used upon oxidation to provide energy (8.3 kcal/g). Other structured lipids such as Caprenin, made of caprylic, capric and behenic acids, or Salatrim, made of stearic and short chain fatty acids have even less energy yield at about 5 kcal/g due to both reduced intestinal absorption and metabolism.

Diglycerides and monoglycerides

Diglycerides (DAGs) are natural components of some edible oils and can be synthesized enzymatically. DAGs, especially 1,3-DAG, result in lower postprandial lipaemia in plasma compared with triglycerides with similar fatty acid composition in healthy or insulin-resistant subjects (Takase *et al.*, 2005; Yasunaga *et al.*, 2007). In fact, the lymphatic transport of chylomicrons is delayed and reduced after ingestion of DAG, probably as the result of poor re-esterification of 1,3-DAG into triglycerides within intestinal mucosa cells (Kondo *et al.*, 2003). Moreover, the postprandial clearance of DAG-rich chylomicrons is accelerated (Yasunaga *et al.*, 2007). DAG-rich oils are already available in some countries and one can expect further functional food developments.

A novel monoglyceride-based gel structure (MAG GEL) has recently been developed, which encapsulates liquid oil in a water matrix stabilized by multilayers made of long-chain saturated monoglycerides (Marangoni *et al.*, 2007). Ingestion of this preparation resulted in a blunted postprandial triglyceride rise compared with that of a comparable oil–water mixture. This is another example of strategies dedicated to manipulate lipid assimilation to improve postprandial lipid metabolism.

3.5.4 Altering the physicochemical properties of lipid supramolecular structures

As mentioned above, the physicochemical properties of the substrate and media are keys to efficient triglyceride hydrolysis catalysed by gut lipases. Thus, another approach to modulate lipolysis efficiency would be to alter the physicochemical characteristics of the system.

Emusion droplet size

As the concentration of emulsion surface area is a key determinant of lipolysis rate, increasing the droplet size should lower lipolysis efficiency. This has already been demonstrated by our group *in vitro* (Armand *et al.*, 1992; Borel *et al.*, 1994b), in rats (Borel *et al.*, 1994a) and in humans (Armand *et al.*, 1999).

Adding soluble viscous dietary fibres such as guar gums or pectins can reduce emulsification and increase lipid droplet size. This results in a viscosity-dependent manner, a lower *in vitro* lipolysis rate in the gastric media (Pasquier *et al.*, 1996a) as well as the intestinal one (Pasquier *et al.*, 1996b), and was confirmed with guar gum *in vivo* in the rat (Lairon, 2001).

Another natural compound such as green tea extract rich in polyphenols can markedly lower lipid digestion (Juhel *et al.*, 2000). An *in vitro* study showed that gastric lipolysis can be fully inhibited, while duodenal lipolysis can only be lowered: overall, a 37% inhibition of the overall lipolysis process has been observed with low amounts of green tea extract (60 mg/g fat). Such an inhibition has been explained by a marked reduction in the extent of emulsification and increase in droplet size.

Further attempts should be developed in that line to slow down and reduce overall lipid digestibility. Conversely, in physiopathological cases with insufficient lipolysis capacity (i.e. pancreatic insufficiency), reducing the droplet size would markedly increase the rate of lipolysis in the stomach and then in the small intestine.

Emulsion stability

Promoting acid-stable vs unstable lipid emulsions in the gastric media can also delay gastric emptying (Marciani *et al.*, 2007), and possibly improve satiety. In fact, intra-gastric lipolysis would be more efficient in the presence of a sustained emulsion area, allowing the release of more free fatty acids. In turn, they stimulate greater cholecystokinine release and act on cells sensitive to fatty acids in the duodenum, resulting in a slowed gastric emptying. Acid-stable lipid emulsions can be prepared using specific emulsifiers whose suitability for chronic human use should be further evaluated.

The native milk fat globule can be disrupted under processing to generate bulk lipids (i.e. butter) so that handling in the gut and triglyceride postprandial occurrence in the circulation can be different from other lipid sources (Mekki *et al.*, 2002; Michalsky *et al.*, 2005; Lairon *et al.*, 2007b).

Emulsion properties

For most long chain saturated fatty acids, the melting point is above room or body temperature. This means that the fatty acid chains are not in a true liquid state but rather in liquid–crystalline or crystalline ones. As shown recently, manipulating this condition can impact lipid digestibility by pancreatic lipase (Bonnaire *et al.*, 2008).

Manipulating the physicochemical properties of the amphipatic monolayer at the emulsion surface should also have marked consequences on lipase efficiency. Indeed, this has largely been demonstrated during *in vitro* studies with all digestive lipases. A practical example is given by the milk globule with a supramolecular structure with specific properties (Lopez, 2005). In premature newborns with limited digestive capacities the native milk fat globule is much better lipolysed in the stomach than a formula (Armand *et al.*, 1996b). In addition, the properties of the milk fat globule can be altered by some physicochemical processes (homogenization, selective separation) that would markedly impact digestibility and resulting postprandial occurrence in the circulation as observed (Michalsky *et al.*, 2005, 2006).

Phospholipids and proteins are amphipathic compounds with a large diversity and there are still lots of unsolved issues in this area. Phospholipids are the main structural component of membranes and globule monolayers as well as bile secretion, and are well-known emulsifiers. We (Lairon *et al.*, 1978, 1980b) and others (Patton and Carey, 1981) have long ago shown *in vitro* the regulatory role of bile phospholipids on the binding of pancreatic lipase onto interfaces. This raised the question of the potential *in vivo* limiting effect of excess phospholipids on lipolysis. More recently, the role of phospholipids on gastric lipase action has been investigated (Favé *et al.*, 2007), indicating that phospholipid species have different effects on *in vitro* gastric lipolysis. This should be more intensively investigated.

Proteins and peptides are present in most foods or can be specifically prepared from protein-rich foodstuffs such as milk or legumes. Depending on their primary and secondary structures, they exhibit variable amphipathic or hydrophobic properties, which can interfere in the emulsification and/or lipolysis process, free fatty acid binding and the resulting lipid postprandial occurrence in the circulation. This field has unfortunately been poorly investigated up to now.

3.5.5 Inhibiting fatty acid and cholesterol intestinal uptake

Phospholipids (mainly phosphatidylcholines, i.e. lecithins) are both provided by bile and diet and take part in the assembly of many lipid structures present in the gut lumen. It has been shown *in vitro* that the presence of intact phospholipids inhibit the absorption of cholesterol, but not of fatty acids (Mackay *et al.*, 1997; Homan and Hamelehle, 1998). Conversely, phospholipid hydrolysis by phospholipase A2 facilitated the incorporation of micellar cholesterol into intestinal Caco-2 cells in a dose-dependent manner (Hamada *et al.*, 2005). In rats, lymphatic recovery of cholesterol infused into the duodenum was accelerated by the co-administration of phospholipase A2. Accelerated cholesterol absorption was also observed when a part of micellar PC was replaced by lysophosphatidylcholine (LysoPC) and oleic acid (Hamada *et al.*, 2005).

It thus clearly appears that phospholipids present in the intestinal lumen in mixed micelles need to be hydrolysed by phospholipsase A2 to ensure efficient cholesterol absorption. Indeed, most phospholipids present in the human duodenum content are in the form of lyso-phospholipids (Armand *et al.*, 1996a). It is therefore tempting to suggest that increasing the amount of dietary phospholipids could be a strategy to reduce cholesterol absorption, but this remains to be demonstrated.

Some kinds of dietary fibres, especially the soluble viscous ones such as beta-glucans (oat, barley), pectins or psyllium, can alter fatty acid and cholesterol uptake in animals and humans as reviewed recently (Lairon *et al.*, 2007a). Indeed, oat bran added to a fat test meal significantly increases lipid output at the end of the small intestine and, as a result, lowers by about 40% the level of chylomicron lipids in the circulation postprandially (Cara *et al.*, 1992; Lia *et al.*, 1997). This is expected to account, at least in part, for the cholesterol lowering of such sources of dietary fibres. In addition, a wheat fraction such as wheat germ can also lower lipid absorption from the small intestine and resulting postprandial lipaemia (Cara *et al.*, 1992).

This highlights the important potential of plant-derived materials for altering lipid uptake from the small intestine. The specific role played by phytosterols is reported in Chapter 7.

3.6 References

ALBERT CM, CAMPOS H, STAMPFER MJ, RIDKER PM, MANSON JE, WILLETT WC, MA J (2002). Blood levels of long-chain n-3 fatty acids and the risk of sudden death. *N Engl J Med* **346**, 1113–18.

ARMAND M (2007). Lipases and lipolysis in the human digestive tract: where do we stand? *Curr Opin Clin Nutr Metab Care* **10**, 156–64.

ARMAND M, BOREL P, YTHIER P, DUTOT G, MELIN C, SENFT M, LAFONT H, LAIRON D (1992). Effects of droplet size, triacylglycerol composition, and calcium on the hydrolysis of complex emulsions by pancreatic lipase: an *in vitro* study. *J Nutr Biochem* **3**, 333–41.

ARMAND M, BOREL P, DUBOIS C, SENFT M, PEYROT J, SALDUCCI J, LAFONT H, LAIRON D (1994). Characterization of emulsions and lipolysis of dietary lipids in human stomach. *Am J Physiol* **266**, G372–81.

ARMAND M, BOREL P, PASQUIER B, DUBOIS C, SENFT M, ANDRE M, PEYROT J, SALDUCCI J, LAIRON D (1996a). Physicochemical characteristics of emulsions during fat digestion in human stomach and duodenum. *Am J Physiol* **271**, G172–83.

ARMAND M, HAMOSH M, MEHTA NR, ANGELUS PA, PHILPOTT JR, HENDERSON TR, DWYER NK, LAIRON D, HAMOSH P (1996b). Effect of human milk or formula on gastric function and fat digestion in the premature infant. *Pediatr Res* **40**, 429–37.

ARMAND M, PASQUIER B, ANDRE M, BOREL P, SENFT M, PEYROT J, SALDUCCI J, PORTUGAL H, JAUSSAN V, LAIRON D (1999). Digestion and absorption of 2 fat emulsions with different droplet sizes in the human digestive tract. *Am J Clin Nutr* **70**, 1096–106.

BANSAL S, BURING JE, RIFAI N, MORA S, SACKS FM, RIDKER PM (2007). Fasting compared with nonfasting triglycerides and risk of cardiovascular events in women. *JAMA* **298**, 309–16.

BERNBACK S, BLACKBERG L, HERNELL O (1989). Fatty acids generated by gastric lipase promote human milk triacylglycerol digestion by pancreatic colipase-dependent lipase. *Biochim Biophys Acta* **1001**, 286–93.

BONNAIRE L, SANDRA S, HELGASON T, DECKER EA, WEISS J, MCCLEMENTS DJ (2008). Influence of lipid physical state on the *in vitro* digestibility of emulsified lipid. *J Agric Food Chem* **56**(10), 3791–7.

BOREL P, ARMAND M, YTHIER P, DUTOT G, MELIN C, SENFT M, LAFONT H, LAIRON D (1994a). Digestion and absorption of tube-feeding emulsions with different droplet sizes and compositions in the rat. *J Parent Ent Nutr* **18**, 534–43.

BOREL P, ARMAND M, YTHIER P, DUTOT G, MELIN C, SENFT M, LAFONT H, LAIRON D (1994b). Hydrolysis of emulsions with different triglycerides and droplet sizes by gastric lipase *in vitro*. Effect on pancreatic lipase activity. *J Nutr Biochem* **5**, 124–33.

BORGSTRÖM B, HILDEBRAND H (1975). Lipase and co-lipase activities of human small intestinal contents after a liquid test meal. *Scand J Gastroent* **10**, 585–91.

BOSNER MS, LANGE LG, STENSON WF, OSTLUND RE JR (1999). Percent cholesterol absorption in normal women and men quantified with dual stable isotopic tracers and negative ion mass spectrometry. *J Lipid Res* **40**, 302–8.

CARA L, DUBOIS C, BOREL P, ARMAND M, SENFT M, PORTUGAL H, PAULI AM, BERNARD PM, LAIRON D (1992). Effects of oat bran, rice bran, wheat fibre and wheat germ on postprandial lipaemia in healthy adults. *Am J Clin Nutr* **55**, 81–8.

CAREY MC, SMALL DM, BLISS CM (1983). Lipid digestion and absorption. *Ann Rev Physiol* **45**, 651–77.

CARRIÈRE F, BARROWMAN JA, VERGER R, LAUGIER R (1993). Secretion and contribution to lipolysis of gastric and pancreatic lipases during a test meal in humans. *Gastroenterology* **105**, 876–88.

CHEN YD, SWAMI S, SKOWRONSKI R, COULSTON AM, REAVEN GM (1993). Effect of variations in dietary fat and carbohydrate intake on postprandial lipaemia in patients with noninsulin dependent diabetes mellitus. *J Clin Endocrinol Metab* **76**, 347–51.

CHUNG HJ, MIN DB (2004). Developments in fat replacers. In *Functional Foods, Cardiovascular Disease and Diabetes*, Ed. A Arnoldi, Boca Raton, FL/Cambridge: CRC/Woodhead Pub., pp. 351–73.

COUILLARD C, BERGERON N, PRUD'HOMME D, BERGERON J, TREMBLAY A, BOUCHARD C, MAURIEGE P, DESPRES JP (1998). Postprandial triglyceride response in visceral obesity in men. *Diabetes* **47**, 953–60.

DUBOIS C, BEAUMIER G, JUHEL C, ARMAND M, PORTUGAL H, PAULI AM, BOREL P, LATGE C, LAIRON D (1998). Effects of graded amounts (0–50 g) of dietary fat on postprandial lipaemia and lipoproteins in normolipidemic adults. *Am J Clin Nutr* **67**, 31–8.

DYERBERG J, BANG HO (1982). A hypothesis on the development of acute myocardial infarction in Greenlanders. *Scand J Clin Lab Invest Suppl* **161**, 7–13.

FAVÉ G, LEVEQUE C, PEYROT J, PIERONI G, COST ETC, ARMAND M (2007). Modulation of gastric lypolysis by the phospholipid species: link to specific lipase–phospholipid interaction at the lipid/water interface. *FASEB J* **21**, A1010-a.

FRAZER AC, SCHULMAN JH, STEWART HC (1944). Emulsification of fat in the intestine of the rat and its relationship to absorption. *J Physiol* **103**, 306–16.

GARGOURI Y, PIERONI G, RIVIERE C, SAUNIÈRE JF, LOWE PA, SARDA L, VERGER R (1986). Kinetic assay of human gastric lipase on short- and long-chain triacylglycerol emulsions. *Gastroenterology* **91**, 919–25.

GILHAM D, LABONTE ED, ROJAS JC, JANDACEK RJ, HOWLES PN, HUI DY (2007). Carboxyl ester lipase deficiency exacerbates dietary lipid absorption abnormalities and resistance to diet-induced obesity in pancreatic triglyceride lipase knockout mice. *J Biol Chem* **282**, 24642–9.

GISSI (1999). Dietary supplementation with *n*-3 polyunsaturated fatty acids and vitamin E after myocardial infarction: results of the GISSI-Prevenzione trial. Gruppo Italiano per lo Studio della Sopravvivenza nell'Infarto miocardico. *Lancet* **354**, 447–55.

GIUGLIANO D, ESPOSITO K (2008). Mediterranean diet and metabolic diseases. *Curr Opin Lipidol* **19**, 63–8.

HAIKAL Z, PLAY B, LANDRIER JF, GIRAUD A, GHIRINGHELLI O, LAIRON D, JOURDHEUIL-RAHMANI D (2008). NPC1L1 and SR-BI are involved in intestinal cholesterol absorption from small-size lipid donors. *lipids* **43**, 401–8.

HAMADA T, IKEDA I, TAKASHIMA K, KOBAYASHI M, KODAMA Y, INOUE T, MATSUOKA R, IMAIZUMI K (2005). Hydrolysis of micellar phosphatidylcholine accelerates cholesterol absorption in rats and Caco-2 cells. *Biosci Biotechnol Biochem.* **9**, 1726–32.

HAMOSH, M (1990). *Lingual and Gastric Lipases: Their Role in Fat Digestion*. Boca Raton, FL: CRC Press.

HAMOSH M, KLAEVEMAN H, WOLF RO, SCOW RO (1975). Pharyngeal lipase and digestion of dietary triglyceride in man. *J Clin Invest* **55**, 908–13.

HANSEN SN, HARRIS WS (2007). New evidence for the cardiovascular benefits of long chain omega-3 fatty acids. *Curr Atheroscler Rep* **9**, 434–40.

HERNELL O, STAGGERS JE, CAREY MC (1990). Physical-chemical behavior of dietary and biliary lipids during intestinal digestion and absorption. 2. Phase analysis and aggregation states of luminal lipids during duodenal fat digestion in healthy adult human beings. *Biochemistry* **29**, 2041–56.

HOFFMAN AF, BORGSTRÖM B (1964). Physicochemical state of lipids in intestinal content during their digestion and absorption. *J Clin Invest* **43**, 43–9.

HOMAN R, HAMELEHLE KL (1998). Phospholipase A2 relieves phosphatidylcholine inhibition of micellar cholesterol absorption and transport by human intestinal cell line Caco-2. *J Lipid Res* **39**, 1197–209.

HUI DY, LABONTÉ ED, HOWLES PN (2007). Development and physiological regulation of intestinal lipid absorption. II. Dietary lipid absorption, complex lipid synthesis, and the intracellular packaging and secretion of chylomicrons. *Am J Physiol Gastrointest Liver Physiol* **293**, G645–50.

JEPPESEN J, HOLLENBECK CB, ZHOU MY, COULSTON AM, JONES C, CHEN YD, REAVEN GM (1995). Relation between insulin resistance, hyperinsulinemia, postheparin plasma lipoprotein lipase activity, and postprandial lipaemia. *Arterioscler Thromb Vasc Biol* **15**, 320–4.

JOURDHEUIL-RAHMANI D, CHARBONNIER M, DOMINGO N, LUCCIONI F, LAFONT H, LAIRON D (2002). Biliary anionic peptide fraction and apoA-I regulate intestinal cholesterol uptake. *Biochem Biophys Res Commun* **292**, 390–5.

JUHEL C, ARMAND M, PAFUMI Y, ROSIER C, VANDERMANDER J, LAIRON D (2000). Green tea extract (AR25) inhibits lipolysis of triglycerides in gastric and duodenal medium *in vitro*. *J Nutr Biochem* **11**, 45–51.

KARPE F, HAMSTEN A (1995). Postprandial lipoprotein metabolism and atherosclerosis. *Curr Opin Lipidol* **6**, 123–9.

KRIS-ETHERTON PM, PEARSON TA, WAN Y, HARGROVE RL, MORIARTY K, FISHELL V, ETHERTON TD (1999). High-monounsaturated fatty acid diets lower both plasma cholesterol and triacylglycerol concentrations. *Am J Clin Nutr* **70**, 1009–15.

KONDO H, HASE T, MURASE T, TOKIMITSU I (2003). Digestion and assimilation features of dietary DAG in the rat small intestine. *Lipids* **38**, 25–30.

LAIRON D (1996). Lipid absorption and metabolism: physiological and molecular aspects. *Proc Nutr Soc* **55**(1B), 1–3.

LAIRON D (2001). Dietary fibers and dietary lipids. In *Advanced Dietary Fibre Technology*, Eds BW McCleary and L Prosky. Wageningen, The Netherlands: Blackwell Science Ltd, pp. 177–85.

LAIRON D (2008). Macronutrient intake and modulation on chylomicron production and clearance. *Atherosclerosis* suppl, **9**, 45–8.

LAIRON D, NALBONE G, LAFONT H, LEONARDI J, DOMINGO N, HAUTON JC, VERGER R (1978). Possible roles of bile lipids and colipase in lipase adsorption. *Biochemistry* **17**, 5263–9.

LAIRON D, NALBONE G, LAFONT H, LEONARDI J, VIGNE JL, CHABERT C, HAUTON JC, VERGER R (1980). Effects of bile lipids on the absorption and activity of pancreatic lipase on triacylglycerol emulsions. *Biochim Biophys Acta* **618**, 119–28.

LAIRON D, PLAY B, JOURDHEUIL-RAHMANI D (2007). Digestible and indigestible carbohydrates: interactions with postprandial lipid metabolism. *J Nutr Biochem* **18**, 217–27.

LAIRON D, LOPEZ-MIRANDA J, WILLIAMS C (2007b). Methodology for studying postprandial lipid metabolism. *Eur J Clin Nutr* **61**, 1145–61.

LIA A, ANDERSSON H, MEKKI N, JUHEL C, SENFT M, LAIRON D (1997). Postprandial lipaemia in relation to sterol and fat excretion in ileostomy subjects given oat-bran and wheat test meals. *Am J Clin Nutr* **66**, 357–65.

LINDSTRÖM M, LJUSBERG-WAHREN H, LARSSON K, BORGSTRÖM B (1981). Aqueous lipid phases of relevance to intestinal fat digestion and absorption. *Lipids* **16**, 749–54.

LINTHORST JM, BENNETT CLARK S, HOLT PR (1977). Triglyceride emulsification by amphipaths present in the intestinal lumen during digestion of fat. *J Coll Interface Sci* **60**, 1–10.

LOPEZ C (2005). Focus on the supramolecular structure of milk fat in dairy products. *Reprod Nutr Dev* **45**, 497–511.

LOPEZ-MIRANDA J, PÉREZ-MARTINEZ P, PÉREZ-RIMENEZ F (2006). Health benefits of monounsaturated fatty acids. In *Improving the Fat Content of Foods*, Eds C Williams & J Buttriss. Boca Raton, FL/Cambridge: CRC/Woodhead Pub., pp. 71–106.

LOPEZ-MIRANDA J, WILLIAMS C, LAIRON D (2007). Dietary, physiological, genetic and pathological influences on postprandial lipid metabolism. *Br J Nutr* **98**, 458–73.

MACKAY K, STARR JR, LAWN RM, ELLSWORTH JL (1997). Phosphatidylcholine hydrolysis is required for pancreatic cholesterol esterase- and phospholipase A2-facilitated cholesterol uptake into intestinal Caco-2 cells. *J Biol Chem* **272**, 13380–9.

MANSBACH CM 2ND, GORELICK F (2007). Development and physiological regulation of intestinal lipid absorption. II. Dietary lipid absorption, complex lipid synthesis, and the intracellular packaging and secretion of chylomicrons. *Am J Physiol Gastrointest Liver Physiol* **293**, G645–50.

MANSBACH CM, COHEN RS, LEFF PB (1975). Isolation and properties of the mixed lipid micelles present in intestinal content during fat digestion in man. *J Clin Invest* **56**, 781–91.

MARANGONI AG, IDZIAK SHJ, VEGA C, BATTE H *et al.* (2007). Encapsulation-structuring of edible oil attenuates acute elevation of blood lipids and insulin in humans. *Soft Matter* **3**, 183–7.

MARCIANI L, WICKHAM M, SINGH G, BUSH D, PICK B, COX E, FILLERY-TRAVIS A, FAULKS R, MARSDEN C, GOWLAND PA, SPILLER RC (2007). Enhancement of intragastric acid stability of a fat emulsion meal delays gastric emptying and increases cholecystokinin release and gallbladder contraction. *Am J Physiol Gastrointest Liver Physiol* **292**, G1607–13.

MEKKI N, CHRISTOFILIS MA, CHARBONNIER M, ATLAN-GEPNER C, DEFOORT C, JUHEL C, BOREL P, PORTUGAL H, PAULI AM, VIALETTES B, LAIRON D (1999). Influence of obesity and body fat distribution on postprandial lipaemia and triglyceride-rich lipoproteins in adult women. *J Clin Endocrinol Metab* **84**, 184–91.

MEKKI N, CHARBONNIER M, BOREL P, LEONARDI J, JUHEL C, PORTUGAL H, LAIRON D (2002). Butter differs from olive oil and sunflower oil in its effects on postprandial lipaemia and triacylglycerol-rich lipoproteins after single mixed meals in healthy young men. *J Nutr* **132**, 3642–9.

MICHALSKI MC, BRIARD V, DESAGE M, GELOEN A (2005). The dispersion state of milk fat influences triglyceride metabolism in the rat – a $^{13}CO_2$ breath test study. *Eur J Nutr* **44**, 436–44.

MICHALSKI MC, SOARES AF, LOPEZ C, LECONTE N, BRIARD V, GELOEN A (2006). The supramolecular structure of milk fat influences plasma triacylglycerols and fatty acid profile in the rat. *Eur J Nutr* **45**, 215–24.

MINIHANE AM, LOVEGROVE JA (2006). Health benefits of polyunsaturated fatty acids (PUFAs). In *Improving the Fat Content of Foods*, Eds C Williams & J Buttriss. Boca Raton, FL/Cambridge: CRC/Woodhead Pub., pp. 107–40.

MIURA S, SAKU K (2008). Ezetimibe, a selective inhibitor of the transport of cholesterol. *Intern Med* **47**, 1165–70.

NALBONE G, LAIRON D, LAFONT H, DOMINGO N, HAUTON JC, JULIEN R, SARDA L (1974). Behavior of biliary phospholipids in intestinal lumen during fat digestion in rat. *Lipids* **9**, 765–70.

NALBONE G, LAIRON D, CHARBONNIER-AUGEIRE M, VIGNE JL, LEONARDI J, CHABERT C, HAUTON JC, VERGER R (1980). Pancreatic phospholipase A2 hydrolysis of phosphatidylcholines in various physicochemical states. *Biochim Biophys Acta* **620**, 612–25.

NORDESTGAARD BG, BENN M, SCHNOHR P, TYBJAERG-HANSEN A (2007). Nonfasting triglycerides and risk of myocardial infarction, ischemic heart disease, and death in men and women. *JAMA* **298**, 299–308.

PAFUMI Y, LAIRON D, DE LA PORTE PL, JUHEL C, STORCH J, HAMOSH M, ARMAND M (2002). Mechanisms of inhibition of triacylglycerol hydrolysis by human gastric lipase. *J Biol Chem* **277**, 28070–9.

PASQUIER B, ARMAND M, CASTELAIN C, GUILLON F, BOREL P, LAFONT H, LAIRON D (1996a). Emulsification and lipolysis of triacylglycerols are altered by viscous soluble dietary fibres in acidic gastric medium *in vitro*. *Biochem J* **314**, 269–75.

PASQUIER B, ARMAND M, GUILLON F, CASTELAIN C, BOREL P, BARRY JL, PIERONI G, LAIRON D (1996b). Viscous soluble dietary fibres alter emulsification and lipolysis of triacylglycerols in duodenal medium *in vitro*. *J Nutr Biochem* **7**, 293–302.

PATSCH JR, MIESENBOCK G, HOPFERWIESER T, MUHLBERGER V, KNAPP E, DUNN JK, GOTTO AM, JR, PATSCH W (1992). Relation of triglyceride metabolism and coronary artery disease. Studies in the postprandial state. *Arterioscler Thromb* **12**, 1336–45.

PATTON JS, CAREY MC (1981). Inhibition of human pancreatic lipase-colipase activity by mixed bile salt-phospholipid micelles. *Am J Physiol* **241**, G328–36.

PEREZ-JIMENEZ F, ALVAREZ DE CIENFUEGOS G, BADIMON L, BARJA G, BATTINO M, BLANCO A, BONANOME A, COLOMER R, CORELLA-PIQUER D, COVAS I, CHAMORRO-QUIROS J, ESCRICH E, GAFORIO JJ, GARCIA LUNA PP, HIDALGO L, KAFATOS A, KRIS-ETHERTON PM, LAIRON D, LAMUELA-RAVENTOS R, LOPEZ-MIRANDA J, LOPEZ-SEGURA F, MARTINEZ-GONZALEZ MA, MATA P, MATAIX J, ORDOVAS J, OSADA J, PACHECO-REYES R, PERUCHO M, PINEDA-PRIEGO M, QUILES JL, RAMIREZ-TORTOSA MC, RUIZ-GUTIERREZ V, SANCHEZ-ROVIRA P, SOLFRIZZI V, SORIGUER-ESCOFET F, DE LA TORRE-FORNELL R, TRICHOPOULOS A, VILLALBA-MONTORO JM, VILLAR-ORTIZ JR, VISIOLI F (2005). International conference on the healthy effect of virgin olive oil. *Eur J Clin Invest* **35**, 421–4.

PRINCE LM (1974). *Emulsions and Emulsion Technology*. New York: Lissant, pp. 125–78.

REBOUL E, BERTON A, MOUSSA M, KREUZER C, CRENON I, BOREL P (2006). Pancreatic lipase and pancreatic lipase-related protein 2, but not pancreatic lipase-related protein 1, hydrolyze retinyl palmitate in physiological conditions. *Biochim Biophys Acta* **176**(1), 4–10.

ROCHE HM, GIBNEY MJ (1995). Postprandial triacylglycerolaemia – nutritional implications. *Prog Lipid Res* **34**, 249–66.

ROCHE HM, ZAMPELAS A, KNAPPER JM, WEBB D, BROOKS C, JACKSON KG, WRIGHT JW, GOULD BJ, KAFATOS A, GIBNEY MJ, WILLIAMS CM (1998). Effect of long-term olive oil dietary intervention on postprandial triacylglycerol and factor VII metabolism. *Am J Clin Nutr* **68**, 552–60.

SARDA L, DESNUELLE P (1958). Actions of pancreatic lipase on esters in emulsions. *Biochim Biophys Acta* **30**, 513–21.

SMALL DM (1986). *The Physical Chemistry of Lipids from Alkanes to Phospholipids*. New York: Plenum Press.

STAGGERS JE, HERNELL O, CAREY MC (1990). Physical-chemical behavior of dietary and biliary lipids during intestinal digestion and absorption. 1. Phase behavior and aggregation states of model lipid systems patterned after aqueous duodenal contents of healthy adult human beings. *Biochemistry* **29**, 2028–40.

TAKASE H, SHOJI K, HASE T, TOKIMITSU I (2005). Effect of diacylglycerol on postprandial lipid metabolism in non-diabetic subjects with and without insulin resistance. *Atherosclerosis* **180**, 197–204.

TORRES IC, MIRA L, ORNELAS CP, MELIM A (2000). Study of the effects of dietary fish intake on serum lipids and lipoproteins in two populations with different dietary habits. *Br J Nutr* **83**, 371–9.

VERGER R (1984). Pancreatic lipases. In: *Lipases*, Ed. B Borgström and HL Brockman. New York: Elsevier, pp. 84–150.

WILLETT WC, SACKS F, TRICHOPOULOU A, DRESCHER G, FERRO-LUZZI A, HELSING E, TRICHOPOULOS D (1995). Mediterranean diet pyramid: a cultural model for healthy eating. *Am J Clin Nutr* **61**, 1402S–6S.

WILLIAMS CM (1997). Postprandial lipid metabolism: effects of dietary fatty acids. *Proc Nutr Soc* **56**, 679–92.

WHITCOMB DC, LOWE ME (2007). Human pancreatic digestive enzymes. *Dig Dis Sci* **52**, 1–17.

YACOOB P, TRICON S (2006). Conjugated fatty acids (CLAs) and health. In *Improving the Fat Content of Foods*, Eds C Williams & J Buttriss. Boca Raton, FL/Cambridge: CRC/Woodhead Pub., pp. 182–212.

YASUNAGA K, SAITO S, ZHANG YL, HERNANDEZ-ONO A, GINSBERG HN (2007). Effects of triacylglycerol and diacylglycerol oils on blood clearance, tissue uptake, and hepatic apolipoprotein B secretion in mice. *J Lipid Res* **48**, 1108–21.

4

Physicochemical basis of the digestion and absorption of triacylglycerol

C. M. Lo and P. Tso, University of Cincinnati, USA

Abstract: Dietary lipids and many lipophilic vitamins and drugs are transported in lymph by chylomicrons which are secreted by the small intestine. This chapter reviews our current understanding of the digestion, uptake, intracellular metabolism, and packaging of dietary lipids into chylomicrons. A number of digestive enzymes are involved in the digestion of triacylglycerol, phospholipids and cholesterol in the lumen. Unilamellar vesicles (liposomes) in the lumen and lipid transporters in the mucosal brush border membrane are both important carriers involved in the uptake of digested fatty acids, monoglycerol, and cholesterol. This chapter also provides detailed information regarding the roles which intracellular fatty acid transporters, cholesterol transporters, and sterol carrier proteins play in lipid metabolism in the small intestine. In addition, the present review illustrates the mechanism by which intracellular assembly and modification occur during the formation of chylomicrons and very low density lipoprotein. Furthermore, clinical disorders related to intestinal lipid transport are discussed. The authors' basic and clinical insights into the processes of intestinal lipid absorption provide valuable information about effective, safe ways to prevent obesity and hyperlipidemia.

Key words: lipase, enterocytes, fatty acid binding protein, transporter, pluronic-L81, acyl-CoA cholesterol acyltransferase.

4.1 Introduction

Since dietary lipids and many lipophilic vitamins and drugs are carried by chylomicrons made by small intestinal epithelial cells (enterocytes) and are transported in lymph, this review is an update of our current understanding of the processes involved in the digestion, uptake, intracellular metabolism, and the packaging of dietary lipids into chylomicrons. The major focus of this chapter will be the digestion, absorption, and transport of triacylglycerol (TG), which is the predominant dietary lipid. Readers interested in cholesterol absorption should also refer to the excellent review published by Dawson and Rudel[1] as well as those by other investigators.[2,3]

Dietary fat constitutes a significant portion of calories in the Western diet – as much as 30% of the total caloric intake, or 90–100 grams per day. Dietary intake of fat has received considerable attention over the last few decades, as diets high in fat have been linked to high blood lipid levels, especially cholesterol, and also an increased risk of coronary heart disease.[4–6] It has generally been accepted that diets rich in saturated FAs are more cholesterolemic (tending to raise blood cholesterol) than diets rich in polyunsaturated FAs.[7] *Trans*-fatty acids have double bonds, yet they behave more like saturated FAs and are considered just as atherogenic as saturated fat.[8,9] The Surgeon General of the United States currently recommends that for any individual, overall fat consumption should be maintained at or below a level of 30% of the total caloric intake, and also that no more than 300 mg cholesterol should be consumed in one day. This standard has also been adopted by the American Heart Association.

Over the past decade, there has been increased effort to modify, either chemically or biologically, the FA profile of naturally occurring TGs in order to obtain a particular physical property or to maximize a physiological function of the TG following ingestion. An exciting new approach to optimize the metabolic benefits of specific lipid mixtures has been the development and manufacture manufacturing of structured triglycerides, or STGs. STGs are produced by the chemical interesterification of both medium and long chain FAs on the same glycerol backbone by hydrolysis and random re-esterification.[10,11] These resultant TG molecules are chemically distinct and offer unique advantages from their constituent physical mixture of medium chain (MCT) and long chain (LCT) triacylglycerides. STGs containing medium chain FAs may provide a useful vehicle for rapid hydrolysis and absorption due to the smaller molecular size and greater water solubility compared with LCTs. STGs are currently being manufactured for their potential clinical benefits. The clinical applications of STGs have been thoroughly reviewed by Heird *et al.*,[12] Bell *et al.*,[13] and Mu and Porsgaard.[14] Although STGs retain some characteristics of MCTs and LCTs, they may be as effective as an alternative lipid source that could overcome the gastrointestinal intolerance related to the sole use of MCT or LCT in patients with malabsorptive diseases. We have demonstrated that STG promotes the lymphatic absorption of both vitamin A and vitamin E better than the constituent physical mixture with similar FA composition. Interestingly, the enhanced delivery of vitamins A and E into lymph by STG was not limited to normal animals, but was also observed in animals with impaired gastrointestinal absorptive functions resulting from ischemia reperfusion-induced injury.[15,16] Ascertaining the capabilities STG may have in enhancing the lymphatic absorption of lipid soluble drugs is an area well worth exploring.

4.2 Luminal digestion of dietary lipids

4.2.1 Gastric lumen

The digestion of dietary lipids in humans begins in the stomach. The enzyme involved is called acid lipase, which is secreted by the gastric mucosa. Acid lipase works best in the acidic environment of the stomach. Human acid (gastric) lipase has a pH optimum ranging from 3.0 to 6.0,[17,18] and it hydrolyzes MCT better than LCT.[19] The main hydrolytic products of gastric lipase are diacylglycerides (DGs) and FAs.[17,18,20] Gastric lipase does not hydrolyze phospholipids (PL) or cholesterol ester. Human gastric lipase has been cloned. It has 379 amino acid residues,[21] and bears considerable homology (78%) to rat lingual lipase. Little homology exists between human gastric lipase and human pancreatic lipase.

In neonates, the digestion of TG by gastric lipase in the stomach plays an important role in lipid digestion. Milk fat, the primary source of nourishment for neonates, is primarily composed of MCT, an ideal substrate for acid lipases. Furthermore, the pancreatic lipase system is not fully developed in the neonate.[22] Gastric lipase is also important in adult lipid digestion, especially evident in cystic fibrosis patients, who maintain the ability to absorb dietary lipid even though pancreatic lipase secretion is markedly or completely inhibited.[23] Gastric lipase activity in the stomach is not compromised in patients with cystic fibrosis, and Armand *et al.*[24] reported that gastric lipase activity is high in patients with cystic fibrosis maintained on moderate and high-fat diets.

The stomach is the major site for the emulsification of dietary fat, an important prerequisite for efficient hydrolysis by pancreatic lipase. Gastric chyme is propelled forward through the antrum to the pylorus via the peristaltic waves of the corpus (Fig. 4.1). Liquid is squirted into the duodenum along with small solid particles in the chyme. The pylorus closes, and the antrum contracts, forcefully grinding the solid particles. These contractions force the antral contents to retropel from the terminal antrum back into the corpus. The combination of the squirting of antral contents into the duodenum, the grinding action of the antrum, and the retropulsion of the antral contents back into the corpus account for most of the mechanical forces involved in the initial emulsification of dietary TG. Emulsification is also aided by the DG and FA resulting from the action of acid lipases in the stomach. The PL that is normally present in the diet further aids the emulsification of dietary fat.

4.2.2 Intestinal lumen

The lipid emulsion enters the small intestine as fine lipid droplets that are less than 0.5 μm in diameter,[26,27] and so the emulsification process occurring in the stomach serves to ensure that lipid is emptied from the stomach efficiently. The combined action of bile and pancreatic juice acting in the small intestine brings about a marked change in the chemical and physical

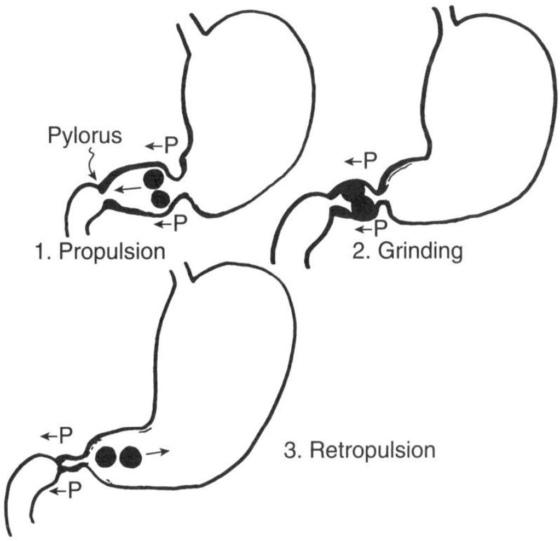

Fig. 4.1 Diagrammatic representation of the consequences of antral peristalsis.[25]

properties of the ingested lipid emulsion. Most of the digestion of TG is brought about by pancreatic lipase acting in the upper part of the intestinal lumen. The pancreatic lipase works at the interface that exists between the oil and aqueous phases.[28–31] The velocity of lipolysis is dependent on the factors that modify both physicochemical properties of the interface as well as the surface area.[32–34] Based on the work of DiMagno *et al.*,[35] it has been generally accepted among gastroenterologists that the pancreas secretes more lipase than what is needed in order to digest the fat ingested by humans.

Pancreatic lipase acts mainly on the sn-1 and sn-3 positions of the TG molecule to release 2-monoacylglycerol (2-MG) and free FAs.[33,36–38] Although 1-monoacylglycerol (1-MG) is formed from 2-MG through isomerization in an aqueous medium, 2-MG is the predominant form of MG absorbed by the small intestine, since the formation of 1-MG occurs slower than the small intestinal uptake of 2-MG.[39] Although there could be further hydrolysis of the 1- or 2-MG by pancreatic lipase to form glycerol and FA,[40] most of the 2-MG is absorbed before degrading or isomerizing to form 1-MG because of the rapid rate of absorption of 2-MG.

Pure pancreatic lipase functions extremely inefficiently when acting in only a bile salt–lipid mixture, yet lipase present in pancreatic juice hydrolyzes TG extremely effectively. This interesting observation led to the discovery of the cofactor known as colipase. In 1969, Morgan *et al.* made the crucial observation that colipase is necessary for efficient lipase activity only if bile salt is present.[41] The laboratories of Professor Borgstrom in Lund and Professor Desnuelle in Marseille have yielded most of the information in our current understanding of the biochemistry of colipase and its interaction with pancreatic lipase. Colipase has been purified from a number of animal species.[42–45] The mechanism of how colipase works has been discussed in detail by Erlanson-Albertsson[46] who observed that TG lipid droplets coated with bile salts are not accessible to pancreatic lipase. However, binding of the colipase to the TG/aqueous interface allows the lipase molecule to gain access to the lipid/aqueous interface.[47,48] Pancreatic lipase binds with colipase with a 1:1 molar ratio.[47]

4.2.3 Digestion of phospholipid

The digestion of PL occurs in the intestinal lumen, and the reaction is catalyzed by pancreatic phospholipase A_2 (PLA_2) (EC 3.1.1.4) at the sn-2 position to yield an FA and lysophosphatidylcholine (LPC).[49,50] The characteristics of PLA_2 have been studied thoroughly. It was first purified and characterized from porcine pancreas.[51] It is secreted as an anionic zymogen, which is activated by tryptic cleavage,[51,52] has a molecular weight of approximately 14 000,[51] requires calcium for activation,[53,54] and its activity requires the presence of bile salts.[55] It has multiple isoforms[56,57] and apparently requires a 2:1 bile salt to PC molar ratio for optimal activity.[58] It is heat stable, and most efficiently acts within a pH range of 8–9.[55] The global deletion of this enzyme does not abolish phospholipid digestion and absorption, suggesting that other enzyme/s compensate for the lack of the PLA_2.[59]

4.2.4 Digestion of cholesteryl ester

Most dietary cholesterol is present as free sterol, with only 10–15% existing as sterol ester.[60] Cholesteryl ester entering the small intestine must first be hydrolyzed before free cholesterol can be absorbed. The enzyme involved in the hydrolysis process is cholesterol esterase (3.1.1.13). It has been purified from porcine,[61,62] rat,[63] and human pancreas.[64,65]

4.3 Importance of micellar solubilization in the uptake of dietary lipids by enterocytes

Much of our current understanding of the micellar solubilization and uptake of dietary lipids comes from the work of Hofmann and Borgstrom, who discovered the importance of micellar solubilization in the uptake of lipid digestion products by enterocytes.[66,67] This concept was later challenged by Carey and his associates, who discovered the co-existence of unilamellar liposomes and bile salt–lipid mixed micelles in the small intestine.[27] Until recently, the uptake of lipid digestion products by enterocytes was considered passive. However, work by several investigators has raised the possibility that some lipids may be taken up by the enterocytes via carrier-mediated processes that are energy dependent. This theory and its implications will be reviewed later.

4.3.1 Importance of micellar solubilization

Understanding the importance of the micellar solubilization of 2-MG and FA prior to their uptake by enterocytes requires an understanding of the role of the unstirred water layer – a concept introduced by Dietschy and his colleagues.[68–70] Shown in Fig. 4.2, the brush border membrane of the enterocytes is separated from the bulk fluid phase in the intestinal lumen by an unstirred water layer. This unstirred water layer mixes poorly with the bulk phase in the intestinal lumen. Consequently, solute molecules in the bulk phase gain access to the brush border membrane by diffusion across this unstirred water layer. Because of the low solubility of FA and MG in the aqueous medium, very few molecules gain access to the brush border membrane (arrow 1). In

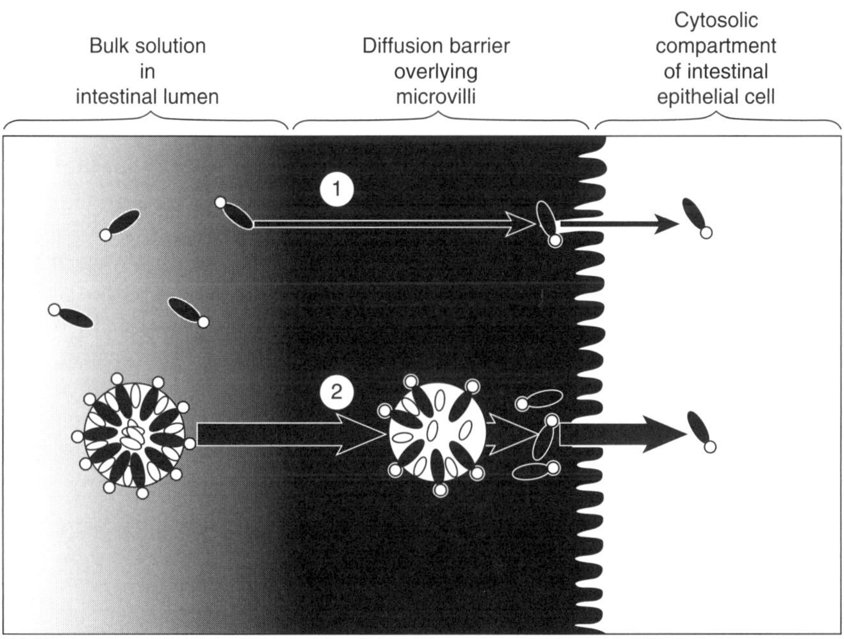

Fig. 4.2 Diagrammatic representation of the effect of bile salt micelles (or vesicles) in overcoming the diffusion barrier resistance by the unstirred water layer. In the absence of bile acids, individual lipid molecules must diffuse across the barriers overlying the microvillus border of the intestinal epithelial cells (arrow 1). Hence, uptake of these molecules is largely diffusion limited. In the presence of bile acids (arrow 2), large amounts of these lipid molecules are delivered directly to the aqueous–membrane interface so that the rate of uptake is greatly enhanced.[70]

contrast, the micellar solubilization of MG and FA greatly enhances the number of molecules available for uptake by the enterocytes (arrow 2). Despite the slower rate of diffusion of the micelle relative to the monomolecular FA molecule (due to size), micellar solubilization markedly enhances the diffusion of FA and MG molecules across the unstirred water layer. The same mechanism applies to the transport of lipid soluble drugs and compounds across the unstirred water layer to the enterocytes.

If micellar solubilization is so important in the absorption of lipid-soluble molecules such as fatty acids and cholesterol, can we explain the absorption of lipid-soluble molecules purely on the basis of the degree of solubilization by micelles? Watt and Simmonds[71] showed a linear relationship between the amount of cholesterol taken up by the small intestine and the micellar cholesterol concentration, thus demonstrating the importance of micellar solubilization in the uptake of cholesterol. Using Pluronic F-68, a non-ionic surfactant capable of promoting micellar solubilization of cholesterol but not its uptake by enterocytes, Watt and Simmonds demonstrated that enterocyte uptake of cholesterol depends on both the solubilization and structure of the bile salt (they proposed it is the planar structure of the bile acid that is important).[71] The function of bile salts in the process of intestinal cholesterol uptake thus extends beyond its role in cholesterol solubilization. Additionally, the role of bile salts on cholesterol absorption may extend beyond the luminal uptake. For instance, chenodeoxycholyl taurine (CDC-tau) is a better micellar solubilizer of cholesterol than cholyl taurine (C-tau), even though cholesterol uptake is significantly greater with C-tau than it is with CDC-tau.[72–74]

Sylven found that the ability of the small intestine to discriminate between cholesterol and beta-sitosterol absorption is energy-dependent and compromised due to the deprivation of blood supply.[75] The possibility that transporters are present at the brush border membrane is illustrated in patients with beta-sitosterolemia, a condition in which the intestine fails to discriminate between cholesterol and beta-sitosterol.[76–78] Is it possible that the importance of bile salts in facilitating the uptake of lipid-soluble nutrients and molecules by the small intestine extends beyond the detergent properties of bile salts? Clearly, this is a question of great interest and potential therapeutic implication. This topic will be again discussed in Section 4.4 on mucosal transporters.

4.3.2 Importance of unilamellar vesicles

After human jejunal contents collected during the digestion of a lipid meal were spun in an ultracentrifuge, a solid particulate layer on the bottom of the tube, a clear micellar layer in the middle, and an oily phase on the top were observed.[67] The oily phase consisted mostly of TG, partial glycerides, and FAs. The clear micellar phase consisted of bile salts, FAs, and MGs. However, when Porter and Saunders[79] carefully analyzed the top oily or aqueous phase by ultracentrifugation as well as passing the intestinal contents through a series of filters with progressively smaller pores (the smallest being 100 nm in diameter), they found that the resultant fraction did not display a clear micellar phase. Instead, a slightly turbid phase was observed. Furthermore, a concentration gradient of lipids in the micellar phase was found. The full implication of these findings was not appreciated by the investigators until later, when Patton and Carey observed the digestion of fat *in vitro* using light microscopy.[80] These investigators observed the constituent presence of at least three phases during fat digestion: (1) the oil phase (mainly TG, partial glycerides and FA); (2) the calcium soap phase (Ca^{2+} ions and protonated long-chain FA); and (3) the viscous isotropic phase (MG and FA), leading to the conclusion that it is an oversimplification to divide the intestinal contents into simply an oil and a micellar phase.

Carey *et al.*[27] proposed that, when the bile salt concentration in the lumen exceeds the critical micellar concentration, the lipid in the intestinal lumen is incorporated into mixed micelles, likely assuming the form of mixed disc-like particles, more or less saturated with lipids, with a hydrodynamic radius of about 200 Å. When the amount of lipid in the aqueous phase increases further, the formation of liquid crystalline vesicles (liposomes) with hydrodynamic radii of 400–600 Å eventually results.[27,81] This finding may have important clinical implications. Patients with low intraluminal bile salt concentrations,[82] or those with bile fistulae,[83] seem to be able to absorb fat quite well. Carey *et al.* provided evidence of the crystalline vesicles leading to their proposal that liquid crystalline vesicles play an important role in the uptake of FA and MG by enterocytes[27] in patients afflicted with these types of diseased conditions. This question was addressed recently by research conducted by Woollett *et al.*[84] Their study was conducted on human subjects with inborn errors of bile acid synthesis who were being treated with supplemental bile acid therapy. The study commenced three weeks after the withdrawal of supplements from the subjects, and involved administration of a lipid meal with or without bile acid added. With the increased polar phospholipids and fatty acids, it would appear that lipid incorporated in either the micelle or the vesicle is taken up by the enterocytes well. In contrast, cholesterol uptake by the enterocytes is dependent strictly on the cholesterol being incorporated into mixed micelles and the uptake from vesicular cholesterol is very poor. The factors that govern the relative importance of vesicular versus micellar uptake of lipid-soluble molecules is a topic well worth exploring, particularly in the context of drug delivery.

4.4 Mucosal brush border membrane lipid transporters

Until very recently, it was generally believed that FA and MG are absorbed by the enterocytes through simple diffusion.[85] Strauss demonstrated quite simply and elegantly that the uptake of FA is passive and not temperature dependent.[86] The idea that FA may be taken up by enterocytes via a carrier-mediated process has been implied in an earlier finding by Chow and Hollander.[87] This group demonstrated that linoleate uptake by the small intestine reflects a concentration-dependent dual mechanism of transport. At low linoleate concentration, FA is taken up via a carrier-dependent process, whereas at a higher lineolate concentration, FA is taken up predominantly by passive diffusion. The MG and FA enter the enterocytes as monomers.[85] Studies by Stremmel first directly showed the existence of a FA binding protein associated with the brush border membrane, and that this protein plays a role in the uptake of FA by enterocytes.[88,89] Although Stremmel mainly focused on FA uptake, he found that this FA binding protein was also capable of transporting cholesterol, but not cholesterol ester. Stremmel *et al.*[89] demonstrated that this protein is mainly present in the apical and lateral regions of the villus (where tight junctions are located) and in the crypt. Consequently, the FA binding protein appears to be a plausible candidate transporter for a whole array of lipid molecules, including cholesterol. This conclusion, however, is of concern for two reasons. First, this transporter was later determined to be the mitochondrial glutamic oxaloacetic transaminase, which is an intracellular enzyme and is not involved in lipid absorption.[90] Second, why do crypt cells express this protein when, at this stage, they are not involved in fat absorption?

Thurnhofer *et al.* first described the presence of a binding protein in the small intestinal brush border membrane that facilitates the uptake of cholesterol by the small intestine.[91–94] The protein has an apparent molecular weight of around 14000 Da as determined by SDS polyacrylamide gel electrophoresis, and a value of 11500 Da (determined by gel filtration on Sephadex G-75SF). Using the brush border membrane, Thurnhofer *et al.*[93] demonstrated that cholesterol uptake is most effective from cholate mixed micelles, and is characterized by short half-times of merely seconds. As expected, proteolytic treatment of the brush border membrane vesicles significantly reduced the capacity of these vesicles to take up cholesterol. When polyclonal antibodies raised against the 14K protein were present in the incubation medium, cholesterol uptake by these vesicles was also significantly reduced. This 14K protein was later identified as SCP-2, which is an intracellular protein;[95] thus, the identity of the plasma membrane-bound cholesterol transport protein was put to question. This series of apparently 'wild goose' chases stemmed from the faulty approach of using the hydrophobic ligands as the bait, which often bind non-specifically to proteins in the brush border preparations. An additional complication is the cross-contamination of the brush border membrane with proteins from other subcellular fractions. Regardless, questions remain, owing to the possibility that some of these plasma membrane proteins may also reside part of the time intracellularly.

A number of other proteins have also been shown to bind lipids. These include GP330 (also called megalin), CD36, and caveolin. GP330, a member of the low density lipoprotein receptor gene family, is an endocytic receptor expressed in many absorptive epithelia, including kidney proximal tubules, type II pneumocytes, mammary epithelium, and thyroid follicular cells.[96] It has been demonstrated that GP330 is involved in the renal uptake of polybasic drugs,[96–98] vitamin B_{12},[98] cholesterol-carrying lipoproteins,[99] albumin,[100] and proteases.[97] The fact that the forebrain of GP330 knockout mice fail to develop has been attributed to the deficient supply of cholesterol for the brain of the fetus through the maternal–fetal lipoprotein transport system.[101] Whether or not GP330 is expressed in the intestine remains uncertain.[96] Moreover, whether or not GP330 participates in cholesterol uptake by the small intestine is still unknown. Lastly, Hauser *et al.*[102] provided evidence that scavenger receptor BI is involved in the intestinal uptake of cholesterol. In their more recent paper, Schulthess *et al.*[103] demonstrated that the uptake of cholesterol mediated by scavenger receptors is inhibited by an amphipathic alpha-helix of 18 amino acids, lending further support to this receptor's involvement in intestinal cholesterol absorption. Van Bennekum *et al.*[104] have provided additional evidence that SR-BI is involved in intestinal cholesterol uptake, and that this uptake can be inhibited by Ezetimibe, a potent inhibitor of cholesterol uptake by enterocytes.

A membrane transporter for FA has been identified in adipocytes. This FA transporter is inhibited by sulfo-*N*-succinimidyl derivatives of long chain FAs[105–109] and by 4,4′-diisothiocyanostilbene-2-2′-sulfonate (DIDS). It has an apparent molecular weight of 88 kDa, an isolectric point of 6.9, and has strong sequence homology to CD36 and PAS IV. PAS IV is a protein enriched in the apical membranes of lipid-secreting mammary cells during lactation, and cloning of this binding protein revealed that it bears 85% homology to CD36, which is present in human platelets and lactating mammary epithelia.[106] Northern blot analysis revealed that this message is abundant in the heart, intestine, fat, muscle, and testis.[107–109] Fatty acid transporters have been localized to the brush border membrane, and expression levels are highest in the jejunum, less abundant in the duodenum, and lowest in the ileum.[109] This same group reported that a high-fat diet rich in long chain FA, but not medium chain FAs, results in increased fatty acid transporter expression.[110] Using the lymph fistula mouse model, Nauli *et al.*[111] have recently demonstrated that CD36 is involved in promoting the uptake of cholesterol by the small intestine and, while it does not seem to be involved in the uptake of fatty acids by the small intestine, it indeed plays an important role in the packaging of absorbed fatty acids as triglycerides into chylomicrons.

Other potential binding proteins have also been identified. One binding protein for long chain FAs has been cloned in adipocytes by Schaffer and Lodish.[112] Recently, Stahl *et al.*[113] identified the presence of FATP4, a member of the large family of FA transport proteins, in the small intestine. Moulson *et al.*[114] reported that a wrinkle-free phenotype is associated with the spontaneous autosomal recessive mutation of the *FATP4* gene, resulting in a very tight and thick-skinned phenotype. This observation was confirmed in a subsequent report by Herrmann *et al.*,[115] which showed that the lack of FATP4, specifically in the epidermis of the skin, resulted in the same phenotype. Hall *et al.*[116] showed that FATP4, in addition to its role in the uptake of FA, may also exhibit acyl-CoA synthetase activity. As of yet, the role of FATP4 in the uptake of FA *in vivo* is unclear. Caveolin is another protein that binds cholesterol.[117] Caveolin was the first reported protein associated with caveolae. Caveolae are non-clathrin-coated invaginations present on the surface to bind glycolipids,[118] cholesterol,[119] glycosylphosphatidylinositol (GPI)-linked proteins,[120] and other proteins for potocytosis.[121] It is currently unknown if caveolin plays a role in the intestinal absorption of cholesterol and FAs.

There have been two extremely exciting developments in recent years in the investigation of transporters involved in cholesterol absorption. The first finding involves the drug Ezetimibe, a compound developed by Schering-Plough that is extremely potent in inhibiting intestinal cholesterol absorption.[122–124] Early studies using photoaffinity derivatives of Ezetimibe specifically labeled the scavenger receptor SR-BI protein.[125] *In vitro* studies from two independent laboratories also showed that mammalian cells transfected with SR-BI cDNA displayed an increased ability for cholesterol uptake from micellar substrates in comparison to mock-transfected cells with constitutively low SR-BI expression.[125–127] Most importantly, the increased capacity for cholesterol uptake by SR-BI transfected cells was indeed subject to Ezetimibe inhibition in both of these studies.[125,127] Taken together, these data can be interpreted as evidence supporting a role of SR-BI on the membrane of enterocytes as the cholesterol transporter solely responsible for cholesterol absorption from the intestinal lumen. The distribution of SR-BI along the gastrocolic axis (mostly in the duodenum and the jejunum) and on the apical side of the brush border membrane is also consistent with the hypothesis that SR-BI participates in cholesterol absorption.[127–129]

Another cholesterol transporter that has been implicated recently in cholesterol absorption is the NPC1-L1 (Niemann-Pick C1 Like 1) protein. In 2004, Altmann *et al.*[130] demonstrated that NPC1-L1 plays an important role in the absorption of cholesterol by the small intestine. NPC1-L1 is expressed mainly in the duodenum and the jejunum, however substantial protein levels are also found in the ileum. Davies *et al.* found that the inactivation of NPC1-L1 results in the reduction of intestinal cholesterol absorption, and the prevention of diet induced hypercholesterolemia.[131] As expected, Davis *et al.* reported that the feeding of cholesterol/cholate results in the down-regulation of intestinal NPC1-L1 mRNA expression in wild-type mice.[132] NPC1-L1 deficiency results in up-regulation of intestinal hydroxymethylglutaryl-CoA synthase mRNA expression, increased intestinal cholesterol synthesis, down-regulation of ABCA1 mRNA, but no change in ABCG5 or ABCG8 mRNA expression. The studies of Altmann *et al.*,[130]

Garcia-Calvo *et al.*,[133] and Iyer *et al.*,[134] hint quite strongly that NPC1-L1 is expressed in the intestinal epithelial cells, probably at the apical membrane. Recent data from Knopfel *et al.*,[135] revealed that cholesterol uptake by brush border membrane vesicles isolated from NPC1L1-knockout and wild-type animals did not differ between groups. Furthermore, they found that Ezetimibe and its analogues reduce cholesterol uptake to the same extent in both wild-type and NPC1L1-knockout mouse brush border membrane vesicles. This observation was also confirmed by Labonte *et al.*[136] Also Knopfel *et al.* determined that NPC1L1 is probably located intracellularly, rather than at the brush border membrane. These interesting observations raise the questions of (1) how NPC1L1 is involved in cholesterol absorption; and (2) whether NPC1L1 is the target of Ezetimibe, or just one of many potential targets.

The second exciting development in the area of cholesterol absorption is the discovery that cholesterol absorption in the small intestine is regulated by ABC transporters. Repa *et al.*[137] reported that the intestinal absorption of cholesterol is regulated by the expression of the reverse cholesterol transporter ABC-A1. In turn, ABC-A1 is regulated by the formation of retinoid X receptor (RXR) heterodimers with either oxysterols (LXRs), or with the bile acid receptor (FXR). Berge *et al.* identified in ß-sitosterolemic patients seven different mutations in two adjacent genes encoding two adenosine triphosphate (ATP)-binding cassette (ABC) transporters (ABCG5 and ABCG8).[138] This same group hypothesized that ABCG5 and ABCG8 normally cooperate to restrict the intestinal uptake and biliary secretion of sterols. Mutation of these genes results in the excess uptake of sterols, including plant sterols such as ß-sitosterol. Lee *et al.*[139] reported the mutation of ABCG5 in nine unrelated sitosterolemic patients. Although these new findings are very exciting and of integral importance in our mechanistic understanding of how the gut discriminates between the uptake of cholesterol and plant sterols, there are still a number of unanswered questions. First, the mechanism by which the various ABC transporters in the gut regulate cholesterol absorption remains unclear. Second, are ABC transporters involved in the reverse transport of other lipid-soluble compounds, including lipid-soluble drugs? Lastly, it would seem that the physiological and the therapeutic manipulation of ABC transporters are potential ways to modify intestinal cholesterol absorption in animals and humans. This subject has recently been reviewed by Wang.[140]

4.5 Intracellular metabolism of dietary lipids

To date, it is not known how the various absorbed lipids migrate from the site of absorption to the endoplasmic reticulum, where the biosynthesis of complex lipids takes place. An FA binding protein (FABP) present in the small intestine has been isolated and characterized by Ockner and

Manning,[141] and it has been suggested that FABP plays an important role in the intracellular transport of absorbed FA. This is partly supported by findings that FABP concentration is greater in the villi than in the crypts, greater in the jejunum than in the ileum, and greater in intestinal mucosae of animals fed a high-fat diet than in those fed a low-fat diet.[141,142] We know there are at least two FABP types in enterocytes (I-FABP and L-FABP). The preceding letter indicates the organ from which the form was first isolated (I = intestine and L = liver). These two FABPs differ in their binding specificity. I-FABP binds strongly with FA, and L-FABP binds with long-chain FAs, LPC, retinoids, bilirubin, carcinogens, and even selenium.[143–145] Based on nuclear magnetic resonance (NMR) binding studies, Cistola *et al.*[146] speculated that the binding of I-FABP is involved in the intracellular transport of FA, while the L-FABP is involved in the intracellular transport of MG and LPC. However, none of these functions of FABP has been tested rigorously in *in vivo* situations. Binding proteins of FAs have been quite well reviewed by Storch and Thumser.[147]

Demonstrating *in vivo* functions of the FABPs has been very difficult. One strategy has been to knock out the gene of a particular FABP. This, however, has not yielded definitive results, since other FABPs are often capable of compensating for the deficit in function of the knocked out FABP. For example, when Shaughnessy *et al.*[148] used the adipocyte FABP knockout mouse model to study its function, the keratinocyte FABP functionally compensated for the absence of the adipocyte FABP. Using the I-FABP knockout mouse model, investigators found that males have higher plasma TG and greater body weight than wild types,[149] thus implying that fat absorption is normal in these genetically modified animals. The female knockouts weighed more than wild types, but less than male knockouts. When the investigators who generated the mouse determined if fat absorption is compromised, they found that I-FABP null animals absorb lipid as well as the wild-type animals.[150] As noted earlier, one cannot conclude from this data that I-FABP is not physiologically important for fat absorption, as other intracellular FABPs may be compensating for the lack of I-FABP. Recently, Newberry *et al.*[151] reported that L-FABP knockout animals did not exhibit fat malabsorption, but that the kinetics of intestinal lipid secretion was slower in the null animals than in the wild types. Investigation of how these FABPs work together in a concerted manner to facilitate fat absorption in the intestine is still ongoing in a number of laboratories, and hopefully we will gain a better understanding of the process in the coming years.

Two sterol carrier proteins, SCP-1 (47 000 Da) and SCP-2 (13 500 Da), have been isolated and characterized.[152,153] SCP-1 is important in the microsomal conversion of squalene to lanosterol,[154] while SCP-2 (also known as the non-specific lipid transfer protein) participates in the microsomal conversion of lanosterol to cholesterol.[155] Additionally, SCP-2 is involved in the intracellular transport of cholesterol from cytoplasmic lipid droplets to mitochondria, and also in the translocation of cholesterol from the outer mitochondrial membrane to the inner mitochondrial membrane.[156] SPC-2 also appears to be involved in the intracellular trafficking of PC and FAs, and it has been suggested to play a role in peroxisomal FA-CoA binding as well.[157–160] Other proteins that may be involved in transcellular sterol transport are NPC-1 (Niemann Pick-C1 protein) and NPC-2. Recently, Dixit *et al.*[161] demonstrated in NPC-1 and NPC-2 knockout animals that each respective mutation does not affect the uptake or the absorption of cholesterol, suggesting that these proteins may not be important in mammalian cholesterol absorption.

4.5.1 Intracellular metabolism of monoglycerides and fatty acid

2-MG and FA are reconstituted to form TG, mainly via the MG pathway. As shown in Fig. 4.3, 2-MG is reacylated into TG by the consecutive action of MG acyl transferase (MGAT) and DG acyltransferase (DGAT).[162,163] The enzymes involved in this MG pathway are present in a complex called 'triglyceride synthetase',[162,164] and this complex has been purified by Lehner and Kuksis.[165] It is thought that the synthesis of TG from DG is catalyzed by the enzyme acyl CoA:DGAT. The gene for this enzyme has been isolated, and a knockout mouse has been generated. Interestingly, this mouse is able to synthesize normal amounts of TG in the intestinal mucosa,[166]

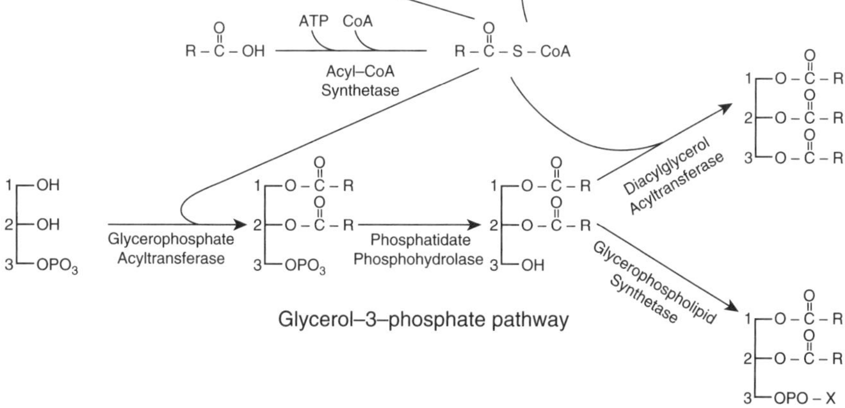

Fig. 4.3 Pathways of triacylglycerol biosynthesis in the intestinal mucosa.

thereby raising the question of whether or not another enzyme(s) is involved in the formation of TG from DG. Data from Oelkers *et al.*[167] shows that a lecithin cholesterol acyltransferase-like gene produces an enzyme that mediates DG esterification in yeast. From the recent data generated using the DGAT knockout animals,[166] it is likely that a related protein is also present in intestinal epithelial cells.

Several studies have demonstrated that the enzymes involved in the MG pathway are located on the cytoplasmic surface of the endoplasmic reticulum.[168] This finding has important implications on our understanding of the intracellular packaging of lipoproteins. It seems to indicate that TG is formed at the cytoplasmic surface of the endoplasmic reticulum, and then enters the cisternae of the organelle. Because TG has a low solubility in PL bilayers (~3 mol%), Atkinson and Small[169] postulated that TG molecules rapidly saturate the membrane. Once the solubility of TG is exceeded, the TG splits the bilayer and forms a small lens. As the lens grows, it bulges into the cytoplasmic or cisternal side of the endoplasmic reticulum. Finally, the protrusion pinches off from the membrane and forms lipid droplets in the cytoplasm or precursors of lipoproteins in the cisternae of the endoplasmic reticulum. Using ultrastructural studies, Wetterau and Zilversmit[170–172] demonstrated that a protein in the liver, small intestine, and several other organs promotes the transfer of TG and cholesterol esterase between membranes. The function of this transfer protein will be discussed later in Section 4.7 on disorders of intestinal lipid absorption.

A second pathway taking place in the intestinal mucosa leading to TG formation is the alpha-glycerophosphate pathway.[162,163] This pathway involves the stepwise acylation of glycerol-3-phosphate to form phosphatidic acid (Fig. 4.3). In the presence of phosphatidate phosphohydrolase, phosphatidic acid is hydrolyzed to form DG, which is then converted to TG. The relative importance of the MG-pathway and the alpha-glycerophosphate pathway depends on the supply of 2-MG and FA. During normal lipid absorption, when 2-MG is sufficiently present, the 2-MG pathway facilitates the conversion of 2-MG and FA to form TG, which aids in inhibiting the alpha-glycerophosphate pathway.[162,163,173] Conversely, when the supply of 2-MG is lacking or insufficient, the alpha-glycerophosphate pathway becomes the major pathway by which TG is formed.

4.5.2 Phospholipids

Some absorbed LPC is reacylated to form PC.[174–177] The remaining absorbed LPC is hydrolyzed to form glycero-3-phosphorylcholine.[178] The liberated FA is used for TG synthesis, while the glycero-3-phosphorylcholine is readily transported to the portal blood to be metabolized in the liver.[179] Another reaction occurring in the intestinal mucosa is the combination of two LPC molecules to yield one PC molecule and one molecule of glycero-3-phosphorylcholine.[66,180]

4.5.3 Cholesterol

Exogenous cholesterol absorbed by enterocytes enters a free cholesterol pool within the enterocytes in which cholesterol from endogenous sources is also stored. Endogenous cholesterol is derived from three sources: (1) non-dietary cholesterol absorbed from the lumen (biliary cholesterol and cholesterol from cells shed from the intestinal mucosa), (2) cholesterol derived from plasma lipoproteins,[181] and (3) cholesterol synthesized *de novo*.[182–184] The enterocytes treat each of these sourced cholesterol types differently. For instance, cholesterol derived from the intestinal lumen does not mix evenly with the free cholesterol pool and is preferentially esterified in enterocytes for export to lymph as TG-rich lipoproteins.[185–187] Stange and Dietschy found that very little newly synthesized cholesterol is tranported to the lymph during fasting.[186] However, during active lipid absorption, significantly more newly synthesized cholesterol is incorporated into TG-rich lipoproteins that are transported to lymph. Readers interested in cholesterol synthesis and the uptake of lipoproteins by the small intestine are referred to the articles and reviews of Stange and Dietschy,[186] Dietschy *et al.*,[188] and Spady *et al.*[181,189]

Cholesterol is transported almost exclusively by the lymphatic system mainly as esterified cholesterol, and the rate of the esterification of cholesterol regulates its lymphatic transport.[190] Two proposed enzymes involved in cholesterol esterification are cholesterol esterase[191,192] and acyl-CoA cholesterol acyltransferase (ACAT).[191,193,194] The distribution and regulation of ACAT in the small intestinal epithelium has been studied in considerable detail. The rat jejunum and ileum have high specific activities of ACAT, the jejunum displaying slightly higher activity than the ileum. Conversely, the specific activity of ACAT in the guinea pig, rabbit, and human is significantly higher in the jejunum than in the ileum.[195–197] This enzyme is stimulated by ingestion of a high-cholesterol diet.[195,196] However, it is not clear whether this increase in ACAT activity is caused by the high-cholesterol diet itself or by the increase in microsomal cholesterol that is isolated from these animals for the purpose of conducting the ACAT bioassay.

Using immunocytochemistry, Gallo *et al.*[198] demonstrated that intracellular cholesterol esterase is derived from pancreatic cholesterol esterase. A later study by Field[199] confirmed the presence of cholesterol esterase in the enterocyte. This interesting concept was further proven by Bruneau *et al.*[200] who demonstrated that the pancreatic bile salt-dependent lipase (cholesterol esterase) transverses across the intestinal epithelial cells to enter into the circulation. The reason why this enzyme is resistant to attack by the various proteases present in the intestinal lumen and enterocytes is unclear and should be explored further.

Most investigators believe that ACAT plays a more important role in mucosal cholesterol esterification than does cholesterol esterase. This is supported by several substantiated observations. First, ACAT displays the highest activity in the segment of the small intestine that is most actively involved in cholesterol absorption.[195–197] Second, the activity that is present in the intestinal epithelium adequately accounts for all of the cholesterol esterase transported by the small intestine.[201] Third, Watt and Simmonds[202] failed to demonstrate an effect of the diversion of pancreatic juice (the origin of mucosal cholesterol esterase) on the absorption and esterification of luminal dietary cholesterol in lymph fistula rats. Finally, through employing a number of specific ACAT inhibitors, several studies have shown a reduction in lymphatic cholesterol output.[191,203–205] ACAT inhibitors continue to be synthesized, and interested readers are referred to Lee *et al.*[206] for additional information.

Chang and associates have played a pivotal role in the purification and identification of ACAT proteins.[207–209] Two have been identified – ACAT1 and ACAT2. Using immunohistochemistry, Chang *et al.*[208] reported that ACAT-1 is present in fetal and adult hepatocytes, and that ACAT-2 is present only in fetal hepatocytes. Furthermore, Chang *et al.*[208] found that the ACAT activity of the small intestine can be immunodepleted by antibodies raised against ACAT-2, and that most of ACAT-2 is located at the apices of the villi. The role of ACAT-2 in intestinal cholesterol absorption is supported by the findings of Buhman *et al.*,[210] who reported that ACAT-2 knockout mice are resistant to diet-induced hypercholesterolemia due to defective cholesterol esterification and poor absorption by the small intestinal epithelial cells.

4.6 Formation of intestinal chylomicrons and very low density lipoproteins

Despite the wealth of information gathered over the past 30 years about intestinal lipid absorption, the mechanism of the intracellular assembly, modification, and secretion of lipoproteins from small intestinal epithelial cells is not fully understood. This is partly due to the complexity of the processes involved and the lack of good experimental models by which to study the various steps. Intestinal cell culture systems (e.g. CaCo-2 cells) have been used extensively to study the formation and secretion of lipoproteins[85,211–214] and the genetic expression and post-translational modification of apolipoproteins.[215] During fasting, very low density lipoproteins (VLDL) are the only lipoproteins produced by the small intestine.[216–218] After a meal, the small intestine produces predominantly chylomicrons (CMs).[218,219] Currently, the separation of intestinal CMs and VLDLs is based on an operational criterion. Lipoproteins that have a Svedberg flotation (S_f) rate exceeding 400 are classified as CMs; those with a S_f rate of 20–400 are defined as VLDLs.[220] Numerous studies support the idea that intestinal CMs and VLDLs represent lipoproteins produced by two separate pathways. Ockner *et al.*[216] demonstrated that the intraduodenal infusion of palmitate causes a marked increase in VLDL transport, but that VLDL output remains unchanged when oleate and linoleate are infused. In contrast, CM output is markedly increased when oleate and linoleate are infused. The FA composition of the VLDL-TG is different from the CM-TG, likely indicative of the presence of two different pathways for VLDL and CM assembly. An ultrastructural and biochemical study conducted by Mahley *et al.*[221] showed that intestinal Golgi vesicles contain either CMs or VLDL particles and that little mixing of particle sizes occurs; thus it was concluded that separate biosynthetic pathways exist for assembly of these distinct lipoproteins. Further evidence is provided by Vahouny *et al.*,[222] who demonstrated that puromycin yields no significant effect on the incorporation of radioactive leucine into VLDL peptides in male rats. In contrast, however, the incorporation of radioactive leucine into CM peptides was markedly inhibited.

Studies conducted by Tso *et al.*[223,224] have shown that rats fed as little as 0.5 mg/h of a hydrophobic surfactant, known as Pluronic L-81 (L-81), display markedly impaired lymphatic transport of TG and cholesterol. Further study showed that L-81 inhibited lipid transport by blocking the formation of intestinal CMs, but not the formation of VLDL particles. Using this unique compund, Tso *et al.* further showed that intraduodenal infusion of egg phosphatidylcholine into rats resulted mostly in the lymphatic transport of VLDLs, and that this transport was not affected by the administration of L-81.[225] However, when triolein was infused, the lymphatic transport of lipid was inhibited because the feeding of triolein resulted primarily in the formation of CMs.[223,224] These results led Tso *et al.* to propose the existence of two pathways for the formation of intestinal lipoproteins – one that forms predominantly CMs, and one that forms predominantly VLDLs (Fig. 4.4).[225] Tso *et al.* proposed that the pathway forming CMs is inhibited by

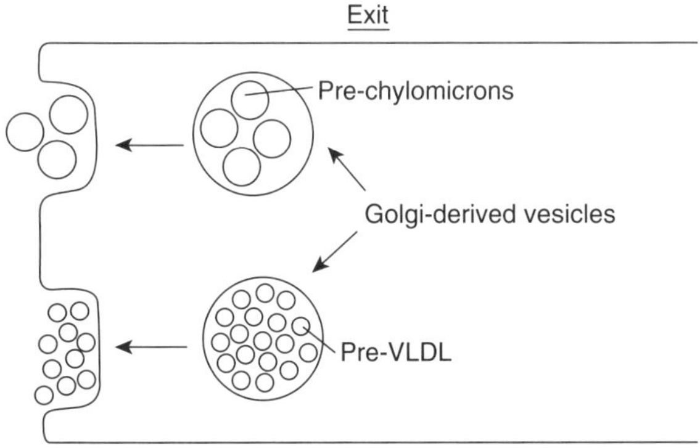

Fig. 4.4 Packaging and secretion of intestinal chylomicrons (CM) and very low density lipoproteins (VLDL). The diagram depicts Golgi-derived vesicles containing either pre-CM or pre-VLDL particles. Little mixing of pre-CM and pre-VLDL particles in these vesicles occurs.

L-81, but the pathway forming VLDLs is not, and that pre-CM and pre-VLDL particles are packaged in the Golgi apparatus into either pre-CM or pre-VLDL-containing vesicles. The Golgi-derived vesicles containing either pre-CMs or pre-VLDLs likely correspond to the two vesicle types observed by Mahley *et al.*[221] This hypothesis is further supported by the study conducted by Nutting *et al.*[226] They measured the appearance time for CMs in control rats and for VLDLs in L-81 treated rats. The appearance time, defined as the time between placement of radioactive FA into the intestinal lumen and the appearance of radioactive lipid in lymph, was 10.8 min in control rats – significantly shorter than the 16.2 min observed in the L-81-treated rats. Thus, it seems to take longer to package the VLDL particles than the CM particles. Finally, it seems that this *in vivo* observation can also be duplicated in cell culture systems. Using CaCo-2 cells, Luchoomun and Hussain[227] demonstrated that L-81 inhibits CM but not VLDL formation by these cells.

Although we are far from clear on exactly how the CMs and VLDLs are put together, recent work by Mansbach and his colleagues begins to shed some light on the mechanism involved. Siddiqi *et al.*[228] showed that a rate-limiting step in the trafficking of CM through the enterocytes involves the exit of CM from the endoplasmic reticulum to the Golgi apparatus through the prechylomicron transport vesicles. They also painstakingly isolated and characterized the prechylomicron transport vesicles and demonstrated the involvement of the SNARE proteins. Recently, Neeli *et al.*[229] showed the liver FABP is involved in the formation as well as the budding of the pre-chylomicron transport vesicles. Interested readers should refer to these excellent papers for additional information.

4.7 Clinical disorders of intestinal lipid transport

In humans, the liver secretes only apolipoprotein B-100 (apo B-100), and the small intestine secretes only apolipoprotein B-48 (apo B-48).[230–232] Both apo B-100 and apo B-48 are encoded by the same gene.[233,234] The biogenesis of apo B-48 involves a unique mechanism by which the CAA codon encoding Gln at 2153 of the apo B-100 mRNA is changed to UAA (a stop codon) and thus forms apo B-48. Rat apo B-48 has a molecular weight of about 240 000 Da[235] and is an extremely hydrophobic protein.[236] Each CM or VLDL particle has one apo B-48.[237] The absolute requirement of apo B for the formation of CM is well illustrated by the apo B knockout animals. We do not know, however, whether the production of apo B is physiologically rate-limiting in the formation of CM by the enterocytes. Data from several laboratories indicate that the supply of apo B is probably not the rate-limiting step for forming CM. Hayashi *et al.*[238] demonstrated that apo B output in lymph, an indication of the relative number of CM produced by the small intestine, does not change after intraduodenal infusion of lipid, despite the fact that lymphatic TG output increases seven- to eight-fold. These data support the finding by Davidson *et al.*[239] that no increase in apo B synthesis results from lipid absorption.

Abetalipoproteinemia is a rare genetic disorder involving the complete failure of the liver and gut to make TG-rich lipoproteins.[240,241] The thought has been that abetalipoproteinemic patients have a problem in synthesizing apo B. Glickman *et al.*[232] reported that apo B synthesis, as determined by ^3H leucine incorporation, is decreased, but not abolished, in abetalipoproteinemic patients, thus suggesting that failure to synthesize apo B by the gut and liver may not be the only reason abetalipoproteinemic patients fail to produce CM and VLDL. This was later confirmed by the finding that abetalipoproteinemia results from the mutation of the microsomal TG transfer protein gene.[242–245] The role of microsomal TG transfer protein in the formation of chylomicrons by the small intestine is well covered in the reviews by Berriot-Varoqueaux *et al.*[246] and Hussain.[85]

Anderson's disease, named after the investigator who first reported it, is another disorder in which there is a deficiency in the ability to form CMs by the small intestine.[246–248] Anderson's disease is also known as chylomicron retention disorder because, although observable CM particles are present in the enterocytes, none is observed in the intercellular space; this suggests that the secretion of CMs is defective among patients who have this disease. In a recent study, Dannoura *et al.* carefully demonstrated that patients with Anderson's disease do not have a defect in the genes that code for known apoproteins or microsomal TG transfer protein, thus suggesting that this diseased condition is caused by an unknown factor crucial for the secretion of chylomicrons.[248] Currently, no animal model is available with which to study this perplexing disorder.

4.8 Conclusions

As we have already discussed at the beginning of this chapter, many dietary lipids and lipophilic compounds (including drugs) are absorbed and transported by the enterocytes packaged as chylomicrons and VLDL. We have reviewed the processes involved in the digestion, uptake, intracellular metabolism, and packaging of dietary lipids into chylomicrons. Hopefully, this chapter has achieved its mission by providing readers with a comprehensive and current review of the subject. More importantly, it is hoped that this chapter will serve as a stimulus to the many investigators exploring basic as well as the clinical aspects of intestinal fat absorption. With obesity and hyperlipidemia existing as common clinical problems that a rapidly growing number of clinicians deal with on a daily basis, inhibition of the gastrointestinal absorption of lipids may prove to be an effective and safe way of dealing with these problems.

4.9 Acknowledgments

This work was supported by the National Institutes of Health, grants DK056863, DK059630, DK076928, ES014464, DK068463.

4.10 References

1. DAWSON PA, RUDEL LL (1999), 'Intestinal cholesterol absorption,' *Curr Opin Lipidol*, **10**, 315.
2. WANG DQ (2003), 'New concepts of mechanisms of intestinal cholesterol absorption,' *Ann Hepatol*, **2**, 113.
3. PLOSCH T, KOSTERS A, GROEN AK, KUIPERS F (2005), 'The ABC of hepatic and cholesterol transport,' *Handb Exp Pharmacol*, **170**, 465.
4. KANNEL WB, DAWBER TR, FRIEDMAN GD *et al.* (1964), 'Risk factors in coronary heart disease. An evaluation of several serum lipids as predictors of CHD,' *Ann Intern Med*, **61**, 888.
5. LEVY D, KANNEL WB (1988), 'Cardiovascular risks: New insights from Framingham,' *Am Heart J*, **116**, 266.
6. AUSTIN MA (1991), 'Plasma triglyceride and coronary heart disease,' *Arteriosclerosis Thrombosis*, **11**, 2.
7. BEYNEN AC, KRITCHEVSKY D (1986), *Nutritional Effects on Cholesterol Metabolism*, Voorthuizen, Transmodial.
8. VALENZUELA A, MORGADO N (1999), 'Trans fatty acid isomers in human health and in the food industry,' *Biol Res*, **32**, 273.
9. KATAN MB (2000), 'Trans fatty acids and plasma lipoproteins,' *Nutr Rev*, **58**, 188.
10. BABAYAN VK (1987), 'Medium chain triglycerides and structured lipids,' *Lipids*, **22**, 417.
11. MASCIOLI EA, BABAYAN VK, BISTRIAN BR, BLACKBURN GL (1988), 'Novel triacylglycerols for special medical purposes,' *J Par Ent Nutr*, **12**, 127S.
12. HEIRD WC, GRUNDY SM, HUBBARD VS (1986), 'Structured lipids and their use in clinical nutrition,' *Am J Clin Nutr*, **43**, 320.
13. BELL SJ, BRADLEY D, FORSE RA, BISTRIAN B (1997), 'The new dietary fats in health and disease,' *J Am Diet Assoc*, **97**, 280.
14. MU H, PORSGAARD T (2005), 'The metabolism of structured triglycerides,' *Prog Lipid Res*, **44**, 430.
15. TSO P, LEE T, DEMICHELE SJ (1999), 'Lymphatic absorption of structured triglycerides vs. physical mix in a rat model of fat malabsorption,' *Am J Physiol*, **277**, G333.
16. TSO P, LEE T, DEMICHELE SJ (2001), 'Randomized structured triglycerides increase lymphatic absorption of tocopherol and retinol compared with the equivalent physical mixture in a rat model of fat malabsorption,' *J Nutr*, **131**, 2157.
17. ABRAMS CK, HAMOSH M, LEE TC *et al.* (1988), 'Gastric lipase: localization in the human stomach,' *Gastroenterology*, **95**, 1460.
18. HAMOSH M, SCANLON JW, GANOT D *et al.* (1981), 'Fat digestion in the newborn: characterization of lipase in gastric aspirates of premature and term infants,' *J Clin Invest*, **67**, 838.
19. LIAO TH, HAMOSH P, HAMOSH M (1984), 'Fat digestion by lingual lipase: mechanism of lipolysis in the stomach and upper small intestine,' *Pediatr Res*, **18**, 402.
20. COHEN M, MORGAN RGH, HOFMANN AF (1971), 'Lipolytic activity of human gastric and duodenal juice against medium- and long-chain triglycerides,' *Gastroenterology*, **60**, 1.

21. BODMER MW, ANGAL S, YARRATON GT *et al.* (1987), 'Molecular cloning of a human gastric lipase and expression of the enzyme in yeast,' *Biochim Biophys Acta*, **909**, 237.
22. GRAND RJ, WATKINS JB, TORTI FM (1976), 'Development of the human gastrointestinal tract: a review,' *Gastroenterology*, **70**, 790.
23. ROSS CAC (1955), 'Fat absorption studies in the diagnosis and treatment of pancreatic fibrosis,' *Arch Dis Child*, **30**, 316.
24. ARMAND M, HAMOSH M, PHILPOTT JR *et al.* (2004), 'Gastric function in children with cystic fibrosis: effect of diet on gastric lipase levels and fat digestion,' *Pediatr Res*, **55**, 457.
25. KELLY KA (1981), *Physiology of the Gastrointestinal Tract*, vol. 1, New York, Raven Press.
26. SENIOR JR (1964), 'Intestinal absorption of fats,' *J Lipid Res*, **5**, 495.
27. CAREY MC, SMALL DM, BLISS CM (1983), 'Lipid digestion and absorption,' *Ann Rev Physiol*, **45**, 651.
28. SARDA L, DESNUELLE P (1958), 'Action de la lipase pancreatique sur les esters en emulsion,' *Biochim Biophys Acta*, **30**, 513.
29. BENZONANA G, DESNUELLE P (1965), 'Etude cinetique de l'action de la lipase pancreatique sur des triglycerides en emulsion. Essai d'une enzymologie en milieu heterogene,' *Biochim Biophys Acta*, **105**, 121.
30. DESNUELLE P (1976), *Lipid Absorption: Biochemical and Clinical Aspects*, Lancaster, MTP Press.
31. SCHÖNHEYDER F, VOLQUARTZ K (1946), 'Gastric lipase in man,' *Acta Physiol Scand*, **11**, 349.
32. BROCKERHOFF H (1968), 'Substrate specificity of pancreatic lipase,' *Biochim Biophys Acta*, **159**, 296.
33. MATTSON FH, BECK LW (1956), 'The specificity of pancreatic lipase on the primary hydroxyl groups of glycerides,' *J Biol Chem*, **219**, 735.
34. SIMMONDS WJ (1972), *Blood Lipids and Lipoproteins: Quantitation, Composition and Metabolism*, New York, Wiley Interscience.
35. DIMAGNO EP, GO VL, SUMMERSKILL WH (1973), 'Relations between pancreatic enzyme outputs and malabsorption in severe pancreatic insufficiency,' *N Engl J Med*, **288**, 813.
36. BORGSTROM B (1953), 'On the mechanism of the hydrolysis of glycerides by pancreatic lipase,' *Acta Chem Scand*, **7**, 557.
37. MATTSON FH, VOLPENHEIN RA (1964), 'The digestion and absorption of triglycerides,' *J Biol Chem*, **239**, 2772.
38. MATTSON FH, VOLPENHEIN RA (1968), 'Hydrolysis of primary and secondary esters of glycerol by pancreatic juice,' *J Lipid Res*, **9**, 79.
39. BORGSTROM B (1964), 'Influence of bile salt, pH, and time on the action of pancreatic lipase; physiological implications,' *J Lipid Res*, **5**, 522.
40. HOFMANN AF, BORGSTROM B (1963), 'Hydrolysis of long-chain monoglycerides in micellar solution by pancreatic lipase,' *Biochim Biophys Acta*, **70**, 317.
41. MORGAN RGH, BARROWMAN J, BORGSTROM B (1969), 'The effect of sodium taurodeoxycholate and pH on the gel filtration behaviour of rat pancreatic protein and lipases,' *Biochim Biophys Acta*, **175**, 65.
42. ERLANSON C, BORGSTROM B (1972), 'Purification and further characterization of colipase from porcine pancreas,' *Biochim Biophys Acta*, **271**, 400.
43. STERNBY B, BORGSTROM B (1979), 'Purification and characterization of human pancreatic colipase,' *Biochim Biophys Acta*, **572**, 235.
44. MAYLIE MF, CHARLES M, GACHE C, DESNUELLE P (1971), 'Isolation and partial identification of a pancreatic colipase,' *Biochim Biophys Acta*, **229**, 286.
45. MAYLIE MF, CHARLES M, GACHE C, DESNUELLE P (1973), 'On porcine pancreatic colipase: large scale purification and some properties,' *Biochem Biophys Res Commun*, **52**, 291.

46. ERLANSON-ALBERTSSON C (1992), 'Pancreatic colipase. Structural and physiological aspects,' *Biochim Biophys Acta*, **1125**, 1.
47. PATTON JS, ALBERTSSON PA, ERLANSON C, BORGSTROM B (1978), 'Binding of porcine pancreatic lipase and colipase in the absence of substrate studies by two-phase partition and affinity chromatography,' *J Biol Chem*, **253**, 4195.
48. ALLOUCHE M, CASTANO S, COLIN D, DESBAT B, KERFELEC B (2007), 'Structure and orientation of pancreatic colipase in a lipid environment: PM-IRRAS and Brewster angle microscopy studies,' *Biochemistry*, **46**, 15188.
49. BORGSTROM B, DAHLQVIST A, LUNDH G, SJÖVALL J (1957), 'Studies of intestinal digestion and absorption in the human,' *J Clin Invest*, **36**, 1521.
50. VAN DEN BOSCH H, POSTEMA NM, DE HAAS GH, VAN DEENEN LLM (1965), 'On the positional specificity of phospholipase A from pancreas,' *Biochim Biophys Acta*, **98**, 657.
51. DE HAAS GH, POSTEMA NM, NIEUWENHUIZEN W, VAN DEENEN LLM (1968), 'Purification and properties of phospholipase A from porcine pancreas,' *Biochim Biophys Acta*, **159**, 103.
52. ARNESJÖ B, BARROWMAN J, BORGSTROM B (1967), 'The zymogen of phospholipase A_2 in rat pancreatic juice,' *Acta Chem Scand*, **21**, 2897.
53. VERHEIJ HM, VOLWERK JJ, JANSEN EH *et al.* (1980), 'Methylation of histidine-48 in pancreatic phospholipase A2. Role of histidine and calcium ion in the catalytic mechanism,' *Biochemistry*, **19**, 743.
54. FERNANDEZ MS, MEJIA R, ZAVALA E (1991), 'The interfacial calcium ion concentration as modulator of the latency phase in the hydrolysis of dimyristoylphosphatidylcholine liposomes by phospholipase A_2,' *Biochem Cell Biol*, **69**, 722.
55. ARNESJÖ B, GRUBB A (1971), 'The activation, purification, and properties of rat pancreatic juice phospholipase A_2,' *Acta Chem Scand*, **25**, 577.
56. TSAO FHC, COHEN H, SYNDER WR *et al.* (1973), 'Multiple forms of porcine pancreatic phospholipase A_2: isolation and specificity,' *J Supramol Structure*, **1**, 490.
57. PUIJK WC, VERHEIJ HM, WIETZES P, DE HAAS GH (1979), 'The amino acid sequence of the phospholipase A_2 isoenzyme from porcine pancreas,' *Biochim Biophys Acta*, **580**, 411.
58. NALBONE G, LAIRON D, CARBONNIER-AUGEIRE M *et al.* (1980), 'Pancreatic phospholipase A2 hydrolysis of phosphatidylcholines in various physicochemical states,' *Biochim Biophys Acta*, **620**, 612.
59. RICHMOND BL, BOILEAU AC, ZHENG S, HUGGINS KW, GRANHOLM NA, TSO P, HUI DY (2001), 'Compensatory phospholipids digestion is required for cholesterol absorption in pancreatic phospholipase A(2)-deficient mice,' *Gastroenterology*, **120**, 1193.
60. MCINTYRE N (1976), *Lipid Absorption: Biochemical and Clinical Aspects*, London, MTP Press Ltd.
61. ALBRO PW, THOMAS RO (1973), 'Enzymatic hydrolysis of di-(2-ethylhexyl) phthalate by lipases,' *Biochim Biophys Acta*, **360**, 380.
62. MOMSEN WE, BROCKMAN HL (1977), 'Purification and characterization of cholesterol esterase from porcine pancreas,' *Biochim Biophys Acta*, **486**, 103.
63. ERLANSON C (1975), 'Purification, properties and substrate specificity of a carboxylesterase in pancreatic juice,' *Scand J Gastroenterology*, **10**, 401.
64. LOMBARDO D, GUY O, FIGARELLA C (1978), 'Purification and characterization of a carboxyl ester hydrolase from human pancreatic juice,' *Biochim Biophys Acta*, **527**, 142.
65. MEYER JG (1989), 'Lipolytic enzymes of the human pancreas. II. Purification and properties of cholesterol ester hydrolase,' *Biochim Biophys Acta*, **1002**, 89.
66. HOFMANN AF, BORGSTROM B (1962), 'Physico-chemical state of lipids in intestinal content during their digestion and absorption,' *Fed Proc*, **21**, 43.

67. HOFMANN AF, BORGSTROM B (1964), 'The intraluminal phase of fat digestion in man: The lipid content of the micellar and oil phases of intestinal content obtained during fat digestion and absorption,' *J Clin Invest*, **43**, 247.
68. DIETSCHY JM, SALLEE VL, WILSON FA (1971), 'Unstirred water layers and absorption across the intestinal mucosa,' *Gastroenterology*, **61**, 932.
69. WILSON FA, SALLEE VL, DIETSCHY JM (1971), 'Unstirred water layers in intestine: rate determinant of fatty acid from micellar solutions,' *Science*, **174**, 1031.
70. WESTERGAARD H, DIETSCHY JM (1976), 'The mechanism whereby bile acid micelles increase the rate of fatty acid and cholesterol uptake into the intestinal mucosal cell,' *J Clin Invest*, **58**, 97.
71. WATT SM, SIMMONDS WJ (1976), 'The specificity of bile salts in the intestinal absorption of micellar cholesterol in the rat,' *Clin Exp Pharmacol Physio*, **3**, 305.
72. REYNIER MO, MONTET JC, GEROLAMI A *et al.* (1981), 'Comparative effects of cholic, chenodeoxycholic, and ursodeoxycholic acids on micellar solubilization and intestinal absorption of cholesterol,' *J Lipid Res*, **22**, 467.
73. COHEN BI, RAICHT RF, MOSBACH EH (1977), 'Sterol metabolism studies in the rat. Effects of primary bile acids (sodium taurochenodeoxycholate and sodium taurocholate) on sterol metabolism,' *J Lipid Res*, **18**, 223.
74. WATT SM, SIMMONDS WJ (1984), 'Effects of four taurine-conjugated bile acids on mucosal uptake and lymphatic absorption of cholesterol in the rat,' *J Lipid Res*, **25**, 448.
75. SYLVEN C (1970), 'Influence of blood supply on lipid uptake from micellar solution by the rat small intestine,' *Biochim Biophys Acta*, **203**, 365.
76. BHATTACHARYYA AK, CONNOR WE (1974), 'Beta-sitosterolemia and xanthomatosis. A newly described lipid storage disease in two sisters,' *J Clin Invest*, **53**, 1033.
77. SHULMAN RS, BHATTACHARYYA AK, CONNOR WE, FREDRICKSON DS (1976), 'Beta-sitosterolemia and xanthomatosis,' *N Engl J Med*, **294**, 482.
78. SALEN G, SHEFER S, NGUYEN L *et al.* (1997), 'Sitosterolemia,' *Subcell Biochem*, **28**, 453.
79. PORTER HP, SAUNDERS DR (1971), 'Isolation of the aqueous phase of human intestinal contents during the digestion of a fatty meal,' *Gastroenterology*, **60**, 997.
80. PATTON JS, CAREY MC (1979), 'Watching fat digestion,' *Science*, **204**, 145.
81. STAFFORD RJ, CAREY MC (1981), 'Physical-chemical nature of the aqueous lipids in intestinal content after a fatty meal: Revision of the Hofmann–Borgstrom Hypothesis,' *Clin Res*, **28**, 511.
82. MANSBACH CM 2nd, NEWTON D, STEVENS RD (1980), 'Fat digestion in patients with bile acid malabsorption but minimal steatorrhea,' *Dig Dis Sci*, **25**, 353.
83. PORTER HP, SAUNDERS DR, TYTGAT G *et al.* (1971), 'Fat absorption in bile fistula man. A morphological and biochemical study,' *Gastroenterology*, **60**, 1008.
84. WOOLLETT LA, WANG Y, BUCKLEY DD *et al.* (2006), 'Micellar solubilisation of cholesterol is essential for absorption in humans,' *Gut*, **55**, 197.
85. THOMSON ABR, KEELAN M, GARG ML, CLANDININ MT (1989), 'Intestinal aspects of lipid absorption: in review,' *Can J Physiol Pharmacol*, **67**, 179.
86. STRAUSS EW (1966), 'Electron microscopic study of intestinal fat absorption *in vitro* from mixed micelles containing linolenic acid, monoolein, and bile salt,' *J Lipid Res*, **7**, 307.
87. CHOW SL, HOLLANDER D (1979), 'A dual, concentration-dependent absorption mechanism of linoleic acid by rat jejunum *in vitro*,' *J Lipid Res*, **20**, 349.
88. STREMMEL W (1988), 'Uptake of fatty acids by jejunal mucosal cells is mediated by a fatty acid binding membrane protein,' *J Clin Invest*, **82**, 2001.
89. STREMMEL W, LOTZ G, STROHMEYER G, BERK PD (1985), 'Identification, isolation, and partial characterization of a fatty acid binding protein from rat jejunal microvillous membranes,' *J Clin Invest*, **75**, 1068.

90. BERK PD, WADA H, HORIO Y *et al.* (1990), 'Plasma membrane fatty acid-binding protein and mitochondrial glutamic-oxaloacetic transaminase of rat liver are related,' *Proc Natl Acad Sci USA*, **87**, 3484.
91. THURNHOFER H, HAUSER H (1990), 'Uptake of cholesterol by small intestinal brush border membrane is protein-mediated,' *Biochemistry*, **29**, 2142.
92. THURNHOFER H, SCHNABEL J, BETZ M *et al.* (1991), 'Cholesterol-transfer protein located in the intestinal brush-border membrane. Partial purification and characterization,' *Biochim Biophys Acta*, **1064**, 275.
93. THURNHOFER H, LIPKA G, HAUSER H (1991), 'Membrane proteins exposed on the external side of the intestinal brush-border membrane have fusogenic properties,' *Eur J Biochem*, **201**, 273.
94. LIPKA G, SCHULTHESS G, THURNHOFER H *et al.* (1995), 'Characterization of lipid exchange proteins isolated from small intestinal brush border membrane,' *J Biol Chem*, **270**, 5917.
95. WOUTERS FS, MARKMAN M, DEGRAAF P *et al.* (1995), 'The immunohistochemical localization of the non-specific lipid transfer protein (sterol carrier protein-2) in rat small intestine enterocytes,' *Biochim Biophys Acta*, **1259**, 192.
96. LUNDGREN S, CARLING T, HJÄLM G *et al.* (1997), 'Tissue distribution of human gp330/megalin, a putative Ca^{2+}-sensing protein,' *J Histochem Cytochem*, **45**, 383.
97. FARQUHAR MG (1995), 'The unfolding story of megalin (gp330): Now recognized as a drug receptor,' *J Clin Invest*, **96**, 1184.
98. MOESTRUP SK, CUI S, VORUM H *et al.* (1995), 'Evidence that epithelial glycoprotein 330/megalin mediates uptake of polybasic drugs,' *J Clin Invest*, **96**, 1404.
99. WILLNOW TE, GOLDSTEIN JL, ORTH K *et al.* (1992), 'Low density lipoprotein receptor-related protein and gp330 bind similar ligands, including plasminogen activator–inhibitor complexes and lactoferrin, an inhibitor of chylomicron remnant clearance,' *J Biol Chem*, **267**, 26172.
100. CUI S, VERROUST PJ, MOESTRUP SK, CHRISTENSEN EI (1996), 'Megalin/gp330 mediates uptake of albumin in renal proximal tubule,' *Am J Physiol*, **271**, F900.
101. WILLNOW TE, HILPERT J, ARMSTRONG SA *et al.* (1996), 'Defective forebrain development in mice lacking gp330/megalin,' *Proc Natl Acad Sci USA*, **93**, 8460.
102. HAUSER H, DYER JH, NANDY A *et al.* (1998), 'Identification of a receptor mediating absorption of dietary cholesterol in the intestine,' *Biochemistry*, **37**, 17843.
103. SCHULTHESS G, COMPASSI S, WERDER M *et al.* (2000), 'Intestinal sterol absorption mediated by scavenger receptor is competitively inhibited by amphipathic peptides and proteins,' *Biochemistry*, **39**, 12623.
104. VAN BENNEKUM A, WERDER M, THUAHNAI ST *et al.* (2005), 'Class B scavenger receptor-mediated intestinal absorption of dietary beta-carotene and cholesterol,' *Biochemistry*, **44**, 4517.
105. HARMON CM, LUCE P, BETH AH, ABRUMAD NA (1991), 'Labeling of adipocyte membranes by sulfo-*N*-succinimidyl derivatives of long-chain fatty acids: inhibition of fatty acid transport,' *J Membr Biol*, **121**, 261.
106. ABUMRAD NA, EL-MAGHRABI MR, AMRI EZ *et al.* (1993), 'Cloning of a rat adipocyte membrane protein implicated in binding or transport of long-chain fatty acids that is induced during preadipocyte differentiation. Homology with human CD36,' *J Biol Chem*, **268**, 17665.
107. VAN NIEUWENHOVEN FA, VERSTIJNEN CPHJ, ABUMRAD NA *et al.* (1995), 'Putative membrane fatty acid-translocase and cytoplasmic fatty acid-binding protein are co-expressed in rat heart and skeletal muscles,' *Biochem Biophys Res Commun*, **207**, 747.
108. SPITSBERG VL, MATITASHIVILI E, GOREWIT RC (1995), 'Association and coexpression of fatty-acid-binding protein and glycoprotein CD36 in bovine mammary gland,' *Eur J Biochem*, **230**, 872.

109. POIRIER H, DEGRACE P, NIOT I *et al.* (1996), 'Localization and regulation of the putative membrane fatty-acid transporter (FAT) in the small intestine. Comparison with fatty acid-binding proteins (FABP),' *Eur J Biochem*, **238**, 368.
110. ABUMRAD NA, SFEIR Z, CONNELLY MA, COBURN C (2000), 'Lipid transporters: membrane transport systems for cholesterol and fatty acids,' *Curr Opin Clin Nutr Metab Care*, **3**, 255.
111. NAULI AM, NASSIR F, ZHENG S *et al.* (2006), 'CD36 is important for chylomicron formation and secretion and may mediate cholesterol uptake in the proximal intestine,' *Gastroenterology*, **131**, 1197.
112. SCHAFFER JE, LODISH HF (1994), 'Expression cloning and characterization of a novel adipocyte long chain fatty acid transport protein,' *Cell*, **79**, 427.
113. STAHL A, HIRSCH DJ, GIMENO RE *et al.* (1999), 'Identification of the major intestinal fatty acid transport protein,' *Mol Cell*, **4**, 299.
114. MOULSON CL, MARTIN DR, LUGUS JJ *et al.* (2003), 'Cloning of wrinkle-free, a previously uncharacterized mouse mutation, reveals crucial roles for fatty acid transport protein 4 in skin and hair development,' *Proc Natl Acad Sci USA*, **100**, 5274.
115. HERRMANN T, GRONE HJ, LANGBEIN L *et al.* (2005), 'Disturbed epidermal structure in mice with temporally controlled fatp4 deficiency,' *J Invest Dermatol*, **125**, 1228.
116. HALL AM, WICZER BM, HERRMANN T *et al.* (2005), 'Enzymatic properties of purified murine fatty acid transport protein 4 and analysis of acyl-CoA synthetase in tissues from FATP4 null mice,' *J Biol Chem*, **280**, 11948.
117. MURATA M, PERÄNEN J, SCHREINER R *et al.* (1995), 'VIP21/caveolin is a cholesterol-binding protein,' *Proc Natl Acad Sci USA*, **92**, 10339.
118. PARTON RG (1994), 'Ultrastructural localization of gangliosides; GM_1 is concentrated in caveolae,' *J Histochem Cytochem*, **42**, 155.
119. ROTHBERG KG, YING YS, KAMEN BA, ANDERSON RGW (1990), 'Cholesterol controls the clustering of the glycophospholipid-anchored membrane receptor for 5-methyltetrahydrofolate,' *J Cell Biol*, **111**, 2931.
120. YING YS, ANDERSON RGW, ROTHBERG KG (1992), 'Each caveola contains multiple glycosyl-phosphatidylinositol-anchored membrane proteins,' *Cold Spring Harb Symp Quant Biol*, **57**, 593.
121. ANDERSON RGW, KAMEN BA, ROTHBERG KG, LACEY SW (1992), 'Potocytosis: sequestration and transport of small molecules by caveolae,' *Science*, **255**, 410.
122. VAN HEEK M, FRANCE CF, COMPTON DS *et al.* (1997), '*In vivo* metabolism-based discovery of a potent cholesterol absorption inhibitor, SCH58235, in the rat and rhesus monkey through the indentification of the active metabolites of SCH48461,' *J Pharmacol Exp Ther*, **283**, 157.
123. VAN HEEK M, COMPTON DS, DAVIS HR (2001), 'The cholesterol absorption inhibitor, ezetimibe, decreases diet-induced hypercholesterolemia in monkeys,' *Eur J Pharmacol*, **415**, 79.
124. THURNHOFER H, HAUSER H (1990), 'Uptake of cholesterol by small intestinal brush border membrane is protein-mediated,' *Biochemistry*, **29**, 2142.
125. THURNHOFER H, SCHNABEL J, BETZ M *et al.* (1991), 'Cholesterol-transfer protein located in the intestinal brush-border membrane. Partial purification and characterization,' *Biochim Biophys Acta*, **1064**, 275.
126. BERK PD, WADA H, HORIO Y *et al.* (1980), 'Plasma membrane fatty acid-binding protein and mitochondrial glutamic-oxaloacetic transaminase of rat liver are related,' *Proc Natl Acad Sci*, **87**, 3484.
127. WOUTERS FS, MARKMAN M, DEGRAAF P *et al.* (1995), 'The immunohistochemical localization of the non-specific lipid transfer protein (sterol carrier protein-2) in rat small intestine enterocytes,' *Biochim Biophys Acta*, **1259**, 192.

128. SCHULTHESS G, COMPASSI S, WERDER M *et al.* (2000), 'Intestinal sterol absorption mediated by scavenger receptors is competitively inhibited by amphipathic peptides and proteins,' *Biochemistry*, **39**, 12623.
129. VAN HEEK M, FARLEY C, COMPTON DS *et al.* (2000), 'Comparison of the activity and disposition of the novel cholesterol absorption inhibitor, SCH58235, and its glucuronide, SCH60663,' *Br J Pharmacol*, **129**, 1748.
130. ALTMANN SW, DAVIS HR, ZHU LJ *et al.* (2004), 'Niemann–Pick C1 like protein is critical for intestinal cholesterol absorption,' *Science*, **303**, 1201.
131. DAVIES JP, SCOTT C, OISHI K *et al.* (2005), 'Inactivation of NPC1L1 causes multiple lipid transport defects and protects against diet-induced hypercholesterolemia,' *J Biol Chem*, **280**, 12710.
132. DAVIS HR JR, ZHU LJ, HOOS LM *et al.* (2004), 'Niemann–Pick C1 Like 1 (NPC1L1) is the intestinal phytosterol and cholesterol transporter and a key modulator of whole-body cholesterol homeostasis,' *J Biol Chem*, **279**, 33586.
133. GARCIA-CALVO M, LISNOCK J, BULL HG *et al.* (2005), 'The target of ezetimibe is Niemann–Pick C1-Like 1 (NPC1L1),' *Proc Natl Acad Sci USA*, **102**, 8132.
134. IYER SP, YAO X, CRONA JH *et al.* (2005), 'Characterization of the putative native and recombinant rat sterol transporter Niemann–Pick C1 Like 1 (NPC1L1) protein,' *Biochim Biophys Acta*, **1722**, 282.
135. KNOPFEL M, DAVIES JP, DUONG PT, KVAERNO L, CARREIRA EM, PHILLIPS MC, IOANNOU YA, HAUSER H (2007), 'Multiple plasma membrane receptors but not NPC1L1 mediate high-affinityy, ezetimibe-sensitive cholesterol uptake into the intestinal brush border membrane,' *Biochim Biophys Acta*, **1771**, 1140–7.
136. LABONTE ED, HOWLES PN, GRANHOLM NA, ROJAS JC, DAVIES JP, IOANNOU YA, HUI DY (2007), 'Class B type I scavenger receptor is responsible for the high affinity cholesterol binding activity of intestinal brush border membrane vesicles,' *Biochim Biophys Acta*, **1771**, 1132.
137. REPA JJ, TURLEY SD, LOBACCARO JMA *et al.* (2000), 'Regulation of absorption and ABC1-mediated efflux of cholesterol by RXR heterodimers,' *Science*, **289**, 1524.
138. BERGE KE, TIAN H, GRAF GA *et al.* (2000), 'Accumulation of dietary cholesterol in sitosterolemia caused by mutations in adjacent ABC transporters,' *Science*, **290**, 1771.
139. LEE MH, LU K, HAZARD S *et al.* (2001), 'Identification of a gene *ABCG5*, important in the regulation of dietary cholesterol absorption,' *Nat Genet*, **27**, 79.
140. WANG DQ (2007), 'Regulation of intestinal cholesterol absorption,' *Annu Rev Physiol*, **69**, 221.
141. OCKNER RK, MANNING JA (1974), 'Fatty acid binding protein in small intestine. Identification, isolation and evidence for its role in cellular fatty acid transport,' *J Clin Invest*, **54**, 326.
142. OCKNER RK, MANNING JA, POPPENHAUSEN RB, HO WK (1972), 'A binding protein for fatty acids in cytosol intestinal mucosa, liver, myocardium, and other tissues,' *Science*, **177**, 56.
143. GLATZ JFC, VEERKAMP JH (1985), 'Intracellular fatty acid-binding proteins,' *Int J Biochem*, **17**, 13.
144. BASS NM (1988), 'The cellular fatty acid-binding proteins: aspects of structure, regulation, and function,' *Int Rev Cytol*, **111**, 143.
145. BANSAL MP, COOK RG, DANIELSON KG, MEDINA D (1989), 'A 14-kilodalton selenium-binding protein in mouse liver is fatty acid-binding protein,' *J Biol Chem*, **264**, 13780.
146. CISTOLA DP, SACCHETTINI JC, BANASZAK LJ *et al.* (1989), 'Fatty acid interactions with rat intestinal and liver fatty acid-binding proteins expressed in *Escherichia coli*. A comparative 13C NMR study,' *J Biol Chem*, **264**, 2700.
147. STORCH J, THUMSER AF (2000), 'The fatty acid transport function of fatty acid-binding proteins,' *Biochim Biophys Acta*, **1486**, 28.

148. SHAUGHNESSY S, SMITH ER, KODUKULA S *et al.* (2000), 'Adipocyte metabolism in adipocyte fatty acid binding protein knockout mice (aP2–/–) after short-term high-fat feeding: functional compensation by the keratinocyte fatty acid binding protein,' *Diabetes*, **49**, 904.
149. VASSILEVA G, HUWYLER L, POIRIER K, AGELLON LB, TOTH MJ (2000), 'The intestinal fatty acid binding protein is not essential for dietary fat absorption in mice,' *FASEB J*, **14**, 2040.
150. AGELLON LB, TOTH MJ, THOMSON AB (2002), 'Intracellular lipid binding proteins of the small intestine,' *Mol Cell Biochem*, **239**, 79.
151. NEWBERRY EP, XIE Y, KENNEDY SM *et al.* (2006), 'Protection against Western diet-induced obesity and hepatic steatosis in liver fatty-acid binding protein knockout mice,' *Hepatology*, **44**, 1191.
152. NOLAND BJ, AREBALO RE, HANSBURG E, SCALLEN TJ (1980), 'Purification and properties of sterol carrier protein$_2$,' *J Biol Chem*, **255**, 4282.
153. SCALLEN TJ, SEETHARAM B, SRIKANTAIAH MV *et al.* (1975), 'Sterol carrier protein hypothesis: requirement for three substrate-specific soluble proteins in liver cholesterol biosynthesis,' *Life Sci*, **16**, 853.
154. SRIKANTAIAH MV, HANSBURY E, LOUGHRAM ED, SCALLEN TJ (1976), 'Purification and properties of sterol carrier protein$_1$,' *J Biol Chem*, **251**, 5496.
155. SCALLEN TJ, NOLAND BJ, GAVEY KL *et al.* (1985), 'Sterol carrier protein 2 and fatty acid-binding protein,' *J Biol Chem*, **260**, 4733.
156. VAHOUNY GV, DENNIS P, CHANDERBHAN R *et al.* (1984), 'Sterol carrier protein 2 (SCP_2) mediated transfer of cholesterol to mitochondrial inner membranes,' *Biochem Biophys Res Commun*, **122**, 509.
157. LEONARD AN, COHEN DE (1998), 'Submicellar bile salts stimulate phosphatidylcholine transfer activity of sterol carrier protein 2,' *J Lipid Res*, **39**, 1981.
158. STARODUB O, JOLLY CA, ATSHAVES BP *et al.* (2000), 'Sterol carrier protein-2 localization in endoplasmic reticulum and role in phospholipid formation,' *Am J Physiol*, **279**, C1259.
159. MURPHY EJ (1998), 'Sterol carrier protein-2 expression increases NBD-stearate uptake and cytoplasmic diffusion in L cells,' *Am J Physiol*, **275**, G237.
160. WIRTZ KW, WOUTERS FS, BASTIAENS PH *et al.* (1998), 'The non-specific lipid transfer protein (sterol carrier protein 2) acts as a peroxisomal fatty acid-CoA binding protein,' *Biochem Soc Trans*, **26**, 374.
161. DIXIT SS, SLEAT DE, STOCK AM, LOBEL P (2007), 'Do mammalian NPC1 and NPC2 play a role in intestinal cholesterol absorption?,' *Biochem J*, **408**, 1.
162. JOHNSTON JM (1976), *Lipid Absorption: Biochemical and Clinical Aspects*, London, MTP Press.
163. KUKSIS A, MANGANARO F (1986), *Fat Absorption*, Boca Raton, CRC Press.
164. RAO GA, JOHNSTON JM (1966), 'Purification and properties of triglyceride synthetase from the intestinal mucosa,' *Biochim Biophys Acta*, **125**, 465.
165. LEHNER R, KUKIS A (1995), 'Triacylglycerol synthesis by purified triacylglycerol synthetase of rat intestinal mucosa. Role of acyl-CoA acyltransferase,' *J Biol Chem*, **270**, 13630.
166. SMITH SJ, CASES S, JENSEN DR *et al.* (2000), 'Obesity resistance and multiple mechanisms of triglyceride synthesis in mice lacking Dgat,' *Nat Genet*, **25**, 87.
167. OELKERS P, TINKELENBERG A, ERDENIZE N *et al.* (2000), 'A lecithin cholesterol acyltransferase-like gene mediates diacylglycerol esterification in yeast,' *J Biol Chem*, **275**, 15609.
168. BELL RM, BALLAS LM, COLEMAN RA (1981), 'Lipid topogenesis,' *J Lipid Res*, **22**, 391.
169. ATKINSON D, SMALL DM (1986), 'Recombinant lipoproteins: implications for structure and assembly of native lipoproteins,' *Annu Rev Biophys Biophys Chem*, **15**, 403.

170. WETTERAU JR, ZILVERSMIT DB (1984), 'A triglyceride and cholesteryl ester transfer protein associated with liver microsomes,' *J Biol Chem*, **259**, 10863.
171. WETTERAU JR, ZILVERSMIT DB (1985), 'Purification and characterization of microsomal triglyceride and cholesteryl ester transfer protein from bovine liver microsomes,' *Chem Phys Lipids*, **38**, 205.
172. WETTERAU JR, ZILVERSMIT DB (1986), 'Localization of intracellular triacylglycerol and cholesteryl ester transfer activity in rat tissues,' *Biochim Biophys Acta*, **875**, 610.
173. POLHEIM D, DAVID JSK, SCHULTZ FM *et al.* (1973), 'Regulation of triglyceride biosynthesis in adipose and intestinal tissue,' *J Lipid Res*, **14**, 415.
174. NILSSON Å (1968), 'Intestinal absorption of lecithin and lysolecithin by lymph fistula rats,' *Biochim Biophys Acta*, **152**, 379.
175. SATO Y (1970), 'The metabolic fate of lysolecithin administered into rat duodenal lumen,' *Tohuku J Exp Med*, **100**, 227.
176. SCOW RO, STEIN Y, STEIN O (1967), 'Incorporation of dietary lecithin and lysolecithin into lymph chylomicrons in the rat,' *J Biol Chem*, **242**, 4919.
177. SUBBAIAH PV, SASTRY PS, GANGULY J (1970), 'Acylation of lysolecithin in the intestinal mucosa of rats,' *Biochem J*, **118**, 241.
178. OTTOLENGHI A (1964), 'Estimation and subcellular distribution of lecithinase activity in rat intestinal mucosa,' *J Lipid Res*, **5**, 532.
179. LE KIM D, BETZING H (1976), 'Intestinal absorption of polyunsaturated phosphatidylcholine in the rat,' *Hoppe-Seylers Z Physiol Chem*, **357**, 1321.
180. ERBLAND JF, MARINETTI GV (1965), 'The enzymatic acylation and hydrolysis of lysolecithin,' *Biochim Biophys Acta*, **106**, 128.
181. SPADY DK, TURLEY SD, DIETSCHY JM (1985), 'Receptor-independent low density lipoprotein transport in the rat *in vivo*. Quantitation, characterization, and metabolic consequences,' *J Clin Invest*, **76**, 1113.
182. TURLEY SD, ANDERSON JM, DIETSCHY JM (1981), 'Rates of sterol synthesis and uptake in the major organs of the rat *in vivo*,' *J Lipid Res*, **22**, 551.
183. ANDERSON JM, TURLEY SD, DIETSCHY JM (1982), 'Relative rates of sterol synthesis in the liver and various extrahepatic tissues of normal and cholesterol-fed rabbits,' *Biochim Biophys Acta*, **711**, 421.
184. SPADY DK, DIETSCHY JM (1983), 'Sterol synthesis *in vivo* in 18 tissues of the squirrel monkey, guinea pig, rabbit, hamster, and rat,' *J Lipid Res*, **24**, 303.
185. FELDMAN EB, RUSSELL BS, CHEN R *et al.* (1983), 'Dietary saturated fatty acid content affects lymph lipoproteins: studies in the rat,' *J Lipid Res*, **24**, 967.
186. STANGE EF, DIETSCHY JM (1985), 'The origin of cholesterol in the mesenteric lymph of the rat,' *J Lipid Res*, **26**, 175.
187. POOL C, NUTTING DF, SIMMONDS WJ, TSO P (1991), 'Effect of Pluronic L-81, a hydrophobic surfactant, on intestinal mucosal cholesterol homeostasis,' *Am J Physiol*, **261**, G256.
188. DIETSCHY JM, SPADY DK, STANGE EF (1983), 'Quantitative importance of different organs for cholesterol synthesis and low-density-lipoprotein degradation,' *Biochem Soc Trans*, **11**, 639.
189. SPADY DK, BILHEIMER DW, DIETSCHY JM (1983), 'Rates of receptor-dependent and -independent low density lipoprotein uptake in the hamster,' *Proc Natl Acad Sci USA*, **80**, 3499.
190. THOMSON ABR, DIETSCHY JM (1981), *Physiology of the Gastrointestinal Tract*, New York, Raven Press.
191. CLARK SB, TERCYAK AM (1984), 'Reduced cholesterol transmucosal transport in rats with inhibited mucosal acyl CoA: cholesterol acyltransferase and normal pancreatic function,' *J Lipid Res*, **25**, 148.
192. GALLO LL, NEWBILL T, HYUN J, VAHOUNY GV (1977), 'Role of pancreatic cholesterol esterase in the uptake and esterification of cholesterol by isolated intestinal cells,' *Proc Soc Exp Biol Med*, **156**, 277.

193. BORJA CR, VAHOUNY GV, TREADWELL CR (1964), 'Role of bile and pancreatic juice in cholesterol absorption and esterification,' *Am J Physiol*, **206**, 223.
194. NORUM KR, HELGERUD P, PETERSON LB *et al.* (1983), 'Influence of diets on acyl-CoA: cholesterol acyltransferase in villous and crypt cells from rat small intestinal mucosa and in the liver,' *Biochim Biophys Acta*, **751**, 153.
195. NORUM KR, LILLJEQVIST AC, DREVON DA (1977), 'Coenzyme-A-dependent esterification of cholesterol in intestinal mucosa from guinea-pig,' *Scand J Gastroenterol*, **12**, 281.
196. FIELD FJ, COOPER AD, ERICKSON SK (1982), 'Regulation of rabbit intestinal acid acyl coenzyme A-cholesterol acyltransferase *in vivo* and *in vitro*,' *Gastroenterology*, **83**, 873.
197. HELGERUD P, SAAREM K, NORUM KR (1981), 'Acyl-CoA:cholesterol acyltransferase in human small intestine: its activity and some properties of the enzymic reaction,' *J Lipid Res*, **22**, 271.
198. GALLO LL, CHIANG Y, VAHOUNY GV, TREADWELL CR (1980), 'Localization and origin of rat intestinal cholesterol esterase determined by immunocytochemistry,' *J Lipid Res*, **21**, 537.
199. FIELD FJ (1984), 'Intestinal cholesterol esterase: intracellular enzyme or contamination of cytosol by pancreatic enzymes,' *J Lipid Res*, **25**, 389.
200. BRUNEAU N, BENDAYAN M, GINGRAS D, GHITESCU L, LEVY E, LOMBARDO D (2003), 'Circulating bile salt-dependent lipase originates from the pancreas via intestinal transcytosis,' *Gastroenterology*, **124**, 470–80.
201. HELGERUD P, HAUGEN R, NORUM KR (1982), 'The effect of feeding and fasting on the activity of acyl-CoA: cholesterol acyltransferase in rat small intestine,' *Eur J Clin Invest*, **12**, 493.
202. WATT SM, SIMMONDS WJ (1981), 'The effect of pancreatic diversion on lymphatic absorption and esterification of cholesterol in the rat,' *J Lipid Res*, **22**, 157.
203. FUKUSHIMA H, AONO S, NAKAMURA Y *et al.* (1969), 'The effect of *N*-(alpha-methylbenzyl) linoleamide on cholesterol metabolism in rats,' *J Athero Res*, **10**, 403.
204. HARNETT KM, WALSH CT, ZHANG L (1989), 'Effects of Bay o 2752, a hypocholesterolemic agent on intestinal taurocholate absorption and cholesterol esterification,' *J Pharmacol Exp Therap*, **251**, 502.
205. TSO P, MORSHED KM, NUTTING DF (1991), 'Importance of acyl CoA–cholesterol acyltransferase (ACAT) in the esterification of cholesterol by enterocytes,' *FASEB J*, **5**, A709.
206. LEE HT, ROARK WH, PICARD JA *et al.* (1998), 'Inhibitors of acyl-CoA:cholesterol *O*-acyltransferase (ACAT) as hypocholesterolemic agents: synthesis and structure–activity relationships of novel series of sulfonamides, acylphosphonamides and acylphosphoramidates,' *Bioorg Med Chem Lett*, **8**, 289.
207. CHANG CC, CHEN J, THOMAS MA *et al.* (1995), 'Regulation and immunolocalization of acyl-coenzyme A:cholesterol acyltransferase in mammalian cells as studied with specific antibodies,' *J Biol Chem*, **270**, 29532.
208. CHANG CC, SAKASHITA N, ORNVOLD K *et al.* (2000), 'Immunological quantitation and localization of ACAT-1 and ACAT-2 in human liver and small intestine,' *J Biol Chem*, **275**, 28083.
209. MIYAZAKI A, SAKASHITA N, LEE O *et al.* (1998), 'Expression of ACAT-1 protein in human atherosclerotic lesions and cultured human monocyte-macrophages,' *Arterioscler Thromb Vas Biol*, **18**, 1568.
210. BUHMAN KK, ACCAD M, NOVAK S *et al.* (2000), 'Resistance to diet-induced hypercholesterolemia and gallstone formation in ACAT-2 deficient mice,' *Nat Med*, **6**, 1341.
211. MURPHY S, ALBRIGHT E, MATHUR SN, FIELD FJ (1990), 'Effect of eicosapentaenoic acid on triacylglycerol transport in CaCo-2 cells,' *Biochim Biophys Acta*, **1045**, 147.

212. KAM NT, ALBRIGHT E, MATHUR SN, FIELD FJ (1989), 'Inhibition of acylcoenzyme A:cholesterol acyltransferase activity in CaCo-2 cells results in intracellular triglyceride accumulation,' *J Lipid Res*, **30**, 371.
213. KAM NT, ALBRIGHT E, MATHUR SN, FIELD FJ (1990), 'Effect of lovastatin on acyl-CoA: cholesterol acyltransferase (ACAT) activity and the basolateral-membrane secretion of newly synthesized lipids by CaCo-2 cells,' *Biochem J*, **272**, 427.
214. TRABER MG, KAYDEN HJ, RINDLER MJ (1987), 'Polarized secretion of newly synthesized lipoproteins by the CaCO-2 human intestinal cell line,' *J Lipid Res*, **28**, 1350.
215. MURPHY S, ALBRIGHT E, MATHUR SN *et al.* (1992), 'Apolipoprotein B mRNA abundance is decreased by eicosapentaenoic acid in CaCo-2 cells. Effect on the synthesis and secretion of apolipoprotein B,' *Arterioscler Thromb*, **12**, 691.
216. OCKNER RK, HUGHES FB, ISSELBACHER KJ (1969), 'Very low density lipoproteins in intestinal lymph: role in triglyceride and cholesterol transport during fat absorption,' *J Clin Invest*, **48**, 2367.
217. OCKNER RK, MANNING JA (1974), 'Fatty acid binding protein in small intestine. Identification, isolation and evidence for its role in cellular fatty acid transport,' *J Clin Invest*, **54**, 326.
218. TSO P, DRAKE DS, BLACK DD, SABESIN SM (1984), 'Evidence for separate pathways of chylomicron and very low density lipoprotein assembly and transport by rat small intestine,' *Am J Physiol*, **247**, G599.
219. ZILVERSMIT DB (1965), 'The composition and structure of lymph chylomicrons in dog, rat, and man,' *J Clin Invest*, **44**, 1610.
220. LINDGREN FT, JENSEN LC, HATCH FT (1972), *Blood, Lipids, and Lipoproteins: Quantitation, Composition and Metabolism*, New York, Wiley.
221. MAHLEY RW, BENNETT BD, MORRE DJ *et al.* (1971), 'Lipoproteins associated with Golgi apparatus isolated from epithelial cells of rat small intestine,' *Lab Invest*, **25**, 435.
222. VAHOUNY GV, BLENDERMANN EM, GALLO LL, TREADWELL CR (1980), 'Differential transport of cholesterol and oleic acid in lymph lipoproteins: sex differences in puromycin sensitivity,' *J Lipid Res*, **21**, 415.
223. TSO P, BALINT JA, BISHOP MB, RODGERS JB (1981), 'Acute inhibition of intestinal lipid transport by Pluronic L-81 in the rat,' *Am J Physiol*, **241**, G487.
224. TSO P, BALINT JA, RODGERS JB (1980), 'Effect of hydrophobic surfactant (Pluronic L-81) on lymphatic lipid transport in the rat,' *Am J Physiol*, **239**, G348.
225. TSO P, DRAKE DS, BLACK D, SABESIN SM (1984), 'Evidence for separate pathways of chylomicrons and very-low density lipoprotein assembly and secretion by rat small intestine,' *Am J Physiol*, **247**, G599.
226. NUTTING D, HALL J, BARROWMAN JA, TSO P (1989), 'Further studies on the mechanism of inhibition of intestinal chylomicron transport by Pluronic L-81,' *Biochim Biophys Acta*, **1004**, 357.
227. LUCHOOMUN J, HUSSAIN MM (1999), 'Assembly and secretion of chylomicrons by differentiated cells: Nascent triglycerides and preformed phospholipids are preferentially used for lipoprotein assembly,' *J Biol Chem*, **274**, 19565.
228. SIDDIQI SA, SIDDIQI S, MAHAN J, PEGGS K, GORELICK FS, MANSBACH CM 2nd (2006), 'The identification of a novel endoplasmic reticulum to Golgi SNARE complex used by the prechylomicron transport vesicle,' *J Biol Chem*, **281**, 20974.
229. NEELI I, SIDDIQI SA, SIDDIQI S, MAHAN J, LAGAKOS WS, BINAS B, GHEYI T, STORCH J, MANSBACH CM 2nd (2007), 'Liver fatty acid-binding protein initiates budding of pre-chylomicron transport vesicles from intestinal endoplasmic reticulum,' *J Biol Chem*, **282**, 17974.

230. EDGE SB, HOEG JM, SCHNEIDER PD, BREWER HB JR (1985), 'Apolipoprotein B synthesis is humans: liver synthesizes only apolipoprotein B-100,' *Metabolism*, **34**, 726.
231. GLICKMAN RM, ROGERS M, GLICKMAN JN (1986), 'Apolipoprotein B synthesis by human liver and intestine *in vitro*,' *Proc Natl Acad Sci USA*, **83**, 5296.
232. GLICKMAN RM, GLICKMAN JN, MAGUN A, BRIN M (1991), 'Apolipoprotein synthesis in normal and abetalipoproteinemic intestinal mucosa,' *Gastroenterology*, **101**, 749.
233. CHEN SH, HABIB G, YANG CY *et al.* (1987), 'Apolipoprotein B-48 is the product of a messenger RNA with an organ-specific in-frame stop codon,' *Science*, **238**, 363.
234. POWELL LM, WALLIS SC, PEASE RJ *et al.* (1987), 'A novel form of tissue-specific RNA processing produces apolipoprotein-B48 in intestine,' *Cell*, **50**, 831.
235. KANE JP, HARDMAN DA, PAULUS HE (1980), 'Heterogeneity of apolipoprotein B: isolation of a new species from human chylomicrons,' *Proc Natl Acad Sci USA*, **77**, 2465.
236. CARDIN AD, WITT KR, BARNHART CL, JACKSON RL (1982), 'Sulfhydryl chemistry and solubility properties of human plasma apolipoprotein B,' *Biochemistry*, **21**, 4503.
237. MARTINS IJ, SAINSBURY AJ, MAMO JC, REDGRAVE TG (1994), 'Lipid and apolipoprotein B-48 transport in mesenteric lymph and the effect of hyperphagia on the clearance of chylomicron-like emulsions in insulin-deficient rats,' *Diabetologia*, **37**, 238.
238. HAYASHI H, FUJIMOTO K, CARDELLI JA *et al.* (1990), 'Fat feeding increases size, but not number of chylomicrons produced by small intestine,' *Am J Physiol*, **259**, G709.
239. DAVIDSON NO, MAGUN AM, BRASITUS TA, GLICKMAN RM (1987), 'Intestinal apolipoprotein A-I and B-48 metabolism: effects of sustained alterations in dietary triglyceride and mucosal cholesterol flux,' *J Lipid Res*, **28**, 388.
240. ISSELBACHER KJ, SCHEIG R, PLOTKIN GR, CAULFIELD JB (1964), 'Congenital beta-lipoprotein deficiency: a hereditary disorder involving a defect in the absorption and transport of lipids,' *Medicine*, **43**, 347.
241. WAYS PO, PARMENTIER CM, KAYDEN HJ *et al.* (1967), 'Studies on the absorptive defect for triglyceride in abetalipoproteinemia,' *J Clin Invest*, **46**, 35.
242. WETTERAU JR, AGGERBECK LP, BOUME ME *et al.* (1992), 'Absense of microsomal triglyceride transfer protein in individuals with abetalipoproteinemia,' *Science*, **256**, 999.
243. GORDON DA, JAMIL H (2000), 'Progress towards understanding the role of microsomal triglyceride transfer protein in apolipoprotein-B lipoprotein assembly,' *Biochim Biophys Acta*, **1486**, 72.
244. SHARP D, RICCI B, KIENZLE B *et al.* (1994), 'Human microsomal triglyceride transfer protein large subunit gene structure,' *Biochemistry*, **33**, 9057.
245. OHASHI K, ISHIBASHI S, OSUGA J *et al.* (2000), 'Novel mutations in the microsomal triglyceride transfer protein gene causing abetalipoproteinemia,' *J Lipid Res*, **41**, 1199.
246. BERRIOT-VAROQUEAUX N, AGGERBECK LP, SAMSON-BOUMA M, WETTERAU JR (2000), 'The role of the microsomal triglyceride transfer protein in abetalipoproteinemia,' *Annu Rev Nutr*, **20**, 663.
247. ROY CC, LEVY E, GREEN PHR, SNIDERMAN A, LETARTE J, BUTS JP *et al.* (1987), 'Malabsorption, hypocholesterolemia and fat filled enterocytes with increased intestinal apo B. Chylomicron retention disease,' *Gastroenterology*, **92**, 390.
248. DANNOURA AH, BERRIOT-VAROQUEAUX N, AMATI P *et al.* (1999), 'Anderson's disease: exclusion of apolipoprotein and intracellular lipid transport genes,' *Art Thromb Vasc Bio*, **19**, 2494.

5

Non-starch polysaccharides in the gastrointestinal tract

A. C. Ouwehand, K. Tiihonen, H. Mäkeläinen and N. Rautonen, Danisco, Finland; O. Hasselwander, Danisco, UK; and G. Sworn, Danisco, France

Abstract: Non-starch polysaccharides (NSPs) are an important part of our diet and play an essential role in the development of functional foods. NSP are a diverse group of carbohydrates consisting primarily of components of plant wall cells, including gums, plant mucilages, algal polysaccharides and other polysaccharides such as inulin and polydextrose. The current chapter describes the physiological effects of NSP; in most cases as prebiotics. Furthermore, NSPs give structure, mouthfeel and bulk to foods, which are relevant properties especially for the formulation of functional foods, which may be foods with reduced fat and/or sugar.

Key words: prebiotics, inulin, polydextrose, galacto-oligosaccharides, gums, cellulose, hemicellulose, pectin, β-glucan, health benefit, application.

5.1 Introduction

Carbohydrates perform important functions in life, owing to their diversity in monomers and their ability to form oligo- and polymers through linkages at different sites on the monomer and through the different orientation of the linkages. In plants, polysaccharides provide strength and structural components (such as cellulose) and serve as an energy source and as stored energy (e.g. starch and inulin). In microorganisms, polysaccharides form structural components of the cell envelope (such as in peptidoglycan and lipopolysacharide) and serve as an energy source (e.g. cellulose and starch). In animals, polysaccharides may function as one of the main sources of energy (e.g. starch) and as limited energy storage (glycogen).

Oligosaccharides function as important recognition sites on the cell's surface and line the gastrointestinal, urogenital and respiratory tract in the form of mucous glycoproteins. With the exception of starch, most oligo- and polysaccharides are poorly digested by animals, including humans. This does not mean that these non-starch polysaccharides (NSPs) are useless to the host; on the contrary. In ruminants, such as cows and sheep, and hind-gut fermenters, such as horses, microbes assist in the degradation of NSP. Also in humans, certain groups of NSP can be degraded by the intestinal microbiota. When such degradation is limited to a small group of microbes and gives rise to specific health benefits, the NSP can be considered a prebiotic. Even when NSP are not degraded by the intestinal microbiota, they are important in providing health benefits, e.g. through faecal bulking and inducing satiety. In addition to the physiological importance of NSPs, some of them are indispensible in the formulation of functional foods. When formulating, for example, sugar-free or fat-free foods, they will provide the appropriate mouthfeel, stability and bulk. NSPs are therefore important components of numerous functional foods; either by being the functional, health-promoting ingredient itself, or a technological component in such foods.

5.2 Types of non-starch polysaccharide

5.2.1 Definition and analysis

The term non-starch polysaccharides describes a group of carbohydrates that are 'macromolecules consisting of a large number of monosaccharides residues joined to each other by glycosidic linkages' (IUB-IUPAC Joint Commission on Biochemical Nomenclature 1982) that do not contain the α-(1,4)-linked glucose characteristic of starch. Generally, a polysaccharide contains ten or more monosaccharide residues.

NSP are a diverse group of carbohydrates consisting primarily of components of plant wall cells such as cellulose, hemicelluloses and pectin, other polysaccharides from plant, algae or seaweed origin and include gums, plant mucilages and algal polysaccharides (Cummings & Stephen 2007; Gray 2006) and other polysaccharides such as inulin and polydextrose.

Although as stated above, NSP are diverse, they are chemically defined and their presence in foods can be analysed. In principle, NSP are hydrolysed and extracted after all starch has been removed following enzymatic hydrolysis. NSP extraction involves precipitation with 80% ethanol to remove the starch and NSP hydrolysis is carried out with sulphuric acid. In some cases, such as for pectin, an additional enzymatic hydrolysis is required. The released sugars can then be quantified by colorimetry or chromatography (Englyst *et al.* 2007).

5.2.2 Types and origin

Cellulose

Cellulose is a linear β-(1,4)-linked glucan containing up to 10000 glucose units per molecule. It is the main structural component of plant wall cells and is hence present in fruits, vegetables and cereals.

Hemicellulose

Hemicellulose is associated with cellulose in plant wall cells. In contrast to cellulose, hemicellulose contains sugars other than glucose such as xylose, mannose, galactose, rhamnose and arabinose as well as carboxylated derivatives of glucose and galactose ('uronic acids'). Hemicelluloses are smaller molecules formed of 50–200 sugar residues and can be both linear and branched. They are also present in fruits, vegetables, legumes and nuts.

Pectin

Pectin is composed of a linear backbone of α-(1,4)-linked galacturonic acid, partially esterified with methanol, interrupted by branched side chains of rhamnose, galactose, xylose, arabinose and galacturonic acid. Pectin is present in the cell walls of fruits and vegetables and is widely used as a food additive for its viscosifying, gelling and protein stabilisation properties.

β-Glucans

β-Glucans are glucose polymers found in the cell wall of cereal grains, particularly oat and barley. β-Glucans are large linear polysaccharides and the glucose units are linked β-(1,3) or β-(1,4). Branched (1,3)/(1,6)-β-glucan is present in yeast, fungi and some mushrooms.

Gums

Gums comprise a diverse group of NSPs and are derived from exudates that form at the sites of injuries to plants such as gum arabic and gum tragacanth or seeds such as guar and locust bean gum. Gums are widely used as food additives for their viscosifying, gelling and protein stabilisation properties.

Gum arabic, also known as gum acacia, is prepared from an exudate from the stems and branches of sub-Saharan *Acacia senegal* and *Acacia seyal* trees (Leguminosae) and produced naturally as large nodules during a process called gummosis to seal wounds in the bark of the tree. It is a highly branched complex of uronic acid containing NSPs.

Guar gum is ground endosperm halves from the seeds of the guar plant *Cyamopsis tetragonoloba* L. The plant has been cultivated in India and Pakistan for centuries, and is also grown in Brazil, Australia and South-Africa. Guar gum is a neutral galactomannan consisting of a linear mannan backbone (β-(1,4)-linked) with the galactose units attached as single side chains by an α-(1,6)-glycosidic linkage.

Locust bean gum is derived from the seed of the leguminous carob tree (*Ceratonia siliqua*), which grows in Mediterranean countries. Like guar gum, locust bean gum is also a galactomannan and consists of a polymeric mannose chain branched with galactose units.

Mucilages

Mucilages are present in cells of the outer layer of seeds of the Plantain family. Psyllium or ispaghula husk is a well-known example.

Algal polysaccharides

Algal polysaccharides include carrageenan, agar and alginates; they replace cellulose in the cell wall. They are extracted from seaweeds or algae and are also used as food additives due to their viscosifying and gelling properties.

Carrageenans are linear polymers of about 25 000 galactose units and are highly sulphated. Alginates are salts of alginic acid, a linear polysaccharide composed of α-L-glucuronic acid and β-mannuronic acid linked through (1,4) glycosidic bonds.

Other non-starch polysaccharides

Other NSP include synthetic derivatives of cellulose such as methylcellulose or hydroxypropylmethylcellulose and also polydextrose and inulin. Polydextrose is a glucose polymer prepared by polycondensation of glucose and sorbitol in the presence of citric acid as a catalyst. Polydextrose is highly branched containing various types of glycosidic bonds with α-(1,6) linkages predominating. Polydextrose comprises of components with a degree of polymerisation of 2 to 35. It has traditionally been used as a low-calorie bulking agent, but is increasingly being used for its physiological effects. Inulin occurs in a variety of plants and is commercially isolated from chicory roots. Inulin is a β-(2,1)-linked fructan with a glucose molecule at the end of each fructose chain and the chains usually consist of between 2 and 60 units.

Dietary fibres according to the suggested definition by the European Food Safety Authority (EFSA) include NSPs, resistant starch, resistant oligosaccharides with three or more monomeric units, and other non-digestible, but quantitatively minor components when naturally associated with dietary fibre polysaccharides, especially lignin (EFSA 2007). NSPs are the main constituents of dietary fibre (Table 5.1).

5.3 Digestion of non-starch polysaccharides

The structural differences between digestible starch and non-digestible cellulose are biologically important. The helical structure formed by the α-linkages in starch is suitable for glucose storing and the straight structure of cellulose formed by β-linkages has a structural role and very limited degradability.

Endogenous α-amylases of vertebrates are important for starch digestibility. Salivary and pancreatic α-amylase hydrolyse the amylose, comprising of glucose chains with α-1,4 linkages, to smaller glucose units. Amylopectin consists of a similar glucose chain, however, with branches of α-1,6 linkages and is hydrolysed partly by α-amylase and partly by small intestinal brush border disaccharidases. Although the pectin molecule consists of a backbone of α-1,4-linkages, its structure of galacturonic acid, which is partially esterified with methanol, makes it highly resistant to α-amylase.

However, α-amylases or disaccharidases are unable to hydrolyse β-1,4 linkages typically found in the main components of NSP; cellulose,

Table 5.1 Summary of non-starch polysaccharides according to the suggested definition of the European Food Safety Authority

Main classes	Subgroups	Monomers	Linkages
Cellulose	–	Glucose	β-(1,4)
Hemicellulose	–	Xylose, galactose, arabinose, mannose, uronic acids	β-(1,4), but also (1,2) and (1,3)
Pectin	–	Galacturonic acid partially esterified with methanol, rhamnose, galactose, xylose, arabinose	α-(1,4)
β-Glucans	Cereal β-glucans	Glucose	β-(1,3) and β-(1,4)
	β-Glucans from yeast, fungi and mushrooms	Glucose	β-(1,3) and β-(1,6)
Gums	Gum arabic	Arabinose, galactose, uronic acids	α-(1,3)
	Guar gum, locust bean gum	Mannose, galactose	β-(1,4) with galactose units attached by α-(1,6)
	Xanthan gum	Glucose, mannose, glucuronic acid, pyruvic acid	β-(1,4)
Mucilages	Psyllium	Arabinose, xylose	β-(1,4) and β-(1,3)
Algal polysaccharides	Carrageenan	Galactose, highly suphated	α-(1,3) and β-(1,4)
	Alginates	Guluronic acid, mannuronic acid	α-(1,4) for guluronic acid and β-(1,4) for mannuronic acid
Others	Polydextrose	Glucose	Various, predominating α-(1,6)
	Inulin	Fructose	β-(1,2)

hemicellulose and pectin. Thus, NSPs reach the colon undigested and become partly or completely fermented by the colonic microbiota to produce short chain fatty acid (SCFA) and gas. In the colon, the digestion of complex NSPs requires the synergistic action of number of enzymes. To understand the digestibility and further the physiological role of different NSPs several *in vitro* and *in vivo* models have been developed.

5.4 Non-starch polysaccharide fermentation in the gastrointestinal tract: research models

The study and sampling of the human gastrointestinal tract, especially the small intestine and proximal large intestine, is very difficult. Thus, the research of NSP fermentation relies heavily on *in vitro* and *in vivo* animal model studies. The effects of different types of NSP on gastrointestinal microbiota and its metabolic activity (e.g. SCFA production) can be easily studied using *in vitro* culture systems, whereas animal models can be used to investigate the ecological and metabolic mechanisms of the microbial populations in different parts of the gut and how NSP affect this gut ecosystem *in vivo* (Rumney & Rowland 1992). However, the relevance of these models for the authentic human gastrointestinal tract needs always to be considered, since substantial differences exist, such as absence of colonocytes, mucous and digestive tract secretions in *in vitro* models and different microbial populations and physiology of animals. Nevertheless, valuable information of the colonic breakdown of complex carbohydrates and the importance of NSP in maintaining gut health has been obtained with both *in vitro* and *in vivo* models (Macfarlane & Macfarlane 2007b).

5.4.1 *In vitro* models

In vitro models that are used in the study of NSP fermentation can be divided into batch cultures, chemostat-type simulators, including semi-continuous and continuous cultures, and non-chemostat-type simulators. All these models use strictly anaerobic conditions to support the growth of colonic microbes. Batch fermenters are generally similarly structured, small-scale bottle fermenters, whereas the different chemostat- and non-chemostat type simulator models have major structural differences. All simulator models, however, use faecal material from a single or several donors and employ artificial intestinal media that originate from media originally published by Gibson and co-workers (Gibson *et al.* 1988b), mimicking the fluid in the end of the human small intestine. These simulators have similar pH set-points (from 5.0 to 7.0), and pH levels and fluid transitions are computer controlled (Mäkivuokko & Nurminen 2006). Samples collected from these models are usually analysed for their microbial composition and metabolites produced through NSP fermentation.

Batch-type models

Batch fermentations are the most commonly used and simplest models to study the fermentation activity of colonic microbes. These batch fermentors are usually anaerobic sealed bottles with pure cultures, defined mixed cultures or faecal slurry, and are used to study the effects of added NSP on the microbes and their fermentation activity. They model a certain part of the gastrointestinal tract and the run-times in batch fermentations range from 2 to 24 hours (Mäkivuokko & Nurminen 2006; Rumney & Rowland 1992). The accumulation of fermentation products (e.g. SCFA) and the depletion of nutrients can alter the conditions and microbiota balance in the fermentor, thus affecting the *in vivo* relevance in longer simulations.

This can be avoided by using more complex simulation models with several vessels and fluid transitions (Mäkivuokko & Nurminen 2006).

Chemostat-type simulators

The first *in vitro* simulator was introduced in 1981 (Miller & Wolin 1981), and several different models have been developed since. All chemostat-type models have three to six sequentially connected anaerobic fermentor vessels representing different compartments of the human gastrointestinal tract (Mäkivuokko & Nurminen 2006).

The Reading simulator, introduced by Gibson and co-workers (Gibson *et al.* 1988), and revised by Macfarlane and co-workers (Macfarlane *et al.* 1998), simulates the human large intestine in three connected vessels with working volumes ranging from 220 to 320 ml. Simulator medium is pumped through the system continuously, and there is a continuous overflow of the material through the three vessels. The Reading model is run for at least 14 days before the actual simulation, in order to achieve microbiological steady-state conditions in the vessels. After the test substrate is added to the model and it is run until a new steady state is achieved, followed by a wash-out period. Samples are collected during and after the different stages of the simulation and subjected to analysis.

Molly and co-workers introduced a Simulator for Human Intestinal Microbiological Ecosystem (SHIME) (Molly *et al.* 1993), which simulates the whole human gastrointestinal tract from stomach to colon. It is a six-stage system, where the first three glass vessels represent the stomach and small intestine, and the subsequent three vessels simulate the colon. Working volumes range from 300 ml to as high as 1600 ml (Alander *et al.* 1999; Kontula *et al.* 1998). The SHIME model is run for 8 days with medium only prior to the actual simulation with the test substance. Feeding of the substrate is continued for 12 days, followed by another period of 8 days of medium only. This 30-day cycle is repeated for all tested substrates and samples are collected after each period.

The EnteroMix® Colon simulator (Fig. 5.1) was introduced by Mäkivuokko and co-workers (Mäkivuokko *et al.* 2005). This model has four parallel units, which all have four connected glass vessels, thus allowing four simulations to be run simultaneously using the same faecal inoculum. This simulation system has small working volumes in its four vessels (from 6 to 12 ml), requiring only 50 ml of faecal slurry. The faecal slurry is pre-incubated for 24 hours before the simulation is started, and it takes 2 days to run a set of four parallel simulations (usually control and three test substrates). During the simulation, the transfer and feeding of the system occurs in 3 hour cycles. The fermented fluids and microbes are transferred semi-continuously in the system (from V1 to V2, V3, V4, and eventually to the waste container), followed by feeding the proximal part (V1) of the artificial colon with fresh simulator medium containing the test substrate. Fermentation and 3 hourly fluid transfers continue for 48 hours, after which

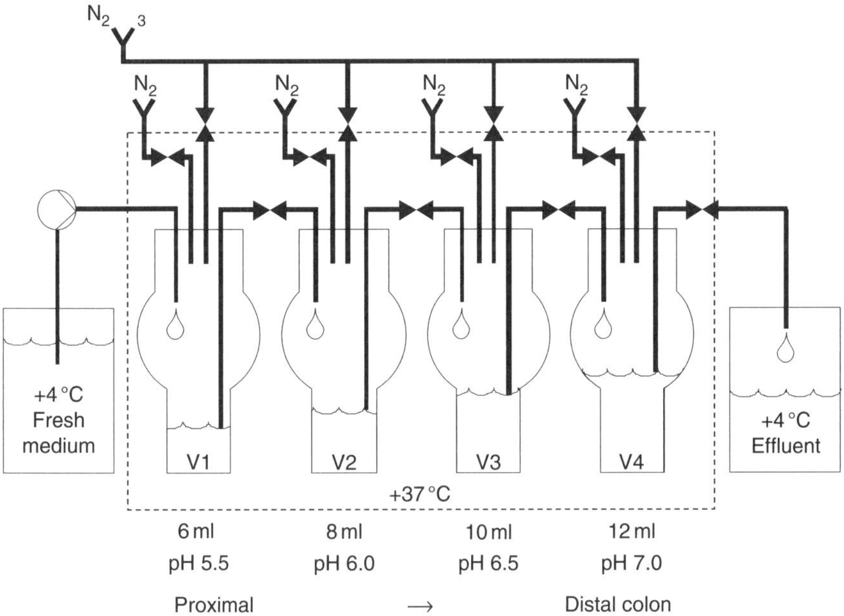

Fig. 5.1 The Enteromix® simulator model. The figure represents the residual volumes of the system after fluid transitions has occurred and fresh medium added to the vessel V1. The vessels V1 to V4 mimic the different regions of the human gastrointestinal tract: caecum + ascending colon, transverse colon, descending colon and the sigmoid + rectum area, respectively. pH controlling and semi-continuous fluid transitions are operated via opening and closing of computer-controlled valves together with nitrogen and ammonia gases. Figure modified from Mäkivuokko *et al.* (2006).

the simulator is stopped and samples collected from the vessels for analysis of microbiota composition and metabolic activity (Mäkeläinen *et al.* 2007; Mäkivuokko *et al.* 2006).

Non-chemostat simulators

The TNO Intestinal Model (TIM) system consists of two parts and was introduced by Minekus and co-workers in 1995 and 1999 (Minekus *et al.* 1995, 1999). The TIM 1 system simulates the stomach and small intestine with its eight sequentially connected glass vessels. The TIM 2 system consists of four glass modules in a loop representing the proximal colon. These dynamic models have peristaltic pumps to transfer the fluid from vessel to vessel, and there is a constant absorption of water and fermentation metabolites (e.g. SCFA) through dialysis membranes. The volume of intestinal fluids in both models is 200 ml and the operation of simulation takes from 1 to 3 days. With the combination of TIM 1 and 2, the digestion and fermentation of a NSP product can be modelled in the whole length of the human gastrointestinal tract.

5.4.2 *In vivo* models

Animal models provide opportunities to study the metabolic and immunological activities of intestinal microbiota in more detail than in the *in vitro* models. Intestinal contents and also tissues and organs can be investigated at autopsy in animals. Conventional, germ-free and human microbiota-associated rodents and piglets have been used as models for the human gastrointestinal tract in health and disease. The gastrointestinal tract of piglets has similarities with the humans in nutritional requirements, and intestinal physiology and metabolism (Fava *et al.* 2007). The effects of non-digestible oligosaccharides and fibre on gut microecology and physiology have been studied in rats (Bielecka *et al.* 2002; Dongowski *et al.* 2002; Henningsson *et al.* 2002; Peuranen *et al.* 2004) and in pigs or piglets in several studies (Correa-Matos *et al.* 2003; Fava *et al.* 2007; Krueger *et al.* 2002; Martinez-Puig *et al.* 2003). Although the usefulness of animal models in studies of the human gastrointestinal tract and microbiota is clear, and there is a wide range of similarities between the two hosts, there are also many morphological and physiological differences between the two species that hinder the straight extrapolation of the results from animal models to humans (Henriksson 2006).

The fermentation of complex carbohydrates in the gut can be studied in humans as well, with healthy volunteers or ileostomy patients, using intubation tubes positioned in the gastrointestinal tract. From samples obtained directly from the gastrointestinal tract, the fermentation of a substrate and the consequences on microbiota can be measured (Englyst & Cummings 1985; Englyst *et al.* 1996; Silvester *et al.* 1995; Stephen *et al.* 1983). Although these investigations involving humans provide the best model for studying the microbiota and fermentation of NSP, they also suffer from many difficulties because of low compliance of the subjects to the study and special practical and ethical limitations (Macfarlane & Macfarlane 2007a). Also, non-invasive methods with human subjects can be used, such as breath hydrogen measurements (Stephen *et al.* 1983) or measuring SCFA in peripheral venous plasma or faeces (Cummings *et al.* 1996). However, since SCFAs are quickly absorbed from the colon and part is used by the colonocytes, these measurements cannot determine the total production of SCFA from NSP without invasive sampling (Cummings & Englyst 1991; Wong *et al.* 2006b).

All *in vitro* and *in vivo* methods have their advantages and disadvantages, and there appears to be no single ideal method for studying the different aspects of NSP fermentation processes in the human gastrointestinal tract. Yet together these models provide a representative view of the ecosystem within the gut, and the suitability of a study model can be decided according to the characteristics studied and the parameters under investigation (Rumney & Rowland 1992).

5.5 Mechanisms of health effects of non-starch polysaccharides

Non-digestible polysaccharides, the main constituents of dietary fibre, can have a major impact on the development of several conditions important for public health. However, mixed results have been published, e.g. of the association between fibre consumption and risk of developing colon cancer (Bingham 2006) and insulin resistance syndrome (Howlett & Ashwell 2008), although most recent consensus acknowledges the need for more detailed classification. The great structural diversity of the polysaccharides is likely to be a major factor explaining the contradictory results. The term 'dietary fibre' is used for a complex mixture of components with varying physiological properties and health effects. The classification of fibres is still in its infancy, and it remains to be determined which specific carbohydrate structures correlate with specific health properties. Thus, the need for understanding the physiological role and health benefits of NSP has increased, especially in Western countries where a low intake of dietary fibre is linked to several metabolic diseases.

The health effects of dietary NSP can be mediated directly, mostly in the upper gastrointestinal tract, where NSP are resistant to digestion and absorption or indirectly, via fermentation in the large intestine and bulking properties. During the passage along the gastrointestinal tract, NSP can influence the digestibility and absorption of nutrients, insulin responses, transit time and food intake. NSP attract water and add bulk to the digestas which increase intestinal peristalsis and soften the stool, preventing constipation and its associated problems such as haemorrhoids. Based on their solubility in water, NSPs can be divided into insoluble (e.g. cellulose and hemicellulose) and soluble (e.g. pectins, gums, mucilages) fibres. The solubility describes mainly the gel-forming properties, which can have nutritional impact but otherwise the difference is not a very distinctive feature. Both soluble and insoluble NSPs can have an effect on fat and glucose responses (Elia & Cummings 2007; Mann 2007; Scheppach *et al.* 2001) and become fermented in the colon (Casci *et al.* 2007). However, current dietary recommendations are based on the epidemiological studies indicating that especially the diet high in water-soluble fibre is inversely associated with the risk of cardiovascular disease (CVD) (Theuwissen & Mensink 2008).

Food intake is regulated in a complex way. The most important satiety signals from the gastrointestinal tract arise from the full stomach and intestine. In addition, several enteric hormones signalling satiety or hunger are secreted by the intestine. The satiety-mediating effects of NSPs are believed to be mediated by either bulking or viscosity. In the stomach the gelling properties of NSPs can contribute to delayed gastric emptying, thus increasing satiety signalling (Hoad *et al.* 2004). The food containing NSPs typically has decreased energy density, which evidently decreases the amount of energy consumed. In the colon, part of the consumed NSP may become fermented, yielding a variety of end products having impact on satiety signalling (Nilsson *et al.* 2008). As an example, consumption of oligofructose has been linked also to modulation of peptide hormones, such as GLP-1, PYY and ghrelin (Cani *et al.* 2004; Delzenne *et al.* 2007). However, the effect of the dietary fibre and glycaemic index on body weight regulation has not been consistent (for review see, e.g. van Dam & Seidell 2007). In the small intestine, NSP can have an effect on the digestion and absorption of the nutrients. Absorption rates of glucose and lipids, such as cholesterol and triglycerides, are important risk factors for developing cardiovascular diseases (Barclay *et al.* 2008; Patsch *et al.* 1992).

The interactions of different carbohydrates with lipid metabolism in the postprandial state have been of special interest in recent years (for review see, e.g. Lairon *et al.* 2007). As NSPs are not digested, they do not contribute to the immediate glucose supply. However, the gelling properties of NSPs can decrease glycaemic response by decreasing the diffusion of sugar and lipid molecules in the gut lumen. As a rule of thumb, the bigger the molecule, the more efficiently it can inhibit absorption (note β-glucan and pectin). This is supported by the observation that high-fibre diets are associated with improved insulin resistance (Liese *et al.* 2005; Ylonen *et al.* 2003). Rye fibre and β-glucans have been shown to decrease insulin reponses by decreasing gastrointestinal polypeptide (GIP) responses (Juntunen *et al.* 2002, 2003). NSPs are also supposed to decrease cholesterol absorption by binding bile acids. Moreover, colonic fermentation of NSP (see below) is known to affect lipid metabolism. Propionate has been shown to inhibit cholesterol synthesis but, on the other hand, fermentation producing high acetate concentrations in peripheral circulation may increase serum cholesterol. Thus, NSP that can decrease the acetate:propionate ratio may reduce serum lipids (Wong *et al.* 2006c). In long-term studies decreased plasma acetate levels and corresponding beneficial blood lipids responses to high fibre intake took several months to occur (Wolever *et al.* 2002).

NSPs can have beneficial effects on mineral absorption. Mineral absorption is believed to be enhanced via fermentation of NSPs by reduction of pH in the large intestine (Heijnen *et al.* 1993; Younes *et al.* 2001). Increased calcium absorption has been described in animal models when diet has been supplemented by fructo-oligosaccharides or other soluble NSPs (Coudray *et al.* 2005; Hara *et al.* 2000; Lopez *et al.* 1999; Zafar *et al.* 2004). In the large intestine, NSPs can have beneficial effects on fermentation and slow down the development of colon carcinoma. Effects of SCFA on gastrointestinal health have been studied extensively (Wong *et al.* 2006a). Microbial fermentation of NSP produces SCFA, primarily acetate, propionate and butyrate. After absorption from the gut lumen, acetate, the principal SCFA in the colon, is taken up by the peripheral tissues and propionate by the liver. Butyrate is essential for the health of colon by providing substrates for epithelial cells (Hamer *et al.* 2008). SCFAs have direct effects on the enterocytes modulating their function and differentiation (Sanderson 2007).

Butyrate has been reported to inhibit cancerous progression both *in vivo* in animal models and *in vitro* in cell models (Scheppach & Weiler 2004). Fermentation of specific NSP may thus inhibit function or growth of cancer cells. Fermented polydextrose has been reported to reduce expression of COX-2 in CaCo-2 cells (Mäkivuokko *et al.* 2005) and reduce tumour size and number in an experimental animal model (Ishizuka *et al.* 2003). With synbiotic treatment consisting of FOS and lactic acid bacteria, beneficial effects on cancer biomarkers have been described also in humans (Rafter et al. 2007).

Many of the health benefits that are linked to NSP relate to the metabolic end products produced by the intestinal microbiota from NSP fermentation, or from direct effects mediated by changes in the composition of the intestinal microbiota. A special subgroup of NSP is therefore formed by prebiotics: non-digestible food ingredients that, when consumed in sufficient amounts, selectively stimulate the growth and/or activity of one or a limited number of microbes in the colon, resulting in documented health benefits (Ouwehand *et al.* 2006). Examples of prebiotics are inulin, fructo-oligosaccharides, galacto-oligosaccharides and polydextrose. Suggested physiological effects of prebiotics include: increase in intestinal *Bifidobacterium* levels (Jie *et al.* 2000), relief of constipation (Macfarlane *et al.* 2006) and modulation of the immune system (Moro *et al.* 2006).

Effects of NSP on immune functions are thought to be mediated mainly via the prebiotic route, by fermentation of the NSP in the large intestine, resulting in modulation of the intestinal microbial community composition and activity. However, direct effects can also be mediated by the binding of NSP on epithelial cells or by the effect on phagocytosing cells, or M-cells and dendritic cells, sampling actively antigens from the gut lumen (Neutra *et al.* 1996). In particular, β-glucans have been suggested to convey direct effects via specific β-glucan receptors on macrophages (Brown *et al.* 2002). Furthermore, direct immune modulating effects of galacto-oligosaccharides have been suggested in caecetomised, antibiotic-treated animals with ovalbumin-specific allergic asthma, although no specific receptor has been identified (Sonoyama *et al.* 2005).

The indirect, prebiotic effects on immune responses can be mediated by the growth of bifidobacteria and lactobacilli, or other beneficial commensal microbes or the suppression of less desirable taxa. Addition of lactic acid bacteria to the diet has been shown to modulate immune responses in many specific gastrointestinal conditions such as diarrhoea (Szajewska *et al.* 2007) and inflammatory bowel disease (Hojsak *et al.* 2007). In addition, extra intestinal effects, such as modulation of allergic disorders (Moro *et al.* 2006) and indications of efficacy against the development of rheumatoid arthritis in animal models have been also reported (Kano *et al.* 2002; So *et al.* 2008). Interaction with the immune system may also occur via metabolites produced by the activated bacteria.

It is noteworthy that specificity of prebiotic polysaccharides should also be perhaps assessed with pathogenic bacteria. Mixed results have been reported on the effect of fructo-oligosaccharides on *Salmonella* infections (ten Bruggencate *et al.* 2003). An important but not very serious side effect is gas produced by the colonic microbes. That is typically recognised as abdominal discomfort.

5.6 Non-starch polysaccharides and mucosal adhesion

Adhesion of microbes to the intestinal mucosa is an important phenomenon. For (potential) pathogenic microbes, it is the first step in pathogenesis (Brumel & Finlay 2000). For non-pathogenic microbes it is also important as it may improve the success for colonisation of the intestine (Vesterlund *et al.* 2005). In addition, the host adhesion may be of benefit as it brings members of the intestinal microbiota in close contact with the immune system. Dendritic cells and M-cells may sample the microbiota present in the mucosa and facilitate in generating oral tolerance to members of the intestinal microbiota and development of the immune system.

With the exception of pathogens, intestinal microbes seem mainly to colonise the mucous layer covering the intestinal epithelium. Probiotics and intestinal pathogens have, for example, been observed to express strain-dependent adhesion to intestinal mucus *in vitro*. The main component of mucus is mucin: a group of glycoproteins excreted by goblet cells that are interspersed between the epithelial cells. In particular, it is the carbohydrate moiety of the molecule that provides receptor sites for microbes. The four primary carbohydrates found in the oligosaccharide moieties of mucin are: *N*-acetylglucosamine, *N*-acetylgalactosamine, fucose and galactose. Mucin oligosaccharide chains are often terminated with sialic acid or sulphate groups (Deplancke & Gaskins 2001).

Oligosaccharides that have similar structures to those found in mucus and in the glycocallix of eukaryotic cells can function as soluble receptor analogues for potential pathogenic microbes, thereby blocking their ability to bind to receptors on host tissues. This has indeed been suggested to be one of the functions of human milk oligosaccharides (Boehm & Stahl 2007). Galacto-oligosaccharides and some other prebiotic substances have also been observed to inhibit the binding of selected pathogens. The question is, however, whether the tested concentrations (16 g/L) have physiological relevance (Shoaf *et al.* 2006). Microbes are also able to bind to fibrous structures from food. Their adhesion to these NSPs improves the ability of the microbes to degrade the fibres. Interestingly, different NSPs appear to be colonised preferably by different microbial communities. Bran was colonised mainly by members of *Clostridium* cluster XIVa (including uncultured bacteria related to *Clostridium hathewayi*, *Eubacterium rectale* and *Roseburia* species). Starch was mainly colonised by uncultured species related to *Ruminococcus bromii*, *Bifidobacterium adolescentis*, *Bifidobacterium breve* and *E. rectale*. The most commonly recovered sequences from mucin were from *Bifidobacterium bifidum* and uncultured bacteria related to *Ruminococcus lactaris* (Leitch *et al.* 2007). The binding property to NSP can also be used for selecting probiotic strains with an affinity to specific prebiotics, e.g. resistant starch, enabling delivery of a combination of pre- and probiotics (Crittenden *et al.* 2001).

5.7 Applications of non-starch polysaccharides in functional foods

As previously described, some NSPs are naturally present in many foods primarily as components of plant cell walls. Cellulose, hemicellulose and pectic substances, for instance, are found in fruit and vegetables, whereas β-glucans are present in cereal grains such as oats and barley. Other NSPs are present in plants and algae or produced by microorganisms that are not traditionally eaten as foods. Many of these have been extracted in purified form for use as gelling and thickening agents and have been used in a wide range of food products for many years (Glicksman 1983; Imeson 1999; Phillips & Williams 2000). This subgroup of NSP is often referred to as hydrocolloids or gums and their functions are summarised in Table 5.2. There is some overlap between the products in terms of functionality, but there is also some specificity as outlined in Table 5.3. More recently, inulin and β-glucans have been available in purified form for use in food products.

The NSPs can be used in two ways in designing functional foods. Firstly, the gums can be used in their traditional sense to stabilise, thicken or gel formulated functional foods. For example, thickeners can be used to replace the mouthfeel lost when sugar is removed from beverages or when fat

Table 5.2 Functionality of non-starch polysaccharides in functional food applications

Functionality	Non-starch polysaccharide
Gelling	Carrageenan, pectin, alginate, xanthan, locust bean gum, agar, gellan gum
Thickening	Xanthan gum, guar gum, locust bean gum, cellulose gum, alginate, carrageenan
Suspension	Xanthan gum, carrageenan, pectin
Emulsification	Gum arabic
Physical stabilisation	Carrageenan, pectin, xanthan gum, cellulose gum, gum arabic
Film formation	Gum arabic, carrageenan, alginate
Mouthfeel	Guar gum, locust bean gum, cellulose gum
Adhesion	Gum arabic
Texturising	All

Table 5.3 Specific functional application of non-starch polysaccharides for functional foods

Non-starch polysaccharide	Specific functionality
Kappa carrageenan	Milk protein reactivity
Cellulose gum, high ester pectin	Protein protection
Alginate	Cold gelation, thermo-irreversibility
Locust bean gum	Synergy with xanthan and kappa carrageenan
Guar gum	Synergy with xanthan gum
Gum arabic	Emulsification, low viscosity
Xanthan gum	Very high low shear viscosity, stability
Gellan gum	Fluid gels

content is reduced. They can also be used to help suspension of added fibre or calcium salts in fortified products.

Secondly, they can be used as the active functional ingredient to provide the physiological benefits described earlier. The increasing trend towards designing functional foods has brought a new focus on NSP and their physiological effects. Traditionally, the gums are used in foods at concentrations well below those required for physiological effects (<1%) to provide mouthfeel, texture and stability. Current European regulations require that a food product contains at least 3g of fibre per 100g or 1.5g of fibre per 100kcal for a claim for it to be a source of fibre. This increases to at least 6g per 100g or 3g per 100kcal for a claim for it to be high in fibre. Simply increasing the concentration of the gum to reach these levels leads to difficulty in processing and undesirable texture due to the high viscosity or gelling properties of the gums. The challenge is to effectively formulate these into appetising food products that are safe and convenient and that provide health benefits for the consumer.

There are essentially two strategies for reducing the impact of high concentrations of gums on food texture and acceptability. The first is to control the molecular weight of the molecule. The second is to control the hydration of the gum in the food product.

The thickening and gelling properties of gums are closely linked to molecular weight and it is generally accepted that, as the molecular weight decreases, thickening and gelling properties decrease (Mitchell 1979). Therefore, by reducing the molecular weight of the polymer, higher concentrations can be added to the food product without decreasing product acceptance. For gums such as pectin, alginate, carrageenan and cellulose derivatives, molecular weight can be controlled to some extent during the normal production process. For other gums such as guar and locust bean gum, which are produced by simple separation from the plant seeds, additional processing with acid or alkali or with specific enzymes is required.

Encapsulation has been used successfully to control the release of ingredients such as flavours and drugs (Ubbink & Kruger 2006) and similar technology can be used to control the hydration of gums. The objective is to delay the hydration of the gum until the desired time. This will be dependent on the application. For example, it may be desirable to minimise hydration during the early part of product preparation to facilitate processing or it may be preferred to limit hydration until the product reaches the stomach. Extrusion technology has also been used to control the dispersion and hydration of gums (Farhat *et al.* 2006; Paeschke & Aimutis 2008). Further development in these areas is needed to provide an effective means of formulating NSPs into food products in sufficient quantities to provide physiological effects.

NSPs such as β-glucans, inulin and polydextrose are not as effective at thickening or gelling as gums and can therefore be used at much higher concentrations without affecting product acceptability. β-Glucans in purified (70–80%) and non-purified (5–10%) form are now available for use in the formulation of functional foods. These can be used in many different applications such as low- or no-fat baked products, and low-fat dressings. The recommended dosage given by the US Food and Drug Administration (FDA) health claim recommendation is 0.75 g of β-glucan per serving and 3 g β-glucan per day for a reduction in LDL cholesterol.

Inulin can be used for sugar reduction in cereal bars, ice cream, chocolate and biscuits, fat replacement in ice cream and meat products, improving the texture of low-fat spreads, mousses and yogurts, fibre enrichment in dairy drinks, cereals and baked goods and for better digestive health in cereals, bakery products and dairy drinks. Inulin has a low molecular weight compared with gums and so does not develop such high viscosity. As a consequence, it is simple to prepare solutions up to 15%. Above this level, it can form a gel or cream, which has been used as a fat replacer (Phillips & Williams 2000).

5.8 Future trends

Non-starch polysaccharides have always been an important part of human nutrition. However, with the introduction of functional foods, their role has been increased. NSPs have important physiological properties, of which the mechanisms are only poorly understood. A better understanding of the physiological properties of NSPs is required for future optimisation of their efficacy. New sources of NSPs, e.g. from side-streams, may become available and enable their potential use in the food industry. Increasing pressure from authorities and consumers for healthy food is likely to increase the role of NSPs as functional ingredients and as technological agents in the reformulation of existing products.

5.9 Sources of further information

Further information on the use and properties of NSPs as prebiotics can be found in the following:

- *Handbook Prebiotics* 2008 Gibson, G.R. and Roberfroid, M. (eds.), CRC Press, Boca Raton, FL.
- *Gastrointestinal Microbiology* 2006 Ouwehand, A.C. and Vaughan, E. (eds.), Taylor and Francis, New York.
- International Probiotic Association (IPA). www.internationalprobiotics.org
- International Scientific Association of Probiotics and Prebiotics (ISAPP). www.isapp.net

5.10 References

ALANDER, M., DE, S., I, NOLLET, L., VERSTRAETE, W., VON WRIGHT, A., & MATTILA-SANDHOLM, T. 1999, 'The effect of probiotic strains on the microbiota of the Simulator of the Human Intestinal Microbial Ecosystem (SHIME)', *Int. J. Food Microbiol.*, vol. 46, no. 1, pp. 71–79.

BARCLAY, A. W., PETOCZ, P., MCMILLAN-PRICE, J., FLOOD, V. M., PRVAN, T., MITCHELL, P., & BRAND-MILLER, J. C. 2008, 'Glycemic index, glycemic load, and chronic disease risk – a metaanalysis of observational studies', *Am. J. Clin. Nutr.*, vol. 87, no. 3, pp. 627–637.

BIELECKA, M., BIEDRZYCKA, E., MAJKOWSKA, A., JUSKIEWICZ, J., & WROBLEWSKA, M. 2002, 'Effect of non-digestible oligosaccharides on gut microecosystem in rats', *Food Res. Int.*, vol. 35, pp. 139–144.

BINGHAM, S. 2006, 'The fibre–folate debate in colo-rectal cancer', *Proc. Nutr. Soc.*, vol. 65, no. 1, pp. 19–23.

BOEHM, G. & STAHL, B. 2007, 'Oligosaccharides from milk', *J. Nutr.*, vol. 137, no. 3 Suppl 2, pp. 847S–849S.

BROWN, G. D., TAYLOR, P. R., REID, D. M., WILLMENT, J. A., WILLIAMS, D. L., MARTINEZ-POMARES, L., WONG, S. Y. C., & GORDON, S. 2002, 'Dectin-1 is a major beta-glucan receptor on macrophages', *J. Exp. Med.*, vol. 196, no. 3, pp. 407–412.

BRUMEL, J. H. & FINLAY, B. B. 2000, 'Bacterial adherence, colonization, and invasion of mucosal surfaces,' in *Virulence Mechanisms of Bacterial Pathogens*, 3rd edn, K. A. Brogden *et al.*, eds., ASM Press, Washington DC, pp. 3–17.

CANI, P. D., DEWEVER, C., & DELZENNE, N. M. 2004, 'Inulin-type fructans modulate gastrointestinal peptides involved in appetite regulation (glucagon-like peptide-1 and ghrelin) in rats', *Br. J. Nutr.*, vol. 92, no. 3, pp. 521–526.

CASCI, T., RASTALL, R. A., & GIBSON, G. R. 2007, *Human Gut Microflora in Health and Disease: Focus on Prebiotics*, in *Functional Foods and Biotechnology*, K. Shetty, G. Paliyat, A. L. Pomelto & R. E. Levin, eds., Taylor and Francis, Oxford, pp. 401–434.

CORREA-MATOS, N. J., DONOVAN, S. M., ISAACSON, R. E., GASKINS, H. R., WHITE, B. A., & TAPPENDEN, K. A. 2003, 'Fermentable fiber reduces recovery time and improves intestinal function in piglets following *Salmonella typhimurium* infection', *J. Nutr.*, vol. 133, no. 6, pp. 1845–1852.

COUDRAY, C., FEILLET-COUDRAY, C., TRESSOL, J. C., GUEUX, E., THIEN, S., JAFFRELO, L., MAZUR, A., & RAYSSIGUIER, Y. 2005, 'Stimulatory effect of inulin on intestinal absorption of calcium and magnesium in rats is modulated by dietary calcium intakes – Short- and long-term balance studies', *European J. Nutr.*, vol. 44, no. 5, pp. 293–302.

CRITTENDEN, R. G., MORRIS, L. F., HARVEY, M. L., TRAN, L. T., MITCHELL, H. L., & PLAYNE, M. J. 2001, 'Selection of a *Bifidobacterium* strain to complement resistant starch in a synbiotic yoghurt', *J. Appl. Microbiol.*, vol. 90, pp. 268–278.

CUMMINGS, J. H. & ENGLYST, H. N. 1991, 'Measurement of starch fermentation in the human large intestine', *Can. J. Physiol. Pharmacol.*, vol. 69, no. 1, pp. 121–129.

CUMMINGS, J. H. & STEPHEN, A. M. 2007, 'Carbohydrate terminology and classification', *Eur. J. Clin. Nutr.*, vol. 61, Suppl 1, pp. S5–18.

CUMMINGS, J. H., BEATTY, E. R., KINGMAN, S. M., BINGHAM, S. A., & ENGLYST, H. N. 1996, 'Digestion and physiological properties of resistant starch in the human large bowel', *Br. J. Nutr.*, vol. 75, no. 5, pp. 733–747.

DELZENNE, N. M., CANI, P. D., & NEYRINCK, A. M. 2007, 'Modulation of glucagon-like peptide 1 and energy metabolism by inulin and oligofructose: experimental data', *J. Nutr.*, vol. 137, no. 11 Suppl, pp. 2547S–2551S.

DEPLANCKE, B. & GASKINS, H. R. 2001, 'Microbial modulation of innate defense: goblet cells and the intestinal mucus layer', *Am. J. Clin. Nutr.*, vol. 73, pp. 1131S–1141S.

DONGOWSKI, G., HUTH, M., GEBHARDT, E., & FLAMME, W. 2002, 'Dietary fiber-rich barley products beneficially affect the intestinal tract of rats', *J. Nutr.*, vol. 132, no. 12, pp. 3704–3714.

EFSA 2007, *Statement of the Scientific Panel on Dietetic Products, Nutrition and Allergies on a Request from the Commission Related to Fibre*, European Food Safety Authority, EFSA-Q-2007–121.

ELIA, M. & CUMMINGS, J. H. 2007, 'Physiological aspects of energy metabolism and gastrointestinal effects of carbohydrates', *European J. Clin. Nutr.*, vol. 61, p. S40–S74.

ENGLYST, H. N. & CUMMINGS, J. H. 1985, 'Digestion of the polysaccharides of some cereal foods in the human small intestine', *Am. J. Clin. Nutr.*, vol. 42, no. 5, pp. 778–787.

ENGLYST, H. N., KINGMAN, S. M., HUDSON, G. J., & CUMMINGS, J. H. 1996, 'Measurement of resistant starch *in vitro* and *in vivo*', *Br. J. Nutr.*, vol. 75, no. 5, pp. 749–755.

ENGLYST, K. N., LIU, S., & ENGLYST, H. N. 2007, 'Nutritional characterization and measurement of dietary carbohydrates', *Eur. J. Clin. Nutr.*, vol. 61 Suppl 1, pp. S19-S39.

FARHAT, I. A., HILL, S. E., MITCHELL, J. R., SCHARF, U. & SERENO, N. M. F. D. 2006, 'Water dispersible xanthan gum composition,' Patent No PCT/WO 2006/065136 A1.

FAVA, F., MAKIVUOKKO, H., SILJANDER-RASI, H., PUTAALA, H., TIIHONEN, K., STOWELL, J., TUOHY, K., GIBSON, G., & RAUTONEN, N. 2007, 'Effect of polydextrose on intestinal microbes and immune functions in pigs', *Br. J. Nutr.*, vol. 98, no. 1, pp. 123–133.

GIBSON, G. R., CUMMINGS, J. H., & MACFARLANE, G. T. 1988, 'Use of a three-stage continuous culture system to study the effect of mucin on dissimilatory sulfate reduction and methanogenesis by mixed populations of human gut bacteria', *Appl. Environ. Microbiol.*, vol. 54, no. 11, pp. 2750–2755.

GLICKSMAN, M. 1983, *Food Hydrocolloids*, Vols I, II and III, CRC Press Inc., Boca Raton, FL.

GRAY, J. 2006, *Dietary Fibre*, 1 edn, ILSI Europe, Brussels.

HAMER, H. M., JONKERS, D., VENEMA, K., VANHOUTVIN, S., TROOST, F. J., & BRUMMER, R. J. 2008, 'Review article: the role of butyrate on colonic function', *Alimentary Pharmacol. Therapeu.*, vol. 27, no. 2, pp. 104–119.

HARA, H., SUZUKI, A., & AOYAMA, Y. 2000, 'Ingestion of the soluble dietary fibre, polydextrose, increases calcium absorption and bone mineralization in normal and total-gastrectomized rats', *Br. J. Nutr.*, vol. 84, pp. 655–661.

HEIJNEN, A. M., BRINK, E. J., LEMMENS, A. G., & BEYNEN, A. C. 1993, 'Ileal pH and apparent absorption of magnesium in rats fed on diets containing either lactose or lactulose', *Br. J. Nutr.*, vol. 70, no. 3, pp. 747–756.

HENNINGSSON, A. M., BJORCK, I. M., & NYMAN, E. M. 2002, 'Combinations of indigestible carbohydrates affect short-chain fatty acid formation in the hindgut of rats', *J. Nutr.*, vol. 132, no. 10, pp. 3098–3104.

HENRIKSSON, A. 2006, 'Animal models for the human gastrointestinal tract,' in *Gastrointestinal Microbiology*, 1st edn, A. Ouwehand & E. E. Vaughan, eds., Francis & Taylor Group, New York, pp. 253–271.

HOAD, C. L., RAYMENT, P., SPILLER, R. C., MARCIANI, L., ALONSO, B. C., TRAYNOR, C., MELA, D. J., PETERS, H. P., & GOWLAND, P. A. 2004, '*In vivo* imaging of intragastric gelation and its effect on satiety in humans', *J. Nutr.*, vol. 134, no. 9, pp. 2293–2300.

HOJSAK, I., JAKLIN KEKEZ, A., & KOLACEK, S. 2007, 'Role of probiotics in the treatment of inflammatory bowel disease (IBD)', *Agrofood Ind. Hi-Tech*, vol. 18, no. 3, pp. 13–16.

HOWLETT, J. & ASHWELL, M. 2008, 'Glycemic response and health: summary of a workshop', *Am. J. Clin. Nutr.*, vol. 87, no. 1, pp. 212S–216S.

IMESON, A. 1999, *Thickening and Gelling Agents for Food*, 2nd edn, Aspen Publishers Inc., Gaithersburg, MD.

ISHIZUKA, S., NAGAI, T., & HARA, H. 2003, 'Reduction of aberrant crypt foci by ingestion of polydextrose in the rat colorectum', *Nutr. Res.*, vol. 23, no. 1, pp. 117–122.

IUB-IUPAC JOINT COMMISSION ON BIOCHEMICAL NOMENCLATURE 1982, 'Polysaccharide nomenclature', *J. Biol. Chem.*, vol. 257, no. 7, pp. 3352–3354.

JIE, Z., BANG-YAO, L., MING-JIE, X., HAI-WEI, L., ZU-KANG, Z., TING-SONG, W., & CRAIG, S. A. S. 2000, 'Studies on the efffects of polydextrose intake on physiologic functions in Chinese people', *Am. J. Clin. Nutr.*, vol. 72, pp. 1503–1509.

JUNTUNEN, K. S., NISKANEN, L. K., LIUKKONEN, K. H., POUTANEN, K. S., HOLST, J. J., & MYKKANEN, H. M. 2002, 'Postprandial glucose, insulin, and incretin responses to grain products in healthy subjects', *Am. J. Clin. Nutr.*, vol. 75, no. 2, pp. 254–262.

JUNTUNEN, M., KIRJAVAINEN, P. V., OUWEHAND, A. C., SALMINEN, S. J., & ISOLAURI, E. 2003, 'Gut microflora changes and probiotics in children in day care centers', *Biosci. Microflora*, vol. 22, pp. 99–107.

KANO, H., KANEKO, T., & KAMINOGAWA, S. 2002, 'Oral intake of *Lactobacillus delbrueckii* subsp *bulgaricus* OLL1073R-1 prevents collagen-induced arthritis in mice', *J. Food Protection*, vol. 65, no. 1, pp. 153–160.

KONTULA, P., JASKARI, J., NOLLET, L., DE, S., I, VON WRIGHT, A., POUTANEN, K., & MATTILA-SANDHOLM, T. 1998, 'The colonization of a simulator of the human intestinal microbial ecosystem by a probiotic strain fed on a fermented oat bran product: effects on the gastrointestinal microbiota', *Appl. Microbiol. Biotechnol.*, vol. 50, no. 2, pp. 246–252.

KRUEGER, M., SCHROEDL, W., ISIK, W., LANGE, W., & HAGEMANN, L. 2002, 'Effects of lactulose on the intestinal microflora of periparturient sows and their piglets', *Eur. J. Nutr.*, vol. 41 Suppl 1, pp. I26–I31.

LAIRON, D., PLAY, B., & JOURDHEUIL-RAHMANI, D. 2007, 'Digestible and indigestible carbohydrates: interactions with postprandial lipid metabolism', *J. Nutr. Biochem.*, vol. 18, no. 4, pp. 217–227.

LEITCH, E. C., WALKER, A. W., DUNCAN, S. H., HOLTROP, G., & FLINT, H. J. 2007, 'Selective colonization of insoluble substrates by human faecal bacteria', *Environ. Microbiol.*, vol. 9, no. 3, pp. 667–679.

LIESE, A. D., SCHULZ, M., FANG, F., WOLEVER, T. M. S., D'AGOSTINO, R. B., SPARKS, K. C., & MAYER-DAVIS, E. J. 2005, 'Dietary glycemic index and glycemic load, carbohydrate and fiber intake, and measures of insulin sensitivity, secretion, and adiposity in the Insulin Resistance Atherosclerosis Study', *Diabetes Care*, vol. 28, no. 12, pp. 2832–2838.

LOPEZ, H. W., LEVRAT, M. A., GUY, C., MESSAGER, A., DEMIGNE, C., & REMESY, C. 1999, 'Effects of soluble corn bran arabinoxylans on cecal digestion, lipid metabolism, and mineral balance (Ca, Mg) in rats', *J. Nutr. Biochem.*, vol. 10, no. 9, pp. 500–509.

MACFARLANE, G. T. & MACFARLANE, S. 2007, 'Models for intestinal fermentation: association between food components, delivery systems, bioavailability and functional interactions in the gut', *Curr. Opin. Biotechnol.*, vol. 18, no. 2, pp. 156–162.

MACFARLANE, G. T., MACFARLANE, S., & GIBSON, G. R. 1998, 'Validation of a three-stage compound continuous culture system for investigating the effect of retention time on the ecology and metabolism of bacteria in the human colon', *Microb. Ecol.*, vol. 35, no. 2, pp. 180–187.

MACFARLANE, S., MACFARLANE, G. T., & CUMMINGS, J. H. 2006, 'Review article: prebiotics in the gastrointestinal tract', *Aliment. Pharmacol. Ther.*, vol. 24, no. 5, pp. 701–714.

MÄKELÄINEN, H., MÄKIVUOKKO, H., SALMINEN, S., RAUTONEN, N., & OUWEHAND, A. C. 2007, 'The effects of polydextrose and xylitol on microbial community and activity in a 4-stage colon simulator', *J. Food Sci.*, vol. 72, no. 5, pp. 153–159.

MÄKIVUOKKO, H. & NURMINEN, P. 2006, '*In vitro* methods to model the gastrointestinal tract,' in *Gastrointestinal Microbiology*, 1st edn, A. C. Ouwehand & E. E. Vaughan, eds., Taylor & Francis Group, New York, pp. 237–252.

MÄKIVUOKKO, H., NURMI, J., NURMINEN, P., STOWELL, J., & RAUTONEN, N. 2005, '*In vitro* effects on polydextrose by colonic bacteria and CaCo-2 cell cyclooxygenase gene expression', *Nutr. Cancer*, vol. 52, no. 1, pp. 94–104.

MÄKIVUOKKO, H., SAARINEN, M., OUWEHAND, A., & RAUTONEN, N. 2006, Effects of lactose on colon microbial community structure and function in a four-stage continuous culture system. *Biosci. Biotechnol. Biochem.*, Vol. 70, pp. 2056–2063.

MANN, J. 2007, 'Dietary carbohydrate: relationship to cardiovascular disease and disorders of carbohydrate metabolism', *European J. Clin. Nutr.*, vol. 61, pp. S100-S111.

MARTINEZ-PUIG, D., PEREZ, J. F., CASTILLO, M., ANDALUZ, A., ANGUITA, M., MORALES, J., & GASA, J. 2003, 'Consumption of raw potato starch increases colon length and fecal excretion of purine bases in growing pigs', *J. Nutr.*, vol. 133, no. 1, pp. 134–139.

MILLER, T. L. & WOLIN, M. J. 1981, 'Fermentation by the human large intestine microbial community in an in vitro semicontinuous culture system', *Appl. Environ. Microbiol.*, vol. 42, no. 3, pp. 400–407.

MINEKUS, M., MARTEAU, P., HAVENAAR, R., & HUIS IN`T VELD, J. H. J. 1995, 'A multicompartmental dynamic computer-controlled model simulating the stomach and small intestine', *ATLA*, vol. 23, pp. 197–209.

MINEKUS, M., SMEETS-PEETERS, M., BERNALIER, A., MAROL-BONNIN, S., HAVENAAR, R., MARTEAU, P., ALRIC, M., FONTY, G., & HUIS IN`T VELD, J. H. J. 1999, 'A computer-controlled system to simulate conditions of the large intestine with peristaltic mixing, water absorption and absorption of fermentation products', *Appl. Microbiol. Biotechnol.*, vol. 53, no. 1, pp. 108–114.

MITCHELL, J. R. 1979, 'Rheology of polysaccharide solutions and gels,' in *Polysaccharides in Foods*, J. M. V. Blanshard and J. R. Mitchell, eds, Butterworth & Co. Ltd, London, pp. 51–52.

MOLLY, K., VANDE, W. M., & VERSTRAETE, W. 1993, 'Development of a 5-step multi-chamber reactor as a simulation of the human intestinal microbial ecosystem', *Appl. Microbiol. Biotechnol.*, vol. 39, no. 2, pp. 254–258.

MORO, G., ARSLANOGLU, S., STAHL, B., JELINEK, J., WAHN, U., & BOEHM, G. 2006, 'A mixture of prebiotic oligosaccharides reduces the incidence of atopic dermatitis during the first six months of age', *Arch. Dis. Child*, vol. 91, no. 10, pp. 814–819.

NEUTRA, M. R., PRINGAULT, E., & KRAEHENBUHL, J. P. 1996, 'Antigen sampling across epithelial barriers and induction of mucosal immune responses', *Annu. Rev. Immunol.*, vol. 14, pp. 275–300.

NILSSON, A. C., OSTMAN, E. M., HOIST, J. J., & BJORCK, I. M. E. 2008, 'Including indigestible carbohydrates in the evening meal of healthy subjects improves glucose tolerance, lowers inflammatory markers, and increases satiety after a subsequent standardized breakfast', *J. Nutr.*, vol. 138, no. 4, pp. 732–739.

OUWEHAND, A. C., MÄKELÄINEN, H., TIIHONEN, K., & RAUTONEN, N. 2006, 'Digestive health,' in *Sweeteners and Sugar Alternatives in Food Technology*, 1st edn, H. Mitchell, ed., Blackwell Publishing Ltd, Oxford, pp. 44–53.

PAESCHKE, T. M. & AIMUTIS, W. R. 2008, 'Controlled hydration of hydrocolloids,' Patent No PCT/WO 2008/045259 A2.

PATSCH, J. R., MIESENBOCK, G., HOPFERWIESER, T., MUHLBERGER, V., KNAPP, E., DUNN, J. K., GOTTO, A. M., & PATSCH, W. 1992, 'Relation of triglyceride-metabolism and coronary-artery disease – studies in the postprandial state', *Arteriosclerosis Thrombosis*, vol. 12, no. 11, pp. 1336–1345.

PEURANEN, S., TIIHONEN, K., APAJALAHTI, J., KETTUNEN, A., SAARINEN, M., & RAUTONEN, N. 2004, 'Combination of polydextrose and lactitol affects microbial ecosystem and immune responses in rat gastrointestinal tract', *Br. J. Nutr.*, vol. 91, no. 6, pp. 905–914.

PHILLIPS, G. O. & WILLIAMS, P. A. 2000, *Handbook of Hydrocolloids*, Woodhead Publishing Ltd, Cambridge.

RAFTER, J., BENNETT, M., CADERNI, G., CLUNE, Y., HUGHES, R., KARLSSON, P. C., KLINDER, A., O'RIORDAN, M., O'SULLIVAN, G. C., POOL-ZOBEL, B., RECHKEMMER, G., ROLLER, M., ROWLAND, I., SALVADORI, M., THIJS, H., VAN LOO, J., WATZL, B., & COLLINS, J. K. 2007, 'Dietary synbiotics reduce cancer risk factors in polypectomized and colon cancer patients', *Am. J. Clin. Nutr.*, vol. 85, no. 2, pp. 488–496.

RUMNEY, C. J. & ROWLAND, I. R. 1992, '*In vivo* and *in vitro* models of the human colonic flora', *Crit. Rev. Food Sci. Nutr.*, vol. 31, no. 4, pp. 299–331.

SANDERSON, I. R. 2007, 'Dietary modulation of GALT', *J. Nutr.*, vol. 137, no. 11, pp. 2557S–2562S.

SCHEPPACH, W. & WEILER, F. 2004, 'The butyrate story: old wine in new bottles', *Curr. Opin. Clin. Nutr. Metab. Care*, vol. 7, pp. 563–567.

SCHEPPACH, W., LUEHRS, H., & MENZEL, T. 2001, 'Beneficial health effects of low-digestible carbohydrate consumption', *Br. J. Nutr.*, vol. 85, no. Suppl. 1, pp. S23–S30.

SHOAF, K., MULVEY, G. L., ARMSTRONG, G. D., & HUTKINS, R. W. 2006, 'Prebiotic galactooligosaccharides reduce adherence of enteropathogenic *Escherichia coli* to tissue culture cells', *Infect. Immun.*, vol. 74, no. 12, pp. 6920–6928.

SILVESTER, K. R., ENGLYST, H. N., & CUMMINGS, J. H. 1995, 'Ileal recovery of starch from whole diets containing resistant starch measured *in vitro* and fermentation of ileal effluent', *Am. J. Clin. Nutr.*, vol. 62, no. 2, pp. 403–411.

SO, J. S., KWON, H. K., LEE, C. G., YI, H. J., PARK, J. A., LIM, S. Y., HWANG, K. C., JEON, Y. H., & IM, S. H. 2008, '*Lactobacillus casei* suppresses experimental arthritis by down-regulating T helper 1 effector functions', *Molecular Immunol.*, vol. 45, no. 9, pp. 2690–2699.

SONOYAMA, K., WATANABE, H., WATANABE, J., YAMAGUCHI, N., YAMASHITA, A., HASHIMOTO, H., KISHINO, E., FUJITA, K., OKADA, M., MORI, S., KITAHATA, S., & KAWABATA, J. 2005, 'Allergic airway eosinophilia is suppressed in ovalbumin-sensitized brown Norway rats fed raffinose and alpha-linked galactooligosaccharide', *J. Nutr.*, vol. 135, no. 3, pp. 538–543.

STEPHEN, A. M., HADDAD, A. C., & PHILLIPS, S. F. 1983, 'Passage of carbohydrate into the colon. Direct measurements in humans', *Gastroenterology*, vol. 85, no. 3, pp. 589–595.

SZAJEWSKA, H., SKORKA, A., RUSZCZYNSKI, M., & GIERUSZCZAK-BIALEK, D. 2007, 'Meta-analysis: *Lactobacillus* GG for treating acute diarrhoea in children', *Aliment. Pharmacol. Ther.*, vol. 25, no. 8, pp. 871–881.

TEN BRUGGENCATE, S. J. M., BOVEE-OUDENHOVEN, I. M. J., LETTINK-WESSINK, M. L. G., & VAN DER MEER, R. 2003, 'Dietary fructo-oligosaccharides dose-dependently increase translocation of *Salmonella* in rats', *J. Nutr.*, vol. 133, pp. 2313–2318.

THEUWISSEN, E. & MENSINK, R. P. 2008, 'Water-soluble dietary fibers and cardiovascular disease', *Physiol. Behav.*, vol. 94, no. 2, pp. 285–292.

UBINK, J. & KRUGER, J. 2006, 'Physical approaches to the delivery of active ingredients in foods,' *Trends Food Sci. Technol.*, vol. 17, pp. 244–254.

VAN DAM, R. M. & SEIDELL, J. C. 2007, 'Carbohydrate intake and obesity', *Eur. J. Clin. Nutr.*, vol. 61 Suppl 1, pp. S75-S99.

VESTERLUND, S., PALTTA, J., KARP, M., & OUWEHAND, A. C. 2005, 'Measurement of bacterial adhesion – *in vitro* evaluation of different methods', *J. Microbiol. Meth.*, vol. 60, pp. 225–233.

WOLEVER, T. M. S., SCHRADE, K. B., VOGT, J. A., TSIHLIAS, E. B., & MCBURNEY, M. I. 2002, 'Do colonic short-chain fatty acids contribute to the long-term adaptation of blood lipids in subjects with type 2 diabetes consuming a high-fiber diet?', *Am. J. Clin. Nutr.*, vol. 75, no. 6, pp. 1023–1030.

WONG, J. M., DE SOUZA, R., KENDALL, C. W., EMAM, A., & JENKINS, D. J. 2006, 'Colonic health: fermentation and short chain fatty acids', *J. Clin. Gastroenterol.*, vol. 40, no. 3, pp. 235–243.

YLONEN, K., SALORANTA, C., KRONBERG-KIPPILA, C., GROOP, L., ARO, A., & VIRTANEN, S. M. 2003, 'Associations of dietary fiber with glucose metabolism in nondiabetic relatives of subjects with type 2 diabetes – The Botnia Dietary Study', *Diabetes Care*, vol. 26, no. 7, pp. 1979–1985.

YOUNES, H., COUDRAY, C., BELLANGER, J., DEMIGNE, C., RAYSSIGUIER, Y., & REMESY, C. 2001, 'Effects of two fermentable carbohydrates (inulin and resistant starch) and their combination on calcium and magnesium balance in rats', *Br. J. Nutr.*, vol. 86, pp. 479–485.

ZAFAR, T. A., WEAVER, C. M., ZHAO, Y., MARTIN, B. R., & WASTNEY, M. E. 2004, 'Nondigestible oligosaccharides increase calcium absorption and suppress bone resorption in ovariectomized rats', *J. Nutr.*, vol. 134, pp. 399–402.

6

Digestion and absorption of proteins and peptides

P. J. Moughan, Riddet Institute, Massey University, New Zealand

Abstract: Aspects of dietary protein quality including the chemical determination of proteins and amino acids, amino acid digestibility and availability and amino acid metabolism are discussed. Information on the role of proteins, peptides and specific amino acids as bioactives is reviewed and the use of proteins, peptides and amino acids in the development of functional foods and nutritionals is introduced.
Key words: protein, amino acids, digestion, absorption, functional foods.

6.1 Introduction

Protein is central to living organisms both structurally and functionally. The mature mammalian body comprises around 16% protein and many regulatory factors, such as enzymes and hormones, are proteins or polypeptides.

Amino acids are the basic building blocks of proteins and, given that there are 20 amino acids commonly used for body protein synthesis, this allows for a myriad of proteins with unique three-dimensional structures and properties. Food proteins not only supply amino acids to allow for the maintenance and growth of proteinaceous structures, but also many amino acids have specific physiological and regulatory functions in their own right. Also, during the digestion of proteins in the alimentary canal, variously sized peptides are released that have a host of physiological effects. It is thus important to have a thorough understanding of the protein and amino acid compositions of foods and as to how proteins are broken down in the digestive tract to allow delivery of amino acids for body protein metabolism.

Of the 20 amino acids deemed to be essential for protein synthesis in animals, some (the dietary essential or indispensable amino acids) must be supplied by the diet pre-formed, while others can be synthesised by the body from other amino acids (transamination or reductive amination) or from simpler precursors (Linder, 1991). Nine amino acids are considered as indispensable in humans (lysine, methionine, threonine, valine, isoleucine, leucine, phenylalanine, tryptophan and histidine). Among these amino acids, lysine and threonine are strictly dietary essential, as there is no precursor allowing for their synthesis after deamination, whereas the remaining dietary essential amino acids can be obtained from their corresponding α-ketoacid and are indispensable for their carbon skeleton. The remaining amino acids are dietary non-essential (arginine, proline, serine, glycine, glutamine, glutamic acid, tyrosine, cysteine, alanine, asparagine and aspartic acid).

Some amino acids normally regarded as being dietary non-essential may become dietary essential under certain metabolic conditions as the cell may not be able to synthesise them at a sufficient rate, and these amino acids are referred to as 'conditionally essential' (Grimble, 1993).

Body proteins are continuously being broken down and replaced (turnover; Schoenheimer, 1942), with an approximate rate of 3–6 grams of protein/kg body weight/day for the adult human. Different body tissues turn over at different rates and body protein turnover is influenced by a number of factors (Waterlow, 2006). It is remarkable to observe, that, in an 80 kg adult human, some 400 grams of body protein are broken down and resynthesised every day, with no long-term change in total body protein. The process of body protein turnover is not completely efficient and there are also losses of body amino acids due to other metabolic processes. The dynamic equilibrium is maintained, of course, by matching losses of body amino acids with intake of dietary protein from food.

In meeting the body's requirement for amino acids, not only the quantity but also the quality of dietary protein is relevant, ushering in the subject of dietary protein quality evaluation (Moughan, 2005a). In a traditional context, dietary protein quality for humans depends upon how closely the array of absorbed dietary amino acids matches the required array of amino acids at the sites of protein synthesis and is thus a function of dietary amino acid composition, dietary amino acid digestibility, amino acid bioavailability and the individual's metabolic requirement for amino acids. These fundamental aspects of protein utilisation are the subject of the following discourse. Quite in addition to its centrality as material for body protein synthesis, dietary protein is important in initiating and maintaining satiety in humans, and many dietary amino acids and peptides have specific biological roles. These latter aspects are also discussed here, before introducing how amino acids, peptides and proteins have been used in the design of functional foods and specialised nutritionals.

6.2 Chemical determination of proteins and amino acids in foods

Amino acids in foods occur as free amino acids or in the form of peptides, proteins or non-peptide bonded polymers. Free amino acids and peptides are particularly important in enhancing flavour, aroma and taste. Free amino acids can be analysed directly after extraction from the food matrix, but hydrolysis is required prior to the analysis of amino acids bound in peptides and proteins.

The crude protein content of foods is calculated based on a determination of the nitrogen present in the food, with the assumption that proteins are the predominant nitrogen-containing compounds in food. Limitations of the crude protein measure are well known (Pomeranz and Meloan, 1980). Whereas crude protein is an important descriptor of foods, more nutritionally – and physiologically – relevant information is given by the food's amino acid composition.

Modern amino acid analysis is capable of providing data with a within-laboratory repeatability of 5% or less, and a reproducibility between laboratories of around 10%. The main methods of amino acid analysis involve acid or alkali hydrolysis of the protein followed by separation and quantification of the released amino acids by ion-exchange, gas-liquid or reverse-phase high-performance liquid chromatography (HPLC). Most of the nutritionally important amino acids can be quantified after acid (hydrochloric) hydrolysis, but separate hydrolysis procedures should be used for methionine, cysteine and tryptophan. Routine amino acid analysis has been in use since the 1950s and in the ensuing decades there has been a very considerable amount of methodological development (Williams, 1988; Rutherfurd and Moughan, 2000; Peace and Gilani, 2005). Despite this, today's methods still bear many of the essential hallmarks of the original Moore and Stein ion exchange chromatography method. Modern liquid chromatography-based methods are faster, more sensitive and more versatile.

Regardless of the method used to separate, derivatise and detect amino acids, a common step faced by the analyst is the conversion from moles of amino acid (as analysed) to a weight basis. It is pertinent to note here that different laboratories adopt different approaches (Rutherfurd and Moughan, 2000), resulting in sizeable differences in the final value calculated. One may view the amino acid after hydrolysis as being present in the free form and use the appropriate molecular weight (including the H_2O added during hydrolysis). Alternatively, the amino acid can be viewed as a constituent of protein (bound) and then the molecular weight used for conversion does not include the molecular weight of water added during hydrolysis.

The hydrolysis step during amino acid analysis is a major source of variation and it has long been recognised that, under standard conditions of hydrolysis (6 M HCl, 110 °C, 24 hr), isoleucine and valine are not fully released from the protein, whereas serine, threonine and other amino acids can be partially destroyed. Thus standard 24 hour hydrolysis amino acid values are approximations. This aspect of amino acid analysis is often overlooked, but can be important where accurate data are required. Accurate estimates of amino acid content can be achieved by using sequential hydrolysis times and by applying curvilinear models of protein hydrolysis (Robel and Crane, 1972). Such techniques have been applied in practice to give accurate absolute data for the amino acid composition of proteins including human milk (Darragh and Moughan, 1998).

Over recent years, interest has turned to determining specific proteins and peptides in foods and physiological fluids including chyme and digesta. Since there may be a large number of different proteins in foods and a potentially huge number of peptides resulting from digestion, their analysis can be an onerous exercise. Consequently, analysis of separation profiles of peptides and proteins is often undertaken rather than the analysis of all individual constituents. Where individual proteins or peptides need to be analysed, however, numerous separation methods are available, including fast protein liquid chromatography (FPLC), HPLC, high-performance capillary electrophoresis (HPCE), gel electrophoresis, chromatofocusing, electrophoresis and gel filtration. Reverse-phase HPLC is the most common method used for peptide separation and liquid chromatography–mass spectrometry (LCMS) allows simultaneous separation and detection. The power of mass spectrometry is being increasingly applied in the field of 'proteomics' to analyse the multitude of proteins present in biological samples simultaneously, in a single analytical platform. Examples of recent work relating to the characterisation of specific food and digesta proteins and peptides are the studies of Salgado *et al.* (2002), Meisel *et al.* (2003) and Fischer *et al.* (2007).

It should be noted that proteomic techniques separate and analyse proteins based on molecular weight and charge, but provide no information on their three-dimensional structure in solution. Protein function is heavily influenced by the three-dimensional structure of the protein, which is modified extensively, post-translationally. The growing field of bioinformatics with computerised databases (Dziuba and Iwaniak, 2006) plays a crucial role in allowing prediction of protein/peptide primary, secondary and tertiary structures as well as deduced functions.

6.3 Protein digestion and amino acid absorption

6.3.1 Overview of digestion

The digestion of food proteins in the alimentary canal is complex, involving interactions among the food matrix, endogenous enzymes, bacterial enzymes and proteinaceous materials secreted and shed into the gut lumen from the gut tissues (endogenous protein). The once held view of digestion as a hydrolytic process occurring solely in the lumen of the stomach and small intestine has been greatly modified. It is now appreciated that protein digestion and amino acid absorption are tightly integrated, implying a highly organised process. The preliminary stages of protein digestion take place in the gut lumen, this being followed by peptide breakdown at the surface or within the enterocyte. Contrary to being essentially a luminal event, digestion can be considered to occur largely at the intestinal surface in close proximity to the sites of absorption. Such a system can be envisaged to facilitate rapid and efficient amino acid absorption. The role of the microflora resident throughout the digestive tract has, in the past, been underemphasised. The microflora play an important part in the digestion of food and the digestion of protein.

Protein digestion and the uptake of amino acids occur throughout the digestive tract. Ingested food is partly broken down by mastication in the mouth and food is mixed with saliva and ingested liquids, creating a medium suitable for the action of digestive enzymes and generating a food bolus that can be swallowed and enter the stomach. Gastric enzymatic digestion of protein is then carried out by the pepsins secreted by the chief cells. The precursors of pepsins, the pepsinogens, are activated by HCl also secreted in the stomach, and the autocatalytic activity of pepsin. The main end product of gastric digestion of proteins is a mixture of proteins and large polypeptides. There is seemingly no absorption of amino acids in the stomach (Zebrowska *et al.*, 1983). Proteins and peptides passing from the stomach are further hydrolysed in the small intestine by enzymes secreted by the pancreas and by intestinal enzymes that are either secreted into the gut lumen, attached to the brush border of the intestine, or are active within the mucosal cells. The pancreatic proteases, secreted as their inactive precursors (zymogens), comprise trypsin, chymotrypsin and elastase (endopeptidases), while the pancreatic exopeptidases comprise carboxypeptidases A and B. The important function of the brush border oliogopeptidases and the intracellular peptidases of the mucosal cells in integrated digestion and absorption has been reviewed by Das and Radhakrishnan (1976). Considerable amounts of amino acids are absorbed as di- and tripeptides, with further intracellular digestion (cytoplasmic aminopeptidases), though some small peptides arising from protein digestion and even small amounts of intact protein may enter the portal circulation directly (Fuller and Tomé, 2005).

In addition to the action of the endogenous enzymes in protein digestion, the proteolytic, deaminative and decarboxylative activities of the intestinal microflora must be considered. Micro-organisms are found throughout the alimentary canal and in particularly high numbers in the large bowel. The microflora undoubtedly play a role in the hydrolysis of proteins during digestion and because of their ability to break down plant fibre (non-starch polysaccharides), afford a greater accessibility of endogenous enzymes to food proteins. Some gut bacteria have ureolytic activity and are involved in body urea recycling. Urea secreted into the intestines from the blood can be synthesised to microbial amino acids or be converted to ammonia and then reabsorbed. It is now clear that gut bacteria in humans can synthesise dietary essential amino acids, which can be absorbed directly and may potentially make a significant contribution towards meeting the metabolic amino acid requirements (Moughan, 2003; Fuller and Tomé, 2005). There is convincing evidence that amino acids are not absorbed as such from the large bowel to any significant extent, so it would appear that the uptake of microbially synthesised amino acids may take place in the small intestine. Although the population of micro-organisms is much lower in the small bowel than in the large bowel, such bacteria have a rapid rate of turnover and may be highly active metabolically.

The metabolic activity of the large intestinal microflora and the observation that amino acids per se are not absorbed in the colon have implications for the determination in practice of protein digestibility. The microflora both degrade and synthesise amino acids extensively in the large intestine. In fact, around 75% of faecal nitrogen is present in microbial bodies (Stephen and Cummings, 1980). The metabolic interference of the microbes and the preponderance of microbial protein in faecal protein mean that only a small proportion of faecal amino acid excretion bears any direct relationship to the flow of undigested amino acids entering the large intestine. With regard to the determination of the digestibility of dietary amino acids, important discrepancies may arise resultant from microbial fermentation in the hindgut. Measurement of amino acids remaining undigested at the end of the small intestine (terminal ileum) is regarded as more appropriate than faecal measurement.

6.3.2 Ileal amino acid digestibility

In monogastric species of animal in general, numerous studies have demonstrated that ileal digestibilities of most amino acids are lower than corresponding digestibilities determined over the entire digestive tract (faecal digestibility). This indicates a net degradation of amino acids in the large intestine. For some amino acids (especially methionine) in some foods, however, a net microbial synthesis is observed. In either case, the faecal digestibility values reflect microbial metabolism rather than being related to absorption of amino acids.

Several studies have been conducted with pigs demonstrating the accuracy of ileal amino acid digestibility values for determining the extent of amino acid uptake from the gut lumen (Moughan, 2003) and the ileal measure is now generally accepted as the most appropriate technique for determining protein and amino acid digestibility.

Ileal digestibility measurement raises the practical problem of how representative samples of digesta flow at the terminal ileum can be obtained. In humans, digesta can be sampled using naso-intestinal intubation (Modigliani *et al.*, 1973) or with the cooperation of ileostomates (Rowan *et al.*, 1994). Neither method can be regarded as routine and for this reason animal models of digestibility have been developed. The growing pig has been shown to be a particularly effective animal model for protein digestion in humans (Moughan *et al.*, 1992, 1994; Rowan *et al.*, 1994). With the pig, digesta may be sampled directly from the intestine from the anaesthetised animal or be collected from animals with surgically implanted gut cannulas.

A consideration when determining ileal amino acid digestibility is the need to correct for ileal endogenous protein. Copious quantities of protein of body origin (endogenous protein) enter the digestive lumen during digestion and although much of this material is digested and reabsorbed, relatively large quantities remain unabsorbed at the terminal ileum. Digestibility should be a measure of ingested amino acids (i.e. diet amino acids in) corrected for undigested dietary amino acids (i.e. diet amino acids out), and thus the endogenous amino acids found in ileal digesta create an artefact. A number of methods have been devised (Moughan, 2003) and can be applied to measure the endogenous protein component and thus make a correction for the endogenous versus undigested dietary amino acid flow. When protein digestibility measures are corrected for the endogenous proteins, they are referred to as 'true' or, when an agreed endogenous correction is used, 'standardised' measures. It is particularly important when determining the protein-digestibility-corrected amino acid score (PDCAAS) for human foods that standardised true ileal digestibility coefficients be used (Darragh *et al.*, 1998).

The sampling of ileal digesta provides data on the digestibility of total nitrogen and amino acids, but also lends itself to the determination of specific proteins, protein fragments and peptides able to withstand digestion in the upper digestive tract. Such compounds found in digesta in small quantities potentially possess bioactive properties (see Section 6.5).

6.3.3 Ileal amino acid digestibility in foods for humans

There is not a great deal of published information on ileal amino acid digestibility determined either directly in humans, or pertaining to human foods determined using animal models. Table 6.1 gives information for some highly and for some more poorly digested protein sources. The true ileal digestibility of crude protein ranged from 51% through 87% to 99%. The variation in actual digestibilities may be greater than that shown in Table 6.1, as many of the more poorly digested vegetable proteins (Gilani *et al.*, 2005) have not yet been subjected to ileal digestibility assay. The data in Table 6.1 also highlight the differences that can occur between the digestibility of protein (total nitrogen) and that of individual amino acids. True ileal amino acid (as opposed to protein) digestibility is the measure of choice for describing the nutritive value of proteins.

Table 6.1 Ileal protein and amino acid digestibility (%) for selected foods

	Mixed diet[1]		Rapeseed isolate[1]	Nutrisoy[2]	Autoclaved Nutrisoy[2]	Soya isolate[3]	Lactic casein[3]	Peas[1]	Lupins[1]	Soya protein isolate[1]	Cows' milk[1]	Cooked egg[1]	Raw egg[1]	Milk[1]	Soya[1]	Soya protein concent rate[1]	Whey protein concent rate[1]
	App	True	True	App	App	True	True	True	True	True	True	True	True	True	True	True	True
Protein	87	98	87	37	77	–	–	89	91	91	96	91	51	95	92	99	98
Arginine	90	98	–	45	90	99	98	–	–	–	–	–	–	–	–	100	99
Histidine	90	99	–	44	83	93	96	–	–	–	–	–	–	95	92	97	89
Isoleucine	91	100	–	40	86	97	95	–	–	–	–	–	–	95	94	97	99
Leucine	92	100	–	37	86	95	99	–	–	–	–	–	–	95	93	97	99
Tryptophan	77	99	–	–	–	–	–	–	–	–	–	–	–	–	–	–	–
Lysine	94	99	–	41	80	99	99	–	–	–	–	–	–	95	95	98	97
Methionine	93	98	–	59	86	100	100	–	–	–	–	–	–	–	–	96	99
Cysteine	86	100	–	35	68	95	99	–	–	–	–	–	–	–	–	99	91
Phenylalanine	90	100	–	39	88	98	100	–	–	–	–	–	–	96	96	97	99
Tyrosine	89	99	–	34	85	99	100	–	–	–	–	–	–	99	97	99	99
Threonine	85	100	–	36	73	92	94	–	–	–	–	–	–	93	89	97	93
Valine	90	100	–	38	84	96	97	–	–	–	–	–	–	96	93	97	98
Glycine	72	92	–	–	–	87	86	–	–	–	–	–	–	92	90	96	98

[1] Human data.
[2] Food grade defatted soya flour (pig data).
[3] Rat data.
App = Apparent.
(Mixed diet, Rowan *et al.*, 1994; rapeseed isolate, AM Deglaire and P J Moughan, unpublished; Nutrisoy and Autoclaved Nutrisoy, from Gilani *et al.*, 2005; soya isolate and lactic casein, Rutherfurd and Moughan, 1998; peas, sweet lupins, soya protein isolate, cows milk, cited by Moughan, 2003; cooked egg and raw egg, Evenepoel *et al.*, 1998; soya protein concentrate and whey protein concentrate, Moughan *et al.*, 2005).

Table 6.2 True ileal digestible total and reactive lysine contents (g/kg air-dry) in selected human foods

	Digestible lysine		% difference
	Total	Reactive[1]	
Heated skim milk powder	19.8	16.6	16
Wheat-based cereal (shredded)	1.3	0.8	39
Corn-based cereal (flaked)	0.4	0.2	50
Rice-based cereal (puffed)	1.1	0.6	46
Mixed cereal (rolled)	3.2	1.9	41

[1] Bioavailable lysine; a difference between total and reactive lysine denotes Maillard damage.
Adapted from Rutherfurd *et al.* 1997, 2006.

6.3.4 Protein-damaged foods

During the processing or prolonged storage of foods, amino acids and especially lysine may undergo structural changes (Moughan, 2003). The presence of such structurally altered amino acids can interfere with conventional methods of amino acid analysis. In brief, early Maillard-type products can revert to the parent amino acid during the strong acid hydrolysis used in amino acid analysis. Such reversion does not occur in the milder acidity of the stomach. This reversion leads to an unpredictable degree of error in the analysis of amino acids both in foods and ileal digesta, and consequently leads to misleading values for amino acid digestibility. For foods whereby protein may have been damaged, specific bioassays based on the measurement of the 'reactive' as opposed to 'total' amounts of an amino acid in the food and digesta have been developed (Moughan and Rutherfurd, 1996). For some human foods, and for the amino acid lysine, nutritionally significant differences have been reported between true ileal digestible 'total' lysine (i.e. conventional methodology) and true ileal digestible 'reactive' lysine (new assay), denoting considerable degrees of Maillard damage (Table 6.2). Such losses of nutritional value may have profound consequences for diets in the developing world, where dietary lysine intakes may be marginal.

6.4 Amino acid metabolism

After their intestinal absorption, dietary amino acids are either used for the synthesis of tissue proteins or as precursors for the synthesis of many nitrogen-containing, sulphur-containing and aromatic compounds with unique biological activities. Amino acids not used for these activities are degraded rapidly, with their nitrogen being released as ammonia or being transferred to keto acids to form alanine, aspartate or glutamate. Ultimately, the nitrogen is incorporated into urea. The carbon skeletons are oxidised directly for energy

Table 6.3 Biological processes underlying amino acid utilisation in the adult human

1. Ingestion of dietary amino acids
2. Amino acid absorption
3. Maintenance processes
• Integumental amino acid loss
• Gut endogenous amino acid loss
• Urinary amino acid loss
• Other miscellaneous amino acid losses
• Synthesis of non-protein nitrogen-containing compounds
• Irreversible modification of amino acids
• Inevitable amino acid catabolism

or are converted to glucose or fatty acids. The balance between the catabolic and anabolic pathways determines the overall dietary nitrogen retention.

Although in reality the absorption and metabolism of amino acids in mammals are complex and highly integrated, with continuous flux within and between body cells, it is useful to conceptualise amino acid metabolism as several discrete physiological processes that underlie or are causative of amino acid utilisation. A concept for amino acid metabolism in the adult human is shown in Table 6.3. For the growing child, net body protein deposition would need to be included, while for pregnant and lactating women, growth of the conceptus and lactational protein synthesis would be additional considerations. The first four maintenance processes listed in Table 6.3 refer to irreversible losses of body amino acids via various routes and are reflective of body protein turnover. The loss of amino acids in the urine and 'other miscellaneous losses' are very small. Integumental losses are small but significant, while gut endogenous amino acid losses are quantitatively important and higher than has been assumed traditionally (Moughan, 2005b). Amino acids are also used to synthesise a wide variety of non-protein compounds essential for normal function (e.g. lysine for carnitine, cysteine for taurine, tryptophan for serotonin and nicotinic acid, arginine for creatine, methionine as a methyl group donor). Further, amino acids may become irreversibly modified and thus unavailable for protein synthesis (e.g. methylation of histidine, methylation and hydroxylation of lysine). These various pathways are expected to constitute a relatively small drain on amino acid fluxes. Of likely greater quantitative significance are the processes described collectively as inevitable amino acid catabolism (Moughan, 2002). This refers to the catabolism of amino acids, not arising from a specific cellular need for energy, or because the amino acid is supplied surplus to metabolic need, but rather because of the very existence of a catabolic machinery. Amino acids enter the free amino acid pool from body protein turnover and from the digestion of food in the digestive tract, and a proportion of the amino acid flux will inevitably be subjected to catabolism. The amino acids of body origin, inevitably catabolised, must be replaced by absorbed dietary amino acids. The degree of inevitable catabolism may be affected by habitual protein intake and thus the set points of the catabolic enzymes.

In humans, food is ingested in discrete meals such that there is a diurnal pattern of food ingestion followed by fasting. This results in prostprandial dietary nitrogen gains followed by postabsorptive body protein losses (Tomé and Bos, 2000). It has been shown, moreover, from phasic studies of body protein turnover (Pacy *et al.*, 1994; Price *et al.*, 1994) that, in the postabsorptive phase, oxidation occurs at a rate determined by the habitual protein intake. This loss has been termed by Millward and co-workers as 'regulatory loss', and the concept of a 'metabolic demand' (obligatory plus regulatory losses) has been extended. The ideas of a 'regulatory loss' of amino acids and that of 'anabolic drive' (Millward and Rivers, 1988; Millward, 1989) assist in providing a biological explanation for 'inevitable catabolism'. The latter authors suggest that there are advantages in consuming amounts of essential amino acids in excess of the amount required to match identifiable needs (obligatory losses), since before their oxidation these amino acids exert a transitory regulating influence (the anabolic drive) on body protein synthesis. Of much recent interest has been the observation (see van Goudoever *et al.*, 2000) that intestinal tissue may be responsible for a not insignificant degree of catabolism of dietary essential amino acids. There appears to be a specific catabolic demand, and 'first-pass' gut amino acid catabolism may contribute to the inevitable catabolism.

Once the metabolic needs (Table 6.3) for amino acids have been met, then surplus absorbed dietary amino acids are oxidised.

6.4.1 Dietary amino acid requirements

The underlying metabolic processes related to body protein maintenance listed in Table 6.3 are what give rise in the adult human to the need for a daily supply of dietary essential amino acids and nitrogen. In the main, the amounts of amino acids and nitrogen required by human subjects have been determined empirically. A common approach has been the conduct of nitrogen balance studies. Determination of the requirement for nitrogen involves a series of studies at different levels of protein intake, each after a period of adaptation to that intake, to find the minimum intake that will produce nitrogen balance. The method has a number of shortcomings (Young *et al.*, 1989). Based on this approach, however, the minimum daily requirement of adult humans for good quality protein is around 0.60 to 0.70 g protein per kg body weight, leading to a current recommended daily allowance of some 0.83 g good quality protein per kg body weight for healthy adult humans. It should be noted that the latter recommendation is for a 'minimal requirement', as individuals are able to adapt metabolically to low dietary protein intakes.

As for protein, the classical approach to determining requirement values for the individual dietary essential amino acids has involved body nitrogen

Table 6.4 Estimates of daily amino acid requirements (mg/kg) for the adult human

	FAO/WHO/UNU (1985)[1]	FAO/WHO/UNU (2007)[2]
Histidine	8–12	10
Isoleucine	10	20
Leucine	14	39
Valine	10	26
Lysine	12	30
Methionine and cysteine	13	15
Phenylalanine and tyrosine	14	25
Threonine	7	15
Tryptophan	3.5	4

[1] Based primarily on N-balance studies.
[2] Estimates revised to account for data from oxidation studies.

balance studies whereby the amount of an amino acid needed to maintain a positive nitrogen balance at a constant balanced total nitrogen intake has been determined. More recently, requirement estimates have been made based on direct or indirect measures of amino acid oxidation and data obtained using these techniques have given rise to much higher estimates of recommended requirement (Table 6.4). In general, the amounts of dietary essential amino acids reported to be required based on amino acid oxidation methods, are some two to three times greater than those calculated based on nitrogen balance. Both empirical approaches can be criticised methodologically (Bos *et al.*, 2000). In the future causation-based models of amino acid metabolism (e.g. Millward and Rivers, 1988) are likely to be developed and will afford a more flexible approach to the estimation of amino acid requirements for humans. Metabolism within and between individuals is highly variable and is affected greatly by both intrinsic and extrinsic factors. Thus amino acid requirements are far from static (Moughan, 2005b).

An important consideration in the estimation of amino acid requirements is the criterion of response. The amounts of amino acid required to maximise muscle function, for example, or to optimise immune responses may be quite different from those needed to achieve nitrogen balance, and future work is likely to emphasise more diverse criteria of response related to longer-term health and optimised organ function.

6.5 Proteins, peptides and amino acids functioning as bioactives

Food proteins provide much more than a supply of amino acids for protein synthesis. Certain proteins, protein fragments, peptides and some free amino acids have specific bioactive properties.

6.5.1 Proteins and protein fragments

A number of native proteins are known to exhibit bioactive properties in the digestive tract. Among these, the antimicrobial activities of immunoglobulins, which may be found in milk, colostrum or animal blood, have been thoroughly researched. Immunoglobins and fragments of the parent immunoglobin molecule are known to resist digestion at least partly (Korhonen and Marnila, 2006) and thus retain biological activity in their passage through the digestive tract. Lactoferrin and its cleaved peptide, lactoferricin, also provide passive and in this case non-specific protection against infection, being active against both bacteria and yeast. The antimicrobial effects may be linked to lactoferrin's ability to bind iron. The bactericidal properties of lactoferrin are often associated with the activities of the milk enzymes lysozyme and lactoperoxidase. Lactoferrin has also been implicated in being involved in cation transport, regulation of immune function and probiotic activity towards Bifidobacteria.

Proteins from plant sources such as phaseolamin, an α-amylase inhibitor from the kidney bean, have found application as digestive (starch) inhibitors. Equally, plant enzymes (e.g. papain from papaya, bromelain from pineapple, actinidin from kiwifruit) have been used as food protein tenderisers, digestive aids and herbal remedies.

Another interesting biological role for protein lies in the area of body weight control and satiety. Dietary protein has specific advantages for inclusion in foods or diets designed for weight loss (Moughan, 2008) and is a satiating nutrient, effective relative to carbohydrate and fat in suppressing voluntary food intake independent of its calorific value (Westerterp-Plantenga and Lejeune, 2005). Whey protein may be particularly satiating.

6.5.2 Bioactive peptides

There has been a considerable research effort, into the bioactive properties of exogenous peptides, and it is now realised that the digestion of food protein gives rise to a myriad of potential bioactivities (see Bos *et al.*, 2000; Rutherfurd-Markwick and Moughan, 2005). Bioactive peptides are generally 3–20 amino acid residues in length and, although both animal and plant proteins are known to contain potential bioactive sequences, most studies to date have involved milk proteins. Bioactive peptides may be present naturally in the food, may be released during the digestion of food protein, or may arise during food processing (e.g. protein hydrolysates, fermented foods).

Bioactive peptides may act as physiological modulators locally in the gut and potentially, systemically. An opioid activity of peptides derived from partial enzymatic digestions of milk proteins and wheat gluten was noted in the late 1970s (Brantl *et al.*, 1979; Ziodrou *et al.*, 1979). Since then, many studies have been undertaken and a large number of bioactive amino acid sequences discovered. It is now understood that bioactive peptides have a

Table 6.5 Some reported physiological effects of natural food-derived peptides

- Modulation of gastrointestinal motility
- Stimulation of secretory processes
- Cholesterol lowering
- Mineral binding and enhanced mineral absorption
- Antimicrobial and antifungal properties
- Immunomodulation
- Antithrombotic activity
- Inhibition of angiotensin converting enzyme (ACE) in the control of hypertension
- Analgesic (pain relief) and other neuroactive effects

wide range of physiological effects, some of which are listed in Table 6.5. Sometimes a peptide may have more than one biological activity. B-casomorphin-7, for example, exhibits opioid, angiotensin converting enzyme inhibitory and immunomodulatory effects (Meisel, 1997).

The generation and identification of bioactive peptides have been performed in a number of ways. Peptides have been produced *in vitro* by enzyme hydrolysis (see Agudelo *et al.*, 2004) and individual peptides isolated and characterised. In some cases peptides have been identified based on comparison of amino acid sequences with those of known biological activity. Identified peptides have been synthesised. *In vivo* studies have been conducted whereby peptides have been isolated from digesta.

Guesdon *et al.* (2006) have recently provided an excellent review on the topic of exogenous opioid peptides, the exorphins. The opioid peptides are known to modulate gastrointestinal function. The authors note that the absorption of peptides larger than di- or tripeptides is usually highly reduced in adults and only the neonatal intestine appears to be permeable to larger food-derived opioid peptides such as the casomorphins. In adults, the intestinal brush border membrane appears to be the main target site for the physiological effects of exogenous opioid peptides. They conclude that there is a growing body of evidence that at least milk proteins and their derivatives serve as more than a food and indeed represent messengers with essential functions.

6.5.3 Specific amino acids

Amino acids may have physiological roles that are unrelated to their direct involvement in protein synthesis. Typically, they are required in small amounts as precursors for the synthesis of other essential compounds or may themselves have a regulatory function. Examples are the role of tryptophan as a precursor for the synthesis of serotonin, potentially impacting mood, sleep and appetite regulation. Arginine leads to the production of nitric oxide. Nitric oxide has several functions including stimulation of the pituitary gland, vasodilation, neurotransmission and immune modulation. The amino acids arginine and leucine are known for their insulinotropic properties. Cysteine is the precursor for taurine, and taurine is abundant in all mammalian cells, particularly neuronal cells, but is not found incorporated in proteins. Taurine is involved in the conjugation of bile acids and plays an important part in the development and maintenance of neuronal and especially retinal cells. Taurine is found in milk, normally in the free form. Cow's milk has low levels of taurine relative to human milk, raising the question as to whether infant formulas based on cow's milk should be supplemented with taurine. Histidine is a precursor for histamine.

Perhaps one of the most studied specific amino acid effects is the role of leucine in regulating the turnover of protein in muscle by inhibiting protein degradation and enhancing protein synthesis (Kimball and Jefferson, 2001). This has led to much interest in the possible use of branch chain amino acids in general and leucine in particular, for metabolic stimulation. It is interesting to note, however, that Waterlow (2006) queries the evidence that leucine acts as a regulator of protein turnover in muscle, at least when given in physiologically normal amounts.

The above are merely selected examples of specific physiological functions of amino acids; there are many others (van de Poll *et al.*, 2006).

6.6 The role of proteins, peptides and amino acids in the development of nutritionals and functional foods

Proteins, often milk proteins but also isolated vegetable proteins (e.g. soya protein isolate), are commonly used to formulate high-value nutritionals for infants or the nutritionally compromised (e.g. elderly, ill, malnourished, individuals recovering from trauma). Peptides and free amino acids also form the basis of highly specialised nutritional preparations for parenteral delivery. Companies such as Abbott and Nutricia market a wide variety of specialised protein-, peptide- or amino acid-based enterals for infants, children and adults. Some of these products are specially formulated for specific medical conditions. Hydrolysates of proteins are used in the manufacture of hypoallergenic formulas and DSM's Pepto Pro® (a mixture of di- and tripeptides) is an example of a peptone that has found wide application in the sports drinks market. DSM has also developed InsuVital™, a preparation of extensively hydrolysed casein, claimed to stimulate the secretion of insulin and targeted at sufferers of Type 2 diabetes. The marketing of nutritionally balanced protein supplements and foods is not a new idea with the brand name Glaxo, for example, originating from New Zealand in the early 1900s. Much unrealised potential exists for developing protein supplements for specific nutritional and health conditions, whereby a particular balance of amino acids may optimise utilisation. The amino acid compositional values given in Table 6.6 serve to highlight the diversity of

Table 6.6 Diversity in the patterns of selected amino acids (expressed relative to lysine base = 100) for a range of milk and animal body proteins

Amino acid	β-Lactoglobulin	α-Lactalbumin	Glyco macro peptide	Whey protein isolate	Muscle	Skin and hair	Liver	Blood
Lysine	100	100	100	100	100	100	100	100
Methionine	28	8	34	33	32	26	31	8
Cysteine	27	53	0	18	15	49	28	15
Arginine	25	10	0	25	77	176	84	47
Histidine	14	27	0	18	43	26	35	75
Isoleucine	59	59	205	50	58	43	65	15
Leucine	130	95	29	124	100	107	128	150
Phenylalanine	31	39	0	32	46	61	69	77
Tyrosine	34	42	0	36	39	37	50	31
Threonine	42	46	288	48	55	63	64	39
Valine	51	39	153	50	58	76	78	96

Adapted from Etzel (2004) and Riis (1983).

amino acid patterns and specific amino acid concentrations available from a range of generally highly digestible natural protein sources.

Whole protein and peptides have also been used to formulate functional foods. The following section provides a brief overview by way of a few selected examples. In general, proteins, peptides and amino acids have been exploited less fully than have some other nutrients and bioactives, in developing functional foods and considerable potential exists for the development of further tailor-made health products.

Functional foods based on bioactive peptides are beginning to appear in the market. The product Recaldent™ contains casein phosphopeptides (CPP) and has been incorporated into chewing gum and gels to assist in the remineralisation of teeth and to protect against tooth decay. Calpis Ltd have brought out a patented milk-derived peptide mixture called AmealPeptide®, which has been clinically shown to assist in blood pressure management.

Even a cursory search on the internet reveals many colostrum products with claims around enhanced immunity, and 'Stollait' milk is sourced from cows that have been regularly vaccinated with antigens (deactivated human pathogens) to produce hyper-immune milk containing antibodies that may confer passive immunity against gut infections. Lactoferrin-supplemented infant formulas and food products are well established and a pepsin hydrolysate of lactoferrin (containing lactoferricin) has been used in infant formulas. There are any number of commercially available foods and beverages based on specific amino acids, peptides or proteins relatively high in particular amino acids and sold around performance and health claims associated with a specific amino acid.

Functional foods are not only developed by adding bioactives to a food matrix, but may also be derived by manipulating the composition of plants and animals, through conventional animal and plant breeding practices, by genetic engineering or by manipulation of the feeding and nutrition of the plant or animal. An example of the latter, is the on-farm production of selenium-enhanced milk (e.g. TATURA-BIO™ Se, Tatura Ltd, Australia), via the nutritional incorporation of selenium into milk protein, a well-digested organic source of selenium. The high-selenium milk can be incorporated into functional foods. An example of the development of a biofortified plant material by genetic means is that of Golden Rice, a variety of rice developed using genetic engineering to contain high levels of β-carotene, a precursor of pro-vitamin A.

Associated with the large number of protein or amino acid-based functional foods is an equally large number of claims, stated or implied, as to effects on health and physiological function. Certainly, not all these claims are adequately 'evidence based', and this should be a matter of concern. If the functional foods industry is to achieve its full potential, it will be critical that regulatory bodies have a clear, consistent and rigorous approach to safety, labelling and health claims issues. There will need to be considerable investment in scientific research to fully establish cause and effect relationships.

Consumer confidence can be eroded by conflicting messages received from the scientific and wider community, underlining the critical role of regulatory authorities in ensuring that sufficient adequate information is available to support sustainable claims. The need for regulatory authorities to be cautious in allowing claims is brought into focus by the recently published conclusion of the American Heart Association (Sacks *et al.*, 2006) that: 'earlier research indicating that soy protein has clinically important favourable effects [decreased blood low-density, lipoprotein cholesterol] as compared with other proteins has not been confirmed'. The US Food and Drug Administration (FDA) had previously (October 1999) approved labelling for foods containing soy protein as protective against heart disease, which in the light of fuller information does not appear to be substantiated. There has been widespread acceptance among consumers of the cholesterol-lowering properties of soy protein, but it would now seem that such an effect is only small even at high intakes of soy protein. There are many other examples in the food and nutrition literature of conflicting information.

6.7 Future trends

Based on the current knowledge base and projections for the worldwide incidence of nutrition-related health disorders, it would seem reasonable to assume that there will be an increasing research emphasis in the medium-term future on the role of proteins, peptides and amino acids in the prevention and treatment of disorders involving the metabolic syndrome. It will be important to understand the role of proteins in developing weight-loss foods, in satiety and for developing low-glycaemic and high-insulinogenic foods and dietary strategems. Higher protein/lower carbohydrate diets have been suggested as being potentially important in the treatment of Type 2 diabetes (Layman and Baum, 2004).

Future work should also emphasise the kinetics of amino acid and peptide uptake vis-à-vis the rates of uptake of other nutrients, allowing a more robust prediction of metabolic outcomes and consequent implications for health. The role of proteins and peptides in influencing stomach emptying rate, digesta transit rate and rate of digestion is of interest.

There is likely to be an increasing recognition of using more advanced health and performance-related response criteria to determine amino acid requirements. Amino acid requirement estimates will become more tailored to specific physiological states (e.g. specific requirements for the elderly or immunologically challenged).

An already very active research front in bioactive peptides will continue into the foreseeable future and increasingly amino acids will be viewed as more than mere substrate for body protein synthesis. An example of a specific amino acid effect attracting much recent attention is that of tryptophan's purported influence on mood.

The effects of dietary amino acids and peptides on gene expression (nutri-genomics) and on the total metabolic cascade (metabolomics) will undoubtedly be buoyant areas for future research.

6.8 Sources of further information and advice

1. FULLER M F and TOME D (2005), '*In vivo* determination of amino acids bioavailability in humans and model animals', *JAOAC Int*, **88**, 923–934.
   An update on the determination of dietary amino acid digestibility and availability.
2. RUTHERFURD S M and MOUGHAN P J (2007), 'Development of a novel bioassay for determining the available lysine content of foods and feedstuffs', *Nutr Res Revs*, **20**, 3–16.
   Implications of chemical alterations to amino acids, sustained during food processing or storage, to the determination of amino acid digestibility.
3. VAN DE POLL M C G, LUIKING Y C, DEJONG C H C and SOETERS P B (2006), 'Amino acids – specific functions'. *Encyclopedia of Human Nutrition*, Boston, MA, Elsevier/Academic Press, 92–100.
   An excellent summary of specific metabolic functions of amino acids and their intermediate products.
4. MARIOTTI F, HUNEAU J-F, MAHÉ S and TOMÉ D (2000), 'Protein metabolism and the gut', *Curr Op Clin Nutr Metab Care*, **3**, 45–50.
   Discussion of the recently appreciated central role of the gut tissues in body protein metabolism.
5. ANDERSON G H and MOORE S E (2004), 'Dietary proteins in the regulation of food intake and body weight in humans', *J Nutr,* **134**, 974S–979S.
   The role of dietary protein in satiety and weight-loss.
6. WOLFE R (2006), 'The underappreciated role of muscle in health and disease', *Am J Clin Nutr*, **84**, 475–482.
   The importance of muscle metabolism in health and disease to overall body protein metabolism, and raising questions concerning relevant end points for recommendations for dietary nutrient intakes.
7. CLARE D A and SWAISGOOD H E (2000) Bioactive milk peptides: a prospectus. *J Dairy Sci*, **83**, 1187–1195.
   An insight into the myriad physiological effects of bioactive peptides from foods.
8. YOUNG V R (2002) '2001 W O Atwater Memorial Lecture and the 2001 ASNS President's Lecture: Human nutrient requirements: The challenge of the post-genome era', *J Nutr*, **132**, 621–629.

A thought-provoking article on the relevance of genomics and proteomics to nutritional research in general and nutrient requirement estimation in particular.

6.9 References

AGUDELO R A, GAUTHIER S F, POULIOT Y, MARIN J and SAVOIE L (2004), 'Kinetics of peptide fraction release during *in vitro* digestion of casein', *J Sci Fd Agric*, **84**, 325–332.

BOS C, GAUDICHON C and TOMÉ D (2000), 'Nutritional and physiological criteria in the assessment of milk protein quality for humans', *J Am Coll Nutr*, **19**, 191S–205S.

BRANTL V H, TESCHEMACHER H, BLASIG J, HENSCHEN A and LOTTSPEICH F (1979), 'Novel opioid peptides derived from casein (-casorphins), I. Isolation from bovine casein peptone'. *Hoppe-Seyler's Z. Physiol Chem*, **360**, 1211–1216.

DARRAGH A J and MOUGHAN P J (1998), 'The amino acid composition of human milk corrected for amino acid digestibility', *Br J Nutr*, **80**, 25–34.

DARRAGH A J, SCHAAFSMA G and MOUGHAN P J (1998), 'Impact of amino acid availability on the protein digestibility corrected amino acid score', *Bull Int Dairy Federation*, **336**, 46–50.

DAS M and RADHAKRISHNAN A N (1976), 'Role of peptidases and peptide transport in the intestinal absorption of proteins', *Wld Rev Nutr Diet*, **24**, 58–87.

DZIUBA J and IWANIAK A (2006), 'Database of protein and bioactive peptide sequences', in Mine Y and Shahidi F, *Nutraceutical Proteins and Peptides in Health and Disease*, Boca Raton, FL, CRC Press, 543–563.

ETZEL M R (2004), 'Manufacture and use of dairy protein fractions', *J Nutr*, **134**, 996S–1002S.

EVENEPOEL P, GEYPENS B, LUYPAERTS A, HIELE M, GHOOS Y and RUTGEERTS P (1998), 'Digestibility of cooked and raw egg protein in humans as assessed by stable isotope techniques', *J Nutr*, **128**, 1716–1722.

FAO/WHO/UNU (1985), *Energy and Protein Requirements*, Report of a Joint FAO/WHO/UNU Expert Consultation, WHO Technical Report Series No. 724, Geneva, World Health Organization.

FAO/WHO/UNU (2007), *Protein and Amino Acid Requirements in Human Nutrition*, Report of a Joint FAO/WHO/UNU Expert Consultation, WHO Technical Report Series No. 935, Geneva, World Health Organization.

FISCHER M, VORAGEN A G J, PIERSMA S R, KOFOD L V, JOERGENSEN C I, GUGGENBUHL P, NUNES C S and GRUPPEN H (2007), 'Presence of indigestible peptide aggregates of soybean meal in pig ileal digesta residue', *J Sci Fd Agric*, **87**, 2229–2238.

FULLER M F and TOMÉ D (2005), '*In vivo* determination of amino acid bioavailability in humans and model animals', *J AOAC Int*, **88**, 923–934.

GILANI G S, COCKELL K A and SEPEHR E (2005), 'Effects of antinutritional factors on protein digestibility and amino acid availability in foods', *J AOAC Int*, **88**, 967–987.

GRIMBLE G K (1993), 'Essential and conditionally-essential nutrients in clinical nutrition', *Nut Res Rev*, **6**, 97–119.

GUESDON B, PICHON L and TOMÉ D (2006), 'Opioid peptides', in Mine Y and Shahidi F, *Nutraceutical Proteins and Peptides in Health and Disease*, Boca Raton, FL, CRC Press, 367–376.

KIMBALL S R and JEFFERSON L S (2001), 'Regulation of protein synthesis by branched-chain amino acids', *Curr Opin Clin Nutr Metab Care*, **4**, 39–43.

KORHONEN H and MARNILA P (2006), 'Bovine milk antibodies for protection against microbial human diseases', in Mine Y and Shahidi F, *Nutraceutical Proteins and Peptides in Health and Disease*, Boca Raton, FL, CRC Press, 137–159.

LAYMAN D K and BAUM J I (2004), 'Dietary protein impact on glycemic control during weight loss', *J Nutr*, **134**, 968S–973S.
LINDER M C (1991), 'Nutrition and metabolism of proteins', in Linder M C, *Nutritional Biochemistry and Metabolism*, Second Edition, New York, Elsevier, 87–109.
MEISEL H (1997), 'Biochemical properties of regulatory peptides derived from milk proteins', *Biopolymers*, **43**, 119–128.
MEISEL H, BERNARD H, FAIRWEATHER-TAIT S, FITZGERALD R J, HARTMANN R, LANE C N, MCDONAGH D, TEUCHER B and WAL J M (2003), 'Detection of casein-phosphopeptides in the distal ileostomy fluid of human subjects', *Br J Nutr*, **89**, 351–358.
MILLWARD D J (1989), 'The endocrine response to dietary protein: the anabolic drive on growth', in Barth C A and Schlimme E, *Milk Proteins*, Darmstadt, Steinkopff, 49–61.
MILLWARD D J and RIVERS J P W (1988), 'The nutritional role of indispensable amino acids and the metabolic basis for their requirements', *Eur J Clin Nutr*, **42**, 367–393.
MODIGLIANI R, RAMBAUD J C and BERNIER J J (1973), 'The method of intraluminal perfusion of the human small intestine I. Principles and technique', *Digestion*, **9**, 176–192.
MOUGHAN P J (2002), 'Simulating the partitioning of dietary amino acids: new directions', *J Anim Sci*, **81**, E60–E67.
MOUGHAN P J (2003), 'Amino acid availability: aspects of chemical analysis and bioassay methodology', *Nutr Res Rev*, **16**, 127–141.
MOUGHAN P J (2005a), 'Dietary protein quality in humans – an overview', *J AOAC Int*, **88**, 874–876.
MOUGHAN P J (2005b), 'Physiological processes underlying the dietary amino acid requirement in humans. The role of the gut', in Vorster H H, Blaauw R, Dhansay M A, Kuzwayo P M N, Moeng T L and Wentzel-Viljoen E, *Proceedings of the 18th International Congress of Nutrition – Nutrition Safari for Innovative Solutions*, Durban, South Africa, 10pp (available on CD).
MOUGHAN P J (2008), 'Milk proteins – a cornucopia for developing functional foods', in Thompson A, Singh H and Boland M, *Milk Proteins: From Expression to Food*, London, Elsevier, 483–499.
MOUGHAN P J and RUTHERFURD S M (1996), 'A new method for determining digestible reactive lysine in foods', *J Agric Fd Chem*, **44**, 2202–2209.
MOUGHAN P J, BIRTLES M J, CRANWELL P D, SMITH W C and PEDRAZA M (1992), 'The piglet as a model animal for studying aspects of digestion and absorption in milk-fed human infants', *Wld Rev Nutr Diet*, **67**, 40–113.
MOUGHAN P J, CRANWELL P D, DARRAGH A J and ROWAN A M (1994), 'The domestic pig as a model animal for studying digestion in humans', in Souffrant W B and Hagemeister H, *Proceedings of the VIth International Symposium on Digestive Physiology in Pigs*, Dummerstorf, Germany, EAAP, 389–396.
MOUGHAN, P J, BUTTS C A, VAN WIJK H, ROWAN A M and REYNOLDS G W (2005), 'An acute ileal amino acid digestibility assay is a valid procedure for use in human ileostomates', *J Nutr*, **135**, 404–409.
PACY P J, PRICE G M, HALLIDAY D, QUEVEDO M R and MILLWARD D J (1994), 'Nitrogen homeostasis in man: the diurnal responses of protein synthesis and degradation and amino acid oxidation to diets with increasing protein intakes', *Clin Sci*, **86**, 103–118.
PEACE R W and GILANI S G (2005), 'Chromatographic determination of amino acids in foods', *J AOAC Int*, **88**, 877–887.
POMERANZ Y and MELOAN C E (1980), 'Nitrogenous compounds', in Pomeranz Y and Meloan C E, *Food Analysis, Theory and Practice*, revised edition, Westport, CT, AVI, 668–691.

PRICE G M, HALLIDAY D, PACY P J, QUEVEDO M R and MILLWARD D J (1994), 'Nitrogen homeostasis in man: influence of protein intake on the amplitude of diurnal cycling of body nitrogen', *Clin Sci*, **86**, 91–102.

RIIS P M (1983), 'The pools of tissue constitutents and products: proteins', in Riis P M, *World Animal Science (3) Dynamic Biochemistry of Animal Production*, Amsterdam, Elsevier, 75–103.

ROBEL E J and CRANE A B (1972), 'An accurate method for correcting unknown amino acid losses from protein hydrolysates', *Anal Biochem*, **48**, 233–246.

ROWAN A M, MOUGHAN P J, WILSON M N, MAHER K and TASMAN-JONES C (1994), 'Comparison of the ileal and faecal digestibility of dietary amino acids in adult humans and evaluation of the pig as a model animal for digestion studies in man', *Br J Nutr*, **71**, 29–42.

RUTHERFURD S M and MOUGHAN P J (1998), 'The digestible amino acid composition of several milk proteins: application of a new bioassay', *J Dairy Sci*, **81**, 909–917.

RUTHERFURD S M and MOUGHAN P J (2000), 'Developments in the determination of protein and amino acids', in Moughan P J, Verstegen M W A and Visser-Reyneveld M I, *Feed Evaluation – Principles and Practice*, Wageningen, The Netherlands, Wageningen Pers, 45–56.

RUTHERFURD S M, MOUGHAN P J and VAN OSCH L (1997), 'Digestible reactive lysine in processed feedstuffs: application of a new bioassay', *J Agric Fd Chem*, **45**, 1189–1194.

RUTHERFURD S M, TORBATINEJAD N M and MOUGHAN P J (2006), 'Available (ileal digestible reactive) lysine in selected cereal-based food products', *J Agric Fd Chem*, **54**, 9453–9457.

RUTHERFURD-MARKWICK K and MOUGHAN P J (2005), 'Bioactive peptides derived from food', *J AOAC Int*, **88**, 955–966.

SACKS F M, LICHTENSTEIN A, VAN HORN L, HARRIS W, KRIS-ETHERTON P and WINSTON M (2006), 'Soy protein, isoflavones, and cardiovascular health': An American Heart Association Science Advisory for Professionals from the Nutrition Committee, *Circulation*, **113**, 1034–1044.

SALGADO P, MONTAGNE L, FREIRE J P, FERREIRA R B, TEIXEIRA A, BENTO O, ABREU M C, TOULLEC R and LALLÈS J P (2002), 'Legume grains enhance ileal losses of specific endogenous serine-protease proteins in weaned pigs', *J Nutr*, **132**, 1913–1920.

SCHOENHEIMER R (1942), *The Dynamic State of Body Constituents*, Cambridge, MA, Harvard University Press.

STEPHEN A M and CUMMINGS J H (1980), 'The microbial contribution to human faecal mass', *J Med Micro*, **13**, 45–56.

TOMÉ D and BOS C (2000), 'Dietary protein and nitrogen utilization', *J Nutr*, **130**, 1868S–1873S.

VAN DE POLL M C G, LUIKING Y C, DEJONG C H C and SOETERS P B (2006), 'Amino acids – specific functions', *Encyclopedia of Human Nutrition*, Boston, MA, Elsevier/Academic Press, 92–100.

VAN GOUDOEVER J B, STOLL B, HENRY J F, BURRIN D G and REEDS P J (2000), 'Adaptive regulation of intestinal lysine metabolism', *Proc Natl Acad Sci*, **97**, 11620–11625.

WATERLOW J C (2006), *Protein Turnover*, Wallingford, UK, CABI.

WESTERTERP-PLANTENGA M S and LEJEUNE M P G M (2005), 'Protein intake and body-weight regulation', *Appetite*, **45**, 187–190.

WILLIAMS A P (1988) 'Determination of amino acids', in Macrae R, *HPLC in Food Analysis*, London, Academic Press, 441–470.

YOUNG, V R, BIER D M and PELLETT P L (1989), 'A theoretical basis for increasing current estimates of the amino acid requirements in adult man, with experimental support', *Am J Clin Nutr*, **50**, 80–92.

ZEBROWSKA T, LOW A G and ZEBROWSKA H (1983), 'Studies on gastric digestion of protein and carbohydrate, gastric secretion and exocrine pancreatic secretion in the growing pig', *Br J Nutr*, **49**, 401–410.

ZIOUDROU C, STREATY R A and KLEE W A (1979), 'Opioid peptides derived from food proteins, the exorphins', *J Biol Chem*, **254**, 2446–2449.

7

Digestion and absorption of lipophilic food micronutrients

M. J. Amiot-Carlin, INSERM, France

Abstract/Key words: This chapter reviews the intake and health benefits of lipophilic micronutrients: vitamins A, E, D and K, carotenoids and phytosterols.

7.1 Introduction

Lipophilic food micronutrients are characterized by octanol–water partition coefficients $\log_{10} p_C > 0$ (Cooper *et al.*, 1997). They are divided into two main classes: micronutrients including vitamins A, D, E and K (Fig. 7.1) and several classes of microconstituents (Fig. 7.2). Among microconstituents, the main lipophilic classes are carotenoids and phytosterols. These microconstituents are also called non-essential micronutrients because no deficiency has been evidenced in relation to the development of pathologies. However, carotenoids and phytosterols, especially in plant-derived foods, have been shown to display beneficial roles to prevent several degenerative chronic diseases. Fat-soluble vitamins (A, E, D and K), carotenoids and phytosterols are highly lipophilic and are characterized by $\log_{10} p_C$ values > 7.6 (Table 7.1). It has been shown that molecules with a $\log_{10} p_C > 7.6$ are incorporated in oil and could behave similarly in the gastrointestinal tract and probably share common transport and regulation pathways.

7.2 Liposoluble micronutrients: main roles, food sources, recommended dietary allowance or adequate intake

7.2.1 Vitamin A and provitaminic A carotenoids

Vitamin A is required for normal vision, gene expression, reproduction, embryonic development and immune function.

The recommended dietary allowance (RDA), or adequate intake (AI), ranges from 300 to 1300 μg/day. Vitamin A has two main origins. The first

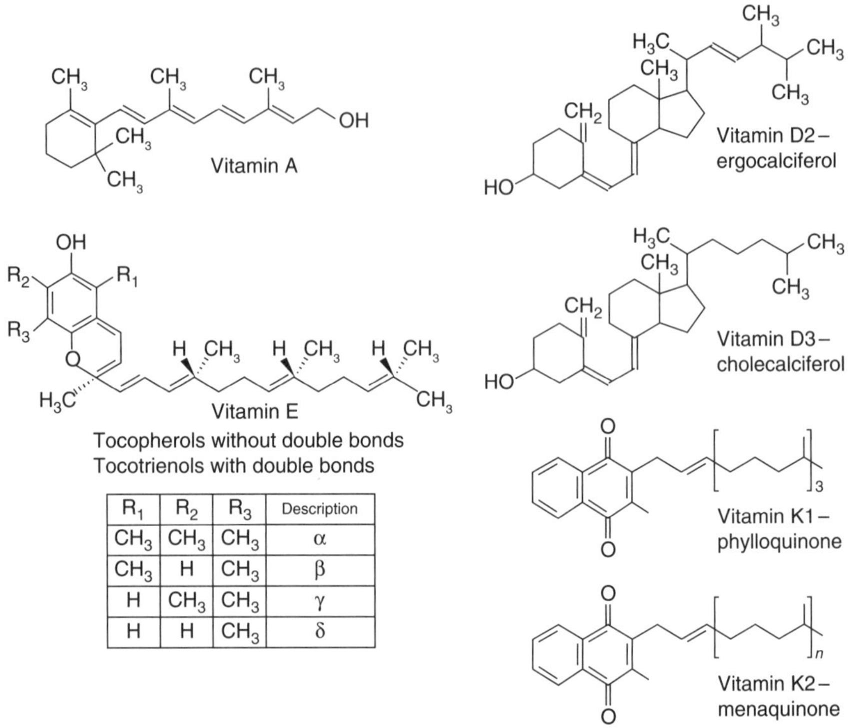

R_1	R_2	R_3	Description
CH_3	CH_3	CH_3	α
CH_3	H	CH_3	β
H	CH_3	CH_3	γ
H	H	CH_3	δ

Fig. 7.1 Structures of liposoluble vitamins.

one is preformed vitamin A, mostly found as retinyl palmitate in liver, dairy products and fish. The second form comes from the provitaminic A carotenoids, present in numerous orange-coloured fruit (mangos, oranges, papaya, apricots), vegetables (carrots, pumpkin, corn, squash, green leafy vegetables) and red palm oil. Carotenoids are lipid-soluble plant pigments containing at least 40 carbons and an extensive conjugated double bond system. Carotenoids are either oxygenated (sub-class of xanthophylls) or non-oxygenated (sub-class of carotenes). Among carotenoids, beta-carotene, alpha-carotene and beta-cryptoxanthin display a provitaminic activity. Because xanthophylls are oxygenated carotenoids, they can be found in plant tissue as esters (conjugated with fatty acids), but also as free forms. Carrots, squash, sweet potato, and spinach are abundant in both beta- and alpha-carotene, and orange is rich in beta-cryptoxanthin.

7.2.2 Vitamin D

Vitamin D is the generic name for compounds exhibiting the biological activity of cholecalciferol (vitamin D3). Vitamin D and its metabolites are essential micronutrients for the skeletal development.

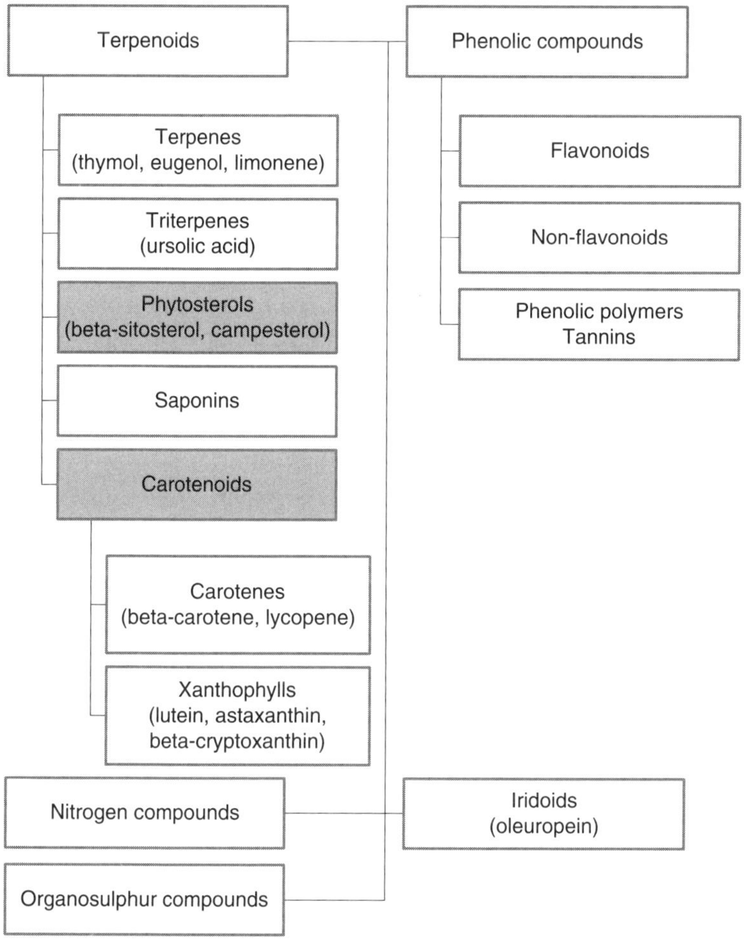

Fig. 7.2 Different classes of non-essential micronutrients.

Table 7.1 Octanol–water partition coefficients ($\log_{10} p_C$) of liposoluble micronutrients (data compiled by Cooper *et al.* 1997)

Micronutrients	$\log_{10} p_C$
α-Carotene	17.6
β-Carotene	17.6
Lycopene	17.6
Zeaxanthin	15.0
Lutein	14.8
α-Tocopherol	12.2
Phylloquinone	11.7
Ergocalciferol	10.4
Retinol	7.6

The RDA remains difficult to determine, and adequate intake values were established in 1997 in order to maintain serum 25(OH)D levels of at least 37.5 nmol/L (15 ng/mL). Thus, AI is 5 μg/day (200 IU) for infants, children and adults until 50 years of age. Intakes are higher from 50 to 70 years (10 μg/day) and 15 μg/day (600 IU) are recommended for people over 70. For pregnant and breast-feeding women, the RDA is 5 μg/day (200 IU) for all ages. Vitamin D3 (cholecalciferol) is the main dietary source of vitamin D provided by the consumption of animal-derived food products, whereas vitamin D2 (ergocalciferol) is present in plants subjected to UV irradiation. Vitamin D3 is also endogenously synthesized by the skin from 7-dehydrocholesterol under the action of sunlight (UVB radiation). Thus, UVB exposure varies according to season, geographic latitude, time of day, etc. affecting vitamin D synthesis in the skin, and it is important for individuals with limited sun exposure to include good dietary sources of vitamin D. For numerous reasons, older people tend to have reduced endogenous production of the vitamin, and thus depend on dietary sources in order to maintain adequate vitamin D status.

7.2.3 Vitamin E

Vitamin E is the name given to a family of eight molecules, named tocopherols and tocotrienols, each structure consisting of a chromanol ring with an aliphatic side chain that is either saturated in the tocopherol group or unsaturated in the tocotrienol group. In each group, there are four isomers, alpha, beta, delta and gamma, corresponding to the methyl substitution of the chromanol ring. Naturally these molecules are found as D-stereoisomers and are not esterified. In our diet, the most commonly found isomers are alpha and gamma tocopherols.

The RDA for vitamin E as *RRR*-alpha-tocopherol (D-alpha-tocopherol) ranges from 5 mg/day (7.5 IU) for infants to 15 mg/day for adults (22.5 IU). RDA reaches 19 mg (28.5 IU) for breast-feeding women. Dietary vitamin E is obtained mainly from plant sources, including sunflower seeds, olive oil and almonds. However, alpha-tocopherol is the main form in supplements and synthetic vitamin E is mostly found as a mixture of esterified stereoisomers as acetate or succinate.

7.2.4 Vitamin K

Vitamin K is used as a generic descriptor of 2-methyl-1,4-naphthoquinone and all its derivatives. In animals fed a vitamin K-deficient diet, this vitamin was shown to exhibit anti-haemorrhagic activity. There are two forms of vitamin K corresponding to the two origins: phylloquinone (vitamin K1) from plants and the menaquinones (vitamin K2) that are bacterially synthesized. Menaquinones are essentially produced by the gut microflora, and a small quantity is found in some foods such as cheeses.

7.2.5 Non-provitaminic A carotenoids

As previously mentioned, carotenoids are the widest distributed group of pigments and occur naturally in large quantities; they are structural diversity, and perform various functions (Fraser and Bramley, 2004). Carotenoids are also important natural sources of orange, yellow and red food colouring for the food and beverage industries. Among non-provitaminic A carotenoids, lycopene and lutein have been particularly studied during the past decade. Dietary supplements providing purified carotenoids and combinations of carotenoids are commercially available.

Lycopene is the predominant nonpolar bioactive carotenoid, mainly provided by the consumption of tomato-derived products. Lycopene is the major pigment in tomatoes and is one of the major carotenoids in the human diet. It has a long hydrocarbon chain with 11 conjugated double bonds, conferring on the one hand easy oxidation in the presence of oxygen and, on the other, isomerisation to *cis* compounds under heat treatment. It must be underlined that lycopene is more stable in the presence of other compounds normally present in tomatoes.

Lutein is a major pigment of many plants. It displays a structure similar to β-carotene with a hydroxyl group on the ionone ring at each end of the molecule and is the major xanthophyll in green and yellow leafy vegetables, such as kale, spinach, mustard greens and green beans. Interest in this carotenoid is growing because it selectively accumulates in the retina and is able to protect photoreceptors against light-initiated oxidative damage and has been associated with a low incidence of age-related macular degeneration (ARMD; Granado *et al.*, 2003). Thus, supplements based on lutein-rich marigold extracts are offered on the market. Apart from the applications to prevent ARMD, new applications are emerging in cosmetics, skin care and, more generally as an antioxidant.

Another xanthophyll lacking provitaminic A activity but being the subject of increasing interest is astaxanthin, which possesses oxygen in its chemical structure. It is naturally derived for commercial use from the microalga *Haematococcus pluralis*. Astaxanthin is a well-known carotenoid that has been marketed as a dietary supplement in Japan and Europe since the late 1990s.

It must be underlined that numerous carotenoids are used as food additives, and thus are mentioned in food products by the E number (E160d: lycopene; E161b: lutein).

7.2.6 Phytosterols

Plant sterols and their conjugated forms (esters and glycosides) are structurally similar to cholesterol. Because of their structural homology with cholesterol and thus their competition with dietary cholesterol in limiting its absorption, an interest in these phytochemicals has grown in developing phytosterol-enriched food products for their hypocholesterolaemic effects (Ostlund, 2002a,b; Tapiero *et al.*, 2003).

In a normal diet, the best food sources include nuts, seeds, unrefined plant oils and legumes. The most common dietary phytosterols are beta-sitosterol, campesterol and stigmasterol. The saturated derivatives of plant sterols are plant stanols, the most common being sitostanol and campestanol. Plant stanols occur naturally in wood pulp, tall oil and soybean oil, but are most commonly obtained in the diet by chemical hydrogenation of plant sterols. Phytosterol intake accounts for 20–25% of the total dietary sterol and greatly differs between non-vegetarians (around 250 mg/day) and vegetarians (over 500 mg/day). Western diets contain approximately 20–50 mg plant stanols. Such an intake remains lower than the recommendation of 2 g that could be reached by enriched food products to achieve a hypocholesterolaemic effect.

7.3 Health roles of liposoluble vitamins, carotenoids and phytosterols

7.3.1 Vitamin A

Combating vitamin A deficiency remains one of the main public health priorities in developing countries. The major consequence of vitamin A deficiency is ocular, with abnormal dark adaptation (night blindness), conjunctival and corneal xerosis (thickening), which can lead to blindness. Besides the vitamin A role in vision, its supplementation was shown to partially improve immune function (Lin *et al.*, 2007). Vitamin A supplementation has been found to decrease both the severity and incidence of deaths related to diarrhoea and measles in developing countries (West, 2000). In addition, it has been reported that children who are only mildly deficient in vitamin A have a higher incidence of respiratory disease and diarrhoea as well as a higher rate of mortality from infectious disease compared with children who consume sufficient vitamin A (Field *et al.*, 2002). However, controversial results have been obtained for vitamin A supplementation in reducing the mother-to-child transmission of HIV.

7.3.2 Vitamin D

Vitamin D deficiency in children leads to rickets and in adults to osteomalacia, both of which are disorders of bone. Numerous epidemiological studies suggest that exposure to sunlight, which enhances the production of vitamin D3 in the skin, is important in preventing many chronic diseases (Holick, 2004). Because very few foods naturally contain vitamin D, sunlight supplies most of our vitamin D requirement. 25-Hydroxyvitamin D or 25(OH)D is the metabolite that should be measured in the blood to determine vitamin D status. A circulating level of 25(OH)D $>$ 75 nmol/L, or 30 ng/mL, is required to maximize the health beneficial effects of vitamin D (Holick and Chen, 2008). In the absence of adequate sun exposure, at least

800–1000 IU vitamin D3/day may be needed to achieve this in children and adults. Vitamin D2 may be equally effective for maintaining circulating concentrations of 25(OH)D when given in physiological concentrations.

More recently, it has been reviewed that low 25(OH)D levels are associated with the cardiovascular disease (CVD) risk factors of hypertension, obesity, diabetes mellitus and the metabolic syndrome, as well as CVD events including stroke and congestive heart failure (Michos and Melamed, 2008). This suggests that vitamin D deficiency may be a contributor to the development of cardiovascular disease potentially through associations with diabetes or hypertension.

In a meta-analysis examining the risk of dying from any cause (Autier and Gandini, 2007) following a vitamin D supplementation and including 18 independent randomized controlled trials with 57 311 participants, the authors reported that intake of ordinary doses of vitamin D supplements seems to be associated with decreases in total mortality rates. Concerning bone health, based on a meta-analysis, Jackson *et al.* (2007) reported a trend towards a reduction in the risk of fall among patients treated with cholecalciferol (vitamin D3) alone compared with placebo. Thus, in order to prevent osteoporosis of older people, vitamin D supplements or vitamin D-enriched food products, in combination with calcium or not, are recommended. However, it is important to redefine the adequate intake of vitamin D for its skeletal roles, taking into account the prevention of hypocalcaemia and toxicity.

7.3.3 Vitamin E

Numerous epidemiological studies have evaluated potential relationships between vitamin E intake and CVD. In several cohort studies involving dietary consumption of vitamin E by food and/or supplements, risk reductions against CVD were observed: the Health Professionals Follow-up Study (Rimm *et al.*, 1993), the Finnish study for women consuming high amounts of vitamin E (Knekt *et al.*, 1994), the Nurses Health study (Stampfer *et al.*, 1993). In the prospective cohort study of 29 092 Finnish male smokers aged 50–69 years (in the Alpha-Tocopherol, Beta-Carotene (ATBC) Cancer Prevention), higher circulating concentrations of alpha-tocopherol within the normal range appeared associated with significantly lower total and cause-specific mortality in older male smokers (Wright *et al.*, 2006). However, in the SENECA study (Survey in Europe on Nutrition and the Elderly, a Concerted Action) including 1168 elderly men and women, plasma concentrations of alpha-tocopherol were not associated with all-cause or cause-specific mortality after a follow-up period of 10 years (Buijsse *et al.*, 2005).

In the excellent meta-analysis recently published by Bjelakovic *et al.* (2007), the authors reported that vitamin E given singly or with other antioxidants did not influence mortality, but when high-bias risk trials were excluded, vitamin E given singly or with other antioxidants significantly increased mortality. Based on the meta-analysis of clinical trials aiming to evaluate the safety and the efficacy of vitamin E supplementation in the prevention of degenerative diseases (Pham and Plakogiannis, 2005a), the available data do not also support the supplementation of vitamin E in cardiovascular disease and cancer prevention. Concerning neurodegenerative diseases (Alzheimer's disease, Parkinson's disease, tardive dyskinesia), and cataract, a reasonable dose of vitamin E (20 mg/day) may be beneficial (Pham and Plakogiannis, 2005b). For all degenerative diseases, high doses of vitamin E supplements should be avoided. This is in agreement with the meta-analysis published by Miller *et al.* (2005), who also reported a possible increase of all-cause mortality with high-dosage vitamin E supplementation.

7.3.4 Vitamin K

Low dietary vitamin K intake has been associated with an increased risk of hip fracture in men and women. In a sub-cohort of participants of the Framingham Heart Study (1996–2000), low dietary vitamin K intake was shown to be associated with low bone mineral density, (Booth *et al.*, 2003). More recently, the same team reported that higher dihydrophylloquinone (a form of vitamin K) intakes are associated with lower bone mineral density in men and women (Troy *et al.*, 2007). Moreover, Yoshida *et al.* (2008) recently found a potential benefit of phylloquinone in glucose homeostasis.

7.3.5 Carotenoids

Numerous epidemiological studies on cardiovascular diseases have been realized in the aim to investigate the relation between carotenoids and CVD, including coronary accident risk and stroke, as rewieved by Tavani and La Vecchia (1999) and Rao (2002). As recently reported by Voutilainen *et al.* (2006), observational studies appeared to converge towards a protective effect of carotenoids on myocardial infarction and stroke, but also on some atherosclerosis markers such as intima media thickness of the common carotid artery or atheromatic plaques formation. Among the 27 observational studies referred, 19 showed an inverse association between some carotenoids and CVD, taking into account dietary intake (6/8 studies) or carotenoids as biomarkers in plasma or serum concentration (11/12 studies), or adipose tissue level (2/2 studies) (Amiot-Carlin *et al.*, 2007).

Intervention trials investigating the effect of β-carotene or lycopene supplementation on CVD have not, however, reported convincing results. Among the seven studies reviewed herein, four primary prevention trials, namely the Multicenter Skin Cancer Prevention Study (Greenberg *et al.*, 1996), the Beta Carotene and Retinol Efficacy Trial (Omenn *et al.*, 1996), the ATBC cancer prevention study (Virtamo *et al.*, 1998), and the Physicians' Health study (Hennekens *et al.*, 1996) have shown no association between a supplementation of β-carotene and risk of death with CVD or non-fatal and fatal myocardial infarction. Recently, findings from the ATBC cancer prevention study even showed that β-carotene supplementation increased the post-trial risk of a first-ever nonfatal myocardial infarction (Tornwall *et al.*, 2004). The Heart Protection Study (2002) also reported significantly increased risk of a fatal coronary event in the β-carotene-supplemented group. Concerning the effect of carotenoids on CVD biomarkers, results from clinical trials are controversial. So, although numerous epidemiological studies reported a protective effect of β-carotene on CVD risk or CVD biomarkers, clinical trials did not agree with this trend. This divergence may depend on several factors. For example, in observational studies, β-carotene is essentially an indicator of a diet rich in fruit and vegetables, which also contain other protective bioactive substances (vitamins, minerals). Thus, in this case, the protective effect of β-carotene may be due to the consumption of β-carotene-rich foods rather than β-carotene alone. So, this compound could act in synergy with and be complementary to other carotenoids or vitamins or polyphenols. Moreover, it is also possible that carotenoids could prevent cellular damage at physiological concentrations, but that their ability to protect against cellular damage disappears at the higher doses used in the supplementation studies (Voutilainen *et al.*, 2006). It was shown by El-Agamey *et al.* (2004) that high doses of carotenoids could produce pro-oxidant effects.

Age-related ocular diseases, such as cataract and ARMD, the leading cause of irreversible blindness, are common problems in the elderly population of western countries. These diseases are thought to result from damages caused, photochemically and nonphotochemically, by oxidative stress to various cell types in the eye (Cruickshanks *et al.*, 1993). The antioxidant properties of lutein and zeaxanthin, recently reviewed by Young and Lowe (2001), may reduce the degree to which oxidative damage promotes these diseases. Otherwise, because these carotenoids also absorb blue light, they may reduce photochemical damage that would otherwise occur in the retina when exposed to light of these wavelengths (Landrum *et al.*, 1997). Eye tissue concentration of lutein/zeaxanthin could reach 1 mmol/l, this concentration being 500 times higher than in other tissues (Schmitz *et al.*, 1993).

7.3.6 Phytosterols

Several clinical trials have demonstrated that a supplementation of plant sterols or stanols can reduce cholesterol absorption (Law, 2000; Volpe *et al.*, 2001; Mensink *et al.*, 2002; Clifton *et al.*, 2004; Thomsen *et al.*, 2004; Korpela *et al.*, 2006). In general, to reduce low-density lipoprotein cholesterol (LDL-C) by 9% to 14%, the recommendation is a daily intake of 2 g of phytosterol, which cannot be reached with a normal diet which generally contains less than 300 mg/day as recently estimated by Jimenez-Escrig *et al.* (2006) and Hearty *et al.* (2008) in two European countries.

7.4 Main biochemical functions of lipophilic micronutrients

In addition to their roles as vitamins, fat-soluble vitamins were shown to display diverse biological actions at different target sites.

Vitamin A, including vitamin A provided by carotenoids, is an essential micronutrient for epithelial cell maintenance, and repair in the respiratory, urinary and intestinal tract, immune response and bone growth and development, vision and immunity (Reichrath *et al.*, 2007). The vitamin A derivative retinoic acid and related compounds (retinoids) are signalling molecules involved in a diverse array of developmental and physiological regulatory processes. Retinoids (retinol, retinal, retinoic acid) interact with receptors of the nuclear receptor family, which act in the nucleus as transcription factors and also mediate the effects of steroid and thyroid hormones.

Vitamin D in humans is essential to regulate calcium and phosphorus metabolism, by promoting their intestinal absorption, and the re-absorption of calcium in kidneys. In addition, the parathyroid glands sense the serum calcium level, and secrete parathyroid hormone (PTH) that promotes the production of calcitriol, the biologically active form of vitamin D3. Increased calcitriol production restores normal serum calcium levels. Many of the biological effects of vitamin D are mediated through the nuclear transcription factor VDR (vitamin D receptor). Vitamin D hormone, $1{,}25(OH)_2D$, associates with VDR and promotes its association with RXR (retinoic acid X receptor). In the presence of $1{,}25(OH)_2D$, the VDR/RXR complex binds VDREs (vitamin D response elements) found in numerous target genes related to calcemic and non-calcaemic functions (deLuca, 2004). As recently reviewed, the functions of vitamin D extend beyond bone to include immune system regulation and anti-proliferative effects on cells (Hewison, 2008).

Vitamin E was thought for years to display only radical scavenging properties, in particular counteracting the oxidation of low-density lipoprotein, suggesting its major preventing role against atherosclerosis. More recently, vitamin E was shown to have non-antioxidant functions including cell signalling and gene regulatory functions (Zingg and Azzi, 2004; Azzi, 2007). Alpha-tocopherol inhibits protein kinase C, 5-lipoxygenase and phospholipase A2 and activates protein phosphatase 2A and diacylglycerol kinase, at the posttranslational level. Some genes (e.g. scavenger receptors, alpha-TTP, alpha-tropomyosin, matrix metalloproteinase-19 and collagenase) are modulated by alpha-tocopherol at the transcriptional level.

Vitamin K is receiving more attention in relation to its role in bone metabolism. Vitamin K is a coenzyme for glutamate carboxylase, which mediates the conversion of glutamate to gamma-carboxyglutamate. Gamma-carboxy glutamic acid (Gla) residues were first identified in prothrombin and coagulation factors in the 1970s; subsequently, extra-hepatic Gla proteins were described, including osteocalcin and matrix Gla protein (MGP). The gamma-carboxylation of the Gla proteins, such as osteocalcin, is essential for the proteins to attract Ca^{2+} and to incorporate these into hydroxyapatite crystals (Bügel, 2008).

Carotenoids are then able to inactivate reactive oxygen species (Krinsky and Yeum, 2003) such as singlet molecular oxygen ($^1O_2$) and peroxyl radicals particularly and protect cellular systems from oxidation. Thus, lutein and zeaxanthin, which mainly accumulate in the macula of the human retina, may be protective against age-related eye diseases. Zeaxanthin is specifically concentrated in the macula, especially in the fovea. Lutein is distributed throughout the retina. The protective effect of lutein and zeaxanthin is due in part to the ability to quench reactive oxygen species and filter out high-energy blue light. By filtering blue light, these pigments protect underlying cell layers from potential light damage. It has been shown that these xanthophylls are located in domains formed from unsaturated lipids suggesting that they could act as antioxidant against lipid oxidation, a mechanism through which lutein and zeaxanthin protect the retina from age-related macular diseases.

The most potent antioxidant among various carotenoids is lycopene (Kris-Etherton *et al.*, 2002; Bhuvaneswari and Nagini, 2005). Lycopene can trap singlet oxygen and reduce mutagenesis in the Ames test. Besides these actions, lycopene was shown to display numerous biological effects, involving anti-inflammatory, antimutagenic and anticarcinogenic activities contributing to the health benefit of lycopene (Heber and Lu, 2002). Lycopene at physiological concentrations can inhibit human cancer cell growth (Wertz *et al.*, 2004). The mechanisms include inhibition of prostatic IGF-I signalling, IL-6 expression and androgen signalling. Moreover, lycopene improves gap-junctional communication, through the up-regulation of connexin 43 and induces phase II drug metabolizing enzymes as well as oxidative defence genes. Interestingly, it has been shown that a combination of low concentrations of lycopene with 1,25-dihydroxyvitamin D exhibits a synergistic effect on cell proliferation and differentiation (Amir *et al.*, 1999). Other potential mechanisms such as stimulation of xenobiotic metabolism, inhibition of cholesterogenesis, modulation of cyclooxygenase pathways and inhibition of inflammation will be considered (Elliott, 2005).

7.5 Bioavailability

Bioavailability is commonly defined as the fraction of ingested lipophilic micronutrient that is absorbed and is available in the bloodstream for mobilization in normal physiological functions and for storage. The bioavailability term covers three main process steps after ingestion. The first one is the bioaccessibility step consisting of the release from the food matrix and its solubilization in the gut lumen. The second one covers the absorption step, which comprises the uptake by intestinal cells followed by the micronutrient secretion into blood circulation. The third is the circulation of micronutrient in the bloodstream and its delivery to different target tissues. During the different steps, micronutrients could be metabolized and metabolites could also display biological actions.

7.5.1 Human assays

Approaches to assess bioavailability

In the **total plasma response approach**, the bioavailability of a micronutrient is determined by measuring its plasma concentrations at different times after single or long-term ingestion of the micronutrient from food meals or from supplements. A curve of 'concentration versus time' is thus obtained allowing the determination of the area-under-curve (AUC) value, which is used as an indicator of the micronutrient absorption. Generally, a relative bioavailability is determined by the comparison of two or more treatments.

The **postprandial chylomicron response approach** is only used for liposoluble micronutrients that follow the same lymphatic route to be transported to the liver. Thus, the bioavailability of the micronutrient is determined by measuring its appearance – or the appearance of metabolites formed at intestinal level – in the postprandial chylomicron fraction of plasma. As previously reported in the plasma response approach, AUC values can be determined from chylomicron curves.

More recent approaches using **stable isotopes** followed in plasma or chylomicrons, faeces or urine samples by mass spectral analysis are promising methods to determine absolute absorption.

Bioavailability data from human studies

Widely variable data have been reported for the absorption efficiency of numerous micronutrients in humans. For vitamin A, retinol absorption efficiency was from 75% (Biesalski, 1997) to almost 100% (Sivakumar and Reddy, 1972); for β-carotene its absorption was shown to range from 3.5% to 90% (Novotny *et al.*, 1995; O'Neill and Thurnham, 1998) and for vitamin E (α-tocopherol) from 10% to 95% (Cohn, 1997; Traber and Sies, 1996). Such discrepancies could be explained by the differences of doses, the formulations given (pills, food products, etc.) and models commonly used to test absorption (postprandial chylomicron response, stable isotopes, ileostomy subjects). Thus, absorption efficiency of vitamin D is not accurately known, but the absorption efficiency of vitamin D3 given as peanut oil is close to 100% in control subjects, while it is only 55% for patients with intestinal malabsorption. It has been reported that the absorption efficiency of natural vitamin K, e.g., vitamin K1 supplied in vegetables, is apparently lower than given as pharmaceutical preparation (Gijsbers *et al.*, 1996). The absorption efficiency of phylloquinone given as a supplement is apparently relatively high, because healthy subjects excrete less than 20% of a 1 mg dose of radiolabelled phylloquinone (Shearer *et al.*, 1974).

7.5.2 Molecular mechanisms governing bioavailability

Models for assessing the bioavailability of liposoluble micronutrients

In addition to animal models, an *in vitro* model was set up, giving promising results. In a first step the model simulates the gastric and duodenal process and evaluates the micellarization of liposoluble micronutrient from a test meal. The amount of micellarized micronutrients is used to estimate bioaccessibility (bioaccessibility of a liposoluble nutrient is the proportion of this micronutrient extracted from food matrix and solubilized in mixed micelles). In a second step, the model uses Caco-2 cells to mimic intestinal uptake. This model was recently used to study the bioavailability of carotenoids and vitamin E (Reboul *et al.*, 2005a, 2006b; Dhuique-Mayer *et al.*, 2007).

Behaviour of lipophilic micronutrients before absorption

At the stomach and duodenum levels, data are scarce on the fate of numerous lipophilic micronutrients. In the stomach, alpha-tocopherol as free form appeared not degraded (Borel *et al.*, 2001), but the hydrolysis of vitamin E esters commonly found in supplements remains unknown. It could be suggested that gastric lipase can cleave esters. By contrast in duodenum, numerous esters could be hydrolysed. Thus, esters of vitamin E were hydrolysed (Borel *et al.*, 2001); sterol and stanol esters were also found hydrolysed in the human upper intestine (Nissinen *et al.*, 2002). However, the hydrolytic enzyme mainly involved remains not determined. Carboxyl ester hydrolase was reported as the enzyme involved in hydrolysis of xanthophyll esters (Breithaupt *et al.*, 2002; Chitchuroonchokchai and Failla, 2006). In the duodenum it is assumed that vitamin D3 esters, if present, are hydrolysed by bile salt-stimulated lipase (Lombardo *et al.*, 1980). Although it has been shown *in vitro* that bile salt-stimulated lipase is able to hydrolyse retinyl esters (Lombardo *et al.*, 1980), more recent studies have shown *in vivo* that this lipase is not significantly involved in the hydrolysis of retinyl palmitate (Weng *et al.*, 1999) and that pancreatic lipase is certainly the main enzyme that hydrolyses this form of vitamin A (Van Bennekum *et al.*, 2000). More recently, it has been shown that classical pancreatic lipase and pancreatic lipase-related proteins 2 were capable of hydrolysing retinyl palmitate in the duodenum, which is the site of pancreatic and biliary secretions (Reboul *et al.*, 2006b). Thus, it is assumed that liposoluble micronutrients as free forms are transferred into micelles before their absorption by intestinal cells.

Absorption molecular mechanisms

Concerning vitamin A, retinol is thought either to be passively diffused, especially at supra-nutritional levels, or to be taken up through a carrier-mediated facilitated mechanism (Noy and Blaner, 1991; Dew and Ong, 1994). For a long time, it was assumed that carotenoids were absorbed by a passive mechanism. However, recent data suggest that carotenoid uptake as well as vitamin E uptake is mediated by the apical transporter Scavenger Receptor class B type I or SR-BI (Borel *et al.*, 2005; Reboul *et al.*, 2006a,b). The involvement of SR-BI in carotenoid uptake was recently confirmed by During and Harrison (2007), while retinol was shown by the same authors to enter intestinal cells by diffusion. They also reported that retinol efflux could occur via the basolateral transporter ABCA1.

Whereas vitamin D is absorbed according to a non-saturable passive mechanism (Hollander *et al.*, 1978), vitamin K1 absorption appears to be mediated by an energy-requiring saturable transport mechanism and vitamin K2 is apparently passively absorbed (Hollander and Rim, 1976; Hollander *et al.*, 1977). However, the possible involvement of transporters in the absorption of these two vitamins should be explored.

Concerning phytosterols, their uptake by enterocytes is apparently energy-independent and facilitated in a similar mechanism to cholesterol, through the involvement of SRBI. In a recent study, Yamanashi *et al.* (2007) demonstrated in CaCo-2 cells that the uptakes of both cholesterol and beta-sitosterol are increased by NPC1L1 overexpression at the apical side. Because very low absorption values of phytosterols ranging from 0.04% to 1.9% have been reported, it is suggested that the limited absorption of phytosterols could be due to the involvement of the two ATP-Binding Cassette (ABC) proteins ABCG5 and ABCG8 responsible for the efflux of phytosterol back to the lumen (Ostlund, 2002a,b; Sudhop *et al.*, 2005).

7.5.3 Factors affecting the bioavailability of the lipophilic micronutrient: food matrix, nutrigenetics

Factors affecting liposoluble micronutrient could be divided into three main categories: the chemical structure, the environment and the individual.

Chemical structure

Hydroxyvitamin D3 was reported to be more bioavailable than vitamin D, either as cholecalciferol or as ergocalciferol (Stamp *et al.*, 1977). Apparently, the study conducted by Traber *et al.* (1992) reports no discrimination between three labelled tocopherols tested (d6-RRR-alpha-tocopheryl acetate, d3-SRR-alpha-tocopheryl acetate, d2-RRR-gamma-tocopherol) during absorption and secretion in chylomicrons, but a preferential enrichment of very low density lipoprotein (VLDL) with RRR-alpha-tocopherol was shown. Apparently absorption of tocotrienols was found similar than tocopherols, but plasma levels were reported to reach 1 μmol/L in humans, which are lower than tocopherol levels (Schaffer *et al.*, 2005). The lower levels of tocotrienols are certainly due to their higher degradation compared with tocopherols.

It has been reported that the bioavailability of carotenoids is related to their polarity (Borel *et al.*, 1998; Reboul *et al.*, 2005b). Borel *et al.* (1996) have reported that more apolar carotenoids are preferentially located in the triacylglycerol core of lipid droplets, while more polar carotenoids such as lutein reside near the surface. In that case, the more apolar lycopene is less available than carotenes, which are less available than xanthophylls. Moreover, lycopene *cis*-isomers are apparently more available than all-*trans* lycopene, because of their probable better transfer into micelles (Boileau *et al.*, 2002). The recent study carried by Unlu *et al.* (2007) confirms a better bioavailability of lycopene in subjects given a tomato sauce rich in lycopene *cis*-isomers.

Because esters of xanthophylls are widely distributed in nature in plant-derived food products, we recently conducted a study in order to evaluate the bioavailability of esters of beta-cryptoxanthin present in citrus juices, by using the '*in vitro* digestion process model coupled to CaCo-2 cell culture' previously described (Dhuique-Mayer *et al.*, 2007). The results showed a preferential uptake of free beta-cryptoxanthin compared to its esters. However, it is supposed that esters are hydrolysed before their micellar uptake by enterocyte. Such hydrolysis is supported by recent data showing no difference in terms of bioavailability between lutein and esters of lutein (Bowen *et al.*, 2002).

Phytosterol are more absorbed than their reduced forms phytostanols: 0.51% for sitosterol versus 0.04% for sitostanol. A ratio close to 10 was also obtained for campesterol versus campestanol (Ostlund *et al.*, 2002a,b).

Environment

Because liposoluble micronutrients can share similar mechanisms of transport and regulation, their interactions could modulate their bioavailability. In general, high doses of a liposoluble micronutrient impair the bioavailability of another one taken at nutritional quantities. In a recent study, plant sterols as free or esters were shown to reduce beta-carotene absorption by 50% (Richelle *et al.*, 2004). Surprisingly, in the same study, whereas plant sterol esters reduced alpha-tocopherol absorption by 20%, free sterols were without effects. The mechanisms for the reductions in the absorption of beta-carotene and alpha-tocopherol by plant sterols and sterol esters were not investigated, but the findings suggest that liposoluble nutrient absorption may be modulated by ABC transporters, nuclear receptors and intracellular trafficking proteins.

Concerning other micronutrients, data are scarce and there is a lack of knowledge to specify the major interactions modulating the bioavailability of liposoluble micronutrients. However, numerous publications reported sparing effects of hydrosoluble dietary components on liposoluble ones. Sparing effects of ascorbic acid and selenium on alpha-tocopherol were recently reported in guinea pig tissues (Bertinato *et al.*, 2007). Tanumihardjo and Dosti (2005) reported that lutein was absorbed faster with simultaneous supplementation of vitamin C, but vitamins C and E did not significantly affect its bioavailability. The absence of effects of vitamin C and E on lutein bioavailability was confirmed in our recent study (Reboul *et al.*, 2007a), whereas lutein absorption was impaired by other carotenoids and the aglycone flavanone naringenin. Naringenin, carotenoids and probably gamma-tocopherol were shown to impair alpha-tocopherol absorption, whereas vitamin C, gallic and caffeic acids (two phenolics) were without effect (Reboul *et al.*, 2007b).

Concerning the influence of macronutrients, it has been reported that lipids and fibres can modulate the bioavailability of liposoluble micronutrients (Borel, 2003). Different mechanisms by which lipids could improve the bioavailability of liposoluble micronutrients were suggested: a better solubilization of liposoluble micronutrient from food matrix to lipidic phase, an increase of their micellarization by a higher micelle production following biliary secretion stimulation, an increase of their incorporation into chylomicrons subsequently by inducing chylomicron synthesis by lipids. Dietary fibres were suspected to affect the absorption of liposoluble micronutrient though several mechanisms: (i) by affecting micelle formation, (ii) by inhibiting lipases and thus affecting the release of liposoluble micronutrients embedded in fat droplets and (iii) by increasing the viscosity of the chyme and thus limiting the diffusion of micelles rich in liposoluble micronutrient to the brush border.

The individual

Numerous human studies report a great variability of micronutrient status, and besides age, sex and physiological state, genetic factors are thought to greatly influence the bioavailability of liposoluble micronutrients. The main documented genetic effect concerns sitosterolaemia (Lee *et al.*, 2001; Kidambi and Patel, 2008). In sitosterolaemia, a rare autosomal recessive disorder, affected individuals hyperabsorb and retain not only cholesterol but also all other sterols, including plant sterols from the intestine. This disorder is caused by mutations in the ABC proteins ABCG5 and ABCG8, which are expressed in the intestine and liver. These mutations increased the net absorption of phytosterols by decreasing the excretion of absorbed phytosterols toward the duodenal lumen.

In a recent work published in our laboratories by Borel *et al.* (2007), the authors suggest that genes involved in lipid metabolism influence the plasma concentrations of liposoluble micronutrients. Genes were genotyped (single nucleotide polymorphisms or SNP): apolipoprotein (apo) A-IV, apo B, apo E, lipoprotein lipase and scavenger-receptor class B type I (SR-BI). Plasma liposoluble micronutrient (alpha-tocopherol, beta-carotene, beta-cryptoxanthin and lycopene) concentrations were significantly different in subjects bearing different SNP in SR-BI. Differences were also evidenced for apo A-IV, apo B, apo E polymorphisms.

It is known that patients suffering from cholestatic liver disease or from cystic fibrosis malabsorb essential fatty acids and liposoluble micronutrients. Strategies able to equilibrate the body level in micronutrients are necessary to prevent dysfunctions or complications associated with micronutrient deficiency. The development of 'intelligent' vectors capable of modulating intracellular distribution of a bioactive micronutrient is an interesting approach.

7.6 Future trends

To warrant the health benefits of liposoluble vitamins and non-essential micronutrients, it is necessary to get more available data based on clinical trials and mechanistic studies. For example, vitamin D (cholecalciferol) supplementation in improving cardiovascular disease risk factors could support potential new application areas. Two areas deserve new application perspectives for liposoluble vitamins: (i) in the prevention of various aspects of neurodegenerative or neuroimmune diseases and (ii) in the early life stages. In fact, vitamin D inadequacy is implicated in the risk of bone disease, autoimmune disease and certain cancers later in life; however, long-term interventional studies do not exist to validate adequate vitamin D intake.

Concerning mechanisms, studies are needed to elucidate health effects at a molecular level. The mechanisms by which liposoluble vitamins are bioactive must be revisited, and to explore gene regulation, microarray technology is a promising tool. With regard to bioavailability studies, it is admitted that liposoluble vitamins, as well other lipophilic dietary microconstituents such as carotenoids, are absorbed and incorporated in chylomicrons for secretion into lymph. However, further studies are needed to elucidate the molecular mechanisms related to their uptake by intestinal cells, their trafficking within the cells and their incorporation into chylomicrons. Specific attention must be given to the competition between these dietary components for their absorption and metabolism, and in general the complexity of the diet must be comprehended in order to optimize the bioavailability of such dietary components.

A big challenge is to better understand the interaction between diet and our genes. It becomes relevant to evaluate the status of liposoluble micronutrients with regard to sub-groups carrying SNPs in genes implied in their bioavailability. In addition, gene regulation mechanisms have to be explored to specify the role of dietary components able to improve the bioavailability of liposoluble micronutrients at gene level. A better knowledge of nutrigenomics and nutrigenetics will allow improvement in formulations and adaptations of them to sub-groups, for example low-responders versus high responders. Thus, companies could offer more personalized functional foods, and personalized recommendations could be communicated in terms of benefit–risk.

7.7 References

M. J. AMIOT-CARLIN, C. BABOT-LAURENT, and F. TOURNIAIRE, Plant pigments as bioactive substances, In: Carmen Socaciu (ed), *Food Colorants, Chemical and Functional Properties*. Boca Raton, FL: CRC Press (2007) 127–146.

H. AMIR, M. KARAS, J. GIAT, M. DANILENKO, R. LEVY, T. YERMIAHU, J. LEVY, and Y. SHARONI, Lycopene and 1,25-dihydroxyvitamin D3 cooperate in the inhibition of cell cycle progression and induction of differentiation in HL-60 leukemic cells, *Nutr Cancer* **33** (1999) 105–112.

P. AUTIER, and S. GANDINI, Vitamin D supplementation and total mortality: a meta-analysis of randomized controlled trials, *Arch Intern Med* **167** (2007) 1730–1737.

A. AZZI, Molecular mechanism of alpha-tocopherol action, *Free Radic Biol Med* **43** (2007) 16–21.

J. BERTINATO, N. HIDIROGLOU, R. PEACE, K. A. COCKELL, K. D. TRICK, P. JEE, A. GIROUX, R. MADERE, G. BONACCI, M. ISKANDAR, S. HAYWARD, N. GILES, and M. R. L'ABBE, Sparing effects of selenium and ascorbic acid on vitamin C and E in guinea pig tissues, *Nutr J* **6** (2007) 7.

V. BHUVANESWARI, and S. NAGINI, Lycopene: a review of its potential as an anticancer agent, *Curr Med Chem Anticancer Agents* **5** (2005) 627–635.

H. K. BIESALSKI, Bioavailability of vitamin A, *Eur J Clin Nutr* **51** Suppl 1 (1997) S71–75.

G. BJELAKOVIC, D. NIKOLOVA, L. L. GLUUD, R. G. SIMONETTI, and C. GLUUD, Mortality in randomized trials of antioxidant supplements for primary and secondary prevention: systematic review and meta-analysis, *JAMA* **297** (2007) 842–857.

T. W. BOILEAU, A. C. BOILEAU, and J. W. ERDMAN, JR., Bioavailability of all-*trans* and *cis*-isomers of lycopene, *Exp Biol Med (Maywood)* **227** (2002) 914–919.

S. L. BOOTH, K. E. BROE, D. R. GAGNON, K. L. TUCKER, M. T. HANNAN, R. R. MCLEAN, B. DAWSON-HUGHES, P. W. WILSON, L. A. CUPPLES, and D. P. KIEL, Vitamin K intake and bone mineral density in women and men, *Am J Clin Nutr* **77** (2003) 512–516.

P. BOREL, Factors affecting intestinal absorption of highly lipophilic food microconstituents (fat-soluble vitamins, carotenoids and phytosterols), *Clin Chem Lab Med* **41** (2003) 979–994.

P. BOREL, P. GROLIER, M. ARMAND, A. PARTIER, H. LAFONT, D. LAIRON, and V. AZAIS-BRAESCO, Carotenoids in biological emulsions: solubility, surface-to-core distribution, and release from lipid droplets, *J Lipid Res* **37** (1996) 250–261.

P. BOREL, V. TYSSANDIER, N. MEKKI, P. GROLIER, Y. ROCHETTE, M. C. ALEXANDRE-GOUABAU, D. LAIRON, and V. AZAIS-BRAESCO, Chylomicron beta-carotene and retinyl palmitate responses are dramatically diminished when men ingest beta-carotene with medium-chain rather than long-chain triglycerides, *J Nutr* **128** (1998) 1361–1367.

P. BOREL, B. PASQUIER, M. ARMAND, V. TYSSANDIER, P. GROLIER, M. C. ALEXANDRE-GOUABAU, M. ANDRE, M. SENFT, J. PEYROT, V. JAUSSAN, D. LAIRON, and V. AZAIS-BRAESCO, Processing of vitamin A and E in the human gastrointestinal tract, *Am J Physiol Gastrointest Liver Physiol* **280** (2001) G95–G103.

P. BOREL, J. DRAI, H. FAURE, V. FAYOL, C. GALABERT, M. LAROMIGUIERE, and G. LE MOEL, [Recent knowledge about intestinal absorption and cleavage of carotenoids], *Ann Biol Clin (Paris)* **63** (2005) 165–177.

P. BOREL, M. MOUSSA, E. REBOUL, B. LYAN, C. DEFOORT, S. VINCENT-BAUDRY, M. MAILLOT, M. GASTALDI, M. DARMON, H. PORTUGAL, R. PLANELLS, and D. LAIRON, Human plasma levels of vitamin E and carotenoids are associated with genetic polymorphisms in genes involved in lipid metabolism, *J Nutr* **137** (2007) 2653–2659.

P. E. BOWEN, S. M. HERBST-ESPINOSA, E. A. HUSSAIN, and M. STACEWICZ-SAPUNTZAKIS, Esterification does not impair lutein bioavailability in humans, *J Nutr* **132** (2002) 3668–3673.

D. E. BREITHAUPT, A. BAMEDI, and U. WIRT, Carotenol fatty acid esters: easy substrates for digestive enzymes? *Comp Biochem Physiol B Biochem Mol Biol* **132** (2002) 721–728.

S. BÜGEL, Vitamin K and bone health in adult humans, *Vitam Horm* **78** (2008) 393–416.

B. BUIJSSE, E. J. FESKENS, D. SCHLETTWEIN-GSELL, M. FERRY, F. J. KOK, D. KROMHOUT, and L. C. DE GROOT, Plasma carotene and alpha-tocopherol in relation to 10-y all-cause and cause-specific mortality in European elderly: the Survey in Europe on Nutrition and the Elderly, a Concerted Action (SENECA), *Am J Clin Nutr* **82** (2005) 879–886.

C. CHITCHUMROONCHOKCHAI, and M. L. FAILLA, Hydrolysis of zeaxanthin esters by carboxyl ester lipase during digestion facilitates micellarization and uptake of the xanthophyll by CaCo-2 human intestinal cells, *J Nutr* **136** (2006) 588–594.

P. M. CLIFTON, M. NOAKES, D. ROSS, A. FASSOULAKIS, M. CEHUN, and P. NESTEL, High dietary intake of phytosterol esters decreases carotenoids and increases plasma plant sterol levels with no additional cholesterol lowering, *J Lipid Res* **45** (2004) 1493–1499.

W. COHN, Bioavailability of vitamin E, *Eur J Clin Nutr* **51** Suppl 1 (1997) S80–85.

D. A. COOPER, R. WEBB, and J. C. PETERS, Evaluation of the potential for Olestrato affect the availability of dietary phytochemicals, *J Nutr* **127** (1997) 1699S–1709S.

K. J. CRUICKSHANKS, R. KLEIN, and B. E. KLEIN, Sunlight and age-related macular degeneration. The Beaver Dam Eye Study, *Arch Ophthalmol* **111** (1993) 514–518.

H. F. DELUCA, Overview of general physiologic features and functions of vitamin D, *Am J Clin Nutr* **80** (2004) 1689S–1696S.

S. E. DEW, and D. E. ONG, Specificity of the retinol transporter of the rat small intestine brush border, *Biochemistry* **33** (1994) 12340–12345.

C. DHUIQUE-MAYER, P. BOREL, E. REBOUL, B. CAPORICCIO, P. BESANCON, and M. J. AMIOT, Beta-cryptoxanthin from citrus juices: assessment of bioaccessibility using an *in vitro* digestion/Caco-2 cell culture model, *Br J Nutr* **97** (2007) 883–890.

A. DURING, and E. H. HARRISON, Mechanisms of provitamin A (carotenoid) and vitamin A (retinol) transport into and out of intestinal Caco-2 cells, *J Lipid Res* **48** (2007) 2283–2294.

A. EL-AGAMEY, G. M. LOWE, D. J. MCGARVEY, A. MORTENSEN, D. M. PHILLIP, T. G. TRUSCOTT, and A. J. YOUNG, Carotenoid radical chemistry and antioxidant/pro-oxidant properties, *Arch Biochem Biophys* **430** (2004) 37–48.

R. ELLIOTT, Mechanisms of genomic and non-genomic actions of carotenoids, *Biochim Biophys Acta* **1740** (2005) 147–154.

C. J. FIELD, I. R. JOHNSON, and P. D. SCHLEY, Nutrients and their role in host resistance to infection, *J Leukoc Biol* **71** (2002) 16–32.

P. D. FRASER, and P. M. BRAMLEY, The biosynthesis and nutritional uses of carotenoids, *Prog Lipid Res* **43** (2004) 228–265.

B. L. GIJSBERS, K. S. JIE, and C. VERMEER, Effect of food composition on vitamin K absorption in human volunteers, *Br J Nutr* **76** (1996) 223–229.

F. GRANADO, B. OLMEDILLA, and I. BLANCO, Nutritional and clinical relevance of lutein in human health, *Br J Nutr* **90** (2003) 487–502.

E. R. GREENBERG, J. A. BARON, M. R. KARAGAS, T. A. STUKEL, D. W. NIERENBERG, M. M. STEVENS, J. S. MANDEL, and R. W. HAILE, Mortality associated with low plasma concentration of beta carotene and the effect of oral supplementation, *JAMA* **275** (1996) 699–703.

HEART PROTECTION STUDY GROUP, MRC/BHF Heart Protection Study of antioxidant vitamin supplementation in 20,536 high-risk individuals: a randomised placebo-controlled trial, *Lancet* **360** (2002) 23–33.

A. P. HEARTY, E. DUFFY, and M. J. GIBNEY, Intake estimates of naturally occurring phytosterols using deterministic and probabilistic methods in a representative Irish population, *Int J Food Sci Nutr* May 21 (2008) 1–14.

D. HEBER, and Q. Y. LU, Overview of mechanisms of action of lycopene, *Exp Biol Med (Maywood)* **227** (2002) 920–923.

C. H. HENNEKENS, J. E. BURING, J. E. MANSON, M. STAMPFER, B. ROSNER, N. R. COOK, C. BELANGER, F. LAMOTTE, J. M. GAZIANO, P. M. RIDKER, W. WILLETT, and R. PETO, Lack of effect of long-term supplementation with beta carotene on the incidence of malignant neoplasms and cardiovascular disease. *N Engl J Med* **334** (1996) 1145–1149.

M. HEWISON, Vitamin D and innate immunity, *Curr Opin Investig Drugs* **9** (2008) 485–490.

M. F. HOLICK, Sunlight and vitamin D for bone health and prevention of autoimmune diseases, cancers, and cardiovascular disease, *Am J Clin Nutr* **80** (2004) 1678S–1688S.

M. F. HOLICK, and T. C. CHEN, Vitamin D deficiency: a worldwide problem with health consequences, *Am J Clin Nutr* **87** (2008) 1080S–1086S.

D. HOLLANDER, and E. RIM, Vitamin K2 absorption by rat everted small intestinal sacs, *Am J Physiol* **231** (1976) 415–419.

D. HOLLANDER, E. RIM, and P. E. RUBLE, JR., Vitamin K2 colonic and ileal *in vivo* absorption: bile, fatty acids, and pH effects on transport, *Am J Physiol* **233** (1977) E124–129.

D. HOLLANDER, K. S. MURALIDHARA, and A. ZIMMERMAN, Vitamin D-3 intestinal absorption *in vivo*: influence of fatty acids, bile salts, and perfusate pH on absorption, *Gut* **19** (1978) 267–272.

C. JACKSON, S. GAUGRIS, S. S. SEN, and D. HOSKING, The effect of cholecalciferol (vitamin D3) on the risk of fall and fracture: a meta-analysis, *QJM* **100** (2007) 185–192.

A. JIMENEZ-ESCRIG, A. B. SANTOS-HIDALGO, and F. SAURA-CALIXTO, Common sources and estimated intake of plant sterols in the Spanish diet, *J Agric Food Chem* **54** (2006) 3462–3471.

S. KIDAMBI, and S. B. PATEL, Sitosterolaemia: pathophysiology, clinical presentation and laboratory diagnosis, *J Clin Pathol* **61** (2008) 588–594.

P. KNEKT, A. REUNANEN, R. JARVINEN, R. SEPPANEN, M. HELIOVAARA, and A. AROMAA, Antioxidant vitamin intake and coronary mortality in a longitudinal population study, *Am J Epidemiol* **139** (1994) 1180–1189.

R. KORPELA, J. TUOMILEHTO, P. HOGSTROM, L. SEPPO, V. PIIRONEN, P. SALO-VAANANEN, J. TOIVO, C. LAMBERG-ALLARDT, M. KARKKAINEN, T. OUTILA, J. SUNDVALL, S. VILKKILA, and M. J. TIKKANEN, Safety aspects and cholesterol-lowering efficacy of low fat dairy products containing plant sterols, *Eur J Clin Nutr* **60** (2006) 633–642.

N. I. KRINSKY, and K. J. YEUM, Carotenoid–radical interactions, *Biochem Biophys Res Commun* **305** (2003) 754–760.

P. M. KRIS-ETHERTON, K. D. HECKER, A. BONANOME, S. M. COVAL, A. E. BINKOSKI, K. F. HILPERT, A. E. GRIEL, and T. D. ETHERTON, Bioactive compounds in foods: their role in the prevention of cardiovascular disease and cancer, *Am J Med* **113** Suppl 9B (2002) 71S–88S.

J. T. LANDRUM, R. A. BONE, and M. D. KILBURN, The macular pigment: a possible role in protection from age-related macular degeneration, *Adv Pharmacol* **38** (1997) 537–556.

M. LAW, Plant sterol and stanol margarines and health, *BMJ* **320** (2000) 861–864.

M. H. LEE, K. LU, and S. B. PATEL, Genetic basis of sitosterolemia, *Curr Opin Lipidol* **12** (2001) 141–149.

J. LIN, F. SONG, P. YAO, X. YANG, N. LI, S. SUN, L. LEI, and L. LIU, Effect of vitamin A supplementation on immune function of well-nourished children suffering from vitamin A deficiency in China, *Eur J Clin Nutr* **62** (2007) 1412–1418.

D. LOMBARDO, P. DEPREZ, and O. GUY, Esterification of cholesterol and lipid-soluble vitamins by human pancreatic carboxyl ester hydrolase, *Biochimie* **62** (1980) 427–432.

R. P. MENSINK, S. EBBING, M. LINDHOUT, J. PLAT, and M. M. VAN HEUGTEN, Effects of plant stanol esters supplied in low-fat yoghurt on serum lipids and lipoproteins, non-cholesterol sterols and fat soluble antioxidant concentrations, *Atherosclerosis* **160** (2002) 205–213.

E. D. MICHOS and M. L. MELAMED, Vitamin D and cardiovascular disease risk, *Curr Opin Clin Nutr Metab Care* **11** (2008) 7–12.

E. R. MILLER, 3RD, R. PASTOR-BARRIUSO, D. DALAL, R. A. RIEMERSMA, L. J. APPEL, and E. GUALLAR, Meta-analysis: high-dosage vitamin E supplementation may increase all-cause mortality, *Ann Intern Med* **142** (2005) 37–46.

M. NISSINEN, H. GYLLING, M. VUORISTO, and T. A. MIETTINEN, Micellar distribution of cholesterol and phytosterols after duodenal plant stanol ester infusion, *Am J Physiol Gastrointest Liver Physiol* **282** (2002) G1009–1015.

J. A. NOVOTNY, S. R. DUEKER, L. A. ZECH, and A. J. CLIFFORD, Compartmental analysis of the dynamics of beta-carotene metabolism in an adult volunteer, *J Lipid Res* **36** (1995) 1825–1838.

N. NOY, and W. S. BLANER, Interactions of retinol with binding proteins: studies with rat cellular retinol-binding protein and with rat retinol-binding protein, *Biochemistry* **30** (1991) 6380–6386.

M. E. O'NEILL, and D. I. THURNHAM, Intestinal absorption of beta-carotene, lycopene and lutein in men and women following a standard meal: response curves in the triacylglycerol-rich lipoprotein fraction, *Br J Nutr* **79** (1998) 149–159.

G. S. OMENN, G. E. GOODMAN, M. D. THORNQUIST, J. BALMES, M. R. CULLEN, A. GLASS, J. P. KEOGH, F. L. MEYSKENS, B. VALANIS, J. H. WILLIAMS, S. BARNHART, and S. HAMMAR, Effects of a combination of beta carotene and vitamin A on lung cancer and cardiovascular disease, *N Engl J Med* **334** (1996) 1150–1155.

R. E. OSTLUND, JR., Phytosterols in human nutrition, *Annu Rev Nutr* **22** (2002a) 533–549.

R. E. OSTLUND, JR., Cholesterol absorption, *Curr Opin Gastroenterol* **18** (2002b) 254–258.

R. E. OSTLUND, JR., J. B. MCGILL, C. M. ZENG, D. F. COVEY, J. STEARNS, W. F. STENSON, and C. A. SPILBURG, Gastrointestinal absorption and plasma kinetics of soy delta(5)-phytosterols and phytostanols in humans, *Am J Physiol Endocrinol Metab* **282** (2002) E911–916.

D. Q. PHAM, and R. PLAKOGIANNIS, Vitamin E supplementation in Alzheimer's disease, Parkinson's disease, tardive dyskinesia, and cataract: Part 2, *Ann Pharmacother* **39** (2005a) 2065–2072.

D. Q. PHAM, and R. PLAKOGIANNIS, Vitamin E supplementation in cardiovascular disease and cancer prevention: Part 1, *Ann Pharmacother* **39** (2005b) 1870–1878.

A. V. RAO, Lycopene, tomatoes, and the prevention of coronary heart disease, *Exp Biol Med (Maywood)* **227** (2002) 908–913.

E. REBOUL, L. ABOU, C. MIKAIL, O. GHIRINGHELLI, M. ANDRE, H. PORTUGAL, D. JOURDHEUIL-RAHMANI, M. J. AMIOT, D. LAIRON, and P. BOREL, Lutein transport by CaCo-2 TC-7 cells occurs partly by a facilitated process involving the scavenger receptor class B type I (SR-BI), *Biochem J* **387** (2005a) 455–461.

E. REBOUL, P. BOREL, C. MIKAIL, L. ABOU, M. CHARBONNIER, C. CARIS-VEYRAT, P. GOUPY, H. PORTUGAL, D. LAIRON, and M. J. AMIOT, Enrichment of tomato paste with 6% tomato peel increases lycopene and beta-carotene bioavailability in men, *J Nutr* **135** (2005b) 790–794.

E. REBOUL, A. BERTON, M. MOUSSA, C. KREUZER, I. CRENON, and P. BOREL, Pancreatic lipase and pancreatic lipase-related protein 2, but not pancreatic lipase-related protein 1, hydrolyze retinyl palmitate in physiological conditions, *Biochim Biophys Acta* **1761** (2006a) 4–10.

E. REBOUL, A. KLEIN, F. BIETRIX, B. GLEIZE, C. MALEZET-DESMOULINS, M. SCHNEIDER, A. MARGOTAT, L. LAGROST, X. COLLET, and P. BOREL, Scavenger receptor class B type I

(SR-BI) is involved in vitamin E transport across the enterocyte, *J Biol Chem* **281** (2006b) 4739–4745.

E. REBOUL, M. RICHELLE, E. PERROT, C. DESMOULINS-MALEZET, V. PIRISI, and P. BOREL, Bioaccessibility of carotenoids and vitamin E from their main dietary sources, *J Agric Food Chem* **54** (2006c) 8749–8755.

E. REBOUL, S. THAP, E. PERROT, M. J. AMIOT, D. LAIRON, and P. BOREL, Effect of the main dietary antioxidants (carotenoids, gamma-tocopherol, polyphenols, and vitamin C) on alpha-tocopherol absorption, *Eur J Clin Nutr* **61** (2007a) 1167–1173.

E. REBOUL, S. THAP, F. TOURNIAIRE, M. ANDRE, C. JUHEL, S. MORANGE, M. J. AMIOT, D. LAIRON, and P. BOREL, Differential effect of dietary antioxidant classes (carotenoids, polyphenols, vitamins C and E) on lutein absorption, *Br J Nutr* **97** (2007b) 440–446.

J. REICHRATH, B. LEHMANN, C. CARLBERG, J. VARANI, and C. C. ZOUBOULIS, Vitamins as hormones, *Horm Metab Res* **39** (2007) 71–84.

M. RICHELLE, M. ENSLEN, C. HAGER, M. GROUX, I. TAVAZZI, J. P. GODIN, A. BERGER, S. METAIRON, S. QUAILE, C. PIGUET-WELSCH, L. SAGALOWICZ, H. GREEN, and L. B. FAY, Both free and esterified plant sterols reduce cholesterol absorption and the bioavailability of beta-carotene and alpha-tocopherol in normocholesterolemic humans, *Am J Clin Nutr* **80** (2004) 171–177.

E. B. RIMM, M. J. STAMPFER, A. ASCHERIO, E. GIOVANNUCCI, G. A. COLDITZ, and W. C. WILLETT, Vitamin E consumption and the risk of coronary heart disease in men, *N Engl J Med* **328** (1993) 1450–1456.

S. SCHAFFER, W. E. MULLER, and G. P. ECKERT, Tocotrienols: constitutional effects in aging and disease, *J Nutr* **135** (2005) 151–154.

H. H. SCHMITZ, C. L. POOR, E. T. GUGGER, and J. W. ERDMAN, JR., Analysis of carotenoids in human and animal tissues, *Methods Enzymol* **214** (1993) 102–116.

M. J. SHEARER, A. MCBURNEY, and P. BARKHAN, Studies on the absorption and metabolism of phylloquinone (vitamin K1) in man, *Vitam Horm* **32** (1974) 513–542.

B. SIVAKUMAR, and V. REDDY, Absorption of labelled vitamin A in children during infection, *Br J Nutr* **27** (1972) 299–304.

T. C. STAMP, J. G. HADDAD, and C. A. TWIGG, Comparison of oral 25-hydroxycholecalciferol, vitamin D, and ultraviolet light as determinants of circulating 25-hydroxyvitamin D, *Lancet* **1** (1977) 1341–1343.

M. J. STAMPFER, C. H. HENNEKENS, J. E. MANSON, G. A. COLDITZ, B. ROSNER, and W. C. WILLETT, Vitamin E consumption and the risk of coronary disease in women, *N Engl J Med* **328** (1993) 1444–1449.

T. SUDHOP, D. LUTJOHANN, and K. VON BERGMANN, Sterol transporters: targets of natural sterols and new lipid lowering drugs, *Pharmacol Ther* **105** (2005) 333–341.

H. TAPIERO, D. M. TOWNSEND, and K. D. TEW, Phytosterols in the prevention of human pathologies, *Biomed Pharmacother* **57** (2003) 321–325.

A. TAVANI, and C. LA VECCHIA, Beta-carotene and risk of coronary heart disease. A review of observational and intervention studies, *Biomed Pharmacother* **53** (1999) 409–416.

A. B. THOMSEN, H. B. HANSEN, C. CHRISTIANSEN, H. GREEN, and A. BERGER, Effect of free plant sterols in low-fat milk on serum lipid profile in hypercholesterolemic subjects, *Eur J Clin Nutr* **58** (2004) 860–870.

M. E. TORNWALL, J. VIRTAMO, P. A. KORHONEN, M. J. VIRTANEN, P. R. TAYLOR, D. ALBANES, and J. K. HUTTUNEN, Effect of alpha-tocopherol and beta-carotene supplementation on coronary heart disease during the 6-year post-trial follow-up in the ATBC study, *Eur Heart J* **25** (2004) 1171–1178.

M. G. TRABER and H. SIES, Vitamin E in humans: demand and delivery, *Ann Rev Nutr* **16** (1996) 321–327.

M. G. TRABER, G. W. BURTON, L. HUGHES, K. U. INGOLD, H. HIDAKA, M. MALLOY, J. KANE, J. HYAMS, and H. J. KAYDEN, Discrimination between forms of vitamin E by humans with and without genetic abnormalities of lipoprotein metabolism, *J Lipid Res* **33** (1992) 1171–1182.

L. M. TROY, P. F. JACQUES, M. T. HANNAN, D. P. KIEL, A. H. LICHTENSTEIN, E. T. KENNEDY, and S. L. BOOTH, Dihydrophylloquinone intake is associated with low bone mineral density in men and women, *Am J Clin Nutr* **86** (2007) 504–508.

N. Z. UNLU, T. BOHN, D. M. FRANCIS, H. N. NAGARAJA, S. K. CLINTON, and S. J. SCHWARTZ, Lycopene from heat-induced *cis*-isomer-rich tomato sauce is more bioavailable than from all-*trans*-rich tomato sauce in human subjects, *Br J Nutr* **98** (2007) 140–146.

A. M. VAN BENNEKUM, E. A. FISHER, W. S. BLANER, and E. H. HARRISON, Hydrolysis of retinyl esters by pancreatic triglyceride lipase, *Biochemistry* **39** (2000) 4900–4906.

J. VIRTAMO, J. M. RAPOLA, S. RIPATTI, O. P. HEINONEN, P. R. TAYLOR, D. ALBANES, and J. K. HUTTUNEN, Effect of vitamin E and beta carotene on the incidence of primary nonfatal myocardial infarction and fatal coronary heart disease, *Arch Intern Med* **158** (1998) 668–675.

R. VOLPE, L. NIITTYNEN, R. KORPELA, C. SIRTORI, A. BUCCI, N. FRAONE, and F. PAZZUCCONI, Effects of yoghurt enriched with plant sterols on serum lipids in patients with moderate hypercholesterolaemia, *Br J Nutr* **86** (2001) 233–239.

S. VOUTILAINEN, T. NURMI, J. MURSU, and T. H. RISSANEN, Carotenoids and cardiovascular health, *Am J Clin Nutr* **83** (2006).

W. WENG, L. LI, A. M. VAN BENNEKUM, S. H. POTTER, E. H. HARRISON, W. S. BLANER, J. L. BRESLOW, and E. A. FISHER, Intestinal absorption of dietary cholesteryl ester is decreased but retinyl ester absorption is normal in carboxyl ester lipase knockout mice, *Biochemistry* **38** (1999) 4143–4149.

K. WERTZ, U. SILER, and R. GORALCZYK, Lycopene: modes of action to promote prostate health, *Arch Biochem Biophys* **430** (2004) 127–134.

C. E. WEST, Meeting requirements for vitamin A, *Nutr Rev* **58** (2000) 341–345.

M. E. WRIGHT, K. A. LAWSON, S. J. WEINSTEIN, P. PIETINEN, P. R. TAYLOR, J. VIRTAMO, and D. ALBANES, Higher baseline serum concentrations of vitamin E are associated with lower total and cause-specific mortality in the Alpha-Tocopherol, Beta-Carotene Cancer Prevention Study, *Am J Clin Nutr* **84** (2006) 1200–1207.

Y. YAMANASHI, T. TAKADA, and H. SUZUKI, Niemann-Pick C1-like 1 overexpression facilitates ezetimibe-sensitive cholesterol and beta-sitosterol uptake in CaCo-2 cells, *J Pharmacol Exp Ther* **320** (2007) 559–564.

M. YOSHIDA, S. L. BOOTH, J. B. MEIGS, E. SALTZMAN, and P. F. JACQUES, Phylloquinone intake, insulin sensitivity, and glycemic status in men and women, *Am J Clin Nutr* **88** (2008) 210–215.

A. J. YOUNG, and G. M. LOWE, Antioxidant and prooxidant properties of carotenoids, *Arch Biochem Biophys* **385** (2001) 20–27.

J. M. ZINGG, and A. AZZI, Non-antioxidant activities of vitamin E, *Curr Med Chem* **11** (2004) 1113–1133.

8

Bioavailability and metabolism of phenolic compounds and glucosinolates

F. A. Tomás-Barberán, A. Gil-Izquierdo, D. A. Moreno, CEBAS-CSIC, Spain

Abstract: The biological activity of dietary polyphenols and glucosinolates is mediated by their bioavailability and metabolism. In the present review, the scientific knowledge regarding the absorption and metabolism of these bioactive compounds is presented. The comparative absorption kinetics of different phenolics and the key role of colonic microbiota on phenolic metabolism are also reviewed. In addition, the physiological changes of glucosinolates after intake and the effect of food matrix on their bioavailability are discussed.

Key words: phenolic compounds, glucosinolates, bioavailability, metabolism.

8.1 Introduction

'Bioactive compounds' are extra-nutritional constituents that typically occur in small quantities in foods. They are being intensively studied to evaluate their effects on health. The impetus sparking this scientific inquiry was the result of many epidemiological studies that have shown protective effects of plant-based diets on cardiovascular disease (CVD) and cancer. Many bioactive compounds have been discovered. These compounds vary widely in chemical structure and function and are grouped accordingly. Phenolic compounds, including their subcategory, flavonoids, are present in all plants and have been studied extensively in cereals, legumes, nuts, olive oil, vegetables, fruits, tea and red wine. Many phenolic compounds have antioxidant properties, and some studies have demonstrated favourable effects on thrombosis and tumourigenesis and promotion. Although some epidemiological studies have reported associations between flavonoids or other phenolics and

CVD and cancer, other studies have not found these associations. Isothiocyanates in cruciferous vegetables have anticarcinogenic actions in experimental models, as well as cardioprotective effects (Kris-Etherton *et al.*, 2002).

Results from epidemiological studies indicate that a high consumption of fruits and vegetables, either alone or as components of a healthy dietary pattern, reduced the risk of obesity, type 2 diabetes and cancer. Adherence to the Mediterranean diet is associated with a high consumption of antioxidant-rich foods such as vegetables and fruits. Polyphenolic compounds and glucosinolates are widely found in characteristic foods of the Mediterranean diet, such as fruits, vegetables, cereals, legumes and wine (Schröder, 2007; Fahey and Kensler, 2007).

As a consequence, a great variety of foods and supplements have been implicated as being sources of protective phytochemical factors. These factors can be used as discrete chemicals, dietary supplements or functional foods. Others have shown that dietary supplements are generally considered to be time-tested but in large part scientifically unproven, whereas functional foods are components of the normal diet that are increasingly shown to have inherent value for maintaining human health (Surh, 2003; Fahey and Kensler, 2007).

Cruciferous vegetables have been studied extensively for their chemoprotective effects. Although they contain many bioactive compounds, the anticarcinogenic actions of cruciferous vegetables are commonly attributed to their content of glucosinolates. Glucosinolates are relatively biologically inert but can be hydrolysed to a range of bioactive compounds such as isothiocyanates (ITC) and indoles by the plant-based myrosinase, or less efficiently by the colonic microflora. A number of mechanisms whereby ITC and indoles may protect against colorectal cancer have been identified. In experimental animals cruciferous vegetables have been shown to inhibit chemically induced cancer. However, the results of epidemiological studies did not provide sufficient explanation or were inconsistent and this disparity may reflect a lack of sensitivity of such studies. Possible explanations for the failure of certain epidemiological studies to detect an effect include: assessment of cruciferous vegetable intake by methods that are subject to large measurement errors; the interaction between diet and genotype has not been considered; the effect that post-harvest treatments may have on biological effects of cruciferous vegetables has not been taken into account (Lynn *et al.*, 2006; Higdon *et al.*, 2007; Lampe and Chang, 2007; Mays *et al.*, 2008).

In order to understand how these compounds exert their action *in vivo*, the changes occurring after their intake during the digestion process, the interaction with human cells and microbiota in the gastrointestinal tract, and the way they are absorbed and metabolised are essential. In the present chapter, the bioavailability and metabolism of the different polyphenols and glucosinolates are reviewed.

8.2 Phenolic compound bioavailability, absorption and tissue distribution

The generally accepted definition of bioavailability is the proportion of the compound that is digested, absorbed and metabolised through normal pathways. In the past few years, the bioavailability and metabolism of polyphenols have been better understood thanks to the health-promoting properties attributed to them (D'Archivio *et al.*, 2007).

In general, polyphenol metabolism follows a common pathway in the gastrointestinal tract. These compounds are not affected by the mouth, oesophagus and stomach physiological conditions and reach the small intestine where some of them are metabolised or absorbed, depending on their conjugation with sugars and their solubility properties. In the small intestine, they are mainly absorbed as aglycones or as simple glucosides and the remaining non-absorbed compounds (olygomers or polymers, rhamnosylglucosides, neohesperidosides, or esters with different compounds) finish in the large intestine, where they are metabolised by the microbiota to render first aglycones and then simple phenolic acids (see below) (Manach *et al.*, 2003, 2005; Lafay and Gil-Izquierdo, 2008).

The phenolic metabolites absorbed at the small or large intestine can be conjugated at the intestine cells to produce glucuronide or methyl conjugates, and are transported by the mesenteric vein up to the liver. The enzymatic armour of this organ additionally conjugates polyphenols by glucuronidation, sulphation or methylation, reactions carried out by the phase II enzymes. This is part of the metabolic detoxification process common to many xenobiotics, which restricts their potential toxic effects and facilitates their biliary and urinary elimination by increasing their hydrophilicity (Manach *et al.*, 2004; Lafay and Gil-Izquierdo, 2008).

Polyphenols are able to be taken up by tissues, particularly those in which they are metabolised. These compounds and their metabolites are eliminated mainly in urine and bile. Polyphenols which are secreted in the bile suffer the enterohepatic recycling. They are secreted via the biliary tract into the duodenum where they are subjected to the action of bacterial enzymes (glucuronidases and sulphatases) in the small intestine and colon, after which they may be reabsorbed. This process allows a longer contact of polyphenols and their metabolites at physiological level (Manach *et al.*, 2003). The activity of this route depends on the nature of the polyphenol (Crespy *et al.*, 2003)

Anthocyanins

Clinical studies carried out with humans consuming different types of fruit containing anthocyanins have shown that these phenolic pigments are poorly absorbed (Lapidot *et al.*, 1998; Felgines *et al.*, 2003). The concentration of anthocyanins in plasma ranged from 10 to 50 nmol/L (after a 50 mg of aglycone equivalent supply) and the mean time to reach the maximum concentration was 1.5h for plasma and 2.5h for urine. At intakes of 188–3570mg total cyanidin glycosides, the maximal plasma anthocyanin concentrations were also very low, in the order of 2.3–96nmol/L (Galvano *et al.*, 2004, 2007). The urinary excretions were found to be in the range between 0.018% and 0.37% of the intake. The time of appearance in the plasma was consistent with absorption at the stomach (24%) but also at the small intestine (23%) (Talavera *et al.*, 2003; Passamonti *et al.*, 2003; Felgines *et al.*, 2005, 2007). Maximal urinary excretion is usually achieved in less than 4h. Some studies revealed that the bioavailability of anthocyanins may be underestimated, since not all of their metabolites may have been identified (Manach *et al.*, 2005).

Anthocyanins are one of the few polyphenols that can be detected in plasma in the native form found in plant foods (glycosides). However, they can also suffer glucuronidation and sulphation reactions and glucuronide and sulphate conjugates are detected in urine in several studies. Kay and co-workers (2004) have also identified an oxidised derivative of anthocyanins. Methylation at the 3′-hydroxyl is also very common in anthocyanins (Felgines *et al.*, 2005; Tian *et al.*, 2006). The rate of metabolites present in plasma or urine varied depending on the experiment, type of food administered, sample conservation, extraction procedures as well as the sensitivity and resolution of the HPLC methods (6% Bitsch *et al.*, 2004, 25% Wu *et al.*, 2002, 68% Kay *et al.*, 2005, 85% Felgines *et al.*, 2005).

Besides the usual organs where the metabolisation and elimination of the anthocyanins take place, such as the liver or kidney, these polyphenols have also been detected, in the course of animal studies, in brain regions that mediate cognitive behaviour (cortex, hippocampus) and eye (Talavera *et al.*, 2005; Andrés-Lacueva *et al.*, 2005; Passamonti *et al.*, 2005).

Flavonols

The bioavailability of flavonols has been extensively studied owing to the high consumption of flavonol-containing foods such as tea, onion or asparagus and the good sensitivity of the analytical techniques used to detect them in biological samples (coulombimetric array detection and mass spectrometry).

The concentration of flavonols in plasma ranged from 0.5 to 3.8µmol/L (after a 50mg of aglycone equivalent supply) and the urinary excretion was found to be in the range 0.31–6.4% of the intake (Manach *et al.*, 2005). This high variability in the absorption may be due to particular polymorphisms for intestinal enzymes or transporters of the volunteers. Another characteristic of the flavonol bioavailability is the slow elimination of the metabolites with half-lives from 11 to 28h (Noroozi *et al.*, 2000; Erlund *et al.*, 2002). The time of appearance in plasma was around 2–4h for flavonol glucosides and around 6h for flavonol rhamnoglucosides, this being consistent with an absorption at the small intestine and the large intestine, respectively (Manach *et al.*, 2005). Glucosides of flavonols are directly absorbed at the small intestine at non-nutritional doses (Sesink *et al.*, 2001) or hydrolysed to render the corresponding aglycone at nutritional doses (Moon *et al.*, 2000). Rhamnosyl-glucosides are led to the colon to be metabolised by the microbiota to render the aglycones first and a number of phenolic acid metabolites after extensive metabolism (Erlund *et al.*, 2000; Manach *et al.*, 2005).

Regarding their transformation at physiological level, flavonols are commonly methylated in the 3′ position and then glucuronidated and/or sulphated, although non-methylated but glucuronidated forms of flavonols were also detected in plasma and urine (Day *et al.*, 2001).

The tissue distribution of flavonols has not yet been extensively studied. They have been detected in the organs responsible for their metabolism, absorption and elimination (liver, small intestine, blood and kidneys) in animal studies (rats and pigs) (Mullen *et al.*, 2002; Bieger *et al.*, 2008). In other studies, although the detection of conjugated forms in tissues is predominant, a variable amount of de-conjugated quercetin aglycone, in the range of 30–100% of total flavonoids, was detected in the organs analysed with the exception of blood (Bieger *et al.*, 2008).

Flavanones

This type of polyphenol is almost exclusively present in citrus fruits and products derived as juices or jams. The popularity of these compounds in the research world lies in the high and regular consumption of orange juice included in the international breakfast. Therefore, the study of the bioavailability of flavanones has been considered of interest (Gil-Izquierdo *et al.*, 2001).

One of the main characteristics of citrus fruits and their products is the high concentration of rhamnosyl-glucosides (rutinosides and neoheperidosides) of flavanones (Felgines *et al.*, 2000; Gil-Izquierdo *et al.*, 2001). This type of polyphenol linked to these disaccharides conditioned their absorption, since the small intestine does not present enzymes able to hydrolyse them (Manach *et al.*, 2003). Therefore, the 5 h time for reaching the maximum concentration in plasma after the intake of these compounds is consistent with absorption of aglycone at the colon after the hydrolysis by the gut microbiota (Felgines *et al.*, 2000). The concentration in plasma varied between 0.1 and 2.2 μmol/L (after a 50 mg of aglycone equivalent supply) and the urinary excretion was 1.1–30.2% of the intake (Erlund *et al.*, 2001; Manach *et al.*, 2003, 2005).

The main circulating metabolites of flavanones are 7-monoglucuronides and 3′ or 4′ monoglucuronides. The sulphated metabolites are also relevant (Manach *et al.*, 2003; Matsumoto *et al.*, 2004; Habauzit *et al.*, 2007). However, methylation, demethylation and transmethylation reactions carried out by the microbiota revealed the appearance of small quantities of other flavanones not originally detected in the fruit product consumed, such as homoeriodictyol from orange juice consumption or hesperetin, homoeriodictyol and isosakuranetin from naringin intake (Horcajada *et al.*, 2006; Silberberg *et al.*, 2006; Habauzit *et al.*, 2007).

Concerning the tissue distribution, only one report describes the detection of flavanone metabolites in different tissues (Silberberg *et al.*, 2006). Kidney and liver, in addition to plasma, were the organs where the occurrence of flavanone metabolites was found. The distribution of flavanone metabolites in tissues from other organs has not been studied so far. The conjugate forms were 98% of the flavanones detected in plasma, and this percentage was a little bit lower in liver and kidney (76 and 65%, respectively).

Procyanidins and flavan-3-ols

The food sources of catechins are very popular and highly consumed (tea, chocolate, apples, pears, grapes and red wine) (de Pascual-Teresa, 1999). The usual models to study their bioavailability have been the intake of cocoa or tea by volunteers (Manach *et al.*, 2005).

The wide nature of procyanidins and flavan-3-ols affects their bioavailability, since they can be detected at different polymerisation degrees and acylations (gallic acid). The galloylation of flavan-3-ols reduces their absorption. Polymerised procyanidins are not absorbed and small amounts of procyanidin dimers B1 and B2 have been detected in plasma (van Amelsvoort *et al.*, 2001; Holt *et al.*, 2002; Sano *et al.*, 2003).

The maximum concentration of flavan-3-ols in plasma varied between 0.03 and 2.7 μmol/L (after a 50 mg aglycone equivalent supply) and the urinary excretion was 0.1–55%. The high interval in the absorption and urinary excretion was due to the wide variability in the nature of flavan-3-ols (Manach *et al.*, 2005).

Epigallocatechin gallate is the only known polyphenol present in plasma in large proportion in a free from. The flavan-3-ols are highly methylated and glucuronidated in the 3′ and 4′ positions (catechin and epicatechin metabolites mainly) (Natsume *et al.*, 2003).

Isoflavones

The almost exclusive supply of isoflavones in our diet is derived from soy and soy products. Contrary to other types of polyphenols, isoflavones can be present in food both as glycosides and aglycones representing two different types of bioavailability (Guy *et al.*, 2008; Steiner *et al.*, 2008).

In general, isoflavones are the second best absorbed polyphenols with a maximum concentration of 2 μmol/L approximately (after a 50 mg aglycone equivalent supply), and urinary excretions of 42% for daidzin and 15.6% for genistin. Apparently, the bioavailability of daidzein is higher than that showed by geninstein. However, the elimination of genistein in bile is higher reflecting a very active enterohepatic recycling (Xu *et al.*, 1994; Sfakianos *et al.*, 1997; Rüfer *et al.*, 2008).

Regarding the nature of the circulating metabolites, aglycones are present in very low rate while the 7-*O*- and 4′-*O*-glucuronides are the main metabolites. The elimination of the metabolites is quite slow as in the case of flavonols (Doerge *et al.*, 2000; Clarke *et al.*, 2002; Shelnutt *et al.*, 2002; Rüfer *et al.*, 2008).

There are some reports describing the accumulation of this polyphenols in breast and prostate tissues (Morton *et al.*, 1997; Hong *et al.*, 2002; Maubach *et al.*, 2003). In fact, glucuronides of genistein and daidzein have been detected in prostate (Guy *et al.*, 2008).

Benzoic acids

These compounds are the best absorbed among the different phenolics reaching up to 4 μmol/L in plasma after administration of 50 mg of pure gallic acid. The main metabolite of benzoic acid in plasma is its methylated form, 4-*O*-methygallic acid (Clifford and Scalbert, 2000; Manach *et al.*, 2005).

Hydroxycinnamates

These phenolic compounds (phenylpropanoids) are ubiquitous in fruits and vegetables of the human diet, but they play a relevant role thanks to the high consumption of coffee. Daily intake of total polyphenol may range from less than 100 mg to an excess of 2 g, and the critical importance of coffee as the major dietary source has been shown by Clifford (2004). A single cup of coffee may contain 70–350 mg of hydroxycinnamates and a coffee drinker could ingest up to 1 g of hydroxycinnamates per day (Clifford, 1999). Owing to the regular consumption of coffee in Western countries, this drink and products derived from it are considered the most efficient and constant contribution of hydroxycinnamic acids supply to the human diet.

Like in the case of anthocyanins, administration of hydroxycinnamic acids in free form implies a rapid absorption from the stomach or the small intestine and they are conjugated by the intestinal and/or hepatic detoxification enzymes (Lafay and Gil-Izquierdo, 2008). In fact, maximal plasma concentration of aglycone and metabolites is reached 30 min and 1 h after the ingestion and the urinary excretion of these molecules ranges between 10 and 40% of the ingested dose. When the hydroxycinnamic acids are esterified with other compounds like araboxylans or hemicelluloses, their absorption and bioavailability decrease (Lafay and Gil-Izquierdo, 2008).

Monocarboxylic acid tranporters (MCT) seem to be implicated in the absorption of some hydroxycinnamates and their microbial metabolites. These transporters are expressed in many tissues (Price *et al.*, 1998; Lafay and Gil-Izquierdo, 2008).

Most biovailability studies concern caffeic acid, ferulic acid and the main chlorogenic acid, the 5-caffeoylquinic acid, although there are other dietary important hydroxycinnamates like rosmarinic acid or caftaric acid. Ferulic acid is rapidly absorbed after half an hour, and this time of absorption is consistent with a high absorption in the stomach. Whatever the form under which ferulic acid was administered, free or combined with different carbohydrates, plasma metabolites were mainly sulphates or sulphoglucuronides of ferulic acid. The free form represented only 5–24% of the total metabolites (Nardini *et al.*, 2002; Rondini *et al.*, 2002, 2004; Zhao *et al.*, 2003, 2004).

Regarding caffeic acid, when volunteers consumed red wine, caffeic acid was rapidly detected in plasma and its concentration varied from 0.084 to 0.3 μmol/L (Abu-Amsha Caccetta *et al.*, 2000; Cartron *et al.*, 2003). Concerning chlorogeninc acid, Olthof and co-workers (2001) showed that the esterification of quinic acid with caffeic acid, as in chlorogenic acid, markedly reduced its absorption in comparison with the previous non-esterified hydroxycynamates cited. In fact, urinary excretion of chlorogenic acid represented 0.3% after a clinical trial with ileostomised patients. Chlorogeninc has also been identified in human urine and plasma by several authors after ingestion of coffee, prune or pure molecule (Olthof *et al.*, 2001; Cremin *et al.*, 2001; Ito *et al.*, 2005). However, other authors failed to detect this phenolic acid in plasma or urine after similar intakes (coffee or pure molecules), suggesting that chlorogenic acid is hydrolysed in the upper part of the gut (Azuma *et al.*, 2000; Rechner *et al.*, 2001; Nardini *et al.*, 2002). Monteiro and co-workers (2007) reported the detection of chlorogenic acid in plasma at 7.66 μmo/L between 0.5–1 h and 1.5–4 h.

Ellagic acid and ellagitannins

These are polyphenols present in our diet thanks to pomegranates, walnuts and other nuts, berries like strawberry, cloudberry, blackberry and raspberry, muscadine grapes and oak-aged wines and spirits, among others (Gil *et al.*, 2000; Mertens-Talcott *et al.*, 2006).

Despite the good consumption of ellagitannins from berries and nuts by humans, the absorption of these phenolics is rather low or non-existent. This behaviour is justified by the large molecular size of these polyphenols, which decreases the transport across the intestinal barrier (Cerdá *et al.*, 2003a, 2005a). However, small amounts of punicalagin, the main ellagitannin of pomegranate with a molecular weight of 1084, were detected in the plasma and urine of rats following long-term administration of pomegranate ellagitannins at high doses (Cerdá *et al.*, 2003b).

Ellagitannins are mainly hydrolysed to release ellagic acid under physiological conditions in the small intestine (Larrosa *et al.*, 2006). Free ellagic acid is rapidly absorbed between 30 min and 1 h, time course after the intake, consistent with an absorption at the stomach or at the upper part of the small intestine to reach maximum concentrations in the range of nmol/L in plasma (109 nmol/L after an acute intake of 800 g pomegranate extract in humans) (Seeram *et al.*, 2004; Stoner *et al.*, 2005, 2006; Mertens-Talcott *et al.*, 2006). The absorption of ellagic acid may be negatively influenced by its binding properties to the intestine epithelium (Whitley *et al.*, 2003).

8.3 Colonic metabolism of dietary phenolic compounds

Most polyphenols are poorly absorbed in the GI tract, and they reach the colon where they are metabolised by the colonic microbiota. The metabolites are often absorbed and may be responsible for biological activities associated with polyphenols. This will also contribute to justify the large inter-individual variability in the effects observed, as this would correlate with differences in the bacterial strains that build up the colonic microbiota.

Gut bacteria can hydrolyse glycosides, glucuronides, sulphates, amides, esters and lactones. They also carry out reduction, ring-cleavage, decarboxylation, demethylation and dehydroxylation reactions. The hydrolysis of glycosides and glucuronides typically results in metabolites that are potentially more biologically active than the parent compounds. In contrast, further bacterial and transformation of aglycones can lead to production of more or less active compounds, depending on the substrate being metabolised and the products formed (Lampe and Chang, 2007).

8.3.1 Microbiota metabolism of flavonoids

Flavonols

These are degraded by colonic microbiota after breaking the flavonoid C ring into simpler phenolic compounds derived from A and B rings (Winter *et al.*, 1989, 1991). Thus, quercetin renders 3,4-dihydroxyphenylacetic acid, 3-hydroxyphenyl acetic acid and 3,4 dihydroxytoluene from the B ring. In addition, phlorogulcinol has also been reported to be produced from the A-ring. 3,4-Dihydroxybenzoic (B ring), 3,4-dihydroxybenzaldehyde; 2,4,6-trihydroxybenzoic acid (A ring), 2-(3,4-dihydroxyphenyl)ethanol; dihydroxyphenylbenzoic acid methyl ester or 4-hydroxy-3-methoxybenzoic acid (vanillic), 3 or 4-hydroxyphenylpropionic have also been reported (Fig. 8.1). Myricetin (which has a 3′,4′,5′-trihydroxy-ring B) releases 3,5-dihydroxy-phenyl acetic acid, 3-hydroxyphenyl acetic acid and 3,4,5-trihydroxyphenyl acetic acid. In the bacterial metabolism of kaempferol (which has a 4′-hydroxy-ring B) only 4-hydroxyphenyl acetic acid has been found (Rechner *et al.*, 2004; Aura, 2005). In the case of quercetin glucosides and rutinosides (rutin), the corresponding aglycone is degraded after release to break down the C ring and then continue with specific dehydroxylations by hydroxylases.

These metabolites are then absorbed and can be detected in plasma and urine as phase II conjugates produced by the human cells, including methyl ethers as a product of COMT (catechol *o*-methyl transferases) and glucuronyl and sulphate transferases. Conjugates with amino acids have also been described in humans and animals. Glucuronidation and methylation occur mainly in the intestinal cells and in the liver, while sulphation takes place mainly in the kidney.

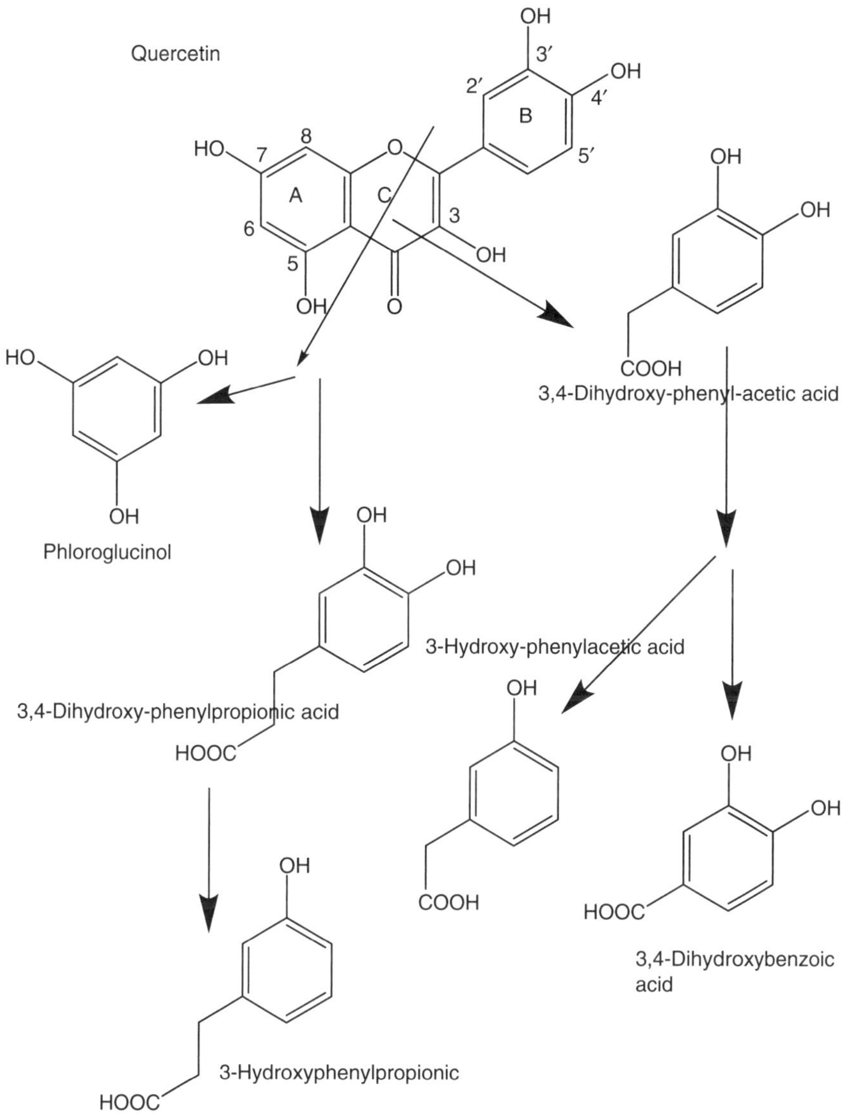

Fig. 8.1 Colonic microbiota metabolism of quercetin.

Anthocyanin pigments

Only a small part of the dietary anthocyanins is absorbed as such or as hydrolysis products in which the sugar moiety is removed (see above). Thus, large amounts of the ingested compounds are likely to enter the colon. Studies looking at the colonic microbiota metabolism of anthocyanins are scarce. Cyanidin 3-rutinoside is first transformed in the corresponding glucoside and then to the aglycone. This is reported to be achieved by gut microbiota (Keppler and Humpf, 2005), and the aglycones, which are chemically unstable, are converted to phenolic acids that then can suffer additional metabolism by the gut microbiota. The anthocyanin nucleus is broken down and protocatechuic acid (3,4-dihydroxybenzoic acid) is detected as a product of human colonic microbiota (Aura *et al.*, 2005). Other metabolites produced *in vitro* by the pig gut microbiota include syringic acid (3,5-dimethoxy, 4-hydroxy-benzoic acid), vanillic acid (3-methoxy, 4-hydroxy-benzoic acid), phloroglucinol aldehyde (2,4,6-trihydroxy benzaldehyde), phloroglucinol acid (2,4,6-trihydroxybenzoic acid), and gallic acid (3,4,5-trihydroxybenzoic acid), depending on the chemical structure of the anthocyanins (Keppler and Humpf, 2005). In the case of methylated anthocyanins, the ring-cleavage degradation products can be de-methylated by the pig gut microbiota. This shows that anthocyanins as flavonoid compounds, also suffer the ring cleavage, to release the B ring and A ring-derived products.

Procyanidins and flavan-3-ols

This is a very complex group of polyphenols including simple flavan-3-ols (catechin and epicatechin; gallocatechin; and epigallocatechin and the corresponding gallate esters) to polymeric procyanidins known as condensed tannins including a whole range of oligomeric intermediates going from dimers to undecamers and dodecamers and then polymers. These polyphenols are one of the main constituents of the phenolic intake in the diet, and are mainly provided by fruits, tea and wine.

The main metabolites detected in urine after intake of catechin and epicatechin are 3-hydroxy-phenyl propionic acid, δ-(3,4,-dihydroxyphenyl-γ-valerolactone; δ-(3-hydroxyphenyl)-γ-valerolactone; 3-hydroxyhippuric acid (both bacterial + human metabolism) (Li *et al.*, 2000; Déprez *et al.*, 2000; Rios *et al.*, 2003; Rechner *et al.*, 2004) (Figs 8.2 and 8.3).

After *in vitro* incubation of epicatechin with human intestinal bacteria, the metabolites pyrogallol, 3′,4′-dihydroxyphenylvaleric acid; 3′-hydroxyphenyl valeric acid; 3,4-dihydroxyphenylpropionic, 3′-hydroxyphenylpropionic; 3′-methoxyphenylvaleric acid and 2″,3″-dihydroxyphenoxyl-3′,4′-dihydroxyphenyl propionic acid were detected (Meselhy *et al.*, 1997). However, epicatechin gallate and epigallocatechin gallate were not degraded by the microbiota (Meselhy *et al.*, 1997).

Studies on the microbial metabolism of dietary condensed tannins (oligomeric and polymeric procyanidins) showed that benzoic, phenylacetic, phenylpropionic and phenyllactic acid derivatives, as well as phloroglucinol, δ-(3-hydroxyphenyl)-γ-valerolactone and 1-(3-hydroxyphenyl)-3-(2,4,6-trihydroxyphenyl)propan-2-ol were produced (Groenewoud and Hundt, 1986). In another study, condensed tannins produced 4-hydroxyphenylacetic, 3-phenylpropionic, 3-hysroxyphenylacetic, 4-hydroxyphenylpropionic, 3-hydroxyphenylvaleric and 3-hydroxyphenylpropionic (Déprez *et al.*, 2000), while valerolactones were not detected.

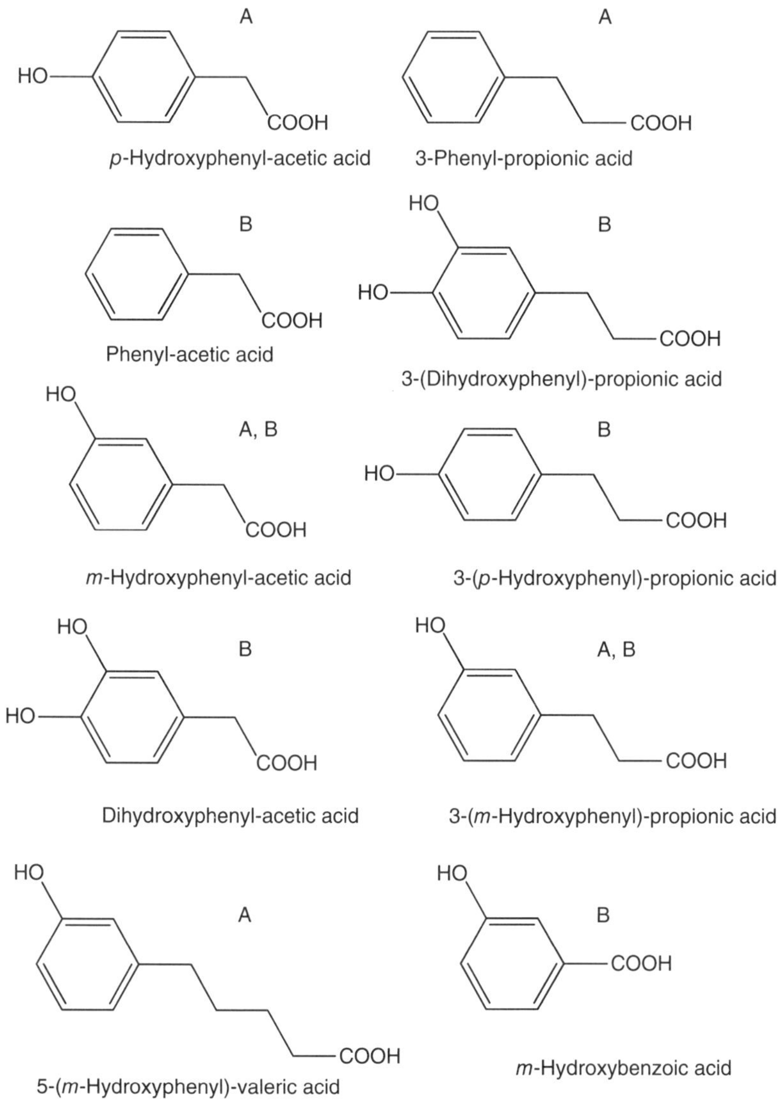

Fig. 8.2 Human colon microbiota metabolites of dietary procyanidins produced *in vitro* (A) (Deprez *et al.*, 2000) and *in vivo* (B) (detected in urine after the intake of chocolate polyphenols; Rios *et al.*, 2003).

Isoflavones

Most of the research on isoflavone bioavailability and metabolism has focused on soybean isoflavones. Isoflavones are absorbed in a small percentage (2–10%), but even so their absorption is higher than that found for other flavonoids, and they are largely transformed in the gut by the

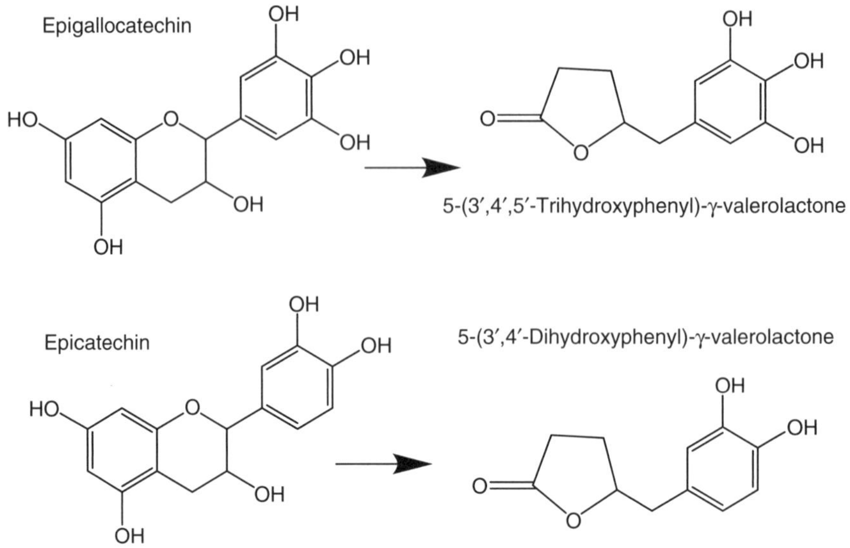

Fig. 8.3 Valerolactone production by colonic microbiota from dietary flavan-3-ols (Li *et al.*, 2000).

microbiota into equol, dihydrodaidzein and *o*-demethyl angolensin (Fig. 8.4). Equol is better as an oestrogenic compound than the precursor isoflavones. The transformation of the native isoflavones in these metabolites, and particularly in equol, depends on the individuals, and both equol 'producers' and 'non-producers' have been reported (Atkinson *et al.*, 2005). The ability of producing equol has been related to the presence in the GI tracts of specific microbiota (Bowey *et al.*, 2003), and therefore, the biological activity of soy isoflavones depends on the colonisation of the GI tract by specific bacteria that modulate the oestrogenic activity of soy-derived foods through the metabolism to render equol or the alternative metabolite *o*-demethylangolensin.

Flavanones

Flavanones seem to be less degraded than other flavonoids by colonic microbiota, and this is probably why these compounds are found to be more bioavailable than other related flavonoids such as flavonols or flavan-3-ols. Flavanone glycosides, such as naringin, suffer first a deglycosylation to render the aglycone, and the aglycone through ring cleavage gives phloroglucinol and 3-(4-hydroxyphenyl) propionic acid. This can be further dehydroxylated to produce 3-phenylpropionic acid. This degradation pathway is similar to that observed in flavonols and other flavonoids (including procyanidins) (Rechner *et al.*, 2004).

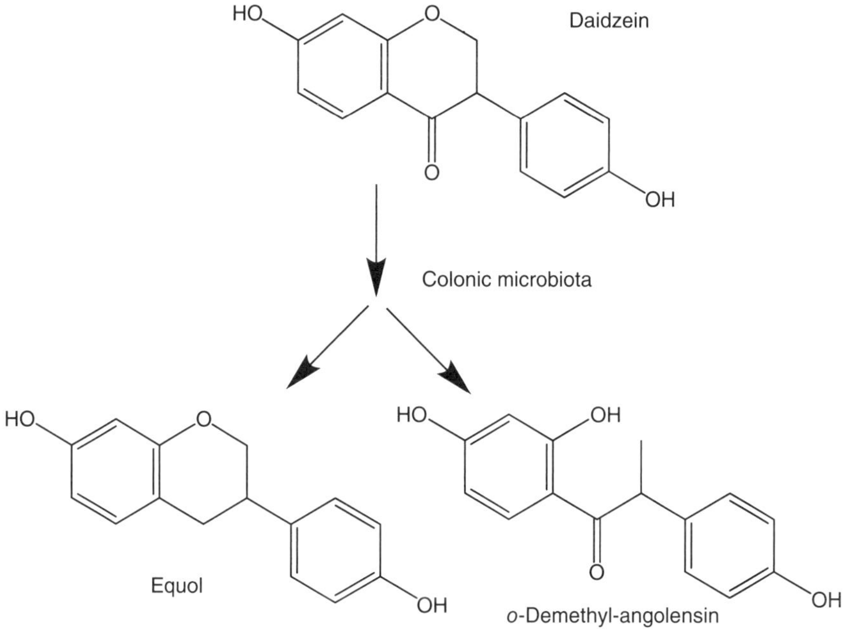

Fig. 8.4 GI microbiota metabolism of daidzein, an estrogenic isoflavone from soy and soy-derived foods and nutraceuticals.

Isoxanthohumol is a prenylated flavanone from hops and beer that has interesting biological activities. *In vivo*, it can be metabolised by colonic microbiota to render 8-prenyl-naringenin (Fig. 8.5) (Possemiers *et al.*, 2005, 2006). This metabolic transformation is carried out by *Eubacterium* species, and particularly by *E. limosum*. In fact, it has recently being demonstrated that this bacterium activates isoxanthohumol from hops (*Humulus lupulus* L.) into the potent phytoestrogen 8-prenylnaringenin *in vitro* and in rat intestine (Possemiers *et al.*, 2008).

8.3.2 Microbiota metabolism of dietary non-flavonoid phenolics

Benzoic acids

These phenolics are often decarboxylated by colonic microbiota when a free hydroxyl group is present in the 4-position. Thus protocatechuic acid (3,4-dihydroxybenzoic) produces catechol (1,2-dihydroxyphenol), and gallic acid (3,4,5-trihydroxy-benzoic acid) produces pyrogallol (1,2,3-trihydroxyphenol). In the same way, vanillic acid (4-hydroxy-3-methoxy benzoic acid) produces methyl catechol (Fig. 8.6) (Aura, 2005). These metabolites are readily absorbed in the gastrointestinal tract.

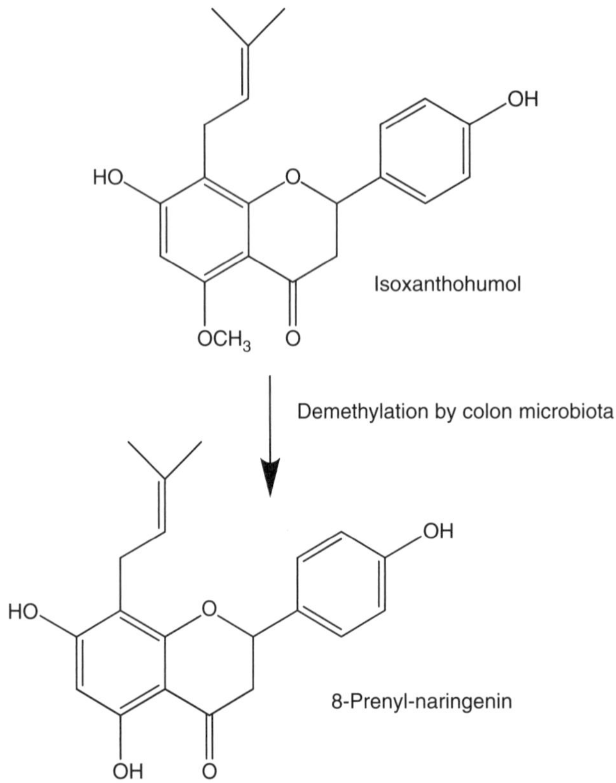

Fig. 8.5 GI microbiota transformation of hop flavanones.

Hydroxycinnamates

Caffeic acid (3,4,dihydroxy-cinnamic acid), as well as *p*-coumaric (4-hydroxy-cinnamic acid), ferulic (4′-hydroxy-3′-methoxy-cinnamic acid) and sinapic (4′-hydroxy-3′,5′-dimethoxycinnamic acid), and their esters with quinic and tartaric acids (chlorogenic, caftaric, etc.), are common dietary phenolics present in a large range of plant-derived food products. *In vitro* studies with human microbiota indicate that the free acids were not detected just after 2 h incubation. The main microbial metabolites of chlorogenic and caftaric acid were 3-hydroxy-phenyl propionic acid and benzoic acid. These were obtained both from caffeic acid, chlorogenic and caftaric acid, suggesting that esterification has no influence on the metabolism of caffeic acid by the gut microbiota (Gonthier *et al.*, 2006). The most frequent metabolites produced by colonic microbiota from ferulic acid are vanillin (3-methoxy-4-hydroxy-benzoic acid) and 3-hydroxy-phenyl propionic acid, and in plasma and urine some conjugated derivatives such as vanilloylglycine and feruloylglycine were detected in addition. In a similar way, *in vivo* Phase II metabolism of the microbiota metabolites produced from caffeic acid

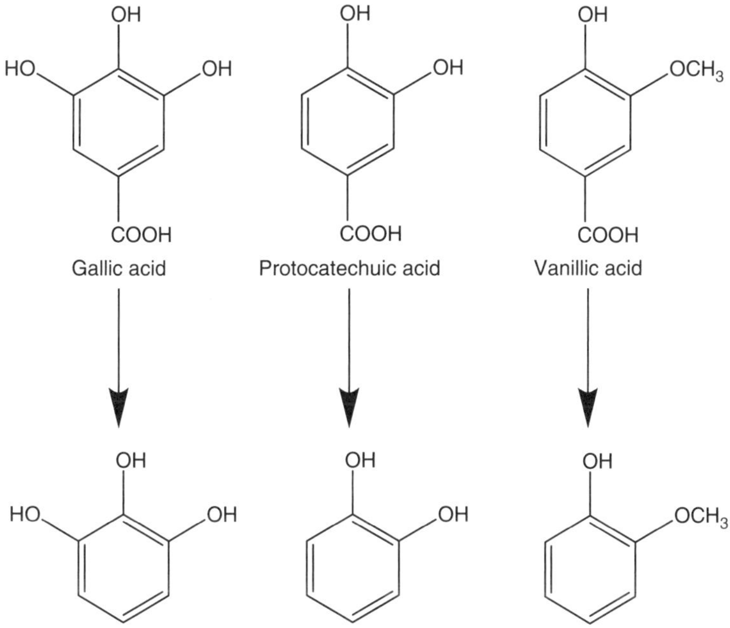

Fig. 8.6 Gut microbiota metabolism of dietary benzoic acid derivatives.

renders the glycynated metabolites, including hippuric acid and 3-hydroxy-hippuric acid (Gonthier *et al.*, 2003; Rechner *et al.*, 2004).

A general trend is that, from esters, the free acid is released by bacterial esterases (Plumb *et al.*, 1999), and the free acid is then metabolised to reduce the double bond to give rise to phenyl-propionic acid and then decarboxylated to produce phenyl-acetic acids. Dehydroxylation occurs first to remove the hydroxyl at the 4-position of the hydroxycinnamic acid residue, and demethylation also occurs at different levels of the degradation pathway.

Ellagic acid and ellagitannins

Both ellagitannins and ellagic acid are largely metabolised by the colon microbiota of different mammals including rats (Cerdá *et al.*, 2004), pigs (Espín *et al.*, 2007) and humans (Cerdá *et al.*, 2005a). In all these cases both ellagic acid and ellagitannins render dibenzopyranones known as urolithins (Fig. 8.7). The main ones reported are urolithin A and B. Nothing is known, however, of the microbiota degradation of ellagitannin-C-glycosides as is the case of castalagin and vescalagin, the main characteristic ellagitannins of oak wood. Ellagitannins are a very interesting group of phenolic metabolites, and their bioavailability and metabolism by colonic microbiota deserve more study.

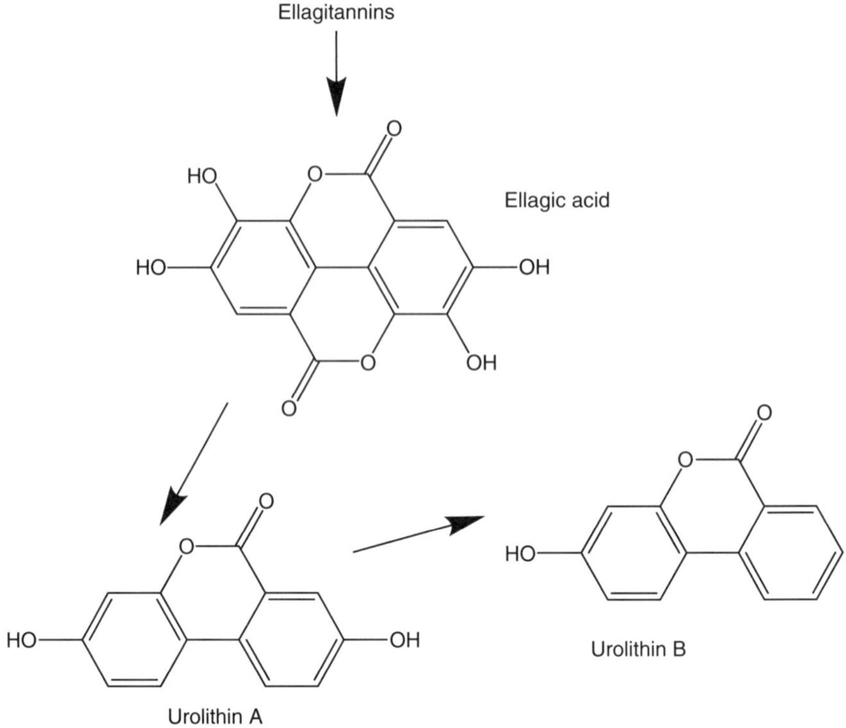

Fig. 8.7 Ellagitannins and ellagic acid metabolism by colonic microbiota.

Lignans
Dietary lignans include a number of phenolic metabolites with different structures (secoisolariciresinol, matairesinol, pinoresinol, lariciresinol, isolariciresinol, syringaresinol). The biological activity of these lignans is related to the production of the known as mammalian phytoestrogens that include the metabolites known as enterolactone and enterodiol (Fig. 8.8) (Glitso *et al.*, 2000; Wang *et al.*, 2000; Bowey *et al.*, 2003). These mammalian phytoestrogens are produced by the gastrointestinal microbiota and the biological activity of lignans depends on the occurrence of these microorganisms able to produce the necessary chemical conversions. Demethylation occurs first from the naturally occurring lignans and dehydroxylation takes place as a second step (Wang, 2002).

8.4 Colonic microbiota responsible for dietary phenolic compound metabolism

The specific microbiota strains responsible for the colonic metabolism of dietary phenolics remain largely unknown, although some species have

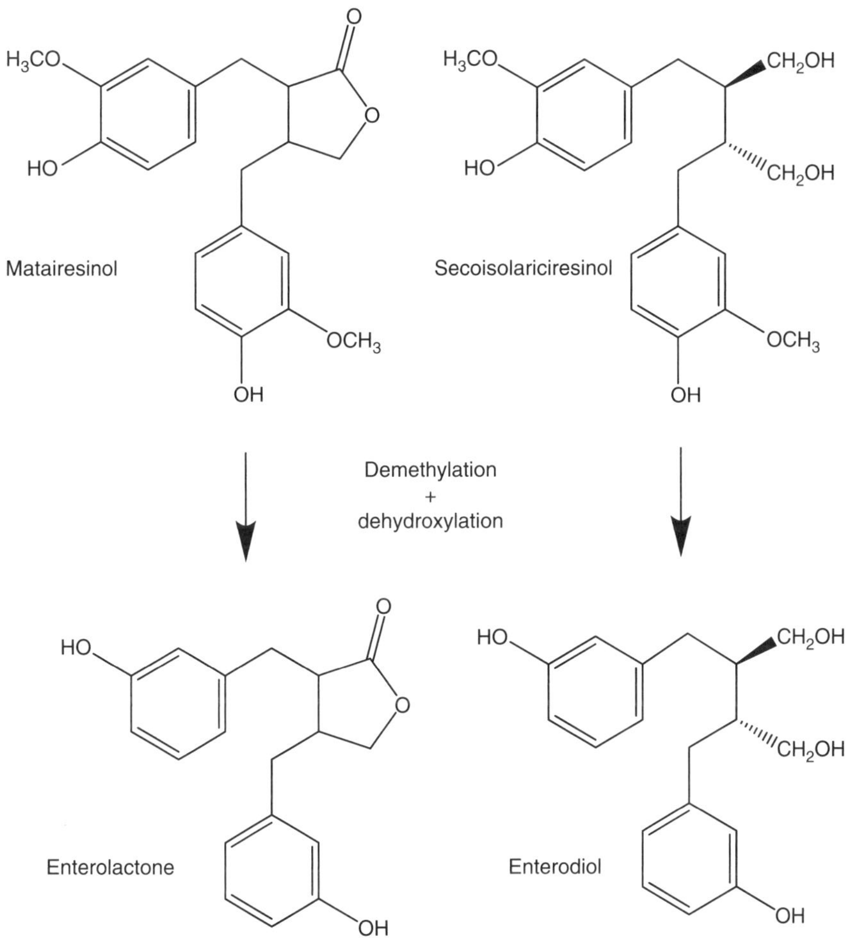

Fig. 8.8 Gut microbiota metabolism of dietary lignans.

been found as responsible for achieving specific steps in the metabolism of different phenolics. Although a large number of microbial species have been identified as constituents of the gut microflora in humans, the colonic strains so far identified as responsible for the phenolic metabolism belong to a limited number of genera, including *Clostridium*, *Butyrovibrio*, *Eubacterium* and *Peptostreptococcus*.

Thus, some *Clostridium* (Winter *et al.*, 1989, 1991), *Butyrovibrio* species (Krishnamurty *et al.*, 1970) and *Eubacterium ramulus* (Schneider *et al.*, 1999) isolated from human faeces are known to break-down the C-ring of flavonols such as quercetin and its glycosides, querecetin 3-glucoside and quercetin 3-rutinoside, to produce phloroglucinol from ring A, and 3,4-dihydroxy-phenyl-acetic acid from the ring B (Fig. 8.1).

The specific removal of the carbonyl group of the flavanone isoxanthohumol to render 8-prenyl naringenin is carried out by *Eubacterium limosum* isolated from humans (Possemiers *et al.*, 2005, 2006). The transformation of dietary lignans into mammalian phytoestrogens is carried out after a demethylation and a dehydroxylation reaction. Two bacterial strains, *Peptostreptococcus* sp. strain SDG-1 and *Eubacterium* sp. strain SDG-2, capable of demethylation and dehydroxylation, respectively, were isolated from a human faecal suspension (Wang *et al.*, 2000). Nothing is known about the colonic microbiota strains responsible for the transformation of ellagitannins and ellagic acid into urolithins, although these metabolites were produced by human faecal bacteria from ellagic acid and the ellagitannin punicalagin (Cerdá *et al.*, 2005b; Espín *et al.*, 2007).

Owing to the poor absorption of dietary phenolics in the small intestine, a relevant part of the phenolic intake should reach the colon where they will be metabolised by the gut microbiota. Thus, the biological activity of dietary phenolics depends largely on their metabolism by colonic microbiota, as these compounds are either metabolically activated to render more bioactive compounds (the case of equol and 8-prenylnaringenin) or less active compounds (a decrease in the number of phenolic hydroxyls decreases the antioxidant activity *in vitro*). This means that, depending on the microbiota present in the gastrointestinal tract of each individual, the phenolics present in the diet can give rise to different phenolic metabolites with different biological activities. Knowledge of the gastrointestinal bacterial strains responsible for specific steps of phenolic metabolism will provide the possibility of producing functional foods in which the phenolic precursors are combined with the desired bacteria, in order to produce specific bioactive metabolites in the colon and therefore modulate and control the biological effects of phenolic compounds in the diet. Of course, other human genetic factors that differentiate the metabolic behaviour of the different individuals should also be considered in order to explain variability in the expected biological effect (Lampe and Chang, 2007).

8.5 Glucosinolates and isothiocyanates

Glucosinolates (β-thioglucoside-*N*-hydroxysulphates), the precursors of isothiocyanates, are present in 16 families of dicotyledonous angiosperms including a large number of edible species. At least 120 different glucosinolates have been identified in these plants, although closely related taxonomic groups typically contain only a small number of such compounds. Glucosinolates and/or their breakdown products have long been known for their fungicidal, bactericidal, nematocidal and allelopathic properties and have recently attracted intense research interest because of their cancer chemoprotective attributes. Numerous reviews have addressed the occurrence of glucosinolates in vegetables, primarily in the family Brassicaceae (syn. Cruciferae; including *Brassica* spp. and *Raphanus* spp.). In addition to the *Brassica* vegetables, these glucosinolates have been found in hundreds of species, many of which are edible or could provide substantial quantities of glucosinolates for isolation, for biological evaluation, and potential application as chemoprotective or other dietary or pharmacological agents (Fahey *et al*., 2001; Mays *et al*., 2008).

There is growing evidence that the protective effects of crucifers against disease may be attributable in large measure to their content of glucosinolates. Glucosinolates in plant cells are accompanied by, but physically segregated from, a β-thioglucosidase (myrosinase), which, when released by crushing of plant cells such as by chewing or food preparation, hydrolyses the glucosinolates, principally to isothiocyanates (mustard oils). This hydrolysis is also mediated by the microflora of the mammalian gastrointestinal tract (Shapiro *et al*., 2001, 2006).

Chemoprevention is an active cancer preventive strategy to inhibit, delay or reverse human carcinogenesis, using naturally occurring or synthetic chemical agents. The term 'chemoprevention' refers to the use of agents to inhibit, reverse or retard tumourigenesis. Numerous phytochemicals derived from edible plants have been reported to interfere with a specific stage of the carcinogenic process. Many mechanisms have been shown to account for the anticarcinogenic actions of dietary constituents, but attention has recently been focused on intracellular-signalling cascades as common molecular targets for various chemopreventive phytochemicals (Surh, 2003; Kwon *et al*., 2007).

A variety of naturally occurring dietary compounds have been shown to possess significant chemopreventive effects and many experimental attempts have been made to address their underlying mechanisms of actions. Numerous cancer cell lines and animal cancer models have been used to evaluate the chemopreventive effects of phytochemicals as well as to elucidate their mechanism of cancer prevention. These studies have resulted in the discovery of several new phytochemicals that possess cancer preventive effects, such as isothiocyanates from cruciferous vegetables, polyphenols and flavonoids (Kwon *et al*., 2007; Cartea and Velasco, 2008).

8.5.1 Bioavailability and metabolism

Although approximately 120 classes of glucosinolates have been identified in plants, each plant species contains up to four different glucosinolates in significant amounts (Fahey *et al*., 2001). Glucosinolates are not bioactive until they have been enzymatically hydrolysed to various bioactive breakdown products by endogenous plant enzyme myrosinase (thioglucoside glucohydrolase, EC3.2.1.147). These breakdown products include isothiocyanates, nitriles, thiocyanates, epithionitriles, oxazolidine-2-thiones and epithioalkanes, depending on the substrate, pH conditions, availability of ferrous ions and the level and activity of specific protein factors such as the epithiospecifier protein (ESP). At physiological pH, isothiocyanates are the major products, whereas nitriles are formed at more acid pH (Grubb and Abel, 2006; Moreno *et al.*, 2006; Cartea and Velasco, 2008).

Glucosinolate–myrosinase system

Isothiocyanates are promising chemopreventive agents that are present in substantial concentrations in *Brassica* cruciferous vegetables; in epidemiological studies, intake of these vegetables was found to afford protection against a number of cancers. Isothiocyanates occur as glucosinolates but are released following exposure to the enzyme myrosinase (thioglucoside glucohydrolase, EC3.2.1.147), which comes into contact with these compounds during harvesting, chopping and mastication of the vegetables. Moreover, microbial myrosinase activity in the human intestine contributes to the release of isothiocyanates from their glucosinolate precursors (Higdon *et al.*, 2007; Hanlon *et al.*, 2008; Mays *et al.*, 2008).

The glucosinolate-defining core structure (the aglycone) is derived from the amino acids alanine, isoleucine, valine, tryptophan, tyrosine, phenylalanine and methionine and from chain elongated derivatives of the latter two amino acids via a biosynthetic pathway whose initial steps correspond to those of cyanogenic glucoside biosynthesis. Further secondary modifications of the core structure significantly increase the number of structurally different glucosinolates found in nature – more than 120 reported structures (Grubb and Abel, 2006; Morant *et al.*, 2008).

The glucosinolates, hydrophilic and stable compounds, are normally sequestered in vacuoles of most plant tissues. Loss of cellular integrity initiates glucosinolate breakdown by myrosinase-catalysed hydrolysis of the glucosidic bond. Myrosinases are specific β-thioglucosidases localised in idioblasts (myrosin cells) scattered throughout most tissues of glucosinolate-producing plants. Thus, plant injury activates the binary glucosinolate–myrosinase system, sometimes called the 'mustard oil bomb', leading to the rapid generation of unstable thiohydroximate-*o*-sulphate intermediates. Subsequent non-enzymatic elimination of the sulphate group and spontaneous rearrangement of the remaining core structure yields a variety of bioactive products, including isothiocyanates, thiocyanates, nitriles, oxazolidine-2-thiones or epithioalkanes. Chemical conditions such as pH, availability of ferrous ions and presence of myrosinase-interacting proteins determine the final composition of the product mix. Some degradation products have potent biocidal activites and are likely to contribute to the plant defence arsenal against pathogens and generalist herbivores; others are believed to play roles as allelochemicals in mediating plant–insect interactions. As components of feed and food, products of glucosinolate hydrolysis are of toxicological and pharmacological importance. Although certain glucosinolate derivatives have antinutritional properties, it is now well established that methionine-derived isothiocyanates can offer substantial protection against cancer, in particular sulphoraphane

(SFN) (Grubb and Abel, 2006; Mays *et al.*, 2008; Morant *et al.*, 2008).

Metabolism and disposition of isothiocyanates

Phytochemicals, in broad terms, are a synonym of plant chemicals (*phyto* is Greek for plant); however, in common usage the term is more limited in scope and usually refers to plant chemicals that are bioactive and are not part of the traditional nutrients, such as vitamins and minerals. Although these compounds are generally viewed as non-essential for normal body functioning, an increasing number of them have been shown to possess disease-fighting activities, including anticarcinogenic and anticancer activities as cancer chemopreventive phytochemicals, e.g. SFN, which was isolated from broccoli in the early 1990s as an inducer of phase 2 enzymes and has since been extensively studied by numerous investigators. It shows a highly promising cancer-fighting ability (Juge *et al.*, 2007; Lampe and Chang, 2007; Zhang and Tang, 2007).

Genetic variation in pathways affecting absorption, metabolism and distribution of phytochemicals is likely to influence exposure at the tissue level, thus modifying disease risk in individuals. Few studies have examined these gene–phytochemical interactions in humans and the sources of variation in phytochemical metabolism and disposition *in vivo*. Two aspects of phytochemical handling that are receiving some attention, particularly in relation to specific phytochemicals, are the impact of intestinal bacteria and genetically polymorphic phase II, conjugating enzymes (Seow *et al.*, 2005; Higdon *et al.*, 2007; Lampe and Chang, 2007).

A prerequisite for bioavailability of any compound is their bioaccessibility in the gut, defined as the amount that is potentially absorbable from the lumen. Depending on the food matrix, for example location in the plant, food processing, gastric and luminal digestion, in addition to the chemical form and properties of nutrients and phytochemicals, a low bioaccessibility may limit their bioavailability significantly (Holst and Williamson, 2008). Gut bacteria can hydrolyse glycosides, glucuronides, sulphates, amides and esters. They also carry out reduction, ring-cleavage, demethylation and dehydroxylation reactions. The hydrolysis of glycosides and glucuronides typically results in metabolites that are more biologically active than the parent compounds. In contrast, further bacterial degradation and transformation of aglycones can lead to production of more or less active compounds, depending on the substrate being metabolised and the products formed. Glucosinolates undergo gut bacterial metabolism. As with other plant compounds, the glucosinolates themselves are not biologically active, but some of their hydrolysis products, e.g. isothiocyanates (ITCs) and indoles, are. The plant enzyme myrosinase, a β-thioglucosidase, co-occurs in plants producing glucosinolates and in intact plant tissues is located in a compartment separate from the glucosinolates. When the cells in plants are damaged (e.g. cut, ground or chewed), enzyme and substrate come in contact, releasing the biologically active ITC. If myrosinase has been inactivated (e.g. with cooking), intestinal microbial metabolism of glucosinolates contributes to ITC exposure, albeit at a lower level. Bacterial strains associated with glucosinolate degradation have been identified and partly characterised and include *Escherichia coli*, *Bacteroides thetaiotaomicron*, *Bacteroides vulgatus*, *Bifidobacterium* spp., *Enterobacter cloacae* and *Lactobacillus agilis* (Lampe and Chang, 2007; Traka and Mithen, 2008).

SFN is considered to be the major anticarcinogenic component in broccoli and the metabolism of SFN is well described and recently reviewed elsewhere (Keck *et al.*, 2003; Bheemreddy and Jeffery, 2007; Zhang and Tang, 2007; Clarke *et al.*, 2008; Hanlon *et al.*, 2008; Traka and Mithen, 2008). The initial reaction involves enzymatic hydrolysis of glucoraphanin by myrosinase, as explained above, with the cleavage of the glycone from the glucosinolate forming glucose, hydrogen sulphate and one of many different aglycones (e.g. thiocyanate, ITC, or a nitrile) depending on the glucosinolate, reaction pH, and availability of ions (Grubb and Abel, 2006; Zhang and Tang, 2007; Clarke *et al.*, 2008).

Intake of a particular isothiocyanate or its precursor glucosinolate does not necessarily equate with exposure at the tissue level. Inter-individual differences in phytochemical metabolism and disposition may be affected by: gut microbial identity and activity; genetic determinants of biotransformation enzyme expression, stability and activity; environmental exposures that influence gut microflora and biotransformation enzymes; variation in levels of endogenous compounds that modulate biotransformation pathways. An enhanced understanding of the factors that contribute to inter-individual differences in the metabolism and disposition of phytochemicals may allow for more comprehensive evaluation of the role of these dietary constituents in cancer prevention. With new molecular techniques available to characterise gut microbial communities, the bacteria involved in the rate-limiting steps of phytochemical metabolism can be characterised. Controlled pharmacokinetic studies that are powered sufficiently to test effects of genotype on phytochemical metabolism may help to identify and quantify the role of specific polymorphisms.

Food matrix effects

Before consumption, cruciferous vegetables are often stored or subjected to a range of treatments such as washing, chopping, blancing, freezing and cooking that may alter their biological effects. Variations in processing and storage may mean that individuals with similar levels of cruciferous vegetable intake are exposed to different levels of bioactive compounds. This variation could mask any association between cruciferous vegetable intake and cancer risk. Most types of post-harvest treatment result in a loss of bioactive compounds. Processing may also beneficially or negatively alter the bioavailability of such compounds (Schenker, 2002; Lynn *et al.*, 2006; Cartea and Velasco, 2008).

For example, the location and production of ITCs in the gastrointestinal tract and the profile of the glucosinolates (GLS)-breakdown products formed is influenced by the extent of thermal processing to which a vegetable is subjected before consumption. When raw or lightly cooked cruciferous vegetables are consumed, most GLS hydrolysis occurs in the proximal gastrointestinal tract, catalysed by the presence of active plant myrosinase. However, the profile of the breakdown products formed after consumption of raw and lightly cooked cruciferous vegetables may vary (Lynn *et al.*, 2006).

Glucosinolate and related isothiocyante contents of *Brassica* vegetables are affected by method of storage and food processing, e.g. cutting, chewing, cooking, fermenting or freezing (Jeffery *et al.*, 2003; Moreno *et al.*, 2006, 2007a,b; Cartea and Velasco, 2008). Nevertheless, given the importance of glucosinolates in terms of their anticarcinogenic activity, few thermal degradation studies have been carried out with regard to food processing. Most of the research has been done in crude extracts and information about the plant myrosinase stability throughout processing is limited. When vegetables are sliced and washed as part of processing, conditions for myrosinase activity are probably optimal. This enzyme is temperature sensitive and consequently, throughout conventional thermal processing, it will be inactivated and it cannot transform glucosinolates into beneficial products. Thereby, it is important to maintain the levels of beneficial glucosinolates after harvest and to provide the correct way of cooking to ensure optimal health benefits.

Consumption of cruciferous vegetables does not pose any genotoxic risk in humans, although it cannot be excluded that consumption of extremely high doses of some glucosinolates could cause adverse effects. The amount of glucosinolates and their degradation products present in vegetables is dependent on processing, preparation and storage conditions (Schenker, 2002). The effect of storage, processing and cooking methods on glucosinolate content has been studied in several *Brassica* vegetables, such as broccoli, Brussels sprouts, cauliflower and cabbage (Jeffery *et al.*, 2003; Moreno *et al.*, 2007a,b; Song and Thornalley, 2007).

Cabbage contains the glucosinolate sinigrin, which is hydrolysed by myrosinase to allyl isothiocyanate; isothiocyanates are thought to inhibit the development of cancer cells by a number of mechanisms. After raw cabbage consumption, allyl isothiocyanates were rapidly excreted in urine. Conversely, healthy human volunteers consumed cooked cabbage and the excretion was delayed. The isothiocyanate production was more extensive after consumption of raw vegetables but isothiocyanates still arise, albeit to a lesser degree, when cooked vegetables are consumed. The lag in excretion on the cooked (microwaved) cabbage treatment suggested that the colon microflora catalyse glucosinolate hydrolysis in that case (Rouzaud *et al.*, 2004).

All the factors and operations through the postharvest chain will activate complex reaction mechanisms, and physical and physiological processes change glucosinolate levels and, subsequently, their breakdown products (Jeffery *et al.*, 2003; Cartea and Velasco, 2008). Prior to consumption, *Brassica* vegetables are subject to different ways of processing. Although some *Brassica* vegetables such as broccoli, cauliflower or cabbage can be eaten raw in salads or pickled form, most of them are cooked before consumption. It has been generally shown that conventional cooking methods such as boiling, steaming, pressure cooking and microwaving reduce the intake of glucosinolates by approximately 20–60%, depending on the method, intensity and type of compound (Rosa and Heaney, 1993; Verkerk and Dekker, 2004; López-Berenguer *et al.*, 2007). Therefore, increased bioavailability of dietary isothiocyanates may be achieved by avoiding boiling of vegetables. Cooking at high temperatures denatures myrosinase into vegetable material, resulting in a lower conversion of glucosinolates to isothiocyanates. Glucosinolate levels can be reduced because of enzymatic breakdown and leaching into the cooking water (Vallejo *et al.*, 2003; López-Berenguer *et al.*, 2007). Leaching of glucosinolates may not represent a dietary loss when culinary practices use this cooking water for soups (Rosa and Heaney, 1993; Moreno *et al.*, 2007b; Cartea and Velasco, 2008).

Steaming, microwaving and stir-fry cooking are popular cooking methods that have a significant effect on the total glucosinolate contents of *Brassica* vegetables. Microwave cooking is an efficient alternative for cooking vegetables owing to the low amount of cooking water required, and it has been used as a good method to inactivate myrosinase with a negligible loss of glucosinolates. The effect of microwave treatment on myrosinase activity and glucosinolate contents has been studied, although the reports are somehow confusing. The possible increased extractability of glucosinolates by using microwave treatment and the leaching of glucosinolates into the cooking water are probable explanations (Verkerk and Dekker, 2004; López-Berenguer *et al.*, 2007).

Stir-fry cooking is gradually becoming one of the major cooking methods used worldwide for *Brassica* vegetables. Song and Thornalley (2007) cooked *Brassica* vegetables by means of the stir-fry method for 3–5 min. Glucosinolate content of several vegetables as broccoli, cabbage, cauliflower or Brussels sprouts did not change significantly through this cooking procedure, presumably because the temperature in the stir-fry process was lower than expected. These authors stated that the stir-fry procedure inhibited myrosinase activity rapidly without any effect on glucosinolate content. This may explain why glucosinolate contents were preserved. Stir-fry cooking with extra virgin olive, soybean, peanut or safflower oil did not reduce the total glucosinolate content of the cooked broccoli compared with that of the uncooked sample (Moreno *et al.*, 2007b).

8.5.2 Experimental evidence of safety and bioactivity

Epidemiological studies support a role for fruits and vegetables, particularly cruciferous vegetables, in decreasing the risk for cancers (Moreno *et al.*,

2006, 2007a; Cornblatt *et al.*, 2007). The factor that sets crucifers apart from other plant foods is a relatively unique family of secondary metabolites termed glucosinolates. Upon hydrolysis glucosinolates give rise to bioactive isothiocyanates (as seen in previous section). A key mechanism of action of dietary anticarcinogens such as SFN is the ability to up-regulate phase II detoxification enzymes such as NAD(P)H-quinone oxidoreductase 1 (NQO1) but also inhibits the enzyme CYP1A, a phase I enzyme that has been associated with activation of a number of pre-carcinogens (Lai *et al.*, 2008). If consumption of three to five servings per week of broccoli can provide a 30–40% decrease in cancer risk, then consumption of more broccoli, or broccoli with higher levels of glucoraphanin (parental glucosinolate of SFN), should theoretically lead to a greater cancer protection. Even though the healthy nature of cruciferous foods is now well recognised, most people eat fewer than one serving a week, pointing out the unpleasant flavour as the reason for eating so little (Engel *et al.*, 2002). For these reasons, a rapid process for production of semi-purified glucosinolate preparations could make possible the development of effective anti-cancer food products and a dietary supplement or fortified food could overcome this aversion (Lai *et al.*, 2008). The highest dose of glucoraphanin provided to rats (30 mg glucoraphanin/kg rat, equivalent to a 10% broccoli diet made from freeze-dried broccoli containing 3 mg glucoraphanin/g DW) provided the greatest NQO1 induction in all tissues evaluated, although the response in the colon was particularly strong. The response to glucoraphanin was similar for purified and semi-purified glucoraphanin preparations, suggesting that semi-purified preparations can be used in supplements and to fortify foods. The dose approximately equivalent to a 10% freeze-dried broccoli diet was effective, and caused no damage to the caecum. It appears that a dose of 60 mg glucoraphanin/kg rat is the optimal bolus dosage which could be used for reducing cancer risk. Future studies should evaluate the mechanism of inflammation in the cecum, in an attempt to control this (Lai *et al.*, 2008).

Cho *et al.* (2006) demonstrated that an extract of broccoli flower had strong antioxidative effect by scavenging radicals and inhibiting protein oxidation induced by radicals. Furthermore, the effect of the broccoli flower against oxidative stress induced by diabetes was also confirmed under an *in vivo* system, demonstrating again that the extract of broccoli flower had a strong antioxidative effect by scavenging radicals and inhibiting protein oxidation induced by radicals. Furthermore, the effect of the broccoli flower against oxidative stress induced by diabetes was also confirmed under an *in vivo* system (100 or 200 mg/kg body weight/day for 20 days) with oral administration of a butanolic fraction of freeze-dried broccoli flower.

Oral administration of either the isothiocyanates or SFN, or its glucosinolate precursor, glucoraphanin, inhibits mammary carcinogenesis in rats with chemically induced cancer. An observed three-fold increase in NQO1 enzymatic activity provides evidence of a pronounced pharmacodynamic action of SFN. In a pilot study, eight healthy women undergoing reduction mammoplasty were given a single dose of a broccoli sprout preparation containing 200 μmol of SFN. Following oral dosing, SFN metabolites were readily measurable in human breast tissue enriched for epithelial cells, providing a strong rationale for evaluating the protective effects of a broccoli sprout preparation in clinical trials for women at risk for breast cancer (Cornblatt *et al.*, 2007).

8.6 Future trends

More needs to be known about the fate of dietary polyphenols after ingestion. Although we know the absorption rate and the metabolic changes occurring *in vivo* for many phenolic compounds and glucosinolates from different food products, the picture is not complete. The bioavailability of several dietary relevant compounds, as is the case of olygomeric procyanidins and ellagitannins, needs to be studied in more detail. The analytical methods available for the detection and quantification of these metabolites in biological fluids and tissues generally underestimate the content of these compounds and their metabolites, as they may interact with proteins and other biological macromolecules, preventing their extraction and presentation in soluble forms necessary for chromatographic analysis.

The study of the effect of the food matrix and the interaction with other food and ingredients in the bioavailability and metabolism of individual phytochemicals also needs to be studied in more detail, and will provide a better knowledge of the events happening *in vivo* once the food phytochemicals have been ingested.

In addition, the role of gut microbiota on the metabolism of the phytochemicals present in food will also need intensive study, as bacterial metabolites are generally quite bioavailable and could be responsible for the biological activity attributed to the metabolites present in food products.

Increasing the knowledge of the food-matrix and food-interaction effects and the role of gut microbiota on the metabolism and activation of the dietary constituents, will provide original ideas for the development of new functional foods, in which a combination of plant-derived food ingredients with the appropriate bacterial strains will lead to a better biological activity for an specific food product.

8.7 Acknowledgements

The authors are grateful to the Spanish MEC for financial support of their work (Programme CONSOLIDER INGENIO 2010, Project FUN-C-FOOD, CSD2007-063).

8.8 References

ABU-AMSHA CACCETTA RA, CROFT KD, BEILIN LJ, PUDDEY IB (2000) Ingestion of red wine significantly increases plasma phenolic acid concentrations but does not acutely affect *ex vivo* lipoprotein oxidizability. *Am. J. Clin. Nutr.* **71**, 67–74.

ANDRÉS-LACUEVA C, SHUKITT-HALE B, GALLI RL, JAUREQUI O, LAMUELA-RAVENTÓS RM, JOSEPH JA (2005) Anthocyanins in aged blueberry-fed rats are found centrally and may enhance memory. *Nutr. Nuerosci.* **8**, 111–120.

ATKINSON C, FRANKENFELD CL, LAMPE JW (2005) Gut bacterial metabolism of the soy isoflavone daidzein: exploring the relevance to human health. *Exp. Biol. Med. (Maywood)* **230**, 155–170.

AURA AM (2005) '*In vitro* digestion models for dietary phenolic compounds', Thesis, VTT, Espoo, Finland.

AURA AM, MARTIN-LOPEZ P, O'LEARY KA, WILLIAMSON G, OKSMAN-CALDENTEY KM, POUTANEN K, SANTOS-BUELGA C (2005) *In vitro* metabolism of anthocyanins by human gut microflora. *Eur. J. Nutr.* **44**, 133–142.

AZUMA K, IPPOUSHI K, NAKAYAMA M, ITO H, HIGASHIO H, TERAO J (2000) Absorption of chlorogenic acid and caffeic acid in rats after oral administration. *J. Agric. Food Chem.* **48**, 5496–5500.

BHEEMREDDY RD, JEFFERY EH (2007) The metabolic fate of purified glucoraphanin in F344 rats. *J. Agric. Food Chem.* **55**, 2861–2866. doi: 10.1021/jf0633544

BIEGER J, CERMAK R, BLANK R, DE BOER VC, HOLLMAN PC, KAMPHUES J, WOLFFRAM S (2008) Tissue distribution of quercetin in pigs after long-term dietary supplementation. *J. Nutr.* **138**, 1417–1420.

BITSCH R, NETZEL M, SONNTAG S, STRASS G, FRANK T, BITSCH I (2004) Urinary excretion of cyanidin clucosides and glucuronides in healthy humans after elderberry juice ingestion. *J. Biomed. Biotechnol.* **4**, 343–345.

BOWEY E, ADLERCREUTZ H, ROWLAND I (2003) Metabolism of isoflavones and lignans by the gut microflora: a study in grem-free and human flora associated rats. *Food Chem. Toxicol.* **41**, 631–636.

CARTEA ME, VELASCO P (2008) Glucosinolates in *Brassica* foods: bioavailability in food and significance for human health. *Phytochem. Rev.* **7**, 213–229. doi: 10.1007/s11101-007-9702-2

CARTRON E, FOURET G, CARBONNEAU MA, LAURET C, MICHEL F, MONNIER L, DESCOMPS B, LEGER CL (2003) Red-wine beneficial long-term effect on lipids but not on antioxidant characteristics in plasma in a study comparing three types of wine – description of two *O*-methylated derivatives of gallic acid in humans. *Free Radic. Res.* **37**, 1021–1035.

CERDÁ B, LLORACH R, CERÓN JJ, ESPÍN JC, TOMÁS-BARBERÁN FA (2003a) Evaluation of the bioavailability and metabolism in the rat of punicalagin and antioxidant polyphenol from pomegranate juice. *Eur. J. Nutr.* **42**, 18–28.

CERDÁ B, CERÓN JJ, ESPÍN JC, TOMÁS-BARBERÁN FA (2003b) The repeated oral administration of high doses of the pomegranate ellagitannin punicalagin to rats for 37 days is not toxic. *J. Agric. Food Chem.* **51**, 3493–3501.

CERDA B, ESPIN J, PARRA, S, MARTINEZ P, TOMAS-BARBERAN FA (2004) The potent *in vitro* antioxidant ellagitannins from pomegranate juice are metabolized into bioavailable but poor antioxidant hydroxyl-6-H-dibenzopyran-6-one derivatives by the colonic microflora of healthy humans. *Eur. J. Nutr.* **43**, 205–220.

CERDÁ B, TOMAS-BARBERAN FA, ESPÍN JC (2005a) Metabolism of antioxidant and chemopreventive ellagitannins from strawberries, raspberries, walnuts and oak-aged red wine in humans: identification of biomarkers and individual variability. *J. Agric. Food Chem.* **53**, 227–235.

CERDÁ B, PERIAGO P, ESPÍN JC, TOMAS-BARBERAN FA (2005b) Identification of urolithin A as a metabolite produced by human colon microflora from ellagic acid and related compounds, *J. Agric. Food Chem.* **53**, 5571–5576.

CHO EJ, LEE YA, YOO HH, YOKOZAWA T (2006) Protective effects of broccoli (*Brassica oleracea*) against oxidative damage *in vitro* and *in vivo*. *J. Nutr. Sci. Vitaminol.* **52**, 437–444.

CLARKE JD, DASHWOOD RH, HO E (2008) Multi-targeted prevention of cancer by sulforaphane. *Cancer Lett.* **269**, 291–304.

CLARKE DB, LLOYD, AS, BOTTING NP, OLDFI MF, NEEDS PW, WISEMAN H (2002) Measurement of intact sulfate and glucuronide phytoestrone conjugates in human urine using isotope dilution liquid chromtatography–tandem mass spectrometry with [13C(3)] isoflavone internal standards. *Anal. Biochem.* **309**, 158–172.

CLIFFORD MN (1999) Chlorogenic acids and other cinnamates – nature, occurrence and dietary burden. *J. Sci. Food Agric.* **79**, 362–372.

CLIFFORD MN (2004) Diet-derved phenols in plasma and tissues and their implications for health. *Planta Med.* **70**, 1103–1114.

CLIFFORD MN, SCALBERT A (2000) Ellagitannins: occurrences in food, bioavailability and cancer prevention. *J. Food Sci. Agric.* **80**, 1118–1125.

CORNBLATT BS, YE L, DINKOVA-KOSTOVA AT, ERB M, FAHEY JW, SINGH NK, CHEN MSA, STIERER T, GARRETT-MAYER E, ARGANI P, DAVIDSON NE, TALALAY P, KENSLER TW, VISVANATHAN K (2007) Preclinical and clinical evaluation of sulforaphane for chemoprevention in the breast. *Carcinogenesis* **28**(7), 1485–1490. doi: 10.1093/carcin/bgm049

CREMIN P, KASIM-KARAKAS S, WATERHOUSE AL (2001) LC/ES-MS detection of hydrxoycinnamates in human plasma and urine. *J. Agric. Food Chem.* **49**, 1747–1750.

CRESPY V, MORAND C, BESSON C, COTELLE N, VÉZIN H, DEMIGNÉ C, RÉMÉSY C (2003) The splanchnic metabolism of flavonoids highly differed according to the nature of the compound. *Am J Physiol Gastrointest Liver Physiol.* **284**, G980–988.

D'ARCHIVIO M, FILESI C, DI BENEDETTO R, GAGIULO R, GIOVANNINI C, MASELLA R (2007) Polyphenols, dietary sources and bioavailability. *Ann Ist. Super Sanitá* **43**, 348–361.

DAY AJ, MELLON F, BARRON D, SARRAZIN G, MORGAN MR, WILLIAMSON G (2001) Human metabolism of dietary flavonoids: identification of plasma metabolites of quercetin. *Free Radic. Res.* **35**, 941–952.

DE PASCUAL-TERESA S (1999) 'Análisis de taninos condensados en alimentos' (Analysis of condensed tannins in food), PhD dissertation. Salamanca, Spain: University of Salalmanca 181.

DÉPREZ S, BREZILLON C, RABOT S, PHILIPPE C, MILA I, LAPIERRE C, SCALBERT A (2000) Polymeric proamthocyanidins are catabolized by human colonic microflora into low-molecular-weight phenolic acids. *J. Nutr.* **130**, 2733–2738.

DOERGE DR, CHANG HC, CHURCHWELL MI, HOLDER CI (2000) Analysis of soy isoflavone conjugation *in vitro* and in human blood using liquid chromatography–mass spectrometry. *Drug Metab. Dipos.* **28**, 298–230.

ENGEL E, BATY C, LE CORRE D, SOUCHON I, MARTIN N (2002) Flavor-active compounds potentially implicated in cooked cauliflower acceptance. *J. Agric. Food Chem.* **50**, 6459–6467.

ERLUND I, KOSONEN T, ALFTHAN G, ALFTHAN G, MÄENPÄÄ J, PERTTUNEN K, KENRAALI J, PARANTAINEN J, ARO A (2000) Pharmcokinetics of quercetin from quercetin aglycone and rutin in healthy volunteers. *Eur. J. Clin. Pharmacol.* **56**, 545–553.

ERLUND I, MERIRINNE E, ALFTHAN G, ARO A (2001) Plasma kinetics and urinary excretion of the flavanones naringenin and hesperetin in humans after ingestion of orange juice and grapefruit juice. *J. Nutr.* **131**, 235–241.

ERLUND I, SILATE ML, ALFTHAN G, RANTAL M, KESANIEMI YA, ARO A (2002) Plasma concentrations of the flavonoids hespertin, naringenin and quercetin in human sungects following their habitual diets, and diets high or low in fruit and vegetables. *Eur. J. Clin. Nutr.* **56**, 891–898.

ESPÍN JC, GONZÁLEZ-BARRIO R, CERDÁ B, LÓPEZ-BOTE C, REY AI, TOMÁS-BARBERÁN FA (2007) Iberian pig as a model to clarify obscure points in the bioavailability and metabolism of ellagitannins in humans. *J. Agric. Food Chem.* **55**, 10476–10485.

FAHEY JW, KENSLER TW (2007) Role of dietary supplements/nutraceuticals in chemoprevention through induction of cytoprotective enzymes. *Chem. Res. Toxicol.* **20**, 572–576.

FAHEY JW, ZALCMANN AT, TALALAY P (2001) The chemical diversity and distribution of glucosinolates and isothiocyanates among plants. *Phytochemistry* **56**, 5–51.

FELGINES C, TEXIER O, MORAND C, MANACH C, SCALBERT A, RÉGERAT F, RÉMÉSY C (2000) Bioavailability of the flavanone naringenin and its glycosides in rats. *Am. J. Physiol Gastrointest. Liver Physiol.* **279**, G1148–1154.

FELGINES C, TALAVERA S, GONTHIER MP, TEXIER O, SCALBERT A, LAMAISON JL, RÉMÉSY C (2003) Strawberry anthocyanins are recovered in urine as glucuro- and sulfoconjugates in humans. *J. Nutr.* **133**, 1296–1301.

FELGINES C, TALAVERA, S., TEXIER O, GIL-IZQUIERDO A, LAMAISON JL, RÉMÉSY C (2005) Blackberry anthocyanins are mainly recovered in urine as methylated and glucuronidated conjugates in humans. *J. Agric. Food Chem.* **53**, 7721–7727.

FELGINES C, TEXIER O, BESSON C, LYAN B, LAMAISON JL, SCALBERT A (2007) Strawberry pelargonidin glycosides are excreted in urine as intact glycosides and glucuronidated pelargonidin derivatives in rats. *Br. J. Nutr.* **98**, 1126–1131.

GALVANO F, LA FAUCI L, LAZZARINO G, GLOGINAO V, TRIIENI A, CIAPPELLANO S, BATTISTINI NC, TAVAZZI B, GLAVANO G (2004) Cyanidins: metabolism and biological properties. *J. Nutr. Biochem.* **15**, 2–11.

GALVANO F, LA FAUCI L, VITAGLIONE P, FOGLIANO V, VANELLA L, FELGINES C (2007) Bioavailability, antioxidant and biological properties of the natuarl free-radical scavengers cyanidin and related glycosides. *Ann. Ist Super Sanitá* **43**, 382–393.

GIL MI, TOMÁS-BARBERÁN FA, HESS-PIERCE B, HOLCROFT DM, KADER AA (2000) Antioxidant activity of pomegranate juice and its relationship with phenolic composition and processing. *J. Agric. Food Chem.* **48**, 4581–4589.

GIL-IZQUIERDO A, GIL MI, FERRERES F, TOMÁS-BARBERÁN, FA (2001) *In vitro* availability of flavonoids and other phenolics in orange juice. *J. Agric. Food Chem.* **49**, 1035–1041.

GLITSO LV, MAZUR WM, ADLERCREUTZ H, WÄHÄLÄ K, MÄKELÄ T, SANDSTRÖM B, BACH KNUDSEN KE (2000) Intestinal metabolism of rye lignans in pigs. *Br. J. Nutr.* **84**, 429–437.

GONTHIER MP, VERNY MA, BESSON C, REMESY C, SCALBERT A (2003) Chlorogenic acid bioavailability largely depends on its metabolism by the gut microflora in rats. *J. Nutr.* **133**, 1853–1859.

GONTHIER MP, REMESY C, SCALBERT A, CHEYNIER V, SOUQUET JM, POUTANEN K, AURA AM (2006) Microbial metabolism of caffeic acid and its esters chlorogenic and caftaric acids by human faecal microbiota *in vitro*. *Biomed. Pharmacother.* **60**, 536–540.

GROENEWOUD G, HUNDT HKL (1986) The microbial metabolism of condensed (+)-catechins bt rat-cecal microflora. *Xenobiotica* **16**, 99–107.

GRUBB CD, ABEL S (2006) Glucosinolate metabolism and its control. *Trends Plant Sci.* **11**(2), 89–100. doi: 10.1016/j.tplants.2005.12.006

GUY L, VÉDRINE N, URPÍ-SARDÁ M, GIL-IZQUIERDO A, AL-MAHARIK N, BOITEAUX JP, SCALBERT A, REMESY C, BOTTING N, MANACH C (2008) Orally administered isoflavones are present as glucuronides in the human prostate. *Nutr. Cancer* **60**, 461–468.

HABAUZIT V, GIL-IZQUIERDO A, NIELSEN IL, MORAND C, WILLIAMSON G, OFFORD E, LEBECQUE P, DAVICCO MJ, COXAM V, HORCAJADA MN (2007) Comparative effect of hesperidin (flavonoid of citrus fruit) and its metabolite hesperetin 7-*O*-glucoside on bone metabolism in adult rats. *Ann. Nutr. Metab.* **51**, 204.

HANLON N, COLDHAM N, GIELBERT A, KUHNERT N, SAUER MJ, KING LJ, IOANNIDES C (2008) Absolute bioavailability and dose-dependent pharmacokinetic behaviour of dietary doses of the chemopreventive isothiocyanates sulforaphane in rat. *British J. Nutr.* **99**, 559–564. doi: 10.1017/S0007114507824093

HIGDON JV, DELAGE B, WILLIAMS DE, DASHWOOD RH (2007) Cruciferous vegetables and human cancer risk: epidemiologic evidence and mechanistic basis. *Pharmacol. Res.* **55**, 224–236. doi: 10.1016/j.phrs.2007.01.009

HOLST B, WILLIAMSON G (2008) Nutrients and phytochemicals: from bioavailability to bioefficacy beyond antioxidants. *Current Op. Biotechnol.* **19**, 73–82. doi: 10.1016/j.copbio.2008.03.003

HOLT RR, LAZARUS SA, SULLARDS MC, ZHU QY, SCHRAMM DD, HAMMERSTONE JF, FRAGA CG, SCHMITZ HH, KEEN CL (2002) Procyanidin dimer B2 [epicatechin-(4beta-8)-epicatechin] in human plasma after the consumption of a flavanol-rich cocoa. *Am. J. Clin. Nutr.* **76**, 798–804.

HONG SJ, KIM SI, KWON SM, LEE JR, CHUNG BC (2002) Comparative study of concentration of isoflavones and lignans in plasma and prostatic tissues of normal control and benign prostatic hyperplasia. *Yonsei Med. J.* **43**, 236–241.

HORCAJADA MN, HABAUZIT V, GIL-IZQUIERDO A, MORAND C, WILLIAMSON G, BARRON D, LEBECQUE P, DAVICCO MJ, OFFORD E, COXAM V (2006) Hesperetin-7-glucose is more effective than hesperidin for improving bone metaholism in the adult rat. *Annales d'Endocrinologie* **67**, 182–183.

ITO H, GONTHIER M, MANACH C, MORAND C, MENNEN L, RÉMÉSY C, SCALBERT A (2005) Polyphenol levels in human uringe after intake of six different polyphenol-rich beverages. *Br. J. Nutr.* **94**, 500–509.

JEFFERY EH, BROWN AF, KURILICH AC, KECK AS, MATUSHESKI N, KELIN BP, JUVIK JA (2003) Variation in content of bioactive components in broccoli. *J. Food Comp. Anal.* **16**, 323–330. doi: 10.1016/S0889-1575(03)00045-0

JUGE N, MITHEN RF, TRAKA M (2007) Molecular basis for chemoprevention by sulforaphane: a chomprehensive review. *Cell. Mol. Life Sci.* **64**, 1105–1127. doi: 10.1007/s00018-007-6484-5

KAY CD, MAZZA GJ, HOLUB BJ (2005) Anthocyanins exist in the circulation primarily as metabolites in adult men. *J. Nutr.* **135**, 2582–2588.

KECK AS, QIAO Q, JEFFERY EH (2003) Food matrix effects on bioactivity of broccoli-derived sulforaphane in liver and colon of F344 rats. *J. Agric. Food Chem.* **51**, 3320–3327. doi: 10.1021/f026189a

KEPPLER K, HUMPF HU (2005) Metabolism of anthocyanins and their phenolic degradation products by the intestinal microflora. *Bioorg. Med. Chem.* **13**, 5195–5205.

KRIS-ETHERTON PM, HECKER KD, BONANOME A, COVAL SM, BINKOSKI AE, KIRSTEN FH, GRIEL AE, ETHERTON TD (2002) Bioactive compounds in foods: their role in the prevention of cardiovascular disease and cancer. *Amer. J. Med.* **113**(9B), 71S–88S.

KRISHNAMURTY HG, CHENG KJ, JONES GA, SIMPSON FJ, WATKIN JE (1970) Identification of products by the anaerobic degradation of rutin and related flavonoids by *Butyrovibrio* sp. C3. *Can. J. Microbiol.* **16**, 759–767.

KWON KH, BARVE A, YU S, HUANG MT, KONG AT (2007) Cancer chemoprevention by phytochemicals: potential molecular targets, biomarkers and animal models. *Acta Pharmacol. Sin.* **28**(9), 1409–1421. doi: 10.1111/j.1745-7254.2007.00694.x

LAFAY S, GIL-IZQUIERDO A (2008) Bioavailability of phenolic acids. *Phytochem. Rev.* **7**, 301–311.

LAI RH, KECK AS, WALLIG MA, WEST LG, JEFFERY EH (2008) Evaluation of the safety and bioactivity of purified and semi-purified glucoraphanin. *Food Chem. Toxicol.* **46**, 195–202. doi: 10.1016/j.fct.2007.07.015

LAMPE JW, CHANG JL (2007) Interindividual differences in phytochemical metabolism and disposition. *Sem. Cancer Biol.* **17**, 347–353. doi: 10.1016/j.semcancer.2007.05.003

LAPIDOT T, HAREL S, GRANI R, KANNAER J (1998) Bioavailability of red wine anthocyanins as detected in human urine. *J. Agric. Food Chem.* **46**, 4297–4302.

LARROSA M, TOMÁS-BARBERÁN FA, ESPÍN JC (2006) The hydrolysable tannin punicalagin releases ellagic acid which induces apoptosis in human colon adenocarcinoma Caco-2-cells by using the mitochondrial pathway. *J. Nutr. Biochem.* **17**, 611–625.

LÓPEZ-BERENGUER C, CARVAJAL M, MORENO DA, GARCÍA-VIGUERA C (2007) Effects of microwave cooking conditions on bioactive compounds present in broccoli inflorescences. *J. Agric. Food Chem.* **55**, 10001–10007. doi: 10.1021/jf071680t

LI C, LEE MJ, SHENG S, MENG X, PRABHU S, WINNIK B, HUANG B, CHUNG JY, YAN S, HO CT, YANG CS (2000) Structural identification of two metabolites of catechins and their kinetics in human urine and blood after tea ingestion. *Chem. Res. Toxicol.* **13**, 177–184.

LYNN A, COLLINS A, FULLER Z, HILLMAN K, RATCLIFFE B (2006) Cruciferous vegetables and colo-rectal cancer. *Proc. Nutr. Soc.* **65**, 135–144. doi: 10.1079/PNS2005486

MANACH C, MORAND C, GIL-IZQUIERDO A, BOUTELOUP-DEMANGE C, RÉMÉSY C (2003) Bioavailability in humans of the flavanones hesperidin and narirutin after the ingestion of two doses of orange juice. *Eur. J. Clin. Nutr.* **57**, 235–242.

MANACH C, SCALBERT, A, MORAND C, RÉMÉSY C, JIMÉNEZ L (2004) Polyphenols: food and biovailability. *Am. J. Clin. Nutr.* **79**, 727–747.

MANACH C, WILLIAMSON G, MORAND C, SCALBERT A, RÉMÉSY C (2005) Bioavailability and bioefficacy of polyphenols in humans. I. Review of 97 bioavailability studies. *Am. J. Clin Nutr.* **81**, 230S–242S.

MATSUMOTO H, IKOMA Y, SUGIURA M, YANO M, HASEGAWA Y (2004) Identification and quantification of the conjugated metabolites derived from orally administered hesperidin in rat plasma. *J. Agric. Food Chem.* **52**, 6653–6659.

MAUBACH J, BRACKE, ME, HEYERICK A, DEPYPERE HT, SERREYN RF, MAREEL MM, DE KEUKELEIRE D (2003) Quantitation of soy-dervied phytoestrogens in human breast tissue and biological fluids by high performance liquid chromlatography. *J Chromatog. B Anal. Techonol. Biomed. Life Sci.* **784**, 137–144.

MAYS JR, WELLER ROSKA RL, SARFARAZ S, MUKHTAR H, RAJSKI SR (2008) Identification, synthesis, and enzymology of non-natural glucosinolate chemopreventive candidates. *ChemBioChem* **9**, 729–747. doi: 10.1002/cbic.200700586

MERTENS-TALCOTT SU, JILMA-STOHLAWETZ P, RIOS J, HINGORANI L, DERENDORF H (2006) Absorption, metabolism, and antioxidant effects of pomegranate (*Punica granatum* l.) polyphenols after ingestion of a standardized extract in healthy human volunteers. *J. Agric. Food Chem.* **54**, 8956–8961.

MESELHY MR, NAKAMURA N, HATTORI M (1997) Biotransformation of (–)-epicatechin-3-*O*-gallate by human intestinal bacteria. *Chem. Pharm. Bull.* **45**, 888–893.

MONTEIRO M, FARAH A, PERRONE D, TRUGO LC, DONANGELO C (2007) Chlorogenic acid compounds from coffee are differentially absorbed and metabolized in humans. *J. Nutr.* **137**, 2196–2201.

MOON JF, NAKATA R, OSHIMA S, INAJUMA T, TERA J (2000) Accumulation of quercetin conjugates in blood plasma after the short-term ingestion of onion by women. *Am. J. Physiol. Regul. Integr. Comp. Physiol.* **279**, R461–467.

MORANT AV, JORGENSEN K, JORGENSEN C, PAQUETTE SM, SÁNCHEZ-PÉREZ R, MOLLER BL, BAK S (2008) β-Glucosidases as detonators of plant chemical defense. *Phytochemistry* **69**, 1795–1813.

MORENO DA, CARVAJAL M, LÓPEZ-BERENGUER C, GARCÍA-VIGUERA C (2006) Chemical and biological characterization of nutraceutical compounds of broccoli. *J. Pharm. Biomed. Anal.* **41**, 1508–1522. doi: 10.1016/j.jpba.2006.04.003

MORENO DA, LÓPEZ-BERENGUER C, CARVAJAL M, GARCÍA-VIGUERA C (2007a) Health benefits of broccoli. Influence of pre- and post-harvest factors on bioactive compounds. *Food* **1**, 297–312.

MORENO DA, LÓPEZ-BERENGUER C, GARCÍA-VIGUERA C (2007b) Effects of stir-fry cooking with different edible oils on the phytochemical composition of broccoli. *J. Food Sci.* **72**, S64–S68. doi: 10.1111/j.1750-3841.2006.00213.x

MORTON MS, CHAN PS, CHENG C, BLACKLOK N, MATOS-FERREIRA A, ABRANCHES-MONTEIRO L, CORREIA L, LLOYD S, GRIFFITHS A (1997) Lignans and isoflavonois in plasma and prostatic fluid in men: samples from Portugal, Hong Kong, and the United Kingdom. *Prostate* **32**, 122–128.

MULLEN W, GRAF, BA, CALDWELL ST, HARTLEY RC, DUTHIE G, EDWARDS CA, LEAN MEJ, CROZIER A (2002) Determination of flavonol metabolites in plasma and tissues of rats by HPLC-radiocounting and tandem mass spectrometry following oral ingestion of [2-^{14}C]Quercetin-4′-glucoside. *J. Agric. Food Chem.* **50**, 6902–6909.

NARDINI M, CIRILLO E, NATELLA F, SCACCINI C (2002) Absorption of phenolic acids in humans after coffee consumption. *J. Agric. Food Chem.* **50**, 5735–5741.

NATSUME M, OSAKABE N, OYAMA M, SASAKI M, BABA S, NAKAMURA Y, OSAWA T, TERAO J (2003) Structures of (−)-epicatechin glucuronide identified from plasma and urine after oral ingestion of (−)-epicatechin: differences between human and rat. *Free Radic. Biol. Med.* **34**, 840–849.

NOROOZI M, BURNS J, CROZIER A, KELLY IE, LEAN ME (2000) Prediction of dietary flavonol consumption from fasting plasma concentration of urinary excretion. *Eur. J. Clin. Nutr.* **54**, 143–149.

OLTHOF MR, HOLLMAN PCH, KATNA MB (2001) Chlorogenic acid and caffeic acid are absorbed in humans. *J Nutr.* **131**, 66–71.

PASSAMONTI S, VRHOVSEK U, VANZO A, MATTIVI F (2003) The stomach as a site for anthocyanins absorption from food. *FEBS Lett.* **544**, 210–213.

PASSAMONTI S, VRHOVSEK U, VANZO A, MATTIVI F (2005) Fast access of some grape pigments to the brain. *J. Agric. Food Chem.* **53**, 7029–7034.

PLUMB GW, GARCIA-CONESA MT, KROON PA, RHODES M, RIDLEY S, WILLIAMSON G (1999) Metabolsim of chlorogenic acid by human plasma, liver, intestine and gut microflora. *J. Sci. Food Agric.* **79**, 390–392.

POSSEMIERS S, HEYERICK A, ROBBENS V, DE KEUKELEIRE D, VERSTRAETE W (2005) Activation of proestrogens from hops (*Humulus lupulus* L.) by intestinal microbiota; conversion of isoxanthohumol into 8-prenylnaringenin. *J. Agric. Food Chem.* **53**, 6281–6288.

POSSEMIERS S, BOLCA S, GROOTAERT C, HEYERICK A, DECROOS K, DHOOGE W, DE KEUKELIERE D, RABOT S, VERSTRAETE W (2006) The prenylflavonoid isoxanthohumol from hops (*Humuls lupulus* L.) is activated into the potent phytoestrogen 8-prenylnaringenin *in vitro* and in the human intestine. *J. Nutr.* **136**, 1862–1867.

POSSEMIERS S, RABOT S, ESPÍN JC, BRUNEAU A, PHILIPE C, GONZALEZ-SARRIAS A, HEYERICK A, TOMAS-BARBERAN FA, DE LEUKELEIRE D, VERSTRAETE W (2008) *Eubacterium limosum* activates isoxanthohumol from hops (*Humulus lupulus* L.) into the potent phytoestrogen 8-prenylnaringenin *in vitro* and in rat intestine. *J. Nutr.* **138**, 1–7.

PRICE N, JACKSON V, HALESTRAP A (1998) Cloning and sequencing of four new mammalian monocarboxylate transporter (MCT) homologes confirmes the existence of a transporter family with an ancient past. *Biochem. J.* **329**, 321–328.

RECHNER A, SPECNCER J, KUHNLE G, HAHN U, RICE-EVANS C (2001) Novel biomarkers of the metabolism of caffeic acid derivatives *in vivo*. *Free Radic. Biol. Med.* **30**, 1213–1222.

RECHNER AR, SMITH MA, KUHNLE G, GIBSON GR, DEBNAM ES, SRAI SKS, MOORE KP, RICE-EVANS CA (2004) Colonic metabolism of dietary polyphenol: influence of structure on microbial fermentation products. *Free Rad. Biol. Med.* **36**, 212–225.

RIOS LY, GONTHIER MP, RÉMÉSY C, MILA I, LAPIERRE C, LAZARUS SA, WILLIAMSON G, SCALBERT A (2003) Chocolate intake increases urinary excretion of polyphenol-derived phenolic acids in healthy human subjects. *Am. J. Clin. Nutr.* **77**, 912–918.

RONDINI L, PEYRAT-MAILLARD MN, MARSSET-BAGLIERI A, BERSET C (2002) Sulfated ferulic acid is the main *in vivo* metabolite found after short-term ingestion of free ferulic acid in rats. *J. Agric. Food Chem.* **50**, 3037–3041.

RONDINI L, PEYRAT-MAILLARD MN, MARSSET-BAGLIERI A, FROMENTIN G, DURAND P, TOME D, PROST M, BERSET C (2004) Bound ferulic acid from bran is more bioavailable than the free compound in rat. *J. Agric. Food Chem.* **52**, 4338–4343.

ROSA EAS, HEANEY RK (1993) The effect of cooking and processing on the glucosinolate content: studies on four varieties of Portuguese cabbage and hybrid white cabbage. *J. Sci. Food Agric.* **62**, 259–265. doi: 10.1002/jsfa.2740620309

ROUZAUD G, YOUNG SA, DUNCAN AJ (2004) Hydrolysis of glucosinolates to isothiocyanates after ingestion of raw or microwaved cabbage by human volunteers. *Cancer Epidemiol. Biomark. Prev.* **13**, 125–131.

RÜFER CE, BUB A, MÖSENEDER J, WINTERHALTER P, STÜRTZ M, KULLING SE (2008) Pharmacokinetics of the soybean isoflavone daidzein in its aglycone and glucoside form: a randomized, double-blind, crossover study. *Am. J. Clin. Nutr.* **87**, 1314–1323.

SANO A, YAMAKOSHI J, TOKUTAKE S, TOBE K, KUBOTA Y, KIKUCHI M (2003) Procyanidin B1 is detected in human serum after intake of proanthocyanidin-rich grape seed extract. *Biosci. Biotechnol. Biochem.* **67**, 1140–1143.

SEERAM NP, LEE R, HEBER D (2004) Bioavailability of ellagic acid in human plasma after consumption of ellagitannins from pomegranate (*Punica granatum* L.) juice. *Clin. Chim. Acta* **348**, 63–68.

SCHENKER S (2002) Broccoli. *Nutr. Bull.* **27**, 159–160.

SCHNEIDER H, SCHWIERTZ A, COLLINS MD, BLAUT M (1999) Anaerobic transformation of quercetin-3-glucoside by bacteria from the human intestinal tract. *Arch. Microbiol.* **171**, 81–91.

SCHRÖDER H (2007) Protective mechanisms of the Mediterranean diet in obesity and type 2 diabetes. *J. Nutr. Biochem.* **18**, 149–160. doi:10.1016/j.jnutbio.2006.05.006

SEOW A, VAINIO H, YU MC (2005) Effect of glutathione-*S*-transferase polymorphisms on the cancer preventive potential of isothiocyanates: an epidemiological perspective. *Mutation Res.* **592**, 58–67. doi: 10.1016/j.mrfmmm.2005.06.004

SESINK AL, O'LEARY KA, HOLLMAN PC (2001) Quercetin glucuronides but not glucosides are present in human plasma after consumption of quercetin-3-glucoside or quercetin-4′-glucoside. *J. Nutr.* **131**, 1938–1941.

SFAKIANOS J, COWARD L, KIRK M, BARNES S (1997) Intestinal auptake and biliary excretion of the isoflavone genistein in rats. *J. Nutr.* **127**, 1260–1268.

SHAPIRO TA, FAHEY JW, WADE KL, STEPHENSON KK, TALALAY P (2001) Chemoprotective glucosinolates and isothiocyanates of broccoli sprouts: metabolism and excretion in humans. *Cancer Epidemiol. Bio. Prev.* **10**, 501–508.

SHAPIRO TA, FAHEY JW, DINKOVA-KOSTOVA AT, HOLTZCLAW WD, STEPHENSON KK, WADE KL, YE L, TALALAY P (2006) Safety, tolerance, and metabolism of broccoli sprout glucosinolates and isothiocyanates: a clinical Phase I study. *Nutr. Cancer* **55**(1), 53–62.

SHELNUTT SR, CIMINO CO, WIGGINS PA, RONIS MJ, BADGER TM (2002) Pharmacokinetics of the glucuronide and sulfate conjugates of genistein and daidzein in men and women after consumption of a soy beverage. *Am. J. Clin. Nutr.* **76**, 588–594.

SILBERBERG M, GIL-IZQUIERDO A, MORAND C, COMBARET L, SCALBERT A, RÉMÉSY C (2006) New data on flavanone bioavailability and metabolism. Influence of cancer. *Biomed. Pharmacotherapy* **60**, 529–535.

SONG L, THORNALLEY PJ (2007) Effect of storage, processing and cooking on glucosinolate content of *Brassica* vegetables. *Food Chem. Toxicol.* **45**, 216–224. doi: 10.1016/j.fct.2006.07.021

STEINER C, ARNOULD S, SCALBERT A, MANACH C (2008) Isoflavones and the prevention of breast and prostate cancer: new perspectives opened by nutrigenomics. *Br. J. Nutr.* **99**, ES78–108.

STONER GD, SARD C, APSELOFF G, JMULLET D, WARGO W, POUND V, SING A, SANDERS J, AZIZ R, CASTO B, SUN XL (2005) Pharmacokinetics of anthocyanins and ellagic acid in healthy volunteers fed freeze-dried black raspberries daily for 7 days. *J. Clin. Pharmacol.* **45**, 1153–1164.

STONER GD, CHEN T, KRESTY LA, AZIZ RM, REINEMANN T, NINES R (2006) Protection against esophageal cancer in rodents with lyophilized berries: potential mechanisms. *Nutr. Cancer* **54**, 33–46.

SURH YJ (2003) Cancer chemoprevention with dietary phytochemicals. *Nature Rev. Cancer* **3**, 768–780. doi: 10.1038/nrc1189

TALAVERA S, FELGINES C, TEXIER O, BESSON C, LAMAISON JL, RÉMÉSY C (2003) Anthocyanins are efficiently absorbed from the stomach in anesthetized rats. *J. Nutr.* **133**, 4178–4182.

TALAVERA S, FELGINES C, TEXIER O, BESSON C, GIL-IZQUIERDO A, LAMAISAON JL, RÉMÉSY C (2005) Anthocyanin metabolism in rats and their distribution to digestive area, kidney, and brain. *J. Agric. Food Chem.* **23**, 3902–3908.

TIAN Q, GIUSTI MM, STONER GD SCHWARTZ SJ (2006) Urinary excretion of black raspberry (*Rubus occidentalis*) anthocyanins and their metabolites. *J. Agric. Food Chem.* **54**, 1467–1472.

TRAKA M, MITHEN R (2008) Glucosinolates, isothiocyanates and human health *Phytochem. Rev.* **8**, 269–282.

VALLEJO F, TOMÁS-BARBERÁN FA, GARCÍA-VIGUERA C (2003) Phenolic compound contents in edible parts of broccoli inflorescences after domestic cooking. *J. Sci. Food Agric.* **83**, 1511–1516. doi: 10.1002/jsfa.1585

VAN AMELSVOORT JM, VAN HOF KH, MATHOT JN, MULDER TP, WIERSMA A, TIJBURG LB (2001) Plasma concentrations of individual tea catechins after a single oral dose in humans. *Xenobiotica* **31**, 891–901.

VERKERK R, DEKKER M (2004) Glucosinolates and myrosinase activity in red cabbage (*Brassica oleracea* L. var. *Capitata* f. *rubra* DC.) after various microwave treatments. *J. Agric. Food Chem.* **52**, 7318–7323. doi: 10.1021/jf0493268

WANG LQ (2002) Mammalian phytoestrogens: enterodiol and enterolactone. *J. Chromatogr. B.* **777**, 289–309.

WANG LQ, MESELHY MR, LI Y, QIN GW, HATTORI M (2000) Human intestinal bacteria capable of transforming secoisolariciresinol diglucoside to mammalian lignans, enterodiol and enetrolactone. *Chem. Pharm. Bull.* **48**, 1601–1610.

WHITLEY AC, STONER GD, DARBY HW, WALLE T (2003) Intestinal epithelial cell accumulation of the cancer preventive polyphenol ellagic acid – extensive binding to protein and DNA. *Biochem. Pharmacol.* **66**, 907–915.

WINTER J, MOORE LH, DOWELL VR, BOKKENHEUSER VD (1989) C-Ring cleavage of flavonoids by human intestinal bacteria. *Appl. Environment. Microbiol.* **55**, 1203–1208.

WINTER J, POPOFF MR, GRIMONT P, BOKKENHEUSER VD (1991) *Clostridium orbiscindens* sp. Nov., a human intestinal bacterium capable of cleaving the flavonoid C-ring. *Int. J. Syst. Bacteriol.* **41**, 355–357.

WU X, CAO G, PRIOR RL (2002) Absorption and metabolism of anthocyanins in elderly women after consumption of elderberry or blueberry. *J. Nutr.* **132**, 1865–1871.

XU S, WANT HJ, MURPHY PA, COOK L, HENDRICH S (1994) Daidzein is a more bioavailable soymilk isoflavone than is genistein in adult women. *J. Nutr.* **124**, 825–832.

ZHANG Y, TANG L (2007) Discovery and development of sulforaphane as a cancer chemopreventive phytochemical. *Acta Pharamcol. Sin.* **28**(9), 1343–1354. doi: 10.1111/j.1745-7254.2007.00679.x

ZHAO Z, EGASHIRA Y, SANDA H (2003) Ferulic acid sugar esters are recovered in rat plasma and urine mainly as the sulfoglucuronide of ferulic acid. *J. Nutr.* **133**, 1355–1361.

ZHAO Z, EGASHIRA Y, SANADA H (2004) Ferulic acid is quickly absorbed from rat stomac as the free form and then conjugated mainly in liver. *J. Nutr.* **134**, 3083–3088.

9

Developing effective probiotic products: bioavailability and other factors

S. Lahtinen, N. Rautonen and A. Ouwehand, Danisco, Finland; A. Henrikson, Danisco, Singapore; and P. Steele, Danisco, USA

Abstract: Probiotics have many suggested health benefits, some of which are better documented than others. This chapter describes the selection of probiotics, the documentation of their health benefits and the suggested mechanisms of these health benefits. Since probiotics are among the main value drivers in the dairy industry and are prime examples of functional foods, the challenges and opportunities of probiotic products (also outside the dairy sector) are discussed. Application of probiotics in (functional) foods is mainly limited by water activity, pH, storage temperature and required shelf-life. The technological solutions for these challenges are discussed. Finally, the potential future trends and opportunities of probiotic functional foods are discussed.

Key words: probiotic, *Lactobacillus*, *Bifidobacterium*, health efficacy, intestinal microbiota, application.

9.1 Introduction

Probiotics have been defined in many ways; currently the most widely accepted definition is the one by the FAO/WHO (FAO/WHO 2002): 'live microorganisms which when administered in adequate amounts confer a health benefit on the host'. The definition indicates that probiotics need to be viable at the moment of consumption and need to be consumed in sufficient amounts; furthermore, there should be a documented health benefit. What amount needs to be consumed for a given health benefit is unclear. However, it is likely that different probiotic strains and different health benefits require specific doses. A study by Shornikova and co-workers demonstrate that a daily dose of 10^{10} CFU *Lactobacillus reuteri* reduced severity of rotavirus infection, and the effect was less significant if the daily dose was reduced 10^7 (Shornikova *et al.* 1997). Most other studies that demonstrate a beneficial effect of probiotics have used a daily dose of

10^9–10^{10} CFU, which suggest that the minimum effective dose is within this range for these strains. Other studies did in general not look at a health benefit, but at differences in faecal recovery (Ahmed *et al.* 2007) and are therefore not dose–response studies.

Probiotics are, by definition, microorganisms. The most commonly used strains belong to the genera *Lactobacillus* and *Bifidobacterium*, although species from other genera are also being used as probiotics (Table 9.1). The use of species from these two genera has historic reasons as probiotics have mainly been included in dairy foods. Even though probiotic foods have been on the market for a considerable time, the market is dynamic and developing continuously, with numerous new product launches annually (Sveje 2008).

As will be discussed below, when developing a probiotic functional food, many elements have to be considered, including strain properties, level of health benefit documentation and stability in the final product. The most desirable scenario for optimal probiotic stability requires that the food matrix, processing and storage do not contribute to excessive loss of probiotic viability during shelf-life while not providing conditions which can lead to undesirable sensory properties. All of these factors are strain and application dependent.

9.2 Selecting probiotics

There are no known specific requirements for the origin of a new probiotic strain. Although some may argue that it should be of human origin when intended for human use, there does not seem to be any rationale for that (Ouwehand & Lahtinen 2008), although one might not like to use strains isolated from diseased tissue. Once strains are isolated, they need to fulfil a number of requirements (Ouwehand *et al.* 1999).

When a probiotic strain is intended to be ingested as part of a (functional) food or as a supplement, it is generally accepted that the strains need to be able to resist the low pH and pepsin exposure of gastric transit. It also needs to resist exposure to bile (Daniel *et al.* 2006). Another property that may be beneficial, but not necessarily, is adhesion to the intestinal mucosa; it may prolong transient colonisation, aid in competitive exclusion against potential pathogens and improve the ability to interact with the intestinal mucosa (Vesterlund *et al.* 2005). If strains do not seem to survive the above conditions, techniques such as microencapsulation can be considered (Crittenden *et al.* 2001). Obviously, for probiotic health targets outside the gastrointestinal tract, such as the urogenital tract, oral cavity and skin, these selection criteria do not apply (Ouwehand 2003).

Strains that are considered as probiotics have to be safe, *primum non nocere*, although safety is a relative property since nothing is without any risk, a substantial degree of safety would have to be provided. Species from the genera *Bifidobacterium* and *Lactobacillus* generally have a satisfactory

Table 9.1 Examples of microorganisms commonly used as probiotics

Genus	Species	Strain	Remark
Bacillus	*clausii*		
	coagulans		Sometimes misclassified as *Lactobacillus sporogenes*
	fragilis		
	licheniformis	31	
	subtilis	3, natto	
Bifidobacterium	*breve*		
	animalis ssp. *lactis*	HN019, Bb-12, Bl-04, Bi-07, 420, DN-173010	Also referred to as *B. lactis*
	longum	46, 2C, BB536, Bl-05	
Enterococcus	*faecium*	SF68	
Escherichia	*coli*	Nissle 1917	
Lactobacillus	*acidophilus*	NCFM™, La-5, La-14	
	brevis	CD-2	
	bulgaricus		Primary use in yogurt
	casei	Shirota, DN-114001, CRL 431	May also be *L. paracasei*
	fermentum		
	johnsonii	La1	
	plantarum	299v, Lp-115	
	reuteri	ATCC 55730, RC-14	
	rhamnosus	HN001, GG, Lr-32, GR-1	
	salivarius	Ls-33	
Lactococcus	*lactis*	L1A	Mainly used as dairy starter
Propionibacterium	*freudenreichii* subsp. *shermanii*	JS	
Saccharomyces	*cerevisiae*	No different strains published	Often referred to as *S. boulardii*
Streptococcus	*thermophilus*	St-21, TH-4	Primary use in yogurt

safety record. They have been consumed for thousands of years as part of our normal diet and they are part of our intestinal and urogenital microbiota. Rare cases of *Lactobacillus* and even *Bifidobacterium* infections have been reported (Cannon *et al.* 2005), even some isolated cases of infections by probiotic strains have been reported (Boyle *et al.* 2006). It should be noted that such infections almost without exception were found in patients with severe underlying diseases. Furthermore, once the infections were diagnosed, they were with few exceptions successfully treated. Consequently, these organisms are generally considered to be safe and there do not seem to be concerns for consumers that are not suffering from serious underlying conditions. This is also indicated by the qualified presumption of safety (QPS) approach, for selected members of these genera, as advocated by the European Food Safety Agency (EFSA) (Barlow *et al.* 2007). Strains belonging to predefined species are assumed to be safe and do not require specific safety documentation. A remaining safety concern is, however, the presence of transferable antibiotic resistance. Although the antibiotic resistance in the probiotic may be of little harm, the fact that it might be transferred to pathogenic microbes is a matter of concern. Strains bearing transferable antibiotic resistance should preferably not be used as probiotics (Vankerckhoven *et al.* 2008). Although most, if not all, commercially used *B. lactis* strains carry *tetW* in their chromosome, the gene does not seem to be flanked by transferable elements and is therefore considered non-transferable.

Once a promising probiotic candidate strain has been identified, the first time it will have to be cultivated on a large scale is often in preparation for a clinical trial. Large-scale cultivation of strains is very different from cultivation at laboratory scale. A commonly used laboratory growth medium for lactic acid bacteria is de Man, Rogosa, Sharpe medium (MRS; de Man *et al.* 1960) but this is too expensive for large-scale cultivation, as it is composed of, among others, meat and yeast extract and casein hydrolysate. Full anaerobicity may not always be achieved upon large-scale cultivation. Likewise, shear forces are stronger, which may affect survival. After cultivation, the strains will need to be harvested and freeze dried, which may further affect viability. In this respect, it is important to realise that growth medium, cryoprotectants and time of harvest (one may get higher yield in the end product when not growing to highest cell density) all affect the quality of the probiotic and thereby of its stability. In addition to stability during production, probiotics will need to remain viable in different product applications with each their own specific challenges, as discussed towards the end of this chapter.

Documented health effects are a prerequisite for the probiotic status (see definition). Before performing a human intervention trial (Gill *et al.* 2001a), it is not uncommon to first perform *in vitro* studies (Prasad *et al.* 1998), followed by animal studies (Gill *et al.* 2000), where it is important that the animal model actually represents what is sought for in the human study. The latter, when well designed (double blind, placebo controlled, randomised) is a prerequisite to establish a strain as a probiotic; see below for further details on health efficacy study strategies. Further documentation is, however, always possible; studies repeated by other groups, multi-centre studies and finally meta-analyses. Regardless of the level of documentation, the health claims that can be made are strictly regulated and may allow only very general statements. In Europe a regulatory framework exists to apply for the use of specific claims on, for example, prevention of disease (European Parliament and the Council of the European Union 2006).

9.3 Experimental methods for efficacy studies

Recent years have seen a steady increase in research on probiotic cultures, which reflects a general increase in demand for efficacy data. Here a more detailed description is given of the type of studies and methodologies that have been used to characterise and select probiotic cultures for different applications.

It is believed that probiotic cultures should possess a number of properties to have a beneficial effect on human health, of which some can be assessed *in vitro* and in animal studies (preclinical). Therefore, it is appropriate to assess cultures in suitable preclinical trials, to ensure that cultures possess such properties before proceeding with clinical studies. The ability to persist the human gastrointestinal (GI) tract, at least transiently, is one such property. Furthermore, a true probiotic culture should have one or more beneficial effects on human health. Such beneficial effects could include anti-tumourogenic, anti-pathogenic and immune-modulating activities. Sections below give examples on preclinical studies that have been carried out to evaluate probiotic cultures *in vitro* and *in vivo*, and human studies that have been conducted to evaluate the effects of cultures on clinical end points and biomarkers for specific health conditions.

9.3.1 Preclinical studies

As mentioned above, survival and persistence are the main selection criteria for new probiotic strains. The ability of a probiotic culture to adhere to mucosal surfaces is generally regarded as a positive attribute and many earlier studies on prospective probiotic cultures focused on their adhesive properties (Henriksson & Conway 1996; Vesterlund *et al.* 2005). A variety of models have been used to assess adhesion of bacteria to mucosal and epithelial surfaces, including direct microscopy (Tuomola & Salminen 1998; Wold *et al.* 1988) and indirect measurements of adhesion using radioactively labelled bacteria (Conway & Adams 1989; Conway & Kjelleberg 1989). The ability to survive in the GI tract is another important probiotic trait, and it is recommended that prospective probiotic cultures are assessed for their ability to survive in conditions of the human GI tract. Several models have been used to evaluate their ability to survive under these conditions, including low pH buffers containing gastric enzymes (Daniel *et al.* 2006; Ding & Shah 2007) and true human gastric juice (Conway *et al.* 1987). Similarly, several methods have been used to assess the effect of bile acids and pancreatic enzymes found in the small intestine (Daniel *et al.* 2006; Ding & Shah 2007).

As for the assessment of anti-pathogen activities, a great variety of methods have been described. Some of these methods use co-cultures of potentially probiotic cultures and model pathogens to monitor anti-pathogen activity (Henriksson & Conway 2001a). This type of method does not discriminate between the effects of different compounds produced by the culture. Instead, fractionated culture supernatant or other culture fractions may be used to investigate the effect of different compounds (Bernet-Camard *et al.* 1997; Hudault *et al.* 1997).

Subsequent to an assessment *in vitro*, the effect of a probiotic culture can be assessed *in vivo* using a variety of animal models. In this type of study, animals are challenged with a pathogen and a potential probiotic culture. A protective culture can be identified by monitoring the incidence and severity of infection, or the levels of pathogen in faeces or blood. Such models usually apply conventional, specific pathogen-free (Gill *et al.* 2001; Henriksson & Conway 2001b; Mahoney & Henriksson 2003) or gnotobiotic animals (Filho-Lima *et al.* 2000; Silva *et al.* 1999).

For assessment of anti-carcinogenic properties, *in vitro* models have been applied to investigate if certain probiotic cultures are capable of degrading or absorbing carcinogens in foods, and thereby reducing the risk of cancer (Turbic *et al.* 2002; Zhang & Ohta 1990). Animal models include assays to investigate the effect of pre- and probiotics on the apoptotic response, which is one of the primary defences against tumour formation (Hughes & Rowland 2001; le Leu *et al.* 2005). Animal models are important tools for investigating if a culture inhibits the actual tumour formation *in vivo*. Such models usually involve challenging of animals with a carcinogen, and monitoring of the subsequent incidence and severity of tumour formation in animals treated with a probiotic culture or a placebo (Goldin & Gorbach 1980; Klinder *et al.* 2004). This type of models are similar to models that can be used to investigate the anti-inflammatory effects of cultures on the gastrointestinal mucosa (Peran *et al.* 2005).

The effect of probiotics on the systemic immune system has been investigated using a wide range of different models, both *in vitro* and *in vivo*. *In vitro* models using human blood cells have been used to investigate the effect of probiotics on secretion of cytokines including TNF-α, IL-10 and IFN-γ (Clancy *et al.* 2006; Kekkonen *et al.* 2008). Animal models have been useful in confirming the effect on secretion of these cytokines *in vivo* (Peng *et al.* 2007), as well as determining if a probiotic culture has an effect on the acquired immunity, such as the formation of immunoglobulins (Kaburagi *et al.* 2007; Olivares *et al.* 2007; Peng *et al.* 2007; Tejada-Simon *et al.* 1999; Zhou & Gill 2005).

9.3.2 Clinical studies

Preclinical studies like these may suggest that a culture has one or several beneficial effects on human health. An observed effect in animals may warrant further investigation in clinical studies. Clinical studies are often classified as phase I, II, III and IV, depending on what is being investigated. As for pharmacological agents, larger clinical studies on probiotics should be placebo controlled, randomised and double blind to improve integrity and reliability of the study outcome. Typically, a potential new probiotic culture would initially be applied in a phase I trial to investigate survival of the culture in the gastrointestinal tract (Ouwehand *et al.* 2008b; Yuki *et al.* 1999), or if the culture has effect on particular biomarkers. Natural killer (NK) cells and immunoglobins in blood are examples of biomarkers that have been assessed in this type of trials (Gill *et al.* 2000, 2001a; Paineau *et al.* 2008).

The effect of a culture on clinical end points, such as the incidence, duration and/or severity of a disease, is assessed in a second phase (phase II). If this type of trial gives an indication of a beneficial effect, then this may warrant further investigation of the culture in a phase III trial, which usually include several hundred subjects. Studies of this type (phases II and III), which monitor specific and appropriate end points, have identified probiotic cultures with beneficial effects on a range of health conditions such as respiratory infections (de Vrese *et al.* 2005b; Winkler *et al.* 2005), allergic disease (Kalliomäki *et al.* 2003; Rosenfeldt *et al.* 2003), recurrence of cancer (Aso *et al.* 1995; Naito *et al.* 2008), digestive disorders (Niedzielin *et al.* 2001; Nobaek *et al.* 2000) and infections (Rosenfeldt *et al.* 2004; Saavedra *et al.* 1994), as will be discussed in more detail below.

The examples given here are only a few of a vast number of methods that have been used to investigate the functionality and efficacy of probiotics and functional foods, from the early explorative and mechanistic studies *in vitro*, to large clinical studies. Together, these studies have generated valuable data on functional foods and their benefits to human health quality of life.

9.4 Health benefits of probiotics

Probiotics have been linked with a range of different health benefits. The level of documentation of different health benefits varies from well-documented effects such as improvement of lactose ingestion (Kim & Gilliland 1983) to certain more hypothetical effects, which hardly have been tested in a clinical setting (Table 9.2). In general, the health benefits of

Table 9.2 The targets of the suggested health benefits of probiotics, and the current level of scientific proof supporting them. Modified from Lahtinen (2007)

Target	Proof	Notes
Diarrhoea	+++	Some types well-documented (e.g. rotavirus diarrhoea), others not (e.g. traveller's diarrhoea)
Constipation	+	Also negative studies
Bowel habits of healthy subjects	+	Dose-dependent
Irritable bowel syndrome	++	Effects mainly on bloating
Crohn's disease	–	Recent large studies negative
Ulcerative colitis	+	Encouraging based on small studies
Pouchitis	+	Encouraging based on small studies
Short bowel syndrome	+	Increased risk of sepsis
Necrotising enterocolitis	+	Encouraging; increased risk of sepsis
Helicobacter pylori: eradication	–	Complete eradication unlikely
H. pylori: enhancement of antibiotic therapies	+	Reduces side effects
Liver diseases: treatment and protection	(+)	No clinical trials
Liver diseases: binding of mycotoxins	+	More clinical studies needed
Kidney diseases: reduction of uremic toxins	+	Limited but encouraging evidence
Calcium oxalate stone disease	+	Based on small studies
Vaginal infections	++	Promising application
Candidiasis	(+)	Experimental data only
Lactose digestion	+++	Pasteurised products less effective
Mineral absorption	±	Prebiotics may be more effective
Blood lipid levels	±	May be strain specific; animal studies more effective
Diabetes	(+)	No clinical data
Prevention of eczema	++	Promising, but also negative results
Treatment of eczema and/or food allergies	±	Effects seen mainly on food-sensitised children
Treatment of pollen allergies, rhinitis	+	More clinical studies needed
Treatment of asthma	–	Limited data
Rheumatoid arthritis	(+)	Mainly experimental data
High blood pressure	++	Mediated by extracellular peptides
Cancer: epidemiological studies	±	Limited and contradicting data
Cancer: recurrence of bladder cancer	+	Some clinical evidence
Cancer: tumour reduction	(+)	Good *in vitro* and animal data
Respiratory tract infections	++	Encouraging results from various countries
Otitis media	–	Very limited evidence
Oral health (caries, gingivitis, halitosis)	+	Most evidence on gingivitis
Autism	(+)	Anecdotal evidence only

+++ Well documented; ++ appears effective; + potential, needs further assessment; (+) anecdotal evidence; ± contradicting evidence; – no effect.

probiotics are strain-specific, require sufficient dose and duration of administration, and largely depend on the health status of the host. The proposed health effects mediated by probiotics are mainly defined by the role of resident microbes in host health. Following birth, all mucosal surfaces are colonised by microbial communities. The resident microbes play an important role on the mucosa by reducing risk of colonisation by pathogens and enhancing the host defence systems. Resident microbes influence not only development of mucosal but also systemic immune responses and regulation. Entirely different functionalities of microbes are mediated by their influence on host nutrition, and especially on host energy metabolism. Even specific behavioural effects of host can be attributed to intestinal signalling mediated by the microbes.

9.4.1 Anti-pathogenic effects

Probiotics have been proposed to influence the health of several mucosal compartments of the host, including the GIT, urogenital tract, nasopharyngeal cavity and oral cavity. Prevention and treatment of infections in the gastrointestinal tract and also on other mucosal surfaces of human body constitute a major target for probiotic therapies. Efficacy of probiotics against acute infectious diarrhoea is well documented, and the most-studied pathogens in this respect are rotavirus and *Clostridium difficile* (Sazawal *et al.* 2006). Other infectious agents such as *Salmonella*, *Shigella*, *Campylobacter*, *Yersinia* and parasites have been studied to lesser extent. Probiotics have been proposed to reduce *Candida* infections on gastrointestinal (Wagner *et al.* 1997), vaginal (Falagas *et al.* 2006) and oral surfaces (Hatakka *et al.* 2007a), but in general the efficacy of probiotics against candidiasis requires further investigation. Beneficial effects of probiotics on bacterial vaginosis shows promise (Reid *et al.* 2001), while the effects on recurrent urinary tract infections are inconclusive.

Probiotics may not always have direct effects on infection. However, they may in addition have effects complementary to conventional drug therapies. For example, probiotics can alleviate the side effects of antibiotic therapies, including shortening of antibiotic-associated diarrhoea (Szajewska *et al.* 2006) and enhanced restoration of normal gut microbiota following antibiotic therapies (Engelbrektson *et al.* 2006). While attempts to eradicate *Helicobacter pylori* from the gut by probiotics alone have yielded inconsistent results, probiotics may still have adjuvant effects on antibiotic therapies against *H. pylori* (Hamilton-Miller 2003). Moreover, probiotics may enhance the immune responses to oral vaccinations (de Vrese *et al.* 2005a; Paineau *et al.* 2008).

9.4.2 Respiratory tract infections

Recent studies have suggested that probiotics are effective in the incidence and/or duration of common respiratory tract infections. The specific strains studied in this respect include *Lactobacillus acidophilus* NCFM™ and *Bifidobacterium lactis* Bi-07 (Ouwehand *et al.* 2008a), *Lactobacillus gasseri* PA 16/8, *Bifidobacterium longum* SP 07/3 and *B. bifidum* MF 20/5 (de Vrese *et al.* 2006), and *Lactobacillus rhamnosus* GG (Hatakka *et al.* 2001). Given the prevalence of the common cold in all age groups, probiotic therapies aiming at the reduction of symptoms or duration of common cold episodes would be very beneficial. However, a study assessing the effect of *L. rhamnosus* GG in the treatment and prevention of acute otitis media did not result in prevention of occurrence of the disease (Hatakka *et al.* 2007b). It may not seem obvious that consuming a probiotic will have a health benefit in the respiratory tract. However, as will be discussed below on mechanisms of probiotic action, specific probiotic strains are able to modulate the mucosal immunity. Since the intestine, respiratory and urogenital tract share a common mucosal immune system; modulation of this part of the immune system in one site, e.g. the intestine, will also affect the immune system in the other sites, e.g. the respiratory tract (Sansonetti 2004). Furthermore, consumption of a combination of probiotics (*L. rhamnosus* GG, *B. lactis* 420, *L. acidophilus* 145 and *Streptococcus thermophilus*) has been shown to modulate the microbiota of the oropharynx (Glück & Gebbers 2003).

9.4.3 Irritable bowel syndrome

Several of the proposed probiotic health benefits relate to improvement of gut function. Irritable bowel syndrome (IBS) is a rapidly emerging target for probiotic therapies. The condition, characterised by chronic functional diarrhoea, constipation or both and accompanied by visceral pain, is of unknown aetiology and is therefore regarded a 'syndrome' and not a 'disease'. Several strains and strain combinations have been suggested to have beneficial effects on IBS (Guyonnet *et al.* 2007; Niedzielin *et al.* 2001), although lack of effect has also been reported (Niv *et al.* 2005). Typically, the beneficial effects are associated with reduced bloating and abdominal distension. It has been suggested that certain probiotics such as *L. acidophilus* NCFM™ may also be capable of reducing intestinal pain by directly influencing expression of intestinal pain receptors (Rousseaux *et al.* 2006). Studies on the effects of probiotics on constipation have yielded contradictory results: for example a study with *Lactobacillus casei* Shirota suggested alleviation of constipation (Koebnick *et al.* 2003), while a study with *L. rhamnosus* GG suggested no effect (Banaszkiewicz & Szajewska 2005). Some studies have also suggested moderate effects on the bowel movements and gut function of healthy subjects (Larsen *et al.* 2006; Olivares *et al.* 2006a), although the clinical significance of such effects is open for discussion.

9.4.4 Inflammatory bowel disease

Reduction of the symptoms of intestinal inflammation and in particular inflammatory bowel disease (IBD) has received much attention. Despite the link between altered gut microbiota composition and Crohn's disease, the most common from of IBD, the clinical trials attempting to use probiotics in the treatment of this disease have not shown an improvement in symptoms or duration of remission (Marteau *et al.* 2006; Prantera *et al.* 2002). In contrast, certain probiotics may be effective in the treatment of other forms of IBD, including pouchitis (Gionchetti *et al.* 2003) and ulcerative colitis (Kruis *et al.* 2004). Some evidence exists for the benefit of probiotics in oral inflammation, including gingivitis (Krasse *et al.* 2006).

9.4.5 Immune function

Treatment and prevention of allergies by probiotics is a promising area of probiotic research. For example, several studies have shown that the probiotic strains *B. lactis* HN019 and *L. rhamnosus* HN001 improve the natural immunity of elderly subjects (Gill *et al.* 2001a, b). Several clinical studies have suggested that probiotic administration from late pregnancy until first months after the birth may reduce the risk of atopic eczema (Kalliomäki *et al.* 2001; Rautava *et al.* 2002) or IgE-sensitised eczema (Abrahamsson *et al.* 2007; Viljanen *et al.* 2005) in children, although some clinical trials have yielded negative results (Kopp *et al.* 2008; Taylor *et al.* 2007). Despite early studies suggesting the efficacy of probiotics in the treatment of allergies, it is now generally agreed that the prevention of allergies with probiotic therapies is more effective than treatment of allergies (Boyle & Tang 2006). Recently, Sistek and others suggested that benefits of treating allergies with probiotics are most likely to occur among food-sensitised children (Sistek *et al.* 2006). Studies on the treatment of pollen allergies with probiotics have yielded inconsistent results (Helin *et al.* 2002; Ishida *et al.* 2005).

9.4.6 Other disease targets

Normal gut microbiota plays an important role in maintaining human health and preventing a number of diseases (Guarner & Malagelada 2003), including kidney diseases (Dunn *et al.* 1998), necrotising enterocolitis (Hoyos 1999), liver diseases (Solga & Diehl 2003) rheumatoid arthritis (Toivanen 2003) and autism (Bingham 2003). Probiotic bacteria may also be helpful in fighting against pathogens on oral surfaces (Caglar *et al.* 2006). The effects of probiotics on skin infections are scarcely documented (Ouwehand *et al.* 2003). Recently, alterations in gut microbiota have been linked with obesity (Kalliomäki *et al.* 2008; Ley *et al.* 2005).

In some of these cases, the role of the gut microbiota and the health status is well established, while in other cases the research is only at its infancy. The connection between gut microbiota and diseases provide rationale for using probiotics as modulators of gut microbiota and immune function in order to prevent and treat diseases related to gut microbiota and to maintain general health and well-being.

Taken together, there is substantial and rapidly increasing evidence suggesting that probiotics and fermented foods have beneficial effects on many aspects of human health. In most cases, the efficacy of probiotics is higher in prevention of diseases rather than in curing the diseases. Efficacy of the prevention of common diseases such as diarrhoea and the common cold suggest that probiotics offer health benefits to everyone and each age group, including healthy individuals.

9.4.7 Health claims

Probiotics have been linked with a plethora of different health benefits. The scientific documentation supporting the suggested health benefits varies greatly between the different benefits as well as between different probiotic strains. By definition, probiotics 'confer a health benefit on the host' (FAO/WHO 2002), and the functionality of the probiotics is the main argument for their sale and consumption. Despite this, regulations regarding health claims of probiotics used in marketing of probiotic products are only now being set up. For example, in Europe, the European Food Safety Agency (EFSA) reviews the health claims submitted to EFSA by the suppliers of probiotics and by the producers of probiotic end products. The first list of approved health claims is set to be published in 2010. The health claims evaluated by EFSA fall under Article 13.1, Article 13.5 and Article 14 of The Regulation on Nutrition and Health Claims on Foods (European Parliament and the Council of the European Union 2006). Article 13.1 consists of 'generic' claims, based on generally accepted scientific evidence. Article 13.5 is for claims based on newly developed scientific data. Article 14 consists of claims relating to reduction of disease risk and also claims related to children's development and health.

In Japan, generic health claims of functional foods and food ingredients are not strictly regulated. More stringent regulation of health claims is offered by the FOSHU (FOod for a Specific Health Use) labelling system, which was set up in 1991. The FOSHU claims are evaluated by an expert committee. The Food with Nutrient Function Claims (FNFC) system, which was set up more recently by the Ministry of Health, Labour and Welfare of Japan, is ingredient-based, and focuses mainly on vitamins and minerals (Hosoya 1998).

9.5 Proposed mechanisms of probiotic health effects

A major issue in the establishment of the clinical health effects of probiotic bacteria is the demonstration of the mechanisms behind the observed beneficial outcomes. This has proved to be a very challenging task as it is likely that multiple mechanisms are involved in most of the host–microbe interactions related to probiotic bacteria.

9.5.1 Modulation of host microbiota and adherence to host tissues

Many diseases and disorders are associated with aberrant gut microbiota (Fooks & Gibson 2002), providing a rationale for the use of probiotics (and prebiotics, see Chapter 5 on non-starch polysaccharides) to treat these disorders through modulation of the intestinal microbiota. Several studies have indicated that administration of probiotic strains can modulate the intestinal microbiota, and this is believed to play a role in certain proposed health benefits of probiotic bacteria. Changes in the levels of intestinal lactobacilli and bifidobacteria have been reported in a number of studies (Ouwehand *et al.* 2008c; Sullivan *et al.* 2001; Tannock *et al.* 2000; Yamano *et al.* 2006), while other studies do not suggest significant changes (Donnet-Hughes *et al.* 1999; Larsen *et al.* 2006). The microbiota of the large intestine of healthy adults is generally very stable, and the possible changes mediated by probiotics are temporary. Administration of probiotic bacteria does not lead to permanent colonisation in humans, although sometimes prolonged re-isolation of administered strains is observed (Alander *et al.* 1999). In infants, the colonisation may be more persistent, although permanent colonisation remains to be demonstrated (Gueimonde *et al.* 2006). Modulation of vaginal microbiota by administration of oral probiotics has also been suggested (Reid *et al.* 2003).

The ability of probiotic bacteria to adhere to intestinal mucus and epithelial cells may serve as a mechanism allowing close and prolonged host–microbe interactions. Many probiotic strains are able to bind to human intestinal mucus *in vitro*, but the adherence is strain-specific (Collado *et al.* 2008; Ouwehand *et al.* 2001; Tallon *et al.* 2007). Clinical evidence demonstrating that exogenously administered probiotics can adhere in the human intestinal mucosa is limited. Nevertheless, some studies have suggested that probiotics may adhere to human mucus *in vivo* (Alander *et al.* 1997; Morelli *et al.* 2006; Valeur *et al.* 2004). Probiotic strains may also reduce the adhesion of pathogenic strains to host mucus (Collado *et al.* 2007; Vesterlund *et al.* 2006). Production of antimicrobial substances by probiotic bacteria may also influence the intestinal microbiota composition. Production of organic acids may lead to lowering of the colonic pH and subsequent alteration of colonic microbiota (Salminen & Salminen 1997). Probiotic bacteria may also produce several other antimicrobial agents, such as hydrogen peroxide, carbon dioxide, diacetyl, low molecular weight substances such as reuterin, and bacteriocins (Ouwehand & Vesterlund 2004). However, the effect of bacteriocins in the gut is not clear, as bacteriocins are peptides, and thus are susceptible to both host and microbial proteases present in the gut (Fuller & Gibson 1997). Indeed, colonisation of mice with nisin-producing *Lactococcus lactis* failed to induce any change in microbiota composition although fragments of nisin (indicating *in situ* production) were detected (Bernbom *et al.* 2006).

9.5.2 Effects on gut permeability

Compromised mucosal barrier and increased gut permeability are typical of several gastrointestinal disorders, and it has been suggested that the restoration and stabilisation of the gut mucosal barrier has a critical role in the mechanisms of the proposed health effects of probiotics. Improvement of gut barrier function by administration of probiotic bacteria has been shown in murine models (Madsen *et al.* 2001). Effects on gut barrier and bacterial translocation have been demonstrated in several experimental settings, including acute liver injury (Adawi *et al.* 1999), thermal injury (Gun *et al.* 2005), biliary obstruction (White *et al.* 2006) and psychological stress (Ait-Belgnaoui *et al.* 2006; Zareie *et al.* 2006). In humans, the current evidence for the improvement of gut barrier function is scarce and somewhat contradictory. Some studies have suggested improvement in gut barrier function (Rosenfeldt *et al.* 2004), while other studies have indicated no improvement in barrier function (Jain *et al.* 2004; McNaught *et al.* 2005). In the case of infections, it has been suggested that probiotic bacteria may counteract the adverse effects of pathogens on the transepithelial resistance (Resta-Lenert & Barrett 2003).

9.5.3 Regulation of the immune system and immune function

The mucosal surface of the gastrointestinal tract provides a huge surface area vulnerable to invasion by pathogens and exposed to potentially noxious components from food and digestion. Furthermore, the lower intestine is also heavily populated by a microbiota (Hooper & Gordon 2001). Thus, it is no wonder that the intestinal immune system is the largest and most complex part of human immune system (Mowat 2003). In fact, maturation of the individual immune system is dependent on intestinal microbial stimulation after birth (Gordon *et al.* 1997; Lanning *et al.* 2000; Sudo *et al.* 1997). A number of studies have shown that diets, supplemented by probiotic bacteria, can also modulate the immune system and its function (Gill & Prasad 2008). Most of the early studies have been conducted using *in vitro* or animal models, but the number of well-conducted clinical studies focusing on the interactions between probiotics and the immune system is increasing. Modulation of the regulation of the immune system is likely to play a role in several of the proposed health benefits of probiotics, such as effects on allergies, gastrointestinal and respiratory tract infections, and intestinal inflammation.

Immune responses consist of innate immune responses and adaptive immune responses. The innate immune system is continuously 'on guard' and provides the first line of defence against harmful agents invading the host or other harmful challenges in the healthy host's environment, such as cancerous changes of host cells. Innate immune responses may be modulated by probiotics in several ways. Enhancement of phagocytic responsiveness by strains *Bifidobacterium lactis* HN019 (Arunachalam *et al.* 2000; Gill *et al.* 2001b) and *Lactobacillus rhamnosus* HN001 (Gill & Rutherfurd 2001; Sheih *et al.* 2001) has been demonstrated in humans. An increase in phagocyte responsiveness has been reported also for other probiotic strains

(Donnet-Hughes *et al.* 1999; Olivares *et al.* 2006b), but some trials have also indicated a lack of response (Christensen *et al.* 2006), suggesting that the immunomodulatory effects may be strain specific. In addition, in some cases reduced immune sufficiency or imbalanced immune regulation is a prerequisite for observing improvement. It is thus possible that the effects of probiotic bacteria on phagocytes are different in, for example, healthy and allergic subjects or in young and elderly subjects (Pelto *et al.* 1998). Probiotic treatments have been shown to increase the proportion and the activity of NK cells in blood in humans. The activity of NK cells may be increased by probiotic intake (Gill *et al.* 2001a; Takeda *et al.* 2006). Probiotic bacteria have also been found to influence faecal and serum cytokine levels (O'Mahony *et al.* 2005; Ouwehand *et al.* 2008b; Pohjavuori *et al.* 2004), and these changes may correlate with changes in gut microbiota (Ouwehand *et al.* 2008c). Toll-like receptors (TLRs) are an integral part of the innate immune system, and a crucial link between innate and adaptive immune responses. Increases in the levels of soluble CD14, a circulating co-receptor for TLR, have been linked with administration of probiotics (Rautava *et al.* 2006).

Adaptive immune responses can be classified into humoral immunity and cell-mediated immunity. Humoral immunity is mediated through antibody-producing plasma cells (B lymphocytes). The enhancement of humoral immune response has been suggested as a possible mechanism for certain health effects of probiotics. By increasing neutralising antibody titres and levels of specific immunoglobulins, specific probiotics or combinations of probiotic strains may be used as adjuvant in combination with vaccinations (de Vrese *et al.* 2005; Kukkonen *et al.* 2006; Paineau *et al.* 2008). Probiotics can also stimulate specific antibody responses during acute rotavirus gastroenteritis, therefore partially explaining the reduced duration of the disease in probiotic-supplemented subjects (Majamaa *et al.* 1995). Studies on the effects of probiotics on IgA levels in serum, faeces or mucosal surface have yielded mixed results, with some studies suggesting an increase and others suggesting no effect (Christensen *et al.* 2006; Olivares *et al.* 2006b; Woodcock *et al.* 2004). In formula-fed infants in particular, early induction of endogenous mucosal IgA antibodies would be especially beneficial in protection against colonisation by pathogens. However, here again mixed results have been obtained with probiotic supplementation (Bakker-Zierikzee *et al.* 2006; Rautava *et al.* 2006).

Cell-mediated adaptive immunity is mediated by T lymphocytes. Consumption of *B. lactis* HN019 has been reported to enhance cellular immune functions in elderly subjects (Arunachalam *et al.* 2000; Gill *et al.* 2001b). The balance between the different types of T-helper cell responses (Th1 and Th2) is thought to play a critical role in the development of atopic and autoimmune diseases, and probiotics may modulate this balance (Rautava *et al.* 2004). Increasing evidence suggests that the first step in the development of many intestinal inflammatory diseases, including IBD, ulcerative colitis or pouchitis, may be the breakdown of the mucosal barrier in the host intestine (Laukoetter *et al.* 2008). Firstly, the improvement of the gut barrier integrity, and secondly, the modulation of the intestinal anti-inflammatory responses in the intestine by modulating the Th3 (TGF-β) responses, are crucial in maintaining the anti-inflammatory status of the intestine.

Probiotic bacteria have also been shown to modulate the cell surface phenotype and cytokine release of dendritic cells. These cells are the most potent antigen-presenting cells (Hart *et al.* 2004; Mohamadzadeh *et al.* 2005), which play a pivotal role in development of tolerance. Modulation of the phenotype and the functions of dendritic cells may be a key mechanism mediating the effects of probiotics on gut homeostasis and on the balance between pro- and anti-inflammatory immune responses, and may also partly explain why certain probiotics appear to be effective as vaccine adjuvants (Mohamadzadeh *et al.* 2005).

The potential of probiotic strains to modulate the immune system and function is well documented, but given the complexity of the immune system and the number of mediators involved in the regulation of the immune function, it is sometimes difficult to draw conclusions on the clinical benefits of the observed modulation of immune system components.

9.5.4 Probiotics and intestinal pain receptors

It has been suggested that probiotics may also have direct effects on the nervous system of the host. Recently, a novel mechanism for probiotic action in regard to intestinal pain was discovered. Rousseaux *et al.* (2006) demonstrated that the probiotic strain *Lactobacillus acidophilus* NCFM may directly modify the opioid pain receptors in the gut, resulting in reduction of pain sensation. This mechanism demonstrates the importance of the gut–brain axis, and may partly explain the efficacy of probiotics in the treatment of IBS.

9.6 Applications with probiotics

Around the world, the sales of food and beverages containing probiotics have shown impressive growth. While traditionally probiotics have been applied in dairy foods, most predominantly yogurt, this market is now expanding to a variety of non-traditional foods including confectionery, baby foods, processed meats, snacks, desserts and breakfast cereals. As mentioned above, probiotics utilised in food applications have been shown to provide a variety of health benefits from improved digestion to enhanced immune health and the list is expanding as research continues on the contribution of probiotics to human health. The human health benefits are known to be strain and dose dependent. So, a manufacturer is recommended to add the specific strain referenced in a clinical trial to have clear substantiated documentation of the health benefit. The dose (bacterial cells per serving) required is dependent on both the dose utilised in the study substantiating the health benefit and on the stability of the probiotic in the food product. Therefore, the health benefit desired, the strain to be utilised, the dose, including consideration of stability in the desired food product, are all critical considerations when delivering probiotics in foods and beverages.

There are key elements in food and food manufacturing which affect probiotic viability. These include product formulation, manufacturing (including packaging) and storage conditions. Understanding these factors in an application is essential to minimising probiotic loss and hence delivering a probiotic dose that has clinically documented efficacy.

Common formulation factors to consider include pH, organic acids, water activity, food additives, carbohydrates (fermentable carbon sources), starter cultures and antimicrobials. Each of these factors has been found to affect probiotic viability. Additionally, interactions between these factors are likely to have significant impact on probiotic stability in foods; this is analogous to hurdle technology employed in the control of food spoilage and pathogenic microorganisms in foods. Obviously, it is not always possible to alter these factors without altering the organoleptic properties and shelf-life of the food, and therefore selection of product-specific probiotics is an essential consideration.

The tolerance of a probiotic to pH is strain and application specific. For example, when selecting a probiotic for (non-fermented) milk, a product with a pH close to neutral, a critical selection criterion is the inability to grow in milk since growth in milk significantly increases the likelihood of producing undesirable flavours. In contrast, when selecting a probiotic for a fermented dairy product, products with relatively low pH (e.g. pH 4.0–4.3), the critical selection criterion is the ability to retain viability in these low pH products throughout shelf-life. Furthermore, it is important that the probiotic does not produce off-flavours during manufacture and storage. In low pH products with high levels of organic acids it is important to consider the relationship between pH and organic acids. It is well recognised that the undissociated form of organic acids is primarily responsible for their antimicrobial properties. As the pH declines, the concentration of the undissociated organic acids increases and hence their bactericidal activity increases (Cotter & Hill 2003). This can be of particular concern when incorporating probiotics into fruit juices and drinks.

Water activity (A_w) plays an important role in probiotic viability, especially in very low moisture, low moisture and intermediate moisture foods. Products with water activity levels below 0.20 (e.g. dietary supplements, dry instant beverages, chocolate or infant formula) can exhibit a shelf-life of greater than 1 year with no appreciable loss of probiotic viability. The choice of excipient, or any other components added to these foods is of prime importance as they may increase the A_w. Foods in the intermediate moisture range (e.g. cereal, confectionery, bars) face significant challenges to probiotic stability. In fact, most commercially available probiotics cannot survive during the long shelf-life (>6 months) at ambient temperatures required by this food category. Solutions for incorporation of probiotics in intermediate moisture foods will likely require additional technologies, such as encapsulation.

There are many ingredients used in food formulation that have been shown to influence the growth and stability of probiotics. In general, the major components of food; such as proteins, fats, and carbohydrates have protective or neutral impacts on probiotic viability. A study conducted by Vinderola and co-workers (2002b) reported no effect on probiotic stability for ingredients such as lysozyme, natomycin, artificial sweeteners (acesulfame and aspartame), many flavours, natural colours (Carmin, Curcuma/Bixin and bixin), diacetyl, and acetoin at levels commonly utilised in foods. However, they also showed that some ingredients commonly used in foods, can have adverse affects on the viability of some probiotic strains at levels used in food; such as some flavours and colourant mixtures (Vinderola *et al.* 2002a). The inconsistency in results obtained with flavours and colours is probably due to the broad range of compounds included within these ingredient categories and the influence of specific food colour and flavour compounds on probiotic viability requires further study. In addition to the neutral to detrimental effects observed with some ingredients on probiotic viability, other ingredients have been shown to enhance the viability of some probiotic strains. One study has shown that the addition of cysteine, whey protein concentrate, acid casein hydrolysates or tryptone can improve stability of some strains of *L. acidophilus* and bifidobacteria in yogurt (Dave & Shah 1998). These ingredients implicate the importance of redox and readily utilisable nitrogen source (peptides and amino acids) in viability of probiotic bacteria.

Starter culture and probiotic interactions can be either detrimental (competition or production of antimicrobial agents) or advantageous (enhanced growth or stability) to probiotic viability depending on the starter culture and probiotic strains utilised. The extent of the interaction between the starter culture and probiotics has been shown to be increased by adding the probiotic at the beginning of fermentation with the starter culture (Heller 2001). Among the detrimental affects, the ability of the starter culture to reduce the pH and increase the level of organic acids are the most common causes of starter-related reductions in probiotic viability. Additionally, production of antimicrobial agents, such as hydrogen peroxide, carbon dioxide, diacetyl, or low molecular weight substances (e.g. reuterin or bacteriocins) are of concern when selecting starter cultures for probiotic-containing fermented foods. Starter culture attributes that may be advantageous for probiotic growth or stability include the production of readily utilisable nitrogen sources (peptides and amino acids), reducing the amount of oxygen present, lowering the redox potential, and relatively small reductions in pH (i.e. reducing the pH of milk from 6.4 to less than 6.0). Vinderola and co-workers (2002b) demonstrated that probiotic bacteria vary in their sensitivity to starter cultures, with *L. acidophilus* strains exhibiting the most sensitivity when compared with strains of *L. casei* and *Bifidobacterium*. Additionally, these researchers noted that some probiotic bacteria could delay or inhibit growth of starter bacteria. These results support the notion starter culture and probiotic interactions need to taken into consideration when formulating fermented foods.

Studies have shown that some probiotic–food combinations can enhance the bioavailability of some food-derived nutrients. For example, Tang and co-workers (2007) reported improved calcium solubility in calcium-fortified soymilk fermented with *L. acidophilus* ATCC 4962 and *L. casei* ASCC290. Additionally, fermentation of the soymilk with some probiotic strains has been demonstrated to enhance the bioavailability of soy isoflavones, a class of phytoestrogens. The conversion of isoflavone glycosides (IG) into their more biologically active aglycones (diadzein, genistein and glycetein) can be catalysed by enzymes derived from some strains of probiotics (Pham & Shah 2008; Tang *et al.* 2007). These studies highlight potential future opportunities to utilise selected probiotics to enhance the nutritional quality of specific foods.

Probiotics have been shown to function as biopreservatives in some food applications. In particular, numerous studies with bifidobacteria and lactobacilli have demonstrated potential in this area. Bifidobacteria have been shown to inhibit spoilage microorganisms in products such as cheese (fresh and hard) and raw meats (catfish, chicken, and shrimp). In studies utilising *B. longum* subsp. *infantis* NCFB 2255 and *B. breve* NCFB 2258 it was shown that incorporation of these probiotics inhibited *Pseudomonas* spp. in cottage cheese, thereby extending shelf-life by 14 days (O'Riordan & Fitzgerald 1998). Several studies have shown the combination of sodium acetate and specific *Bifidobacterium* ssp. retard the growth of spoilage microorganisms and improve overall sensory properties in raw meats (Al Dagal & Bazaraa 1999). Clearly, the primary reason for adding probiotic to foods is to provide a specific health benefit; however, extending product shelf-life may be a secondary consideration in some applications.

Finally, manufacturing and storage conditions are critical considerations. Manufacturing steps that incorporate excessive oxygen or elevated temperatures have been shown to contribute to loss of probiotic viability throughout shelf-life. Selection of equipment that minimises shear and oxygen incorporation during mixing and movement of the product through the processing plant is essential. In fact, oxygen toxicity is considered a primary factor responsible for probiotic loss during storage (Talwalkar & Kailasapathy 2004). With the exception of spore-forming probiotics, probiotics must be added after thermal processes such as pasteurisation, as the vast majority of probiotics would be killed during these processes. It has been suggested that pre-treatments, such as encapsulation, could be developed to protect probiotics during thermal processing. Concerns during storage and distribution are primarily related to controlling temperature and temperature fluctuation. In general, lower temperatures improve probiotic stability. Controlling temperature fluctuation during storage and distribution improves probiotic stability in products as diverse as ice cream and powdered beverages. The optimisation of manufacturing and storage of a specific probiotic-containing food is frequently specific to the process, product and manufacturing plant.

Foods containing efficacious doses of clinically documented probiotics can now be found commercially available in many regions of the world. Numerous researchers have proven that probiotics can be successfully delivered, at efficacious levels, in many foods including cheese (Ong & Shah 2008; Phillips *et al.* 2006; Vinderola *et al.* 2000; Yilmaztekin *et al.* 2004) and cereals (Charalampopoulos *et al.* 2002; Ouwehand *et al.* 2004). Recently published product surveys by researchers show that, although many manufacturers are meeting targets for dose (cell count per serving) with clinically documented strains, some manufacturers are not (Masco *et al.* 2005; Perea *et al.* 2007). The presence of products in the marketplace that do not contain an efficacious probiotic dose has the potential to undermine consumer confidence in this product category and hence should be of concern to those interested in promoting the development and sale of probiotic-containing foods. The list of foods containing probiotics is likely to expand greatly in the next decade; additional research on the factors that affect probiotic stability in foods and methods for enhancing their survival will be required to meet consumer demand for these products.

9.7 Future trends

Probiotics have been one of the driving factors in the functional foods area with, as best example, the yogurt drinks. In the short term, this is likely to continue. However, there are other possibilities for probiotics applications. One example is, of course, the combination with other functional ingredients, such as prebiotics. Such 'synbiotic' products are already on the market but are marketed as probiotics and prebiotics/fibre or do not mention the prebiotics. The term synbiotic seems to be too challenging for the consumer.

New potential targets may lie outside the traditional areas as intestinal health and immune modulation (Ouwehand 2003). Cosmetic applications ('cosmeceuticals') could be one such area; this may still relate the traditional target of immune function as the skin and the intestinal mucosa share the same immune system. Weight management is likely to remain a hot topic for probiotics; especially with the observed correlations between obesity and the intestinal microbiota (Turnbaugh *et al.* 2006). Other new potential targets may relate to mental health or stress; probiotics have been suggested to reduce the negative effects of stress (Logan & Katzman 2005). Hence, there is no lack of new potential health targets for probiotics.

Another new target for probiotics could be in the field that traditionally is associated with pharmaceuticals; delivery of bioactive compounds. Although there is a rather general resistance to genetically modified organisms (GMO), at least in Europe, There could very well be acceptance of GMO microbes that deliver pharmaceuticals in diseases that are otherwise difficult to treat (Braat *et al.* 2006). Mucosal delivery of vaccines has long been explored, but application has been up to now been without success (Wells & Mercenier 2008).

The success of probiotics in many of these new, but also existing, targets, depends on legislation. If and what claims are allowed, what are the requirements for pharmaceutical probiotics, etc. The FOSHU legislation in Japan set the tone very early on (Hosoya 1998). The Regulation on health claims made on foods will set the frame for what is allowed in Europe; opening opportunities for functional ingredients with general health properties and aimed at reduction of disease risk (European Parliament and the Council of the European Union 2006). With clear guidelines on what can be claimed, there will be an incentive and requirement for manufacturers to investigate the health benefits of their ingredients, including probiotics, if they intend to make a health claim.

9.8 Sources of further information

- *Handbook Prebiotics* 2008 GIBSON, G.R. and ROBERFROID, M. (eds.), CRC Press, Boca Raton, FL.
- *Gastrointestinal Microbiology* 2006 OUWEHAND, A.C. and VAUGHAN, E. (eds.), Taylor and Francis, New York.
- *Lactic Acid Bacteria* 2004 SALMINEN, S., VON WRIGHT, A. and OUWEHAND, A.C. (eds.), Marcel Dekker, New York.
- International Scientific Association of Probiotics and Prebiotics (ISAPP), www.isapp.net
- Gut Flora Foundation, www.gutflora.org
- International Probiotics Association, www.internationalprobiotics.org

9.9 References

ABRAHAMSSON, T. R., JAKOBSSON, T., BÖTTCHER, M. F., FREDRIKSON, M., JENMALM, M. C., BJÖRKSTEN, B., & OLDAEUS, G. 2007, 'Probiotics in prevention of IgE-associated eczema: a double-blind, randomized, placebo-controlled trial', *J Allergy Clin Immunol*, vol. 119, no. 5, pp. 1174–1180.

ADAWI, D., MOLIN, G., AHRNE, S., & JEPPSSON, B. 1999, 'Modulation of the colonic bacterial flora affects differently bacterial translocation and liver injury in an acute liver injury model', *Microb Ecol Health D*, vol. 11, pp. 47–54.

AHMED, M., PRASAD, J., GILL, H., STEVENSON, L., & GOPAL, P. 2007, 'Impact of consumption of different levels of *Bifidobacterium lactis* HN019 on the intestinal microflora of elderly human subjects', *J Nutr Health Aging*, vol. 11, no. 1, pp. 26–31.

AIT-BELGNAOUI, A., HAN, W., LAMINE, F., EUTAMENE, H., FIORAMONTI, J., BUENO, L., & THEODOROU, V. 2006, '*Lactobacillus farciminis* treatment suppresses stress induced visceral hypersensitivity: a possible action through interaction with epithelial cell cytoskeleton contraction', *Gut*, vol. 55, no. 8, pp. 1090–1094.

AL DAGAL, M. M. & BAZARAA, W. A. 1999, 'Extension of shelf life of whole and peeled shrimp with organic acid salts and bifidobacteria', *J Food Prot.*, vol. 62, no. 1, pp. 51–56.

ALANDER, M., KORPELA, R., SAXELIN, M., VILPPONEN-SALMELA, T., MATTILA-SANDHOLM, T., & VON WRIGHT, A. 1997, 'Recovery of *Lactobacillus rhamnosus* GG from human colonic biopsies', *Lett Appl Microbiol*, vol. 24, no. 5, pp. 361–364.

ALANDER, M., SATOKARI, R., KORPELA, R., SAXELIN, M., VILPPONEN-SALMELA, T., MATTILA-SANDHOLM, T., & VON WRIGHT, A. 1999, 'Persistence of colonization of human colonic mucosa by a probiotic strain, *Lactobacillus rhamnosus* GG, after oral consumption', *Appl Environ Microbiol*, vol. 65, no. 1, pp. 351–354.

ARUNACHALAM, K., GILL, H. S., & CHANDRA, R. K. 2000, 'Enhancement of natural immune function by dietary consumption of *Bifidobacterium lactis* (HN019)', *Eur J Clin Nutr*, vol. 54, no. 3, pp. 263–267.

ASO, Y., AKAZA, H., KOTAKE, T., TSUKAMOTO, T., IMAI, K., NAITO, S., & GROUP, B. S. 1995, 'Preventive effect of a *Lactobacillus casei* preparation on the recurrence of superficial bladder cancer in a double-blind trial', *Eur Urol*, vol. 27, pp. 104–109.

BAKKER-ZIERIKZEE, A. M., TOL, E. A., KROES, H., ALLES, M. S., KOK, F. J., & BINDELS, J. G. 2006, 'Faecal SIgA secretion in infants fed on pre- or probiotic infant formula', *Pediatr Allergy Immunol*, vol. 17, no. 2, pp. 134–140.

BANASZKIEWICZ, A. & SZAJEWSKA, H. 2005, 'Ineffectiveness of *Lactobacillus* GG as an adjunct to lactulose for the treatment of constipation in children: a double-blind, placebo-controlled randomized trial', *J Pediatr*, vol. 146, no. 3, pp. 364–369.

BARLOW, S., CHESSON, A., COLLINS, J. D., DYBING, E., FLYNN, A., FRUIJTIER-PÖLLOTH, C., HARDY, A., KNAP, A., KUIPER, H., LE NEIDRE, P., SCHANS, J., SCHLATTER, J., SILANO, V., & SKERFVING, S. V. P. 2007, *Introduction of a Qualified Presumption of Safety (QPS) Approach for Assessment of Selected Microorganisms Referred to EFSA*, European Food Safety Authority, EFSA-Q-2005–293.

BERNBOM, N., LICHT, T. R., BROGREN, C. H., JELLE, B., JOHANSEN, A. H., BADIOLA, I., VOGENSEN, F. K., & NORRUNG, B. 2006, 'Effects of *Lactococcus lactis* on composition of intestinal microbiota: role of nisin', *Appl Environ Microbiol*, vol. 72, no. 1, pp. 239–244.

BERNET-CAMARD, M.-F., LIÉVIN, V., BRASSART, D., NEESER, J.-R., SERVIN, A. L., & HUDAULT, S. 1997, 'The human *Lactobacillus acidophilus* strain La1 secretes a nonbacteriocin antibacterial substance(s) active *in vitro* and *in vivo*', *Appl Environ Microbiol*, vol. 63, no. 7, pp. 2747–2753.

BINGHAM, M. 2003, 'Functional foods: dietary intervention strategies in autistic spectrum disorders', *Food Sci Tech Bull*, vol. 1, no. 4, pp. 1–11.

BOYLE, R. J. & TANG, M. L. 2006, 'The role of probiotics in the management of allergic disease', *Clin Exp Allergy*, vol. 36, no. 5, pp. 568–576.

BOYLE, R. J., ROBINS-BROWNE, R. M., & TANG, M. L. 2006, 'Probiotic use in clinical practice: what are the risks?', *Am J Clin Nutr*, vol. 83, no. 6, pp. 1256–1264.

BRAAT, H., ROTTIERS, P., HOMMES, D. W., HUYGHEBAERT, N., REMAUT, E., REMON, J. P., VAN DEVENTER, S. J., NEIRYNCK, S., PEPPELENBOSCH, M. P., & STEIDLER, L. 2006, 'A phase I trial with transgenic bacteria expressing interleukin-10 in Crohn's disease', *Clin Gastroenterol Hepatol*, vol. 4, no. 6, pp. 754–759.

CAGLAR, E., KAVALOGLU CILDIR, S., ERGENELI, S., SANDALLI, N., & TWETMAN, S. 2006, 'Salivary mutans streptococci and lactobacilli levels after ingestion of the probiotic bacterium *Lactobacillus reuteri* ATCC 55730 by straws or tablets', *Acta Odontol Scand*, vol. 64, no. 5, pp. 314–318.

CANNON, J. P., LEE, T. A., BOLANOS, J. T., & DANZIGER, L. H. 2005, 'Pathogenic relevance of *Lactobacillus*: a retrospective review of over 200 cases', *Eur J Clin Microbiol*, vol. 24, no. 1, pp. 31–40.

CHARALAMPOPOULOS, D., WANG, R., PANDIELLA, S. S., & WEBB, C. 2002, 'Application of cereals and cereal components in functional foods: a review', *Int J Food Microbiol*, vol. 79, pp. 131–141.

CHRISTENSEN, H. R., LARSEN, C. N., KAESTEL, P., ROSHOLM, L. B., STERNBERG, C., MICHAELSEN, K. F., & FROKIAER, H. 2006, 'Immunomodulating potential of supplementation with probiotics: a dose–response study in healthy young adults', *FEMS Immunol Med Microbiol*, vol. 47, no. 3, pp. 380–390.

CLANCY, R. L., GLEESON, M., COX, A., CALLISTER, R., DORRINGTON, M., D'ESTE, C., PANG, G., PYNE, D., FRICKER, P., & HENRIKSSON, A. 2006, 'Reversal in fatigued athletes of a defect in interferon gamma secretion after administration of *Lactobacillus acidophilus*', *Br J Sports Med*, vol. 40, no. 4, pp. 351–354.

COLLADO, M. C., MERILUOTO, J., & SALMINEN, S. 2007, 'Role of commercial probiotic strains against human pathogen adhesion to intestinal mucus', *Lett Appl Microbiol*, vol. 45, no. 4, pp. 454–460.

COLLADO, M. C., MERILUOTO, J., & SALMINEN, S. 2008, 'Adhesion and aggregation properties of probiotic and pathogen strains', *Eur Food Res Technol*, vol. 226, no. 5, pp. 1065–1073.

CONWAY, P. L. & ADAMS, R. F. 1989, 'Role of erythrosine in the inhibition of adhesion of *Lactobacillus fermentum* strain 737 to mouse stomach tissue', *J Gen Microbiol*, vol. 135, pp. 1167–1173.

CONWAY, P. L. & KJELLEBERG, S. 1989, 'Protein-mediated adhesion of *Lactobacillus fermentum* strain 737 to mouse stomach squamous epithelium', *J Gen Microbiol*, vol. 135, pp. 1175–1186.

CONWAY, P. L., GORBACH, S. L., & GOLDIN, B. R. 1987, 'Survival of lactic acid bacteria in the human stomach and adhesion to intestinal cells', *J Dairy Sci*, vol. 70, pp. 1–12.

COTTER, P. D. & HILL, C. 2003, 'Surviving the acid test: responses of gram-positive bacteria to low pH', *Microbiol Mol Biol Rev*, vol. 67, no. 3, pp. 429–453.

CRITTENDEN, R., LAITILA, A., FORSSELL, P., MÄTTÖ, J., SAARELA, M., MATTILA-SANDHOLM, T., & MYLLÄRINEN, P. 2001, 'Adhesion of bifidobacteria to granular starch and its implications in probiotic technologies', *Appl Environ Microbiol*, vol. 67, no. 8, pp. 3469–3475.

DANIEL, C., POIRET, S., GOUDERCOURT, D., DENNIN, V., LEYER, G., & POT, B. 2006, 'Selecting lactic acid bacteria for their safety and functionality by use of a mouse colitis model', *Appl Environ Microbiol*, vol. 72, no. 9, pp. 5799–5805.

DAVE, R. I. & SHAH, N. P. 1998, 'Ingredient supplementation effects on viability of probiotic bacteria in yogurt', *J Dairy Sci*, vol. 81, no. 11, pp. 2804–2816.

DE MAN, J. C., ROGOSA, M., & SHARPE, M. E. 1960, 'A medium for the cultivation of lactobacilli', *J Appl Bact*, vol. 23, no. 1, pp. 130–135.

DE VRESE, M., RAUTENBERG, P., LAUE, C., KOOPMANS, M., HERREMANS, T., & SCHREZENMEIR, J. 2005, 'Probiotic bacteria stimulate virus-specific neutralizing antibodies following a booster polio vaccination', *Eur J Nutr*, vol. 44, no. 7, pp. 406–413.

DE VRESE, M., WINKLER, P., RAUTENBERG, P., HARDER, T., NOAH, C., LAUE, C., OTT, S., HAMPE, J., SCHREIBER, S., HELLER, K., & SCHREZENMEIR, J. 2005b, 'Effect of *Lactobacillus gasseri* PA 16/8, *Bifidobacterium longum* SP 07/3, *B. bifidum* MF 20/5 on common cold episodes: a double blind, randomized, controlled trial', *Clin Nutr*, vol. 24, no. 4, pp. 481–491.

DE VRESE, M., WINKLER, P., RAUTENBERG, P., HARDER, T., NOAH, C., LAUE, C., OTT, S., HAMPE, J., SCHREIBER, S., HELLER, K., & SCHREZENMEIR, J. 2006, 'Probiotic bacteria reduced duration and severity but not the incidence of common cold episodes in a double blind, randomized, controlled trial', *Vaccine*, vol. 24, pp. 6670–6674.

DING, W. K. & SHAH, N. P. 2007, 'Acid, bile, and heat tolerance of free and micro-encapsulated probiotic bacteria', *J Food Sci*, vol. 72, no. 9, p. M446–M450.

DONNET-HUGHES, A., ROCHAT, F., SERRANT, P., AESCHLIMANN, J. M., & SCHIFFRIN, E. J. 1999, 'Modulation of nonspecific mechanisms of defense by lactic acid bacteria: effective dose', *J Dairy Sci*, vol. 82, no. 5, pp. 863–869.

DUNN, S. R., SIMENHOFF, M. L., AHMED, K. E., GAUGHAN, W. J., ELTAYEB, B. O., FITZPATRICK, M. E. D., EMERY, S. M., AYRES, J. W., & HOLT, K. E. 1998, 'Effect of oral administration of freeze-dried *Lactobacillus acidophilus* on small bowel bacteria overgrowth in patients with end stage kidney disease: reducing uremic toxins and improving nutrition', *Int Dairy J*, vol. 8, pp. 545–553.

ENGELBREKTSON, A. L., KORZENIK, J. R., SANDERS, M. E., CLEMENT, B. G., LEYER, G., KLAENHAMMER, T. R., & KITTS, C. L. 2006, 'Analysis of treatment effects on the microbial ecology of the human intestine', *FEMS Microbiol Ecol*, vol. 57, no. 2, pp. 239–250.

EUROPEAN PARLIAMENT AND THE COUNCIL OF THE EUROPEAN UNION 2006, 'Regulation (EC) No 1924/2006 of the European Parliament and the Council of 20 December 2006 on nutrition and health claims made on foods', *Off J Eur Union*, vol. L404, pp. 9–25.

FALAGAS, M. E., BETSI, G. I., & ATHANASIOU, S. 2006, 'Probiotics for prevention of recurrent vulvovaginal candidiasis: a review', *J Antimicrob Chemother*, vol. 58, no. 2, pp. 266–272.

FAO/WHO 2002 'Guidelines for the evaluation of probiotics in food', http://www.who.int/foodsafety/publications/fs_management/probiotics2/en/, pp. 1–11.

FILHO-LIMA, J. V. M., VIEIRA, E. C., & NICOLI, J. R. 2000, 'Antagonistic effect of *Lactobacillus acidophilus*, *Saccharomyces boulardii* and *Escherichia coli* combinations against experimental infections with *Shigella flexneri* and *Salmonella enteritidis* subsp. *typhimurium* in gnotobiotic mice', *J Appl Microbiol*, vol. 88, pp. 365–370.

FOOKS, L. J. & GIBSON, G. R. 2002, 'Probiotics as modulators of the gut flora', *Br J Nutr*, vol. 88 Suppl 1, p. S39–S49.

FULLER, R. & GIBSON, G. R. 1997, 'Modification of the intestinal microflora using probiotics and prebiotics', *Scand J Gastroenterol Suppl*, vol. 222, pp. 28–31.

GILL, H. & PRASAD, J. 2008, 'Probiotics, immunomodulation, and health benefits', *Adv Exp Med Biol*, vol. 606, pp. 423–454.

GILL, H. S. & RUTHERFURD, K. J. 2001, 'Probiotic supplementation to enhance natural immunity in the elderly: effects of a newly characterized immunostimulatory strain *Lactobacillus rhamnosus* HN001 (DR20™) on leucocyte phagocytosis', *Nutr Res*, vol. 21, pp. 183–189.

GILL, H. S., RUTHERFURD, K. J., PRASAD, J., & GOPAL, P. K. 2000, 'Enhancement of natural and acquired immunity by *Lactobacillus rhamnosus* (HN001), *Lactobacillus acidophilus* (HN017) and *Bifidobacterium lactis* (HN019)', *Br J Nutr*, vol. 83, pp. 167–176.

GILL, H., RUTHERFURD, K. J., & CROSS, M. L. 2001a, 'Dietary probiotic supplementation enhances natural killer cell activity in the elderly: an investigation of age-related immunological changes', *J Clin Immunol*, vol. 21, no. 4, pp. 264–271.

GILL, H. S., RUTHERFURD, K. J., CROSS, M. L., & GOPAL, P. K. 2001b, 'Enhancement of immunity in the elderly by dietary supplementation with the probiotic *Bifidobacterium lactis* HN019', *Am J Clin Nutr*, vol. 74, no. 6, pp. 833–839.

GILL, H. S., SHU, Q., LIN, H., RUTHERFURD, K. J., & CROSS, M. L. 2001c, 'Protection against translocating *Salmonella typhimurium* infection in mice by feeding the immuno-enhancing probiotic *Lactobacillus rhamnosus* strain HN001', *Med Microbiol Immunol*, vol. 190, pp. 97–104.

GIONCHETTI, P., RIZZELLO, F., HELWIG, U., VENTURI, A., LAMMERS, K. M., BRIGIDI, P., VITALI, B., POGGIOLI, G., MIGLIOLI, M., & CAMPIERI, M. 2003, 'Prophylaxis of pouchitis onset with probiotic therapy: a double-blind, placebo-controlled trial', *Gastroenterology*, vol. 124, no. 5, pp. 1202–1209.

GLÜCK, U. & GEBBERS, J.-O. 2003, 'Ingested probiotics reduce nasal colonization with pathogenic bacteria (*Staphylococcus aureus, Streptococcus pneumoniae*, and β-hemolytic streptococci)', *Am J Clin Nutr*, vol. 77, pp. 517–520.

GOLDIN, B. R. & GORBACH, S. L. 1980, 'Effect of *Lactobacillus acidophilus* dietary supplements on 1,2-dimethylhydrazine dihydrochloride-induced intestinal cancer in rats', *J Natl Cancer Inst*, vol. 64, no. 2, pp. 263–265.

GORDON, J. I., HOOPER, L. V., MCNEVIN, M. S., WONG, M., & BRY, L. 1997, 'Epithelial cell growth and differentiation. III. Promoting diversity in the intestine: conversations between the microflora, epithelium, and diffuse GALT', *Am J Physiol*, vol. 273, no. 3 Pt 1, pp. G565–G570.

GUARNER, F. & MALAGELADA, J. R. 2003, 'Gut flora in health and disease', *Lancet*, vol. 361, no. 9356, pp. 512–519.

GUEIMONDE, M., KALLIOMÄKI, M., ISOLAURI, E., & SALMINEN, S. 2006, 'Probiotic intervention in neonates – will permanent colonization ensue?', *J Pediatr Gastroenterol Nutr*, vol. 42, no. 5, pp. 604–606.

GUN, F., SALMAN, T., GURLER, N., & OLGAC, V. 2005, 'Effect of probiotic supplementation on bacterial translocation in thermal injury', *Surg Today*, vol. 35, no. 9, pp. 760–764.

GUYONNET, D., CHASSANY, O., DUCROTTE, P., PICARD, C., MOURET, M., MERCIER, C. H., & MATUCHANSKY, C. 2007, 'Effect of a fermented milk containing *Bifidobacterium animalis* DN-173 010 on the health-related quality of life and symptoms in irritable bowel syndrome in adults in primary care: a multicentre, randomized, double-blind, controlled trial', *Aliment Pharmacol Ther*, vol. 26, no. 3, pp. 475–486.

HAMILTON-MILLER, J. M. 2003, 'The role of probiotics in the treatment and prevention of *Helicobacter pylori* infection', *Int J Antimicrob Agents*, vol. 22, no. 4, pp. 360–366.

HART, A. L., LAMMERS, K., BRIGIDI, P., VITALI, B., RIZZELLO, F., GIONCHETTI, P., CAMPIERI, M., KAMM, M. A., KNIGHT, S. C., & STAGG, A. J. 2004, 'Modulation of human dendritic cell phenotype and function by probiotic bacteria', *Gut*, vol. 53, no. 11, pp. 1602–1609.

HATAKKA, K., SAVILAHTI, E., PONKA, A., MEURMAN, J. H., POUSSA, T., NÄSE, L., SAXELIN, M., & KORPELA, R. 2001, 'Effect of long term consumption of probiotic milk on infections in children attending day care centres: double blind, randomised trial', *Brit Med J*, vol. 322, no. 7298, pp. 1327–1331.

HATAKKA, K., AHOLA, A. J., YLI-KNUUTTILA, H., RICHARDSON, M., POUSSA, T., MEURMAN, J. H., & KORPELA, R. 2007a, 'Probiotics reduce the prevalence of oral candida in the elderly – a randomized controlled trial', *J Dent Res*, vol. 86, no. 2, pp. 125–130.

HATAKKA, K., BLOMGREN, K., POHJAVUORI, S., KAIJALAINEN, T., POUSSA, T., LEINONEN, M., KORPELA, R., & PITKÄRANTA, A. 2007b, 'Treatment of acute otitis media with probiotics in otitis-prone children-a double-blind, placebo-controlled randomised study', *Clin Nutr*, vol. 26, no. 3, pp. 314–321.

HELIN, T., HAAHTELA, S., & HAAHTELA, T. 2002, 'No effect of oral treatment with an intestinal bacterial strain, *Lactobacillus rhamnosus* (ATCC 53103), on birch-pollen allergy: a placebo-controlled double-blind study', *Allergy*, vol. 57, no. 3, pp. 243–246.

HELLER, K. J. 2001, 'Probiotic bacteria in fermented foods: product characteristics and starter organisms', *Am J Clin Nutr*, vol. 73, pp. 374S–379S.

HENRIKSSON, A. & CONWAY, P. L. 1996, 'Adhesion of *Lactobacillus fermentum* 104-S to porcine stomach mucus', *Curr Microbiol*, vol. 33, no. 1, pp. 31–34.

HENRIKSSON, A. & CONWAY, P. L. 2001a, 'Colonization resistance induced in mice orogastrically dosed with human faecal homogenates from different donors', *Microb Ecol Health Dis*, vol. 13, pp. 96–99.

HENRIKSSON, A. & CONWAY, P. L. 2001b, 'Isolation of human faecal bifidobacteria which reduce signs of *Salmonella* infection when orogastrically dosed to mice', *J Appl Microbiol*, vol. 90, pp. 223–228.

HOOPER, L. V. & GORDON, J. I. 2001, 'Commensal host–bacterial relationships in the gut', *Science*, vol. 292, no. 5519, pp. 1115–1118.

HOSOYA, N. 1998, 'Health claims in Japan – Foods for specified health uses and functional foods', *J Nutr Food*, vol. 1, no. 3/4, pp. 1–11.

HOYOS, A. B. 1999, 'Reduced incidence of necrotizing enterocolitis associated with enteral administration of *Lactobacillus acidophilus* and *Bifidobacterium infantis* to neonates in an intensive care unit', *Int J Infect Dis*, vol. 3, no. 4, pp. 197–202.

HUDAULT, S., LIÉVIN, V., BERNET-CAMARD, M.-F., & SERVIN, A. L. 1997, 'Antagonistic activity exerted *in vitro* and *in vivo* by *Lactobacillus casei* (strain GG) against *Salmonella typhimurium* C5 infection', *Appl Environ Microbiol*, vol. 63, pp. 513–518.

HUGHES, R. & ROWLAND, I. R. 2001, 'Stimulation of apoptosis by two prebiotic chicory fructans in the rat colon', *Carcinogenesis*, vol. 22, no. 1, pp. 43–47.

ISHIDA, Y., NAKAMURA, F., KANZATO, H., SAWADA, D., YAMAMOTO, N., KAGATA, H., OH-IDA, M., TAKEUCHI, H., & FUJIWARA, S. 2005, 'Effect of milk fermented with *Lactobacillus acidophilus* strain L-92 on symptoms of Japanese cedar pollen allergy: a randomized placebo-controlled trial', *Biosci Biotechnol Biochem*, vol. 69, no. 9, pp. 1652–1660.

JAIN, P. K., MCNAUGHT, C. E., ANDERSON, A. D., MACFIE, J., & MITCHELL, C. J. 2004, 'Influence of synbiotic containing *Lactobacillus acidophilus* La5, *Bifidobacterium lactis* Bb 12, *Streptococcus thermophilus*, *Lactobacillus bulgaricus* and oligofructose on gut barrier function and sepsis in critically ill patients: a randomised controlled trial', *Clin Nutr*, vol. 23, no. 4, pp. 467–475.

KABURAGI, T., YAMANO, T., FUKUSHIMA, Y., YOSHINO, H., MITO, N., & SATO, K. 2007, 'Effect of *Lactobacillus johnsonii* La1 on immune function and serum albumin in aged and malnourished aged mice', *Nutrition*, vol. 23, no. 4, pp. 342–350.

KALLIOMÄKI, M., SALMINEN, S., ARVILOMMI, H., KERO, P., KOSKINEN, P., & ISOLAURI, E. 2001, 'Probiotics in primary prevention of atopic disease: a randomised placebo-controlled trial', *Lancet*, vol. 357, no. 9262, pp. 1076–1079.

KALLIOMÄKI, M., SALMINEN, S., POUSSA, T., ARVILOMMI, H., & ISOLAURI, E. 2003, 'Probiotics and prevention of atopic disease: 4-year follow-up of a randomised placebo-controlled trial', *Lancet*, vol. 361, pp. 1869–1871.

KALLIOMÄKI, M., CARMEN, C. M., SALMINEN, S., & ISOLAURI, E. 2008, 'Early differences in fecal microbiota composition in children may predict overweight', *Am J Clin Nutr*, vol. 87, no. 3, pp. 534–538.

KEKKONEN, R. A., KAJASTO, E., MIETTINEN, M., VECKMAN, V., KORPELA, R., & JULKUNEN, I. 2008, 'Probiotic *Leuconostoc mesenteroides* ssp. *cremoris* and *Streptococcus thermophilus* induce IL-12 and IFN-gamma production', *World J Gastroenterol*, vol. 14, no. 8, pp. 1192–1203.

KIM, H. S. & GILLILAND, S. E. 1983, '*Lactobacillus acidophilus* as a dietary adjunct for milk to aid lactose digestion in humans', *J Dairy Sci*, vol. 66, no. 5, pp. 959–966.

KLINDER, A., FORSTER, A., CADERNI, G., FEMIA, A. P., & POOL-ZOBEL, B. L. 2004, 'Fecal water genotoxicity is predictive of tumor-preventive activities by inulin-like oligofructoses, probiotics (*Lactobacillus rhamnosus* and *Bifidobacterium lactis*), and their synbiotic combination', *Nutr Cancer*, vol. 49, no. 2, pp. 144–155.

KOEBNICK, C., WAGNER, I., LEITZMANN, P., STERN, U., & ZUNFT, H. J. 2003, 'Probiotic beverage containing *Lactobacillus casei* Shirota improves gastrointestinal symptoms in patients with chronic constipation', *Can J Gastroenterol*, vol. 17, no. 11, pp. 655–659.

KOPP, M. V., HENNEMUTH, I., HEINZMANN, A., & URBANEK, R. 2008, 'Randomized, double-blind, placebo-controlled trial of probiotics for primary prevention: no clinical effects of *Lactobacillus* GG supplementation', *Pediatrics*, vol. 121, no. 4, pp. e850–e856.

KRASSE, P., CARLSSON, B., DAHL, C., PAULSSON, A., NILSSON, A., & SINKIEWICZ, G. 2006, 'Decreased gum bleeding and reduced gingivitis by the probiotic *Lactobacillus reuteri*', *Swed Dent J*, vol. 30, no. 2, pp. 55–60.

KRUIS, W., FRIC, P., POKROTNIEKS, J., LUKAS, M., FIXA, B., KASCAK, M., KAMM, M. A., WEISMUELLER, J., BEGLINGER, C., STOLTE, M., WOLFF, C., & SCHULZE, J. 2004, 'Maintaining remission of ulcerative colitis with the probiotic *Escherichia coli* Nissle 1917 is as effective as with standard mesalazine', *Gut*, vol. 53, no. 11, pp. 1617–1623.

KUKKONEN, K., NIEMINEN, T., POUSSA, T., SAVILAHTI, E., & KUITUNEN, M. 2006, 'Effect of probiotics on vaccine antibody responses in infancy – a randomized placebo-controlled double-blind trial', *Pediatr Allergy Immunol*, vol. 17, no. 6, pp. 416–421.

LAHTINEN, S. 2007, 'New insights into the viability of probiotic bacteria', Department of Biochemistry and Food Chemistry, University of Turku, Turku.

LANNING, D., SETHUPATHI, P., RHEE, K. J., ZHAI, S. K., & KNIGHT, K. L. 2000, 'Intestinal microflora and diversification of the rabbit antibody repertoire', *J Immunol*, vol. 165, no. 4, pp. 2012–2019.

LARSEN, C. N., NIELSEN, S., KAESTEL, P., BROCKMANN, E., BENNEDSEN, M., CHRISTENSEN, H. R., ESKESEN, D. C., JACOBSEN, B. L., & MICHAELSEN, K. F. 2006, 'Dose–response study of probiotic bacteria *Bifidobacterium animalis* subsp *lactis* BB-12 and *Lactobacillus paracasei* subsp *paracasei* CRL-341 in healthy young adults', *Eur J Clin Nutr*, vol. 60, no. 11, pp. 1284–1293.

LAUKOETTER, M. G., NAVA, P., & NUSRAT, A. 2008, 'Role of the intestinal barrier in inflammatory bowel disease', *World J Gastroenterol*, vol. 14, no. 3, pp. 401–407.

LE LEU, R. K., BROWN, I. L., HU, Y., BIRD, A. R., JACKSON, M., ESTERMAN, A., & YOUNG, G. P. 2005, 'A synbiotic combination of resistant starch and *Bifidobacterium lactis* facilitates apoptotic deletion of carcinogen-damaged cells in rat colon', *J Nutr*, vol. 135, no. 5, pp. 996–1001.

LEY, R. E., BACKHED, F., TURNBAUGH, P., LOZUPONE, C. A., KNIGHT, R. D., & GORDON, J. I. 2005, 'Obesity alters gut microbial ecology', *Proc Natl Acad Sci USA*, vol. 102, no. 31, pp. 11070–11075.

LOGAN, A. C. & KATZMAN, M. 2005, 'Major depressive disorder: probiotics may be an adjuvant therapy', *Med Hypoth*, vol. 64, pp. 533–538.

MADSEN, K., CORNISH, A., SOPER, P., MCKAIGNEY, C., JIJON, H., YACHIMEC, C., DOYLE, J., JEWELL, L., & DE SIMONE, C. 2001, 'Probiotic bacteria enhance murine and human intestinal epithelial barrier function', *Gastroenterology*, vol. 121, no. 3, pp. 580–591.

MAHONEY, M. & HENRIKSSON, A. 2003, 'The effect of processed meat and meat starter cultures on gastrointestinal colonization and virulence of *Listeria monocytogenes* in mice', *Int J Food Microbiol*, vol. 84, pp. 255–261.

MAJAMAA, H., ISOLAURI, E., SAXELIN, M., & VESIKARI, T. 1995, 'Lactic acid bacteria in the treatment of acute rotavirus gastroenteritis', *J Pediatr Gastroenterol Nutr*, vol. 20, no. 3, pp. 333–338.

MARTEAU, P., LEMANN, M., SEKSIK, P., LAHARIE, D., COLOMBEL, J. F., BOUHNIK, Y., CADIOT, G., SOULE, J. C., BOURREILLE, A., METMAN, E., LEREBOURS, E., CARBONNEL, F., DUPAS, J. L., VEYRAC, M., COFFIN, B., MOREAU, J., ABITBOL, V., BLUM-SPERISEN, S., & MARY, J. Y. 2006, 'Ineffectiveness of *Lactobacillus johnsonii* LA1 for prophylaxis of post-operative recurrence in Crohn's disease: a randomised, double blind, placebo controlled GETAID trial', *Gut*, vol. 55, no. 6, pp. 842–847.

MASCO, L., HUYS, G., DE BRANDT, E., TEMMERMAN, R., & SWINGS, J. 2005, 'Culture-dependent and culture-independent qualitative analysis of probiotic products claimed to contain bifidobacteria', *Int J Food Microbiol*, vol. 102, no. 2, pp. 221–230.

MCNAUGHT, C. E., WOODCOCK, N. P., ANDERSON, A. D., & MACFIE, J. 2005, 'A prospective randomised trial of probiotics in critically ill patients', *Clin Nutr*, vol. 24, no. 2, pp. 211–219.

MOHAMADZADEH, M., OLSON, S., KALINA, W. V., RUTHEL, G., DEMMIN, G. L., WARFIELD, K. L., BAVARI, S., & KLAENHAMMER, T. R. 2005, 'Lactobacilli activate human dendritic cells that skew T cells toward T helper 1 polarization', *Proc Natl Acad Sci USA*, vol. 102, no. 8, pp. 2880–2885.

MORELLI, L., GARBAGNA, N., RIZZELLO, F., ZONENSCHAIN, D., & GROSSI, E. 2006, '*In vivo* association to human colon of *Lactobacillus paracasei* B21060: Map from biopsies', *Dig Liver Dis*, vol. 38, no. 12, pp. 894–898.

MOWAT, A. M. 2003, 'Anatomical basis of tolerance and immunity to intestinal antigens', *Nat Rev Immunol*, vol. 3, no. 4, pp. 331–341.

NAITO, S., KOGA, H., YAMAGUCHI, A., FUJIMOTO, N., HASUI, Y., KURAMOTO, H., IGUCHI, A., & KINUKAWA, N. 2008, 'Prevention of recurrence with epirubicin and lactobacillus casei after transurethral resection of bladder cancer', *J Urol*, vol. 179, no. 2, pp. 485–490.

NIEDZIELIN, K., KORDECKI, H., & BIRKENFELD, B. 2001, 'A controlled, double-blind, randomized study on the efficacy of *Lactobacillus plantarum* 299V in patients with irritable bowel syndrome', *Eur J Gastroenterol Hepatol*, vol. 13, no. 10, pp. 1143–1147.

NIV, E., NAFTALI, T., HALLAK, R., & VAISMAN, N. 2005, 'The efficacy of *Lactobacillus reuteri* ATCC 55730 in the treatment of patients with irritable bowel syndrome – a double blind, placebo-controlled, randomized study', *Clin Nutr*, vol. 24, no. 6, pp. 925–931.

NOBAEK, S., JOHANSON, M.-L., MOLIN, G., AHRNÉ, S., & JEPSSON, B. 2000, 'Alteration of intestinal microflora is associated with reduction in abdominal bloating and pain in patients with irritable bowel syndrome', *Am J Gastroenterol*, vol. 95, no. 5, pp. 1231–1238.

O'MAHONY, L., MCCARTHY, J., KELLY, P., HURLEY, G., LUO, F., CHEN, K., O'SULLIVAN, G. C., KIELY, B., COLLINS, J. K., SHANAHAN, F., & QUIGLEY, E. M. 2005, '*Lactobacillus* and *Bifidobacterium* in irritable bowel syndrome: symptom responses and relationship to cytokine profiles', *Gastroenterology*, vol. 128, no. 3, pp. 541–551.

O'RIORDAN, K. & FITZGERALD, G. F. 1998, 'Evaluation of bifidobacteria for the production of antimicrobial compounds and assessment of performance in cottage chees at refrigeration temperature', *J Appl Microbiol*, vol. 85, pp. 103–114.

OLIVARES, M., DIAZ-ROPERO, M. A., GOMEZ, N., LARA-VILLOSLADA, F., SIERRA, S., MALDONADO, J. A., MARTIN, R., LOPEZ-HUERTAS, E., RODRIGUEZ, J. M., & XAUS, J. 2006a, 'Oral administration of two probiotic strains, *Lactobacillus gasseri* CECT5714 and *Lactobacillus coryniformis* CECT5711, enhances the intestinal function of healthy adults', *Int J Food Microbiol*, vol. 107, no. 2, pp. 104–111.

OLIVARES, M., DIAZ-ROPERO, M. P., GOMEZ, N., LARA-VILLOSLADA, F., SIERRA, S., MALDONADO, J. A., MARTIN, R., RODRIGUEZ, J. M., & XAUS, J. 2006b, 'The consumption of two new probiotic strains, *Lactobacillus gasseri* CECT 5714 and *Lactobacillus coryniformis* CECT 5711, boosts the immune system of healthy humans', *Int Microbiol*, vol. 9, no. 1, pp. 47–52.

OLIVARES, M., DIAZ-ROPERO, M. P., SIERRA, S., LARA-VILLOSLADA, F., FONOLLA, J., NAVAS, M., RODRIGUEZ, J. M., & XAUS, J. 2007, 'Oral intake of *Lactobacillus fermentum* CECT5716 enhances the effects of influenza vaccination', *Nutrition*, vol. 23, no. 3, pp. 254–260.

ONG, L. & SHAH, N. P. 2008, 'Influence of probiotic *Lactobacillus acidophilus* and *L. helveticus* on proteolysis, organic acid profiles, and ACE-inhibitory activity of cheddar cheeses ripened at 4, 8 and 12 °C', *J Food Sci*, vol. 73, pp. 111–120.

OUWEHAND, A. C. 2003, 'Probiotics: time to move beyond Metchnikoff?', *Drug Disc Today*, vol. 8, no. 23, p. 1063.

OUWEHAND, A. & LAHTINEN, S. 2008, 'The (non-)sense of human origin of probiotics', *NutraCos*, vol. 7, no. 1, pp. 8–10.

OUWEHAND, A. C. & VESTERLUND, S. 2004, 'Antimicrobial components from lactic acid bacteria,' in *Lactic Acid Bacteria – Microbiological and Functional Aspects*, Third edition edn, S. Salminen, A. von Wright, & A. Ouwehand, eds., Marcel Dekker, Inc., New York, pp. 375–395.

OUWEHAND, A. C., KIRJAVAINEN, P. V., SHORTT, C., & SALMINEN, C. 1999, 'Probiotics: mechanisms and established effects', *Int Dairy J*, vol. 9, pp. 43–52.

OUWEHAND, A. C., TUOMOLA, E. M., TÖLKKÖ, S., & SALMINEN, S. 2001, 'Assessment of adhesion properties of novel probiotic strains to human intestinal mucus', *Int J Food Microbiol*, vol. 64, no. 1–2, pp. 119–126.

OUWEHAND, A. C., BÅTSMAN, A., & SALMINEN, S. 2003, 'Probiotics for the skin: a new area of potential application?', *Lett Appl Microbiol*, vol. 36, no. 5, pp. 327–331.

OUWEHAND, A. C., KURVINEN, T., & RISSANEN, P. 2004, 'Use of a probiotic *Bifidobacterium* in a dry food matrix, an *in vivo* study', *Int J Food Microbiol*, vol. 95, pp. 103–106.

OUWEHAND, A., LEYER, G., & CARCANO, D. 2008a, 'Probiotics reduce incidence and duration of respiratory tract infection symptoms in 3- to 5-year-old children', *Pediatrics*, vol. 121, no. Suppl. 2, p. S115.

OUWEHAND, A., TIIHONEN, K., SAARINEN, M., PUTAALA, H., & RAUTONEN, N. 2008b, 'Influence of a combination of *Lactobacillus acidophilus* NCFM and lactitol on healthy elderly: Intestinal and immune parameters', *Br J Nutr*, vol. 101, pp. 367–375.

OUWEHAND, A. C., BERGSMA, N., PARHIALA, R., LAHTINEN, S., GUEIMONDE, M., FINNE-SOVERI, H., STRANDBERG, T., PITKÄLÄ, K., & SALMINEN, S. 2008c, '*Bifidobacterium* microbiota and parameters of immune function in elderly subjects', *FEMS Immunol Med Microbiol*, vol. 53, pp. 18–25.

PAINEAU, D., CARCANO, D., LEYER, G., DARQUY, S., ALYANAKIAN, M. A., SIMONEAU, G., BERGMANN, J. F., BRASSART, D., BORNET, F., & OUWEHAND, A. C. 2008, 'Effects of seven potential probiotic strains on specific immune responses in healthy adults: a double-blind, randomized, controlled trial', *FEMS Immunol Med Microbiol*, vol. 53, no. 1, pp. 107–113.

PELTO, L., ISOLAURI, E., LILIUS, E. M., NUUTILA, J., & SALMINEN, S. 1998, 'Probiotic bacteria down-regulate the milk-induced inflammatory response in milk-hypersensitive subjects but have an immunostimulatory effect in healthy subjects', *Clin Exp Allergy*, vol. 28, no. 12, pp. 1474–1479.

PENG, S., LIN, J. Y., & LIN, M. Y. 2007, 'Antiallergic effect of milk fermented with lactic acid bacteria in a murine animal model', *J Agric Food Chem*, vol. 55, no. 13, pp. 5092–5096.

PERAN, L., CAMUESCO, D., COMALADA, M., NIETO, A., CONCHA, A., DIAZ-ROPERO, M. P., OLIVARES, M., XAUS, J., ZARZUELO, A., & GALVEZ, J. 2005, 'Preventative effects of a probiotic, *Lactobacillus salivarius* ssp. *salivarius*, in the TNBS model of rat colitis', *World J Gastroenterol*, vol. 11, no. 33, pp. 5185–5192.

PEREA, V. M., HERMANS, K., VERHOEVEN, T. L., LEBEER, S. E., VANDERLEYDEN, J., & DE KEERSMAECKER, S. C. 2007, 'Identification and characterization of starter lactic acid bacteria and probiotics from Columbian dairy products', *J Appl Microbiol*, vol. 103, no. 3, pp. 666–674.

PHAM, T. T. & SHAH, N. P. 2008, 'Effects of lactulose supplementation on the growth of bifidobacteria and biotransformation of isoflavone glycosides to isoflavone aglycones in soymilk', *J Agric Food Chem*, vol. 56, no. 12, pp. 4703–4709.

PHILLIPS, M., KAILASAPATHY, K., & TRAN, L. 2006, 'Viability of commercial probiotic cultures (*L. acidophilus*, *Bifidobacterium* sp., *L. casei*, *L. paracasei* and *L. rhamnosus*) in cheddar cheese', *Int J Food Microbiol*, vol. 108, no. 2, pp. 276–280.

POHJAVUORI, E., VILJANEN, M., KORPELA, R., KUITUNEN, M., TIITTANEN, M., VAARALA, O., & SAVILAHTI, E. 2004, '*Lactobacillus* GG effect in increasing IFN-gamma production in infants with cow's milk allergy', *J Allergy Clin Immunol*, vol. 114, no. 1, pp. 131–136.

PRANTERA, C., SCRIBANO, M. L., FALASCO, G., ANDREOLI, A., & LUZI, C. 2002, 'Ineffectiveness of probiotics in preventing recurrence after curative resection for Crohn's disease: a randomised controlled trial with *Lactobacillus* GG', *Gut*, vol. 51, no. 3, pp. 405–409.

PRASAD, J., GILL, H., SMART, J., & GOPAL, P. K. 1998, 'Selection and characterisation of *Lactobacillus* and *Bifidobacterium* strains for use as probiotics', *Int Dairy J*, vol. 8, pp. 993–1002.

RAUTAVA, S., KALLIOMÄKI, M., & ISOLAURI, E. 2002, 'Probiotics during pregnancy and breast-feeding might confer immunomodulatory protection against atopic disease in the infant', *J Allergy Clin Immunol*, vol. 109, no. 1, pp. 119–121.

RAUTAVA, S., RUUSKANEN, O., OUWEHAND, A., SALMINEN, S., & ISOLAURI, E. 2004, 'The hygiene hypothesis of atopic disease – an extended version', *J Pediatr Gastroenterol Nutr*, vol. 38, no. 4, pp. 378–388.

RAUTAVA, S., ARVILOMMI, H., & ISOLAURI, E. 2006, 'Specific probiotics in enhancing maturation of IgA responses in formula-fed infants', *Pediatr Res*, vol. 60, no. 2, pp. 221–224.

REID, G., BRUCE, A. W., FRASER, N., HEINEMANN, C., OWEN, J., & HENNING, B. 2001, 'Oral probiotics can resolve urogenital infections', *FEMS Immunol Med Microbiol*, vol. 30, no. 1, pp. 49–52.

REID, G., CHARBONNEAU, D., ERB, J., KOCHANOWSKI, B., BEUERMAN, D., POEHNER, R., & BRUCE, A. W. 2003, 'Oral use of *Lactobacillus rhamnosus* GR-1 and *L. fermentum* RC-14 significantly alters vaginal flora: randomized, placebo-controlled trial in 64 healthy women', *FEMS Immunol Med Microbiol*, vol. 35, no. 2, pp. 131–134.

RESTA-LENERT, S. & BARRETT, K. E. 2003, 'Live probiotics protect intestinal epithelial cells from the effects of infection with enteroinvasive *Escherichia coli* (EIEC)', *Gut*, vol. 52, no. 7, pp. 988–997.

ROSENFELDT, V., BENFELDT, E., NIELSEN, S. D., MICHAELSEN, K. F., JEPPESEN, D. L., VALERIUS, N. H., & PAERREGAARD, A. 2003, 'Effect of probiotic *Lactobacillus* strains in children with atopic dermatitis', *J Allergy Clin Immunol*, vol. 111, no. 2, pp. 389–395.

ROSENFELDT, V., BENFELDT, E., VALERIUS, N. H., PAERREGAARD, A., & MICHAELSEN, K. F. 2004a, 'Effect of probiotics on gastrointestinal symptoms and small intestinal permeability in children with atopic dermatitis', *J Pediatr*, vol. 145, no. 5, pp. 612–616.

ROUSSEAUX, C., THURU, X., GELOT, A., BARNICH, N., NEUT, C., DUBUQUOY, L., DUBUQUOY, C., MEROUR, E., GEBOES, K., CHAMAILLARD, M., OUWEHAND, A., LEYER, G., CARCANO, D., COLOMBEL, J. F., ARDID, D., & DESREUMAUX, P. 2006, '*Lactobacillus acidophilus* modulates intestinal pain and induces opioid and cannabinoid receptors', *Nat Med*, vol. 13, no. 1, pp. 35–37.

SAAVEDRA, J. M., BAUMAN, N. A., OUNG, I., PERMAN, J. A., & YOLKEN, R. H. 1994, 'Feeding of *Bifidobacterium bifidum* and *Streptococcus thermophilus* to infants in hospital for prevention of diarrhoea and shedding of rotavirus.', *Lancet*, vol. 344, no. October 15, pp. 1046–1049.

SALMINEN, S. & SALMINEN, E. 1997, 'Lactulose, lactic acid bacteria, intestinal microecology and mucosal protection', *Scand J Gastroenterol Suppl*, vol. 222, pp. 45–48.

SANSONETTI, P. J. 2004, 'War and peace at mucosal surfaces', *Nat Rev Immunol*, vol. 4, no. 12, pp. 953–964.

SAZAWAL, S., HIREMATH, G., DHINGRA, U., MALIK, P., DEB, S., & BLACK, R. E. 2006, 'Efficacy of probiotics in prevention of acute diarrhoea: a meta-analysis of masked, randomised, placebo-controlled trials', *Lancet Infect Dis*, vol. 6, no. 6, pp. 374–382.

SHEIH, Y. H., CHIANG, B. L., WANG, L. H., LIAO, C. K., & GILL, H. S. 2001, 'Systemic immunity-enhancing effects in healthy subjects following dietary consumption of the lactic acid bacterium *Lactobacillus rhamnosus* HN001', *J Am Coll Nutr*, vol. 20, no. 2 Suppl, pp. 149–156.

SHORNIKOVA, A.-V., CASAS, I., MYKKÄNEN, H., SALO, E., & VESIKARI, T. 1997, 'Bacteriotherapy with *Lactobacillus reuteri* in rotavirus gastroenteritis', *Pediatr Infect Dis J*, vol. 16, pp. 1103–1107.

SILVA, A. M., BAMBIRRA, E. A., OLIVEIRA, A. L., SOUZA, P. P., GOMES, D. A., VIEIRA, E. C., & NICOLI, J. R. 1999, 'Protective effect of bifidus milk on the experimental infection with *Salmonella enteritidis* subsp. *typhimurium* in conventional and gnotobiotic mice', *J Appl Microbiol*, vol. 86, pp. 331–336.

SISTEK, D., KELLY, R., WICKENS, K., STANLEY, T., FITZHARRIS, P., & CRANE, J. 2006, 'Is the effect of probiotics on atopic dermatitis confined to food sensitized children?', *Clin Exp Allergy*, vol. 36, no. 5, pp. 629–633.

SOLGA, S. F. & DIEHL, A. M. 2003, 'Non-alcoholic fatty liver disease: lumen–liver interactions and possible role for probiotics', *J Hepatol*, vol. 38, no. 5, pp. 681–687.

SUDO, N., SAWAMURA, S., TANAKA, K., AIBA, Y., KUBO, C., & KOGA, Y. 1997, 'The requirement of intestinal bacterial flora for the development of an IgE production system fully susceptible to oral tolerance induction', *J Immunol*, vol. 159, no. 4, pp. 1739–1745.

SULLIVAN, Å., PALMGREN, A. C., & NORD, C. E. 2001, 'Effect of *Lactobacillus paracasei* on intestinal colonisation of *Lactobacilli*, *Bifidobacteria* and *Clostridium difficile* in elderly persons', *Anaerobe*, vol. 7, pp. 67–70.

SVEJE, M. 2008, 'A new era for gut health?' *NutraCos* vol. 7, no. 3, pp. 8–11.

SZAJEWSKA, H., RUSZCZYNSKI, M., & RADZIKOWSKI, A. 2006, 'Probiotics in the prevention of antibiotic-associated diarrhea in children: A meta-analysis of randomized controlled trials', *J Pediatr*, vol. 149, no. 3, pp. 367–372.

TAKEDA, K., SUZUKI, T., SHIMADA, S. I., SHIDA, K., NANNO, M., & OKUMURA, K. 2006, 'Interleukin-12 is involved in the enhancement of human natural killer cell activity by *Lactobacillus casei* Shirota', *Clin Exp Immunol*, vol. 146, no. 1, pp. 109–115.

TALLON, R., ARIAS, S., BRESSOLLIER, P., & URDACI, M. C. 2007, 'Strain- and matrix-dependent adhesion of *Lactobacillus plantarum* is mediated by proteinaceous bacterial compounds', *J Appl Microbiol*, vol. 102, no. 2, pp. 442–451.

TALWALKAR, A. & KAILASAPATHY, K. 2004, 'The role of oxygen in the viability of probiotic bacteria with reference to *L. acidophilus* and *Bifidobacterium* spp', *Curr Issues Intest Microbiol*, vol. 5, no. 1, pp. 1–8.

TANG, A. L., SHAH, N. P., WILCOX, G., WALKER, K. Z., & STOJANOVSKA, L. 2007, 'Fermentation of calcium-fortified soymilk with *Lactobacillus*: effects on calcium solubility, isoflavone conversion, and production of organic acids', *J Food Sci*, vol. 72, no. 9, pp. M431–M436.

TANNOCK, G. W., MUNRO, K., HARMSEN, H. J., WELLING, G. W., SMART, J., & GOPAL, P. K. 2000, 'Analysis of the fecal microflora of human subjects consuming a probiotic product containing *Lactobacillus rhamnosus* DR20', *Appl Environ Microbiol*, vol. 66, no. 6, pp. 2578–2588.

TAYLOR, A. L., DUNSTAN, J. A., & PRESCOTT, S. L. 2007, 'Probiotic supplementation for the first 6 months of life fails to reduce the risk of atopic dermatitis and increases the risk of allergen sensitization in high-risk children: A randomized controlled trial', *J Allergy Clin Immunol*, vol. 119, no. 1, pp. 184–191.

TEJADA-SIMON, M. V., USTUNOL, Z., & PESTKA, J. J. 1999, 'Effects of lactic acid bacteria ingestion on basal cytokine mRNA and immunoglobulin levels in the mouse', *J Food Prot*, vol. 62, no. 3, pp. 287–291.

TOIVANEN, P. 2003, 'Normal intestinal microbiota in the aetiopathogenesis of rheumatoid arthritis', *Ann Rheum Dis*, vol. 62, no. 9, pp. 807–811.

TUOMOLA, E. M. & SALMINEN, S. J. 1998, 'Adhesion of some probiotic and dairy *Lactobacillus* strains to Caco-2 cell cultures', *Int J Food Microbiol*, vol. 41, no. 1, pp. 45–51.

TURBIC, A., AHOKAS, J. T., & HASKARD, C. A. 2002, 'Selective *in vitro* binding of dietary mutagens, individually or in combination, by lactic acid bacteria', *Food Add. Contam.*, vol. 19, no. 2, pp. 144–152.

TURNBAUGH, P. J., LEY, R. E., MAHOWALD, M. A., MAGRINI, V., MARDIS, E. R., & GORDON, J. I. 2006, 'An obesity-associated gut microbiome with increased capacity for energy harvest', *Nature*, vol. 444, no. 7122, pp. 1027–1031.

VALEUR, N., ENGEL, P., CARBAJAL, N., CONNOLLY, E., & LADEFOGED, K. 2004, 'Colonization and immunomodulation by *Lactobacillus reuteri* ATCC 55730 in the human gastrointestinal tract', *Appl Environ Microbiol*, vol. 70, no. 2, pp. 1176–1181.

VANKERCKHOVEN, V., HUYS, G., VAN CANNEYT, M., VAEL, C., KLARE, I., ROMOND, M.-B., ENTENZA, J. M., MOREILLON, P., WIND, R. D., KNOL, J., WIERTZ, E., POT, B., VAUGHAN, E. E., KAHLMETER, G., & GOOSSENS, H. 2008, 'Biosafety assessment of probiotics used for human consumption: recommendations from the EU-PROSAFE project', *Trends Food Sci Technol*, vol. 19, pp. 102–114.

VESTERLUND, S., PALTTA, J., KARP, M., & OUWEHAND, A. C. 2005, 'Measurement of bacterial adhesion – *in vitro* evaluation of different methods', *J Microbiol Meth*, vol. 60, pp. 225–233.

VESTERLUND, S., KARP, M., SALMINEN, S., & OUWEHAND, A. C. 2006, '*Staphylococcus aureus* adheres to human intestinal mucus but can be displaced by certain lactic acid bacteria', *Microbiology*, vol. 152, no. Pt 6, pp. 1819–1826.

VILJANEN, M., SAVILAHTI, E., HAAHTELA, T., JUNTUNEN-BACKMAN, K., KORPELA, R., POUSSA, T., TUURE, T., & KUITUNEN, M. 2005, 'Probiotics in the treatment of atopic eczema/dermatitis syndrome in infants: a double-blind placebo-controlled trial', *Allergy*, vol. 60, no. 4, pp. 494–500.

VINDEROLA, C. G., PROSELLO, W., GHIBERTO, T. D., & REINHEIMER, J. A. 2000, 'Viability of probiotic (*Bifidobacterium*, *Lactobacillus acidophilus* and *Lactobacillus casei*) and nonprobiotic microflora in Argentinian Fresco cheese', *J Dairy Sci*, vol. 83, no. 9, pp. 1905–1911.

VINDEROLA, C. G., COSTA, G. A., REGENHARDT, S., & REINHEIMER, J. A. 2002a, 'Influence of compounds associated with fermented dairy products on the growth of lactic acid starter and probiotic bacteria', *Int Dairy J*, vol. 12, no. 7, pp. 579–589.

VINDEROLA, C. G., MOCCHIUTTI, P., & REINHEIMER, J. A. 2002b, 'Interactions among lactic acid starter and probiotic bacteria used for fermented dairy products', *J Dairy Sci*, vol. 85, no. 4, pp. 721–729.

WAGNER, R. D., PIERSON, C., WARNER, T., DOHNALEK, M., FARMER, J., ROBERTS, L., HILTY, M., & BALISH, E. 1997, 'Biotherapeutic effects of probiotic bacteria on candidiasis in immunodeficient mice', *Infect Immun*, vol. 65, no. 10, pp. 4165–4172.

WELLS, J. M. & MERCENIER, A. 2008, 'Mucosal delivery of therapeutic and prophylactic molecules using lactic acid bacteria', *Nat Rev Microbiol*, vol. 6, no. 5, pp. 349–362.

WHITE, J. S., HOPER, M., PARKS, R. W., CLEMENTS, W. D., DIAMOND, T., & BENGMARK, S. 2006, 'The probiotic bacterium *Lactobacillus plantarum* species 299 reduces intestinal permeability in experimental biliary obstruction', *Lett Appl Microbiol*, vol. 42, no. 1, pp. 19–23.

WINKLER, P., DE VRESE, M., LAUE, C., & SCHREZENMEIR, J. 2005, 'Effect of a dietary supplement containing probiotic bacteria plus vitamins and minerals on common cold infections and cellular immune parameters', *Int J Clin Pharmacol Ther*, vol. 43, no. 7, pp. 318–326.

WOLD, A. E., THORSSÉN, M., HULL, S., & SVANBORG EDÉN, C. 1988, 'Attachment of *Escherichia coli* via mannose- or Galα1-4Galβ-containing receptors to human colonic epithelial cells', *Infect Immun*, vol. 56, no. 10, pp. 2531–2537.

WOODCOCK, N. P., MCNAUGHT, C. E., MORGAN, D. R., GREGG, K. L., & MACFIE, J. 2004, 'An investigation into the effect of a probiotic on gut immune function in surgical patients', *Clin Nutr*, vol. 23, no. 5, pp. 1069–1073.

YAMANO, T., IINO, H., TAKADA, M., BLUM, S., ROCHAT, F., & FUKUSHIMA, Y. 2006, 'Improvement of the human intestinal flora by ingestion of the probiotic strain *Lactobacillus johnsonii* La1', *Br J Nutr*, vol. 95, no. 2, pp. 303–312.

YILMAZTEKIN, M., OZER, B. H., & ATASOY, F. 2004, 'Survival of *Lactobacillus acidophilus* LA-5 and *Bifidobacterium bifidum* BB-02 in white-brined cheese', *Int J Food Sci Nutr*, vol. 55, no. 1, pp. 53–60.

YUKI, N., WATANABE, K., MIKE, A., TAGAMI, Y., TANAKA, R., OHWAKI, M., & MOROTOMI, M. 1999, 'Survival of a probiotic, *Lactobacillus casei* strain Shirota, in the gastrointestinal tract: Selective isolation from faeces and identification using monoclonal antibodies', *Int J Food Microbiol*, vol. 48, pp. 51–57.

ZAREIE, M., JOHNSON-HENRY, K. C., JURY, J., YANG, P. C., NGAN, B. Y., MCKAY, D. M., SODERHOLM, J. D., PERDUE, M. H., & SHERMAN, P. M. 2006, 'Probiotics prevent bacterial translocation and improve intestinal barrier function in rats following chronic psychological stress', *Gut*, vol. 55, no. 11, pp. 1553–1560.

ZHANG, X. B. & OHTA, Y. 1990, 'Antimutagenicity and binding of lactic acid bacteria from chinese cheese to mutagenic pyrolyzates', *J Dairy Sci*, vol. 73, no. 10, pp. 2702–2710.

ZHOU, J. S. & GILL, H. S. 2005, 'Immunostimulatory probiotic *Lactobacillus rhamnosus* HN001 and *Bifidobacterium lactis* HN019 do not induce pathological inflammation in mouse model of experimental autoimmune thyroiditis', *Int J Food Microbiol*, vol. 103, no. 1, pp. 97–104.

Part II

Advances in research methods to study food sensory perception, digestion and adsorption

10

Measuring the oral behaviour of foods

I. A. M. Appelqvist, CSIRO, Australia

Abstract: The interactions between biological surfaces (in the mouth) and product materials under physiological oral processing conditions play an important role in generating sensory attributes and determining sensory perception. This chapter reviews measurement techniques that probe oral food processing either directly *in vivo* or *ex vivo* (including artificial mouths), discusses the techniques in context of the in-mouth process or mechanism that they probe (break down and fracture mechanics, food–saliva and food–biological surface interactions) and describes the results in relation to sensory perception. Some aspects of flavour release in relation to use of artificial mouths are also described.

Key words: measurement techniques of oral food processing, food material properties, food behaviour and sensory perception, food–saliva interactions, artificial mouths.

10.1 Introduction

Studying and elucidating the interactions between biological surfaces (in the mouth) and product materials under physiological oral processing conditions has been difficult and until recently has not been very systematic. This difficulty is partly due to the complex nature of both physical and mechanical 'measurement' within such physiological environments, and because the physical/mechanical responses of food is highly time dependent through both the 'openness' of the product materials (swelling, dissolving, etc.) and the dynamic nature of biological surfaces and fluids. It is, however, through these complex domains that our products interact, change physically and chemically, and eventually elicit the sensory response that consumers perceive.

The interaction between food materials and physiological surfaces and fluids, which plays an important role in generating sensory attributes, is still not well understood in terms of the physics and biophysics of the interfacial properties between product materials and biological surfaces and fluids.

This aspect of measurement and the inclusion of knowledge about structural changes that occur after processing in the mouth are important to progress our understanding of sensory behaviour and to predict and quantify the stimuli generated during eating (van Aken *et al.*, 2007). The technical challenges for the food material scientists are to be able to measure the dynamic nature of material changes, which for many breakdown mechanisms can be very fast, and to measure these changes under relevant physiological conditions. Added to this is the complexity in which a number of changes to the materials properties of food during mastication occur simultaneously, and as yet what mechanisms dominate in terms of sensory perception are not fully known. Further complexity is in how multimodel features of food are integrated and is a fundamental neuroscientific question in food perception (Verhagen and Engelen, 2006).

The aim of this chapter is to outline and discuss a range of techniques that have been used by food material scientists and engineers to try to probe some of the aspects of oral processing identified above. The chapter will attempt to review the techniques in context of the in-mouth process or mechanism that they probe and how this information has been used to relate to sensory perception. The techniques and measurement approaches identified fall into a number of categories: those that use *in vivo* techniques that measure and visualise changes in food during mastication directly; those that use the mouth as a 'rheometer', the analysis of which is directed on the expectorated food; and those that measure *ex vivo*, but have taken into account some of the physiological and mechanical characteristics relevant to the mouth under which food gets processed. The type of technique selected has largely been determined by the 'texture' of the food, so that solid foods such as meat, cheese and nuts have been measured in terms of their breakdown and fracture mechanics whereas soft-solids such as cream cheese, yoghurt and mayonnaise are measured primarily through their interaction with saliva and/or the biological oral surfaces.

Conceptually, it is clear that the product dynamics and mouth interaction must also have a role to play in the delivery of small molecules and the release of ingredients at specified target sites, which offer novel routes to control texture and taste. Some aspects of flavour release will be briefly covered in Section 10.6 on artificial mouths.

10.2 *In vivo* visualisation measurements for understanding food behaviour in the mouth

The importance of measuring the impact of oral processing on the structural changes of food in the mouth, how these dynamic aspects of food interact with sensory receptors and finally the relationship to sensory perception has long been recognised. Understanding the various mechanisms involved with oral processing of food and quantifying the in-mouth structuring and disassembly of food materials, as well as their interaction with oral surfaces, will support the establishment of engineering rules to control these mechanisms by the design of the structure and composition of food.

Recently food research studies have focused on investigating *in vivo* the product interaction with the structures of the oral apparatus and surfaces. A range of visualisation techniques has been used to gain a better understanding of the mouth movements, to visualise the surface oral structures and to monitor the complex interactions of food materials during eating. The most relevant techniques for measuring oral behaviour of food are described in the next section.

10.2.1 X-ray-based imaging for visualising oral movements

Attempts have been made to quantify tongue movements using videofluorography of lead markers glued to the tongue (Hiiemae and Palmer, 2003). Limitations of this technique are that only a small number of markers can be used and the radio-opacity of the mandible and teeth obscure the tongue, so that the complexity of the tongue movement is not captured. In addition having to use a radio opaque contrast medium in the food and because exposure to X-rays must be kept to a minimum, this technique has been replaced by more modern visualisation techniques. However, X-ray imaging has been used to visualise chewing action and swallowing of solid and semi-solid foods in real time (Hiiemae *et al.*, 2002), and has contributed to our understanding of the sequences of activity and processes that are undergone during eating of food. Videofluoroscopy, a dynamic X-ray technique, has been applied to observe the process of swallowing food and fluids using a fluid medium contrast (Buettner *et al.*, 2001) and results were analysed according to the stages of swallowing (bolus uptake, beginning of bolus transport, velopharyngeal closure, triggering of the swallowing reflex, propulsion of the bolus towards the oesophagus and original position) defined by Hannig (1995). The X-ray images showed that, during mastication of solid food, intermittent opening of the connection of the oral cavity to the naso- and dorsal oropharynx can be observed and that food residue is left on the back of the tongue after swallowing, which provides an after-taste and a reservoir for aroma molecules to be detected long after the food bolus has left the oral cavity.

10.2.2 Echo-sonography for measuring tongue movement

Ultrasonic echo-sonography has been used extensively in speech research (Green and Wang, 2003; Stone, 2005) and in studies of dysphagia (Casa *et al.*, 2003) as it has an adequate rate of data capture and it is non-invasive. Two forms of display are commonly used: B-mode imaging which shows a two-dimensional slice through the body (De Wijk *et al.*, 2006b) and M-mode which depicts movement as a function of time (Hashimoto and Shinoda, 1999). The sonograph is based on the time of flight of high-frequency pulses emitted from the probe and is sensitive to changes in the acoustic impedance of the tissues. Thus the interface between the tongue surface and air generates a strong reflection but when the tongue touches the hard palate some energy passes through the interface, allowing the hard palate to be visualised and tongue palate contacts to be identified. De Wijk *et al.* (2006b) recently explored the use of ultrasonic imaging for the quantification of oral movements, especially tongue movements, during oral processing of semi-solid foods. Their interest was in determining the effects of specific food properties, such as taste (sweetness and bitterness) and texture (viscosity and creaminess) on the oral movements. These movements were characterised into three time periods corresponding to different processing phases, the bulk phase when the food is taken into the mouth and eaten, the swallow phase when the food is being swallowed and the clearance phase when the food is being cleared. The ultrasound study demonstrated that oral movements were determined by food properties, such as taste and texture as well as the rated attribute.

10.2.3 Magnetic resonance imaging

Magnetic resonance imaging (MRI) and functional MRI (fMRI) have a number of advantages over other imaging techniques in that they provide direct quantitative and non-invasive measurements of body tissues such as the brain, skin, oral cavity and the gastrointestinal tract (Marciani *et al.*, 2001a,b; Fillery-Travis *et al.*, 2002). fMRI has had most success in producing *in vivo* high-resolution images of static tissues such as the brain to measure for example, the response as a bold signal in a specific part of the brain to sensory stimulus like taste (O'Doherty *et al.*, 2001; De Araujo *et al.*, 2003a; Schoenfeld *et al.*, 2004; Rolls 2005), smell (Marciani *et al.*, 2006a), pleasant touch (Francis *et al.*, 1999) and texture (Zald and Pardo, 2000; De Araujo *et al.*, 2003b, De Araujo and Rolls, 2004; Miyamoto *et al.*, 2006; Alonso *et al.*, 2007). MRI has been used to determine morphological characteristics of skin tissue (Mirrashed and Sharp, 2004) and skin hydration/drying (Ablett *et al.*, 1988; Loden, 1992; Zemtsov, 1993). However, most MRI studies have been conducted for the diagnosis of pretherapeutic stages of tumours of the oropharynx, the oral cavity and the floor of the mouth (Lenz *et al.*, 2000) and it is in the clinical setting that the technique of MRI and that of computed tomography has developed as non-invasive methods for diagnostic evaluations.

The process of eating and drinking has been observed *in vivo* by application of time resolved MRI (Buettner *et al.*, 2001). The study was aimed at elucidating the timing and performance of the physiological organs involved in mastication and swallowing. It was shown that, during the sequence of mastication, the mouth protects the airways from obstruction by food particles by setting up a physiological barrier that is capable of retaining volatile molecules within the oral cavity. These barriers allow access of odorants to the nasal cavity only at certain times during the eating process, which is controlled by the texture of the food and the amount of food present in the mouth. Although potentially ideal, MRI is currently too slow to resolve some of the more rapid movements of the tongue made during mastication.

MRI is being used extensively to measure real-time processes in the gastrointestinal (GI) tract (Marciani *et al.*, 2001a, 2006b; Fillery-Travis *et al.*, 2002; Hoad *et al.*, 2006, 2007) and the first basic engineering models for digestion (Stoll *et al.*, 2000; Spratt *et al.*, 2005) are starting to appear. Results show that the stomach behaves as a poorly mixed system in which the walls oscillate, causing some surface mixing and erosion. *In vivo* imaging of intergastric gelation of model food (Hoad *et al.*, 2004) and gastric emptying (Marciani *et al.*, 2001b) have demonstrated that the time taken for complete digestion depends on the original food structure, with more highly structured food taking longer to digest.

10.2.4 Video rate endoscopy for visualisation of surface structures

Adams and co-workers (2007) applied video rate endoscopy for the visualisation of food materials in the mouth and reported on the distribution of food material in the oral cavity and clearance behaviour due to salivary flow. They were able to collect sub-millimetre resolution, real-time images of the oral mucosal surfaces from around the mouth from people both before and after eating, with the advantage that the subject could sit in a natural sitting position, which is more realistic. The principles of video rate confocal endoscopy have been described by Watson *et al.* (2002), who also verified the safety and flexibility of the technique to probe soft tissues in the body. Both fluorescent imaging/spectroscopy and reflectance imaging are possible and, as the soft tissues can generate contrast, it is also possible to use confocal imaging. Fluorescent labelling of the mouth structures was found to produce greater differentiation between the features of interest, and the images revealed information on both the structures within the oral cavity and on the product residue after eating. Analysis of the fluorescence emission spectra could give quantitative information about the food residue left after eating. Fluorescent images collected from the surface of the tongue after processing different viscosity oils (Adams *et al.*, 2007) showed evidence of emulsification and indicated that droplet break-up is a function of viscosity.

White light reflectance imaging was used to visualise the near-surface aspects of arterioles and capillary loops supplying blood to the mouth. The response of the blood flow to cold thermal stimulus (Adams *et al.*, 2007) and to trigeminal stimulus from a cooling agent such as menthol (Appelqvist,

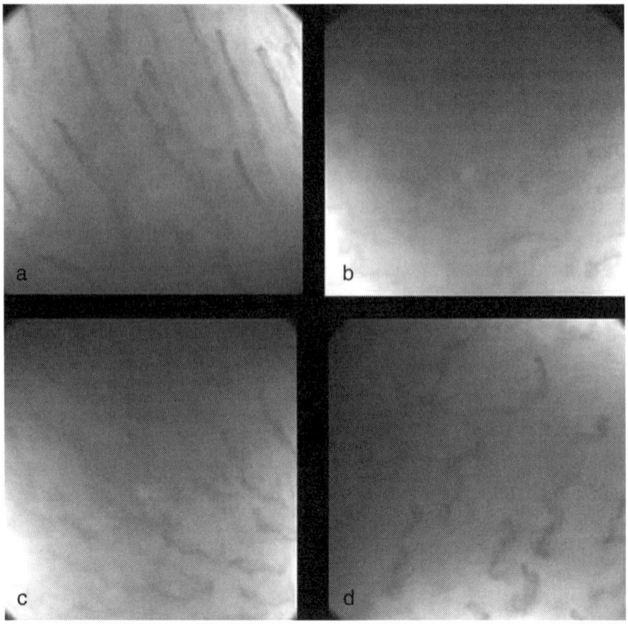

Fig. 10.1 Incoherent epi-illumination white light images from the inner cheek before (a) and after (b) application of ice, and after (c) direct application of a menthol mint and 5 min (d) after application. The capillary network is clearly visible under the oral mucosa in image (a) whereas the capillary structures virtually disappear due to reduction in blood flow after the ice was applied in image (b). Image (c) shows a slight reduction in contrast and a change to the capillary characteristics which increase as shown in image (d) where the structures appear more dilated probably because the oral mucosa has been slightly irritated by the menthol in the mint. The image width is about 1.5 mm. (Images based on Adams *et al.*, 2007, modified from Appelqvist, 2005.)

2005) was observed (see Fig. 10.1). This imaging mode was used to compare the response of blood flow on the cheek after placing either a block of ice or a menthol mint against the cheek surface. It can be seen that the contrast of the blood capillaries diminishes in Fig. 10.1(b) after the ice has been applied compared with pre-treatment (Fig. 10.1a) because the capillaries constrict and the blood flow reduces, which returns to normal shortly (Fig. 10.1a). In comparison, the capillaries after having a menthol mint against the cheek surface initially show a reduction in contrast associated with reduced blood flow (Fig. 10.1c), but then increase in contrast beyond the initial state, suggesting slight irritation of the oral mucosa (Fig. 10.1d). For highly detailed tissue structural information and to collect data on the food residues remaining on the tissue surfaces, non-confocal fluorescence imaging in combination with a strong contrast agent such as sodium fluorescein was used, which gave good spatial and temporal resolution. The results from model biopolymer solutions that were swirled and spat out indicate that there is inhomogeneous coverage of the mouth, that this is related to the underlying structure of the tongue and that the rate of material clearance is dependent on the surface contact that occurs.

Adams *et al.* (2007) also confirmed that an increase in viscosity also increased the amount of residue left (Goulet and Brudevold, 1986) and that the rate the mouth processed the residue and cleared it from the oral cavity was influenced by salivary flow rates and rheological properties. Previous results have reported a bi-phasic clearance for solutions (Bashir *et al.*, 1995); however, Adams *et al.* (2007) found that they could fit a single exponential to their clearance data. As techniques improve in resolution and can measure the processes that occur directly, more accurate quantitative data will be obtained, which will challenge both some data in the literature and conclusions that have been accepted in the past.

Direct measurement of the food left in the mouth after eating without further disrupting it will be important to increase our understanding of food material behaviour in use and its impact on sensory perception. The potential for this technique is that it will be able to examine a wide variety of food materials ranging from aqueous solutions to solid foods, including multi-component food. Dual channel imaging and different fluorescent labels will enable simultaneous investigation of two or more components in complex food. The technique also allows the determination of the spatial distribution of residue and the visualisation of structures that make up the mouth coating.

Imaging modalities currently used to diagnose disease in the oral cavity could potentially be used to visualise the oral processing of food. These include plain radiography (panoramic radiography and intraoral radiography), nuclear medicine scintigraphy, ultrasound (US), computed tomography (CT), MRI and positron emission tomography (PET) (Rumboldt *et al.*, 2003; Ng *et al.*, 2005). It will be the advancement in the visualisation techniques in the medical sciences that will ultimately be used by the food researchers to understand the mechanisms of oral processing and food behaviour.

10.3 Measuring solid food fracture breakdown upon oral processing

The effect of oral processing on solid food materials and the elucidation of the mechanisms by which food such as chocolate, nuts, meat and hard cheese fracture and breakdown during mastication has been widely investigated (Szczesniak, 1963; Lucus *et al.*, 2002; Öhgren *et al.*, 2004; Loren *et al.*, 2007; Van den Berg, 2007; Brink *et al.*, 2007). Models such as the three-dimensional model for the processing of solid and semi-solid food, based on analysis of expectorated food, have been proposed (Hutchings and Lillford, 1988). The breakdown model based on meat products has three principal dimensions, which were loosely defined as the ‘degree of structure’, 'degree of lubrication' and 'time'. The model describes the processing of a solid food through these dimensions as a food-specific 'breakdown path' in which the bolus travels until a physiological trigger is met, which determines swallowing or not. The nature of the mechanical breakdown of these solids is dependent on the microstructure and the oral movements of the mouth in response to the changes in physical structure of the food. Having the ability to measure these variables from the mastication process, the fracture behaviour and the change in food microstructure is important to improve our understanding of oral behaviour of food and its relation to sensory perception.

10.3.1 Electromyography for texture characterisation

Electromyography (EMG) is the recording of the electrical phenomena that determine muscle health, muscle excitation and contraction. Electromyographic and jaw movement: (kinematic) recordings are commonly used to study mastication, from which several variables can be measured, such as amplitude of jaw opening during chewing and speed of jaw movements. Other factors that can be measured are the mastication force needed to break down solid food and the duration of mastication and rate of chewing (Perlman, 2006). Surface EMG is a technique based on attaching bipolar electrodes onto the four main masticatory muscles (masseter and temporal) and measuring the activity of the muscles during mastication of solid-like food where considerable activity from chewing using large mandibular movements can be generated in the jaw closing muscles. This technique has been used to compare activity in the jaw in subjects to evaluate oral processing of model foods with different hardness (Veyrune *et al.*, 2007) and tenderness of meat (Veyrune and Mioche, 2000). Since mastication is a physiological process controlled by the central nervous system and modulated by inputs from the mouth, information gained from EMG has shown that the mastication process adapts to changes in characteristics of the food. For example, the masticatory forces measured during chewing of solid food decreased as the food started to break down and the initial force required fracturing solid foods increased with increased hardness. A number of studies using EMG have been conducted to assess texture characteristics such as tenderness, hardness, crunchiness and juiciness, on products such as carrots, biscuits, cooked meat, cooked rice and cheese, and close-fitting correlations have been found between texture sensory attributes and EMG measurements (Gonzalez *et al.*, 2001).

10.3.2 Microscopy and large deformation measures to probe structure–mechanical relations

Techniques that have been used to determine the effect of oral processing on soft-solids such as mixed protein–polysaccharide gels have included large deformation measures and visualisation techniques simultaneously to allow structural changes such as failure points and crack propagation in composite food to be followed directly under dynamic conditions (Loren *et al.*, 2007).

Confocal laser scanning microscopy and large deformation measurements
Commercially, tensile stages have been developed with sensitive load cells, which can be placed under the confocal laser scanning microscope (CLSM) because of their small size. Analyses of solid materials (George *et al.*, 2003) and visualisation of stress concentration in polymers (Olmos *et al.*, 2002) can be conducted and time resolved measurements of structure and consistency can be used to explore material failure characteristics in both tension and compression.

Van den Berg (2007) used CSLM imaging under uniaxial compression and showed that protein–polysaccharide phase separated gels fractured through the protein network and only at a few places, whereas stranded gels fractured in many places, which was accompanied by coarsening of the protein network. The number of fracture sites and the rate of crack propagation in a food material have great impact on the perceived sensory properties. The way a structure deforms and breaks under stress is crucial for properties such as flow and fracture behaviour, sensory perception of structure, water release and mobility and release of active compounds. The perceived texture of foods is largely determined by structural rearrangements during the deformation process (Lillford, 2000, 2001) and having the ability to measure food failure behaviour under relevant physiological parameters such as time, temperature, stress and shear is important, since it mimics to some extent the breakdown of a food during consumption. Understanding the mechanism by which food deforms and breaks down at the microstructure length scale gives the food industry important knowledge about the structure–mechanical relationship of their ingredients so that better prediction of food sensory behaviour can be determined and foods can be designed with the desired texture and functionality.

Analysing fractures in food systems by means of microscopy techniques is a relatively new approach and has been useful in demonstrating the influence of the microstructure on material failure properties. Plucknett and co-workers (Plucknett and Normand, 2000, Plucknett *et al.*, 2001) carried out some of the first dynamic experiments on the fracture behaviour of gelatin/maltodextrin and gelatin/agarose gels using CLSM in combination with a tensile stage. They observed that these materials fractured differently because of the interfacial properties such as the bonding energy between the two components and the mechanical strength of the networks in the two phases which determine their ability to deform and flow. For example, Rizzieri and co-workers demonstrated ductile behaviour in a gelatin/maltodextrin system using a specially built tensile stage in combination with an environmental scanning electron microscope (ESEM) (Rizzieri *et al.*, 2003).

Hermansson and co-workers have extensively used CLSM to follow transient changes in natural food that have been manipulated directly through, for example, applying a notch in complex structured foods such as cheese, in order to monitor the fracture line through the food microstructure and the rate at which the crack tip moves (Loren *et al.*, 2007). For practical reasons a small notch is made in the sample, so that the start of the crack can be induced and the microscope can be focused directly on that part of the sample. As the material is deformed, the notch widens and starts to move through the sample following the weakest part of the structure. The tensile stage makes it possible to simultaneously measure the microstructure and the stress–strain properties on the micron scale. CLSM combined with time-dependent image analysis allows data from the tensile stage to be related to the individual sequential micrographs, which capture the progress of the crack tip, which allows comparison of the required deformation for the same crack length. The importance of investigating the effect of microstructure on the breakdown behaviour of food materials is that it will provide information on the relationship between the sensory perception of texture and the mechanical behaviour of the food.

Øiseth and Lundin (2008) have used CLSM in combination with deformation measurements to investigate the fracture mechanics of plant tissues such as carrots both raw and after processing to determine the effect of processing on failure performance of whole pieces of vegetable. Figure 10.2 shows the force–distance curves from raw and blanched carrots during tensile testing and indicates that the raw carrot withstands more stress before it fractures compared to the heat treated sample. The CLSM micrographs (Fig. 10.2b–d) show how cracks propagate through the heated carrot tissue and the last two images (Fig. 10.2e and f) show CLSM 3D representations of the fractured tissue of (e) raw and (f) blanched carrot strips. In the raw sample, the crack has propagated through the cell walls as can be seen by ruptured cells, whereas in the heat-treated samples the tissue has separated mostly between the cells due to the weakening of the middle lamella after heating. These studies of microstructure-failure behaviour for plant materials provide the potential to determine the relationship between agronomic environment, processing and mechanical behaviour on sensory perception of texture and breakdown.

In order to fully map the structural dynamics of composite foods leading to failure and breakdown there is a need for sophisticated measurement techniques for fracture dynamics at the microscopic level in addition to traditional large-scale rheological methods. It is clear that there are advantages in combining large deformation and/or rheological measures while viewing the behaviour of food materials directly under such stresses in real time, to simulate oral processing conditions. It should be noted that for very rapid fracture mechanics, CLSM may not be sufficient to follow the structural changes because of the limitations in scanning rate and so other microscopy techniques such as optical, video and new techniques such as

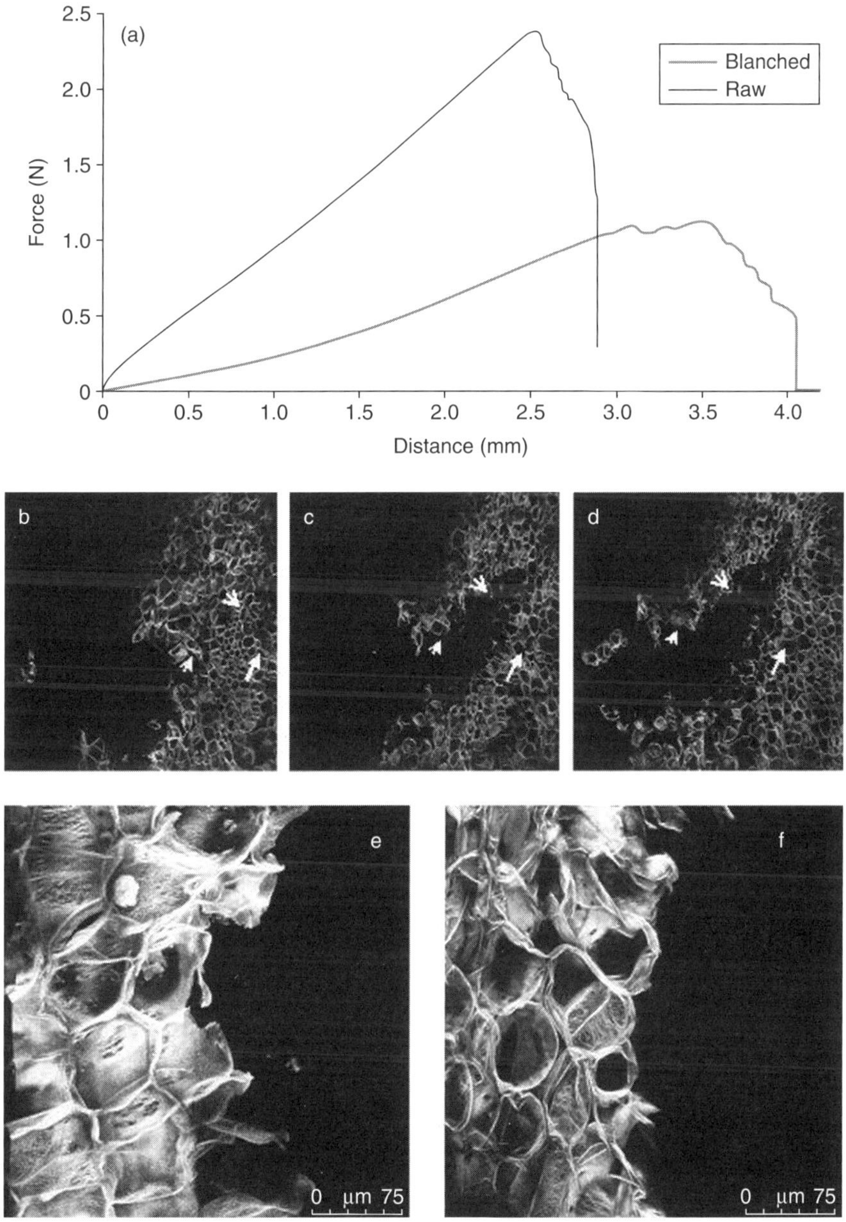

Fig. 10.2 Tensile testing of carrot strips. (a) Force–distance curves from raw and blanched carrots during tensile testing. The raw carrot withstands more stress before it fractures compared with the heat-treated sample. (b)–(d) Confocal laser scanning micrographs showing how the crack propagates through the heat-treated carrot tissue. The arrows serve as viewing guidance to three different cells during the testing process. Image size 1.55 × 1.55 mm². The last two images show CLSM 3D representations of the fractured tissue of (e) raw and (f) blanched carrot strips. In the raw sample, the crack has propagated through the cell walls as can be seen by ruptured cells, whereas in the heat-treated samples the tissue has separated mostly between the cells. (Unpublished results, Sofia Kihlman Øiseth, with permission from CSIRO.)

multifocal multiphoton microscopy, which allows fast acquisition of 3D data may need to be considered (Egner *et al.*, 2004; Egner and Hell, 2005). For an excellent review of the modern CLSM and how it can be used to examine and control the microstructure of complex foods, including measuring mass transport and analysis of CLSM images, the reader is referred to Loren, *et al.* (2007).

10.3.3 Chew and expectorate analysis

Chew and expectorate experiments have been used to measure the process of diminution of solid food materials such as peanuts and characterised visually using light microscopy. Figure 10.3 shows light micrographs of five peanuts having been chewed to different degrees in the mouth before being spat out. It is clear that, as the number of chews increases to about 5, the peanuts are continually being fragmented into smaller pieces, after which further chewing starts to produce a bolus between the peanut fragments

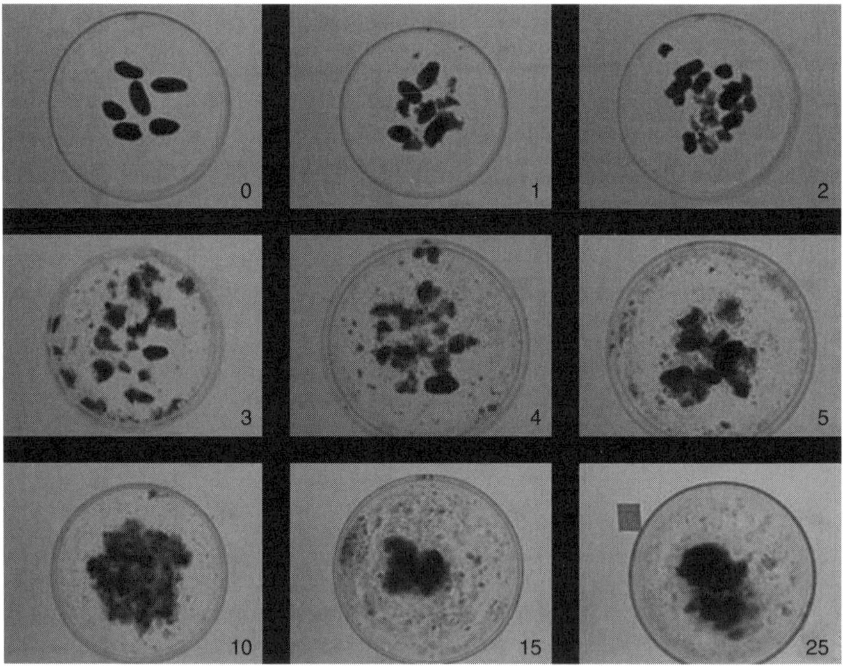

Fig. 10.3 Spat out samples of five peanuts with increased levels of mastication ranging from 1 chew to 25 chews. It is clear that the peanuts are fragmented into small pieces by chew 4 and there after a bolus starts to form with the saliva from chew 5 up to chew 10, which indicates time to swallow. Forced chewing beyond time to swallow causes the peanut fragments to disperse (Zerdin and Kelly, 2008 with permission from CSIRO.)

and saliva (chews 5 to 10) and at this point the food is ready to be swallowed. Chewing beyond this point seems to cause increased dispersion of the peanut pieces from the main bolus mass and was reported to be 'uncomfortable' (Zerdin and Kelly, 2008). The advantage of this approach is that all the mouth physiology, mechanics and dynamics are inherent in the characterisation of the spat-out bolus, which provides direct information on the impact of oral processing on the fracture and breakdown of solid foods and on the changes in soft material structures due to mixing with saliva and shearing by oral movements. The latter is discussed further in the next section.

10.4 Measuring soft-solid food breakdown and interaction with saliva

Crucial in the oral processing of soft-solid foods such as sour cream, yoghurt, custard and soft cheeses are the structural and phase changes that occur from heating or cooling to mouth physiological temperature, mixing with saliva, the contact with the oral surfaces and the flow involved in squeezing and shearing between palate and tongue. In general the oral behaviour important for mouthfeel in soft materials is the rate of breakdown delivered primarily through tongue movement and mixing with saliva (De Wijk *et al.*, 2006a) and film-forming and binding on the oral surfaces delivered through squeezing the food between surfaces (Sala *et al.*, 2008). In the following sections the measurements used to determine structural changes of key food components (starch and emulsions) after oral processing and mixing with saliva and the film-forming and binding of food emulsions on oral surfaces will be discussed.

10.4.1 Measurement of physiological effects of saliva on food components

Human whole saliva (HWS) is a complex physiological secretion that performs essential functions such as protection of oral health and lubrication of mouth tissues, as well as pre-digestion of food through dilution, enzyme hydrolysis and ionic interaction (buffering) which impact on food structure and breakdown rates. The interaction between saliva and food components both *in vitro* by adding saliva to food or *in vivo* by mixing the food in mouth and spitting out has been extensively studied particularly for starch-based (Appelqvist *et al.*, 1995; De Wijk *et al.*, 2003, 2006a) and emulsion-based foods (van Aken *et al.*, 2005, 2007; Vingerhoeds *et al.*, 2005; Silletti *et al.*, 2007a,b,c).

Saliva and starch

Mixing of saliva with food that contains amylase-sensitive starches often induces fast breakdown of food. When starch is heated, the granules hydrate

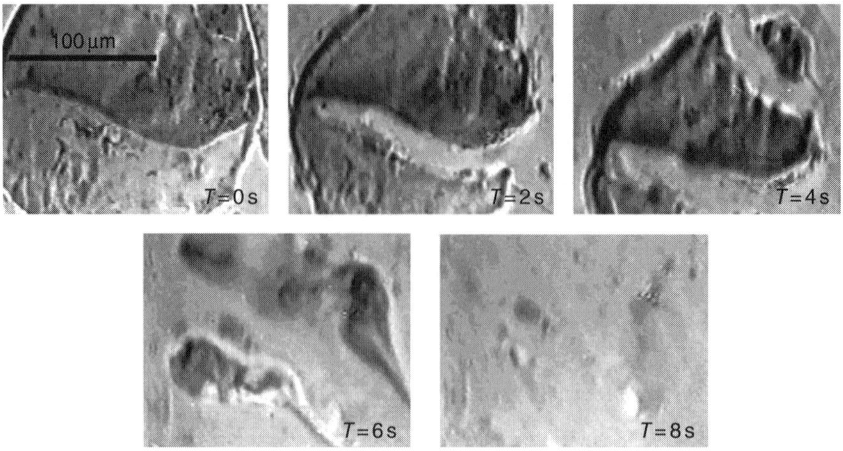

Fig. 10.4 Light micrographs of cooked starch being digested by human saliva on an optical slide in real time. The micrographs clearly show the starch granule being hydrolysed as the saliva imbibes from right to left in each image. (Adapted with modification from Appelqvist *et al.*, 1995.)

and swell to provide texture, and become highly sensitive to the enzyme alpha amylase found in human saliva. This leads to fast digestion of starch in which the granule structure breaks down and disappears as shown in Fig. 10.4, resulting in a loss in viscosity of the product in the mouth (Engelen *et al.*, 2003a,b; De Wijk *et al.*, 2004). The rate of hydrolysis of starch granules can be altered by the type of starch selected (e.g. chemically modified) and the food matrix that surrounds it, by reducing the accessibility of the amylase enzyme to the starch granule (Appelqvist *et al.*, 1995). The importance of amylase action on controlling texture attributes such as creaminess was demonstrated in a range of custards where slowing the enzymic breakdown increased the creaminess ratings in a sensory test (Janssen *et al.*, 2007).

Saliva and emulsions

Saliva has been shown to interact with other food components through shear induced mixing generated by the tongue moving against the hard palate, which can induce shear thinning and can cause coalescence of oil droplets (van Aken *et al.*, 2005, 2007; Vingerhoed, *et al.*, 2005; van Aken, 2007). The oil droplets in unflocculated emulsions mixed with saliva either in the mouth or *in vitro* were found to aggregate (Vingerhoeds *et al.*, 2005; Silletti *et al.*, 2007a) and the flocculation mechanism (Silletti *et al.*, 2007b) characterised by CLSM and turbidity measurement is believed to be regulated by a balance of forces including depletion, van der Waals forces and/ or electrostatic interactions between emulsion droplets and salivary proteins. It is possible that the large bulky proteins such as the glycoproteins in saliva could cause depletion between the oil drops driving the droplets together and flocculation. On the other hand, salts in the saliva could act as a charge screen reducing the interaction between salivary proteins and the oil drops. Finally, displacement of emulsifier at the oil surface could potentially take place, causing destabilisation of the emulsion. Having a better understanding of these potential mechanisms at play in the physiological environment gives potential for food scientists to design the emulsion interface by selecting, for example, the appropriately charged emulsifier to stabilise the emulsion so that the tendency to flocculate can be controlled (Silletti *et al.*, 2007c).

To gain better understanding of the mechanisms underlying food performance under oral conditions, a number of researchers have started to integrate *in vitro* and *in vivo* instrumental measurements with sensory studies on a systematic set of food samples (De Wijk *et al.*, 2006b). These workers used *in vitro* and *in vivo* instrumental tests to determine the surface and bulk-related properties of the food bolus that relate to the perceived oral texture of products such as starch-containing custards. Measurements included the food's infrared reflectance to determine oil distribution, turbidity measures of spat-out rinse water to assess precipitation and flocculation effects, digital imaging of spat-out foods, which were analysed with respect to homogeneity and the friction (lubrication) between the food and the oral tissue, using tribology (De Wijk and Prinz, 2005, 2006; De Wijk *et al.*, 2006a). A model for custard products was proposed based on the results characterised by three main sensory dimensions: roughness to creaminess driven by lubrication due to fat, melting to thickness driven by viscosity due to starch hydrolysis, and airiness to heterogeneity primarily driven by mixing with saliva. The approach of integrating 'instrumental-sensory-ingredient' relationships firstly will facilitate an understanding of what instrumental techniques actually measure and secondly will provide the product developer with information on ingredient functionality to optimise specific product ranges that have been investigated.

10.5 Measuring soft-solid food interactions with oral surfaces: lubrication and binding

Friction at the interface of the food with the oral mucosa is detected by mechanoreceptors in the oral mucosa. Friction forces depend on factors such as the rheology and lubricious properties of the saliva (Bongaerts *et al.*, 2007b), the food and mucosa and the speed with which the two surfaces, e.g. the food bolus and tongue, move across each other. The force exerted by the tongue on the food bolus also contributes to the friction coefficient of the food. Oral friction also depends on the difference between sliding and rolling motions as well as on the shear rate. It is likely that during mastication there are different rolling and sliding motions dependent on the food eaten.

10.5.1 Tribology measurement

Friction between two sliding surfaces in general depends on (a) the properties of the lubricating substance in the contact zone separating the surfaces (Cassin *et al.*, 2001) and the presence of an adsorbed layer, (b) the pressure exerted pushing the two surfaces together which is dependent on the relative speed and (c) the initial roughness and mechanical properties of the surfaces in contact. Friction has been measured over a wide range of entrainment speeds and Stribeck curves have been obtained spanning the boundary, mixed and hydrodynamic lubrication regimes (Cassin *et al.*, 2001; Butt *et al.*, 2003). The boundary regime is representative of where the surfaces are in contact with each other and the entrainment speed of fluid into the contact zone is slow and depends on the fluid constituents to form boundary films. In this regime the coefficient of friction is not dependent on the speed and the load. Boundary lubrication is characterised by an 'immobile layer' adsorbed to the surface that does not take part in the hydrodynamic flow of the bulk fluid (Georges *et al.*, 1993; Spikes, 1996). At high speed the hydrodynamic regime operates where a lubricant film entrained into the contact zone produces sufficiently high fluid pressure to fully separate the surfaces. The film thickness and friction generated in this type of lubrication are dependent on the viscosity of the fluid at high shear rate present in the lubricant film. Between the boundary and hydrodynamic regime lies the mixed regime of lubrication. Here the asperities on the surfaces are on the same length scale as the thickness of the lubricant film, so the contact load is borne in part by fluid pressure and in part by asperity contact pressure. In this regime the coefficient of friction decreases with increasing speed.

10.5.2 Rheology and tribology of saliva

The rheology and lubricating properties of saliva are highly important owing to its influence on oral health and physiochemical processes within the oral environment. Rheological measurement of HWS until recently has often been performed erroneously and/or limited to the viscosity at a single shear rate.

Stokes and Davies (2007) have re-examined the rheological measurement of whole saliva and have demonstrated the importance of controlling the environment of the rheological measurement and the timing. The recommendation is that saliva is tested immediately after expectoration and that a thin layer of surfactant solution is applied around the rim of the rheometer plates to reduce protein migrating to the air–liquid interface.

Stokes and Davies showed that the viscosity and viscoelasticity of HWS depended on the method of stimulation where mechanical action stimulated slightly shear-thinning and relatively inelastic saliva, while acidic solutions (e.g. citric acid) stimulated saliva that was highly elastic and shear-thinning. For acid-stimulated saliva, the results showed a high ratio between the primary normal stress and the shear stress which, for such a low viscosity fluid, indicated that saliva's elastic properties dominated its flow behaviour and indicated its lubrication role within the oral cavity. The boundary lubrication properties of mechanically stimulated HWS was demonstrated by Bongaerts *et al.* (2007a), who measured the lubricating properties of saliva in a soft hydrophobic contact and investigated the impact of applied load, entrainment speed and surface roughness on lubrication. It was found that an increase in surface roughness decreased the lubricating properties of saliva while it was increased for water. They also showed that the boundary lubricating properties of HWS did not change with time, whereas the bulk viscoelastic properties degraded over time. This suggests that the large bulky glycoproteins responsible for the rheology of saliva are not responsible for its boundary lubricating properties, being too large to fit the gap.

Recently, interfacial shear rheology was used to probe the relationship between surface shear elasticity of saliva and loss of lubricity when compounds such as polyphenols are added, resulting in astringent mouthfeel (Rossetti *et al.*, 2008). The glycoproteins contained in saliva are highly surface active and tend to migrate to the air–liquid interface, forming a solid-like surface film that is responsible for the lubricating properties of saliva (in the mixed regime) during mastication. The addition of citric acid and polyphenols appears to disrupt this surface film reducing the interfacial shear elasticity G' of saliva and thereby reducing lubrication of oral tissues. Another explanation by the investigators was suggested in which the added food components cause the glycoproteins to aggregate and thereby reduce the interfacial shear elasticity. However, in general, aggregation of protein often results in an increase in G' and therefore what might be occurring is that the proteins in the saliva are being displaced by surface active components in the food which provide a new surface with different lubricating properties.

10.5.3 Tribology measurements of soft-solid food emulsions *ex vivo*

Tribological measurements have been used as a tool to predict the lubrication and sensory mouth feel of model biological fluids (Cassin *et al.*, 2001; de Vincente *et al.*, 2006a,b; Bongaerts *et al.*, 2007a) and model food emulsions (Dresselhuis *et al.*, 2008a,b). In general, the sensory perception of soft-solid food during mastication is dependent on its frictional behaviour as a thin film under high shear rates in the gap between the tongue and hard palate. Sensory attributes such as slipperiness, smoothness, fattiness, astringency and creaminess have been shown to correlate with the frictional behaviour of emulsions between oral surfaces (Malone *et al.*, 2003a; Lee *et al.*, 2004; De Hoog *et al.*, 2006) and certain rheological parameters such as viscoelasticity (Jellema *et al.*, 2005).

The lubricating behaviour of foods has commonly been analysed with standard tribological equipment such as the pin-on-disc or ball-on-disc set-up (de Vicente *et al.*, 2006a,b). However, the problem has been to select a suitable surface that will mimic the key characteristics of oral mucosa for generating relevant friction measurements *ex vivo*. Important characteristics of the oral surface, which are thought to influence the behaviour of lubricating substances, are the roughness of the surface, the deformability and the wetting characteristics (De Hoog *et al.*, 2006; Dresselhuis *et al.*, 2008a). It has been shown by De Hoog *et al.* (2006) that the load-dependent behaviour of the kinetic friction measured for food emulsions changed depending on the surfaces used when they compared hard glass–metal smooth surfaces with mucosal surfaces from pig tongue or oesophagus (Prinz *et al.*, 2007). They found that the friction decreased with increasing load for the mucosal surfaces, but was constant for glass-metal surfaces.

In the lubrication of oral surfaces, such as the tongue and palate, it has been suggested that the boundary and mixed regime dominate (Malone *et al.*, 2003a) and that the lubricating nature of saliva is most effective in the mixed and boundary regime (Bongaerts *et al.*, 2007b). While this can be demonstrated *ex vivo* on artificial mucosal surfaces, it has been questioned whether the boundary regime in the mouth can be obtained (Lundin, 2008) since the mastication process involves the tongue compressing food between surfaces rather than having food entrained into the soft contact zone as in the tribological experiments. In addition, it is important to note that in the oral cavity the surfaces are mostly soft and deformable, and the food fluids are often non-Newtonian (van Aken *et al.*, 2005) so that the shear viscosity is high at low shear rates, unlike water in which the shear viscosity remains low for most shear rates relevant to oral processing of soft food and therefore does not act as a good lubricant.

Typically, the oral regime is characterised by a mean contact pressure and a low traction speed during eating (Chojnicka *et al.*, 2008). The contact pressure in the mouth is estimated to be approximately 30 kPa and the shear rate applied in the mouth during mastication varies between 1 and 1000 s^{-1} (Sharma and Sherman, 1973). Recent studies on lubricating properties of emulsions (Dresselhuis *et al.*, 2008b) and protein aggregates (Chojnicka *et al.*, 2008) have tried to mimic more closely the relevant oral conditions in which lubrication due to the oral processing of soft-solid foods occurs and have tried to take into account the changes that occur to saliva during eating (Bongaerts *et al.*, 2007b), and the amount and properties of the adhered food. The surface roughness changes as a result of abrasion during eating and the traction speed that is relevant for the oral regime (Malone *et al.*, 2003a; Lee *et al.*, 2004). Eating itself also induces changes both in the structure of the food (Malone *et al.*, 2003b; de Wijk and Prinz, 2005) and on the oral tissue that can have an effect on the lubrication properties sensed.

10.5.4 Evanescence wave spectroscopy

Evenescent wave technology has been used to investigate specific and non-specific adsorption of biomolecules to surfaces without the need for labelling (Jonsson *et al.*, 1991; Knoll, 1991). Optical biosensors based on this technology allow *in situ* observations of real-time kinetics of the processes of molecular physi- or chemisorption. Information gained from this measurement includes association equilibrium constants, the timescales of the deposition processes and the adsorbed amount per unit surface, so that binding isotherms of biomolecules to specific surfaces can be obtained. Cassin *et al.* (2001) investigated the adsorption properties of polymers onto biomimics of oral mucosa using evanescent wave spectroscopy (EWS) and showed that the polymer that adsorbed onto solid surfaces was able to reduce friction in the boundary lubrication regime from tribology measurements. Biopolymers such as guar, which does not adsorb on surfaces, showed high friction in boundary lubrication but still promoted the onset of mixed lubrication; thus friction started to fall from its boundary values at low speeds.

Further studies by Appelqvist *et al.* (2004) using EWS demonstrated that the residence time of food coatings could be controlled by the level of binding to the oral mucosa, which was dependent on the overall charge of the surface of the food component. Emulsions were designed with a stabiliser that interacted with the oral mucosa to enhance surface deposition and increase the residence time of the oil droplets. The interfacial interactions between various emulsions and a mucin-covered solid substrate were investigated using EWS, and the influence of different emulsifiers on the extent of oil deposition onto oral mucosa was evaluated (see Fig. 10.5). The data showed that the chitosan emulsion adsorbed to the greatest extent onto the mucin film surface due to electrostatic interaction between the positively charged emulsifier and the negatively charged mucin film. The egg yolk stabilised emulsion which was slightly positively charged adsorbed to the mucin surface to a lesser extent and tween 60, which is non-ionic, did not interact with the mucin film. Increased binding increased the residence time for food films and impacted on the sensory properties perceived. Specifically, it was shown that emulsions that remained longer in the mouth increased the after-taste and flavour release after swallowing, which was measured directly in the headspace of the nasal cavity of subjects using atmospheric pressure chemical ionisation mass spectroscopy (APCI-MS).

10.6 Artificial mouth models

A review of the literature reveals that a wide range of artificial mouths have been developed to mimic some aspect of oral processes during eating (van Ruth *et al.*, 2000; Salles *et al.*, 2007) and to measure the flavour released from food components as a function of mastication and food breakdown (Roberts and Acree, 1995; van Ruth and Roozen, 2000; Rabe *et al.*, 2002).

It is clear that, while these artificial mouths have had some success in replicating specific areas of oral processing, there are no systems as yet available

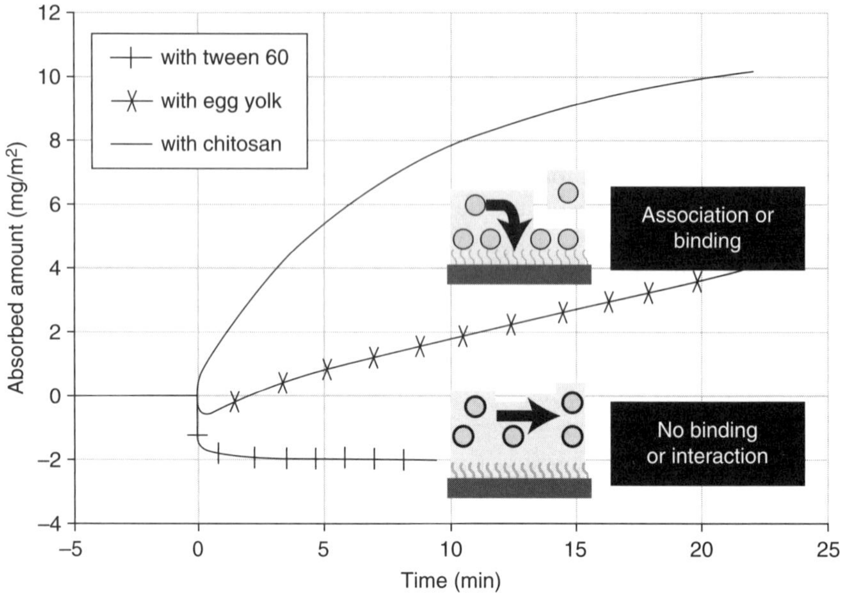

Fig. 10.5 Deposition of oil droplets in emulsions on mucous glycoprotein surface stabilised with different emulsifiers that adsorb to a mucin-covered surface to different degrees. Chitosan is the most positively charged emulsifier and is electrostatically attracted to the negatively charged mucin film. The proteins in the egg yolk are slightly positively charged and interact with the mucin surface to some degree, while the tween 60, owing to its non-ionic nature, did not show any adsorption onto the mucin covered surface. Measurements carried out at 35 °C. (Adapted and modified from Appelqvist *et al.*, 2004.)

that can mimic the complex nature of the real mouth and therefore there will still be reliance on methodologies such as time intensity, descriptive analysis and discrimination tests in which key attributes can be extracted from real-time sensory data based on real consumption of food by subjects. The quantification of sensory perception is, however, difficult since oral processing of food is strongly coupled to changes in food texture and taste via a feedback mechanism. Sensory perception is also dependent on a hedonic aspect, which relates to cultural background and experience and the interpretation and integration of information from receptors via complex neural pathways in the brain provide a challenging investigation.

The focus in this section will be on the artificial mouth designs that are commonly used by a number of researchers and have had some validation in their simulation of real mouth conditions and processes. The most commonly used artificial mouth is that developed by van Ruth and Roozen (2000). This is based on a plunger that is hemispherical, which crushes food against the bottom of a glass test tube and is mostly suitable for soft-solid food. The device allows for the introduction of saliva and the breakdown of soft foods at mouth temperature and head space sampling of aroma compounds. Results of aroma release from a range of foods (Hansson *et al.*, 2003; Mayr *et al.*, 2003) using this device appear to be similar to those measured *in vivo* monitored by proton-transfer-reaction mass spectroscopy. Roberts and Acree (1995) developed an artificial mouth based on a blender, which incorporated a purge and trap and allowed the addition of saliva and temperature control at 37 °C. The blender speed was controlled to reproduce shear rates reported to occur during eating. The retronasal aroma simulator is a flavour analysis method that more closely simulates mouth conditions than existing headspace methods. The feature of the device (saliva addition, temperature regulation and shearing) allowed foods in different formats to be analysed and indicated different headspaces from dynamic headspace trapping.

Prinz *et al.* (2007) used an apparatus that simulated oral mixing that consisted of an electric motor that rotated the sample (semi-solid food). Also attached, which remained fixed, were a mixing vane, video camera, laser, optical sensor and temperature probe. This system was developed to measure changes in the viscosity of food due to physiological changes that are relevant in the mouth such as temperature, shear, dilution and structure breakdown. Samples recovered from the *in vivo* mouth were compared with those from the mouth simulator using an image processing technique which demonstrated that the simulator could mimic oral processing of soft-solids in real time. Finally, the most sophisticated artificial mouth is the one based on a design by Salles *et al.* (2007) in which they developed a chewing simulator that faithfully reproduces most of the functions of the human mouth. The active part of the system is a special cell that is fully actuated and computer controlled and can accurately reproduce shear and compression strengths and tongue function in real time. *In vivo* measures using the breakdown of peanuts in the mouth was compared with the results produced from the chewing simulator and found to be super-imposable.

10.7 Conclusions

Clearly, the structural changes in food that occur in the mouth and how they interact with the sensory receptors are important for delivering sensory perception. However, the challenge will be to both gain a deeper understanding of the various mouth processing mechanisms and to integrate this knowledge with the neural bases on which the multimodel aspect of food perception is delivered. The development of techniques that can probe and quantify in-mouth structuring and breakdown of food materials in either a realistic biological mouth environment *ex vivo*, or measure non-invasively food–mouth interaction *in vivo*, will lead to establishing engineering rules that can be used to design food. The starting point for the design of structured foods is an understanding of the science underpinning the various performance functions, which is driven by the food microstructure. The response of structural changes in food to oral processing is also very dependent on the mouth conditions, such as the composition of the saliva and the mouth movements which are different for individuals, so that, within the context of food design models, these variations will need to be considered. Finally it will be the integration between our understanding of oral processing and neuroscience that will progress our understanding of how food is perceived, since interaction within and among the multisensory modalities are common and are highly relevant to food perception.

10.8 Future trends

For the future, direct quantitative and non-invasive measurement of oral tissues and the breakdown of food in real time will be possible. A framework of techniques used in an integrated manner to elucidate the mechanisms of food–oral tissue interactions and mechanical breakdown under a physiological environment will be possible, which will allow complete analysis of food behaviour and the ability of food technologists to design food more effectively with the desired performance and consumer benefits.

Already hand-held I-scan pressure mapping systems are available (from Tekscan) that use a laminated plastic film with up to 2288 pressure sensing areas. The sensor is very thin and flexible and can be designed to different shapes including the shape of the oral soft surfaces or the teeth. The technique will generate 2D and 3D pressure maps and can record as a movie up to 100 frames per second. This potentially can capture the changes in pressure induced as food is processed in the mouth, giving the investigator a real-time sequence of pressures produced during eating, and can identify the pressures required for solid food to fracture and components such as encapsulated actives to be broken, releasing their contents in the mouth.

Innovative techniques such as capsule endoscopy, which involves a tiny imaging camera (Hartmann *et al.*, 2004) have opened up new horizons for early diagnosis of disease but the potential for such technology to measure and visualise in real time the inter-oral and digestive processes in humans is possible. The SmartPill (SmartPill GI monitoring system, Anon. 2008) is a wireless capsule which measures pressure, pH and temperature as it transits the GI tract and has already been tested in clinical trials to determine the effect of food structure and composition on gastric emptying and ileal/caecal transit time. This technique also has potential for monitoring the physiological changes that occur in oral processing of food.

10.9 Sources of further information and advice

The review article by van Aken *et al.* (2007) on 'Food colloids under oral conditions' gives a very comprehensive overview of the structural and rheological changes of food during eating that are important in sensory perception. The review covers key aspects of the oral cavity, the physiology of saliva and, the interaction of food with the oral surfaces and salivary components, and introduces the reader to modern techniques for measuring oral processing. It discusses a selection of oral processing mechanisms relevant for soft solids, with an emphasis on oil-in-water emulsions.

Understanding and Controlling the Microstructure of Complex Foods published by Woodhead Publishing in 2007 (McClements, 2007) provides a review of the current understanding of significant aspects of food structure and methods for its control. It focuses on the fundamental structural elements present in foods such as proteins and fats and the forces that hold them together. The book discusses novel analytical techniques that provide information on the morphology and behaviour of food materials and examines how the principles of structural design can be employed to improve the performance and functionality of foods.

10.10 References

ABLETT S, CARPENTER T A, HALL L D, HODGSON R J and SLATER D C (1988), 'MRI microscopy of human skin'. In: *Society of Magnetic Resonance in Medicine Book of Abstracts*, San Francisco, CA, 3, 1063.

ADAMS S, SINGLETON S, JUSKAITIS, R and WILSON, T (2007), '*In-vivo* visualisation of mouth–material interactions by video rate endoscopy', *Food Hydrocolloids*, **21**, 986–995.

ALONSO B C, MARCIANI L, HEAD K, CLARK P, SPILLER R C, RAYMENT P, ABLETT S, FRANCIS S and GOWLAND P A (2007), 'Functional magnetic resonance imaging assessment of the cortical representation of oral viscosity', *J. Texture Studies*, **38**, 725–737.

ANON. (2008), 'Tekscan I-scan pressure-mapping systems now have Hi speed USB sensor connectivity', *Sensor Rev.*, **28** (1), 78–79.

APPELQVIST I A M (2005), 'I am what I eat' – The biomechanics of eating', Research Prize brochure, Unilever, The Netherlands

APPELQVIST I A M, BROWN C R T, GOFF T C, LANE S J and NORTON I T (1995), 'Application of hydrocolloids in frozen sauces', in 8th Conference on Gums and Stabilisers for the Food Industry, E Wales Inst Wrexham Wales, *Gums and Stabilisers for the Food Industry*, **8**, 99–114.

APPELQVIST I A M, MALONE M E, GOFF T C, HEINRICH E and NANDI A (2004), 'Controlled deposition and release of flavour to control aftertaste in-mouth': 12th Conference on Gums and Stabilisers for the Food Industry, Date: Jun 23–27, 2003 N E Wales Inst Wrexham Wales, *Gums and Stabilizers for the Food Industry*, **12**, 294, 43–53.

BASHIR E, GUSTAVSSON A and LAGERLOF F (1995), 'Site specificity of citric acid retention after an oral rinse', *Caries Res.*, **29**, 467–469.

BONGAERTS J H H, FOURTOUNI K and STOKES J R (2007a), 'Soft-tribology: lubrication in a compliant PDMS-PDMS contact', *Tribology International*, **40**, 10–12, 1531–1542.

BONGAERTS J H H, ROSETTI D and STOKES J R (2007b), 'The lubricating properties of whole saliva', *Tribol. Lett.*, **27**, 277–287.

BRINK J, LANGTON M, STADING M and HERMANSSON A-M (2007), 'Simultaneous analysis of the structural and mechanical changes during large deformation of whey protein isolate/gelatin gels at the macro and micro levels,' *Food Hydrocoll.*, **21**, 409–419.

BUETTNER A, BEER A, HANNIG C and SETTLES M (2001), 'Observation of the swallowing process by application of videofluoroscopy and real-time magnetic resonance imaging – consequences for retronasal aroma stimulation', *Chem. Senses*, **26**, 1211–1219.

BUTT H J, GRAFF K and KAPPL M (2003), *Physics and Chemistry of Interfaces*, Weinheim, Wiley VCH, 225.

CASA M J, KENNY D J and MACMILLAN R E (2003), 'Buccal and lingual activity during mastication and swallowing in typical adults', *J. oral Rehabil.*, **30**, 9–16.

CASSIN G, HEINRICH E and SPIKES H A (2001), 'The influence of surface roughness on the lubrication properties of adsorbing and non-adsorbing biopolymers', *Tribol. Lett.*, **11** (2) 95–102.

CHOJNICKA A, DE JONG S, DE KRUIF C G and VISSCHERS R W (2008), 'Lubrication properties of protein aggregate dispersions in a soft contact', *J. Agric. Food Chem.*, **56**, 1274–1282.

DE ARAUJO I E and ROLLS E T (2004), 'Representation in the human brain of food texture and oral fat', *J. Neurosci.*, **24** (12), 3086–3093.

DE ARAUJO I E, KRINGLEBACH M L, ROLLS E T and HOBDEN P (2003a), 'Representation of umami taste in the human brain', *J. Neurophysiol.*, **90**, 313–319.

DE ARAUJO I E, KRINGLEBACH M L, ROLLS E T and MCGLONE F (2003b), 'Human cortical responses to water in the mouth, and the effects of thirst', *J. Neurophysiol.*, **90**, 1865–1876.

DE HOOG E H A, PRINZ J F, HUNTJENS L, DRESSELHUIS D M and VAN AKEN G A (2006), 'Lubrication of oral surfaces by food emulsions: the importance of surface characteristics', *J. Food Sci.*, **71** (7), 337–341.

DE VICENTE J, STOKES J R and SPIKES H A (2006a), 'Soft lubrication of model hydrocolloids', *Food Hydrocolloids*, **20**, 483–491.

DE VICENTE J, SPIKES H A and STOKES J R (2006b), 'Viscosity ratio effect in the emulsion lubrication of soft EHL contact', *J Tribol.-T Asme*, **128** (4), 795–800.

DE WIJK R A and PRINZ J F (2005), 'The role of friction in perceived oral texture', *Food Quality Prefer.*, **16** (2), 121–129.

DE WIJK R A and PRINZ J F (2006), 'Mechanisms underlying the role of friction in oral texture', *J. texture studies*, **37**, 413–427.

DE WIJK R A, ENGELEN L and PRINZ J F (2003), 'The role of intra-oral manipulation in the perception of sensory attributes', *Appetite*, 40, 1–7.

DE WIJK R A, PRINZ J F and ENGELEN L (2004), 'The role of alpha amylase in the perception of oral texture and flavour in custards', *Physiol. Behaviour*, **83**, 81–91.

DE WIJK R A, PRINZ J F and JANSSEN A M (2006a), 'Explaining perceived oral texture of starch-based custard desserts from standard and novel instrumental tests', *Food Hydrocolloids*, **20**, 24–34.

DE WIJK R A, WULFERT F and PRINZ J F (2006b), 'Oral processing assessed by M-mode ultrasound imaging varies with food attribute', *Physiol. Behaviour*, **89**, 15–21.

DRESSELHUIS, D M, STUART, M A C, VAN AKEN, GA, SCHIPPER R G and DE HOOG E H A (2008a), 'Fat retention at the tongue and the role of saliva: Adhesion and spreading of 'protein-poor' versus 'protein-rich' emulsions,' *J. Colloid Interface Sci.*, **321** (1), 21–29.

DRESSELHUIS DM, DE HOOG EHA, STUART MAC, VINGERHOEDS M H and VAN AKEN G A (2008b), 'The occurrence of in-mouth coalescence of emulsion droplets in relation to perception of fat', *Food Hydrocolloids*, **22** (6), 1170–1183.

EGNER A and HELL S W (2005), 'Fluorescence microscopy wiyth super-resolved optical sections', *Trends Cell Biol.*, **15** (4), 207–215.

EGNER A, VERRIER S, GOROSHKOV A, SOLING H-D and HELL S W (2004), '4Pi-microscopy of the Golgi apparatus in live mammalian cells', *J. Structure Biol.*, **147**, 70–76.

ENGELEN L, DE WIJK R A, PRINZ J F, JANSSEN A M, VAN DER BILT A and BOSMAN F (2003a), 'A comparison of the effects of added saliva, alpha amylase and water on texture perception in semisolids', *Physiol. Behaviour*, **78**, 805–811.

ENGELEN L, DE WIJK R A, PRINZ J F, VAN DER BILT A, and BOSMAN F (2003b), 'The relationship between saliva flow after different stimulations and the perception of flavour and texture attributes in custard desserts', *Physiol. Behaviour*, **78**, 165–169.

FILLERY-TRAVIS A, MARCIANI L, GOWLAND P A and SPILLER R C (2002), 'The role of polysaccharides in the gastric processing of foods', in Williams P A and Phillips G O, *Gums and Stabilisers for the Food Industry 11*, Cambridge, N E Wales Inst Wrexham Wales, **11**, 342–348.

FRANCIS S, ROLLS E T, BOTWELL R, MCGLONE F, O'DOHERTY J, BROWNING A, CLARE S and SMITH E (1999), 'The representation of pleasant touch in the brain and its relationship with taste and olfactory areas', *Neuroreport*, **10**, 453–459.

GEORGE M, COUPEAU C, COLIN J and GRILLHÉ J (2003), 'Atomic force microscopy observations of successive damaging mechanisms of thin films on substrates under tensile stress', *Thin Solid Films*, **429**, 267–272.

GEORGES J M, MILLOT S, LOUBET J L and TONCK J (1993), 'Drainage of thin liquid films between relatively smooth surfaces', *J Chem. Phys*, **98** (9), 7345–7360.

GONZALEZ R, MONTOYA I and CARCEL J (2001), ' The use of electromyography on food texture assessment', *Food Sci. Technol. Int.*, **7** (6), 461–471.

GOULET D and BRUDEVOLD F (1986), 'The effects of viscosity on oral clearance of glucose', *J. Dental Res.*, **65**, 283.

GREEN J R and WANG Y T (2003), 'Tongue-surface movement patterns during speech and swallowing', *J. Acoust. Soc. Am.*, **113**, 20–33.

HANNIG C (1995), *Radiologische Funktionsdiagnostik des Pharynx und Oesophagus*, Springer-Verlag, Berlin.

HANSSON A, GIANNOULI P and VAN RUTH S (2003), 'The influence of gel strength on aroma release from pectin gels in a model mouth and *in vivo*, monitored with proton transfer reaction mass spectroscopy', *J. Agric. Food Chem.*, **51**, 4732–4740.

HARTMANN D, SCHILLING D, BOLZ G and RIEMANN J F (2004), 'Capsule endoscopy, technical impact, benefits and limitations', *Langenbecks Arch Surg.*, **389**, 225–233.

HASHIMOTO K and SHINODA K (1999), 'Development of X-ray TV M-mode and reconstructed ultrasound M-mode methods for investigating tongue movement during swallowing in humans', *J. Oral Sci.*, **41** (1), 1–4.

HIIEMAE K M and PALMER J B (2003), 'Tongue movements in feeding and speech', *Crit. Rev. Oral Biol. Med.*, **14**, 413–429.

HIIEMAE K M, PALMER J B, MEDICIS S W, HEGENER J JACKSON B S and LIEBERMAN D E (2002), 'Hyoid and tongue surface movements in speaking and eating', *Arch. Oral Biol.*, **47**, 11–27.

HOAD C L, RAYMENT P, SPILLER R C, MARCIANI L, ALONSO B D, TRAYNOR C, MELA D J, PETERS H P F and GOWLAND P A (2004) '*In vivo* imaging of intra-gastric gelation and its effect on satiety in humans', *J. Nutr.*, **134** (9), 2293–2300.

HOAD C L, COX E F, RAYMENT P, SPILLER R C, WRIGHT P J, BUTLER M, MARCIANI L and GOWLAND P A (2006) 'Gastric emptying, transit times and visualisation of alginate beads in the gastrointestinal tract', 14th Scientific Meeting and Exhibition of the International Society for Magnetic Research in Medicine, Seattle, 8–12 May 2006.

HOAD C L, MARCIANI L, FOLEY S, TOTMAN J J, WRIGHT J, BUSH D, COX E F, CAMPBELL E, SPILLER R C and GOWLAND P A (2007), 'Non-invasive quantification of small bowel water content by MRI: a validation study', *Phys. Med. Biol.*, **52** (23), 6909–6922.

HUTCHINGS J B and LILLFORD P J (1988), 'The perception of food textures – the philosophy of the breakdown path', *J. Texture Studies*, **19** (2), 103–115.

JANSSEN A M, TERPSTRA M E J, DE WIJK R A and PRINZ J F (2007), 'Relations between rheological properties, saliva induced structure breakdown and sensory texture attributes of custard', *J. Texture Studies*, **38** (1), 42–69.

JELLEMA R H, JANSSEN A M, TERPSTRA M E J, DE WIJK R A and SMILDE A K (2005), 'Relating the sensory sensation "creamy mouthfeel" in custards to rheological measurements', *J. Chemometrics*, **19**, 191–200.

JONSSON U, FAGERSTAM L, IVARSSON B and MALMQVIST M, (1991), 'Real-time biospecific interaction analysis using surface-plasmon resonance and a sensor chip technology', *Biotechniques*, **11**, 620–626.

KNOLL W (1991), 'Polymer thin-films and interfaces characterised with evanescent light', *Makromolekulare Chemie – Macromolecular Chem. Phys.*, **192** (12), 2827–2856.

LEE S, HEUBERGER M, ROUSSET P and SPENCER N D (2004), 'A tribological model for chocolate in the mouth: general implications for slurry-lubricated hard/soft sliding counterfaces', *Tribol. Lett.*, **16** (3), 239–249.

LENZ M, GREESS H, BAUM U, DOBRITZ M and KERSTING-SOMMERHOFF B (2000), 'Oropharynx, oral cavity, floor of the mouth: CT and MRI', *European J. Radiol.*, **33**, 203–215.

LILLFORD P J (2001), 'Mechanisms of fractures in foods', *J. Texture Studies*, **32**, 397–417.

LILLFORD P J (2000), 'The materials science of eating and food breakdown', *MRS Bull.*, 38–43.

LODEN M (1992), 'The increase in skin hydration after application of emollients with different amounts of lipids', *Acta Derm. Venereol.*, **72**, 327–330.

LOREN N, LANGTON M and HERMANSSON A-M (2007), 'Confocal fluorescence microscopy (CLSM) for food structure characterisation: in *Understanding and Controlling the Microstructure in Complex Foods* edited by D J McClements, Woodhead Publishing Limited, Cambridge, UK, 232–260.

LUCAS P W, PRINZ J F, AGRAWAL K R and BRUCE I C (2002), 'Food physics and oral physiology', *Food Quality Pref.*, **13**, 203–213.

LUNDIN L (2008), Personnel communication, CSIRO.

MALONE M E, APPELQVIST I A M and NORTON I T (2003a), 'Oral behaviour of food hydrocolloids and emulsions. Part 1, Lubrication and deposition considerations', *Food Hydrocolloids*, **17** (6), 763–773.

MALONE M E, APPELQVIST I A M and NORTON I T (2003b), 'Oral behaviour of food hydrocolloids and emulsions. Part 2. Taste and Aroma release', *Food Hydrocolloids*, **17** (6), 775–784.

MARCIANI L, GOWLAND P A, FILLERY-TRAVIS A, MANOJ P, WRIGHT J, SMITH A, YOUNG P, MOORE R and SPILLER R C (2001a), 'Assessment of antral grinding of model solid meals with echo-planar imaging', *Am. J. Physiol. Gastrointest. Liver Physiol.*, **280** (5), 844–849.

MARCIANI L, GOWLAND P A, SPILLER R C, MANOJ P, MOORE R J, YOUNG P and FILLERY-TRAVIS A J (2001b), 'Effect of meal viscosity and nutrients on satiety, intragastric dilution, and emptying assessed by MRI', *Am. J. Physiol. Gastrointest. Liver Physiol.*, **280** (6), 1227–1233.

MARCIANI L, PFEIFFER J, HORT J, HEAD K, BUSH D, TAYLOR A J, SPILLER R C, FRANCIS S and GOWLAND P A (2006a), 'Improved methods for fMRI studies of combined taste and aroma stimuli', *J. Neurosci. Methods*, **158**, 186–194.

MARCIANI L, WICKHAM M S J, BUSH D, FAULKS R, WRIGHT J, FILLERY-TRAVIS A J, SPILLER R C and GOWLAND P A (2006b), 'Magnetic resonance imaging of the behaviour of oil-in-water emulsions in the gastric lumen of man,' *Bri. J. Nutr.*, **95** (2), 331–339.

MAYR D, VAN RUTH S and MARK T D (2003), 'Evaluation of the influence of mastication on temporal aroma release of ripe and unripe bananas, using a model mouth system and gas chromatography-olfactometry', *Eur. Food Res. Technol.*, **217**, 291–295.

MCCLEMENTS J D (2007), *Understanding and Controlling the Microstructure of Complex Foods,* Woodhead Publishing Limited, Cambridge, UK.
MIOCHE L and MARTIN J F (1998), 'Training and sensory judgement effects on mastication as studied by electromyography', *J. Food Sci.*, **63** (2), 1.
MIRRASHED F and SHARP J C (2004), '*In vivo* morphological characterisation of skin by MRI micro-imaging methods', *Skin Res. Technol.*, **10**, 149–160.
MIYAMOTO J J, HONDA M, SAITO D N, OKADA T, ONO T, OHYAMA K and SADATO N (2006), 'The representation of the human oral area in the somatosensory cortex: a functional MRI study', *Cereb. Cortex*, **16** (5), 669–675.
NG S H, YEN T C, LIAO C T, CHANG J T T, CHAN S C, KO S F , WANG H M and WONG H F (2005), 'F-FDG PET and CT/MRI in oral cavity squamous cell carcinoma: a prospective study of 124 patients with histologic correlation', *J. Nuclear Med.*, **44** (7), 1136–1143.
O'DOHERTY J, ROLLS E T, FRANCIS S, BOTWELL R and MCGLONE F (2001), 'Representation of pleasant and aversive taste in the human brain', *J. Neurophysiol.,* **85**, 1315–1321.
ÖHGREN C, LANGTON M and HERMANSSON A M (2004), 'Structure–fracture measurements of particulate gels', *J. Mater. Sci.*, **39**, 6473–6482.
OISETH S L and LUNDIN L (2008) Personal communication and unpublished data, CSIRO.
OLMOS D, AZNAR J, BENITO-GONZÁLEZ J and BASELGA J (2002), 'A fluorescence method to estimate the distribution of stresses in polymer materials', *J. Mater. Proc. Technol.*, **143–144**, 495–500.
PERLMAN A L (2006), 'Electromyography in oral and pharyngeal motor disorders; Part 1 Oral cavity, pharynx and esophagus, *GI Motilit*, **10**, 1038.
PLUCKNETT K P and NORMAND V (2000), 'Plane stress essential work of fracture of 'pseudo-ductile' gelatin/maltodextrin biopolymer gel composites', *Polymer*, **41**, 6833–6841.
PLUCKNETT K P, POMFRET S J, NORMAND V, FERDINANDO D, VEERMAN C and FRITH W J (2001), 'Dynamic experimentation on the confocal laser scanning microscope: Application to soft-solid, composite food materials', *J. Microscopy*, **201**, 279–290.
PRINZ J F, DE WIJK R A and HUNTJENS L (2007), 'Load dependency of the coefficient of friction of oral mucosa', *Food Hydrocolloids*, **21** (3), 402–408.
RABE S, KRINGS U, BANAVARA D S and BERGER R G (2002), 'Computerised apparatus for measuring dynamics flavour release from liquid food matrices', *J. Agric. Food Chem.*, **50**, 6440–6447.
RIZZIERI R, BAKER F S and DONALD A (2003), 'A study of the large strain deformation and failure behaviour of mixed biopolymer gels via *in situ* ESEM', *Polymer*, **44**, 5927–5935.
ROBERTS D D and ACREE T E (1995), 'Simulation of retronasal aroma using a modified head space technique: investigating the effects of saliva, temperature, shearing and oil on flavour release', *J. Agric. Food Chem.*, **43**, 2179–2186.
ROLLS E T (2005), 'Taste, olfactory, and food texture processing in the brain, and the control of food intake', *Physiol. Behav.*, **85** (1), 45–56.
ROSSETTI D, YAKUBOV G E, STOKES J R, *et al.* (2008), 'Interaction of human whole saliva and astringent dietary compounds investigated by interfacial shear rheology, *Food Hydrocolloids*, **22**, (6), 1068–1078.
RUMBOLDT Z , DAY T and MICHEL M (2003), 'Imaging of oral cavity cancer', *Oral Oncology*, 42 (9), 854–865.
SALA G, DE WIJK R A, VAN DE VELDE F and VAN AKEN G A (2008), 'Matrix properties affect the sensory perception of emulsion-filled gels', *Food Hydrocolloids*, **22**, 353–363.

SALLES C, TARREGA A, MIELLE P, MARATRAY J, GORRIA P, LIABOEUF J and LIODENOT J-J (2007), 'Development of a chewing simulator for food breakdown and the analysis of *in vitro* flavour compound release in a mouth environment', *J. Food Eng.*, **82**, 189–198.

SCHOENFELD M A, NEUER G, TEMPLEMANN C, SCHUBLER K, NOESSELT T, HOPF J M and HEINZE H J (2004), 'Functional magnetic resonance tomography correlates of taste perception in the human primary taste cortex', *J. Neuroscience*, **127**, 347–353.

SHARMA F and SHERMAN P (1973), 'Identification of stimuli controlling the sensory evaluation of viscosity. II Oral methods', *J. Textural Studies*, **4** (1), 111–118.

SILLETTI E, VINGERHOEDS M H, NORDE W and VAN AKEN G A (2007a), 'The role of electrostatics in saliva-induced emulsion flocculation', *Food Hydrocolloid*, **21** (4), 596–606.

SILLETTI E, VINGERHOEDS M H, NORDE W and VAN AKEN G A (2007b), 'Saliva-induced emulsion flocculation: the role of droplet charge': in edited by Dickinson E and M Leser; Royal Society of Chemistry, Cambridge, UK, *Food Colloids: Self Assembly and Material Science*, 463–472.

SILLETTI E, VINGERHOEDS M H, NORDE W and VAN AKEN G A (2007c), 'Complex formation in mixtures of lysozyme-stabilised emulsions and human saliva', *J Colloid Interfaces Sci.*, **313**, 485–493.

SPIKES H A (1996), 'Direct observation of boundary layers', *Langmuir*, **12** (19), 4567–4573.

SPRATT P, NICOLELLA C and PYLE D L (2005), 'An engineering model of the human colon', *Trans IChemE C*, **85**, 147–157.

STOKES J R and DAVIES G A (2007), 'Viscoelasticity of human whole saliva collected after acid and mechanical stimulation', *Biorheology*, **44** (3), 141–160.

STOLL B R, BATYCKY R P, LEIPOLD H R, MILSTEIN S and EDWARDS D A (2000), 'A theory of molecular absorption from the small intestine', *Chem. Eng. Sci.*, **55**, 473–489.

STONE M (2005), 'A guide to analysing tongue motion from ultrasound images', *Clin. Linguist Phon.*, **19**, 455–501.

SZCZESNIAK A S (1963), 'Objective measurements of food texture', *J. Food Sci.*, **28** (4), 410–420.

VAN AKEN G A (2007) 'Relating food microstructure to sensory quality': in *Understanding and Controlling the Microstructure of Complex Foods*, Woodhead Publishing, Cambridge, UK, 449–482.

VAN AKEN G A, VINGERHOEDS M H and DE HOOG E H A (2005), 'Colloidal behaviour of food emulsions under oral conditions': in *Food hydrocolloids, interactions, microstructure and processing*, The Royal Society of Chemistry, Cambridge, UK, 356–366.

VAN AKEN G A, VINGERHOEDS M H and HOOG E H A (2007) 'Food colloids under oral conditions', *Curr. Opin. Colloid Interface Sci.*, **12**, 251–262.

VAN DEN BERG L, VAN VLEIT T, VAN DER LINDEN E, VAN BOEKEL M A J S and NAN DE VELDE F (2007), 'Microstructure affects breakdown properties and sensory perception of whey proteins/polysaccharides mixed gels', *Food Hydrocolloids*, **21** (5), 961–976.

VAN RUTH S M and ROOZEN J P (2000), 'Influence of mastication and saliva on aroma release in a mouth model system', *Food Chem.*, **71**, 339–345.

VAN RUTH S M, O'CONNOR C H and DELAHUNTY C M (2000), 'Relationships between temporal release of aroma compounds in a model mouth system and their physico-chemical characteristics', *Food Chem.*, **71**, 393–399.

VERHAGEN J V and ENGELEN L (2006), 'The neurocognitive bases of human multimodal food perception: sensory integration', *Neurosci. Biobehavioural Rev.*, **30**, 613–650.

VEYRUNE J L and MIOCHE L (2000), 'Complete denture wearers: electromyography of mastication and texture perception whilst eating meat', *European J. Oral Sci.*, **108** (2), 83–92.

VEYRUNE J L, LASSAUZAY C, NICOLAS E, PEYRON M A and WODA A (2007), 'Mastication of model products in complete denture wearers, *Archives Oral Biol.* **52** (12), 1180–1185.

VINGERHOEDS M H, BLIJDENSTEIN T B J, ZOET F D and VAN AKEN G A (2005), 'Emulsion flocculation induced by saliva and mucin', *Food Hydrocolloids*, **19**, 915–922.

WATSON T F, NEIL M A A, JUSKAITIS R, COOK R J and WILSON T (2002), 'Video-rate confocal endoscopy', *J. Microscopy*, **207**, 37–42.

ZALD D H and PARDO J V (2000), 'Cortical activation induced by intraoral stimulation with water in humans', *Chem. Senses*, **25** (3), 267–275.

ZEMTSOV A (1993), 'P-31 magnetic-resonance spectroscopy to study noninvasively metabolism in cutaneous tissue', *Plastic Reconstructive Surgery*, **92** (7), 1411–1412.

ZERDIN K and KELLY M (2008), Personnel communication and unpublished data, CSIRO.

11

Measurement and simulation of flavour release from foods

A. J. Taylor, University of Nottingham, UK

Abstract: Unless foods taste good, humans will not consume them and any nutritional benefits will be lost. Understanding the mechanisms involved in human flavour perception has led to the development of analyses that measure flavour at different stages of the perception process. Release of flavour chemicals from food can be monitored using *in vivo* and *in vitro* systems and the effect of food structure on release can be assessed. The complexity of oral processing has hindered progress in modelling the release processes *in vivo* but *in vitro* experiments can be better controlled and the basic physicochemical principles established.

Key words: aroma, tastant, release, measurement, modelling, food structure, mechanism, *in vivo*.

11.1 Introduction

Flavour is a complex sensation which is associated both with the pleasurable aspects of food and the need to eat food to maintain nutritional status. The sensation of flavour determines our choice of foods and therefore determines our *intake* of nutrients. Whether the pleasure aspect is linked to nutritional needs or whether pleasure is a learned, but separate, component is still unclear (Blake, 2006). However, the perception of taste by higher levels of the brain occurs only under conditions of hunger (Rolls, 1997), further demonstrating the role of flavour in controlling food intake. Recent research has shown that the same flavour receptors may also play a role in the gut by regulating the *uptake* of some nutrients (Margolskee *et al.*, 2007). Because of the link between flavour and nutrient intake and uptake, it is of interest to understand the basis of flavour, and its perception in the body, so that we can deliver appropriate nutrition through healthy foods that are acceptable to consumers.

There is no doubt that human activities in the last hundred or so years have accelerated the pace of change and there is concern that evolution (to adapt to these changes) will not take place over these short timescales and that intervention is necessary to address the situation. Although this may seem new, it appears that changes in diet have had significant effects on humans in the past, albeit over longer timescales. Data from the fossil record show that the teeth, jaw muscles and salivary amylase characteristics of *Homo sapiens* changed significantly two million years ago as the diet changed to utilise cooked starchy foods (Lucas *et al.*, 2006). It is postulated that the ability to react to dietary changes is one of the characteristics that separates human behaviour from that of other species. Seen in this light, our current attempts to influence dietary intake may just be part of a long (several million years) journey to adapt to the situations that humans make for themselves through their actions.

Over the last five or so years, attempts by food manufacturers to meet nutritional targets, by reformulating foods with less fat, sugar and salt, have been limited by the significant flavour changes that arise. It is now well established that reformulation changes a range of flavour modalities such as taste, aroma, viscosity and mouthfeel and, unless these changes can be addressed to produce an acceptable flavour, the food product is unlikely to be consumed on a regular basis. Thus, although nutrition and flavour have been treated as two separate subjects in the past, it is becoming evident that integration of the disciplines is necessary to meet the needs of consumers in their quest for a healthy diet, especially in situations where food is plentiful.

11.2 Measuring flavour

The ultimate measurement of flavour is through human perception and sensory analytical techniques (Stone and Sidel, 2004). There are well-established protocols for measuring flavour perception in human subjects using statistically designed methods to take into account the natural variation within the population and to avoid the 'noise' in panels due to the difficulty of judging the presence of a flavour or assessing the intensity of a flavour sensation. The strength of sensory analysis is that it indicates the performance of a food product when consumed by people, but its weakness is the difficulty in determining which components of the food are responsible for specific flavour characteristics. To overcome this weakness, instrumental analysis of food flavour is an obvious, complementary step. However, to choose the appropriate instrumental analyses, it is essential to understand how humans perceive flavour.

It is now agreed that flavour creates a 'multi-modal construct' in the brain when food is consumed (Dalton *et al.*, 2000; Driver and Spence, 2000;

Calvert, 2001). In other words, flavour perception involves input from different senses (multi-modal inputs) and the inputs can interact during processing of signals in the brain, leading to the idea of 'cross-modality' (Small, 2004). The earlier notion that the flavour of complex foods could be represented by 'parallel' inputs from the senses has been replaced by the multi-modal and cross-modal concepts. Thus tastants like sugar and acid can affect the perception of a fruit aroma both in terms of intensity and in character (Pfeiffer *et al.*, 2006). Similarly, the viscosity of a food can affect the overall flavour perception (Hollowood *et al.*, 2000; Visschers *et al.*, 2006). For these reasons, instrumental flavour analyses need to measure the volatile aroma components of flavour, the non-volatile tastants and the physical properties of the food.

11.3 Methods to measure the flavour profile during eating and drinking

Choosing suitable measurement methods depends on the purpose of the analysis. To establish the flavour content of a food, classical extraction techniques are used and the extract is then subjected to separation and identification techniques using gas chromatography–mass spectroscopy (GC-MS) for the volatile components (Reineccius, 2006) and liquid chromatography-MS (LC-MS) for the non-volatile components. However, the flavour profile that is sensed by the aroma and taste receptors is often different from the total flavour composition and the profile changes with time. Methods to measure these profiles close to the receptors, and during the eating process, have been developed (Soeting and Heidema, 1988; Davidson *et al.*, 2000; Linforth and Taylor, 2003).

11.3.1 Aroma analyses

For aroma analyses, air is sampled close to the exit from the nose and the volatile components can be analysed in real time using various mass spectrometric techniques. All the techniques operate by ionising the aroma compounds and analysing them using mass detectors. Initial methods used electron impact ionisation (Soeting and Heidema, 1988), but this approach produced a complex spectrum in which it was difficult to assign ions to compounds. Given the common structures found in many aroma compounds, a single ion could be produced by several compounds and the task of deconvoluting the spectra in mixtures was the limiting factor. Alternative ionisation methods were developed to overcome these issues. Chemical ionisation methods initially generate a reagent ion such as H_3O^+ or NO^+ and these reagent ions then react with volatile aroma molecules (M) in the sample to give ions of the form $[M + H]^+$ or M^+. This 'soft' ionisation generates the protonated molecular ion or molecular ion with little fragmentation.

The commonly available soft ionisation techniques are atmospheric pressure chemical ionisation (APCI) (Linforth *et al.*, 1996; Linforth and Taylor, 2003), proton transfer reaction (PTR) (Lindinger *et al.*, 1998) and selected ion flow tube (SIFT) (Spanel and Smith, 1999; Freeman and McEwan, 2002). When coupled to a mass spectrometer (quadrupoles or time of flight), the combination of soft ionisation and ion monitoring leads to a read-out of ion intensity against time – the so-called 'real time' profile. Each technique has its advantages and disadvantages. APCI and PTR perform well for fast-moving changes such as the conditions found in breath by breath analysis; APCI is less sensitive to changes in moisture content, while SIFT and PTR offer the choice of different reagent ions to help assign compounds to ions by the different ionisation patterns. PTR can potentially provide better sensitivity over longer sampling times (periods of several minutes). The differences in sensitivity between the ionisation techniques are relatively small and are compound dependent, so the choice of ionisation depends on availability of equipment, the type of application and the nature of the compounds to be monitored. Typically, sensitivities are in the order of μL to nL of aroma per L of air (ppmv to ppbv) although, under certain special conditions, pL of aroma per L of air can be detected (pptv) (Lindinger *et al.*, 1998). It should be emphasised that all the techniques are best suited to monitoring of known compounds, which give unique ions so that there is no confusion over assignment of ions to compounds. Various approaches have been reported to overcome the assignment problem when unknowns are involved. These include the use of GC-MS (Taylor *et al.*, 2003; Lindinger *et al.*, 2005) or the use of stable isotope labelled precursors (Channell *et al.*, 2008).

Figure 11.1 shows a typical 'clean' mass spectrum obtained from the headspace (the air above the sample) of fresh banana at a single time point, using the soft ionisation from APCI. The ion peaks can be assigned to the known banana aroma compounds identified by conventional extraction and GC-MS.

Figure 11.2 shows the release of volatile compounds from fresh orange over a period of a few minutes. The mass analysers are operating at high frequencies so that detail of breath by breath aroma release can be seen. Acetone is often monitored as it is a by-product of the human liver and serves as a marker for exhalation and indicates the subject's breathing patterns. The initial trace (up to the 77 min mark) shows the absence of any ions in the limonene, ethyl butanoate and ethanol ion channels, indicating the subject is 'clean' and there is no carry-over from previous samples. The acetone peaks represent exhalations. The 'noise' on the breathing peaks is partly due to the chewing action of the subject (which pumps small volumes of air from the mouth to the nose) as well as the inconsistent mass transfer

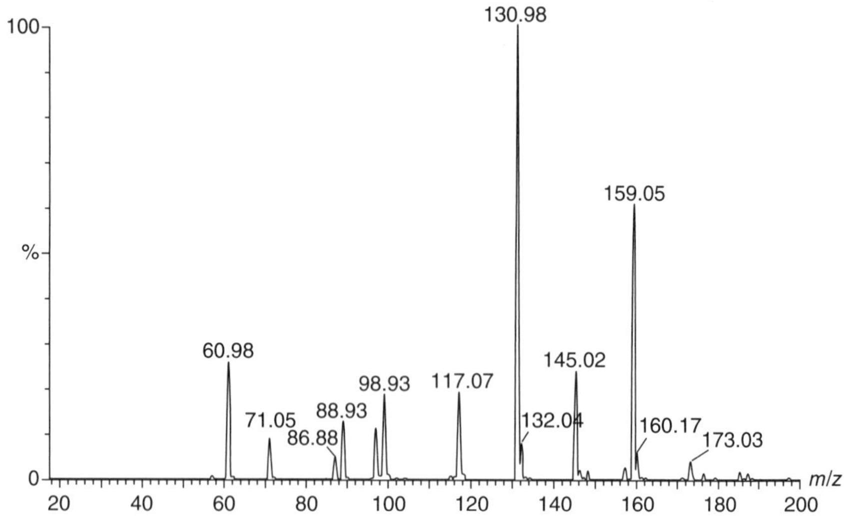

Fig. 11.1 APCI-MS headspace analysis of fresh banana. The ions can be assigned to known banana volatiles, e.g. *m/z* 117 and 131 are the protonated molecular ions of ethyl butyrate and isoamyl acetate, respectively.

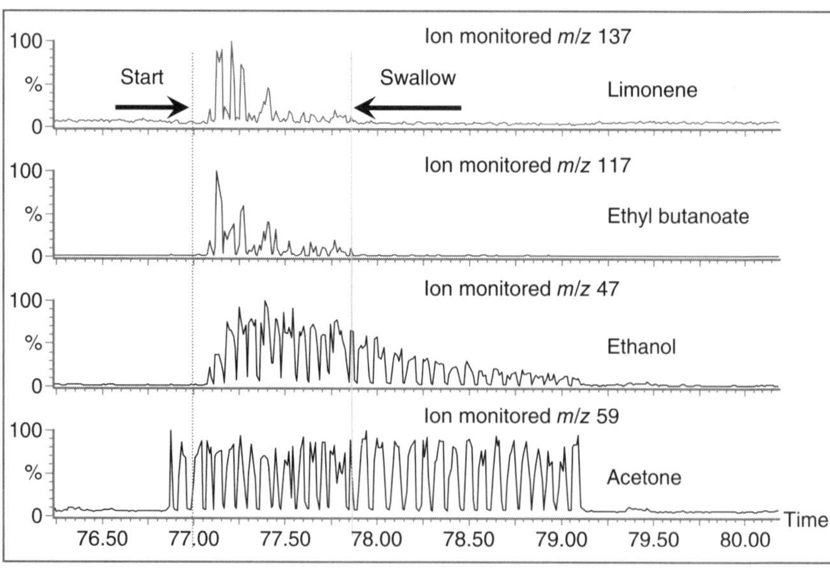

Fig. 11.2 APCI-MS traces obtained by monitoring exhaled air from the nose of a subject during eating of a segment of fresh orange.

of aroma from mouth to nose. The three compounds monitored are released when the orange is placed in the mouth (start) but the release profiles are different and are related to the physicochemical properties of the compounds. Some compounds persist in the exhaled breath even after the orange has been swallowed (swallow).

11.3.2 Tastant analyses

At first sight, analysing tastants in close proximity to the taste buds appears an easier task than analysing aromas in the nose. Access to the taste buds is certainly easier, but the difficulty is in sampling the phase that is in contact with the taste buds rather than sampling the masticated food which coats the tongue. In-mouth sensors have been developed and tested *in vivo* by mounting microelectrodes in dental plates and then monitoring the release of ionic compounds (Jack *et al.*, 1995). Release of salt from food has been achieved by measuring Na^+ concentrations in the mouth while acid release can be followed using a micro pH electrode (Davidson *et al.*, 1998). The advantage of the dental plate is the provision of real-time monitoring but the disadvantages of dental plates and electrodes are obvious: a unique dental plate has to be made for each subject, the electrodes can monitor only a limited range of the tastants found in food, the electrodes can break and cause a hazard to the subject, wires have to be led out of the mouth, which makes eating uncomfortable, and the plate location in the roof of the mouth does not represent the location of the taste buds on the tongue.

Alternatives have been developed based on 'off-line' sampling followed by LC-MS analysis. Typically, a cosmetic 'cotton bud' is pre-weighed and used to sample the saliva phase from the tongue of a subject eating the food sample at different time intervals. The cotton bud is re-weighed to calculate the saliva content and then extracted with methanol–water and an aliquot analysed by direct liquid phase MS (Davidson *et al.*, 2000). The sampling process is usually replicated to obtain a fuller range of time points and a time–release curve can be constructed from the samples to show both release and persistence of tastants in the mouth. A typical result showing the release of sodium, calcium and potassium ions during eating of cheese is shown in Fig. 11.3.

The trace is 'noisy' as it consists of points obtained from one person who consumed a portion of cheese on several occasions; the data were then aggregated from the different occasions. The technique works best with food samples that form a discrete bolus so that the saliva phase sampled represents the chemical signals reaching the taste buds. Chewing gum gives excellent results for sugar and sweeteners release but successful results have also been obtained from potato crisps (chips), gelled foods, biscuits (cookies), cheese, beer (hop acid release and persistence) and fruits such as oranges (acid and sugar release).

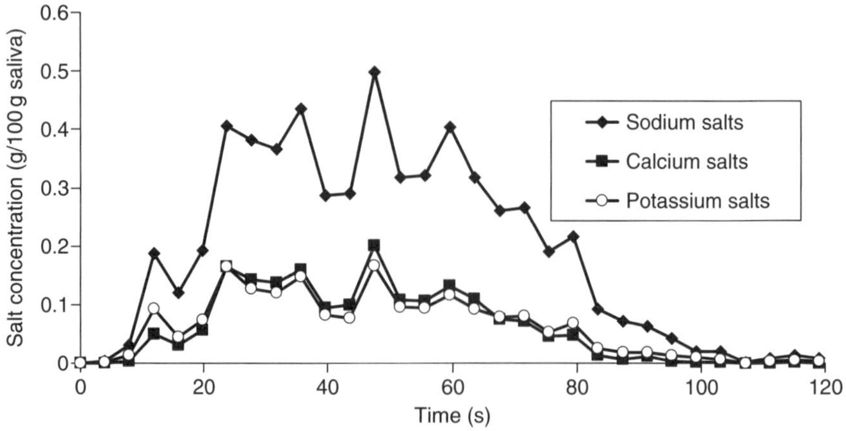

Fig. 11.3 Tastant release during eating of cheese. Swabs were taken from the tongue of a subject, extracted with water and the ion content measured off-line.

11.3.3 Viscosity and material properties measurements

There are well-established methods for measuring material properties of foods but, again, an appreciation of how they behave during eating is required to develop appropriate tests. Hutchings and Lillford described the approaches needed (Hutchings and Lillford, 1988; Lillford, 1991) and the example of cookie consumption highlights the many changes that occur during eating. Initially, cookie texture is perceived during the first bite which could be described by fracture mechanics. The cookie fragments then undergo size reduction as chewing proceeds, while simultaneously becoming hydrated which increases the adhesive properties and, with mechanical manipulation by the tongue and mouth, forms a bolus of hydrated cookie, ready for swallowing. A key question is which of these processes are important in the perception of biscuit texture and overall flavour acceptability. There is some preliminary evidence from our laboratory that a decrease in cookie crispness affects the overall flavour perception even though the aroma and tastant release is minimally affected. This suggests that fracture mechanics and the measurement of the sensory attribute, crispness, is one route to follow but the 'mouthfeel' aspects (due to hydration of the cookie matrix, the dissolution of sugar from the matrix and the melting of the fat component) should not be ignored. The difficulty in understanding complex systems such as cookies is the fact that the components interact significantly and attempts to formulate samples with, say, reduced sweetness inevitably result in changes to texture and hydration properties. It is therefore difficult to deconvolute the effect of one particular attribute from the overall effects.

Viscous foods represent simpler structured food systems and some progress has been made in understanding the links between their material properties and the effects on flavour perception (Cutler *et al.*, 1983). It is well established that, for the same tastant and aroma content, an increase in food viscosity will decrease flavour perception (Pangborn and Szczesniak, 1974; Baines and Morris, 1988; Guinard and Mazzucchelli, 1996). The observation was followed by various hypotheses, which have since been tested using the *in vivo* techniques described earlier in this section. A change in viscosity could affect flavour perception through three potential mechanisms:

1. Viscosity is a stimulus in its own right and it affects overall flavour perception through a cross-modal interaction with the tastant and aroma signals.
2. The viscosity of the solution decreases the release of aroma during eating and therefore the overall flavour intensity will be decreased.
3. The viscosity of the food delays tastant release to the taste buds and this decrease in tastant signal then causes a decrease in overall perceived flavour.

Option two is the easiest to address experimentally and several studies have shown that the maximum intensity of aroma release is not significantly affected by sample viscosity (Hollowood *et al.*, 2000, 2002; Cook *et al.*, 2002; Weel *et al.*, 2002). Buettner and Montserrat (2005) studied the release data from Weel's paper and proposed that slight differences in the initial rate of release might account for the perceptual differences but no evidence (for or against) has yet been produced to further this idea.

Option three, that viscosity affects tastant release, has been studied indirectly by comparing perceived flavour intensity with the ability of the hydrocolloid samples to mix with water. The hypothesis is based on the observation that some viscous starch solutions seem to have good flavour release properties compared with other hydrocolloids (Ferry *et al.*, 2006b) and this is related not to viscosity but to the ability of the hydrocolloid solution to mix with the saliva layer in mouth so that mass transfer of tastants from the solution to the taste buds occurs (Ferry *et al.*, 2006a).

Option 1, that viscosity is a stimulus in it own right and acts through a cross-modal pathway, has been partly addressed in experiments which attempted to produce emulsion samples which were iso-viscous, iso-sweet and which delivered the same aroma profile (iso-release) which were then assessed for their sensory flavour properties (Bayarri *et al.*, 2007). Despite the apparent similarities of the samples, a trained panel perceived differences in some samples. The results are difficult to interpret as the system contained different fat levels and viscosity was maintained by adding hydroxy propyl methyl cellulose (HPMC), which imparts a slight taste to the samples. This demonstrates the difficulty in designing suitable experiments to probe the origins of flavour as there are many interacting and confounding factors which are difficult to exclude. Although a full understanding has yet to be achieved, the author's opinion is that viscosity acts mainly through changing tastant release, although there may also be some subtle effects on mouthfeel in certain systems.

Since viscosity measurements depend on the shear conditions used, research has been carried out to estimate shear conditions in mouth. One obvious hypothesis is that the mechanoreceptors in our mouths can detect shear forces. There are currently two different but complementary ideas on the perception of shear in mouth. The first concept involves 'bulk' rheology and the perception of viscosity under conditions where in-mouth shear is around 50 s^{-1} (Shama and Sherman, 1973). This basic concept was adapted by Kokini who proposed that shear perception in the mouth was due to compression of the sample against the palate by the tongue and that the resulting 'oral shear stress' could be modelled and values extrapolated from conventional *in vitro* rheological measurements of the sample (Elejalde and Kokini, 1992). In some applications, the Kokini value seems to explain the effects of viscosity on flavour perception better than the 50 s^{-1} values (Cook *et al.*, 2003) but other workers using other hydrocolloid systems have found good agreement with the 50 s^{-1} values (Baines and Morris, 1989).

The second concept is that many parts of the mouth experience thin films of saliva mixed with viscous materials and that, under these conditions, the shear rate is many orders of magnitude higher (de Vicente *et al.*, 2006). This latter paper also introduces the idea that the mouth may sense lubricating properties as well as shear forces and so measurements of the tribological properties of foods in thin food/saliva films are another way of measuring the textural properties of foods.

Given the wide range of material properties found in foods, generalisations and extrapolations should be avoided. Each food needs to be considered on its own to identify the material properties that may impact on sensory perception of the food. It should be noted from the above discussions that even minor reformulation changes, e.g. the substitution of one hydrocolloid by another, can have significant effects on perceived flavour and therefore product developers need to be aware of these issues.

If the key attributes determining flavour can be identified and measured, then it should be possible to use these values as an instrumental benchmark of flavour and test any new formulations or variants of a product against this benchmark. There are no published reports from real foods but some laboratory-scale experiments have shown that the principles can be successfully employed. To illustrate the point, APCI-MS was used to measure aroma release from regular and low-fat milks in a group of 90 people (Shojaei *et al.*, 2006). The aroma content was then altered, based on the first trial, and the low- and regular fat milks re-presented to the panellists who were unable to distinguish them on the basis of flavour, despite the slightly lower viscosity of the low-fat samples. In this simple example, the aroma content of milk was the key flavour factor, as low- and regular fat milk have very similar colour, appearance, viscosity and tastant contents. Applying these concepts to real foods to produce reduced fat, salt and sugar analogues which 'taste' the same as the regular products will indicate the general directions needed to create the same 'taste' but still requires the input of flavourists to balance the flavour for those factors which cannot be measured.

11.4 Flavour release: mechanisms, effects of food structure and oral processing

To be sensed, flavour molecules need to be transported from the food to the receptors located in the mouth and nose. These processes are classically explained by mass transfer using well-known principles such as diffusion, partition and convection depending on the physical state of the food (Darling *et al.*, 1986; Overbosch *et al.*, 1991; Taylor, 1998; Boelrijk *et al.*, 2006; Linforth and Taylor, 2006; Voilley, 2006). To appreciate how flavours are released *in vivo*, a consideration of some basic physical chemistry is necessary. Figure 11.4 shows the classical *in vitro* system which describes mass transfer mechanisms between a liquid and a gas phase. It is hypothesised that the behaviour of compounds close to, or at, the interface between the two phases is different from that in the bulk phases. The thickness of the liquid boundary layers in an aqueous and in a viscous system were calculated at 3.8 and 28 μm, respectively (Taylor, 2002) from a release model proposed by de Roos and Wolswinkel (1994).

These basic mechanisms (and the associated length scales) assist in understanding the effects of oral processing and food structure on flavour release. Tastants and aromas will be rapidly lost from the surfaces of food whether in solution or in its intact state. Diffusion is a slow process and will

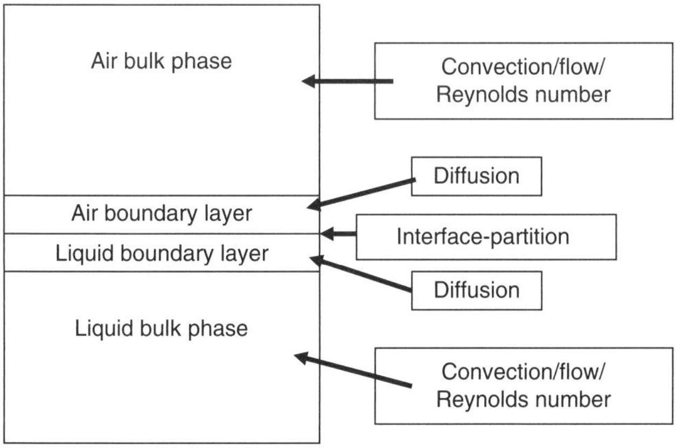

Fig. 11.4 Schematic representation of the food, water and interfacial phases, and the physicochemical processes, involved in mass transfer of aromas from food to air.

only transport these flavour compounds over distances of 1–10 μm (depending on the viscosity of the phase) in the time the food is in the mouth, prior to swallowing. Mechanisms such as surface generation/re-generation would seem to be important and will depend on mechanical agitation by the tongue, teeth and cheeks. However, in-mouth mass transfer is particularly difficult to model using basic physicochemical concepts as they are based on standard geometries such as spheres and plane surfaces, whereas the mouth geometry is not well defined. Although several models for flavour release have been proposed (see, for example, deRoos and Wolswinkel, 1994; Hills and Harrison, 1995; deRoos, 2000; Weel *et al.*, 2003; Normand *et al.*, 2004; Pionnier *et al.*, 2004), not all of the models have been tested against *in vivo* release measurements. The successful models usually contain a semi-empirical approach, e.g. deRoos and Wolswinkel (1994), as pure theory cannot yet describe adequately the complexity of mixing and mass transfer in mouth.

Emulsions represent a well-defined and common food structure, and flavour release has been studied in a range of emulsions using theoretical and experimental approaches. A series of papers was published by McNulty (McNulty and Karel, 1973a, b, c; McNulty, 1987) describing the theoretical effects of phase volume on the partitioning and ultimate release of volatile compounds from emulsions. These papers provide a good grounding in the physic-chemical aspects of flavour release in emulsions but interpretation of the information requires an appreciation of the methods used. There are three basic systems for measuring flavour release, two *in vitro* systems and the *in vivo* methods discussed previously. The simplest situation involves equilibrating the sample with air in a sealed system, which provides useful data on partition coefficients or the ratio of aroma compound in the air and liquid phases (Taylor, 1998). The other *in vitro* method used is dynamic headspace dilution, where the air above the sample is diluted with a stream of clean air, simulating the aroma profile above a food prior to consumption. This latter system delivers some dynamic information about aroma release but there is no dilution of the liquid phase (as happens in-mouth when saliva flows) and the sample size tends to represent the bulk phase situation rather than the thin layers found in the mouth. These limitations of *in vitro* systems will be addressed again in Section 11.5 when model mouth design is discussed.

Reviews of the effects of lipids and emulsions on flavour release have been published (Dumont, 2006; Ollivon, 2006). Generally, the presence of lipid causes a change in partition coefficient with the greatest effects observed for the most hydrophobic compounds. The result is that the aroma profile above an aqueous sample and a sample containing lipid shows little change in hydrophilic compounds but a decrease for the hydrophobic aroma compounds in the lipid sample. The profile of the aroma mixture is therefore 'skewed' and it is well known that flavours need to be reformulated for fat-containing products to overcome this effect and restore the flavour. Thus flavour companies produce many variants of common flavours such as strawberry, each variant designed to function optimally in a particular food matrix like milk shake, yoghurt or ice cream.

A long-standing question has been whether the composition of emulsions causes differences in flavour release. Reports in the literature on the effect of fat type, emulsifiers and fat content suggest some common findings (Shamil *et al.*, 1992; Plug and Haring, 1993; Hort and Cook, 2007). Flavour release seems to be fairly independent of fat content until a certain, critical fat content is reached, when significant changes in flavour release occur. The critical fat content is product dependent with values for yoghurt and biscuits reported as <3.5 g/100 g (Brauss *et al.*, 1999) and between 4 and 18 g/100 g fat (Brauss *et al.*, 2000) respectively. At low fat levels, interactions with other food components such as proteins can become significant (Seuvre *et al.*, 2000). The effect of other compositional factors such as pH, particle size and oil/emulsifier fraction have been reported (van Ruth *et al.*, 2002a, b, c) but the analyses were mainly *in vitro* and some of the differences noted may not translate into the situation found *in vivo*.

More sophisticated structures have been developed as ingredients for fat reduction in food. For example, a patent (Appelqvist *et al.*, 2000) describes the use of composite particles which can deliver the viscosity and aroma delivery associated with regular fat foods from matrices containing low fat levels. The ability to make multiple emulsions (e.g. water-in-oil-in-water) using cross-flow emulsification equipment provides another route to structures that may behave like fat while significantly reducing the fat content of food. This technique has potential for the food industry, providing suitable food-grade emulsifiers can be found to stabilise the structures. Another feature of flavour release is the need to stabilise flavour in the food during shelf-life but release flavour on eating. Encapsulation is the most popular choice of flavour manufacturers (Benczedi, 2002) although various microemulsion systems have been proposed to fulfil this role as these structures are thermodynamically stable (Yaghmur *et al.*, 2002) but undergo phase transition and release flavour when diluted with water either during food preparation or in the mouth (Taylor *et al.*, 1999). Liposome structures have also been investigated as food compatible systems for controlled release in food (Reineccius, 1995). Empty yeast cells have also been used as natural structures for the stabilisation and release of food ingredients (Bishop *et al.*, 1998) and are effective for some types of flavours (Dardelle *et al.*, 2007).

Aroma release from gels has been studied to determine the factors that control aroma release. A thermo-reversible gelatine–sucrose gel was loaded with a dye and its release into a 'saliva' phase was monitored to simulate flavour release (Harrison and Hills, 1996). From these studies, it was found that the bulk melting temperature of the gel controlled dye release. However, *in vivo*, release would depend on whether melting temperature was above or below mouth temperature as heat transfer would then become the issue. The situation was further complicated by the fact that sucrose was solubilised from the surface of the gel and this decreased the melting temperature of the sucrose-depleted gelatin layer.

11.5 Simulating flavour release from foods *in vitro*

Simulation of flavour release has been carried out using two methods, *in vitro* experimental systems, often referred to as 'model mouths', and mathematical models incorporating fundamental principles of heat and mass transfer. The experimental systems have typically mimicked some of the functionality found in human mouths, but it has been very difficult to fully recreate all conditions until recently (Salles *et al.*, 2007). The 'Dijon' mouth mimics chewing in 3 D and provides opportunities for on-line monitoring of aroma release as well as sampling of the 'saliva' phase for off line analysis. The introduction to the paper by Salles *et al.* clearly lays out the limitations of existing model mouths, a detailed specification covering ratios of food, saliva and air phase as well as the operating conditions (speed of 'jaw' movement, forces applied, etc.). To date, no validation tests have been published to compare flavour release in the model and in human mouths.

Another recent development is a system to simulate mixing in mouth which occurs largely through tongue action and is thought to be related to sensory perception of food texture (Prinz *et al.*, 2007). Mixing in the system is monitored using image analysis and the simulator can also study the 'effects of shear, dilution, and alpha-amylase concentration on the rheology and heterogeneity of the product ... in real time'. Other model mouths include the simple homogeniser-based device developed by van Ruth and Roozen (van Ruth *et al.*, 1995) and the retronasal aroma simulator developed by Roberts, Deibler and Acree based on rapid mixing of large amounts of sample and saliva using an electric motor to generate sufficient amounts of volatiles in the headspace for analysis (Roberts and Acree, 1995; Deibler *et al.*, 2001).

As with many food-related topics, the decision on whether to use model mouths or human subjects to measure flavour release depends very much on the question that research is trying to answer. Human oral processing is variable and people's flavour release and perception are also variable. However, this variability reflects the real situation when groups of consumers eat foods and can give useful information on performance in the marketplace. Model mouths reduce variability and can compare flavour release from different matrices to develop an understanding of the processes involved in flavour release and ultimately, flavour perception. Making a machine to join these two ideals together is a long-term goal but requires much work and validation.

Mathematical modelling of flavour release finds itself in a similar position to model mouths. It can be applied to food samples with well-defined geometry and under controlled conditions, such as those used by *in vitro* flavour release systems where the fundamental scientific principles of heat and mass transfer can be applied. The difficulty is in deciding how oral processing, anatomy and physiology affect the parameters associated with these well-established rules and how to deal with the variability in the mouth and between human panellists. Several theoretical models have been developed to describe flavour release from different foods such as emulsions (Harrison *et al.*, 1997) and gels (Harrison and Hills, 1996) as well as models that describe the general principles (Harrison *et al.*, 1998). There is evidence that some factors are important, e.g. mastication behaviour which drives aroma release (Buettner and Schieberle, 2000), but not enough is known to be categoric about which effects to take into consideration. Some of the issues are very demanding, for instance, trying to estimate the diameter of the throat to establish air flow seems straightforward until it is realised that the throat diameter is variable and can change with flow rate. Estimating particle size during mastication is also a major task (Agrawal *et al.*, 2000). Even basic values, such as determining the surface area of a food during eating, or the thickness of the saliva layers in different parts of the mouth, become excessively complicated and the pragmatic solution is to abandon mathematical modelling and carry out a series of *in vivo* analyses to measure flavour release.

11.6 Future trends

The relatively recent discovery of flavour receptors elsewhere in the body and particularly in the digestive tract has opened up a whole new area for flavour studies (Katz *et al.*, 2000). The receptors were found using molecular biology screening techniques and their potential functions are now being studied. A report that the sweet taste receptor in the gut acts as the sensor for glucose uptake (Margolskee *et al.*, 2007) has led to much speculation that flavour molecules may affect both food intake and uptake and has further enhanced the need for flavour to be part of nutritional and digestive studies. These findings may help explain previous results, e.g. the reported effect of sweetness on glucose uptake (Teff and Engelman, 1996) and have already led to patents on the potential use of sweetness inhibitors as food additives to reduce glucose uptake in the gut (Shirazi-Beechey and Iserentant, 2007). The hunt is on to understand the roles of other taste and aroma receptors in the body. While the potential for nutrient control through flavour receptors is obvious and attractive, we should bear in mind that, if nutrients are consumed but not absorbed, they will affect gut function and may cause unpleasant side effects, such as those experienced with high levels of Olestra in the diet.

In summary, the sense of flavour is key to the intake of foods so that nutritional benefits can be delivered. If flavour is also shown to be involved in the uptake of macronutrients such as sugars and proteins, researchers will need to develop new techniques for the assessment of flavours. For instance, methods for measuring flavours in the gut will be required along with delivery systems that can stimulate receptors in the mouth and the appropriate part of the gut.

11.7 References

AGRAWAL, K. R., LUCAS, P. W. and BRUCE, I. C. (2000), 'The effects of food fragmentation index on mandibular closing angle in human mastication', *Archives of Oral Biology*, **45**, 577–584.

APPELQVIST, I. A., BROWN, C. R., HOMAN, J. E., JONES, M. G., MALONE, M. E. and NORTON, I. T. (2000), 'Low-fat food emulsions for e.g. spreads, dressing or mayonnaise, have gel particles for delaying the release of the flavor molecules'. WO200007462-A; EP1102548-A; WO200007462-A1; AU9951601-A; BR9912775-A; EP1102548-A1; EP1102548-B1; DE69904053-E; ES2188206-T3; US6703062-B1.

BAINES, Z. V. and MORRIS, E. R. (1988), Effect of polysaccharide thickeners on organoleptic attributes. *Gums and stabilisers for the food industry*. Phillips, G. O., Williams, P. A. and Wedlock, D. J. Oxford, IRL Press: 192–201.

BAINES, Z. V. and MORRIS, E. R. (1989), Suppression of perceived flavour and taste by food hydrocolloids. *Food Colloids*. Bee, R. D., Richmond, P. and Mingens, J. Cambridge, Royal Society of Chemistry. **75**, 184–192.

BAYARRI, S., SMITH, T., HOLLOWOOD, T. and HORT, J. (2007), 'The role of rheological behaviour in flavour perception in model oil/water emulsions', *European Food Research and Technology*, **226**, 161–168.

BENCZEDI, D. (2002), Flavour encapsulation using polymer-based delivery systems. *Food Flavour Technology*. Taylor, A. J. Sheffield, Sheffield Academic Press: 153–166.

BISHOP, J. R. P., NELSON, G. and LAMB, J. (1998), 'Microencapsulation in yeast cells', *Journal of Microencapsulation*, **15**, 761–773.

BLAKE, A. (2006), The learning of human flavour preferences. *Flavour in food*. Voilley, A. and Etievant, P. X. Boca Raton, FL, CRC Press: 369–402.

BOELRIJK, A. E. M., SMIT, G. and WEEL, K. G. C. (2006), Flavour release from liquid food products. *Flavour in Food*. Voilley, A. and Etievant, P. X. Cambridge, Woodhead Publishing: 260–286.

BRAUSS, M. S., LINFORTH, R. S. T., CAYEUX, I., HARVEY, B. and TAYLOR, A. J. (1999), 'Altering the fat content affects flavour release in a model yogurt system', *Journal of Agricultural and Food Chemistry*, **47**, 2055–2059.

BRAUSS, M. S., BALDERS, B., LINFORTH, R. S. T., AVISON, S. and TAYLOR, A. J. (2000), 'Fat content, baking time, hydration and temperature affect flavor release from biscuits in model and real systems', *Flavour Fragrance Journal*, **14**, 351–357.

BUETTNER, A. and MONTSERRAT, M. (2005), Retronasal aroma perception – a closer look at psychophysical interaction phenomena. *State-of-the-Art in Flavour Chemistry and Biology*. Hofmann, T., Rothe, M. and Schieberle, P. Garching, Deutsche Forschungsanstalt für Lebensmittelchemie: 3–11.

BUETTNER, A. and SCHIEBERLE, P. (2000), 'Influence of mastication on the concentrations of aroma volatiles – some aspects of flavour release and flavour perception', *Food Chemistry*, **71**, 347–354.

CALVERT, G. A. (2001), 'Crossmodal processing in the human brain: insights from functional neuroimaging studies', *Cerebral Cortex*, **11**, 1110–1123.

CHANNELL, G. A., WULFERT, F. and TAYLOR, A. J. (2008), 'Identification and monitoring of intermediates and products in the acrylamide pathway using on-line analysis', *Journal of Agricultural and Food Chemistry*, **56**, 6097–6104.

COOK, D. J., HOLLOWOOD, T. A., LINFORTH, R. S. T. and TAYLOR, A. J. (2002), 'Perception of taste intensity in solutions of random coil polysaccharides above and below c*', *Food Quality and Preference*, **13**, 473–480.

COOK, D. J., HOLLOWOOD, T. A., LINFORTH, R. S. T. and TAYLOR, A. J. (2003), 'Oral shear stress predicts flavour perception in viscous solutions', *Chemical Senses*, **28**, 11–23.

CUTLER, A. N., MORRIS, E. R. and TAYLOR, L. J. (1983), 'Oral perception of viscosity in fluid foods and model systems', *Journal of Texture Studies*, **14**, 377–395.

DALTON, P., DOOLITTLE, N., NAGATA, H. and BRESLIN, P. A. S. (2000), 'The merging of the senses: integration of subthreshold taste and smell', *Nature Neuroscience*, **3**, 431–432.

DARDELLE, G., NORMAND, V., STEENHOUDT, M., BOUQUERAND, P. E., CHEVALIER, M. and BAUMGARTNER, P. (2007), 'Flavour-encapsulation and flavour-release performances of a commercial yeast-based delivery system', *Food Hydrocolloids*, **21**, 953–960.

DARLING, D. F., WILLIAMS, D. and YENDLE, P. (1986), Physico-chemical interactions involved in aroma transport processes from solution. *Interactions of Food Components*. Birch, G. G. and Lindley, M. G. London, Elsevier Applied Science: 165–188.

DAVIDSON, J. M., LINFORTH, R. S. T. and TAYLOR, A. J. (1998), 'In-mouth measurement of pH and conductivity during eating', *Journal of Agricultural and Food Chemistry*, **46**, 5210–5214.

DAVIDSON, J. M., LINFORTH, R. S. T., HOLLOWOOD, T. A. and TAYLOR, A. J. (2000), Release of non-volatile flavor components *in vivo*. *Flavor release: Linking experiments, theory and reality*. Roberts, D. D. and Taylor, A. J. Washington D.C, American Chemical Society. **763**, 99–111.

DE VICENTE, J., STOKES, J. R. and SPIKES, H. A. (2006), 'Soft lubrication of model hydrocolloids ', *Food Hydrocolloids*, **20**, 483–491.

DEIBLER, K. D., ACREE, T. E., LAVIN, E. H., TAYLOR, A. J. and LINFORTH, R. S. T. (2001), Flavor release measurements with retronasal aroma simulator. *Flavour 2000*. Rothe, M. Bergholz Rehbrucke, Eigenverlag M Rothe: 41–48.

DEROOS, K. B. (2000), Physicochemical models of flavor release from foods. *Flavor release*. Roberts, D. D. and Taylor, A. J. Washington, DC, American Chemical Society. **763**, 126–141.

DEROOS, K. B. and WOLSWINKEL, K. (1994), Non-equilibrium partition model for predicting flavour release in the mouth. *Trends in Flavour Research*. Maarse, H. and Van der Heij, D. G. Amsterdam, Elsevier Science: 15–32.

DRIVER, J. and SPENCE, C. (2000), 'Multisensory perception: beyond modularity and convergence', *Current Biology*, **10**, R731–R735.

DUMONT, J.-P. (2006), Emulsion flavour interactions. *Flavour in Food*. Voilley, A. and Etievant, P. X. Boca Raton, FL, CRC Press: 156–171.

ELEJALDE, C. C. and KOKINI, J. L. (1992), 'The psychophysics of pouring, spreading and in-mouth viscosity', *Journal of Texture Studies*, **23**, 315–336.

FERRY, A.-L. S., MITCHELL, J. R., HORT, J., HILL, S. E., TAYLOR, A. J., LAGARRIGUE, S. and VALLÈS-PÀMIES, B. (2006a), 'In-mouth amylase activity can reduce perception of saltiness in starch-thickened foods', *Journal of Agricultural and Food Chemistry*, **54**, 8869–8873.

FERRY, A. L., HORT, J., MITCHELL, J. R., COOK, D. J., LAGARRIGUE, S. and PAMIES, B. V. (2006b), 'Viscosity and flavour perception: Why is starch different from hydrocolloids?', *Food Hydrocolloids*, **20**, 855–862.

FREEMAN, C. G. and MCEWAN, M. J. (2002), 'Rapid analysis of trace gases in complex mixtures using selected ion flow tube-mass spectrometry', *Australian Journal of Chemistry*, **55**, 491–494.

GUINARD, J. X. and MAZZUCCHELLI, R. (1996), 'The sensory perception of texture and mouthfeel', *Trends in Food Science & Technology*, **7**, 213–219.

HARRISON, M. and HILLS, B. P. (1996), 'A mathematical model to describe flavour release from gelatine gels', *International Journal of Food Science and Technology*, **31**, 167–176.

HARRISON, M., HILLS, B. P., BAKKER, J. and CLOTHIER, T. (1997), 'Mathematical models of flavor release from liquid emulsions', *Journal of Food Science*, **62**, 653–659.

HARRISON, M., CAMPBELL, S. and HILLS, B. P. (1998), 'Computer simulation of flavor release from solid foods in the mouth', *Journal of Agricultural and Food Chemistry*, **46**, 2736–2743.

HILLS, B. P. and HARRISON, M. (1995), 'Two-film theory of flavour release from solids', *International Journal of Food Science and Technology*, **30**, 425–436.

HOLLOWOOD, T. A., LINFORTH, R. S. T. and TAYLOR, A. J. (2000), The relationship between volatile release and perception. *Flavor release: Linking experiments, theory and reality*. Roberts, D. D. and Taylor, A. J. Washington D.C., American Chemical Society. **763**, 370–380.

HOLLOWOOD, T. A., LINFORTH, R. S. T. and TAYLOR, A. J. (2002), 'The effect of viscosity on the perception of flavour', *Chemical Senses*, **27**, 583–591.

HORT, J. and COOK, D. J. (2007), Formulating low fat foods: the challenge of retaining flavour quality. *Modifying Flavour in Food*. Taylor, A. J. and Hort, J. Cambridge, Woodhead Publishing: 131–145.

HUTCHINGS, J. B. and LILLFORD, P. J. (1988), 'The perception of food texture – the philosophy of the breakdown path', *Journal of Texture Studies*, **19**, 103–115.

JACK, F. R., PIGGOTT, J. R. and PATERSON, A. (1995), 'Cheddar cheese texture related to salt release during eating, measured by conductivity – a preliminary study', *Journal of Food Science*, **60**, 213–217.

KATZ, D. B., NICOLELIS, M. A. L. and SIMON, S. A. (2000), 'Nutrient tasting and signaling mechanisms in the gut IV. There is more to taste than meets the tongue', *American Journal of Physiology – Gastrointestinal and Liver Physiology*, **278**, G6–G9.

LILLFORD, P. J. (1991), Texture and the acceptability of food. *Feeding and the Texture of Food*. Vincent, P. J. F. and Lillford, P. J. New York, Cambridge University Press: 231–243.

LINDINGER, W., HANSEL, A. and JORDAN, A. (1998), 'On-line monitoring of volatile organic compounds at pptv levels by means of proton-transfer-reaction mass spectrometry (PTR-MS) – medical applications, food control and environmental research', *International Journal of Mass Spectrometry*, **173**, 191–241.

LINDINGER, C., POLLIEN, P., ALI, S., YERETZIAN, C., BLANK, I. and MARK, T. (2005), 'Unambiguous identification of volatile organic compounds by proton-transfer reaction mass spectrometry coupled with GC/MS', *Analytical Chemistry*, **77**, 4117–4124.

LINFORTH, R. S. T. and TAYLOR, A. J. (2003), 'Direct mass spectrometry of complex volatile and non-volatile flavour mixtures', *International Journal of Mass Spectrometry*, **223–224**, 179–191.

LINFORTH, R. S. T. and TAYLOR, A. J. (2006), The process of flavour release. *Flavour in Food*. Voilley, A. and Etievant, P. X. Cambridge, Woodhead Publishing: 287–307.

LINFORTH, R. S. T., INGHAM, K. E. and TAYLOR, A. J. (1996), Time course profiling of volatile release from foods during the eating process. *Flavour Science: Recent Developments*. Taylor, A. J. and Mottram, D. S. Cambridge, Royal Society Chemistry: 361–368.

LUCAS, P. W., ANG, K. Y., SUI, Z., AGRAWAL, K. R., PRINZ, J. F. and DOMINY, N. J. (2006), 'A brief review of the recent evolution of the human mouth in physiological and nutritional contexts', *Physiology & Behavior*, **89**, 36–38.

MARGOLSKEE, R. F., DYER, J., KOKRASHVILI, Z., SALMON, K. S. H., ILEGEMS, E., DALY, K., MAILLET, E. L., NINOMIYA, Y., MOSINGER, B. and SHIRAZI-BEECHEY, S. P. (2007), 'T1R3 and gustducin in gut sense sugars to regulate expression of Na^+-glucose cotransporter 1', *Proceedings of the National Academy of Sciences of the United States of America*, **104**, 15075–15080.

MCNULTY, P. B. (1987), Flavor release – elusive and dynamic. *Food Structure and Behavior*. Blanshard, J. M. V. and Lillford, P. London, Academic Press: 245–248.

MCNULTY, P. B. and KAREL, M. (1973a), 'Factors affecting flavor release and uptake in O/W emulsions. I. Release and uptake models', *Journal of Food Technology*, **8**, 309–318.

MCNULTY, P. B. and KAREL, M. (1973b), 'Factors affecting flavor release and uptake in O/W emulsions. II Stirred cell studies', *Journal of Food Technology*, **8**, 319–331.

MCNULTY, P. B. and KAREL, M. (1973c), 'Factors affecting flavor release and uptake in O/W emulsions. III. Scale-up model and emulsion studies', *Journal of Food Technology*, **8**, 415–427.

NORMAND, V., AVISON, S. and PARKER, A. (2004), 'Modeling the kinetics of flavour release during drinking', *Chemical Senses*, **29**, 235–245.

OLLIVON, M. (2006), Lipid–flavour interactions. *Flavour in Food*. Voilley, A. and Etievant, P. X. Boca Raton, FL, CRC Press: 133–171.

OVERBOSCH, P., AFTEROF, W. G. M. and HARING, P. G. M. (1991), 'Flavor release in the mouth', *Food Reviews International*, **7**, 137–184.

PANGBORN, R. M. and SZCZESNIAK, A. S. (1974), 'Effect of hydrocolloids and viscosity on aromatic flavour compounds', *Journal of Texture Studies*, **4**, 467–482.

PFEIFFER, J., HORT, J., HOLLOWOOD, T. A. and TAYLOR, A. J. (2006), 'Taste–aroma interactions in a ternary system: a model of fruitiness perception in sucrose/acid solutions', *Perception & Psychophysics*, **68**, 216–227.

PIONNIER, E., CHABANET, C., MIOCHE, L., TAYLOR, A. J., LE QUERE, J. L. and SALLES, C. (2004), '*In vivo* nonvolatile release during eating of a model cheese: relationships with oral parameters', *Journal of Agricultural and Food Chemistry*, **52**, 565–571.

PLUG, H. and HARING, P. G. M. (1993), 'The role of ingredient–flavour interactions in the development of fat-free foods', *Trends in Food Science and Technology*, **4**, 150–152.

PRINZ, J. F., JANSSEN, A. M. and DE WIJK, R. A. (2007), '*In vitro* simulation of the oral processing of semi-solid foods', *Food Hydrocolloids*, **21**, 397–401.

REINECCIUS, G. A. (1995), Liposomes for controlled-release in the food-industry. *Encapsulation and Controlled Release of Food Ingredients*. Risch, S. J. and Reineccius, G. A. Washington, DC, American Chemical Society. **590**, 113–131.

REINECCIUS, G. A. (2006), *Flavor Chemistry and Technology*, Boca Raton, FL, Taylor & Francis.

ROBERTS, D. D. and ACREE, T. E. (1995), 'Simulation of retronasal aroma using a modified headspace technique – investigating the effects of saliva, temperature, shearing, and oil on flavor release', *Journal of Agricultural and Food Chemistry*, **43**, 2179–2186.

ROLLS, E. T. (1997), 'Taste and olfactory processing in the brain and its relation to the control of eating', *Critical Reviews in Neurobiology*, **11**, 263–287.

SALLES, C., TARREGA, A., MIELLE, P., MARATRAY, J., GORRIA, P., LIABOEUF, J. and LIODENOT, J. J. (2007), 'Development of a chewing simulator for food breakdown and the analysis of *in vitro* flavor compound release in a mouth environment', *Journal of Food Engineering*, **82**, 189–198.

SEUVRE, A. M., DIAZ, M. A. E. and VOILLEY, A. (2000), 'Influence of the food matrix structure on the retention of aroma compounds', *Journal of Agricultural and Food Chemistry*, **48**, 4296–4300.

SHAMA, F. and SHERMAN, P. (1973), 'Identification of stimuli controlling the sensory evaluation of viscosity. II Oral methods', *Journal of Texture Studies*, **4**, 111.

SHAMIL, S., WYETH, L. J. and KILCAST, D. (1992), 'Flavour release and perception in reduced fat foods', *Food Quality and Preference*, **3**, 51–60.

SHIRAZI-BEECHEY, S. and ISERENTANT, D. (2007), 'Method to control body weight'. WO/2007/085593.

SHOJAEI, Z. A., LINFORTH, R. S. T., HORT, J., HOLLOWOOD, T. A. and TAYLOR, A. J. (2006), 'Measurement and manipulation of aroma delivery allows control of perceived fruit flavour in low and regular fat milks', *International Journal of Food Science and Technology*, **41**, 1192–1196.

SMALL, D. M. (2004), 'Crossmodal integration – insights from the chemical senses', *Trends in Neurosciences*, **27**, 120–123.

SOETING, W. J. and HEIDEMA, J. (1988), 'A mass-spectrometric method for measuring flavor concentration–time profiles in human breath', *Chemical Senses*, **13**, 607–617.

SPANEL, P. and SMITH, D. (1999), 'Selected ion flow tube – mass spectrometry: detection and real-time monitoring of flavours released by food products', *Rapid Communications in Mass Spectrometry*, **13**, 585–596.

STONE, H. and SIDEL, J. L. (2004), *Sensory Evaluation Practices*, Amsterdam, Elsevier.

TAYLOR, A. J. (1998), 'Physical chemistry of flavour', *International Journal of Food Science and Technology*, **33**, 53–62.

TAYLOR, A. J. (2002), 'Release and transport of flavours *in vivo*: physico chemical, physiological and perceptual considerations', *Comprehensive Reviews in Food Safety and Food Science*, **1**, 45–57.

TAYLOR, A. J., ALSTON, M. J., HEMINGWAY, K. M., CHAPPELL, C. G. and MLOTKIEWICZ, J. A. (1999), 'A flavor-delivering system for foods and beverages'. WO9962357-A; WO9962357-A1; AU9940521-A.

TAYLOR, A. J., SIVASUNDARAM, L. R., LINFORTH, R. S. T. and SURAWANG, S. (2003), Identification of volatile compounds using combined GC-EI-API-MS. *Handbook of Flavor Characterization. Sensory Analysis, Chemistry and Physiology*. Deibler, K. D. and Delwiche, J. New York, Marcel Dekker: 411–422.

TEFF, K. L. and ENGELMAN, K. (1996), 'Oral sensory stimulation improves glucose tolerance in humans: effects on insulin, C-peptide, and glucagon', *American Journal of Physiology – Regulatory Integrative and Comparative Physiology*, **39**, R1371–R1379.

VAN RUTH, S. M., ROOZEN, J. P. and COZIJNSEN, J. L. (1995), 'Comparison of flavor release from rehydrated French beans in the mouth and in a mouth model system', *Chemical Senses*, **20**, 146.

VAN RUTH, S. M., DE VRIES, G., GEARY, M. and GIANNOULI, P. (2002a), 'Influence of composition and structure of oil-in-water emulsions on retention of aroma compounds', *Journal of the Science of Food and Agriculture*, **82**, 1028–1035.

VAN RUTH, S. M., KING, C., DELARUE, M. and GIANNOULI, P. (2002b), 'Release of volatile compounds from emulsions: influence of beta-lactoglobulin and pH', *Italian Journal of Food Science*, **14**, 145–158.

VAN RUTH, S. M., KING, C. and GIANNOULI, P. (2002c), 'Influence of lipid fraction, emulsifier fraction, and mean particle diameter of oil-in-water emulsions on the release of 20 aroma compounds', *Journal of Agricultural and Food Chemistry*, **50**, 2365–2371.

VISSCHERS, R. W., JACOBS, M. A., FRASNELLI, J., HUMMEL, T., BURGERING, M. and BOELRIJK, A. E. M. (2006), 'Cross-modality of texture and aroma perception is independent of orthonasal or retronasal stimulation', *Journal of Agricultural and Food Chemistry*, **54**, 5509–5515.

VOILLEY, A. (2006), Flavour retention and release from the food matrix: an overview. *Flavour in Food*. Voilley, A. and Etievant, P. X. Boca Raton, CRC Press: 117–132.

WEEL, K. G. C., BOELRIJK, A. E. M., ALTING, A. C., VAN MIL, P., BURGER, J. J., GRUPPEN, H., VORAGEN, A. G. J. and SMIT, G. (2002), 'Flavor release and perception of flavored whey protein gels: perception is determined by texture rather than by release', *Journal of Agricultural and Food Chemistry*, **50**, 5149–5155.

WEEL, K. G. C., BOELRIJK, A. E. M., BURGER, J. J., GRUPPEN, H., VORAGEN, A. G. J. and SMIT, G. (2003), 'A protocol for measurement of *in vivo* aroma release from beverages', *Journal of Food Science*, **68**, 1123–1128.

YAGHMUR, A., ASERIN, A. and GARTI, N. (2002), 'Phase behavior of microemulsions based on food-grade nonionic surfactants: effect of polyols and short-chain alcohols', *Colloids and Surfaces A – Physicochemical and Engineering Aspects*, **209**, 71–81.

12

Improving *in vitro* simulation of the stomach and intestines

K. Venema, R. Havenaar and M. Minekus, TNO Quality of Life, The Netherlands

Abstract: This chapter describes the application of well-established *in vitro* models of the gastrointestinal (GI) tract. Such models can be used to perform simplified experiments under uniform and well-controlled conditions. However, the models should mimic the *in vivo* conditions to a high degree in order to be used for functional foods design. If this is accomplished, mechanisms can be studied that underlie some of the processes occurring in the lumen of the GI tract. Several examples are given in this chapter.

Key words: *in vitro* model, stomach, small intestine, colon, functional food.

12.1 Introduction

This chapter describes the application of well-established *in vitro* models of the gastrointestinal (GI) tract. Models can be used to perform simplified experiments under uniform and well-controlled conditions. However, simulating such a complex system as the GI tract carries the risk of oversimplification. Most models of the GI tract do not successfully simulate the dynamic conditions in its lumen (Boisen and Eggum, 1991; Rumney and Rowland, 1992; Savoie, 1994), which is necessary to answer the variety of questions that have been raised by specialists in various fields, for example in the food, feed and pharmaceutical industries. Increased knowledge of food processing, molecular biology and nutrition has resulted in the production of functional foods and novel foods. The health claims used for functional foods require the establishment of efficacy, while the safety of novel foods has to be assessed before they can be marketed (Schaafsma, 1997). The feed industry aims at improving the bioavailability of their products, introducing alternative protein and fat sources and reducing the faecal output of environmental pollutants such as phosphates. Finally, the pharmaceutical industry has an interest in studying the dissolution of drugs, slow-release systems and drug–nutrient interactions. An *in vitro* model that would successfully simulate the relevant conditions of the GI tract can therefore be used for a broad range of applications. Several models will be highlighted in this chapter, with emphasis on the system from TNO (the TIM systems), which have the highest predictive value towards events occurring in the lumen of the gut of monogastric species, including man. The development of such a model involved a multi disciplinary approach, combining microbiology, physiology, gastroenterology, process technology and automation.

12.1.1 Parts of the gastrointestinal tract and their functions

The main function of the GI tract is to break down food and to transport nutrients into the body. This is performed in a system of cavities and tubes that starts with the stomach and ends with the rectum, each of which has a specific task (Table 12.1). Although the GI tract is situated inside the body, the interior (lumen) of the GI tract can be regarded as the outside world. The wall of the GI tract forms the barrier between lumen and body, similar in function to the skin. The walls of the separate sections of the GI tract are highly differentiated with regard to their specific task in the digestive process. There are cells that secrete hydrochloric acid, mucus or enzymes, and those that absorb specific nutrients through active transport across the cell membrane, and cells with immunological functions. Furthermore, the GI tract harbours numerous microorganisms which interact with the host as well as with foods. Several models have been developed that aim to mimic especially what happens in the lumen of the GI tract (see below).

12.1.2 Important aspects to simulate gastrointestinal functions

The digestive tract consists of separate compartments, dedicated to a specific step in digestion (Table 12.1). To study the fate of ingested compounds,

Table 12.1 Main functions of the separate parts of the digestive tract

Stomach	Storage Particle reduction Digestion by pepsin and lipase Acidification Barrier to microorganisms
Small intestine	Emulsification of fat by bile Digestion and absorption of protein, carbohydrates and fat Absorption of nutrients and water
Large intestine	Fermentation of undigested materials by the microbiota Absorption of water, fermentation products and sodium

it is important to expose the meal to each step of digestion with a realistic transit time for each compartment. Because of secretion, transit of the meal and absorption of nutrients and water, the composition of the chyme is changing in time. In other words, different fractions of the meal are exposed to different conditions in each part of the GI tract. The effect of gastric transit depends on the interaction between different parameters such as gastric emptying, secretion of enzymes, hydrochloric acid and water. The digestion of milk protein is a good example to illustrate the interaction of gastric parameters. Gastric pH after ingestion of the milk decreases slowly. The meal is gradually delivered from the stomach and thus portions of the meal escape exposure to low pH and consequently to peptic activity. The gradual delivery of a meal can be described by mathematical equations that calculate the cumulative amount of meal delivered in time, expressed as a percentage of intake (Decuypere *et al.*, 1986; Elashoff *et al.*, 1982). Liquids and semi-liquids show an exponential gastric delivery pattern, while solids have a more linear pattern of gastric delivery (Notivol *et al.*, 1984). To obtain a realistic gastric delivery of the meal, especially when there are particles in the meal, the sieving activity of the pylorus should be mimicked. To mimic the grinding of particles and to mix and transport the chyme in a physiological fashion, it is important to reproduce the characteristics of the motility of the gut. The peristaltic movements are a very efficient way to propagate the concentrated chyme through the gut.

Digestive processes such as gastric emptying, secretion of digestive fluids and mucus, and motility are highly controlled by hormonal and neural regulation mechanisms, influenced by the food and external factors (Burks *et al.*, 1985). Often the absorption of nutrients is controlled to meet the body's requirements, or depending on the properties of the gut wall or on the presence of specific transport mechanisms. For study of the behaviour of microorganisms in the gut, also the interaction between microbiota and the host needs to be consided (Umesaki *et al.*, 1997). The immunological response of the host is a major determinant of the microbiota's composition.

The aspects described above may lead to the following criteria to design a realistic GI tract model, as have been proposed by Longland (1991):

- sequential use of digestive enzymes;
- appropriate pH and co-factors, co-enzymes, bile salts, etc.;
- removal of end products of enzyme or microbial activity to prevent product inhibition and death in the case of the microbiota;
- mixing appropriately in each step of the digestion process;
- physiological residence times for each digestive step.

Not mentioned by Longland, but very important, is the influence of the body on digestion of the food, resulting in important feedback mechanisms.

12.2 Models of gastrointestinal function

This section will give an overview of GI tract models developed to date and discuss them in relation to the criteria for an adequate simulation of gastrointestinal functions, as described in the previous section.

12.2.1 Models to study digestion

Several models for estimating digestibility have been described and evaluated by Boisen and Eggum (1991) and Savoie (1994). The methods described generally involve a single, two- or three-step digestion, simulating gastric digestion, gastric/small intestinal digestion and gastric/small intestinal/large intestinal digestion, respectively. The models are static models: the steps of digestion are simulated by exposing the test material to an enzyme solution at a fixed pH and temperature during a fixed period of time. In static gastric models, the test material is exposed to pepsin at a pH below 2.5 during a period that ranges from 0.5 to 48h (Boisen and Eggum, 1991). A gastric model that incorporates a flow of secretion has been described by Vatier *et al.* (1988) to assess the characteristics of an antacid. A similar model by Savalle *et al.* (1989) was dedicated to the study of gastric digestion and evacuation of milk proteins. Gastric juice is pumped into a vessel, while the gastric contents are removed from the vessel to simulate gastric emptying. The gastric pH is not kept at a fixed value, but controlled by the addition of hydrochloric acid. These gastric models can be described as dynamic models since liquid flows and the pH are controlled and change over time.

After gastric digestion, the test material is generally exposed to digestion with pancreatic enzymes at around pH 7.5. Incubation times ranged from 1h (Babinszky *et al.*, 1990) to 18h (Boisen and Fernadez, 1991a). Small intestinal digestion is most frequently simulated with pancreatin as a source of pancreatic enzymes (Babinszky *et al.*, 1990; Boisen and Eggum, 1991; Savoie, 1994), or with intestinal fluid (Furuya *et al.*, 1979). Some methods include an extraction step to avoid the interference of fat with the determination of protein digestibility (Babinszky *et al.*, 1990). The digestive mixtures are generally mixed with a magnetic stirrer (Savoie, 1994) or in a shaker. Englyst *et al.* (1992) used marbles to mimic small intestinal peristalsis in a system that determines the digestible fraction of resistant starch.

The most advanced digestion system described to date is the dialysis cell method (Gauthier *et al.*, 1982, 1986), which uses a dialysis tube to remove (enzyme-inhibiting) products of digestion. To evaluate degradation, several methods have been used such as measurement of acid production during proteolysis (Pedersen and Eggum, 1983), colorimetric measurement of the products of starch digestion (Holm *et al.*, 1988), and determination of undissolved nutrients by filtration or centrifugation after treatment with a precipitating agent such as trichloroacetic acid (Büchmann, 1979). The large intestinal digestion step is used to simulate microbial degradation of dietary fibre. This step is simulated with rumen fluid (Vervaeke *et al.*, 1979) or fibre-degrading enzymes (Boisen and Fernadez, 1991a, b).

12.2.2 Models to study microorganisms

The behaviour of microorganisms is generally studied in models of the large intestine. Only few models include the micro-ecology of the stomach and the small intestine (Coutts *et al.*, 1987; Molly *et al.*, 1993).

Models that simulate fermentation by colonic microbiota are reviewed by Rumney and Rowland (1992). Three types of models have been described to study different aspects of colonic microbiota: batch culture systems, semi-continuous culture systems and continuous culture systems. Batch cultures are mainly used for simple short-term carbohydrate fermentation experiments (1 to 2 days) and only involve incubation of test material with faeces or colonic contents (Barry *et al.*, 1995; Van Hoeij *et al.*, 1997; Vince *et al.*, 1990). The experiments are generally performed in closed vessels under anaerobic conditions. Semi-continuous cultures need a more sophisticated set-up. The microbiota is fed while some of the contents are removed from the fermentation vessel intermittently to mimic the entry of chyme from the ileum and a flow of chyme to the next part of the gut. Continuous cultures have the same set-up as the semi-continuous cultures, except that they have a regular feeding of microbiota and removal of contents. This approach results in a steady-state situation in which the growth rate of the microorganisms is determined by the dilution rate. To simulate the consecutive parts of the colon, different systems have been designed with two, three or five vessels in series (Gibson *et al.*, 1988; Miller and Wolin, 1981; Molly *et al.*, 1993). These systems generally allow for growth of strictly anaerobic microorganisms by flushing with anaerobic gas. The pH is measured and controlled within the physiological range through addition of acid or alkali. Both continuous and semi-continuous cultures have been used to study the micro-ecology of the microbiota, degradation of undigested materials, enzyme activities and production of interesting metabolites such as short chain fatty acids (SCFA), gases and toxic compounds.

12.2.3 Limitations of the gastrointestinal tract models developed to date

This section will discuss the limitations of the GI tract models described above with respect to a realistic simulation of the aspects that influence the fate of ingested compounds. It will bridge to the next section that describes the most sophisticated models to date, the TNO TIM systems, in which most of these limitations are taken into account.

Composition of the chyme

The composition of the chyme is influenced by the transit of the meal, secretion of digestive fluids, and absorption of nutrients and water. None of the models described above simulates these combined aspects and obtains a physiological chyme composition for the different digestive stages in time.

Enzyme, bile and electrolyte concentrations are not physiological (Boisen and Eggum, 1991). Especially the single enzyme methods are limited in their use since enzymes usually work together to digest a meal (Savoie, 1994). Pancreatin or intestinal fluid is relatively cheap and contains a mixture of relevant enzymes. A disadvantage of these preparations is that their composition is not well defined, with a batch-to-batch variation of enzyme activities. Also, pancreatin contains a considerable amount of non-enzyme material. Generally, the gastric pH profile after ingestion of the meal is not simulated, which may result in an unrealistic exposure to peptic and acidic conditions.

None of the colonic models described so far includes removal of metabolites and water (Rumney and Rowland, 1992). This results in lower microbial density than found in the colonic content *in vivo*.

Motility and transit

All of the models are mixed with an impellor, a magnetic stirrer, on a shaker or are not mixed at all. The kneading type of mixing as occurs *in vivo* cannot be mimicked with one of these devices. A realistic gastric residence time could be simulated only in the gastric models of Vatier *et al.* (1988) and Savalle *et al.* (1989). All other models mimicked gastric passage as a static batch process. The difference between the exposure to sequential steps of digestion in a static system and in a dynamic system is presented in Fig. 12.1. Small intestinal transit is also generally mimicked as a batch process, which is slightly more physiological than simulating gastric passage as a batch process. The start of the experiment can be regarded as the beginning of the small intestine, where bile and pancreatic secretion are mixed with the gastric output. Incubation time can be regarded as the time needed for this mixture to travel through the small intestine. It has been suggested by McNeill Alexander (1994) that the small intestine can be best described as a plug flow reactor (PFR), which is a tube along which the contents flow with only radial mixing. However, in the small intestine there is also extensive longitudinal mixing by segmentation, especially when the chyme is liquid.

Probably the most realistic way to simulate the transit of the meal is to model the small intestine as a series of small continuously stirred tank reactors (CSTRs). The size of the compartments determines the extent of longitudinal mixing. A large number of small compartments assumes little longitudinal axial mixing and acts together as a PFR. Larger compartments assume homogeneous chyme along a section of the gut due to longitudinal mixing. The extent of mixing and propagation of the meal are determined by its bulk and viscosity. An ingested capsule travelled through the small intestine in 8 hours (Evans *et al.*, 1988), which perfectly fits the PFR model with no longitudinal mixing. A typical gastric and ileal delivery of a solid meal is

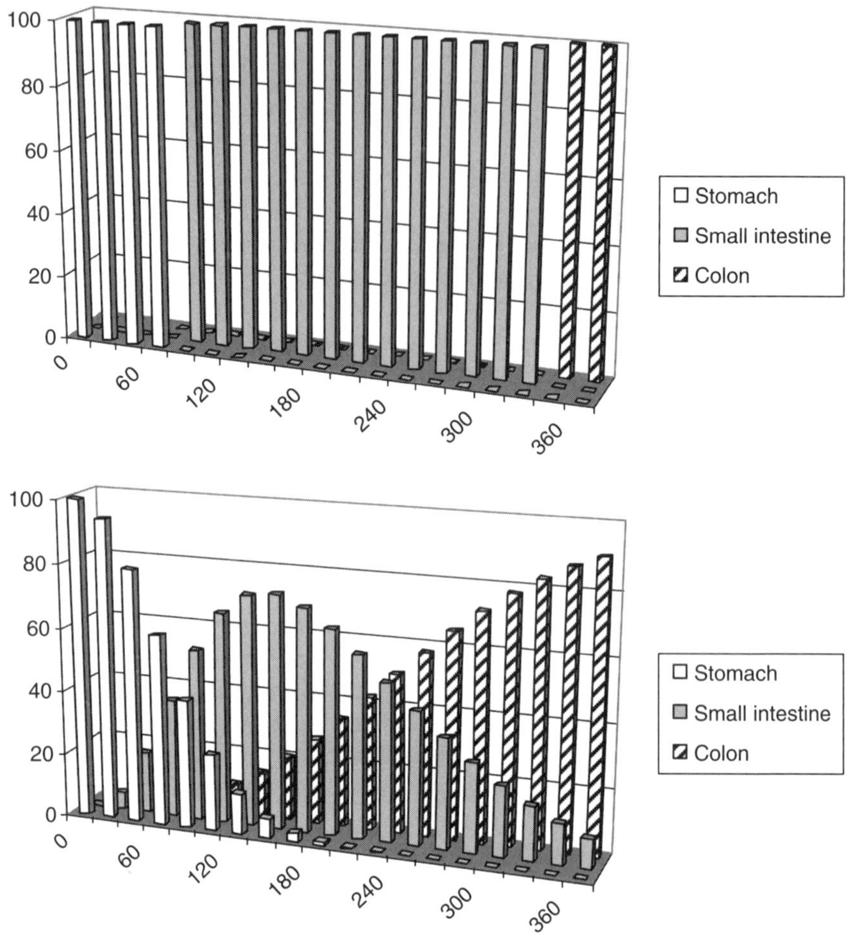

Fig. 12.1 Exposure of a meal to successive steps of digestion in a static system (top) and in a dynamic system (bottom).

shown in Fig. 12.2. The delay and pattern of ileal delivery show that in this case the small intestine also approximates to a PFR. Liquid meals, however, may have a much shorter transit time through the small intestine.

Marteau *et al.* (1993) demonstrated that 50% of a milk meal, and also of a yogurt meal, was evacuated from the small intestine ca. 1.5 h after ingestion. The addition of indigestible components such as lactulose can decrease the small intestinal transit time (Holgate and Read, 1983) because it retains fluid in the lumen of the small intestine through osmotic activity. The transit of lactulose can best be simulated in a model based on a cascade of CSTRs. The study with lactulose shows that water absorption is an important determinant for small intestinal transit.

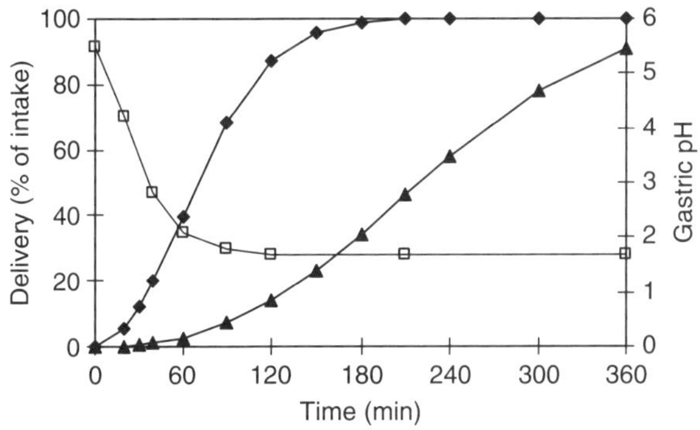

Fig. 12.2 Example of gastric pH curve (□) and gastric (♦) and ileal (▲) delivery curves in TIM-1 during the passage of a solid meal through the upper GI tract.

Colon models are generally CSTRs connected together to mimic sequential regions of the colon. However, the colon can act as a CSTR only if the chyme is liquid enough to be mixed. Owing to water absorption, mixing of the chyme decreases as it travels down the colon, causing the colon to act increasingly like a PFR. Microorganisms cannot be maintained in a PFR because they wash out with the plug flow. In the large intestine resident microorganisms resist the flow of chyme because they are attached to the gut wall. In fact, attachment to the gut wall is regarded as a prerequisite for invading microorganisms to overcome their lag phase in the new environment and to colonise the intestine (Freter, 1992). Experiments in continuous flow fermenters have shown that attachment to the glass wall of the vessel is also necessary for invading microorganisms to overcome the colonisation barrier. Although the ecological principles might be similar, the mechanisms of adherence in a CSTR are very different from *in vivo* conditions. Therefore, an *in vitro* model may be useful to study microbial ecology, but not mechanistic aspects of gut colonisation (Freter, 1992).

Response of the body

The fact that *in vitro* models cannot simulate the reaction of the body to compounds in the food can be regarded as an important limitation of *in vitro* models in general. Also, the rate of absorption of nutrients is difficult to predict *in vivo*, since *in vivo* absorption occurs often by facilitated or active transport systems that involve carrier proteins to transport the molecules across the enterocyte membrane. The complex interactions of microorganisms with the body cannot be simulated in any colon model to date.

It should be noted that the absence of feedback mechanisms can also be an advantage because it improves the reproducibility of the system and allows studies to be carried out with the variation of only selected parameters.

12.3 The TNO *in vitro* models of the gastrointestinal tract (TIM systems)

12.3.1 TIM-1 – the TNO *in vitro* model of the stomach and small intestine

The TNO *in vitro* model of the stomach and small intestine (nicknamed TIM-1) consists of four successive compartments (Fig. 12.3) simulating the stomach, duodenum, jejunum and ileum (Minekus *et al.*, 1995). Each compartment is formed by two connected basic units consisting of a glass jacket with a flexible wall inside.

Water is pumped from a water bath around the flexible walls to control the temperature inside the units and the pressure on the flexible walls. Changes in water pressure are achieved by computer-activated rotary pumps. This enables mixing of the chyme by alternating compression and relaxation of the flexible walls, simulating the peristaltic movements. The

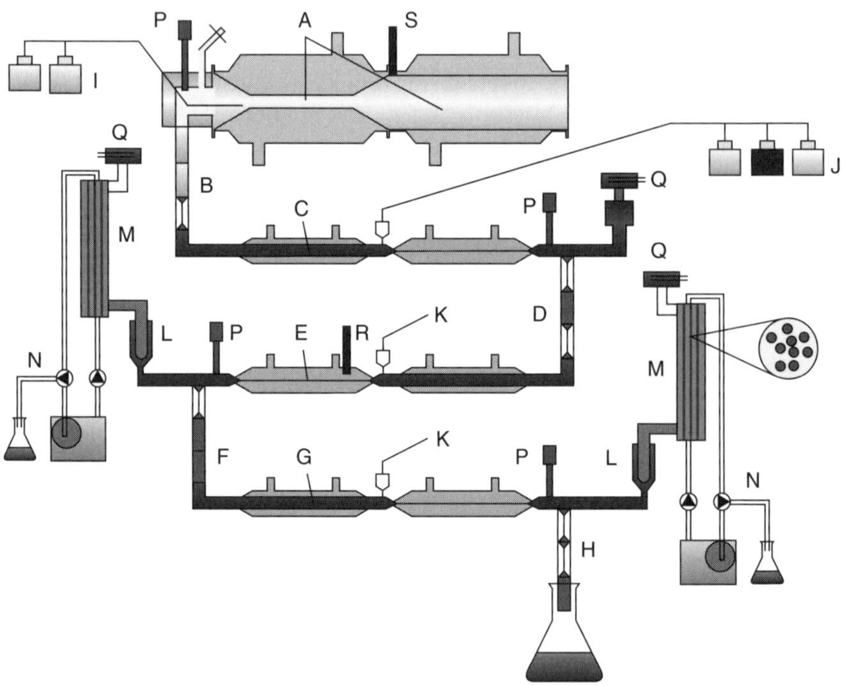

Fig. 12.3 Schematic representation of diagram of the dynamic, multi-compartmental model of the stomach and small intestine (TIM-1): A stomach compartment; B pyloric sphincter; C duodenum compartment; D peristaltic valve; E jejunum compartment; F peristaltic valve; G ileum compartment; H ileo-caecal sphincter; I stomach secretion; J duodenum secretion; K jejunum/ileum secretion; L pre-filter; M semi-permeable membrane; N water absorption; P pH electrodes; Q level sensors; R temperature sensor; S pressure sensor.

compartments are connected by peristaltic valve-pumps consisting of three connected T-tubes, each with a separate tube-like flexible wall inside. If pressure is applied to the outside of the flexible wall, the valve is closed. In the open position the flexible walls facilitate unhindered passage of the chyme through the valves. Peristaltic pumping is achieved by regulating the sequence of opening and closing of the three parts of the valve-pump. During each peristaltic cycle, a constant volume of chyme is transferred. The frequency of peristaltic cycles is dictated by a computer, allowing the flow rate of the chyme to be controlled, enabling the passage of different types of a 'meal' to be mimicked, as a glass of water needs to travel through the system much quicker than, for instance, a breakfast. The volume in each compartment is monitored with a level sensor connected to the computer.

A predetermined quantity of the meal is introduced into the gastric compartment within a pre-set period of time, with a peristaltic pump. The gastric and duodenal compartments are equipped with pH electrodes. The pH values are controlled via the computer by secreting either water or 1 M HCl into the stomach, or by secreting either water or 1 M $NaHCO_3$ into the duodenum. To avoid irregular pH values in the stomach due to incomplete mixing, HCl is secreted through a perforated tube. Secretions of all gastrointestinal juices are regulated by using computer-controlled syringe pumps. The jejunal and ileal compartments are connected with hollow-fibre devices to absorb digestion products and water from the chyme and to control electrolyte and bile salt concentrations in the chyme. The model is computer controlled and the computer program has been designed to accept parameters and data obtained from *in vivo* studies in animals or human volunteers, such as the quantity and duration of a meal, the pH curves in the stomach and duodenum, secretion rates into the different compartments, water absorption from the small intestine and gastric and ileal delivery into the duodenum and colon.

To control the transit of chyme, a power exponential formula for gastric and ileal delivery is used as described by Elashoff *et al.* (1982) (Equation 12.1).

$$f = 1 - 2^{-\left(\frac{t}{t_{1/2}}\right)^{\beta}} \qquad [12.1]$$

where f represents the fraction of meal marker delivered, $t_{½}$ the half-time of delivery, t the time, and β a parameter describing the shape of the curve. This formula offers a method for controlling the gastric and ileal delivery in the model with only two parameters ($t_{½}$, β) to describe the curve.

12.3.2 TIM-2 – TNO's *in vitro* model of the large intestine

The large intestinal model (Minekus *et al.*, 1999) consists of units based on the same concept as that developed for the gastric/small intestinal model.

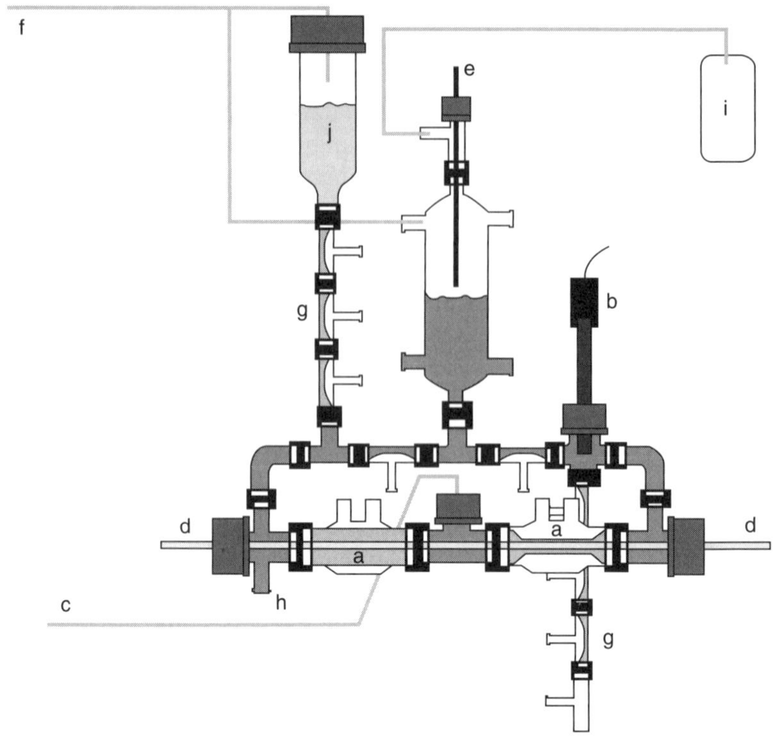

Fig. 12.4 Schematic diagram of the dynamic, multi-compartmental model of the large intestine (TIM-2): a peristaltic compartments; b pH-electrode; c alkali pump; d dialysis liquid circuit with hollow fibres; e level-sensor; f N_2 gas inlet; g in- or outlet valves; h sampling-port; i gas outlet; j 'ileal delivery' container.

Four glass units (Fig. 12.4a), each with a flexible wall inside, are connected to each other. Peristaltic movements are achieved by pumping water into the space between the glass jacket and the flexible wall. The computer controls the sequential squeezing of these walls, thus causing a peristaltic wave which forces the chyme to circulate through the loop-shaped model. The tubular shape of the lumen of the model prevents 'obstipation'. The pH is measured with a pH electrode (b) and controlled by the addition of a 5 M NaOH solution (c). The dialysis liquid is pumped through hollow-fibre membranes (molecular weight cut-off 50 000) positioned in the lumen of the model (d). Used dialysis liquid is collected in another bottle for analysis. The amount of chyme in the model is monitored with a pressure sensor (e) and kept on a pre-set level through the absorption of water with a pump in the dialysis circuit. The ileal effluent medium (j) is mixed and kept anaerobic with nitrogen (f), and is introduced into the large intestinal model with the peristaltic valve system (g) as described for TIM-1. Samples can be taken from a sample port (h). Gas is collected in a gas-bag (i).

The system is inoculated with a standardised microbiota. For this, ten healthy adult individuals donate a faecal sample, which is subsequently mixed and used to inoculate a fed-batch fermentor and grown to 5 litres during a period of 40 h. Subsequently, this microbial suspension is aliquoted and snap-frozen in liquid nitrogen using a cryoprotectant. The aliquots are then stored at −80 °C and used as inocula for TIM-2. This results in the ability to use a standardised microbiota in several (approximately 100) experiments over time, and allows the comparison of different substrates with the same standardised microbiota (Venema *et al.*, 2000). Alternatively, the faecal donations of different individuals can be inoculated in different TIM-2 models, to allow for the comparsion between individuals on the same substrate (Venema *et al.*, 2003).

12.4 Model validation

Validation of the TIM systems has been an integral part of the development of the systems. After all, what good is a model if it does not mimic the real world? The stomach and small intestinal model (TIM-1) has been validated with respect to the digestion of carbohydrate, protein and fat (Minekus 1998), survival of probiotic microorganisms (Marteau *et al.*, 1997), availability for uptake by the body of both fat- and water- soluble vitamins (Minekus and van de Berg, personal communication), and the availability of minerals, such as calcium, iron and phopshorus (Larsson *et al.*, 1997).

TIM-2 has been been more difficult to validate, owing to the limited accessibility of the colon in humans. For this, use has been made of so-called sudden-death individuals, who died because of a heart attack, road accident or gun shot wound and had given prior written consent for their bodies to be used for research (Cummings *et al.*, 1987; Macfarlane *et al.*, 1992). Using those data, TIM-2 was developed and validated with respect to the activity and composition of the microbiota (Minekus *et al.*, 1999; Venema *et al.*, 2000). Concentrations of microbial metabolites, such as SCFA, lactate, ammonia and other protein fermentative compounds are within the physiological range.

12.5 Models for different applications

The various dynamic GI tract models developed by TNO so far simulate the gastrointestinal conditions of babies, young adults and the elderly, as well as those of dogs (Smeets-Peeters 2000; Smeets-Peeters *et al.*, 1998, 1999), pigs and calves (Minekus, 1998). Besides the average physiological conditions and the biological variation, abnormal or specific conditions can also be simulated in a reproducible way. Selected examples are given below.

12.5.1 Infant model

Compared with adults and the elderly, infants have a different physiology of the GI tract (Ménard, 1994). This means that these different parameters, such as transit through the gastric compartment, secretion of gastric acid and concentrations of enzymes need to be adjusted when the physiology of infants is to be mimicked properly. Also when mimicking the large intestine, the inoculum needs to be collected from infants. Here, differences in microbiota between breast-fed infants and those fed an infant formula have to be taken into account.

12.5.2 Simulation of patients

In most instances, physiological parameters reported in literature reflect those of healthy individuals. In TIM the two extremes in a population can be mimicked to test the effect of the extremes on the process of interest (e.g. probiotic survival under conditions of slow versus fast gastric transit, or high versus low bile salt concentrations in the duodenum). The system allows specific change to one parameter while all others are kept constant. In this manner also several patient populations can be mimicked (e.g. those with a pancreatic insufficiency, secreting only low amounts of pancreatic enzymes; http://www.hacres.com/diet/research/Enzyme_TNO_Brochure.pdf). However, to properly mimic the conditions and parameters of patients, we depend on the available literature data.

For the large intestine, experiments have been carried out with a microbiota collected from patients with inflammatory bowel disease (IBD) (Van Nuenen *et al.*, 2004, 2005). Changes in the kinetics and amount of SCFA produced by the microbiota from IBD patients in comparison with that of healthy individuals have led to the identification of possible mechanisms that underlie relapse in these patients, based on the activity of the microbiota (Van Nuenen *et al.*, 2004, 2005).

12.5.3 Animal models

So far, the development of the TIM models has been restricted to monogastrics. However, besides human systems, systems have also been developed for dogs, pigs and calves (which at a young age can also be considered monogastric) for TIM-1, and dogs, pigs and ducks for TIM-2. The development of FIDO (the dog-equivalent of TIM) was initiated as an alternative for animal experiments (Smeets-Peeters 2000; Smeets-Peeters *et al.*, 1998, 1999). Besides the ethical reason to reduce the number of anmials used in experiments, it was also recognised that the *in vitro* model enabled study of certain mechanisms that could not be revealed in the animal experiments, such as the bioavailability of calcium from various sources (Smeets-Peeters 2000; Smeets-Peeters *et al.*, 1999). An interesting example of how the *in vitro* model provides data that cannot be obtained even in

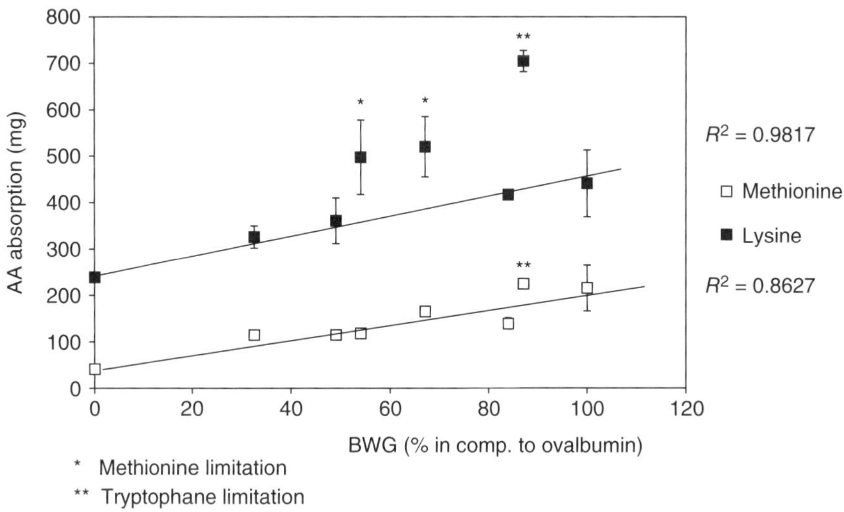

Fig. 12.5 Body weight gain (BWG) of chickens plotted against the amino acids (AA) absorbed in TIM-1 on different feeds.

animal experiments is exemplified in Fig. 12.5. This shows the body weight gain (BWG) of chickens plotted against the availability for uptake of amino acids from different feeds (in the figure only methionine and lysine are plotted, which are usually limiting for growth in various feeds). When a data-point is on the solid line, the amino acid is limiting for growth; when it is above the line it is not. The figure shows that several feeds are limiting in both methionine and lysine; some only in one of the two amino acids. One feed (indicated with **) is not limiting in either of these two amino acids, but appeared to be limiting in tryptophan. It is not possible to get this type of data from animal experiments alone, except by trial and error, since even if the animals are sampled a mass-balance cannot be made, owing to the use of the amino acids by the animal. TIM does allow to make a full mass-balance, and thus allows the study of underlying mechanisms of the processes occuring in the GI tract with respect to digestion, solubility of minerals, etc.

12.6 Applications

The *in vitro* models can be used for numerous applications. Some have already been mentioned in the paragraphs above. Apart from obvious applications in food digestion and functional food development, which will be exemplified below, pharmaceutical applications are numerous. However, also with respect to the availability of heavy metals when a baby takes a mouthful of polluted soil, the models have been shown to be powerful tools to determine risk of exposure to these toxic compounds. The following examples will be limited in number and restricted to functional foods. For a full overview of possibilities, we refer to Section 12.8.

12.6.1 Survival of probiotics

In a validation study with volunteers who had a nasal tube until the end of the small intestine (terminal ileum; Marteau *et al.*, 1997) the survival of probiotic strains after passage through the upper GI tract was compared. The data showed an excellent correlation between the *in vitro* results and those from clinical studies for nine different probiotic isolates (Marteau *et al.*, 1997 and unpublished results). This has led us to conclude that the *in vitro* model is predictive for establishing the survival of probiotics. Apart from the average physiological parameters in a population, the extremes can also be tested. When this is done for gastric transit and bile concentrations, the model can predict not only the average survival in a population, but also the extremes, allowing food companies to optimise the dose in their product to reach efficicay in the whole study population (Marteau *et al.*, 1997). Owing to the predictive nature of the system, it has been used to develop enteric-coated capsules containing probiotics (Rudolph *et al.*, 2005), and even chewable tablets (Venema *et al.*, 2008).

12.6.2 Prebiotics, the production of butyrate and changing the composition of the microbiota

SCFA (acetate, propionate and butyrate) are the major end products of bacterial fermentation in the large intestine and affect key functions of the colonic epithelium *in vivo*. These compounds are key participants in gut maintenance (Bergman, 1990; Kruh *et al.*, 1991; Mariadason *et al.*, 2000) and may also be beneficial contributors to the peripheral metabolism in humans (Macfarlane and Cummings, 1991). Therefore, SCFA have been the subject of numerous investigations. Butyrate is considered the most important of the SCFA (Hamer *et al.*, 2008). In the large intestine, butyrate is present in millimolar concentrations. Butyrate is metabolised by epithelial cells and is responsible for 70% of their energy need (Roediger, 1982; Scheppach, 1994). In addition, butyrate has been shown to influence numerous processes, such as epithelial cell proliferation and differentiation, cancer suppression and mucosal inflammation (Hamer *et al.*, 2008).

Prebiotics are defined as components in the food that stimulate health-beneficial microbes in the endogenous microbiota (Gibson and Roberfroid, 1995). Since practically all prebiotics commercialised to date are carbohydrates, they are fermented by the colonic microbiota and lead to the production of SCFA (and consequently might lower putrefactive fermentation of proteins; Van Nuenen *et al.*, 2003). TIM-2 allows the study of the effect of prebiotics on both SCFA production as well as changes in the composition of the microbiota (Maathuis *et al.*, submitted; Van Nuenen *et al.*, 2003; Venema *et al.*, 2003, 2005, submitted). In TIM-2 all the SCFA that are produced are collected, while *in vivo* no mass-balance can be made and production of SCFA can be highly underestimated. For instance, in faeces only ~5% of estimated daily production of SCFA can be found, because >95% of the SCFA are taken up by the colonic epithelium. Faecal concentrations of SCFA therefore only reflect local production of SCFA (Venema *et al.*, 2003). Also, when sampling blood, most of the SCFA are extracted by the colonic epithelium (for butyrate) or the liver (for acetate and propionate). However, novel technologies using stable isotope techniques have been developed recently to study the processes in the colon in more detail (see Section 12.7).

12.6.3 Safety evaluation studies related to genetically modified foods

TIM-1 has also been used to study gene stability and gene transfer of genetically modified (GM) foods (Van der Vossen and Havenaar, 1997). These results showed that free DNA from GM crops was rapidly degraded in the stomach and particularly in the duodenum within minutes, but that the genes could still be found in the ileum when present in the crop itself, indicting that the genes were protected from degradative enzymes through their presence within the cell-structure of the plant. Also, transfer of antibiotic-resistance markers between different microorganisms could be shown, albeit at a very low frequency. The models also allow the stability of new (GM) proteins to be studied, in terms of risk of allergenicity of these proteins.

12.6.4 Bioconversion of polyphenols

Flavonoids and other polyphenolic dietary compounds are studied, for instance, for their antioxidant capacity and/or effects on colon cancer (e.g. for quercetin). However, the colonic microbiota is capable of fermenting these polyphenolic compounds and producing all kinds of other phenolic metabolites (Gao *et al.*, 2006). Some of these microbial metabolites have interesting activities (Gao *et al.*, 2006), although for most metabolites this has not been studied. It is clear, however, that the polyphenols are rapidly converted by the microbiota and, therefore, that it may be necessary to focus on the microbial metabolites and their bioactivity rather than on the polyphenols itself. It is also clear that studies in rodents do not reflect what could happen in the colon of humans, as rodents have a different microbiota with different activity. Hence, the use of *in vitro* models mimicking the large intestine of human individuals is imperative in these kinds of studies.

Application of the model has also been shown to speed up the development of a novel clinical food (Zeijdner and Mohede, 1999). These are just a few examples of the multiple applications of *in vitro* models. The interested reader is referred to Section 12.8 for more information.

12.7 Future trends

12.7.1 Stable isotope technologies

The importance of the human large intestine for nutrition, health and disease, is becoming increasingly realised. There are numerous indications of a distinct role of the gut in such important issues as immune disorders and obesity-linked diseases. Research on this long-neglected organ, which is colonised by a myriad of bacteria, is a rapidly growing field that is currently providing fascinating new insights in the processes going on in the colon, and their relevance for the human host due to the use of stable-isotope technologies (De Graaf and Venema, 2007; Egert *et al.*, 2007). Use of stable isotopes for bioavailability studies are discussed elsewhere in this book. Here we will focus on the use of stable isotopes to study the processes in the large intestine. Perhaps one of the greatest difficulties in research of intestinal metabolism and function is the requirement for adequate minimally invasive experimental techniques that allow for *in vivo* research in humans. Such techniques will have to cope with severely limited possibilities for manipulation of experimental conditions as well as for material sampling. The use of stable isotopes may prove to be a key factor to success here. Stable isotope-labelled molecules follow the same metabolic routes, and function identically in physiological processes as their natural unlabelled counterparts. The isotopic label, however, allows for their specific detection at any desired stage after their administration, allowing the processes in which they are involved to be indirectly monitored. We have set out to use stable-isotope labelled substrates (primarily ^{13}C-labelling) in combination with TIM-2, to shed some light on the processes that happen in the dark environment of the colon. The principle of the use of stable-isotope labelled substrates is shown in Fig. 12.6 (Venema *et al.*, 2007). The substrate is incubated with a microbiota, either in a test tube, a sophisticated *in vitro* model such as TIM-2, or even a human being. Subsequently, some members of the microbiota ferment the substrate. Hence, the label ends up in microbial metabolites, but also in the biomass of those members of the microbiota that have fermented the substrate. Both metabolites (with metabolomics) and biomass (with stable isotope probing) can be analysed specifically with respect to the presence of the label (see below).

Metabolomics

Of the functional genomics toolbox, metabolomics is the most recent addition. The technique involves the non-targeted, holistic analysis of changes in the total set of metabolites in a sample (the metabolome) in response to environmental or cellular changes. Only now is the metabolomics approach technically feasible, owing to the enormous improvements made in the past few years in analytical chemistry and bioinformatics. There have been enormous improvements in the separation and detection of metabolites. Moreover, progress in bioinformatics now makes it possible to process and

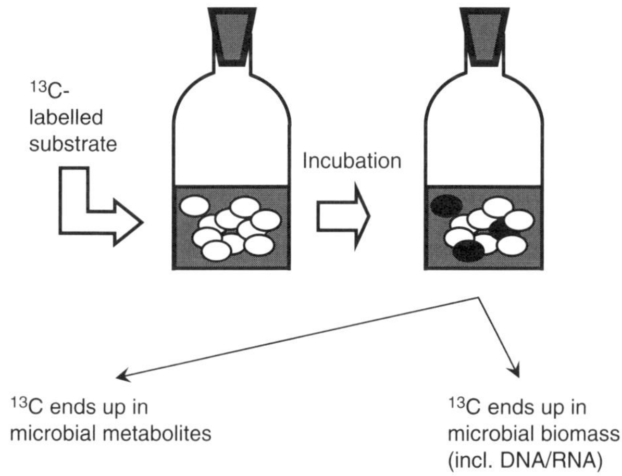

Fig. 12.6 The principle of stable-isotope use. A ^{13}C-labelled substrate is added to a microbiota. Certain members of the microbiota (indicated by the black circles) will ferment the substrate and consequently produce metabolites from the substrate which become labelled, as well as incorporate the label in their biomass.

interpret large sets of biochemical data generated through this non-biased holistic approach.

Most measurements on microbiota and metabolites in humans are performed in faeces, which is basically the only non-invasive material that can be obtained from healthy volunteers. A drawback of analysing faecal samples is the fact that they do not represent quantitatively what happens in the proximal part of the colon where fermentation of most prebiotics takes place. SCFAs from prebiotic fermentation are predominantly produced in the proximal part of the colon and will be absorbed by the body to a considerable extent (>95%) during subsequent transit of the chyme to the distal colon and rectum, which may take anywhere from 24 to >72 hours depending on the individual. Consequently, the amount of SCFA recovered in the faeces will not reflect those resulting from fermentation of the prebiotics in the proximal colon, but rather that of local production in the distal colon. In an attempt to clarify what happens in the colon and to set up the tools to study this, TIM-2 was fed with 1 gram of ^{13}C-labelled glucose (as a model substrate) (Egert *et al.*, 2007). In this study RNA-stable isotope probing (SIP) and nuclear magnetic resonance (NMR)-based metabolic profiling of fermentation products were combined to identify bacteria fermenting carbohydrates under conditions simulating the human GI tract. In the experiment using 40 mM of uniformly labelled ^{13}C-glucose, NMR analysis revealed ^{13}C-labelled lactate, acetate, butyrate and formate as the principal fermentation products, while also ethanol and glycerol were detected. Glycerol was absent from the dialysate spectra, suggesting a cytoplasmic origin.

Within the colon a complex foodweb exists, comprising microbe–microbe and host–microbe metabolite exchange. Singly labelled acetate (a 2-carbon molecule) and doubly labelled butyrate (a 4-carbon molecule) were found. This is indicative of mixing of labelled metabolites with an unlabelled pool present before introduction of the substrate (e.g. for doubly labelled butyrate, the coupling of a fully labelled acetate with a non-labelled acetate). This, and the kinetics of butyrate production, have led the authors to conclude that cross-feeding occurred between different members of the microbiota. The study showed that stable isotope-based techniques hold great potential to couple the fermentation of carbohydrates in the human GI tract – including those with a prebiotic character – with phylogenetic identities of distinct intestinal bacteria (Egert *et al.*, 2006). With the advent of this technology, we are currently testing more relevant carbohydrates to test their fermentation characteristics.

Stable isotope probing

Clearly, a deeper understanding of their role in health and disease requires unravelling the *in situ* functionality of the microorganisms colonising the human GI tract. For this, researchers have to cope with the individuality and complexity of a community in a hardly accessible habitat. On the other hand, since there are only a limited number of biochemical routes leading from a given substrate (e.g. glucose) to a product (e.g. acetate), it is probable that there is an enormous functional redundancy in this system. Nevertheless, many of the conversions carried out by individual species of the GI tract microbiota and the resulting metabolic fluxes are not known, or knowledge is anecdotal. Since little is know about the actual *in situ* functions of human colonic microorganisms, SIP techniques appear particularly promising. SIP approaches involve incubation of microorganisms with a stable isotope labelled substrate under conditions resembling the environmental situation (Fig. 12.6 above). Only the actively metabolising microbes incorporate the label into their biomass, including phylogenetic biomarkers. After incubation, identification of active microbes is achieved by molecular analysis of labelled vs. unlabelled biomarkers. Here, nucleic acids clearly have the highest phylogenetic resolution and allow identification of active, but not-yet-cultured species (De Graaf and Venema, 2007; Egert *et al.*, 2006). RNA is the most responsive (sensitive) biomarker for SIP analyses, since it occurs in higher cellular copy numbers, has a higher turnover rate than DNA, and is produced independent of cellular replication (Manefield *et al.*, 2002). In the experiments in TIM-2 eluded to above using uniformly labelled glucose (Egert *et al.*, 2007), 16S rRNA T-RFLP was used to assess the microbes that used the labelled glucose. Labelling of various microbial species could be detected. Specifically, bacteria that were active after glucose addition were related to *Streptococcus bovis*, *Enterococcus faecium* and *E. faecalis*, and *Clostridium perfringens*, because they had incorporated glucose-derived ^{13}C into their rRNA. *S. bovis* and *C. perfringens* were regarded as the most active glucose-fermenters in the gut model under these circumstances. Again, these experiments show the power of stable-isotope technology, and it is our belief that this technology holds great promise for the future.

12.7.2 DNA micro-arrays to study the composition of the microbiota

Another exciting new area of development is the use of DNA micro-arrays to study the composition of the intestinal microbiota. To date, two platforms have been developed independently (Rajilić-Stojanović, 2007; Schuren *et al.*, submitted). The study of the composition of the (intestinal) microbiota has recently gained enormous momentum through the development of such DNA micro-array methods to study the presence of hundreds of species at the same time. Like other molecular approaches that have been used in the recent past, the micro-array platform also relies on the species-specific DNA signatures in the 16S rDNA. Owing to the high-throughput DNA sequencing possibilities of this decade, these micro-arrays can be customised for every conceivable complex microbiota. Shifts in the composition of the microbiota – for instance, before and after intake of prebiotics – can be quickly addressed using this technology. The DNA-microarray platform developed by TNO (Schuren *et al.*, submitted), named the Intestinal-Chip (or I-Chip), contains over 350 probes that detect in a semi-quantitative way different bacteria at the level of individual species, genera, and larger phylogenetic groups. The array developed by the Wageningen University (Rajilić-Stojanović, 2007), the HITChip, is a high-density phylogenetic microarray targeting small subunit ribosomal RNA sequences of all microbial phylotypes hitherto described for the human GI tract, and contains close to 1200 probes. It was used to assess the impact of faecal inoculum preparation and operation conditions of TIM-2. This study revealed that propagation of mixed faecal donations as is used for the preparation of a standardised inoculum for TIM-2 (Venema *et al.*, 2000) has only a limited effect on the microbiota composition, with slight changes observed mainly within the Firmicutes. Hierarchical cluster analysis showed that samples taken throughout the inoculum preparation grouped with microbiota profiles observed for faecal samples of healthy adults. The changes detected with the HITChip could be confirmed, although at low resolution, by denaturing gradient gel electrophoresis of small subunit rRNA amplicons.

Combining metabolomics, stable isotope probing and DNA micro-arrays

The ultimate use of the new technologies described above would be a combination of them. Analysing fractions with high incorporation of label with high-throughput array-platforms allows the functionality of the intestinal microbiota to be studied in more detail. Certainly, if that can be done on the level of mRNA to reveal which genes are active under the given conditions, coupled to production of metabolites, and biochemical pathways, in

Table 12.2 List of colonic *in vitro* models and (selected; most relevant) Pubmed authors that have published on them

SHIME (simulator of the human intestinal microbial ecosystem)	Verstraete W, Van de Wiele TR, De Boever P
A 4-stage colon simulator	Mäkeläinen HS, Ouwehand AC
A multistage continuous culture simulator of the human colonic microbiota	Macfarlane S, Macfarlane GT
A three-stage continuous culture system	Gibson GR, Rastall RA, Tuohy KM, Tzortzis G
An *in vitro* colonic model with immobilised cells	Lacroix C, Fliss I

the near future we will see a systems biology approach to this complex microbial community that, in addition, has several interactions with its host. Apart from *in vitro* models, these techniques can be used in a clinical setting, allowing study of the microbiota in its natural habitat. Combined with other disciplines such as gastro-enterology, and progress in totally unrelated fields such as nanotechnology, it is clear that exciting times are ahead for those people active in this research field.

12.8 Sources of further information and advice

For further reading with respect to the future developments in *in vitro* models, the interested reader is referred to reviews by De Graaf and Venema (2007) and Egert *et al.* (2006) for stable isotope technology. An excellent review on the state-of-the-art of the microbiota in the GI tract has recently been published (Rajilić-Stojanović *et al.*, 2007). For combinations of *in vitro* models with cell cultures the reader is referred to Verwei *et al.* (2006). Only a limited number of examples have been given with respect to the application of *in vitro* models. For more examples, the interested reader is advised to search Pubmed for the authors of this contribution.

For more information on other colonic *in vitro* models, Table 12.2 gives a list of models, with corresponding authors that can be searched in Pubmed.

12.9 References

BABINSZKY L, VAN DER MEER JM, BOER H, and DEN HARTOG LA (1990), 'An *in-vitro* method for the prediction of the digestible crude protein content in pig feeds', *J Sci Food Agric*, **50**, 173–178 **doi: 10.1002/jsfa.2740500205**

BARRY JL, HOEBLER C, MACFARLANE GT, MACFARLANE S, MATHERS JC, REED KA, MORTENSEN PB, NORDGAARD I, ROWLAND IR, and RUMNEY CJW (1995), 'Estimation of the fermentability of dietary fibre *in vitro*: a European interlaboratory study', *Br J Nutr*, **74**, 303–332 **doi: 10.1079/BJN19950137**

BERGMAN EN (1990), 'Energy contributions of volatile fatty acids from the gastrointestinal tract in various species', *Physiol Rev*, **70**, 567–590

BOISEN S, and EGGUM BO (1991), 'Critical evaluation of *in vitro* methods for estimation digestibility in simple-stomach animals', *Nutr Res Rev*, **4**, 141–162

BOISEN S, and FERNADEZ JA (1991a), '*In vitro* digestibility of energy and amino acids in pig feeds' pp 231–236 In: Verstegen MWA, Huisman J and Hartog LA (Eds) *Digestive Physiology in Pigs*, PuDoc, Wageningen, the Netherlands

BOISEN S, and FERNADEZ JA (1991b), '*In vitro* digestion as a basis for the prediction of energy and protein value in pig feeds'. 42nd Annual Meeting of European Association of Animal Production, Berlin, Germany

BÜCHMANN NB (1979), '*In vitro* digestibility of protein from barley and other cereals', *J Sci Food Agric*, **30**, 583–589

BURKS TF, GALLIGAN JJ, PORRECA F, and BARBER WD (1985), 'Regulation of gastric emptying', *Fed Proc*, **44**, 2897–2901

COUTTS TM, ALDRICK AJ, and ROWLAND IR (1987), 'Use of continuous culture to study the gastric microflora of a hypochlorhydric patient', *Toxicity in Vitro*, **1**, 17–21

CUMMINGS JH, POMARE EW, BRANCH WJ, NAYLOR CP, and MACFARLANE GT (1987), 'Short chain fatty acids in human large intestine, portal, hepatic and venous blood', *Gut*, **28**, 1221–1227 **doi: 10.1136/gut.28.10.1221**

DECUYPERE JA, DENHOOVEN RM, and HENDERICKX HK (1986), 'Stomach emptying of milk diets in pigs. A mathematical model allowing description and comparison of the emptying pattern, *Arch Animal Nutr*, **36**, 679–696

DE GRAAF AA, and VENEMA K (2007), 'Gaining insight in microbial physiology in the large intestine: a special role for stable isotopes', *Adv Microb Physiol*, **53**, 73–168 **doi: 10.1016/S0065–2911(07)53002-X**

EGERT M, DE GRAAF AA, SMIDT H, DE VOS WM, and VENEMA K (2006), 'Beyond diversity: functional microbiomics of the human colon', *Trends Microbiol*, **14**, 86–91 **doi: 10.1016/j.tim.2005.12.007**

EGERT M, DE GRAAF AA, MAATHUIS A, DE WAARD P, PLUGGE CM, SMIDT H, DEUTZ NEP, DIJKEMA C, DE VOS WM, and VENEMA, K (2007), 'Identification of glucose-fermenting bacteria present in an *in-vitro* model of the human intestine by RNA-stable isotope probing', *FEMS Microbiol Ecol*, **60**, 126–135 **doi: 10.1111/j.1574–6941.2007.00281.x**

ELASHOFF JD, REEDY TJ and MEYER JH (1982), 'Analysis of gastric emptying data', *Gastroenterology*, **83**, 1306–1312

ENGLYST HN, KINGMAN SM, and CUMMINGS JH (1992), 'Classification and measurement of nutritionally important starch fractions', *Eur J Clin Nutr*, **46**, s33–s50

EVANS DF, PYE G, BRAMLEY R, CLARK AG, DYSON TJ, and HARDCASTLE JD (1988), 'Measurements of gastrointestinal pH profiles in normal ambulant subjects', *Gut*, **29**, 1035–1041 **doi:10.1136/gut.29.8.1035**

FRETER R (1992), 'Factors affecting the microecology of the gut', pp 111–144 In: Fuller R (Ed) *Probiotics*, Chapman and Hall, London, UK

FURUYA S, SAKAMOTO K, and TAKAHASHI S (1979), 'A new *in vitro* method for the estimation of digestability using the intestinal fluid of the pig', *Br J Nutr*, **41**, 511–520

GAO K, XU A, KRUL C, VENEMA K, LIU Y, NIU Y, LU J, BENSOUSSAN L, SEERAM NP, HEBER D, and HENNING SM (2006), 'Of major phenolic acids formed during human microbial fermentation of tea, citrus, and soy flavonoid supplements only 3,4-dihydroxyphenylacetic acid has antiproliferative activity', *J Nutr*, **136**, 52–57

GAUTHIER SF, VACHON C, JONES JD, and SAVOIE I (1982), 'Assessment of protein digestibility by *in vitro* enzymatic hydrolysis with simultaneous dialysis', *J Nutr*, **112**, 1718–1725

GAUTHIER SF, VACHON C, and SAVOIE I (1986), 'Enzymatic conditions of an *in vitro* method to study protein digestion', *J Food Sci*, **51**, 960–964 **doi: 10.1111/j.1365–2621.1986.tb11208.x**

GIBSON GR, and ROBERFROID MB (1995), 'Dietary modulation of the human colonic microbiota, introducing the concept of prebiotics', *J Nutr*, **125**, 1401–1412

GIBSON GR, CUMMINGS JH, and MACFARLANE GT (1988), 'Use of three-stage continuous culture system to study the effect of mucin on dissimilatory sulfate reduction and methanogenesis by mixed populations of human gut bacteria', *Appl Environm Microbiol*, **54**, 2750–2755

HAMER HM, JONKERS D, VENEMA K, VANHOUTVIN S, TROOST FJ, and BRUMMER R-J (2008), 'Review article, the role of butyrate on colonic function', *Aliment Pharmacol Ther*, **27**, 104–119 **doi: 10.1111/j.1365–2036.2007.03562.x**

HOLGATE AM, and READ NW (1983), 'Relation between small bowel transit time and absorption of a solid meal', *Dig Dis Sci*, **28**, 812–819 **doi: 10.1007/BF01296904**

HOLM J, LUNDQUIST I, BJÖRCK I, ELIASSON A, and ASP NG (1988), 'Degree of starch gelatinization, digestion rate of starch *in vitro*, and metabolic response in rats', *Am J Clin Nutr*, **47**, 1010–1016

KRUH J, DEFER N, and TICHONICKY L (1991), 'Molecular and cellular effects of sodium butyrate', In: pp 45–50 Roche AF, (Ed) *Short-chain Fatty Acids, Metabolism and Clinical Importance*, Report of the tenth Ross conference on medical research. Ross Laboratories, Columbus, Ohio

LARSSON M, MINEKUS M, and HAVENAAR R (1997), 'Estimation of the bio-availability of iron and phosphorus in cereals using a dynamic *in-vitro* gastrointestinal model', *J Sci Food Agric*, **74**, 99–106 **doi: 10.1002/(SICI)1097–0010(199705)74:1<99::AID-JSFA775>3.0.CO;2-G**

LONGLAND AC (1991), 'Digestive enzyme activities in pigs and poultry', pp 3–18 In: Fuller MF (Ed) *In vitro Digestion for Pigs and Poultry*, CAB International, Wallingford, UK

MAATHUIS A, HOFFMAN A, EVANS A, SANDERS L, and VENEMA K (submitted), 'The effect of maize based fibres on the activity and composition of the microbiota determined in a dynamic in vitro model of the human large intestine'

MACFARLANE GT, and CUMMINGS JH (1991), 'The colonic flora, fermentation and large bowel digestive function', In: pp 51–92 Phillips SF, Pemberton JH and Shorter RG (Eds), *The large intestine, physiology, pathophysiology, and disease* Raven Press, New York

MACFARLANE GT, GIBSON GR, and CUMMINGS JH (1992), 'Comparison of fermentation reactions in different regions of the human colon', *J Appl Bacteriol*, **72**, 57–64

MANEFIELD M, WHITELEY AS, OSTLE N, INESON P, and BAILEY MJ (2002), 'RNA stable isotope probing, a novel means of linking microbial community function to Phylogeny', *Appl Environ Microbiol*, **68**, 5367–5373 **doi: 10.1128/AEM.68.11.5367–5373.2002**

MARIADASON JM, CORNER GA, and AUGENLICHT LH (2000), 'Genetic reprogramming in pathways of colonic cell maturation induced by short chain fatty acids: comparison with trichostatin A, sulindac, and curcumin and implications for chemoprevention of colon cancer', *Cancer Res*, **60**, 4561–4572

MARTEAU P, POCHART P, BOUHNIK Y, and RAMBAUD JC (1993), 'Fate and effects of some transiting microorganisms in the human gastrointestinal tract', *World Rev Nutr Diet*, **74**, 1–21

MARTEAU P, MINEKUS M, HAVENAAR R, and HUIS IN'T VELD JHJ (1997), 'Survival of lactic acid bacteria in a dynamic model of the stomach and small intestine: validation and the effects of bile', *J Dairy Sci*, **80**, 1031–1037

MCNEILL ALEXANDER R (1994), 'Optimum gut structure for specified diets', pp 54–62 In: Chivers DJ and Langer P (Eds), *The Digestive System in Mammals*, Cambridge University Press, Cambridge

MÉNARD D (1994), 'Development of human intestinal and gastric enzymes', *Acta Paediatr Suppl*, **405**, 1–6

MILLER TL, and WOLIN MJ (1981), 'Fermentation by the human large intestine microbial community in an *in vitro* semi continuous culture system', *Appl Environm Microbiol*, **42**, 400–407

MINEKUS M (1998), 'Development and validation of a dynamic model of the gastrointestinal tract', PhD Thesis, University of Utrecht, Elinkwijk bv, Utrecht, Netherlands

MINEKUS M, MARTEAU P, HAVENAAR R, and HUIS IN'T VELD JHJ (1995), 'A multi compartmental dynamic computer-controlled model simulating the stomach and small intestine', *Alternat Lab Animals*, **23**, 197–209

MINEKUS M, SMEETS-PEETERS M, BERNALIER A, MAROL-BONNIN S, HAVENAAR R, MARTEAU P, ALRIC M, FONTY G, and HUIS IN'T VELD JH (1999), 'A computer-controlled system to simulate conditions of the large intestine with peristaltic mixing, water absorption and absorption of fermentation products', *Appl Microbiol Biotechnol*, **53**, 108–114 **doi: 10.1007/s002530051622**

MOLLY K, VAN DE WOESTYNE M, and VERSTRAETE W (1993), 'Development of a 5-step multichamber reactor as a simulation of the human intestinal microbial ecosystem', *Appl Microbiol Biotechnol*, **39**, 254–258 **doi: 10.1007/BF00228615**

NOTIVOL R, CARRIO I, CANO L, ESTORCH M, and VILARDELL F (1984), 'Gastric emptying of solid and liquid meals in healthy young subjects', *Scand J Gastroenterol*, **19**, 1107–1113

PEDERSEN B, and EGGUM BO (1983), 'Prediction of protein digestibility by an *in vitro* enzymatic pH-stat procedure', *Zeitschrift für Tierphysiology, Tierernährung und Futtrmittelkunde*, **45**, 190–200

RAJILIĆ-STOJANOVIĆ M (2007), 'Diversity of the human gastrointestinal microbiota, novel perspectives from high throughput analyses', PhD thesis, Wageningen University, the Netherlands

RAJILIĆ-STOJANOVIĆ M, SMIDT H, and DE VOS WM (2007), 'Diversity of the human gastrointestinal tract microbiota revisited', *Environ Microbiol*, **9**, 2125–2136 **doi: 10.1111/j.1462–2920.2007.01369.x**

ROEDIGER WE (1982), 'Utilization of nutrients by isolated epithelial cells of the rat colon', *Gastroenterology*, **83**, 424–429

RUDOLPH MW, MANNECK I, and HENKE S (2005), 'Development of a novel controlled release tablet formulation for the site specific delivery of probiotic strains', In: *Proceedings of the CRS Annual Meeting*, Miami, FL

RUMNEY CJ, and ROWLAND IA (1992), '*In vivo* and *in vitro* models of the human colonic flora' *Crit Rev Food Sci Nutr*, **31**, 299–331

SAVALLE B, MIRANDA G, and PELISSIER, JP (1989), '*In vitro* simulation of gastric digestion of milk proteins', *J Agric Food Chem*, **37**, 1336–1340 **doi: 10.1021/jf00089a028**

SAVOIE, L (1994), 'Digestion and absorption of food, usefulness and limitations of *in vitro* models', *Can J Physiol Pharmacol*, **72**, 407–414 **doi:10.1139/y94–060**

SCHAAFSMA, G (1997), 'Nutritional evaluation of novel and functional foods', pp 81–95 In: *The Western Diet with a Special Focus on Dairy Products*, Institue Danone, Bruxelles, Belgium

SCHEPPACH W (1994), 'Effects of short chain fatty acids on gut morphology and function', *Gut*, 35, S35–S38

SCHUREN F, DE VLIEGER A, CASPERS M, KIERS J, NAUTA A, VAN DER VOSSEN J, and TE BIESEBEKE R (submitted), 'PCR and microarray analysis of infant microbiota composition in a double-blinded placebo-controlled clinical trial'

SMEETS-PEETERS MJE (2000), 'Feeding FIDO, Development, validation and application of a dynamic *in vitro* model of the gastrointestinal tract of the dog', PhD Thesis Wageningen University Universal Press, Veenendaal, The Netherlands

SMEETS-PEETERS MJE, WATSON T, MINEKUS M, and HAVENAAR R (1998), 'A review of the physiology of the canine digestive tract related to the development of *in vitro* systems', *Nutr Res Rev*, **11**, 45–69

SMEETS-PEETERS MJE, MINEKUS M, HAVENAAR R, SCHAAFSMA G, and VERSTEGEN MWA (1999), 'Description of a dynamic *in vitro* model of the dog gastrointestinal tract and an evaluation of various transit times for protein and calcium', *Alternat Lab Animals*, **27**, 935–949

UMESAKI Y, OKADA Y, IMAOKA A, SETOYAMA H, and MATSUMOTO S (1997), 'Interactions between epithelial cells and bacteria, normal and pathogenic', *Science*, **276**, 964–965 **doi**: **10.1126/science.276.5314.964**

VAN DER VOSSEN J, and HAVENAAR R (1997), 'Gene stability and gene transfer of genetically modified foods in the TNO gastro-intestinal model', pp 22–23 In: van der Kamp JW and Havenaar R (Eds), *Safety Evaluation Methods of Novel and Transgenic Food Crops*, Proceedings Sixth SABAF Workshop AIR Concerted Action CT 94 2342, Vienna, Austria, TNO, Zeist, the Netherlands

VAN HOEIJ KA, GREEN CJ, PIJNEN A, SPECKMANN A, and BINDELS JG (1997), 'A novel *in vitro* method to asess colonic short chain fatty acid (SCFA) and gas production of indigestible carbohydrates', p 131 In: *Proceedings of the International Symposium 'Non-digestible oligosaccharides: healthy food for the colon*?', Wageningen, the Netherlands

VAN NUENEN HMC, MEYER PD, and VENEMA K (2003), 'The effect of various inulins and *Clostridium difficile* on the metabolic activity of the human colonic microbiota *in vitro*', *Microb Ecol Health Dis*, **15**, 137–144 **doi**: **10.1080/08910600310018959**

VAN NUENEN HMC, VENEMA K, VAN DER WOUDE JCJ, and KUIPERS EJ (2004), 'The metabolic activity of fecal microbiota from healthy individuals and patients with inflammatory bowel disease', *Dig Dis Sci*, **49**, 485–491 **doi**: **10.1023/B:DDAS.0000020508.64440.73**

VAN NUENEN M, DE LIGT RA, DOORNBOS RP, VENEMA K, VAN DER WOUDE CJ, and KUIPERS EJ (2005), 'The influence of microbial metabolites on human intestinal epithelial cells and macrophages *in vitro*', *FEMS Immunol Med Microbiol*, **45**, 183–189 **doi**: **10.1016/j.femsim.2005.03.010**

VATIER J, LIONNET F, VITRE MT, and MIGNON M (1988), 'A model of an artificial stomach for assessing the characteristics of an antacid', *Aliment Pharmacol Therap*, **2**, 461–470 **doi**: **10.1111/j.1365–2036.1988.tb00719.x**

VENEMA K, VAN NUENEN HMC, SMEETS-PEETERS M, MINEKUS M, and HAVENAAR R (2000), 'TNO's *in vitro* large intestinal model, an excellent screening tool for functional food and pharmaceutical research', *Ernährung/Nutrition*, **24**, 558–564

VENEMA K, VAN NUENEN H, VAN DEN HEUVEL E, POOL W, and VAN DER VOSSEN J (2003), 'The effect of lactulose on the composition of the intestinal microbiota and short-chain fatty acid production in human volunteers and a computer-controlled model of the proximal large intestine', *Microb Ecol Health Dis*, **15**, 94–105 **doi**: **10.1080/08910600310019895**

VENEMA K, VERMUNT SHF, and BRINK EJ (2005), 'D-Tagatose increases butyrate production by colonic microbiota in healthy men and women', *Microb Ecol Health Dis*, **17**, 47–57 **doi**: 10.1080/08910600510035093

VENEMA K, DE GRAAF AA, and DEUTZ NEP (2007), 'Metabolic conversions of dietary carbohydrates by gut microbes', pp 145–156 In: Salovaara H, Gates F and Tenkanen M (Eds) *Proceedings of DF2006, Dietary Fibre components and functions*, Wageningen Academic Publishers, Wageningen, the Netherlands.

VENEMA K, MAATHUIS A, GIESBRECHT I, BOHNHORST P, and CHRIST A (2008), 'Use of a dynamic, computer-controlled *in vitro* model of the stomach and small intestine (TIM-1) to study survival of probiotics in a chewable tablet', In: *Proceedings of the TNO Beneficial Microbes Conference*, Amsterdam, The Netherlands.

VENEMA K, MAATHUIS A, MENON R, MURPHY M and BOILEAU T (submitted), 'Survival of probiotics and functionality of probiotics and prebiotics during passage through a dynamic, computer-controlled *in vitro* model simulating the conditions in the human gastrointestinal tract'

VERVAEKE IJ, DECUYPERE JA, DIERICK NA, and HENDRICKX HK (1979), 'Quantitative *in vitro* evaluation of the energy metabolism influenced by virginiamycin and spiramycin used as growth promotors in pig nutrition', *J Animal Sci*, **49**, 846–856

VERWEI M, FREIDIG AP, HAVENAAR R, and GROTEN JP (2006), 'Predicted serum folate concentrations based on *in vitro* studies and kinetic modeling are consistent with measured folate concentrations in humans', *J Nutr*, **136**, 3074–3078

VINCE AJ, MCNIEL NI, WAGER JD, and WRONG OM (1990), 'The effect of lactulose, pectin, arabinogalactan and cellulose on the production of organicacids and metabolism of ammonia by intestinal bacteria in a faecal incubation system', *Br J Nutr*, **63**, 17–26 **doi**: **10.1046/j.1443–9611.2003.00110.x**

ZEIJDNER EE, and MOHEDE ICM (1999), 'Latest tool for screening new clinical foods A dynamic, computer-controlled model of the human gastrointestinal tract is the most up-to-date technology for testing new foods', *New World Health*, **1999/2000**, 105

13

The use of Caco-2 cells in defining nutrient bioavailability: application to iron bioavailability of foods

R. Glahn, USDA-ARS Cornell University, USA

Abstract: *In vitro* models can be useful tools in developing objectives that warrant testing in animal and human subjects. For nutrient absorption studies, Caco-2 cell monolayers have been widely used for defining certain aspects of nutrient uptake and transfer across epithelial cells. For a practical example, Caco-2 cell monolayers have been applied as a screening tool to address the food factors associated with iron deficiency anemia (IDA). IDA is the most common micronutrient deficiency worldwide and is primarily due to poor dietary Fe bioavailability. Development of foods with improved iron bioavailability is essential to alleviating this critical deficiency. Human and animal studies of iron absorption from food are time-consuming, expensive and offer limited capacity to address luminal interactions of iron and food ingredients. These factors have led scientists to pursue rapid, high-throughput *in vitro* methods that enable analysis of food–iron interactions and prediction of Fe bioavailability for humans. As a result, a simulation of *in vitro* digestion combined with Caco-2 cell monolayers was developed. The primary reason for this evolution of methodology is the fact that Fe solubility does not always correlate with Fe availability. Addition of the Caco-2 cell monolayer adds a living component to the model system that in theory should reflect the key step in iron bioavailability (i.e. uptake of iron by the enterocyte). *In vitro* digestion and Caco-2 cell culture conditions can vary significantly, and if proper physiological and cell culture principles are not applied, then the *in vitro* method can generate results that are not a true reflection of *in vivo* effects. Therefore, it is critical that an *in vitro* model be assessed under a broad range of conditions and validated against known effects in humans. This review summarizes the development, validation, and application of currently the most broadly applied *in vitro* digestion/Caco-2 cell culture model, providing it as an example of how epithelial cell lines can be used in practical nutrition research.

Key words: Caco-2, bioavailability, *in vitro*, cell culture, food iron.

13.1 Introduction

In vitro models can be a useful and productive approach in many if not all of the life sciences. Furthermore, coupling *in vitro* studies with *in vivo* testing can be even more productive as *in vitro* studies are by nature less expensive, rapid, and often allow greater manipulation and simplification for mechanistic studies of physiological processes at the level of the cell. These cellular observations often give clues to *in vivo* effects and thus allow researchers to design more definitive animal and human trials. However, as with any *in vitro* model, care must be taken to accurately reproduce the physiological conditions relevant to the experimental objectives; otherwise, one runs the risk of generating information that is merely an artifact of the conditions, and not representative of the *in vivo* physiology it was designed to replicate.

For studies of intestinal absorption of nutrients, the use of intestinal cell cultures has facilitated our understanding of the mechanisms of absorption of many nutrients. Of the major cell lines used in nutrition research, the Caco-2 cell line has become widely used and characterized for a broad range of nutrient uptake studies. In most cases, the use of Caco-2 cell monolayers has proven useful for elucidating mechanisms of nutrient uptake; however, Caco-2 cell monolayers may not always be useful, necessary, or appropriate as a tool to predict bioavailability of nutrients. This is because the Caco-2 cell monolayer is merely a layer of cells, and there are a multitude of other factors that can regulate and influence absorption in the intestinal lumen. Not all of these factors such as the intestinal microflora, nutritional status, disease states, nutrient interactions, etc. can be replicated *in vitro*. There are definite limitations for intestinal cell monolayers and these should always be considered for each nutrient of study.

As stated previously, there is a multitude of literature demonstrating that this cell line is useful in defining mechanisms of uptake of various nutrients. Hence this chapter will focus on an example of the next level of use for cell culture models, which is the use of the cell line as a high-throughput screening tool for food iron bioavailability. Iron represents a unique challenge in nutrition as it is an essential nutrient but often poor in bioavailability and thus Fe deficiency affects more than a third of the world's population. Given the complexity of iron bioavailability in foods, the use of an *in vitro* model is particularly essential for developing foods with more bioavailable Fe.

This chapter is organized into the following sections: (1) the origin of the Caco-2 cell line; (2) *in vitro* measurement of Fe bioavailability; (3) the physiology of the *in vitro* digestion/Caco-2 cell model; (4) validation of the *in vitro* digestion/Caco-2 cell model; and (5) the justification for using the cell line to measure Fe availability.

13.2 Origin of the Caco-2 cell line

The Caco-2 cell line was established from a human colon adenocarcinoma in the late 1970s.[1] The most common source of obtaining the Caco-2 cell line is the American Type Culture Collection (ATCC, Manassas, VA; see http://www.atcc.org). The primary clone of the Caco-2 cell line that is available through ATCC is known as HTB-37; however, numerous other clones are known to exist in various laboratories worldwide, some of which are more useful or unique to the study of certain nutrients or pharmaceuticals.[2,3] The Caco-2 cell line has been highly characterized for morphology, functional differentiation, and uptake of a broad range of nutrients and pharmaceuticals. Although colonic in origin, in culture the Caco-2 cell differentiates and closely resembles mature intestinal absorptive cells.[4,5]

For many nutrients, the Caco-2 cell has been observed to be a useful model for measurement of uptake and perhaps transfer across the epithelial cell layer.[6–8] In regards to Fe, early studies of Caco-2 cell monolayers documented greater Fe uptake and transepithelial transfer from Fe^{+2}-ascorbate versus Fe^{+3}-citrate or Fe^{+3}-NTA (nitrilotriacetic acid), and also observed greater iron uptake and transfer in iron-deficient versus iron-loaded cells.[9–11] Subsequent studies demonstrated the need to utilize an iron removal solution to accurately quantify Caco-2 cell iron uptake.[12] Han *et al.* demonstrated that inositol phosphates inhibit Fe and Zn uptake and transfer across Caco-2 monolayers; that ascorbate offsets the inhibitory effect of phytate on Caco-2 cell iron absorption; and that reduction of Fe^{+3} to Fe^{+2} dramatically increases Fe uptake.[13–15] The first evidence of transporter-mediated uptake of Fe in Caco-2 cells was demonstrated by Gangloff *et al.*[16] Subsequent studies identified the intracellular proteins and intestinal iron uptake transporters present in the brush border membrane of Caco-2 cells which contributed to more in-depth knowledge of the molecular mechanisms of iron absorption enjoyed today.[17–20]

Iron balance is primarily regulated by absorption as there is no excretory mechanism for Fe, merely loss through fecal excretion. Given this fact, the first step in Fe bioavailability depends on whether the Fe is in a form that can be taken up by the intestinal epithelial cell. It is at this level that the Caco-2 cell line can be used as an effective, first-level screening tool.

As an example of how Caco-2 models can be applied to nutrient bioavailability, this chapter will also feature the development, validation, and application of a specific *in vitro* digestion/Caco-2 cell model of Fe availability.[21] As evident in the literature, this model appears to be the most widely applied *in vitro* model in the field of Fe availability. It is a robust model as it has demonstrated the capability to be a high-throughput system with relatively low cost, has shown the capability to examine a broad range of foods and meal conditions, and produces results that, in general, agree with human studies. Indeed, with the recent increase in global biofortification programs such as HarvestPlus®, this model has the potential to offer key information to bioavailability studies and deserves an in depth evaluation and review.

13.3 *In vitro* measurement of iron bioavailability

In vitro estimation of iron bioavailability dates back to the mid-1930s and has been reviewed a number of times over the past 25 years.[22–24] The first widely used *in vitro* technique for measuring iron bioavailability was published by Miller and Schricker and co-worker[25] and involved the use of pepsin, pancreatic, and bile extracts to simulate intestinal digestion of foods. The intestinal 'digests' were then incubated in the presence of a 'dialysis bag.' Iron bioavailability was estimated by the amount of Fe that dialyzed into the bag, hence Fe bioavailability from this method primarily reflects Fe solubility and molecular size.

The potential pitfall of simply using Fe dialyzability or Fe solubility as a marker of Fe availability is that it can significantly overestimate availability. For example, Fe–citrate is a highly soluble complex, yet it has relatively low iron availability as shown in both human studies and cell culture.[26,27] Monoferric phytate is another highly soluble form of Fe, yet in single meal feeding studies it is clearly a poor source of available Fe in many foods, particularly when phytate exists in great molar excess relative to Fe.[28–33] Therefore, given the potential pitfalls of using iron dialyzability as a marker of availability, it is clear that *in vitro* methods for measuring iron availability need to include a component that is more closely correlated with intestinal iron uptake.

The first publications on coupling *in vitro* digestion with culture of Caco-2 cell monolayers appeared in the mid-1990s.[34,35] This methodology simply placed the radiolabeled dialysate from the Miller method on top of Caco-2 cell monolayers. This study and subsequent studies documented the enhancing effect of ascorbic acid and meat and demonstrated that the combination of *in vitro* digestion and Caco-2 cell culture offered significant advantages over measurement of iron dialyzability.[36,37] However, these early attempts at combining *in vitro* digestion with Caco-2 cell culture were complicated by the need to use radioactive Fe to measure Caco-2 cell uptake. Radioisotopes are useful in the measurement of cell iron uptake and manageable when used at low volumes; however, there is a safety issue with radioisotope use, handling radioisotopes is inconvenient and tedious, and the extrinsic radiolabel may not fully equilibrate with all of the food iron. For example, it is very likely that extrinsic radioiron will not equilibrate with heme iron or ferritin iron under certain food conditions. Also, for the extrinsic radioiron to equilibrate with the intrinsic food iron, it must be subject to the same processing, cooking and *in vitro* digestion steps. This results in potential contamination of workspace and equipment, and for *in vitro* digestion studies, requires the use of relatively large volumes of radiolabeled solutions. Another concern of using radioisotopes is that the cell-associated Fe may not be truly taken up by the cell, but merely bound to the surface; however, use of a technique to remove surface bound Fe minimizes this concern.[12]

As a result of these disadvantages, Glahn *et al.*[21] developed a method whereby formation of ferritin, an intracellular protein that stores Fe to protect against oxidative damage, could serve as the marker of Caco-2 cell iron uptake (Fig. 13.1). This method negates the need for use of

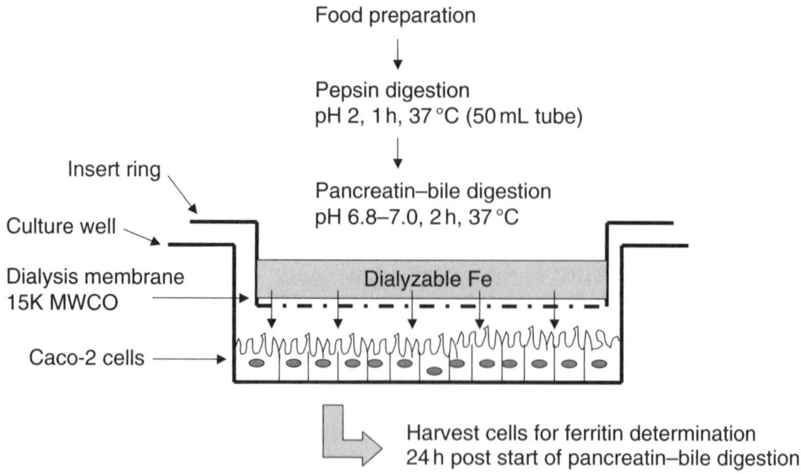

Fig. 13.1 Diagram of the *in vitro* digestion/Caco-2 cell culture model developed by Glahn *et al.*[21] (MWCO = molecular weight cut off).

radioisotopes, and is a sensitive and clear marker of cell Fe uptake as it is well known that cells produce ferritin in response to increases in intracellular iron.[38] Caco-2 cell ferrritin is easily measured via radio-immunoassay (RIA) or enzyme-linked immunosorbent assay (ELISA) from commercially available kits, the same kits used for human ferritin measurements in clinical practice. Moreover, this method enables measurement of iron availability from foods direct from the producer or supermarket shelf and requires no special preparation for use in the cell model.

The *in vitro* digestion conditions developed by Glahn *et al.*[21] involve a dual chamber system that does not require a dialysis bag or centrifugation of the food digest. This model uses a simple method of attaching a dialysis membrane (15 000 Da molecular weight cutoff) to a plastic insert, thus enabling digestion to occur simultaneously with uptake which is the condition present in the intestine. This methodology saves the time of centrifugation or handling of the dialysis bags, thus enabling very high sample throughput at low cost. As a result, this model has been the most widely applied model for foods. It has found applications in development of infant foods;[39,40] in agriculture for screening plant cultivars for bioavailable iron;[41–43] in the pharmaceutical industry for developing improved iron supplements;[44] for studies of human milk and infant formula;[45–48] in fortified ready-to-eat cereals;[49] in assessing elemental iron powders baked into breads;[50] in assessing the bioavailability of Fe from raisins and the effects of raisins on fortified Fe in foods;[51,52] in food science for comparison of fortified iron in milk and breads;[53,54] in assessing the effects of caseinates and casein phosphopeptides;[55,56] and in fundamental studies designed to investigate factors in digests of animal tissue (i.e. meat) that promote iron uptake.[57]

13.4 The physiology of the *in vitro* digestion/Caco-2 model

As an enhancement of the dialysis method to assess Fe bioavailability, Caco-2 cell monolayers have been added to the *in vitro* digestion. In designing an appropriate model for gastrointestinal digestion coupled with culture of intestinal epithelial cells, it is essential to reproduce the physiological conditions of the intestinal lumen as closely as possible. For studies of Fe availability, this involves reproducing the conditions of the duodenum where most Fe absorption is thought to occur. The amounts of pepsin, pancreatin, and bile salts used by Miller and Schricker and co-worker[25] for *in vitro* digestion have generally been maintained throughout many studies and are well accepted by the nutrition community. Only minor variations in pH titration methods and treatment of the enzymes have been necessary to remove contaminant Fe and refine the titration of foods to more closely reproduce *in vivo* conditions.[21] Indeed, the initial studies involving centrifugation steps, dialysis 'bags' and the use of PIPES as a buffer of the digest were certainly less physiological than the subsequent employment of a dialysis membrane insert, buffering with $NaHCO_3$, and the elimination of centrifugation of the digest.[21,25,31,36]

Recent research using inductively coupled plasma mass spectrometry has shown that Caco-2 cell ferritin formation is highly correlated with cell Fe content, thus indicating that Caco-2 ferritin formation remains proportionate to cell Fe uptake over a broad range of Fe availability (Glahn *et al.*, unpublished observations; Fig. 13.2).

The use of a dialysis membrane attached to plastic insert fulfilled a couple of key conditions that facilitated the coupling of *in vitro* digestion with enterocyte culture and measurement of Fe uptake. It protects the cells from the digestive enzymes and bile salts; it allows digestion to occur simultaneously with uptake, which could be important given the low stability of promoters such as ascorbic acid. It protects the cells from significant microbial contamination thus accommodating the overnight incubation of the digest with the epithelial cells and allowing adequate time for ferritin formation to occur. The overnight incubation of the digests with the cells enables a comfortable schedule for laboratory personnel as it negates the need to work outside of normal working hours. Such a factor is essential if high throughput of samples is a goal of the research project.

There has been concern about the effect of the dialysis membrane on limiting the bioavailability of certain forms of Fe such as ferritin and possibly heme–Fe complexes. The ferritin molecule has a molecular weight well in excess of the molecular weight cutoff of the dialysis membrane. Thus, if ferritin can be absorbed intact by intestinal cells, then this form of Fe would not be absorbed under the conditions shown in Fig. 13.1. However, there are several physiological reasons why ferritin is not likely to be absorbed intact, at least not to any significant extent. Under *in vivo* conditions, the surface of the enterocyte is covered with a mucin layer that is permeable to

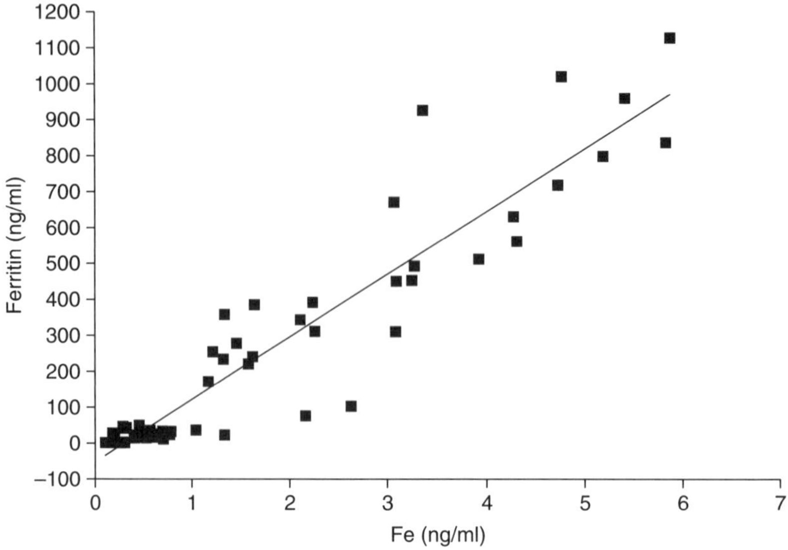

Fig. 13.2 The relationship between Caco-2 cell ferritin formation and cell Fe content ($R = 0.94$, $P < 0.0001$). Cell samples were measured for ^{56}Fe content via inductively coupled plasma emission mass spectroscopy. Ferritin was measured by radioimmunoassay from 59 samples of two separate sets of experiments.

ions and molecules of relatively small size (i.e. a molecular weight of 1000 Da), but impermeable to large proteins such as pepsin and pancreatic enzymes.[58] This permeability cutoff seems to occur around a molecular weight of 17 000, which makes it unlikely that the ferritin molecule could be absorbed intact by the enterocyte, as its molecular weight is well over 500 000. It is important to note that the molecular weight cutoff of the mucin layer is close to that of the dialysis membrane (i.e. 15 000) chosen by Glahn *et al.*[21] and in this respect appears to be a good substitute for the mucin layer. Therefore, iron availability from ferritin most likely results from release of Fe from the molecule due to the presence of ascorbic acid, digestive enzymes, or other compounds in foods. Overall, the conditions originally developed for this method have remained unchanged and, at present, appear to be the most physiological and appropriate for *in vitro* screening.

13.5 Validation of the *in vitro* digestion/Caco-2 cell culture model: comparison with human studies of Fe availability

For an *in vitro* model to be considered a useful tool, it should be consistent with the physiology of the human gastrointestinal tract and exhibit qualitative agreement with human studies. If such is the case, and if the model is capable of handling a broad range of Fe concentration and availability in foods, then it is possible to develop conversion factors for quantitative prediction of human Fe absorption from the same meal. As the reader will see later in this chapter, a conversion equation for predicting human Fe biovailability based on Caco-2 data has been developed.

Studies involving human subjects appear to support the use of Caco-2 cell ferritin formation as an index of Fe availability. For example, a positive correlation between ferritin concentrations in feces collected from human subjects and iron bioavailability has been reported.[59,60] Presumably, fecal ferritin concentrations reflect enterocyte ferritin levels formed in response to uptake of bioavailable dietary iron, and it is this step that is reproduced by the model featured in this manuscript.

Many facets of iron bioavailability observed in humans have also been observed in this model system. For example, studies using the model showed that heme iron uptake is higher than non-heme iron uptake in the presence of phytate;[33] that iron in human milk is more available than iron in bovine milk;[27,46,48] the availability of iron from $FeSO_4$ is higher than from a polysaccharide–Fe complex;[44] that NaFeEDTA is more available than $FeSO_4$ in the presence of polyphenolics;[49,52] and that ascorbic acid and meat enhance uptake[31,57] while phytic acid, tannic acid, and zinc inhibit Fe uptake.[33] Qualitatively similar effects have all been shown in humans and the corresponding human studies are cited in the above-mentioned articles.

This model system has been compared with several human studies by reproducing the meals of the human trials. The most notable comparison involved two human studies that encompass a broad range of iron availability.[61] The first human study documented promotion of iron absorption by ascorbic acid in a semi-synthetic diet.[62] The second human study documented the inhibitory effects of tannic acid on Fe added to a simple bread meal.[63] In the study by Cook and Monsen,[62] increasing levels of ascorbic acid were added to an extrinsically radiolabeled semi-synthetic diet and iron absorption was measured from radioactivity in a blood sample 2 weeks after ingestion of the test meal. The study by Brune *et al.*[63] appears to be the primary study used to generate the widely used algorithm developed by Hallberg and Hulthén[64] to calculate the inhibitory effect of polyphenolics. This study added increasing amounts of tannic acid to a wheat roll meal and measured iron absorption by blood sampling 2 weeks post-consumption of the test meal. In order to compare the *in vitro* and *in vivo* results, the data were expressed as absorption ratios (AR). For the human studies, this calculation represents the percent absorption of iron in the presence of each ascorbic acid or tannic acid level, divided by the percent absorption of iron with no ascorbic acid or tannic acid. From the *in vitro* study, the corresponding Caco-2 cell ferritin formation values were used to calculate the absorption ratio as cell ferritin was used as the measure of Fe uptake. The *in vitro* results correlated well with the human studies (Figs 13.3 and 13.4).

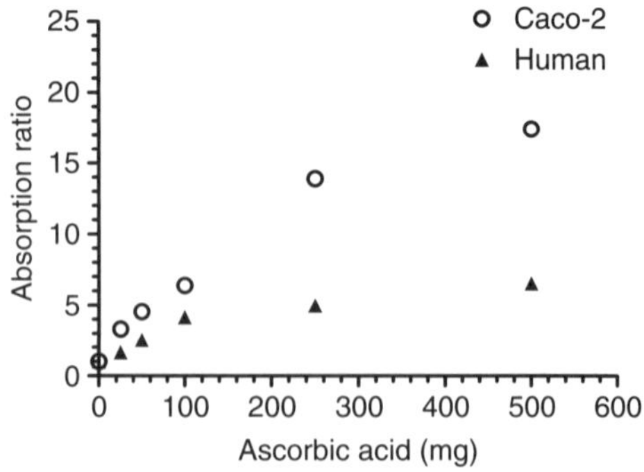

Fig. 13.3 Iron absorption ratios (AR) calculated from Caco-2 and human data for semisynthetic meals containing varying levels of ascorbic acid. Values represent the geometric mean of iron absorption at a given level of ascorbic acid divided by the geometric mean of iron absorption without ascorbic acid. Iron absorption in the Caco-2 cell model was indexed by ferritin formation. The natural log of the Caco-2 cell values and that of human studies were correlated at $R = 0.934$, $P = 0.012$. Adapted from Yun *et al.*[61].

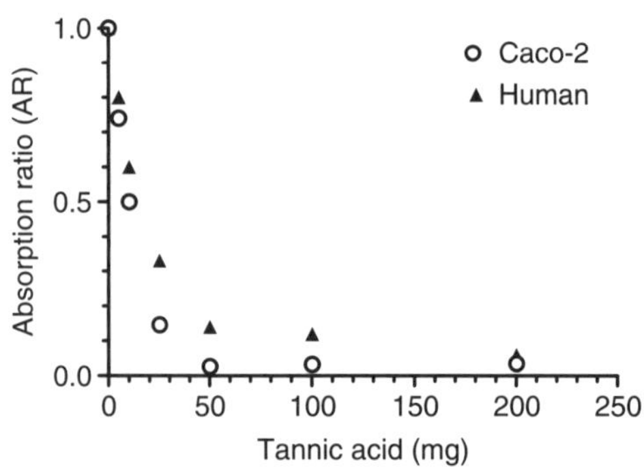

Fig. 13.4 Iron absorption ratios (AR) from Caco-2 cell and human studies on the effects of tannic acid on iron absorption. Values represent the geometric mean of iron absorption at a given level of tannic acid divided by the geometric mean of iron absorption without tannic acid. The natural log of the Caco-2 cell values and that of human studies were correlated at $R = 0.927$, $P = 0.007$. Adapted from Yun *et al.*[61].

Yun *et al.*[61] also demonstrated the quantitative potential of this model to predict Fe absorption in humans. To do so, the authors observed that the combined data from the above-mentioned studies could be plotted on a single graph, thus encompassing a wide range of Fe availability (Fig. 13.5). The equation generated by this plot is $\hat{H} = 0.6401 \times C$. In this equation, $\hat{H}$ is the estimate of human iron absorption, expressed as ln(AR), and C represents the ln(AR) of the corresponding Caco-2 cell data. The publication

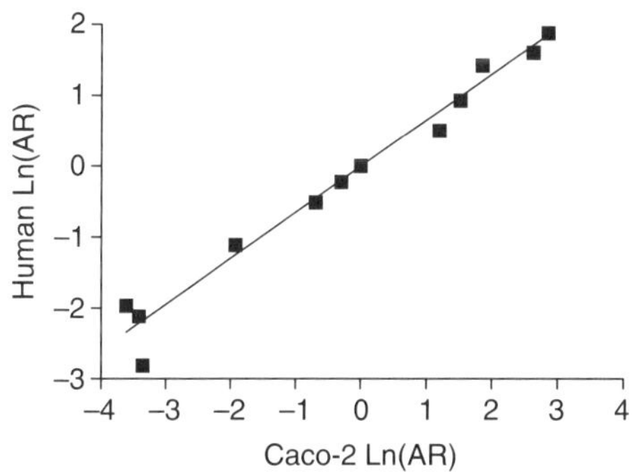

Fig. 13.5 The log–log relationship between absorption ratios (AR) from human and the parallel Caco-2 cell studies of this study. Caco-2 cell values represent the mean ln(AR), calculated from six replicates in the Caco-2 cell model. Human values represent the mean ln(AR), calculated from data for 12–13 subjects in a human study. Values were correlated at $R = 0.986$, $P < 0.001$. Adapted from Yun *et al.*[61]

by Yun *et al.* can form the basis for applying this Caco-2 model as a quantitative predictor of human iron absorption; however, it is reasonable to expect that the conversion factors may change as the model is applied in future studies. The following comparisons are examples to illustrate the predictive power of this model.

Iron absorption from mutant low-phytate maize varieties has been measured relative to wild-type varieties in human subjects.[65] In this study the maize varieties were harvested, the flour was 'nixtamilized' (i.e. soaked in lime) and prepared as tortillas. The tortillas were then extrinsically radiolabeled with Fe and fed to human subjects. Iron absorption was measured via blood collection. Iron uptake from the low phytate maize was 49% higher than from the wild-type maize. A close comparison of these maize samples has also been generated with the *in vitro* digestion/Caco-2 cell model (Table 13.1).

In March of 2003, Dr Victor Raboy, the scientist who developed the mutant maize and co-author on the human study, sent samples to the laboratory of Dr Glahn at the US Plant, Soil and Nutrition Lab, Ithaca, NY. These samples were cooked (i.e. autoclaved), lyophilized, and ground to a powder, and tested for available Fe via the *in vitro* model. The maize samples were from the same lines used in the human study and were of similar iron and phytic acid content. The primary difference between this experiment and the human study was that the maize samples were not nixtamalized (i.e. soaked in lime) and baked into tortillas. The nixtamilization process is essentially an alkaline solution of calcium hydroxide that softens the kernel and adds considerable calcium and other minerals to the samples. The added calcium and the alkaline conditions may certainly decrease the iron availability from the maize. This process could explain

Table 13.1 Comparison of iron availability from mutant low-phytate maize and wild type maize in humans and Caco-2 cells

	Wild-type maize	Low phytate maize	AR[1]	Caco-2 predicted AR[2]
Human iron absorption (%)	5.48	8.15	1.49	1.67
Caco-2 cell ferritin (ng ferritin/mg cell protein)	9.69	21.73	2.24	–

[1] Absorption ratio, i.e. the percent iron absorption of low phytate maize divided by that of the wild-type maize.
[2] The predicted AR based on the conversion equation of $\hat{H} = 0.6401 \times C$, published by Yun *et al.*,[61] where $\hat{H}$ is the predicted ln(AR) for humans and C is an observed ln(AR) for Caco-2 cells.

Table 13.2 Comparison of human and Caco-2 cell iron absorption from corn tortillas and black bean paste meals fortified with FeSO4 or NaFeEDTA

	Test meal with $FeSO_4$	Test meal with NaFeEDTA	AR[1]	Caco-2 predicted AR[2]
Human iron absorption (%)	5.5	9.0	1.64	1.77
Caco-2 cell ferritin (ng ferritin/mg cell protein)	2.46	6.02	2.45	–

[1] Absorption ratio, i.e. the percent iron absorption from the meal with NaFeEDTA divided by that of the meal with $FeSO_4$.
[2] The predicted AR based on the conversion equation of $\hat{H} = 0.6401 \times C$, published by Yun *et al.*,[61] where $\hat{H}$ is the predicted ln(AR) for humans and C is an observed ln(AR) for Caco-2 cells.

why the human iron absorption (AR = 1.49) was lower than that predicted by the Caco-2 model (AR = 1.67). Alternatively, the human study could be different because of the extrinsic labeling method, as it may not have completely equilibrated with the intrinsic iron of the maize. However, despite these differences, the *in vitro* model prediction is reasonably close to the human results.

Davidsson *et al.*[66] measured iron bioavailability from iron-fortified Guatemalan meals based on corn tortillas and black bean paste. One comparison of this study involved the addition of $FeSO_4$ versus NaFeEDTA to a tortilla and black bean paste meal. Significantly more iron was available to the human subjects from the NaFeEDTA (9%) than from the $FeSO_4$-fortified meal (5.5%). These same meal conditions were reproduced as closely as possible for *in vitro* studies (Glahn *et al.*, unpublished observations). A comparison of the results are summarized in Table 13.2. Clearly,

Table 13.3 Comparison of the dose-dependent effects of phytic acid on Fe uptake by human subjects and a similar study using the *in vitro* digestion/Caco-2 cell model.[1]

	AR[2] (phytate:Fe molar ratio)	
	1:1	5:1
Human iron absorption (%)	0.31	0.18
Caco-2 cell ferritin (ng ferritin/mg cell protein)	0.30	0.18

[1] The cited studies are Hallberg *et al.*[32] and Glahn *et al.*[33]
[2] Absorption ratio; for human subjects this equals the percent iron absorption from the meal with phytate divided by that of the meal without phytate; for Caco-2 cells, this equals cell ferritin formation from an *in vitro* digest with phytate divided by that from a digest without phytate.

the Caco-2 cell model provides a slightly higher, but reasonable, estimation of the human results after use of the conversion factor reported by Yun *et al.*[61].

A human study by Hallberg *et al.*[32] documented the dose-dependent effects of phytic acid on Fe availability from a wheat roll meal. The meal consisted of rolls made from white wheat flour and that were low in endogenous phytate and Fe. Various molar ratios of phytate:Fe were consumed by human subjects and the absorption ratios were calculated. A similar study was also done using the *in vitro* digestion/Caco-2 cell model.[33] The *in vitro* study did not 'feed' a wheat roll to the cells, but merely added corresponding amounts of phytic acid and Fe to the *in vitro* digest. There were two molar ratios of phytate:Fe in common between the two studies, at 1:1 and 5:1. The absorption ratios are summarized in Table 13.3 and the values match almost exactly. In reviewing the recent literature, this author notes that there appears to be a discrepancy in the molar amounts of phytate:Fe as calculated by Hurrell[67] where the Hallberg *et al.*[32] paper is cited. The text of the Hallberg *et al.*[32] paper states 'Sodium phytate (sodium inositol hexaphosphate, Sigma Chemical Company, St. Louis, MO) was added in various amounts (2–250 mg expressed as phytate phosphorous) to the rolls before the margarine was spread.' The results in Table 13.3 are based on the interpretation that 2–250 mg of Sigma sodium inositol hexaphosphate product (formula weight = 660) were added to the rolls. The publication by Hurrell[67] presents different numbers for conversion of the ARs and phytate:Fe molar ratios of the Hallberg *et al.* data.[32] This results in different molar ratios and higher AR values in the human subjects (i.e. approximately 0.35 and 0.30 at 0.7:1 and 4.5:1 phytate:Fe molar ratio, respectively). Still, even if the calculations by Hurrell[67] are correct, then at worst case the *in vitro* pattern of inhibition by phytic acid remains qualitatively similar to the human results and a simple conversion factor may be needed.

A relatively recent study by Besiegel *et al.*[68] demonstrated some differences in Fe uptake from beans between the *in vitro* digestion/Caco-2 cell model and human subjects. In this study, extrinsically labeled samples of red and white beans were compared in a single meal feeding trial. The subjects were of varying levels of Fe status and absorbed Fe equally from both the red and white bean samples. These results were in contrast to the *in vitro* results where the white beans gave significantly higher Fe uptake relative to the red beans. The interpretation of the results from this study was that the polyphenols present in the seed coat of the red beans, which are absent in the white beans, were the primary difference in Fe uptake from these samples. Also, the results suggest that the *in vitro* model is more sensitive to the effects of the polyphenols. However, there is a key point that must be considered when examining this study. The samples were extrinsically labeled, and a follow-up study observed that the extrinsic radiolabel did not equilibrate well with the intrinsic Fe of the red bean sample;[69] hence, it is questionable that the extrinsic label accurately measured Fe bioavailability from these samples. It should also be noted in this paper that corn samples were also compared *in vitro* with the human subjects and the corn results were in agreement. Further research is needed to define these conflicting results between the *in vitro* and *in vivo* systems.

There are other striking similarities in results between studies in humans and the *in vitro* digestion/Caco-2 cell model featured in this paper. Baech *et al.*[70] documented the effects of adding pork meat to a phytate-rich, low ascorbic acid meal. They observed that relatively small amounts of meat (<50 g) significantly enhanced non-heme iron absorption from the meal. Using the Caco-2 cell model, similar studies have been observed using a phytate and polyphenolic-rich meal. In this study, small amounts of beef increased Caco-2 cell iron uptake from a tortilla and bean paste meal (Fig. 13.6; Glahn *et al.*, unpublished observations). The basal meals were obviously different in these two studies. The human study meal consisted of boiled polished rice, tomato sauce, pea purée, rapeseed oil, and a wheat roll that was made partially from whole wheat and presumably a refined wheat flour. The meal of the *in vitro* study consisted of 50 g maize tortilla and 50 g black bean paste, the same meal used in a human study and compared previously with the *in vitro* model.[66] In both studies there were significant amounts of phytic acid; however, the meal for the *in vitro* study likely contained greater amounts of polyphenolics. Also, the *in vitro* meal used beef which increased the total Fe content of the meal by 200% at the full serving size. For the human study, the pork sample was relatively low in total iron content and only increased Fe content by approximately 8% at the highest level of meat. These contrasts between the studies negate the usefulness of closer comparison; however, both studies arrive at the same conclusion, that relatively low amounts of meat can improve iron absorption from a meal with low Fe availability.

In conclusion, the above-mentioned comparisons between the *in vitro* digestion/Caco-2 cell model and human studies should represent only the

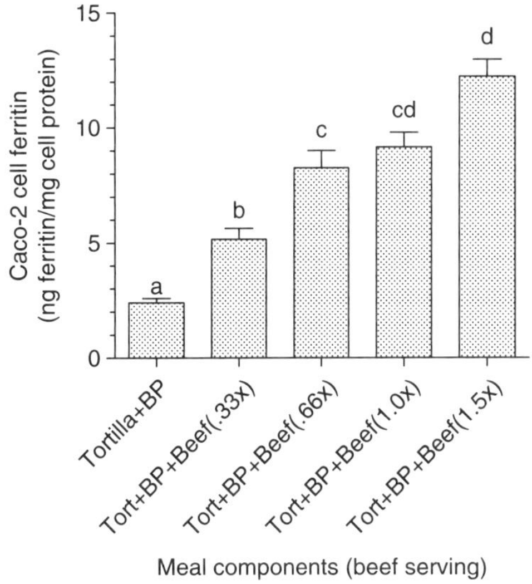

Fig. 13.6 Caco-2 cell iron uptake as measured via cell ferritin formation from a meal containing 50 g tortilla (tort), 50 g bean paste (BP), and cooked beef. The beef serving size was defined as 3 ounces (85 g) wet weight. Text on column labels within parentheses indicate the fraction of the beef serving (i.e. 0.33× equals 1 ounce of beef added to the meal. Column values with no letters in common are significantly different ($P < 0.05$).

beginning of this level of validation. More direct comparisons from the same meals should be pursued in order to refine the conversion factor for *in vitro* predictions of human iron absorption via this model. One should expect that conflicting results will be observed in these types of studies, and recognize that in those differences may lie clues to the actual mechanisms of uptake that occur in the human intestine.

13.6 Justification for use of the *in vitro* digestion/Caco-2 cell model as a screening tool

One of the primary factors that determines an experimental approach is cost. The costs associated with application of this *in vitro* model are far below those of animal and human trials. A laboratory with one or two personnel trained in the use of this *in vitro* model can easily conduct two sets of experiments per week, comparing eight to ten different samples with six independent replications, and process the cell samples for Fe uptake measurement within a few days after the experiment. The US dollar values associated with such costs are difficult to estimate due to potential differences in technician salary and overhead; however, it has been demonstrated in US Department of Agriculture (USDA) facilities that the *in vitro* approach can assess Fe availability of eight to ten samples for approximately \$5000 which includes personnel salary, supplies, and overhead costs (R.P. Glahn, personal observations). Studies in humans comparing this number of samples or conditions are seldom done as it is cost-prohibitive. For example, at USDA facilities, a single or two meal feeding trial of two to four extrinsically radiolabeled food samples would cost \$50000 and would require a minimum of 6–12 months to resolve paperwork, recruit subjects, and collect data (Dr Janet Hunt, USDA-ARS, Grand Forks, ND, personal correspondence). Obviously, performing human studies on more than a handful of samples is very costly for most research programs investigating Fe availability. Given the high cost of human studies it becomes imperative that these studies provide definitive results that advances the field. The *in vitro* digestion/Caco-2 cell culture model featured in this chapter has been developed for precisely that application. Used properly, it can accelerate knowledge of food Fe availability by refining experimental objectives and thereby increase the effectiveness of the human studies. Furthermore, *in vitro* studies can explore intralumenal interactions, effects, and mechanisms that are not possible or cost-effective to address *in vivo*.

The fact that concentration of Fe, the concentration of promoters and inhibitors of Fe uptake, and Fe solubility are not reliable predictors of Fe availability is also a key justification for use of this model. The coupling of Caco-2 cell culture model with *in vitro* digestion essentially makes *in vitro* Fe biovailability screening plausible as it adds a living component to the process and completes the components necessary to model the initial steps in Fe uptake by the enterocyte. From a bioavailability standpoint, the primary step in determining availability is whether or not the form of Fe in the food is accessible for uptake by the enterocyte. After that step, the fate of the Fe is then dependent on the Fe status and physiology of the individual. The conditions defined by Glahn *et al.*[21] were developed with this physiological approach, and were also designed to be cost-effective, easy to use, and able to accommodate a relatively large number of samples.

The following is an example as to how screening by concentration of Fe, promoters, and inhibitors alone can lead to costly mistakes and wasted resources. Mamiro *et al.*[71] tested a complementary food for its effect on alleviating Fe deficiency anemia in 6–12-month-old infants in Tanzania. The objective of the study was to determine if a processed complementary food, estimated to provide more bioavailable Fe, improved the Fe status of infants relative to those consuming the unprocessed meal. The effects of processing were designed to lower antinutrient levels (i.e. phytate and polyphenolics), thereby improving Fe absorption from the meal. The meal had been previously analyzed and exhibited greater Fe solubility with marked decreases in phytate and polyphenolic concentration.[72] After 6 months of feeding, the processed meal provided no additional benefit for growth, hemoglobin formation or Fe status, essentially indicating that no significant additional bioavailable Fe was present in the meal.

On a dry matter basis, this meal contained dried finger millet (65%), kidney beans (19%), peanuts (8%) and mango puree (8%). In the processed meal used by Mamiro *et al.*,[71] phytate levels were reduced by 34%, yielding phytate:Fe molar ratios of 16.6:1 and 11.8:1 in the unprocessed and processed foods, respectively. The nutritional analysis of the same foods conducted by Mbithi-Mwikya *et al.*[72] observed phytate:Fe molar ratios of 16.7:1 and 3.3:1 for the unprocessed and processed foods, respectively. Mamiro *et al.* measured Fe solubility at 19% in the processed meal versus 5% in the unprocessed meal. Also, Mbithi-Mwikya *et al.*[72] did not find any detectable tannins in the processed meal and tannin measurement was not reported in the Mamiro *et al.*[71] study.

Clearly, the results of these two studies indicate that Fe solubility and content of inhibitors would not have been adequate predictors of Fe availability in these meals. One likely explanation for no improvement of Fe availability could be due to the presence of phenolic acids or flavanoids that constitute the tannins of the unprocessed ingredients. Tannins in foods are known to break down during cooking and storage of staple foods such as rice, yet the inhibitory effect on Fe availability remains, probably due to the phenolic acids.[33] The assay used by Mbithi-Mwikya *et al.*[72] may not have detected the phenolic compounds as certain methods for measuring tannins do not accurately measure the breakdown products.[73] Hence, even though phytate levels were reduced in these foods, the polyphenolic effect remains and dramatically inhibited Fe availability. The *in vitro* digestion/Caco-2 cell model would likely detect the inhibitory effect of the phenolics and therefore prevent the waste of resources for an unproductive human study. Moreover, the *in vitro* model could be used to develop a low-cost complementary food that shows significantly higher Fe availability and thus has greater chance for success in the human efficacy trials. Such screening studies to define affordable and consumer-acceptable complementary foods are currently underway in this author's laboratory.[74]

Another key advantage of the *in vitro* digestion/Caco-2 cell model is that it can detect previously unknown or new interactions of foods or ingredients that can promote or inhibit Fe availability. An example of such is the observed effect of sweet potato on Fe availability.[75] In this study orange flesh sweet potatoes were observed to have a strong promotional effect on Fe extrinsically added to a sweet potato sample. The implication of this research is: that developing sweet potatoes with higher Fe density could provide a better source of Fe as well as being an excellent source of provitamin A. Alternatively, as sweet potato flesh is relatively low in Fe content, these observations suggest that fortifying a popular complementary food such as a sweet potato pureé could provide an excellent source of Fe for infants.

Recent *in vitro* screening studies have also documented higher Fe availability in white beans relative to pinto, red, brown or black beans.[76] In this study the levels of phytate varied significantly and was not correlated with

Fe availability. The primary correlation with Fe availability appears to be related to the polyphenolic profile of the bean samples. Significant differences in Fe availability were observed among the white bean genotypes and among the colored bean samples. The analysis of the bean varieties indicates that such differences would not be predicted based on nutritional content of Fe and inhibitors of Fe absorption. This represents another example as to how an *in vitro* model can provide useful insight to identify foods with improved Fe availability, as there are no published studies that suggest white bean varieties may be a better source of Fe. At present, studies are under way to confirm these observations in human subjects. If true, then white beans may represent a practical and effective component for complementary foods such as used in the aforementioned study by Mamiro *et al.*[71]

Further justification for the advent and application of the *in vitro* digestion/Caco-2 model is due to the specific needs of plant breeders and nutritionists in biofortification programs such as HarvestPlus. HarvestPlus is an international, interdisciplinary, research program that seeks to reduce micronutrient malnutrition by utilizing the powers of agriculture and nutrition research to breed staple food crops (e.g. rice, wheat, maize, beans, sweet potatoes, and cassava) with higher levels of Fe, Zn, and provitamin A.

From the very beginning, bioavailability issues have been a major concern for HarvestPlus. Throughout the 10 years of planning, research, and development of HarvestPlus, it became apparent that measuring only the content of iron and zinc and the levels of inhibitors (i.e. phytate, tannins) would not be a viable option for this program for many reasons. First, as stated previously, concentration of Fe and Zn in seeds does correlate with the bioavailability of Fe or Zn in seeds. Second, there is a very large environmental effect on phytate concentration in cereal, grain and legume as the phytate concentration is greatly influenced by the levels of available phosphorous in the soil.[77] This factor makes it practically impossible for plant breeders to use phytate content of breeding lines in their screening for genotypes with high levels of bioavailable iron and zinc. To do so as a breeding strategy would make the process enormously complicated and expensive as it would require development of numerous lines for numerous environments. Moreover, it does not appear that screening crop varieties via phytate content will be useful, as both animal and Caco-2 models show no correlation with Fe availability among genotypes.[33,41,42,78] Although phytate is an inhibitor of Fe availability, these observations indicate that other factors in the seed appear to be responsible for the ultimate bioavailable levels of Fe and Zn. The most likely factors are polyphenolics and the nature of the complexes formed between Fe, Zn and this huge group of compounds. Relatively little is known as to how these compounds react with Fe and Zn to limit the bioavailability of these minerals; however, such studies are in progress within the breeding and bioavailability objectives of HarvestPlus. Finally, aside from screening numerous genotypes to identify those with high and low bioavailability of these nutrients, HarvestPlus must also investigate how such foods interact within the typical diets and meals of the targeted regions; hence, there is a profound need in such a program for a screening tool that can assess the effects of processing, cooking and food interactions in typical meals. Such assessment is not possible using algorithms, as it would require a data set that has measured these effects over a broad range of foods and cooking procedures. A data set of this magnitude using human subjects would be enormously expensive to produce and thus is not likely to ever exist. An *in vitro* model appears to be the only feasible approach to begin to explore these factors and interactions.

13.7 Conclusion

In conclusion, it is clear that over the past decade the advances in knowledge of molecular mechanisms of Fe absorption have been profound, and that the Caco-2 cell line has been a valuable tool in defining those mechanisms. Thus, it is logical to incorporate this cell line into applied research as a tool to measure bioavailable Fe in foods. As evident by the examples in this chapter, the conditions established by Glahn *et al.*[21] have broad applications, from screening genotypes of staple food crops to development of improved forms of Fe for food fortification. However, although the degree to which these *in vitro* conditions agree with human studies is remarkable, it is reasonable to suspect that this *in vitro* system will have limitations on predicting Fe availability. Only direct testing of this model with human studies will enable further refinement and define the limitations of this *in vitro* system.

13.8 References

1. FOGH, J., FOGH, J.M., and ORFEO, T. (1977) One hundred and twenty seven cultured human tumor cell lines producing tumors in nude mice. *J. Nat. Cancer Inst.* **59**:221–226.
2. CARO, I., BOULENC, X., ROUSSET, M., MEUNIER, V., BOURRIE, M., JULIAN, B., JOYEUX, H., ROQUES, C., BERGER, Y., ZWEIBAUM, A., and FABRE, G. (1995) Characterization of a newly isolated Caco-2 clone (TC-7), as a model of transport processes and biotransformation of drugs. *Int. J. Pharmaceut.* **116**(2):147–158.
3. WALTER, E. and KISSEL, T. (1994) Transepithelial transport and metabolism of thyrotropin-releasing hormone (TRH) in monolayers of a human intestinal cell line (Caco-2): evidence for an active transport component? *Pharmaceut. Res.* **11**(11):1575–1580.
4. PINTO, M., ROBINE-LEON, S., APPAY, M.-D., KEDINGER, M., TRIADOU, N., DUSSAULX, E., LACROIX, B., SIMON-ASSMANN, P., HAFFEN, K., FOGH, J., and ZWEIBAUM, A. (1983) Enterocyte-like differentiation and polarization of the human colon carcinoma cell line Caco-2 in culture. *Biol. Cell.* **47**:323–330.
5. VACHON, P.H. and BEAULIEU, J. (1992) Transient mosaic patterns of morphological and functional differentiation in the Caco-2 cell line. *Gastroenterology* **1013**: 414–423.

6. MOHRMANN, I., MOHRMANN, M., BIBER, J., and MURER, H. (1986) Sodium-dependent transport of Pi by an established intestinal epithelial cell line (CaCo-2) *Am. J. Physiol. Gastrointest. Liver Physiol.* **250**:323–330.
7. SAITO, H. and INUI, K. (1993) Dipeptide transporters in apical and basolateral membranes of the human intestinal cell line Caco-2. *Am. J. Physiol. Gastrointest. Liver Physiol.* **265**:289–294.
8. OSYPIW, J.C., GLEESON, D., LOBLEY, R.W., PEMBERTON, P.W., and MCMAHON, R.F.T. (1994) Acid–base transport systems in a polarized human intestinal cell monolayer: Caco-2. *Exp. Physiol.* **79**:723–739.
9. ALVAREZ-HERNANDEZ, X., NICHOLS, G.M., and GLASS, J. (1991) Caco-2 cell line: a system for studying intestinal iron transport across epithelial cell monolayers. *Biochim. Biophys. Acta* **1070**:205–208.
10. HALLEUX, C. and SCHNEIDER, Y.J. (1991) Iron absorption by intestinal epithelial cells: 1. Caco-2 cells cultivated in serum-free medium, on polyethyleneterephthalate microporous membranes, as an *in vitro* model. *In Vitro Cell Dev. Biol.* **274**: 293–302.
11. HALLEUX, C. and SCHNEIDER, Y.J. (1994) Iron absorption by Caco-2 cells cultivated in serum-free medium as an *in vitro* model of the human intestinal epithelial barrier. *J. Cell. Physiol.* **158**:17–28.
12. GLAHN, R.P., GANGLOFF, M.B., MILLER, D.D., VAN CAMPEN, D.R., NORVELL, W.A., and WIEN, E.M. (1995) Bathophenanthroline disulfonic acid and sodium dithionite effectively remove surface-bound iron from Caco-2 cell monolayers. *J. Nutr.* **125**:1833–1840.
13. HAN, O., FAILLA, M.L., HILL, A.D., MORRIS, E.R., and SMITH, J.C. (1994) Inositol phosphates inhibit uptake and transport of iron and zinc by a human intestinal cell line. *J. Nutr.* **124**:580–587.
14. HAN, O., FAILLA, M.L., HILL, A.D., MORRIS, E.R., and SMITH, J.C. (1995a) Reduction of Fe(III) is required for uptake of nonheme iron by Caco-2 cells. *J. Nutr.* **125**:1291–1299.
15. HAN, O., FAILLA, M.L., HILL, A.D., MORRIS, E.R., and SMITH, J.C. (1995b) Ascorbate offsets the inhibitory effect of inositol phosphates on iron uptake and transport by Caco-2 cells. *Proc. Soc. Exp. Biol. Med.* **210**:50–56.
16. GANGLOFF, M.B., LAI, C., VAN CAMPEN, D.R., MILLER, D.D., NORVELL, W.A., and GLAHN, R.P. (1996) Ferrous iron uptake but not transfer is down-regulated in Caco-2 cells grown in high iron serum-free medium. *J. Nutr.* **126**:3118–3127.
17. WOOD, R.J. and HAN, O. (1998) Recently identified molecular aspects of intestinal iron absorption. *J. Nutr.* **128**:1841–1844.
18. HAN, O., FLEET, J.C., and WOOD, R.J. (1999) Reciprocal regulation of HFE and Nramp2 gene expression by iron in human intestinal cells. *J. Nutr.* **129**:98–104.
19. TANDY, S., WILLIAMS, M., LEGGETT, A., LOPEZ-JIMENEZ, M., DEDES, M., RAMESH, B., SRAI, S.K., and SHARP, P. (2000) Nramp2 expression is associated with pH-dependent iron uptake across the apical membrane of human intestinal Caco-2 cells. *J. Biol. Chem.* **275**:1023–1029.
20. MORGAN, E.H. and OATES, P.S. (2002) Mechanisms and regulation of intestinal iron absorption. *Blood, Cells, Mol. Diseases* **29**:384–399.
21. GLAHN, R.P., LEE, O.A., YEUNG, A., GOLDMAN, M.I., and MILLER, D.D. (1998) Caco-2 cell ferritin formation predicts nonradiolabeled food iron availability in an *in vitro* digestion/Caco-2 cell culture model. *J. Nutr.* **128**:1555–1561.
22. MILLER, D.D. and SCHRICKER, B.R. (1982) In *Nutritional Bioavailability of Iron*, C. Kies, ed., American Chemical Society, Washington, DC, pp. 9–26.
23. MILLER, D.D. and SCHRICKER, B.R. (1989) Is solubility *in vitro* a reliable predictor of Fe bioavailability? *Biol. Trace Element Res.* **19**:11–24.
24. VAN CAMPEN, D.R. and GLAHN, R.P. (1999) Micronutrient bioavailability techniques: accuracy, problems and limitations. *Field Crops Res.* **60**:93–113.

25. MILLER, D.D., SCHRICKER, B.R., RASMUSSEN, R.R., and VAN CAMPEN, D. (1981) An *in vitro* method for estimation of iron availability from meals. *Am. J. Clin. Nutr.* **34**(10):2248–2256.
26. HEINRICH, H.C. (1987) Intestinal absorption of 59Fe from neutron-activated commercial oral iron(III)–citrate and iron(III)–hydroxide polymaltose complexes in man. *Arzneim.-Forsch./Drug. Res.* **37**:105–107.
27. GLAHN, R.P., LAI, C., HSU, J., THOMPSON, J.F., and VAN CAMPEN, D.R. (1998) Decreased citrate improves iron availability from infant formula: application of an *in vitro* digestion/Caco-2 cell culture model. *J. Nutr.* **128**:257–264.
28. MORRIS, E.R. and ELLIS, R. (1976) Isolation of monoferric phytate from wheat bran and its biological value as an iron source to the rat. *J. Nutr.* **106**(6):753–760.
29. LIPSCHITZ, D.A., SIMPSON, K.M., COOK, J.D., and MORRIS, E.R. (1979) Absorption of monoferric phytate by dogs. *J. Nutr.* **109**:1154–1160.
30. ELLIS, R. and MORRIS, E. (1979) Effect of sodium phytate on stability of monoferric phytate complex and the bioavailability of the iron to rats. *Nutr. Rep. Int.* **20**(5):739–747.
31. SIMPSON, B.S., MORRIS, E.R., and COOK, J.D. (1981) The inhibitory effect of bran on iron absorption in man. *Am. J. Clin. Nutr.* **34**:1469–1478.
32. HALLBERG, L., BRUNE, M., and ROSSANDER, L. (1989) Iron absorption in man: ascorbic acid and dose dependent inhibition by phytate. *Am. J. Clin. Nutr.* **49**:140–144.
33. GLAHN, R.P., WORTLEY, G.M., SOUTH, P.K., and MILLER, D.D. (2002) Inhibition of iron uptake by phytic acid, tannic acid, and $ZnCl_2$: studies using an *in vitro* digestion/Caco-2 cell model. *J. Agric. Food Chem.* **50**:390–395.
34. GLAHN, R.P., GANGLOFF, M.B., MILLER, D.D., WIEN, E.M., KAPSOKEFALOU, M., and VAN CAMPEN, D.R. (1994) Use of *in vitro* digestion and Caco-2 cell culture to study iron uptake/bioavailability. *FASEB J.* **8**:A712.
35. GANGLOFF, M.B., GLAHN, R.P., MILLER, D.D., NORVELL, W.A., and VAN CAMPEN, D.R. (1996) Assessment of iron availability using combined *in vitro* digestion and Caco-2 cell culture. *Nutr. Res.* **16**:479–487.
36. GLAHN, R.P., WIEN, E.M., VAN CAMPEN, D. R., and MILLER, D.D. (1996) Caco-2 cell iron uptake from meat and casein digests parallels *in vivo* studies: use of a novel *in vitro* method for rapid estimation of iron bioavailability. *J. Nutr.* **126**:332–339.
37. GARCIA, M.N., FLOWERS, C., and COOK, J.D. (1996) The Caco-2 cell culture system can be used as a model to study food iron availability. *J. Nutr.* **126**:251–258.
38. HENTZE, M.W. and KUHN, L.C. (1996) Molecular control of vertebrate iron metabolism: mRNA-based regulatory circuits operated by iron, nitric oxide and oxidative stress. *Proc. Natl. Acad. Sci. USA*, **93**:8175–8182.
39. GLAHN, R.P., LEE, O.A., and MILLER, D.D. (1999) *In vitro* digestion/Caco-2 cell culture model to determine optimal ascorbic acid to Fe ratio in rice cereal. *J. Food Sci.* **64**:925–928.
40. BOATO, F., WORTLEY, G.M., LIU, R., and GLAHN, R.P. (2002) Red grape juice inhibits iron availability: application of an *in vitro* digestion/Caco-2 cell model. *J. Agric. Food Chem.* **50**:6935–6938.
41. OIKEH, S.O., MENKIR, A., MAZIYA-DIXON, B., WELCH, R., and GLAHN, R.P. (2003) Assessment of concentrations of iron and zinc and bioavailable iron in grains of early-maturing tropical maize varieties. *J. Agric. Food Chem.* **51**:3688–3694.
42. OIKEH, S.O., MENKIR, A., MAZIYA-DIXON, B., WELCH, R.M., and GLAHN, R.P. (2004) Assessment of iron bioavailability from 20 elite late-maturing tropical maize varieties using an *in vitro* digestion/Caco-2 cell model. *J. Sci. Food Agric.* **84**:1202–1206.
43. GLAHN, R.P., CHENG, Z., WELCH R.M., and GREGORIO, G.B. (2002) A comparison of iron bioavailability from 15 rice genotypes: studies using an *in vitro* digestion/Caco-2 cell culture model. *J. Ag. Food Chem.* **50**:3586–3591.

44. GLAHN, R.P., RASSIER, M., GOLDMAN, M.I., LEE, O.A., and CHA, J. (2000) A comparison of iron availability from commercial iron preparations using an *in vitro* digestion/ Caco-2 cell culture model. *J. Nutr. Biochem.* **11**:62–68.
45. ETCHEVERRY, P., WALLINGFORD, J.C., MILLER, D.D., and GLAHN, R.P. (2002) Simul taneous determination of (45)calcium and (65)zinc uptake by Caco-2 cells. *J. Agric. Food Chem.* **50**:6287–6294.
46. ETCHEVERRY, P., MILLER, D.D., and GLAHN, R.P. (2004a) A low molecular-weight factor in human milk whey promotes iron uptake by Caco-2 cells. *J. Nutr.* **134**:93–98.
47. ETCHEVERRY, P., WALLINGFORD, J., MILLER, D.D., and GLAHN, R.P. (2004b) Calcium, zinc and iron bioavailabilities from a commercial human milk fortifier: a comparison study. *J. Dairy Sci.* **87**:3629–3637.
48. ETCHEVERRY, P., WISSLER, J., WORTLEY, G., and GLAHN, R.P. (2004c) Caco-2 cell iron uptake from human milk and infant formula. *Nutr. Res.* **24**:573–579.
49. WORTLEY, G., LEUSNER, S., GOOD, C., GUGGER, E., and GLAHN, R.P. (2005) Iron bioavailability of a fortified processed wheat cereal: a comparison of fourteen iron forms using an *in vitro* digestion/human colonic adenocarcinoma (CaCo-2) cell model. *Br. J. Nutr.* **93**:65–71.
50. YEUNG, C.K., MILLER, D.D., CHENG, Z., and GLAHN, R.P. (2005) Bioavailability of elemental iron powders in bread assessed with an *in vitro* digestion/Caco-2 cell culture model. *J. Food Sci.* **70**:199–203.
51. YEUNG, C.K., GLAHN, R.P., WU, X., LIU, R.H., and MILLER D.D. (2002) *In vitro* iron bioavailability and antioxidant activity of raisins. *J. Food Sci.* **68**:701–705.
52. YEUNG, C.K., GLAHN, R.P., and MILLER, D.D. (2003) Iron bioavailability from common raisin-containing foods assessed with an *in vitro* digestion/Caco-2 cell culture model: effects of raisins. *J. Food Sci.* **68**:1866–1870.
53. YEUNG, A.C., GLAHN, R.P., and MILLER, D.D. (2002) Comparison of the availability of various iron fortificants in bread and milk using an *in vitro* digestion/Caco-2 cell culture method. *J. Food Sci.* **67**:2357–2361.
54. YEUNG, C.K., GLAHN, R.P., and MILLER, D.D. (2005) Inhibition of iron uptake from iron salts and chelates by divalent metal cations in intestinal epithelial cells. *J. Agric. Food Chem.* **53**:132–136.
55. YEUNG, A.C., GLAHN, R.P., and MILLER, D.D. (2001) Dephosphorylation of sodium caseinate, enzymatically hydrolyzed casein and casein phosphopeptides by intestinal alkaline phosphatase: implications for iron availability. *J. Nutr. Biochem* **12**:292–299.
56. YEUNG, A.C., GLAHN, R.P., and MILLER, D.D. (2002) Effects of iron source on iron availability from casein and casein phosphopeptides. *J. Food Sci.* **67**:1271–1275.
57. HUH, E.C., HOTCHKISS, A., BROUILLETTE, J., and GLAHN, R.P. (2004) Carbohydrate fractions from cooked fish promote iron uptake by Caco-2 cells. *J. Nutr.* **134**:1681–1689.
58. ALLEN, A. and CARROLL, N.J.H. (1985) Adherent and soluble mucus in the stomach and duodenum. *Digestive Dis. Sci.* **30**:55S–62S.
59. HUNT, J.R. and ROUGHHEAD, Z.K. (1999) Nonheme-iron absorption, fecal ferritin excretion, and blood indexes of iron status in women consuming controlled lactoovovegetarian diets for 8 wk. *Am. J. Clin. Nutr.* **69**:944–952.
60. ROUGHHEAD, Z.K. and HUNT, J.R. (2000) Adaptation in iron absorption: iron supplementation reduces nonheme-iron but not heme-iron absorption from food. *Am. J. Clin. Nutr.* **72**:982–989.
61. YUN, S., HABICHT, J.P., MILLER, D.D., and GLAHN, R.P. (2004) An *in vitro* digestion/ Caco-2 cell culture system accurately predicts the effects of ascorbic acid and polyphenolic compounds on iron bioavailability in humans. *J. Nutr.* **134**: 2717–2721.

62. COOK, J.D. and MONSEN, E.R. (1977) Vitamin C, the common cold, and iron absorption. *Am. J. Clin. Nutr.* **30**:235–241.
63. BRUNE M., ROSSANDER L., and HALLBERG, L. (1989) Iron absorption and phenolic compounds: importance of different phenolic structures. *Eur. J. Clin. Nutr.* **43**:547–558.
64. HALLBERG, L. and HULTHÉN, L. (2000) Prediction of dietary iron absorption: an algorithm for calculating absorption and bioavailability of dietary iron. *Am. J. Clin. Nutr.* **71**:1147–1160.
65. MENDOZA, C., VITERI, F., LÖNNERDAL, B., YOUNG, K.A., RABOY, V., and BROWN, K.H. (1998) Effect of genetically modified, low phytic acid maize on absorption of iron from tortillas. *Am. J. Clin. Nutr.* **68**:1123–1127.
66. DAVIDSSON, L., DIMITRIOU, T., BOY, E., WALCZYK, T., and HURRELL, R.F. (2002) Iron bioavailability from iron-fortified Guatemalan meals based on corn tortillas and black bean paste. *Am. J. Clin. Nutr.* **75**:535–539.
67. HURRELL, R.F. (2004) Phytic acid degradation as a means of improving iron absorption. *Int. J. Vitam. Nutr. Res.* **74**:445–452.
68. BEISEIGEL, J.M., HUNT, J.R., GLAHN, R.P., WELCH, R.M., MENKIR, A., and MASIYA-DIXON, B. (2007) Iron bioavailability from maize and beans: a comparison of human measurements with Caco-2 cell and algorithm predictions. *Am. J. Clin. Nutr.* **86**:388–396.
69. JIN, F., CHENG, Z., RUTZKE, M., WELCH, R.M., and GLAHN, R.P. (2008) Extrinsic labeling method may not accurately measure iron absorption from cooked pinto beans (*Phaseolus vulgaris*); comparison of extrinsic and intrinsic labeling of beans. *J. Agric. Food Chem.* **56**:6881–6885.
70. BAECH, S.B., HANSEN, M., BUKHAVE, K., JENSEN, M., SØRENSON, S.S., KRISTENSEN, L., PURSLOW, P.P., SKIBSTED, L.H., and SANDSTRÖM, B. (2003) Nonheme-iron absorption from a phytate-rich meal is increased by the addition of small amounts of pork meat. *Am. J. Clin. Nutr.* **77**:173–179.
71. MAMIRO, P.S., KOLSTEREN, P.W., VAN CAMP, J.H., ROBERFROID, D.A., TATALIA, S., and OPSOMER, A.S. (2004) Processed complementary food does not improve growth or hemoglobin status of rural Tanzanian infants from 6–12 months of age in Kilosa District, Tanzania. *J. Nutr.* **134**:1084–1090.
72. MBITHI-MWIKYA, S., VAN CAMP, J., MAMIRO, P.R.S., OOGHIE, W., KOLSTEREN, P., and HUYGHEBAERT, A. (2002) Evaluation of the nutritional characteristics of a finger millet based complementary food. *J. Agric. Food Chem.* **50**:3030–3036.
73. SCHOFIELD, P., MBUGUA, D.M., and PELL, A.N. (2001) Analysis of condensed tannins: a review. *Animal Feed Sci. Technol.* **91**:21–40.
74. PACHON, H., STOLTZFUS, R.J., and GLAHN, R.P. (2005) Experimental Biology 2005, San Diego, CA. Abstract. Identifying infant food combinations that maximize iron uptake: application of the Caco-2 cell/*in vitro* model.
75. ARIZA-NIETO, M., HU, Y., WELCH, R.M., GLAHN, R.P., BONIERBALE, M., BURGOS, G., and KAPINGA, R. (2005) Experimental Biology 2005, San Diego, CA. Abstract. Iron bioavailability and sweet potatoes (*Ipomea batatas*).
76. GLAHN, R.P., CHENG, Z., HU, Y., ARIZA-NIETO, M., WELCH, R.M., BEEBE, S., BLAIR, M., and KIMANI, P. (2005) Experimental Biology 2005, San Diego, CA. Abstract. Iron availability from beans of East Africa.
77. LOTT, J.N.A., OCKENDEN, I., RABOY, V., and BATTEN, G.D. (2000) Phytic acid and phosphorous in crop seeds and fruits: a global estimate. *Seed Science Res.* **10**:11–33.
78. WELCH, R.M., HOUSE, W.A., BEEBE, S., GREGORIO, G.B., and CHENG, Z. (2000) Testing iron and zinc bioavailability in genetically enriched beans (*Phaseolus vulgaris* L.) and rice (*Oryza sativa* L.) in a rat model. *Food Nutr. Bull.* **21**(4):428–433.

14

Techniques for assessing the functional response to food of the stomach and small and large intestine

R. Spiller, P. Gowland and L. Marciani, University of Nottingham, UK

Abstract: Functional foods are foods designed to have properties which enhance health. However, the key link between the design of the foods and the measurement of outcomes such as satiety and blood parameters, namely the digestive processes, are often neglected. In order to relate appropriately food properties to health outcomes, the physiological impact of the meal on the gastrointestinal tract needs to be assessed. Magnetic resonance imaging provides an ideal tool for such assessment without disturbing normal physiology. This chapter presents the evolution of different methods used to study these processes focusing particularly on our work with magnetic resonance imaging over the last decade.

Key words: magnetic resonance imaging (MRI), stomach, small bowel, colon, food.

14.1 Introduction

Functional foods are foods designed to have properties which enhance health. Although in the past this has focused on ensuring adequate intake and bioavailability of micronutrients, in this era of rising obesity and diabetes, a major aim is to improve satiety, target delivery of actives and reduce overconsumption. There may also be a desire to regulate gastric emptying of nutrients, while at the same time avoiding side effects such as bloating and diarrhoea. In a world driven by consumer choice, real foods need to be tasty and satisfying and hence are complex, mixed nutrient and multiphasic, with both solid, aqueous and lipid components. However, when trying to assess the effect of manipulating meal components, the journey of the meal through the gastrointestinal (GI) tract (the interface) is often neglected between the design of the foods (the input) and the measurement of outcomes such as satiety and blood parameters (the output). In order to relate these appropriately, there is a clear need to assess the transit and the macroscopic, physiological impact of the meal on the gastrointestinal tract. Such assessment requires techniques which can assess complex meals inside the gut without disturbing the physiology. Previous assessments which involved intubation or dosing with ionising radiation are rapidly being replaced with non-invasive, high-resolution, dynamic imaging techniques such as magnetic resonance imaging (MRI). This chapter presents a brief overview of different methods used to study GI function and reviews some of the results that we have obtained using MRI over the last decade.

14.2 Evolution of techniques to study the gastrointestinal response to feeding

14.2.1 Early studies of the gastrointestinal response to feeding

Gastric emptying

The early studies of gastric emptying performed by Hunt and colleagues (Hunt and Macdonald, 1954) involved using a large bore tube to empty the gastric contents at intervals, thereby assessing the change in gastric volume. This very crude technique, which was extremely arduous for both investigators and subjects and undoubtedly disturbed gastric emptying, was rapidly superseded by the marginally less invasive dye dilution technique of George (1968). This involved adding successively increasing concentration of dye and measuring the residual gastric volume by the dilution as assessed by aspirating a small aliquot. This limited the studies to low-viscosity meals, largely dextrose and amino acid solutions which could be easily aspirated from the stomach. Subsequent studies were done with liquid meals using similar techniques which involved aspiration and assessment of non-absorbable markers to calculate volumes remaining (Malagelada *et al.*, 1976). These tests were highly invasive and uncomfortable to the subjects and limited to meals of low viscosity, which were highly unrepresentative of normal food.

Scintigraphy

A non-invasive approach utilising gamma scintigraphy soon followed and techniques were developed for labelling both solid and liquid phases. Being non-invasive, scintigraphic techniques were suitable for studying patients and were used initially to evaluate the effects of gastric surgery or autonomic neuropathy (Heading *et al.*, 1976; Campbell *et al.*, 1977). These studies clearly showed the differential emptying of liquids and solids, with liquids following an exponential curve, while solid emptying was more linear (Heading *et al.*, 1976). Subsequent labelling of chicken liver particles was used to demonstrate that particles less than 2 mm in diameter emptied faster than larger-sized particles (Meyer *et al.*, 1988). Early studies also indicated that fat often separated from other components of the meal by virtue of its lower density, floating in the gastric fundus ensuring its delayed emptying. The development of a radio-isotope marker for liquid fat, ^{99m}Tc-thiocyanate, allowed the demonstration of this selective retention of fat in the proximal stomach (Edelbroek *et al.*, 1992b). Such scintigraphic studies were used to demonstrate the effect of meal composition and drugs on gastric emptying in healthy volunteers. However, these methods involve exposure of subjects to doses of ionising radiation which, depending on the markers used, could be substantial. The National Radiation Protection Board's limit for members of the general public of 5 mSv per annum restricts the use of these isotopes in any individual to just a few studies per year. Since in many cases it will be desirable to perform serial measurements, this is not an insignificant limitation and efforts have been made to develop other techniques.

Other imaging techniques

While ultrasonography is capable of imaging solid organs such as the liver or heart with great fidelity and in real time, ultrasound waves are reflected by liquid–gas interfaces. The normal stomach and the closely apposed transverse colon often contain such interfaces, which severely limit the use of ultrasound in assessing gastric volumes. By imaging through the liver, some of these problems can be overcome and ultrasound has been used by a small number of investigators. In many cases, however, the assessment must be limited to single dimensions such as the antral diameter in the midline (Hausken and Berstad, 1992). The volume and flow of the antrum can be assessed in real time (Berstad *et al.*, 1994) and a detailed description of antral contractions and trans-pyloric flow have been provided for liquid meals using this technique (Hausken *et al.*, 1998). However, imaging of the events in the gastric fundus is more difficult owing to the air–fluid interface often seen there.

Electrical impedance tomography has also been used to monitor gastric emptying. It is highly non-invasive and inexpensive, but it has limited spatial resolution or sensitivity to meal distribution and can only be used with high-conductivity meals such as salty soups (Chaw *et al.*, 2001). Although X-rays were used in the past to follow the emptying of radio-opaque markers with good spatial resolution, such studies provide limited information on emptying of nutrients, use non-physiological meals for adequate contrast and give unacceptably high radiation doses to subjects.

Manometry

Measuring pressure within the stomach has been used to identify the migrating motor complex (MMC), which is clearly seen in the fasting state but, once the stomach is full with viscous food, the ability to detect movement of the gastric wall is severely impaired and mostly only antral contractions can be registered in the fed state. Manometry cannot predict emptying rates nor identify different handling of complex meals with multiple phases. The gastric barostat has been used to assess gastric tone (Kuiken *et al.*, 1999) and is useful in identifying the receptive relaxation seen after a meal, but the large balloon distended in the stomach and associated nasogastric tube are highly invasive and artificial and are likely to disturb normal postprandial physiology, making extrapolation to the natural situation uncertain. The technique is, however, useful for defining the effect of drugs on gastric tone (Tack *et al.*, 1998, 2000).

Intestinal response to food beyond the pylorus

Studying motility and secretion/absorption in the intestine has been even more difficult. Most reports of intestinal function in the literature are based on invasive animal models with intestinal stomas allowing collection of whole chyme. Until recently, the methods available to use in humans had severe limitations. Oro-intestinal intubation was used, but it is highly invasive and is limited to studying liquid meals that can easily be aspirated. Intraluminal manometry also requires intubation, and although it can be used to evaluate antral motility, it can fail to detect non-occlusive contractions and its utility in assessing the response to different nutrients is limited. Gamma scintigraphy is useful for monitoring multiphase meals, by radioactively labelling different food components with different isotopes. However, this technique yields poor resolution and cannot detect any secretions added to the digesta, though it can measure intestinal transit time since, when the isotope reaches the caecum, it adopts a distinctive shape and position.

14.2.2 Magnetic resonance imaging studies of the gastrointestinal response to feeding

Overview

High-image quality and excellent soft tissue contrast have led to the widespread use of MRI as a tool for clinical diagnosis. However, MRI can also study normal gastrointestinal function in humans with the advantages of having high resolution, being non-invasive and using no ionising radiation, and thus allowing serial, dynamic studies. Since the early 1980s the speed of imaging using MRI has improved so that now high-quality images of the body can be obtained in a matter of hundreds of milliseconds. Over the past 15 years MRI methods have been developed to study the handling of food in the stomach and intestine as well as the brain's response to visceral perception, taste and aroma of food. MRI can measure movement, volumes, flow, parameters related to viscosity and fat content, and has therefore been used to study the effect of meal viscosity and fat content on the handling of food in the gut.

The stomach is an important site for the processing of food, being responsible for its initial storage, dilution, chemical breakdown, mixing, trituration and transport to the small intestine at a rate regulated to avoid overwhelming its absorptive capacity. Gastric secretion and motility are controlled by both the brain and the enteric nervous system via neural and endocrine feedback loops including both the 'duodenal' and 'ileal brakes'. These signals from the gut are generated by the arrival of nutrients at various sites in the GI tract, which stimulate release of neuropeptides such as cholecystokinin, glucagon-like peptide 1 (GLP-1), Peptide YY (PYY) and serotonin (5HT), which have a crucial role in determining the sense of satiety (Bray, 2000; Berthoud, 2002). The factors affecting satiety can be broken down into cephalic effects (such as the perceived texture and flavour of food in response to oral stimulation), gastric effects (such as viscosity and texture, gastric distension, emulsion stability and fat distribution) and intestinal effects (such as the nutrient delivery profile, entero-endocrine signalling and intestino-intestinal reflexes).

Imaging sequences for studying gastric processing

Motion artefacts have limited the use of MRI in the assessment of GI physiology in the past. These arise mainly from the contractions of the gastric wall movements of the diaphragm associated with breathing. In recent years there have been promising advances in the use of fast MRI sequences which largely overcome this problem. Work carried out in Nottingham showed that echo-planar magnetic resonance imaging (EPI) at low field (0.5 T) is well suited for dynamically assessing gastric physiology (Evans *et al.*, 1988). EPI acquires images very rapidly (in under 130 ms) overcoming artefacts due to abdominal motion. Furthermore, the EPI pulse sequence gives intrinsically T_2* weighted images, and hence provides excellent contrast between water-based liquid meals and surrounding tissues, and between the liquid and solid components of a meal (Stehling *et al.*, 1989; Evans *et al.*, 1993), without the need for the addition of MRI contrast agents. EPI can be particularly conveniently combined with other nuclear magnetic resonance (NMR) pulse sequences for quantifying various physical parameters. More recently, we have also started to use other ultrafast imaging sequences including the fast spin echo sequences such as HASTE (an example is shown in Fig. 14.1a), FISP and spoiled gradient echo sequences such as FLASH, which provide complementary information about anatomy and composition of gut contents.

It is important to be able to assess the intragastric distribution of the liquid, viscous and solid components of a multiphase meal, in order to understand the process of digestion. The different proton densities and relaxation times of the liquid, viscous and solid components of a meal make it possible to serially monitor the fate of different phases separately, accurately and non-invasively using EPI. Furthermore, the chemical shift between the resonances of the water and the fat protons can be exploited to image fat and water components separately by suppressing the signal arising from the other component as shown in Fig. 14.1b.

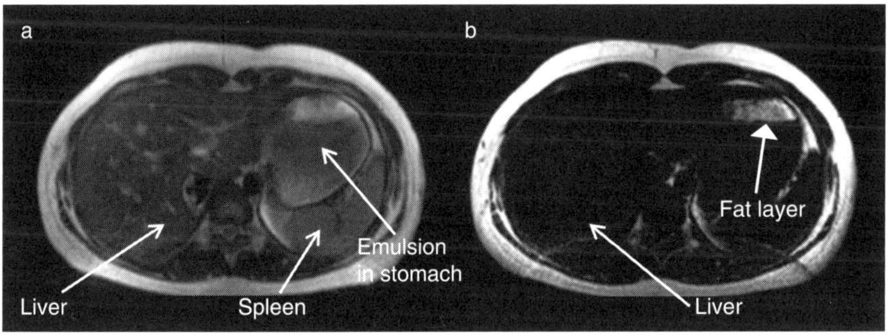

Fig. 14.1 (a) A HASTE water-selective axial section across the stomach of a volunteer who ingested a fat emulsion. Excellent contrast between the test meal and the surrounding organs is shown. (b) The corresponding fat selective image in which only the fat in the body and in the digesta is imaged, showing a clear layer of fat floating on top of the stomach.

We have used MRI to investigate the intragastric mixing and the gastric emptying of multi-phase meals consisting of oil and water, porridge and water, model solid particulates in a model meal matrix and nutrient and non-nutrient viscous polysaccharides and alginates. We have studied the intragastric layering of a mixed-phase fatty meal and used NMR relaxometry to study the fat content of a meal at 0.5 T.

Effect of physical form of food on gastric emptying

Early experiments in animal models suggested that meal viscosity influences gastric function (Prove and Ehrlein, 1982; Cherbut *et al.*, 1990). Human studies also indicated that meal viscosity might slow gastric emptying (Sandhu *et al.*, 1987). However, the degree to which these observed changes are simply a passive result of changes in the physical properties of the gastric contents has proved difficult to study in humans using conventional modalities. We have used EPI to investigate the changes induced in the rate of gastric emptying by varying the physical properties of food. From the rapid, multi-slice, volume data sets, it was also possible to assess fundal volumes (Coleman *et al.*, 2003b), as well as to investigate gastric accommodation, by measuring the circumference of the antrum (Marciani *et al.*, 2001a).

14.3 Imaging specific regions of the gut using magnetic resonance imaging

14.3.1 General methods, subjects and magnetic resonance imaging techniques

This section briefly summarises the methods that are common to most of the studies described in this chapter.

Subjects
Depending on the power calculations for the main outcome of interest, the studies usually required 8–18 volunteers. The subjects were required to be healthy, with no history of gastrointestinal disorders and within the normal range of body mass index. They were asked to avoid alcohol consumption the day before the study, to avoid concomitant medications which altered gastrointestinal motility and to fast overnight before each experiment. Serial experiments were performed more than 1 day apart, generally 7 days apart. The same applied for the patients who were recruited from the Nottingham University Hospitals gastroenterology clinics. We excluded volunteers and patients with metal implants in their body for safety reasons. The length of the scanning sessions varied from a few minutes for fasting studies to several hours, as this is the time scale of GI processing of a meal. During the studies the image data acquisition occurred at intervals between 20 and 45 min depending on the study. The subjects had to lie supine (or sometimes on their side) only for the short time required to take the images, but in-between each period of data acquisition, the subjects were made to sit upright.

Test meals
Several test meals were used in these experiments, ranging from tap water that simply filled the gastric lumen and gave contrast, to elaborate viscous nutrient polysaccharide meals, fat emulsions and gels of varying properties. The test meals were given using Latin square designs to avoid order effects.

Magnetic resonance imaging
We used a variety of MRI sequences and with varying parameters depending on the food material and organ to be imaged, optimising the protocols *in vitro* on the food materials first. Our early work was carried out using EPI on a whole-body 0.5 T purpose-built EPI scanner. This was used to measure gastric volumes and motility and single slice images could be repeated at around 0.3 Hz for dynamic studies. We also used inversion recovery EPI, spin echo EPI and pulsed gradient spin echo (PGSE) EPI to measure, respectively, the relaxation times of the chyme and flow rates in the gastric lumen. More recent work was carried out at higher field, on 1.5 and 3 T Philips Achieva machines using sequences such as transverse balanced TFE (TrueFISP) to measure volumes of the gastric lumen and the relaxation times of the GI contents, coronal TSE (MRCP) to assess water volumes in the small bowel and coronal Dual Echo FFE (gradient echo) to measure colonic volumes. During each image acquisition we asked the subjects to hold their breath for about 15–20 s to avoid motion artefacts.

Satiety assessment
In most of our studies we asked the subjects to score their subjective feelings of fullness, hunger and appetite at various time points throughout the

experiment. Patients and controls were also asked to score symptoms such as bloating and abdominal pain. We subsequently compared the means and the area under the curves of each score against time with the MRI findings on gastric function.

Ethics approvals
The appropriate Ethics Committees approved the research protocols described here and all volunteers and patients gave informed written consent prior the experiments.

14.3.2 Gels in the gastric lumen

Many types of processed foods contain gels, which are added either to provide desirable textures or to stabilise emulsions and complex mixtures to ensure long shelf-life. Several animal studies have indicated that meal viscosity is a key physical factor in influencing gastric motor function (Cherbut *et al.*, 1990). However, the techniques to measure intra-gastric viscosity have been invasive and it is not clear that the results can be directly applied to humans under normal conditions. Human studies have suggested that increased viscosity will slow gastric emptying (Wilmshurst and Crawley, 1980; Krotkiewski, 1984) and that high-viscosity meals increase satiety (Dilorenzo *et al.*, 1988). It has also been proposed that increased meal viscosity might slow absorption of nutrients, and thus improve the management of glucose intolerance and obesity (Zavoral *et al.*, 1983; Blackburn *et al.*, 1984; Haskell *et al.*, 1992).

We investigated the details of meal dilution initially for a high-nutrient, fatty, porridge meal, followed by water. Analysis of signal intensity ratios in the EPI images showed that the porridge hydrated and mixed slowly, and that the meal remained in two phases for more than 90 min. We then aimed to measure the viscosity of model polysaccharide test meal non-invasively *in vivo* within the gastric lumen by calibrating the transverse relaxation rate (T_2^{-1}) of a simple polysaccharide model, locust bean gum, meal against its viscosity *in vitro*. The NMR parameter T_2 is the time constant describing the decline in signal intensity on the images as a function of another specific time delay in the imaging sequence (called the echo-time). T_2 depends on the magnetic environment of the water protons that are being imaged and also on their mobility, hence it is a sensitive probe of the physicochemical environment of the water present in the foods imaged.

Subsequently, we validated the method *in vivo* by aspirating samples of the gastric contents via naso-gastric tubes and measuring the viscosity of the samples, *in vitro*, using a viscometer (Marciani *et al.*, 1998, 2000a). The EPI *in vivo* viscosity measurements correlated well with aspirate viscosity (r^2 = 0.88). We also found that the stomach responded to ingestion of a viscous meal by rapid intragastric dilution leading to a reduction in (zero-shear η_0) viscosity, which was greatest for the most viscous meal. It was

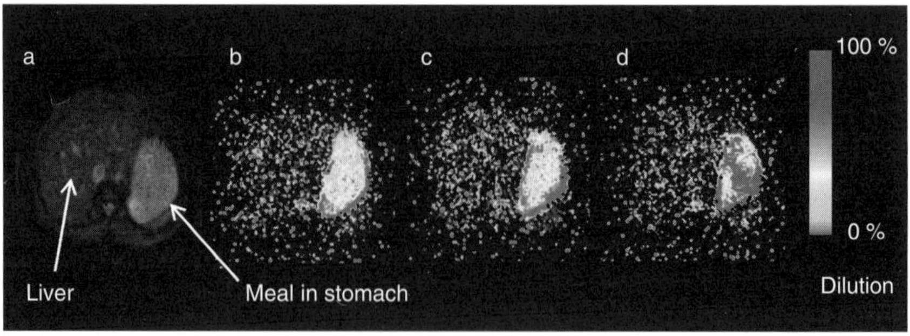

Fig. 14.2 (a) EPI axial section across the stomach of a volunteer who ingested 500 ml of a locust bean gum viscous meal, shown as anatomical reference. The images are dilution maps whereby the greyscale corresponds to the viscosity (for the stomach contents here, bright is viscous and dark is liquid). (b) Acquired 36 min, (c) 48 min and (d) 72 min after feeding, thus showing that gastric secretion progressively diluted the outer boundaries of the viscous meal, while the inner bolus remained viscous for longer. The viscous meals appeared more diluted and mixed at later times. Adapted from Marciani *et al.* (2001b).

found that a 1000-fold increase in the initial meal viscosity induced only a small delay in gastric emptying (Marciani *et al.*, 2000a). This implies an adaptation of gastric propulsive activity to meal viscosity since, if emptying were purely passive, it would be expected that a more viscous meal would be emptied more slowly. We have later used this technique to assess the effect of meal viscosity and nutrient content on intragastric dilution, gastric emptying and motility (Marciani *et al.*, 2001b). We found that the gastric contents of a fluid which, although viscous, was still pourable, were nevertheless relatively poorly mixed up to 45 min after ingestion with secreted fluid imaged surrounding the viscous mass as shown in Fig. 14.2. This also suggested that the more dilute, peripheral components of the meal bolus left the stomach selectively by a process of elution from the outside of the bolus. Increasing meal viscosity did not induce any changes in the frequency and velocity of antral contractions, suggesting that the force of gastric contractions had increased to account for the virtually unchanged rate of emptying. Most importantly, it was confirmed that increased meal viscosity was associated with increased satiety. This was probably due to the stimulation of tension receptors in the antrum.

In a separate study using agar spheres of defined breaking strength as model solid meals (Marciani *et al.*, 2001a), we found that increasing meal viscosity impaired gastric sieving of model solid food, that is to say the agar spheres emptied more rapidly when the matrix of the meal was more viscous. The presence of nutrients delayed gastric emptying, having a stronger effect than meal viscosity, showing that the negative feedback effect of nutrients in the small intestine had a dominant effect in controlling gastric emptying compared with the effect of intragastric viscosity. We also

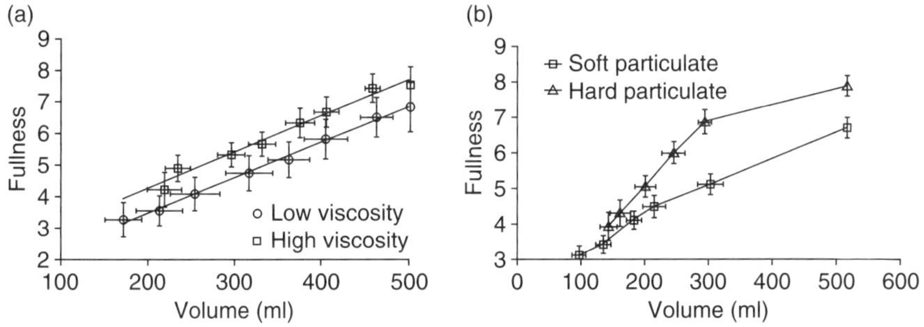

Fig. 14.3 (a) Self-assessment scores for the sense of fullness plotted versus the volume of a low- and high-viscosity locust bean gum test meal remaining in the stomach at different time points during emptying. The data are from 12 volunteers. It can be seen that the sense of fullness increased linearly with gastric volumes and that the fullness scores for the more viscous meal are higher than the controls throughout digestion. Adapted from Marciani *et al.* (2001b). (b) A similar plot but in this study the volunteers were fed low (0.15 N) and high (0.90 N) fracture strength agar beads with a low-viscosity locust bean gum test meal. It can be seen that the linear relationship between fullness feeling and gastric volume was reproduced for the 0.15 N fracture force (soft) beads but that, when the 0.90 N fracture force (hard) beads were fed, this induced higher fullness earlier in gastric emptying. Adapted from Marciani *et al.* (2001a).

demonstrated a linear relationship between gastric volumes and the subjective sense of satiety with low- and high-viscosity, nutrient meals (Fig. 14.3a). This was confirmed when using low-viscosity meals fed together with soft particulate but not with hard particulate, which induced greater satiety (Fig. 14.3b). We also observed that the volume of secretions within the stomach at one hour after ingestion was higher for the nutrient meal than for the non-nutrient meal. The nutrient contents of the meals did not affect the frequency and velocity of antral contractions but likely altered the pyloric contractions and relaxations which determine whether gastric chyme propelled towards the pylorus escapes into the duodenum. This relatively slow process of intragastric meal dilution and mixing with viscous meals may help to understand why dietary fat hydrolysis and starch digestion initiated in the mouth continues in the stomach despite such enzymes being inactivated at the pH characteristic of pure gastric secretion.

Gelling alginates

Achieving increased meal viscosity *in vivo* using food additives may offer one approach to controlling satiety responses. Animal experiments have shown that meal viscosity influences gastric motor function and human studies have suggested that high-viscosity meals are more satisfying but the precise mechanisms are not entirely clear. We have studied the fate of materials designed to gel in the gastric lumen (Hoad *et al.*, 2004). Biopolymers like alginate and pectin may form aggregates or gelled networks in

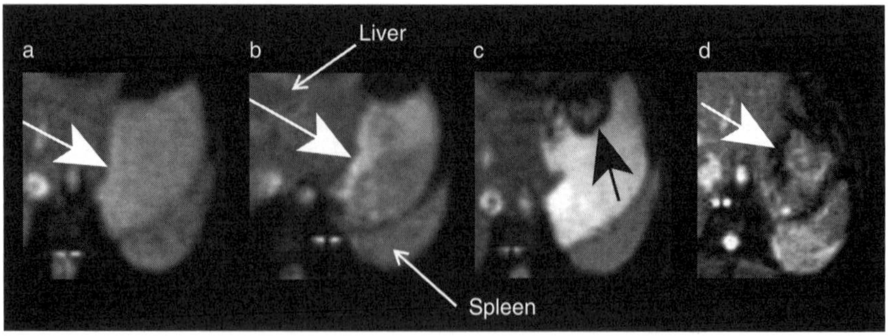

Fig. 14.4 EPI axial sections across the stomach of volunteers who ingested milk-based test meals that were either control or contained different biopolymer gelling alginates. (a) Image of the control meal (arrow) taken 10 min after ingestion, showing that, at that time, the meal in the stomach retained a single homogeneous phase. (b) An image of the same control meal taken 40 min after ingestion, showing that by this time the meal has separated into an upper liquid (brighter) and a lower thicker (darker) phase in the stomach. By contrast, (c) shows an image of a meal containing a gelling alginate that formed a large liquid-filled gel lump in the stomach, visible as a dark edge with a lighter centre and (d) shows an image of a different alginate-containing meal that formed a large solid lump in the stomach identifiable as a homogeneous dark region. Adapted from Hoad *et al.* (2004).

the stomach depending on pH and on the ionic species present. In our studies we demonstrated the formation *in vivo* of alginate biopolymer gels. Such observations are pivotal to understanding *in vivo* meal behaviour. Indeed, we found that meals containing strong-gelling alginates increased the sense of fullness as much as a meal that was already viscous on ingestion. This suggests that agents that gel on contact with acid may be useful additions to weight-reducing diets. This effect may be due to either distension in the gastric antrum or altered transport of nutrients to the small intestine in the gel. The images shown in Fig. 14.4 are an example of the powerful insights that MRI gives into the behaviour of such agents *in vivo*. Alginates are also used in established formulations used as gastric acid reflux suppressants. The mode of action of these formulations is thought to be the formation of an alginate raft that floats on top of the stomach contents, thus providing a physical barrier to reflux into the lower oesophagus in the treatment of gastro-oesophageal reflux disease. The ability to study the alginate raft formation and retention *in vivo* allows investigation of the effect of formulation modification on product performance. We studied two such formulations and monitored the formation of alginate rafts in the stomach (Marciani *et al.*, 2002). We were able to produce three-dimensional volume reconstructions of the rafts that showed the spatial distribution of the rafts within the gastric lumen. T_2 measurement showed also potential for assessment of dynamic changes in the physicochemical properties of rafts in the gastric lumen with time.

14.3.3 Solids and particulates in the gastric lumen

Shear rates in the mouth are high and estimated to average at around 50/s (Wood, 1968) and this is where most breakdown of food occurs. By contrast, the shear in the stomach in the postprandial period is much lower but when combined with the proteolytic action of pepsin and acid this does allow the stomach to break down digestible meal solids into the smaller particles required before they can be emptied via the pylorus. This occurs in the antro-pyloric region, where the pyloric sphincter acts as a sieve to impede large particles from leaving the stomach, its contraction causing retropulsion of larger particulates into the antrum. MRI can easily discriminate between the solid and liquid components of a meal, and therefore monitor the fate of mixed phase (a creamed rice pudding and orange juice example is given in Fig. 14.5a) and particulate and liquid meals.

We have imaged the intragastric fate of a range of solid foods such as roasted chicken (an example is shown in Fig. 14.5b) and model particulates such as agar gel beads (Marciani *et al.*, 2001a), alginate gels (Hoad *et al.*, 2004; Marciani *et al.*, 2002), coarse wheat bran (Marciani *et al.*, 2006b), almonds and sunflower seed oil-bodies (Hoad *et al.*, 2008). Using model, well-characterised particulates the antral grinding forces and shear can be assessed indirectly using MRI. We have carried out this assessment by monitoring the breakdown and emptying of sets of solid agar gel beads, each designed to have a different fracture force (Marciani *et al.*, 2001a). We found that beads with a fracture force >0.9 N showed much delayed emptying, suggesting that this exceeded the maximum grinding force exerted by the human antrum, which is therefore 0.65–0.9 N. (Marciani *et al.*, 2001a).

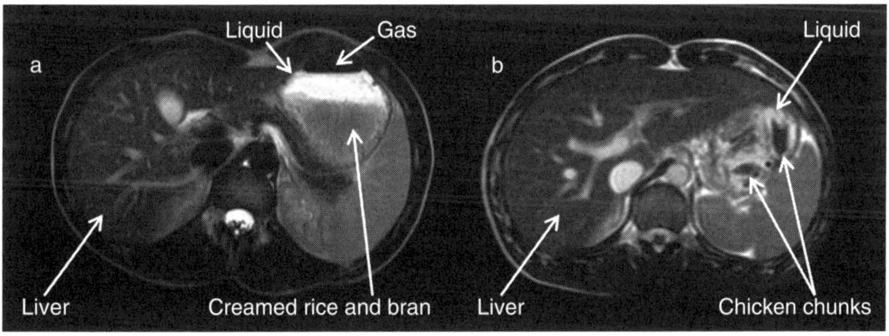

Fig. 14.5 (a) A balanced TFE (TrueFISP) axial section across the stomach of a volunteer who ingested a cream rice pudding with orange juice. These images show excellent contrast between the test meal and the surrounding organs. Additionally, different phases of the meal in the stomach can be observed, with a supernatant liquid phase (appearing bright in these T2 weighted images) and a thicker rice pudding and bran phase at the bottom of the lumen (appearing darker with this MRI sequence). (b) A similar image taken when a volunteer ate a roasted chicken and vegetables meal with a water drink. The chicken chunks appear very dark owing to their solid nature.

In the presence of model solid particles the gastric emptying curves for the total meal volume were exponential and increasing particle fracture strength delayed emptying with both a liquid and a viscous meal. Hard particulates also increased maximum antral diameters and increased the sense of satiety as shown in Fig. 14.3b. We have also observed the persistence of beads in the small intestine and have used this to draw conclusions about the efficiency of gastric sieving.

14.3.4 Fat emulsions in the gastric lumen

Fat, being less dense than water, tends to float above water when free from a solid food matrix and in the normal upright position this leads to delayed gastric emptying compared to water (Boulby *et al.*, 1999). This in turn affects the rate of fat absorption and metabolism and the signalling between the gut and brain (Read *et al.*, 1994). Gamma scintigraphy studies have confirmed the delayed gastric emptying of fat from liquid and solid food phases (Edelbroek *et al.*, 1992a, Cunningham *et al.*, 1991, Jian *et al.*, 1982). Recent MRI studies have exploited the ability of MRI to discriminate between changes in the proton environment of water and fat components of a meal, allowing visualisation and measurement of the gastric emptying of these different components (Howseman *et al.*, 1988; Stehling *et al.*, 1989; Schwizer *et al.*, 1992; Evans *et al.*, 1993; Fraser *et al.*, 1993; Boulby *et al.*, 1997, 1999; Kunz *et al.*, 2005). We used initially a multiphase aqueous and oil meal to measure the emptying rates of oil and water components separately and to observe how posture altered gastric emptying (Boulby *et al.*, 1997). When the subject was lying with the right side down, the lipid phase was observed to float in the fundus and emptying of the aqueous phase was rapid. With the subject lying with the right side up, the lipid layer filled the duodenum, where it could stimulate the duodenal receptors, and gastric emptying was significantly slower. In a subsequent experiment we confirmed that fat delays gastric emptying and using a pulsed gradient spin echo (PGSE) EPI sequence we were able to assess intragastric flow non-invasively (Boulby *et al.*, 1999). High-calorie fatty meals were found to be associated with substantially greater forward and backward flow-events in the antrum, compared with high-calorie, non-fatty meals (Fig. 14.6a). This antral retropulsion could aid fat emulsification by increasing shear.

We have validated a method to assess the fat fraction in an oil-in-water emulsion both *in vitro* and *in vivo* within the gastric lumen using inversion recovery EPI and a two non-exchanging compartments empirical model (Marciani *et al.*, 2004). We have evaluated the intragastric behaviour of emulsions designed to be stable or break in the acidic gastric environment, showing that fat is emptied slower from the stomach for meals that layer and that this can have an effect on the sense of satiety (Marciani *et al.*, 2003). We have also recently shown that acid stable emulsions stimulate greater cholecystokinin release and are associated with delayed gastric emptying

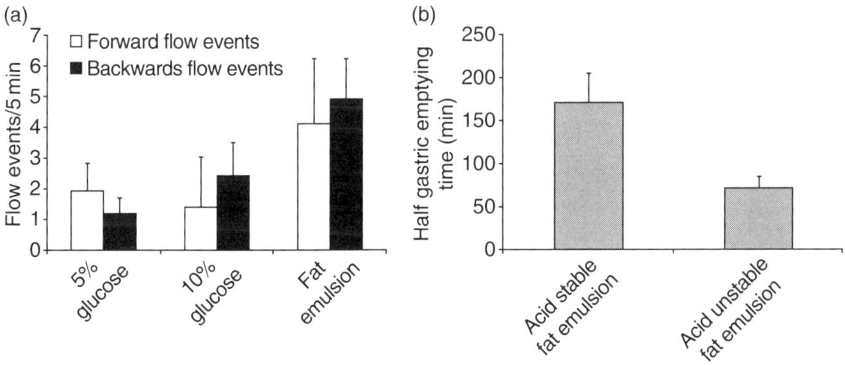

Fig. 14.6 (a) The chart shows the results of flow measurements carried out in the gastric antrum using a flow-sensitive version of the high-speed magnetic resonance imaging technique, echo planar imaging (EPI). The eight volunteers were fed 800 ml of either 5% glucose, 10% glucose or an isotonic fat emulsion nutrient meal. The end point was the number of forward and backwards flow events observed in the antropyloric region over 5 min. Despite delayed gastric emptying, the fat-containing meal was associated with a higher number of substantial to and fro movements which may be important for meal trituration and fat emulsification. (b) The chart shows the results of a gastric emptying study in nine volunteers who were fed 500 ml of a 15% oil emulsion which was either stable or unstable in the acid gastric environment. The acid unstable emulsion meal layered rapidly in the stomach due to fat emulsion breakdown. The gastric half-emptying time of the aqueous phase was three-fold faster for the acid unstable fat emulsion meal than for the acid stable fat emulsion meal.

(Fig. 14.6b) (Marciani *et al.*, 2007d) compared with acid unstable emulsions in which the fat layer empties after the aqueous phase.

14.3.5 Antral motility and flow

The motility of the gastric antrum plays an important role in mixing and transport of food. Antral motility can, to a limited extent, be monitored using naso-gastric manometric catheters. The intubation procedure is invasive and may cause discomfort to the subjects. MRI offers the possibility of non-invasively investigating antral motility (Wright *et al.*, 1999; Marciani *et al.*, 2001c; Schwizer *et al.*, 1994). The gastric lumen can be imaged serially at rapid intervals allowing detection and measurement of the periodic contractions of the antral walls (Schwizer *et al.*, 1994; Marciani *et al.*, 2000b, 2001c). We used in-house analysis software that measures in each dynamic image the antral cross-sectional area by counting the number of pixels perpendicular to the antral axis and displays this information compressed in a two-dimensional motility plot from which the antral contraction frequency, speed and percentage occlusion can be measured. We have validated this technique against manometry, and have found that more contractions are detected using MRI, which would be consistent with manometry failing to detect non-occlusive contractions (Wright *et al.*, 1999). We have used the MRI motility measurements to investigate the effect of liquid and mixed liquid/solid and viscous/solid meals on antral motility (Marciani *et al.*, 2001c). No change was observed in the frequency and velocity of antral contractions which at three contractions/min prove to be remarkably resistant to change.

As already mentioned in the Introduction, Doppler ultrasound studies have shown backward and forward flow events in the antrum using liquid meals (Hausken *et al.*, 1998). Using MRI we have shown that the flow of the meal within the antrum can also be assessed using the PGSE EPI technique (Boulby *et al.*, 1999), and also using 'tagging' in which a grid is magnetically superimposed onto the image by spatially modulating the longitudinal magnetisation prior to imaging (Issa *et al.*, 1994).

14.3.6 Gall bladder contraction

The contraction of the gall bladder is largely driven by the release of cholecystokinin (CCK) from duodenal enteroendocrine cells within the upper small intestine which is thus co-ordinated with gastric emptying and the delivery of nutrients to the duodenum (Lawson *et al.*, 1983). As for gastric emptying, studies on gall bladder contraction have been conducted previously using gamma scintigraphy techniques (Baxter *et al.*, 1985) and ultrasound (Portincasa *et al.*, 2001), suffering from the same limitations previously mentioned. Recently, MRI has been shown to be able to measure the emptying of the gall bladder accurately, non-invasively and with high spatial resolution (Vyas *et al.*, 2002; Inoue *et al.*, 2003). We have assessed the potential of MRI for the simultaneous assessment of gall bladder and gastric emptying in order to be able to study gall bladder and gastric co-ordination in relation to foods without using contrast agents. Using olive oil fat emulsion test meals we observed an exponential correlation between gall bladder and gastric volumes for the first 90 min (Marciani *et al.*, 2005a) and the contraction of the gall bladder in relation to the intragastric stability of fat emulsions (Marciani *et al.*, 2007d). In Fig. 14.7 an example of MRI imaging of gall bladder contraction is shown.

14.3.7 Imaging of small bowel water content

Digestion of food stimulates fluid secretions which include pancreatico-biliary and intestinal secretions that, in addition to the liquids ingested with the food, dilute the chyme, aiding digestion by pancreatic enzymes and equilibrating the osmotic gradients generated by the nutrient molecules in the small bowel. The amount of secretion (salivary, gastric and pancreatic) totals up to 3 litres of water that, in addition to jejunal secretion and fluid ingested with the food, contributes to the total sodium-rich secretion

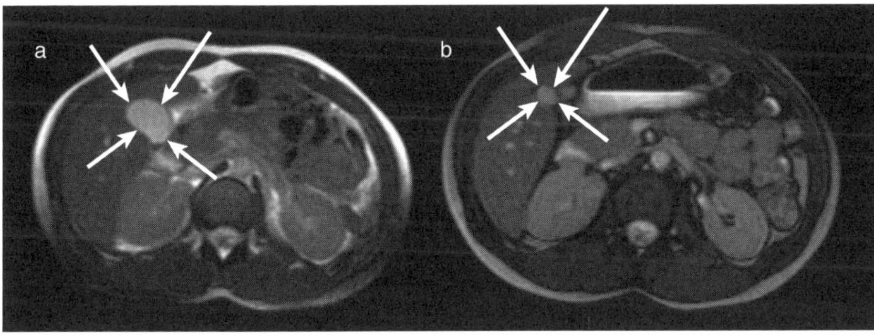

Fig. 14.7 (a) A balanced TFE (TrueFISP) axial section across the gall bladder (indicated by the arrows) of a fasted volunteer. (b) The corresponding image taken 75 min after the subject was fed a chicken and vegetables soup, showing the extent to which the gall bladder contracted releasing bile in the small bowel.

flow through the upper small bowel, which amounts to up to 9 litres per day (Spiller, 1994). Most water and sodium are re-absorbed due to co transport of nutrients and sodium. Subsequent movement to the distal intestine is regulated by numerous GI neurotransmitters, which act on visceral afferents to modulate secreto-motor reflexes. Earlier methods to evaluate small bowel water fluxes involved perfusion via oro-jejunal tubes (Krag and Phillips, 1974; Spiller *et al.*, 1987b). Such techniques are invasive and only allow assessment of limited tracts of the bowel. MRI has good sensitivity for mobile water pools and can assess the water content of the entire small bowel serially and non-invasively, enabling study of the effects of various foods on the small bowel water content. We have explored previously the evaluation of small bowel water content using MRI at low field (Adkin *et al.*, 1995; Hykin *et al.*, 1994), but recent improvements in hardware and imaging sequences have allowed significant improvements since these early studies (Hoad *et al.*, 2007). We now carry out serial, non-invasive monitoring of postprandial changes in small bowel water content using a magnetic resonance cholangiopancreatography (MRCP) sequence that was originally designed to study the pancreato-biliary region (Barish *et al.*, 1996; Takehara, 1996) and is strongly T_2 weighted and sensitive mainly to free mobile water only. We have optimised and validated our MRI small bowel water content measurements against naso-duodenal bolus infusions in healthy volunteers and we are now using them to study the effect of various foods on the function of the small intestine.

An example of the importance of monitoring the small bowel water content is given by bran. Bran is a dietary fibre known to alter small bowel transit, and previous studies in Nottingham using gamma scintigraphy have shown that both bran and plastic pellets were equally effective in increasing bowel transit, suggesting mechanical stimulation of the gut (McIntyre *et al.*,

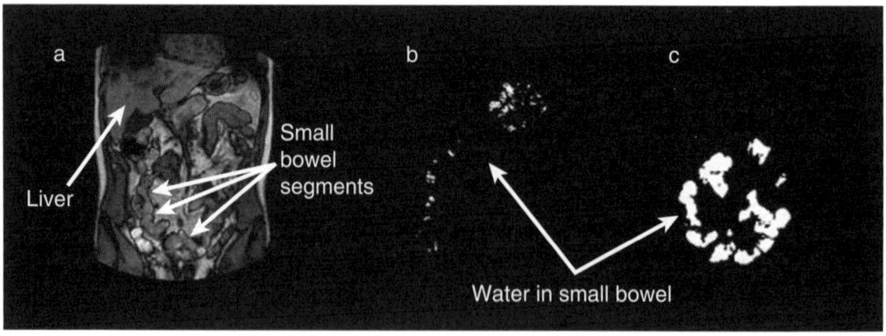

Fig. 14.8 (a) A coronal dual echo FFE (gradient echo) image showing small bowel segments in the abdomen of a healthy volunteer as an anatomical reference. (b) and (c) MRCP images of the water in the small bowel. Using this kind of sequence most of the signal from the body disappears and only bright signal from mobile water is left. (b) Taken 225 min after the volunteer was fed a creamed rice pudding without any bran. Little small bowel water can be detected. (c) The corresponding image taken when the same volunteer was fed, on a separate occasion, the creamed rice pudding together with 15 g coarse wheat bran. This shows a much higher volume of water in the small bowel.

1997). Bran can exacerbate bloating, distension and pain in patients suffering from irritable bowel syndrome (IBS) but the mechanisms are poorly understood. We aimed to define changes in gastric emptying and small bowel water content following ingestion of a standard rice pudding test meal in healthy volunteers. We found that bran significantly delayed the gastric half empting time by up to 20 min and increased small bowel water content as shown in Fig. 14.8 (Marciani *et al.*, 2006c). The most likely mechanism for small bowel water secretion is via mechanical stimulation of the gut mucosa causing serotonin release which stimulates secretion and propulsive motor patterns. Such studies may also help understand the clinical effects of bran supplementation in patients with IBS and/or constipation.

14.3.8 Colonic volumes

MRI can also be used to image the colonic volume response to feeding. This is measured by outlining the colon on every slice of a gradient echo image and then summing these to obtain total colonic volumes. We have already observed a postprandial increase in colonic volume that returns to baseline 90 min after feeding, whilst the size of the left colon did not change significantly. The increase in size of the right side of the colon is likely to be caused by gastro-ileal reflex shifting the contents of the distal small bowel into the ascending colon in preparation for the arrival of the current meal (Read *et al.*, 1986; Spiller *et al.*, 1987a).

14.3.9 Relating magnetic resonance imaging findings with the metabolic response and satiety

MRI can also be used to assess other parameters related to the effects of the gastrointestinal response to food such as blood flow and the cerebral response to feeding. This provides additional information on the metabolic response to the delivery of actives to the gut. We have studied the blood flow changes in the superior mesenteric artery in response to glucose ingestion, finding a substantial variation between individuals in the amplitude and the time to peak of the superior mesenteric artery blood flow response to the oral glucose challenge test, which correlated positively with body mass index (Totman *et al.*, 2007). We also have investigated the CCK response to feeding fat emulsion, finding that acid stable fat emulsions shown to remain homogeneous on MRI released more CCK than acid unstable (layering) fat emulsions (Marciani *et al.*, 2007d). The same studies found that increased CCK release correlated with increased satiety, which could also be achieved by increased meal viscosity and the presence of strong gelling alginates (Hoad *et al.*, 2004; Marciani *et al.*, 2001b, 2007d).

14.4 Compromised gastrointestinal function and gastrointestinal drugs studies

When discussing functional foods and imaging techniques one must remember that there are many GI conditions that compromise gastrointestinal function and cause symptoms postprandially. As described above for investigations of the physiology of normal subjects, MRI offers a non-invasive insight into GI pathology and the relation of symptoms with the transit of food. Furthermore, this would make it possible to avoid in many cases the use of radioactive tracers or of intubation, which is often problematic in such patients. Our early studies assessed gastric emptying and antral motility using a low-viscosity polysaccharide meal containing lipids and carbohydrate in selected patients with suspected compromised gastric function (Marciani *et al.*, 2000c). We recently started a wider programme imaging fasted and postprandially patients suffering from irritable bowel syndrome, coeliac disease and Crohn's disease (Coleman *et al.*, 2003a; Marciani *et al.*, 2005b, 2007b, c). These studies provide useful clinical information in terms of emptying rates, motility and transit abnormalities. We also carried out a range of studies investigating the fasted and postprandial GI tract using drugs designed for the GI tract such as mannitol (Adkin *et al.*, 1995), serotonin receptor agonists (Coleman *et al.*, 2003b) and antagonists (Marciani *et al.*, 2007a), and gelling alginates (Marciani *et al.*, 2002).

14.5 Future trends

As we have shown here, MRI studies are capable of simultaneously assessing multiple parameters and providing unique insights into the passage of food through the human gut. Therefore, despite being perceived as relatively expensive, MRI looks likely to be an increasingly important part of the future assessments of the impact of functional foods on gut physiology. Developments will include improved small and large bowel imaging, with higher temporal and spatial resolution; physicochemical characterisation of digesta *in vivo* using relaxation times and also magnetic resonance spectroscopy (MRS); assessment of fluid flows with phase contrast MRI and evaluation of shear rates using specialised MRI sequences. Water protons are not the only nuclei visible to MRI and MRS. For example one can investigate sodium (^{23}Na), phosphorus (^{31}P), carbon (^{13}C) and fluorine (^{19}F) nuclei. Labelling drugs and meals with fluorine-containing substances is also likely to develop to replace some of the radio-isotope techniques as a means of locating the position of drugs and meal components within the GI tract and timing their transit. Combining imaging with carbon^{13} labelled substrates will allow assessment of absorption, distribution and subsequent metabolism of lipids and monitoring of energy metabolites such as liver glycogen stores. Another important development will be the application of these methods to patients, since many gastrointestinal symptoms precipitate upon feeding but mechanisms are unclear. The MRI methods allow also monitoring of brain function, hence it can be expected that this field will also develop, including monitoring of visceral perception and gastrointestinal distension as well as the cortical representation of taste and aroma, which we have started investigating (Marciani *et al.*, 2005c, 2006a), and ultimately of satiety.

14.6 Conclusion

This chapter has shown the wealth of information that it is possible to extract from a non-invasive MRI feeding study. Many different imaging sequences are available with a range of contrasts that can highlight volumes, multiphase meal components and transit. After years of development and proof of concept studies, we now consider MRI to be a 'one stop shop' for the assessment of the impact of foods on many parameters of GI physiology, health outcomes and pathology. The alternative techniques are generally invasive or involve a radiation dose, and often only measure a single parameter of interest. Surprisingly little is known about the GI tract function and the interaction of different food properties with it: this interaction is far from simple and there is plenty of scope for further work.

14.7 Acknowledgements

We thank the Biotechnology and Biological Sciences Research Council (Swindon, UK) for funding most of the work described in this paper. Dr

Annette Fillery-Travis, Dr Martin Wickham, Mr Richard Faulks, Dr Caroline Hoad, Dr Phil Boulby, Dr Paul Young, Dr Pretima Manoj, Dr Jeff Wright, Mrs Barbara Pick and Mrs Debbie Bush made considerable contributions to the work reviewed here. Dr Ron Coxon, Mr Paul Clark, Dr Rachel Moore, Dr Damien Tyler, Dr Bashar Issa and Professor Sir Peter Mansfield also made contributions to the work reviewed.

14.8 References

ADKIN D A, GOWLAND P, SPILLER R C, FREEMAN A, HYKIN J, ISSA B, HUCKLE P D and WILDING I R (1995) Echo-planar magnetic resonance imaging to assess water volume in the distal small bowel. *Pharmaceutical Research,* **12**, 1134–1139.

BARISH M A, SOTO J A and YUCEL E K (1996) Magnetic resonance cholangiopancreatography of the biliary ducts: techniques, clinical applications, and limitations. *Topics in Magnetic Resonance Imaging,* **8**, 302–311.

BAXTER J N, GRIME J S, CRITCHLEY M and SHIELDS R (1985) Relationship between gastric-emptying of solids and gall-bladder emptying in normal subjects. *Gut,* **26**, 342–351.

BERSTAD A, HAUSKEN T, GILJA O H, THUNE N, MATRE K and ODEGAARD S (1994) Volume measurements of gastric antrum by 3-D ultrasonography and flow measurements through the pylorus by duplex technique. *Digestive Diseases and Sciences,* **39**, S97–S100.

BERTHOUD H R (2002) Multiple neural systems controlling food intake and body weight. *Neuroscience and Biobehavioral Reviews,* **26**, 393–428.

BLACKBURN N A, REDFERN J S, JARJIS H, HOLGATE A M, HANNING I, SCARPELLO J H B, JOHNSON I T and READ N W (1984) The mechanism of action of guar gum in improving glucose-tolerance in man. *Clinical Science,* **66**, 329–336.

BOULBY P, GOWLAND P, ADAMS V and SPILLER R C (1997) Use of echo planar imaging to demonstrate the effect of posture on the intragastric distribution and emptying of an oil/water meal. *Neurogastroenterology and Motility,* **9**, 41–47.

BOULBY P, MOORE R, GOWLAND P and SPILLER R C (1999) Fat delays emptying but increases forward and backward antral flow as assessed by flow-sensitive magnetic resonance imaging. *Neurogastroenterology and Motility,* **11**, 27–36.

BRAY G A (2000) Afferent signals regulating food intake. *Proceedings of the Nutrition Society,* **59**, 373–384.

CAMPBELL I W, HEADING R C, TOTHILL P, BUIST T A S, EWING D J and CLARKE B F (1977) Gastric emptying in diabetic autonomic neuropathy. *Gut,* **18**, 462–467.

CHAW C S, YAZAKI E and EVANS D F (2001) The effect of pH change on the gastric emptying of liquids measured by electrical impedance tomography and pH-sensitive radiotelemetry capsule. *International Journal of Pharmaceutics,* **227**, 167–175.

CHERBUT C, ALBINA E, CHAMP M, DOUBLIER J L and LECANNU G (1990) Action of guar gums on the viscosity of digestive contents and on the gastrointestinal motor function in pigs. *Digestion,* **46**, 205–213.

COLEMAN N S, HOLMES G K T, DUNLOP S P, MARCIANI L, GOWLAND P A, SINGH G, MARSDEN C A and SPILLER R C (2003a) Delayed gastric emptying: new insights into postprandial symptoms in untreated coeliac disease. *Gut,* **52**, A15– A15.

COLEMAN N S, MARCIANI L, BLACKSHAW E, WRIGHT J, PARKER M, YANO T, YAMAZAKI S, CHAN P Q, WILDE K, GOWLAND P A, PERKINS A C and SPILLER R C (2003b) Effect of a novel 5-HT3 receptor agonist MKC-733 on upper gastrointestinal motility in humans. *Alimentary Pharmacology & Therapeutics,* **18**, 1039–1048.

CUNNINGHAM K M, BAKER R J, HOROWITZ M, MADDOX A F, EDELBROEK M A L and CHATTERTON B E (1991) Use of technetium-99m(V)thiocyanate to measure gastric-emptying of fat. *Journal of Nuclear Medicine,* **32**, 878–881.

DILORENZO C, WILLIAMS C M, HAJNAL F and VALENZUELA J E (1988) Pectin delays gastric-emptying and increases satiety in obese subjects. *Gastroenterology,* **95**, 1211–1215.

EDELBROEK M, HOROWITZ M, MADDOX A and BELLEN J (1992a) Gastric-emptying and intragastric distribution of oil in the presence of a liquid or a solid meal. *Journal of Nuclear Medicine,* **33**, 1283–1290.

EDELBROEK M, HOROWITZ M, MADDOX A and BELLEN J (1992b) Gastric emptying and intragastric distribution of oil in the presence of a liquid or a solid meal. *Journal of Nuclear Medicine,* **33**, 1283–1290.

EVANS D F, STEHLING M K, LAMONT G, COXON R, HOWSEMAN A M, ORDRIDGE R J, HARDCASTLE J D and MANSFIELD P (1988) Investigation of gastrointestinal motility with echo planar magnetic-resonance imaging (Epi). *Gut,* **29**, A1452-A1452.

EVANS D F, LAMONT G, STEHLING M K, BLAMIRE A M, GIBBS P, COXON R, HARDCASTLE J D and MANSFIELD P (1993) Prolonged monitoring of the upper gastrointestinal tract using echo-planar magnetic resonance imaging. *Gut,* **34**, 848–852.

FRASER R, BOROVICKA J, SCHWIZER W, ASAL K, CRELIER G, BOESIGER P, BLUM A L, GONVERS J J and FRIED M (1993) Magnetic resonance imaging (MRI) to measure proximal and distal gastric motility during emptying of a liquid meal. *Gastroenterology,* **104**, A509–A509.

GEORGE J D (1968) New clinical method for measuring the rate of gastric emptying: the double sampling test meal. *Gut,* **9**, 237–242.

HASKELL W L, SPILLER G A, JENSEN C D, ELLIS B K and GATES J E (1992) Role of water-soluble dietary fiber in the management of elevated plasma-cholesterol in healthy-subjects. *American Journal of Cardiology,* **69**, 433–439.

HAUSKEN T and BERSTAD A (1992) Wide gastric antrum in patients with non-ulcer dyspepsia – effect of cisapride. *Scandinavian Journal of Gastroenterology,* **27**, 427–432.

HAUSKEN T, GILJA O H, UNDELAND K A and BERSTAD A (1998) Timing of postprandial dyspeptic symptoms and transpyloric passage of gastric contents. *Scandinavian Journal of Gastroenterology,* **33**, 822–827.

HEADING R C, TOTHILL P, MCLOUGHLIN G P and SHEARMAN D J C (1976) Gastric emptying rate measurement in man. A double isotope scanning technique for simultaneous study of liquid and solid components of a meal. *Gastroenterology,* **71**, 45–50.

HOAD C L, RAYMENT P, SPILLER R C, MARCIANI L, ALONSO B D, TRAYNOR C, MELA D J, PETERS H P F and GOWLAND P A (2004) *In vivo* imaging of intragastric gelation and its effect on satiety in humans. *Journal of Nutrition,* **134**, 2293–2300.

HOAD C L, MARCIANI L, FOLEY S, TOTMAN J J, WRIGHT J, BUSH D, COX E F, CAMPBELL E, SPILLER R C and GOWLAND P A (2007) Non-invasive quantification of small bowel water content by MRI: a validation study. *Physics in Medicine and Biology,* **52**, 6909–6922.

HOAD C L, MARCIANI L, GRAY D A, FISK I D, SAKUNKHUN M, COX E F, PLACIDI E, TOTMAN J J, SPILLER R C and GOWLAND P A (2008) Non-invasive imaging of different physical forms of dietary fat during digestion in humans. 16th ISMRM. Toronto.

HOWSEMAN A M, STEHLING M K, CHAPMAN B, COXON R, TURNER R, ORDIDGE R J, CAWLEY M G, GLOVER P, MANSFIELD P and COUPLAND R E (1988) Improvements in snap-shot nuclear magnetic resonance imaging. *British Journal of Radiology,* **61**, 822–828.

HUNT J N and MACDONALD I (1954) The influence of volume on gastric emptying. *Journal of Physiology,* **126**, 459–474.

HYKIN J, FREEMAN A, GOWLAND P, BOWTELL R W, WORTHINGTON B S, SPILLER R and MANSFIELD P (1994) Measurement of GI water content using EPI at 0.5 tesla. *MAGMA,* **2**, 471–473.

INOUE Y, KOMATSU Y, YOSHIKAWA K, AKAHANE M, ISAYAMA H, OHTOMO K and OMATA M (2003) Biliary motor function in gallstone patients evaluated by fatty-meal MR cholangiography. *Journal of Magnetic Resonance Imaging,* **18**, 196–203.

ISSA B, FREEMAN A, BOULBY P, WRIGHT J, GOWLAND P, BOWTELL R, SPILLER R and MANSFIELD P (1994) Gastric motility by tagged EPI. *Magnetic Resonance Materials in Physics, Biology and Medicine (MAGMA),* **2**, 295–298.

JIAN R, VIGNERON N, NAJEAN Y and BERNIER J J (1982) Gastric-emptying and intra-gastric distribution of lipids in man – a new scintigraphic method of study. *Digestive Diseases and Sciences,* **27**, 705–711.

KRAG E and PHILLIPS S F (1974) Active and passive bile acid absorption in man: perfusion studies of ileum and jejunum. *Journal of Clinical Investigation,* **53**, 1686–1694.

KROTKIEWSKI M (1984) Effect of guar gum on body-weight, hunger ratings and metabolism in obese subjects. *British Journal of Nutrition,* **52**, 97–105.

KUIKEN S D, SAMSOM M, CAMILLERI M, MULLAN B P, BURTON D D, KOST L J, HARDYMAN T J, BRINKMANN B H and O'CONNOR M K (1999) Development of a test to measure gastric accommodation in humans. *American Journal of Physiology – Gastrointestinal and Liver Physiology,* **277**, G1217–G1221.

KUNZ P, FEINLE-BISSET C, FAAS H, BOESIGER P, FRIED M, STEINGOTTER A and SCHWIZER W (2005) Effect of ingestion order of the fat component of a solid meal on intragastric fat distribution and gastric emptying assessed by MRI. *Journal of Magnetic Resonance Imaging,* **21**, 383–390.

LAWSON M, EVERSON G T, KLINGENSMITH W and KERN F (1983) Coordination of gastric and gallbladder emptying after ingestion of a regular meal. *Gastroenterology,* **85**, 866–870.

MALAGELADA J R, LONGSTRETH G F, SUMMERSKILL W H J and GO V L W (1976) Measurement of gastric functions during digestion of ordinary solid meals in man. *Gastroenterology,* **70**, 203–210.

MARCIANI L, MANOJ P, HILLS B P, MOORE R J, YOUNG P, FILLERY-TRAVIS A, SPILLER R C and GOWLAND P A (1998) Echo-planar imaging relaxometry to measure the viscosity of a model meal. *Journal of Magnetic Resonance,* **135**, 82–86.

MARCIANI L, GOWLAND P A, SPILLER R C, MANOJ P, MOORE R J, YOUNG P, AL-SAHAB S, BUSH D, WRIGHT J and FILLERY-TRAVIS A J (2000a) Gastric response to increased meal viscosity assessed by echo-planar magnetic resonance imaging in humans. *Journal of Nutrition,* **130**, 122–127.

MARCIANI L, SPILLER R C, GOWLAND P A, WRIGHT J, MOORE R J and YOUNG P (2000b) Magnetic resonance imaging (MRI) assessment of gastric emptying and antral motility in clinical practice: Preliminary results on patients. *Gastroenterology,* **118**, 2056.

MARCIANI L, YOUNG P, WRIGHT J, MOORE R J, EVANS D F, SPILLER R C and GOWLAND P A (2000c) Echo-planar imaging in GI clinical practice: assessment of gastric emptying and antral motility in four patients. *Journal of Magnetic Resonance Imaging,* **12**, 343–346.

MARCIANI L, GOWLAND P A, FILLERY-TRAVIS A, MANOJ P, WRIGHT J, SMITH A, YOUNG P, MOORE R and SPILLER R C (2001a) Assessment of antral grinding of a model solid meal with echo- planar imaging. *American Journal of Physiology – Gastrointestinal and Liver Physiology,* **280**, G844–G849.

MARCIANI L, GOWLAND P A, SPILLER R C, MANOJ P, MOORE R J, YOUNG P and FILLERY-TRAVIS A J (2001b) Effect of meal viscosity and nutrients on satiety, intragastric dilution, and emptying assessed by MRI. *American Journal of Physiology,* **280**, G1227–G1233.

MARCIANI L, YOUNG P, WRIGHT J, MOORE R, COLEMAN N, GOWLAND P A and SPILLER R C (2001c) Antral motility measurements by magnetic resonance imaging. *Neurogastroenterology and Motility,* **13**, 511–518.

MARCIANI L, LITTLE S L, SNEE J, COLEMAN N S, TYLER D J, SYKES J, JOLLIFFE I G, DETTMAR P W, SPILLER R C and GOWLAND P A (2002) Echo-planar magnetic resonance imaging of Gaviscon alginate rafts *in-vivo*. *Journal of Pharmacy and Pharmacology,* **54**, 1351–1356.

MARCIANI L, WICKHAM M, WRIGHT J, BUSH D, FAULKS R, FILLERY-TRAVIS A, GOWLAND P and SPILLER R C (2003) Magnetic resonance imaging (MRI) insights into how fat emulsion stability alters gastric emptying. *Gastroenterology,* **124**, A581– A581.

MARCIANI L, WICKHAM M, HILLS B P, WRIGHT J, BUSH D, FAULKS R, FILLERY-TRAVIS A, SPILLER R C and GOWLAND P A (2004) Intragastric oil-in-water emulsion fat fraction measured using inversion recovery echo-planar magnetic resonance imaging. *Journal of Food Science,* **69**, E290–E296.

MARCIANI L, BUSH D, WRIGHT P, WICKHAM M, PICK B, WRIGHT J, FAULKS R, FILLERY-TRAVIS A, SPILLER R C and GOWLAND P A (2005a) Monitoring of gallbladder and gastric coordination by EPI. *Journal of Magnetic Resonance Imaging,* **21**, 82–85.

MARCIANI L, COLEMAN N S, DUNLOP S P, SINGH G, MARSDEN C A, HOLMES G K, SPILLER R C and GOWLAND P A (2005b) Gallbladder contraction, gastric emptying and antral motility: single visit assessment of upper GI function in untreated celiac disease using echo-planar MRI. *Journal of Magnetic Resonance Imaging,* **22**, 634–638.

MARCIANI L, PFEIFFER J, HORT J, HEAD K, BUSH D, TAYLOR A J, SPILLER R C, FRANCIS S and GOWLAND P A (2005c) Towards fMRI of physiological taste and aroma perception. 12th Annual Scientific Meeting and Exibition of the International Society for Magnetic Resonance in Medicine. Miami.

MARCIANI L, PFEIFFER J C, HORT J, HEAD K, BUSH D, TAYLOR A J, SPILLER R C, FRANCIS S and GOWLAND P A (2006a) Improved methods for fMRI studies of combined taste and aroma stimuli. *Journal of Neuroscience Methods,* **158**, 186–194.

MARCIANI L, TOTMAN J J, HOAD C L, EVANS S, MISTRY A, GOWLAND P A and SPILLER R C (2006b) Bran-induced small bowel secretion: assessment by novel non-invasive MRI technique. *Gastroenterology,* **130**, A743–A743.

MARCIANI L, TOTMAN J J, HOAD C L, EVANS S, MISTRY A, SPILLER R C and GOWLAND P A (2006c) Gastrointestinal effects of bran: a MRI study. *Proceedings of International Society of Magnetic Resonance in Medicine 14.* Seattle, USA.

MARCIANI L, FOLEY S, HOAD C L, CAMPBELL E, ARMSTRONG A, MANBY P, GOWLAND P A and SPILLER R C (2007a) Effects of Ondansetron on small bowel water content: a magnetic resonance imaging study. *Gut,* **56**, A333.

MARCIANI L, FOLEY S, HOAD C L, CAMPBELL E, TOTMAN J J, COX E, GOWLAND P A and SPILLER R C (2007b) Abnormalities of small bowel and colonic water content in diarrohea-predominant irritable bowel syndrome: novel insights from magnetic resonance imaging. *Gut,* **56**, A65–A65.

MARCIANI L, FOLEY S, HOAD C L, CAMPBELL E, TOTMAN J J, COX E, GOWLAND P A and SPILLER R C (2007c) Accelerated small bowel transit and contracted transverse colon in diarrhoea-predominant irritable bowel syndrome (IBS-D): novel insights from magnetic resonance imaging (MRI). *Gastroenterology,* **132**, A141–A141.

MARCIANI L, WICKHAM M, SINGH G, BUSH D, PICK B, COX E, FILLERYTRAVIS A, FAULKS R, MARSDEN C, GOWLAND P A and SPILLER R C (2007d) Enhancement of intragastric acid stability of a fat emulsion meal delays gastric emptying, increases cholecystokinin release and gallbladder contraction. *American Journal of Physiology,* **292**, G1607–G1613.

MCINTYRE A, VINCENT R M, PERKINS A C and SPILLER R C (1997) Effect of bran, ispaghula, and inert plastic particles on gastric emptying and small bowel transit in humans: the role of physical factors. *Gut,* **40**, 223–227.

MEYER J H, ELASHOFF J, PORTERFINK V, DRESSMAN J and AMIDON G L (1988) Human postprandial gastric emptying of 1–3 millimeter spheres. *Gastroenterology,* **94**, 1315–1325.

PORTINCASA P, MOSCHETTA A, DI CIAULA A, PALMIERI V O, MILELLA M, PASTORE G and PALASCIANO G (2001) Changes of gallbladder and gastric dynamics in patients with acute hepatitis A. *European Journal of Clinical Investigation,* **31**, 617–622.

PROVE J and EHRLEIN H J (1982) Motor function of gastric antrum and pylorus for evacuation of low and high-viscosity meals in dogs. *Gut,* **23**, 150–156.

READ N W, ALJANABI M N, HOLGATE A M, BARBER D C and EDWARDS C A (1986) Simultaneous measurement of gastric-emptying, small-bowel residence and colonic filling of a solid meal by the use of the gamma-camera. *Gut,* **27**, 300–308.

READ N, FRENCH S and CUNNINGHAM K (1994) The role of the gut in regulating food-intake in man. *Nutrition Reviews,* **52**, 1–10.

SANDHU K S, ELSAMAHI M M, MENA I, DOOLEY C P and VALENZUELA J E (1987) Effect of pectin on gastric-emptying and gastroduodenal motility in normal subjects. *Gastroenterology,* **92**, 486–492.

SCHWIZER W, MAECKE H and FRIED M (1992) Measurement of gastric emptying by magnetic resonance imaging in humans. *Gastroenterology,* **103**, 369–376.

SCHWIZER W, FRASER R, BOROVICKA J, CRELIER G, BOESIGER P and FRIED M (1994) Measurement of gastric emptying and gastric motility by magnetic resonance imaging (MRI). *Digestive Diseases and Sciences,* **39**, S101–S103.

SPILLER R C (1994) Intestinal absorptive function. *Gut,* **35**, S5–S9.

SPILLER R C, BROWN M L and PHILLIPS S F (1987a) Emptying of the terminal ileum in intact humans – influence of meal residue and ileal motility. *Gastroenterology,* **92**, 724–729.

SPILLER R C, JONES B J M and SILK D B A (1987b) Jejunal water and electrolyte absorption from two proprietary enteral feeds in man: importance of sodium content. *Gut,* **28**, 681–687.

STEHLING M K, EVANS D F, LAMONT G, ORDIDGE R J, HOWSEMAN A M, CHAPMAN B, COXON R, MANSFIELD P, HARDCASTLE J D and COUPLAND R E (1989) Gastrointestinal tract – dynamic MR studies with echo-planar imaging. *Radiology,* **171**, 41–46.

TACK J, BROECKAERT D, COULIE B and JANSSENS J (1998) The influence of cisapride on gastric tone and the perception of gastric distension. *Alimentary Pharmacology and Therapeutics,* **12**, 761–766.

TACK J, COULIE B, WILMER A, ANDRIOLI A and JANSSENS J (2000) Influence of sumatriptan on gastric fundus tone and on the perception of gastric distension in man. *Gut,* **46**, 468–473.

TAKEHARA Y (1996) MR pancreatography: technique and applications. *Topics in Magnetic Resonance Imaging,* **8**, 290–301.

TOTMAN J J, MARCIANI L, FOLEY S, HOAD C L, CAMPBELL E, SPILLER R C and GOWLAND P A (2007) Characterisation of the time course of the superior mesenteric, aorta and internal carotid arteries' blood flow response to the Oral Glucose Challenge Test. 15th ISMRM. Berlin.

VYAS P K, VESY T L, KONEZ O, CIAVELLARA D P, HUA K D and GAISIE G (2002) Estimation of gallbladder ejection fraction utilizing cholecystokinin-stimulated magnetic resonance cholangiography and comparison with hepatobiliary scintigraphy. *Journal of Magnetic Resonance Imaging,* **15**, 75–81.

WILMSHURST P and CRAWLEY J C W (1980) The measurement of gastric transit-time in obese subjects using Na-24 and the effects of energy content and guar gum on gastric-emptying and satiety. *British Journal of Nutrition,* **44**, 1–6.

WOOD F W (1968) Psychophysical studies on the consistency of liquid foods. In Wood, F. W. (Ed.) *Rheology and Texture of Foodstuffs.* London, Staples Printers Ltd.

WRIGHT J, EVANS D, GOWLAND P and MANSFIELD P (1999) Validation of antroduodenal motility measurements made by echo-planar magnetic resonance imaging. *Neurogastroenterology and Motility,* **11**, 19–25.

ZAVORAL J H, HANNAN P, FIELDS D J, HANSON M N, FRANTZ I D, KUBA K, ELMER P and JACOBS D R (1983) The hypolipidemic effect of locust bean gum food-products in familial hypercholesterolemic adults and children. *American Journal of Clinical Nutrition,* **38**, 285–294.

15

Advances in the use of animal models for analysing intestinal cancers and protective effects of dietary components

H. Xiao, University of Massachusetts, USA

Abstract: This chapter begins by discussing the development and features of two of the most widely used rodent models for human colorectal cancer, namely azoxymethane-induced rat colon carcinogenesis and *Apc*$^{Min/+}$ mice models. Then it reviews the results from the studies using these rodent models that have identified many potential preventive dietary components against colon cancer. The major dietary components discussed are (1) dietary fat such as fish oil, alpha-linolenic acid, conjugated linoleic acid, and conjugated linolenic acid; (2) dietary fiber such as inulin-type of fructans, resistant starch, and wheat bran; and (3) tea polyphenols.

Key words: colon cancer prevention, animal models, dietary fat, dietary fiber, tea polyphenols.

15.1 Introduction

Cancer is one of the leading causes of human death around the world, especially in the industrialized Western countries including the United States. It was estimated there were 1 444 920 new cases and 559 650 deaths from cancers in the United States in 2007.[1] The mortality from some major chronic diseases, such as heart diseases, has decreased substantially during the past half century in the United States. However, the mortality from cancer has just begun to show a slight decrease, despite the advances in diagnostic and therapeutic procedures. Cancer has become the number one killer of both men and women under 85 years of age in the United States.[1]

Accumulating evidence has indicated that cancer is a preventable disease. A promising approach to controlling cancer is to prevent it before malignant events have occurred.[2] It was estimated that more than two-thirds of human cancers could be prevented through appropriate modification in lifestyle.[3] Epidemiological evidence has indicated that diet abundant in fruits and vegetables may reduce the risk of cancer, and this effect has been attributed to bioactive components present in these foods. The National Cancer Institute has launched several campaigns to urge people to eat at least five servings of fruit and vegetables a day to fight off cancer. Much effort has been made in understanding the cancer preventive effects of bioactive dietary components.

Colorectal cancer (CRC) is the second leading cause of cancer death in the United States, and it was estimated that 52 180 people would die from CRC in 2007.[1] The intestine may be a promising site for cancer chemoprevention with dietary components that have direct contact and may result in high level of exposure after ingestion. This chapter summarizes the important animal models used in CRC prevention studies and results from these models on representative dietary components with preventive potential against CRC.

15.2 Human colorectal cancer

The majority of human CRC cases are sporadic in origin, and the rest are due to two autosomal dominant inherited conditions including hereditary non-polyposis CRC (HNPCC) and familial adenomatous polyposis (FAP). HNPCC accounts for about 2% of human CRC cases, while FAP is associated with less than 1% of CRC cases.[4,5] CRC development is a multiple step process, and generally follows the adenoma-carcinoma sequence. Aberrant crypt foci (ACF) are thought to be putative precursors of CRC.

Multiple gene mutations have been identified during colorectal carcinogenesis. *Apc* gene mutations are important early events during the development of CRC,[6–12] and among the colon tumors without *Apc* mutation, half of them carry mutations of β-*catenin* gene.[13] The *Apc* gene was identified on human chromosome 5q and encodes a protein of about 2850 amino acid residues.[14,15] APC protein can form a complex with axin and GSK-3β, which facilitates the phosphorylation of β-catenin by GSK-3β. This phosphorylation of β-catenin can accelerate its degradation through ubiquitylation.[16,17] Mutations in *Apc* gene and GSK-3β phosphorylation consensus motif of β-*catenin* gene can lead to hypo-phosphorylation of β-catenin, and this, in turn, stabilizes β-catenin in the cytoplasm. Accumulated cytoplasmic β-catenin can translocate to the nucleus and activate TCF/LEF transcription factors, which induces a set of potential oncogenic genes.[18–20] *K-ras* is another important gene that frequently mutated during colorectal carcinogenesis.[9–12] Oncogenic mutations of *Ras* result in activation of its downstream signaling pathways, such as the Raf/Mek/Erk and PI3K/Akt pathways.[21,22]

15.3 Intestinal carcinogenesis models in rodents

15.3.1 Chemically induced colon carcinogenesis models

In order to study the mechanism of colon carcinogenesis and evaluate protective effects of potential cancer preventive agents, such as bioactive dietary components, it is critical to establish reliable preclinical animal models that recapitulate the major characteristics of human CRC. However, there is a low incidence of spontaneous CRC in experimental animals.[23] Several chemically induced colon carcinogenesis models have been developed,[24] such as: (1) rat colon tumorigenesis induced by aromatic amine, 3,2′-dimethyl-4-aminobiphenyl; (2) rat and mouse colon tumorigenesis induced by derivatives and analogues of cycacin, e.g., methylazoxymethanol (MAM), 1,2-dimethylhydrazine (DMH), and azoxymethane (AOM); (3) rat and mouse colon tumorigenesis induced by direct-acting carcinogens, e.g., methylnitrosourea (MNU) and *N*-methyl-*N*′-nitro-*N*-nitrosoguanidine; and (4) rat and mouse colon tumorigenesis induced by heterocyclic amines found in broiled meat and fish, e.g., 2-amino-1-methyl-6-phenylimidazol (4,5-b) pyridine (PhIP).

Azoxymethane-induced colon carcinogenesis in rats

The AOM-induced colon carcinogenesis in rats is the most widely used model for human colon carcinogenesis.[24–26] Many colon cancer preventive agents have been identified by using this model.[24,27–34] In rats, AOM is a potent carcinogen for the large intestine. AOM can be metabolized to MAM by cytochrome P450 enzymes in the liver, and then be transported to intestine via the bile immediately after its conjugation with glucuronic acid. The glucuronic acid conjugate of MAM can be hydrolyzed by bacterial glucuronidase to form free MAM, which produces a relatively high concentration of MAM in the colon. MAM can be further oxidized to methylazoxyformaldehyde that yields a methyldiazonium ion that is highly reactive and can methylate DNA. Two major DNA adducts that can be formed by methylation are O^6-methylguanine and 7-methylguanine.[35,36] The most important feature of AOM-induced colon carcinogenesis in rats is that this model not only mimics the adenoma–carcinoma sequence observed in human colon carcinogenesis,[37] but also shares many molecular events of pathogenesis with the human situation.[38]

Molecular alterations in azoxymethane-induced colon carcinogenesis

K-Ras mutations are early and frequent events in AOM-induced colon carcinogenesis in rats.[37,39] Similar to the situation in human colon carcinogenesis,[40] AOM causes O^6-methylguanine adduct formation and leads to $G \rightarrow A$ transition in *K-Ras* codon 12 and 13 mutations.[41] Total Ras protein levels, its membrane localization, and farnesyl protein transferase protein levels are significantly elevated in colon tumors in AOM-treated rats.[22,42]

Mutations of the β-catenin gene are found in 75% of AOM-induced rat colon adenocarcinomas,[38] and these mutations are located in codons 33 and 41, encoding serine and threonine residues essential for phosphorylation by GSK-3β, as well as in adjacent codons 32 and 34.[43] These mutations lead to insensitivity to APC-mediated down-regulation and in turn stabilize β-catenin in the cytoplasm.[18,19] We and others have showed that β-catenin is predominantly localized in the cytoplasm and nucleus in rat colon adenomas and carcinomas, but β-catenin is only localized to membranes at the intercellular borders in normal rat colon epithelial cells.[43,44] This is similar to the situation in humans.[45] However, unlike human tumors, AOM-induced tumors in rats seldom carry mutations in *Apc* or *p53* genes, and have a low tendency of metastasis.[38]

Similar to the human situation, cyclooxygenase-2 (COX-2) is markedly elevated in AOM-induced rat colon cancers.[46,47] In AOM-treated rats, increased expression of COX-2 has been found both in stromal elements of adenomas and adenocarcinomas and in epithelial cells in large adenocarcinomas.[29,47] Moreover, cyclin D1 expression is significantly increased by either *K-Ras* or β-catenin mutations,[48] and c-Myc mRNA expression is elevated in the early stage of colon carcinogenesis in AOM-treated rats.[49] Increased expression of inducible nitric oxide synthase (iNOS) in epithelial cells is frequently observed in dysplastic aberrant crypt foci (ACF), adenomas, and adenocarcinomas in rats treated with AOM.[47] Mutational activation of *K-Ras* has been shown to elevate iNOS expression in rat intestinal epithelial cells in the presence of inflammatory stimuli, such as interleukin-1β and lipopolysaccharide.[50]

Aberrant crypt foci as early markers of colon carcinogenesis

Since its first description by Bird[51] in 1987, ACF have been recognized as useful biomarkers for short-term colon carcinogenesis and chemoprevention studies in AOM-treated rats.[25,52] Under the light microscope, ACF can be identified in formalin-fixed colonic tissues stained with methylene blue. ACF have the following morphological characteristics: (1) more enlarged and elevated crypts than normal mucosa and (2) increased pericryptal space and irregular lumens.[44] As pre-neoplastic lesions, ACF occur in rats as early as 2 weeks after AOM administration,[53] and they are more frequent in distal colon where colon tumors develop eventually.[54–56]

ACF in rats shared several phenotypic changes with colon tumors induced by AOM, which includes a decreased expression level of hexosaminidase, reduced α- naphthyl butyrate esterase activities, increased expression level of periodic acid-Schiff reactive material, and increased levels of glutathione-*S*-transferase isoforms.[57] Moreover, ACF also share certain genetic alterations with colon tumors, such as *K-Ras* mutations,[37] which may play an important role in colon carcinogenesis.

Recently, other pre-neoplastic lesions, such as β-catenin-accumulated crypts (BCAC)[58,59] and mucin-depleted foci (MDF),[60,61] have been introduced as early biomarkers for colon carcinogenesis in AOM-treated rats. Both BCAC and MDF were reported to better correlate with colon tumors than ACF in certain cases.[59–61] We believe that, in comparison with all ACF, dysplastic ACF are more predictive biomarkers to study the effect of chemopreventive agents when the AOM-induced rat colon carcinogenesis model is used. This is based on the following:

1. We and others have demonstrated that dysplastic ACF share similar patterns with adenomas and adenocarcinomas on aberrant β-catenin expression.[44,47]
2. We demonstrated that the expression of RXRα, a potential negative regulator of β-catenin, is decreased in ACF with high-grade dysplasia, and it is further decreased in adenomas and adenocarcinomas. The decreased expression of RXRα occurs in parallel with the increased nuclear accumulation of β-catenin in colonic lesions during AOM-induced rat colon carcinogenesis.
3. We successfully used dysplastic ACF as early markers to study inhibitory effects of green tea polyphenols, and subsequently demonstrated their strong protective effects against adenoma and adenocarcinoma formation in AOM-treated rats.[44,62]
4. Both BCAC and MDF are dysplastic in nature.

15.3.2 The Apc$^{Min/+}$ mouse model

Genetically altered rodents are important preclinical models to evaluate the efficacy and mechanisms of action of potential cancer preventive agents. Several genetically altered mouse strains have been developed to mimic the colon carcinogenesis in humans. The loss of APC function has been recognized as a pivotal factor in colon carcinogenesis, especially in FAP patients. The first mouse mutant in the *Apc* gene was identified from a pedigree derived from a mouse treated with the mutagen ethylnitrosourea.[63] The mutant mouse linage carries a non-sense mutation in the murine *Apc* gene and is predisposed to multiple intestinal neoplasms (Min); thus is called *Apc*$^{Min/+}$ mouse. These mice develop multiple intestinal polyps at early age, most of which are adenomas. Adenocarcinomas are seldom observed in *Apc*$^{Min/+}$ mice. Histologically, adenomas in *Apc*$^{Min/+}$ mice show well-delineated, tubular and/or villous structures that are lined by dysplastic mucosal epithelium.[64] Invasion beyond the muscularis mucosa and desmoplasia is not observed.

The *Apc*$^{Min/+}$ mouse model has been used by many researchers to study cancer preventive activities of dietary components. The major drawback of the *Apc*$^{Min/+}$ mouse model is that most of the polyps occur in the small intestine, which is different from human FAP patients where most of polyps develop in the colon. Nevertheless, this model provides an important tool to evaluate the effects of test agents on the Apc-driven tumorigenesis.

Recently, Yamada *et al.*[65] found a number of microadenomas together with a few tumors in the colon of aged *Apc*$^{Min/+}$ mice. These microadenomas have lost the remaining allele of *Apc*, indicating a loss of heterozygosity. In support of these findings, they observed accumulation of β-catenin in all microadenomas found in the colon of *Apc*$^{Min/+}$ mice. These microadenomas may be direct precursors of colon tumors in *Apc*$^{Min/+}$ mice. Efforts have been made to increase the colon tumorigenesis in *Apc*$^{Min/+}$ mice. For example, Issa *et al.*[66] treated the *Apc*$^{Min/+}$ mice with AOM, and induced a four-fold increase in the number of colon tumors. Subsequently, they successfully utilized the AOM-treated *Apc*$^{Min/+}$ mouse model to investigate the possible mechanisms of inhibition of colon carcinogenesis by dietary components.[66]

Several new *Apc* mutant mice, such as *Apc*$^{\Delta 716}$ and *Apc*^{1638N}, have been constructed.[67,68] *Apc*$^{\Delta 716}$ carries a truncating mutation at codon 716, while *Apc*^{1638N} contains a mutation at codon 1638. Similar to *Apc*$^{Min/+}$ mice, these mutant mice develop polyp adenomas mainly in small intestine, but the numbers of polyps developed are largely different.[69] *Apc*$^{\Delta 716}$ develops about 300 polyps, whereas *Apc*^{1638N} forms only about 3 polyps. Introduction of other genes that are thought to have modifying effects on intestinal tumorigenesis can have dramatic influence on the polyp formation in *Apc* mutant mice. For example, introduction of COX-2 gene (*Ptgs2*) knockout mutation into *Apc*$^{\Delta 716}$ mice dramatically reduced the number and size of intestinal polyps.[70] Similarly, cytosolic phospholipse A_2 ($cPLA_2$) gene knockout rendered *Apc*$^{\Delta 716}$ mice reduced polyp size in the intestine.[71] Compound mice with both Smad4 and *Apc*$^{\Delta 716}$ genes developed very invasive adenocarcinomas with histology similar to that of human colon cancer.[72]

15.4 Dietary components in colon cancer prevention

Evidence from epidemiological studies has suggested that dietary factors play important roles in the inhibition of colon cancer development. Numerous preclinical studies have demonstrated the cancer preventive efficacy of various dietary components against colon carcinogenesis in different animal models. Herein, results from laboratory animal studies on several types of dietary factors are summarized. The main focus is on the studies utilizing AOM-treated rats and *Apc*$^{Min/+}$ mice.

15.4.1 Dietary fat

Fish oil

Some epidemiological studies have shown a positive association between increased risk of colon cancer and high intake of animal fat in diet, whereas fish oil and fish consumption was associated with protection against the colon carcinogenesis.[73,74] However, a recent review on human studies challenged the role of fish oil in reducing colon cancer risk.[75] In a double-blind phase II clinical trial involving 60 patients with sporadic colonic adenomas, low-dose fish oil supplementation was found to have both short-term and long-term normalizing effects on the abnormal rectal proliferation patterns associated with increased colon cancer risk.[76] Courtney *et al.* found that dietary supplementation with eicosapentaenoic acid (EPA), a major fish oil fatty acid, decreased cell proliferation and increased apoptosis in colonic mucosa of patients with colorectal adenomas.[77]

Animal studies have amply demonstrated the protective effects of fish oil against colon carcinogenesis. Rao *et al.*[30] compared the effect of mixed lipids rich in saturated fatty acids (HFML) with that of fish oil rich in polyunsaturated fatty acids during the different stages of colon carcinogenesis in AOM-treated rats. Rats fed fish oil in diet (17%) had much lower number of ACF during early stage of colon tumorigenesis (8 weeks after AOM administration), and had much lower tumor incidence and multiplicity in colon at 23 weeks after AOM administration in comparison to the rats fed 20% HFML in diet. Moreover, rats treated with fish oil showed significant reduced multiplicity of adenocarcinomas at 38 weeks after AOM administration in comparison to the rats fed 20% HFML in diet. Fujise *et al.*[78] showed that long-term dietary fish oil treatment decreased ACF multiplicity, tumor incidence, and tumor multiplicity in AOM-treated rats, and in contrast, both corn oil and beef tallow (10% in diet) treatments increased these markers. Several other studies have also demonstrated inhibitory effects of fish oil on chemically induced colon carcinogenesis in rats.[79–81] Moreover, fish oil and its active components have demonstrated protective effects against intestinal tumorigenesis in $Apc^{Min/+}$ mice.[82–85]

The colon cancer preventive effects of fish oil have been ascribed to the *n*-3 polyunsaturated fatty acids (PUFAs) such as eicosapentaenoic acid (EPA; 20:5*n*-3) and docosahexaenoic acid (DHA; 22:6*n*-3). Mechanisms of action of *n*-3 PUFAs from fish oil have been intensively studied (see Roynette *et al.*[86] for review). One of the important roles of *n*-3 PUFAs is to modulate the pathway that produces prostaglandin E2 (PGE2), a known colon tumor promoter. In rodents, dietary *n*-3 PUFAs decreased the activity of PLA2, PLC, and COX-2 in colonic mucosa, which in turn decrease arachidonic acid and PGE2 synthesis.[30,87,88] Ras proteins are critical regulators of cell growth, differentiation, and apoptosis, and their membrane localization is required for activation and malignant transformation. *Ras* gene is frequently mutated in colon cancer and thought to promote colon carcinogenesis. N-3 PUFAs reduced Ras localization to the plasma membrane, which may suppress tumor promoting effects of Ras during colon carcinogenesis.[22,89] Treatment with fish oil inhibited the activity of 7-α-dehydroxylase, one of the enzymes responsible for the formation of secondary bile acids that can be genotoxic to colonocyte.[87] Fish oil-derived *n*-3 PUFAs also induced apoptosis by modulating the levels of multiple factors involved in apoptosis, such as COX-2, PKCbII, Bcl2, PPARδ, PGE2, and PEG3.[86,90,91]

Alpha-linolenic acid

Bedsides the long chain *n*-3 PUFAs such as EPA and DHA, other *n*-3 PUFAs have also been shown to be potential cancer preventive agents. Several studies have demonstrated inhibitory effects of α-linolenic acid (ALA) on colon carcinogenesis. Onogi *et al.*[92] found that dietary treatment with 3–12% perilla oil rich in ALA inhibited ACF formation in AOM-treated rats in a dose-dependent fashion in comparison to the olive oil and safflower oil treatments, and these protective effects were associated with reduction in Ras expression, cell proliferation, and PGE2 levels by perilla oil in colonic mucosa. Using MNU-treated rats, Narisawa *et al.*[93,94] showed that in comparison to safflower oil and palm oil, perilla oil in the diet (3–12%) caused decreases in colon tumor incidence. Their results further suggested that the tumor-suppressing effects of perilla oil were due to decreased sensitivity of colonic mucosa to tumor promoters arising from the altered fatty acid composition in membrane phospholipids of colonic epithelial cells, and were not a result of a decrease of promoters such as bile acid. Moreover, dietary perilla oil (10%) was also found to be tumor-inhibitory on colon carcinogenesis in DMH-treated rats.[95] Another rich source of ALA is flaxseed whose oil has been studied for colon cancer prevention. Williams *et al.*[96] demonstrated that AOM-treated rats fed flaxseed oil (7 or 14% in diet) had both lower numbers of ACF and lower numbers of ACs/ACF in the colon in comparison to the rats fed soybean oil at the same levels. Using the same model, Dwivedi *et al.*[97] investigated the effect of flaxseed oil (15% in diet) on rat colon carcinogenesis in a long-term feeding study that showed suppression on incidence, multiplicity, and size of the colon tumors by flaxseed oil. In *Apc*$^{Min/+}$ mice, dietary flaxseed oil was found to decreased median tumor number and size in one study,[98] while dietary ALA showed no effect on intestinal tumorigenesis in other studies.[82,85]

Conjugated linoleic acid

Conjugated linoleic acid (CLA) refers to a mixture of positional geometric isomers of linoleic acid (LA; *cis*-9, *cis*-12-octadecadienoic acid).[99] The major source of CLA is the food derived from ruminants, such as beef and lamb, as well as the dairy products from these sources. Studies have showed preventive effects of CLA against several cancers, such as colon, forestomach, mammary, and skin.[99] In 2-amino-3-methylimidazo[4,5-f] quinoline (IQ)-treated F344 rats, oral gavage of CLA decreased the number of ACF/colon by 74%, and also lowered IQ-DNA adducts in the colon by 41%.[100] The protective effects of CLA were associated with inhibition of carcinogen activation. Administration of CLA at 1.0% in the diet was also found to reduce colon tumor incidence in DMH-treated rats by induction of apoptosis.[101] In big blue rats, dietary administration of CLA (0.5%) modulate PhIP-induced mutagenesis in a tissue-specific manner, e.g., CLA decreased mutation frequency in the distal colon, but increased mutation frequency in the cecum.[102] However, CLA treatment did not inhibit ACF formation induced by AOM in male Sprague–Dawley rats.[103] Yasui *et al.*[104] investigated effect of 9-*trans*, 11-*trans* CLA, a minor CLA isomer, on the AOM-induced ACF formation during both initiation and post-initiation stages of rat colon carcinogenesis. It was found that administration of 9-*trans*, 11-*trans* CLA at 0.01% and 0.1% in diet significantly reduced the total number of ACF per rat by 37% and 60%, respectively. Dietary treatments with 9-*trans*, 11-*trans* CLA also decreased the total number of aberrant crypts (ACs) per rat and the number of ACs per focus. Most importantly, 9-*trans*, 11-*trans* CLA treatments dose-dependently decreased percentage of ACF containing four or more ACs. Further biochemical and immunohistochemical analysis revealed that treatments with 9-*trans*, 11-*trans* CLA increased apoptosis, suppressed cell proliferation, decreased mRNA expression level of COX-2, decreased protein expression level of cyclin D1, and increased mRNA expression level of PPARγ.

Conjugated linolenic acid

Bioactive conjugated PUFAs, such as conjugated linolenic acid (CLN) isomers, have been found as abundant components in some plant seed oils.[105] Tung, bitter gourd, pomegranate, catalpa, and pot marigold seed oils contain 42–83% of α-eleostearic (*c*9, *t*11, *t*13-CLN), punicic (*c*9, *t*11, *c*13-CLN), catalpic (*t*9, *t*11, *c*13-CLN), and calendic (*t*8, *t*10, *c*12-CLN) acids, respectively.[106] Kohno *et al.*[105] studied effects of CLN isolated from the seeds of bitter gourd (*Momordica charantia*) on colonic ACF formation induced by AOM in rats, and found that feeding of CLN at the levels of 0.01%, 0.1% and 1% in diet dose-dependently decreased the number of ACF per rat. These inhibitory effects were associated with lowered cell proliferation and enhanced apoptosis in ACF of CLN-treated rats. In a subsequent long-term study by the same group, CLN from bitter gourd was shown to inhibit both incidence and multiplicity of colon tumors in AOM-treated rats.[107] Kohno *et al.*[108] also investigated the effect of dietary pomegranate seed oil rich in CLN on the development of AOM-induced colonic cancer and compared it with that of CLA. Administration of CLN as pomegranate seed oil significantly decreased both incidence and multiplicity of colonic adenocarcinomas, while CLA feeding showed a slight, but not significant decrease on multiplicity of adenocarcinomas. Dietary administration of CLN was found to enhance the expression of PPARγ protein in the nonlesional colonic mucosa, which was thought to contribute to the inhibitory effect of CLN on colon carcinogenesis. Moreover, in AOM-treated rats, dietary feeding of CLN as catalpa seed oil has been shown to inhibit colonic ACF formation, in terms of the number of ACF per rat, the number of ACs per rat, the number of ACs per focus, and the percentage of ACF containing four or more ACs.[109] Feeding catalpa

CLN also decreased serum triglyceride level and the expression of COX-2 mRNA in the colonic mucosa.

15.4.2 Dietary fiber

Dietary fiber has been subjected to intensive studies because of its potential inhibitory action on colon cancer development. However, overall results from epidemiological and clinical studies have been controversial, and it remains premature to make a strong recommendation for a protective effect of dietary fiber against colon cancer.[110] Nevertheless, the current recommendation is still to increase daily consumption of dietary fiber especially in the form of whole grains. Various dietary fibers have been investigated in experimental animals where they showed suppressing effects on colon carcinogenesis. These effects are generally thought to be associated with their ability to yield short chain fatty acids in the colon after fermentation by colonic flora. One of the most important short chain fatty acids generated from dietary fiber is butyrate, which plays important roles in the integrity and function of the colonic epithelial cells.[111] *In vitro* studies have shown that butyrate inhibited cell proliferation, stimulated cell differentiation, induced apoptosis, and reduced metastasis in colon cancer cells. Dietary fiber may also provide beneficial effect by alterations of gut microflora composition, reducing bile acid metabolism, increasing fecal bulk, decreasing transit time, and lowering pH levels in the colon.[112] Dietary fiber consists of non-starch polysaccharides such as cellulose, dextrins, inulin, lignin, waxes, chitins, and pectins. Resistant starch is also considered as dietary fiber because it can reach the colon undigested.

Inulin-type of fructans

Inulin-type of fructans exist in relatively high levels in common food stuffs such as leeks, onions, garlic, artichoke, and asparagus,[113] and can be obtained in large quantity from chicory roots for commercial use. The daily per capita intake of inulin-type of fructans in the average Western diet is estimated to range from 1 to 10 g, depending on geographic, demographic, and other related parameters (age, sex, season, etc.). The β(2–1) bond in these fructans cannot be hydrolyzed by the pancreatic or by the brush border hydrolytic enzymes of humans, which render inulin-type of fructans indigestible allowing them to pass through upper intestinal tract to the colon.[114,115]

The effects of inulin on colon carcinogenesis in rodents have been investigated by several research groups, which have been comprehensively reviewed by Pool-Zobel.[111] The majority of these studies have demonstrated protective effects of inulin. Reddy *et al.*[116] compared the effects of oligofructose (average degree of polymerization (DP), 4.5) with those of inulin (average DP, 25) on ACF formation induced by AOM in rats. Their results demonstrated that treatments with inulin or oligofructose at 10% in diet during initiation and post-initiation stages inhibited ACF formation. In comparison to oligofructose, dietary inulin showed stronger inhibitory effects, which may be related to the higher amount of fermentation in distal colon due to slower fermentation rate of inulin (longer chain). These results were consistent with the findings by Poulsen *et al.* that the long-chained inulin Raftiline showed more potent inhibitory effects on ACF formation induced by DMH in rats than did short-chained fructan Raftilose.[117] In contrast, Jacobsen *et al.*[118] found that Raftiline inhibited tumor formation in AOM-treated rats, but the effect was not stronger than that produced by Raftilose. Moreover, either Raftiline or Raftilose showed inhibitory effects on ACF formation. In AOM-treated rats, Rao *et al.*[119] observed that dietary inulin (10%) reduced the number of ACF/cm^2, but had no significant effect on total ACF number. In another study, the treatment with inulin (5%) incorporated into a high-fat diet during post-initiation decreased the number of ACF in AOM-treated rats.[120]

Rowland *et al.*[121] also observed the inhibitory effect of inulin (5%) in a high-fat diet on ACF formation and, more interestingly, their results indicated that the combination treatment with inulin and *Bifidobacterium longum* produced enhanced protective effects against ACF formation, which were associated with potentially beneficial changes in colonic physiology and bacterial metabolic activity in relation to tumor risk. This enhanced protection from combination of inulin and probiotics was further supported by Femia *et al.*[122] whose results showed that a combined administration of Raftilose, *Lactobacillus rhamnosus*, and *Bifidobacterium lactis* was able to further reduce the occurrence of malignant tumors in AOM-treated rats in comparison to the administration of either Raftilose or probiotics alone. Verghese *et al.*[123] determined the effect of 10% dietary inulin on the AOM-induced colon carcinogenesis in rats at initiation, post-initiation, and initiation plus post-initiation stages. Their results showed that dietary inulin treatments at all three stages inhibited formation of ACF and colonic tumors, especially at the post-initiation stage. The effects of inulin were also tested in AOM-induced colon carcinogenesis model in mature rats (12 months old), and dietary treatments with inulin at 2.5, 5.0, and 10% showed dose-dependent suppression on ACF formation.[124]

In comparison to the aforementioned studies using chemically induced rat colon carcinogenesis models, the studies using *Apc*$^{Min/+}$ mice did not provide the consistent support for the protective effects of inulin-type fructans. Several studies even showed enhancing effects of inulin-type fructans on intestinal carcinogenesis in *Apc*$^{Min/+}$ mice, and these effects were associated with activated Wnt signaling in intestinal mucosa.[125] Further studies are needed to clarify the effect of inulin-type fructans on Wnt signaling, which plays an important role in colon carcinogenesis.

Resistant starch

Resistant starch (RS) is the type of starch that is resistant to the digestion in the small intestine and thus reaches the colon undigested, similar to other dietary fiber. RS can be categorized into four types. RS_1 consists of physically entrapped starch within whole plant cells and food matrices (e.g., coarsely milled grain). RS_2 consists of native starch granulates that are highly resistant to digestion by α-amylase (e.g., green banana, high amylase maize starch). RS_3 comprises regarded starches, formed when starchy food are cooked and cooled. RS_4 comprises chemically modified starches (e.g., esterified starches) where the modification interferes with the amylolytic activity of digestive enzymes.[126]

Feeding of RS_2 (potato starch) to rats during the post-initiation stage of colon carcinogenesis was shown to inhibit colonic ACF formation induced by AOM[127] and DMH,[128] while feeding of RS_3, retrograde high-amylose maize, did not protect DMH-treated rats against colonic ACF formation.[129] Liu *et al.*[130] investigated the effects of feeding RS_2 (potato starch) either during the initiation or post-initiation stages of colon carcinogenesis induced by AOM in rats. Their results demonstrated suppressive effects of post-initiation feeding of RS on ACF formation, but a promoting effect of initiation feeding of RS. These results are consistent with the findings by Ferguson *et al.*[131] that feeding of high amylase maize starch or native potato starch during the initiation stage of carcinogenesis induced by IQ in rats caused increased bioavailability of the carcinogen. Bauer-Marinovic *et al.*[132] studied 10% hydrothermally modified Novelose 330, a RS_3, by giving it to the rats during both the initiation and post-initiation stages of colon carcinogenesis induced by DMH. It was observed that the RS treatment abolished the tumor formation, decreased cell proliferation, and enhanced apoptosis of damaged cells in the colon. Le Leu *et al.*[112] fed 10 or 20% high amylase cornstarch, a RS_2, to rats at both the initiation and post-initiation stages of colon carcinogenesis induced by AOM, and found that dietary RS treatment decreased incidence and multiplicity of colonic adenocarcinomas. In another study with AOM-treated rats, they further demonstrated that 10% high amylase cornstarch in diet not only inhibited intestinal neoplasms and colonic adenocarcinomas, but also ameliorated the tumor-enhancing effects of feeding indigestible protein.[133] However, other studies did not find protective effects of RS on colonic tumor formation in rats treated with DMH[134] or on intestinal tumorigenesis in *Apc*$^{Min/+}$ mice.[135] Moreover, RS2 (potato starch) was shown to promote ACF and tumor formation in DMH-treated rats,[136] and to increase intestinal tumor formation in *Apc*1638N mice.[137]

Taken together, further investigations are needed to clarify the effects of RS on colon carcinogenesis, although some studies showed a protective role of RS. The reasons for the inconsistent results on the colon cancer preventive effects of RS may include: different RS used (type and dose), different protocols for carcinogenesis (carcinogen type, dose, and frequency), different feeding regimen (timing and duration) of RS diet, different control diet (fat and fiber content), and different intestinal microflora in the animals used.

Wheat bran

Wheat bran (WB) fiber is a non-starch type of insoluble dietary fiber. The most important physiological effect of WB is probably its dilution potential on carcinogens and tumor promoters such as bile acids, long chain fatty acids, and ammonium.[138] WB was found to be the best carcinogen dilutor in comparison to pectin, guar gum, oat bran, and cellulose.[139] Moreover, WB can accelerate the transit through colon, which can decrease exposure time of colon mucosa to potential hazardous materials. Radiography revealed that WB was the best accelerator of colon transit in comparison with cellulose, guar gum, pectin, and oat bran.[140] Ferguson and co-workers[141] have shown that wheat bran decreased the amount of dietary carcinogens partially through enhanced carcinogen excretion in the feces. Another possible mechanism for protection against carcinogenesis by WB is to enhance the apoptotic deletion of colonic cells suffering DNA damage induced by carcinogens, which in turn, removes the cells with tumorigenic mutations. Hu *et al.*[142] examined the acute apoptotic response to genotoxic carcinogen (AOM) in the colonic epithelium of AOM-treated rats after dietary WB treatment, and their results showed that distal colonic acute apoptotic response to AOM in rats fed WB was twice that in rats fed methylcellulose. WB treatment also lowered luminal pH and increased short chain fatty acids, including butyrate.

Reddy *et al.*[143] observed protective effects of 15% dietary WB against the development of both adenomas and adenocarcinomas in the colon of AOM-treated rats. Similarly, the treatment with WB at 15% in diet for a longer period time was shown to inhibit colon tumor formation in the same model.[144] In DMH-treated rats, WB was shown to have stronger inhibition on colon tumor formation than did rice, corn, or soybean bran.[145] Alabaster *et al.*[146] compared the effects of unprocessed WB with those of processed commercial WB formulations used in breakfast cereals, and found that both types of WB inhibited ACF formation in AOM-treated rats, and that there is no difference between their protective effects. WB can interact with other dietary components. For example, WB and psyllium fiber alone can inhibit AOM-induced colon tumors in rats, whereas the combination of WB and psyllium fiber offered enhanced protection.[147] Furthermore, WB and beta-carotene, individually and in combination, were shown to protect the colon in rats consuming high-fat Western diets from AOM-induced ACF and tumor formation.[148]

15.4.3 Tea polyphenols

Tea, made from dried leaves of the plant *Camellia sinensis*, is the second most popular beverage worldwide next to water. In many different animal models, tea and its constituents have been demonstrated to inhibit tumorigenesis in different organ sites including the lung, oral cavity, esophagus, stomach, small intestine, colon, skin, prostate, mammary glands, liver, pancreas, and bladder.[149–153] Tea polyphenols, which account for about a third of the water-extractable materials in dry weight, are the most abundant bioactive components in tea, among which (−)-epigallocatechin-3-gallate (EGCG) is the most bioactive compound. The intestine may be a promising site for cancer chemoprevention with tea polyphenols, because the absorption of tea polyphenols is low and thus the intestine is exposed to high levels of tea polyphenols after ingestion.[154,155]

The relationship between tea consumption and CRC risk in human has been studied by many investigators, but no clear-cut conclusions can be drawn because of confounding factors.[150,156–159] Sun *et al.*[160] recently conducted a meta-analysis on 21 relevant papers and indicated a reduced risk of CRC risk with intake of green tea (summary odds ratio 0.82, 95% confidence interval = 0.69–0.98). A prospective study on women in Shanghai indicated a negative association between tea consumption and the risk of CRC.[161] A nested case-control study within the Shanghai Cohort Study, involving 18244 men, investigated the association between prediagnostic urinary tea polyphenols and CRC risk.[162] After 16 years of follow-up, the results showed that high prediagnostic urinary levels of epigallocatechin (EGC) and 4′-methylEGC, markers of tea consumption, were significantly associated with a reduced risk of developing CRC in men. These results provide a strong rationale for conducting human intervention trials on the prevention of human CRC with well-defined tea polyphenol preparations. In such trials, ACF can be utilized as a surrogate endpoint biomarker, which is detected and characterized by magnifying chromoendoscopy.[163,164]

The inhibitory effects of tea and tea polyphenols on intestinal tumorigenesis in mice have been consistently observed in different laboratories. Yin *et al.*[165] showed that tea catechins inhibited 1,2-dimethylhydrazine-induced colon carcinogenesis in mice. Suganuma *et al.*[166] and Orner *et al.*[167] both demonstrated an inhibition of tumorigenesis in the *Apc*$^{Min/+}$ mouse model by orally administered green tea and a greater inhibition by its combination with sulindac. In AOM-treated *Apc*$^{Min/+}$ mice, green tea polyphenols given in drinking fluid significantly decreased the number of colon tumors by 50%, and this effect was mainly due to a reduction in the number of small tumors.[66] Recently, Ju *et al.*[168] systematically investigated the effect of two key constituents of green tea, EGCG and caffeine, on intestinal tumorigenesis in *Apc*$^{Min/+}$ mice, and found that intestinal tumor formation was inhibited in a dose-dependent manner by oral administration of EGCG, but not by caffeine. The previous study from the same group also showed that oral administration of green tea inhibited the formation of azoxymethane (AOM)-induced aberrant crypt foci (ACF) in female CF-1 mice on a high-fat diet.[169] In another study, a dietary green tea polyphenol preparation was found to inhibit intestinal tumor formation in *Apc*$^{Min/+}$ mice, while the same preparation given in drinking fluid did not produce significant inhibitory effects.[170] Chemical analysis revealed that administration of green tea polyphenols in the diet delivered two-fold more EGCG to the small intestine compared with delivery in drinking fluid. These results may suggest that diet appears to be a better route of administration for green tea polyphenols than drinking fluid in terms of intestinal cancer prevention.

The inhibitory effects of tea preparation on colon tumorigenesis in rats have also been demonstrated. Colon cancer formation induced by AOM in rats was inhibited by green tea polyphenols in the drinking fluid.[171] Green tea extract (2%) in drinking fluid also significantly inhibited ACF formation in 2-amino-3-methylimidazo[4,5-f]quinoline-treated F344 rats.[172] In another study in AOM-treated F344 rats, however, green tea extract (1 or 2% in drinking fluid) only had a marginal inhibitory effect on ACF formation.[173] In a similar model, when different tea preparations were given to F344 rats after AOM treatment, EGCG was found to inhibit ACF formation, but the effect of green tea polyphenols was marginal.[52] There are also studies that did not observe an inhibitory effect of tea polyphenol preparations in 1,2-dimethylhydrazine- or in AOM-induced rat colon tumorigenesis models.[174–177] The reasons for the inconsistency among the different studies in rats may be related to several factors: (1) the diet used; (2) the protocol of tumor initiation; and (3) the type and dose of tea or polyphenol preparations used, when they were given, and whether they were administered through drinking fluid or the diet.

To investigate the potential protective effects of green tea polyphenols against CRC, we recently conducted a study in the AOM-induced rat colon cancer model using ACF as an end point.[44] F344 rats were given two weekly injections of AOM (15 mg/kg), and then fed a 20% high-fat diet with or without 0.12% or 0.24% Polyphenon E (PPE, a standardized green tea preparation consisting of 65% of EGCG and 22% other catechins) for 8 weeks. Colorectal ACF were analyzed under a microscope after methylene blue staining. It was found that dietary PPE administration significantly and dose-dependently decreased the total number of ACF per rat and the total number of aberrant crypt per rat. Moreover, treatment with 0.24% PPE also significantly decreased the percentage of large ACF (four or more crypts) and the percentage of ACF with high-grade dysplasia in total ACF. The high-grade dysplastic ACF from the 0.24% PPE-treated group had increased apoptosis and decreased nuclear expression levels of β-catenin and cyclin D1. Retinoid X receptor α (RXRα) expression was reduced in high-grade dysplastic ACF, adenoma, and adenocarcinoma during AOM-induced colon carcinogenesis, and the PPE treatment partially prevented the loss of RXRα expression in high-grade dysplastic ACF. These results strongly suggest the colon cancer preventive activity of PPE and identified possible molecular markers for future colon cancer prevention studies.

Based on the above promising results, we conducted another study with PPE in the AOM-induced rats using the colorectal tumor as an end point.[62] Similarly, F344 rats were given two weekly injections of AOM (15 mg/kg), and then fed a 20% high-fat diet with or without 0.24% PPE for 34 weeks. In the positive control group, 96% of rats developed colorectal tumors with multiplicity of 3.64 ± 0.31, and tumor tissues showed highly elevated levels of Akt and phospho-Akt, and decreased levels of caspase-3 activation, in comparison with the normal colorectal mucosa. Dietary PPE treatment did not change liver or kidney weight, but decreased body weight by 5% in the treated group compared with the control. The decrease in body weight may be due to inhibition of lipid absorption by tea polyphenols. Dietary PPE treatment significantly decreased tumor multiplicity and tumor size by 55% ($p < 0.01$) and 45% ($p < 0.05$), respectively. Moreover, treatment with 0.24% PPE also significantly decreased the incidence of adenocarcinoma (from 61% to 27%, $p < 0.05$), the multiplicity of adenoma (by 45%, $p < 0.05$), and the multiplicity of adenocarcinoma (by 80%, $p < 0.01$). Dietary PPE treatment significantly increased the levels of major tea polyphenols, i.e., EGC, EC, EGCG, and ECG, in both plasma and colorectal mucosa of treated rats. The results also showed that PPE treatment decreased levels of PGE2 and LTB4 in plasma of treated rats. Taken together, the results demonstrated convincingly the inhibition of rat colon carcinogenesis by dietary treatment with green tea polyphenols.

15.5 Conclusion

Evidence from epidemiological, clinical, and preclinical studies has indicated the environmental factors and diet in particular are important determinants of colon cancer risk in humans. Prevention of colon cancer by dietary components is a practical and promising approach to controlling this disease. Suitable animal models are critical to evaluate potential cancer preventive effects of dietary components. Both chemically and genetically induced rodent models have been developed to recapitulate major characteristics of human CRC. Although with their own limitations, AOM-treated rats and $Apc^{Min/+}$ mice are two most widely used models for human CRC, and provided valuable tools to identify potential colon cancer preventive dietary components. The major dietary components such as dietary fat and fiber, as well as minor dietary components such as tea polyphenols have been shown to exert inhibitory effects on intestinal carcinogenesis in these rodent models. In order to possibly extend these findings to humans, many more studies are needed to elucidate molecular mechanisms underlying the protective effects of these dietary components, although some mechanisms have been proposed, based on the results observed in cell culture and animal studies.

Abbreviations

AC, aberrant crypt; ACF, aberrant crypt foci; ALA, α-linolenic acid; AOM, azoxymethane; BCAC, β-catenin-accumulated crypts; CLA, conjugated linoleic acid; CLN, conjugated linolenic acid; COX-2, cyclooxygenase-2; CRC, colorectal cancer; DHA, docosahexaenoic acid; DMH, 1,2-dimethylhydrazine; EGC, epigallocatechin; EGCG, (−)-epigallocatechin-3-gallate; FAP, familial adenomatous polyposis; EPA, eicosapentaenoic acid; HNPCC, hereditary non-polyposis CRC; IQ, 2-amino-3-methylimidazo[4,5-f] quinoline; iNOS, inducible nitric oxide synthase; LTB4, leukotriene B4; MAM, methylazoxymethanol; MDF, mucin-depleted foci; MNU, methylnitrosourea; PGE2, prostaglandin E2; PhIP, 2-amino-1-methyl-6-phenylimidazol (4,5-b) pyridine; PLA2, phospholipase A2; PUFAs, polyunsaturated fatty acids; RS, resistant starch; RXRα, retinoid X receptor α; WB, wheat bran.

15.6 References

1. JEMAL, A., SIEGEL, R., WARD, E., MURRAY, T., XU, J., and THUN, M.J., Cancer statistics, 2007. *CA Cancer J Clin*, 2007. **57**(1): p. 43–66.
2. SPORN, M.B. and SUH, N., Chemoprevention: an essential approach to controlling cancer. *Nat Rev Cancer*, 2002. **2**(7): p. 537–43.
3. SURH, Y.J., Cancer chemoprevention with dietary phytochemicals. *Nat Rev Cancer*, 2003. **3**(10): p. 768–80.
4. MECKLIN, J.P., JARVINEN, H.J., HAKKILUOTO, A., HALLIKAS, H., HILTUNEN, K.M., HARKONEN, N., KELLOKUMPU, I., LAITINEN, S., OVASKA, J., TULIKOURA, J., *et al.*, Frequency of hereditary nonpolyposis colorectal cancer. A prospective multicenter study in Finland. *Dis Colon Rectum*, 1995. **38**(6): p. 588–93.
5. BISGAARD, M.L., FENGER, K., BULOW, S., NIEBUHR, E., and MOHR, J., Familial adenomatous polyposis (FAP): frequency, penetrance, and mutation rate. *Hum Mutat*, 1994. **3**(2): p. 121–5.
6. VOGELSTEIN, B., FEARON, E.R., HAMILTON, S.R., KERN, S.E., PREISINGER, A.C., LEPPERT, M., NAKAMURA, Y., WHITE, R., SMITS, A.M., and BOS, J.L., Genetic alterations during colorectal-tumor development. *N Engl J Med*, 1988. **319**(9): p. 525–32.
7. POWELL, S.M., ZILZ, N., BEAZER-BARCLAY, Y., BRYAN, T.M., HAMILTON, S.R., THIBODEAU, S.N., VOGELSTEIN, B., and KINZLER, K.W., APC mutations occur early during colorectal tumorigenesis. *Nature*, 1992. **359**(6392): p. 235–7.
8. MIYAKI, M., KONISHI, M., KIKUCHI-YANOSHITA, R., ENOMOTO, M., IGARI, T., TANAKA, K., MURAOKA, M., TAKAHASHI, H., AMADA, Y., FUKAYAMA, M., *et al.*, Characteristics of somatic mutation of the adenomatous polyposis coli gene in colorectal tumors. *Cancer Res*, 1994. **54**(11): p. 3011–20.
9. ICHII, S., TAKEDA, S., HORII, A., NAKATSURU, S., MIYOSHI, Y., EMI, M., FUJIWARA, Y., KOYAMA, K., FURUYAMA, J., UTSUNOMIYA, J., *et al.*, Detailed analysis of genetic alterations in colorectal tumors from patients with and without familial adenomatous polyposis (FAP). *Oncogene*, 1993. **8**(9): p. 2399–405.
10. KONISHI, M., KIKUCHI-YANOSHITA, R., TANAKA, K., MURAOKA, M., ONDA, A., OKUMURA, Y., KISHI, N., IWAMA, T., MORI, T., KOIKE, M., USHIO, K., CHIBA, M., *et al.*, Molecular nature of colon tumors in hereditary nonpolyposis colon cancer, familial polyposis, and sporadic colon cancer. *Gastroenterology*, 1996. **111**(2): p. 307–17.
11. JEN, J., POWELL, S.M., PAPADOPOULOS, N., SMITH, K.J., HAMILTON, S.R., VOGELSTEIN, B., and KINZLER, K.W., Molecular determinants of dysplasia in colorectal lesions. *Cancer Res*, 1994. **54**(21): p. 5523–6.
12. SMITH, A.J., STERN, H.S., PENNER, M., HAY, K., MITRI, A., BAPAT, B.V., and GALLINGER, S., Somatic APC and K-ras codon 12 mutations in aberrant crypt foci from human colons. *Cancer Res*, 1994. **54**(21): p. 5527–30.
13. SPARKS, A.B., MORIN, P.J., VOGELSTEIN, B., and KINZLER, K.W., Mutational analysis of the APC/beta-catenin/Tcf pathway in colorectal cancer. *Cancer Res*, 1998. **58**(6): p. 1130–4.

14. KINZLER, K.W., NILBERT, M.C., VOGELSTEIN, B., BRYAN, T.M., LEVY, D.B., SMITH, K.J., PREISINGER, A.C., HAMILTON, S.R., HEDGE, P., MARKHAM, A., *et al.*, Identification of a gene located at chromosome 5q21 that is mutated in colorectal cancers. *Science*, 1991. **251**(4999): p. 1366–70.
15. GRODEN, J., THLIVERIS, A., SAMOWITZ, W., CARLSON, M., GELBERT, L., ALBERTSEN, H., JOSLYN, G., STEVENS, J., SPIRIO, L., ROBERTSON, M., *et al.*, Identification and characterization of the familial adenomatous polyposis coli gene. *Cell*, 1991. **66**(3): p. 589–600.
16. RUBINFELD, B., SOUZA, B., ALBERT, I., MULLER, O., CHAMBERLAIN, S.H., MASIARZ, F.R., MUNEMITSU, S., and POLAKIS, P., Association of the APC gene product with beta-catenin. *Science*, 1993. **262**(5140): p. 1731–4.
17. MUNEMITSU, S., ALBERT, I., SOUZA, B., RUBINFELD, B., and POLAKIS, P., Regulation of intracellular beta-catenin levels by the adenomatous polyposis coli (APC) tumor-suppressor protein. *Proc Natl Acad Sci USA*, 1995. **92**(7): p. 3046–50.
18. YOST, C., TORRES, M., MILLER, J.R., HUANG, E., KIMELMAN, D., and MOON, R.T., The axis-inducing activity, stability, and subcellular distribution of beta-catenin is regulated in *Xenopus* embryos by glycogen synthase kinase 3. *Genes Dev*, 1996. **10**(12): p. 1443–54.
19. MORIN, P.J., SPARKS, A.B., KORINEK, V., BARKER, N., CLEVERS, H., VOGELSTEIN, B., and KINZLER, K.W., Activation of beta-catenin-Tcf signaling in colon cancer by mutations in beta-catenin or APC. *Science*, 1997. **275**(5307): p. 1787–90.
20. KORINEK, V., BARKER, N., MORIN, P.J., VAN WICHEN, D., DE WEGER, R., KINZLER, K.W., VOGELSTEIN, B., and CLEVERS, H., Constitutive transcriptional activation by a beta-catenin-Tcf complex in APC–/– colon carcinoma. *Science*, 1997. **275**(5307): p. 1784–7.
21. ROY, H.K., OLUSOLA, B.F., CLEMENS, D.L., KAROLSKI, W.J., RATASHAK, A., LYNCH, H.T., and SMYRK, T.C., AKT proto-oncogene overexpression is an early event during sporadic colon carcinogenesis. *Carcinogenesis*, 2002. **23**(1): p. 201–5.
22. DAVIDSON, L.A., LUPTON, J.R., JIANG, Y.H., and CHAPKIN, R.S., Carcinogen and dietary lipid regulate ras expression and localization in rat colon without affecting farnesylation kinetics. *Carcinogenesis*, 1999. **20**(5): p. 785–91.
23. REDDY, B.S., NARISAWA, T., MARONPOT, R., WEISBURGER, J.H., and WYNDER, E.L., Animal models for the study of dietary factors and cancer of the large bowel. *Cancer Res*, 1975. **35**(11 Pt. 2): p. 3421–6.
24. REDDY, B.S., Studies with the azoxymethane-rat preclinical model for assessing colon tumor development and chemoprevention. *Environ Mol Mutagen*, 2004. **44**(1): p. 26–35.
25. CORPET, D.E. and TACHE, S., Most effective colon cancer chemopreventive agents in rats: a systematic review of aberrant crypt foci and tumor data, ranked by potency. *Nutr Cancer*, 2002. **43**(1): p. 1–21.
26. BOONE, C.W., KELLOFF, G.J., and MALONE, W.E., Identification of candidate cancer chemopreventive agents and their evaluation in animal models and human clinical trials: a review. *Cancer Res*, 1990. **50**(1): p. 2–9.
27. RAO, C.V., NEWMARK, H.L., and REDDY, B.S., Chemopreventive effect of farnesol and lanosterol on colon carcinogenesis. *Cancer Detect Prev*, 2002. **26**(6): p. 419–25.
28. REDDY, B.S., HIROSE, Y., LUBET, R., STEELE, V., KELLOFF, G., PAULSON, S., SEIBERT, K., and RAO, C.V., Chemoprevention of colon cancer by specific cyclooxygenase-2 inhibitor, celecoxib, administered during different stages of carcinogenesis. *Cancer Res*, 2000. **60**(2): p. 293–7.
29. REDDY, B.S., HIROSE, Y., COHEN, L.A., SIMI, B., COOMA, I., and RAO, C.V., Preventive potential of wheat bran fractions against experimental colon carcinogenesis:

implications for human colon cancer prevention. *Cancer Res*, 2000. **60**(17): p. 4792–7.
30. RAO, C.V., HIROSE, Y., INDRANIE, C., and REDDY, B.S., Modulation of experimental colon tumorigenesis by types and amounts of dietary fatty acids. *Cancer Res*, 2001. **61**(5): p. 1927–33.
31. RAO, C.V., WANG, C.Q., SIMI, B., RODRIGUEZ, J.G., COOMA, I., EL-BAYOUMY, K., and REDDY, B.S., Chemoprevention of colon cancer by a glutathione conjugate of 1,4-phenylenebis(methylene)selenocyanate, a novel organoselenium compound with low toxicity. *Cancer Res*, 2001. **61**(9): p. 3647–52.
32. RAO, C.V., INDRANIE, C., SIMI, B., MANNING, P.T., CONNOR, J.R., and REDDY, B.S., Chemopreventive properties of a selective inducible nitric oxide synthase inhibitor in colon carcinogenesis, administered alone or in combination with celecoxib, a selective cyclooxygenase-2 inhibitor. *Cancer Res*, 2002. **62**(1): p. 165–70.
33. REDDY, B.S., KAWAMORI, T., LUBET, R., STEELE, V., KELLOFF, G., and RAO, C.V., Chemopreventive effect of *S*-methylmethane thiosulfonate and sulindac administered together during the promotion/progression stages of colon carcinogenesis. *Carcinogenesis*, 1999. **20**(8): p. 1645–8.
34. REDDY, B.S., KAWAMORI, T., LUBET, R.A., STEELE, V.E., KELLOFF, G.J., and RAO, C.V., Chemopreventive efficacy of sulindac sulfone against colon cancer depends on time of administration during carcinogenic process. *Cancer Res*, 1999. **59**(14): p. 3387–91.
35. FIALA, E.S., Investigations into the metabolism and mode of action of the colon carcinogens 1,2-dimethylhydrazine and azoxymethane. *Cancer*, 1977. **40**(5 Suppl): p. 2436–45.
36. FIALA, E.S., SOHN, O.S., PUZ, C., and CZERNIAK, R., Differential effects of 4-iodopyrazole and 3-methylpyrazole on the metabolic activation of methylazoxymethanol to a DNA methylating species by rat liver and rat colon mucosa *in vivo*. *J Cancer Res Clin Oncol*, 1987. **113**(2): p. 145–50.
37. VIVONA, A.A., SHPITZ, B., MEDLINE, A., BRUCE, W.R., HAY, K., WARD, M.A., STERN, H.S., and GALLINGER, S., K-ras mutations in aberrant crypt foci, adenomas and adenocarcinomas during azoxymethane-induced colon carcinogenesis. *Carcinogenesis*, 1993. **14**(9): p. 1777–81.
38. TAKAHASHI, M. and WAKABAYASHI, K., Gene mutations and altered gene expression in azoxymethane-induced colon carcinogenesis in rodents. *Cancer Sci*, 2004. **95**(6): p. 475–80.
39. ERDMAN, S.H., WU, H.D., HIXSON, L.J., AHNEN, D.J., and GERNER, E.W., Assessment of mutations in Ki-ras and p53 in colon cancers from azoxymethane- and dimethylhydrazine-treated rats. *Mol Carcinog*, 1997. **19**(2): p. 137–44.
40. FEARON, E.R. and VOGELSTEIN, B., A genetic model for colorectal tumorigenesis. *Cell*, 1990. **61**(5): p. 759–67.
41. LUCERI, C., DE FILIPPO, C., CADERNI, G., GAMBACCIANI, L., SALVADORI, M., GIANNINI, A., and DOLARA, P., Detection of somatic DNA alterations in azoxymethane-induced F344 rat colon tumors by random amplified polymorphic DNA analysis. *Carcinogenesis*, 2000. **21**(9): p. 1753–6.
42. SINGH, J., HAMID, R., and REDDY, B.S., Dietary fat and colon cancer: modulating effect of types and amount of dietary fat on *ras-p21* function during promotion and progression stages of colon cancer. *Cancer Res*, 1997. **57**(2): p. 253–8.
43. TAKAHASHI, M., FUKUDA, K., SUGIMURA, T., and WAKABAYASHI, K., Beta-catenin is frequently mutated and demonstrates altered cellular location in azoxymethane-induced rat colon tumors. *Cancer Res*, 1998. **58**(1): p. 42–6.
44. XIAO, H., HAO, X., SIMI, B., JU, J., JIANG, H., REDDY, B.S., and YANG, C.S., Green tea polyphenols inhibit colorectal aberrant crypt foci (ACF) formation and prevent

oncogenic changes in dysplastic ACF in azoxymethane-treated F344 rats. *Carcinogenesis*, 2008. **29**(1): p. 113–19.
45. HAO, X., TOMLINSON, I.P., ILYAS, M., PALAZZO, J.P., and TALBOT, I.C., Reciprocity between membranous and nuclear expression of β-catenin in colorectal tumours. *Virchows Arch*, 1997. **431**(3): p. 167–172.
46. DUBOIS, R.N., RADHIKA, A., REDDY, B.S., and ENTINGH, A.J., Increased cyclooxygenase-2 levels in carcinogen-induced rat colonic tumors. *Gastroenterology*, 1996. **110**(4): p. 1259–62.
47. TAKAHASHI, M., MUTOH, M., KAWAMORI, T., SUGIMURA, T., and WAKABAYASHI, K., Altered expression of beta-catenin, inducible nitric oxide synthase and cyclooxygenase-2 in azoxymethane-induced rat colon carcinogenesis. *Carcinogenesis*, 2000. **21**(7): p. 1319–27.
48. BISSONNETTE, M., KHARE, S., VON LINTIG, F.C., WALI, R.K., NGUYEN, L., ZHANG, Y., HART, J., SKAROSI, S., VARKI, N., BOSS, G.R., and BRASITUS, T.A., Mutational and nonmutational activation of *p21ras* in rat colonic azoxymethane-induced tumors: effects on mitogen-activated protein kinase, cyclooxygenase-2, and cyclin D1. *Cancer Res*, 2000. **60**(16): p. 4602–9.
49. KISHIMOTO, Y., MORISAWA, T., HOSODA, A., SHIOTA, G., KAWASAKI, H., and HASEGAWA, J., Molecular changes in the early stage of colon carcinogenesis in rats treated with azoxymethane. *J Exp Clin Cancer Res*, 2002. **21**(2): p. 203–11.
50. TAKAHASHI, M., MUTOH, M., SHOJI, Y., KAMANAKA, Y., NAKA, M., MARUYAMA, T., SUGIMURA, T., and WAKABAYASHI, K., Transfection of K-rasAsp12 cDNA markedly elevates IL-1beta- and lipopolysaccharide-mediated inducible nitric oxide synthase expression in rat intestinal epithelial cells. *Oncogene*, 2003. **22**(48): p. 7667–76.
51. BIRD, R.P., Observation and quantification of aberrant crypts in the murine colon treated with a colon carcinogen: preliminary findings. *Cancer Lett*, 1987. **37**(2): p. 147–51.
52. WARGOVICH, M.J., JIMENEZ, A., MCKEE, K., STEELE, V.E., VELASCO, M., WOODS, J., PRICE, R., GRAY, K., and KELLOFF, G.J., Efficacy of potential chemopreventive agents on rat colon aberrant crypt formation and progression. *Carcinogenesis*, 2000. **21**(6): p. 1149–55.
53. MCLELLAN, E.A. and BIRD, R.P., Aberrant crypts: potential preneoplastic lesions in the murine colon. *Cancer Res*, 1988. **48**(21): p. 6187–92.
54. TUDEK, B., BIRD, R.P., and BRUCE, W.R., Foci of aberrant crypts in the colons of mice and rats exposed to carcinogens associated with foods. *Cancer Res*, 1989. **49**(5): p. 1236–40.
55. PRETLOW, T.P., O'RIORDAN, M.A., KOLMAN, M.F., and JURCISEK, J.A., Colonic aberrant crypts in azoxymethane-treated F344 rats have decreased hexosaminidase activity. *Am J Pathol*, 1990. **136**(1): p. 13–16.
56. DESCHNER, E.E., Experimentally induced cancer of the colon. *Cancer*, 1974. **34**(3): p. suppl: 824–8.
57. PRETLOW, T.P. and PRETLOW, T.G., Mutant KRAS in aberrant crypt foci (ACF): initiation of colorectal cancer? *Biochim Biophys Acta*, 2005. **1756**(2): p. 83–96.
58. YAMADA, Y., YOSHIMI, N., HIROSE, Y., KAWABATA, K., MATSUNAGA, K., SHIMIZU, M., HARA, A., and MORI, H., Frequent beta-catenin gene mutations and accumulations of the protein in the putative preneoplastic lesions lacking macroscopic aberrant crypt foci appearance, in rat colon carcinogenesis. *Cancer Res*, 2000. **60**(13): p. 3323–7.
59. HIROSE, Y., KUNO, T., YAMADA, Y., SAKATA, K., KATAYAMA, M., YOSHIDA, K., QIAO, Z., HATA, K., YOSHIMI, N., and MORI, H., Azoxymethane-induced beta-catenin-accumulated crypts in colonic mucosa of rodents as an intermediate biomarker for colon carcinogenesis. *Carcinogenesis*, 2003. **24**(1): p. 107–11.

60. CADERNI, G., FEMIA, A.P., GIANNINI, A., FAVUZZA, A., LUCERI, C., SALVADORI, M., and DOLARA, P., Identification of mucin-depleted foci in the unsectioned colon of azoxymethane-treated rats: correlation with carcinogenesis. *Cancer Res*, 2003. **63**(10): p. 2388–92.
61. FEMIA, A.P., DOLARA, P., and CADERNI, G., Mucin-depleted foci (MDF) in the colon of rats treated with azoxymethane (AOM) are useful biomarkers for colon carcinogenesis. *Carcinogenesis*, 2004. **25**(2): p. 277–81.
62. XIAO, H., HAO, X., SIMI, B., JU, J., LEE, M.-J., LU, G., REDDY, B.S., and YANG, C.S., Inhibition of colorectal tumorigenesis in azoxymethane (AOM)-treated rats by green tea polyphenols (proffered paper). Proceedings Abstract for 2007 Frontiers in Cancer Prevention Research Meeting, Philadelphia, PA, 5–8 December.
63. MOSER, A.R., PITOT, H.C., and DOVE, W.F., A dominant mutation that predisposes to multiple intestinal neoplasia in the mouse. *Science*, 1990. **247**(4940): p. 322–4.
64. GERNER, E.W., IGNATENKO, N.A., and BESSELSEN, D.G., Preclinical models for chemoprevention of colon cancer. *Recent Results Cancer Res*, 2003. **163**: p. 58–71; discussion 264–6.
65. YAMADA, Y., HATA, K., HIROSE, Y., HARA, A., SUGIE, S., KUNO, T., YOSHIMI, N., TANAKA, T., and MORI, H., Microadenomatous lesions involving loss of *Apc* heterozygosity in the colon of adult $Apc^{Min/+}$ mice. *Cancer Res*, 2002. **62**(22): p. 6367–70.
66. ISSA, A.Y., VOLATE, S.R., MUGA, S.J., NITCHEVA, D., SMITH, T., and WARGOVICH, M.J., Green tea selectively targets initial stages of intestinal carcinogenesis in the AOM-Apc^{Min} mouse model. *Carcinogenesis*, 2007. **28**(9): p. 1978–84.
67. FODDE, R., EDELMANN, W., YANG, K., VAN LEEUWEN, C., CARLSON, C., RENAULT, B., BREUKEL, C., ALT, E., LIPKIN, M., KHAN, P.M., *et al.*, A targeted chain-termination mutation in the mouse *Apc* gene results in multiple intestinal tumors. *Proc Natl Acad Sci USA*, 1994. **91**(19): p. 8969–73.
68. OSHIMA, M., OSHIMA, H., KITAGAWA, K., KOBAYASHI, M., ITAKURA, C., and TAKETO, M., Loss of Apc heterozygosity and abnormal tissue building in nascent intestinal polyps in mice carrying a truncated *Apc* gene. *Proc Natl Acad Sci USA*, 1995. **92**(10): p. 4482–6.
69. TAKETO, M.M., Mouse models of gastrointestinal tumors. *Cancer Sci*, 2006. **97**(5): p. 355–61.
70. OSHIMA, M., DINCHUK, J.E., KARGMAN, S.L., OSHIMA, H., HANCOCK, B., KWONG, E., TRZASKOS, J.M., EVANS, J.F., and TAKETO, M.M., Suppression of intestinal polyposis in $Apc^{delta716}$ knockout mice by inhibition of cyclooxygenase 2 (COX-2). *Cell*, 1996. **87**(5): p. 803–9.
71. TAKAKU, K., SONOSHITA, M., SASAKI, N., UOZUMI, N., DOI, Y., SHIMIZU, T., and TAKETO, M.M., Suppression of intestinal polyposis in $Apc^{(delta\ 716)}$ knockout mice by an additional mutation in the cytosolic phospholipase A(2) gene. *J Biol Chem*, 2000. **275**(44): p. 34013–16.
72. TAKAKU, K., OSHIMA, M., MIYOSHI, H., MATSUI, M., SELDIN, M.F., and TAKETO, M.M., Intestinal tumorigenesis in compound mutant mice of both *Dpc4* (Smad4) and *Apc* genes. *Cell*, 1998. **92**(5): p. 645–56.
73. CAYGILL, C.P. and HILL, M.J., Fish, *n*-3 fatty acids and human colorectal and breast cancer mortality. *Eur J Cancer Prev*, 1995. **4**(4): p. 329–32.
74. CAYGILL, C.P., CHARLETT, A., and HILL, M.J., Fat, fish, fish oil and cancer. *Br J Cancer*, 1996. **74**(1): p. 159–64.
75. MACLEAN, C.H., NEWBERRY, S.J., MOJICA, W.A., KHANNA, P., ISSA, A.M., SUTTORP, M.J., LIM, Y.W., TRAINA, S.B., HILTON, L., GARLAND, R., and MORTON, S.C., Effects of omega-3 fatty acids on cancer risk: a systematic review. *JAMA*, 2006. **295**(4): p. 403–15.

76. ANTI, M., ARMELAO, F., MARRA, G., PERCESEPE, A., BARTOLI, G.M., PALOZZA, P., PARRELLA, P., CANETTA, C., GENTILONI, N., DE VITIS, I., *et al.*, Effects of different doses of fish oil on rectal cell proliferation in patients with sporadic colonic adenomas. *Gastroenterology*, 1994. **107**(6): p. 1709–18.
77. COURTNEY, E.D., MATTHEWS, S., FINLAYSON, C., DI PIERRO, D., BELLUZZI, A., RODA, E., KANG, J.Y., and LEICESTER, R.J., Eicosapentaenoic acid (EPA) reduces crypt cell proliferation and increases apoptosis in normal colonic mucosa in subjects with a history of colorectal adenomas. *Int J Colorectal Dis*, 2007. **22**(7): p. 765–76.
78. FUJISE, T., IWAKIRI, R., KAKIMOTO, T., SHIRAISHI, R., SAKATA, Y., WU, B., TSUNADA, S., OOTANI, A., and FUJIMOTO, K., Long-term feeding of various fat diets modulates azoxymethane-induced colon carcinogenesis through Wnt/beta-catenin signaling in rats. *Am J Physiol Gastrointest Liver Physiol*, 2007. **292**(4): p. G1150–6.
79. MINOURA, T., TAKATA, T., SAKAGUCHI, M., TAKADA, H., YAMAMURA, M., HIOKI, K., and YAMAMOTO, M., Effect of dietary eicosapentaenoic acid on azoxymethane-induced colon carcinogenesis in rats. *Cancer Res*, 1988. **48**(17): p. 4790–4.
80. NELSON, R.L., TANURE, J.C., ANDRIANOPOULOS, G., SOUZA, G., and LANDS, W.E., A comparison of dietary fish oil and corn oil in experimental colorectal carcinogenesis. *Nutr Cancer*, 1988. **11**(4): p. 215–20.
81. LATHAM, P., LUND, E.K., and JOHNSON, I.T., Dietary *n*-3 PUFA increases the apoptotic response to 1,2-dimethylhydrazine, reduces mitosis and suppresses the induction of carcinogenesis in the rat colon. *Carcinogenesis*, 1999. **20**(4): p. 645–50.
82. PETRIK, M.B., MCENTEE, M.F., JOHNSON, B.T., OBUKOWICZ, M.G., and WHELAN, J., Highly unsaturated (*n*-3) fatty acids, but not alpha-linolenic, conjugated linoleic or gamma-linolenic acids, reduce tumorigenesis in $Apc^{(Min/+)}$ mice. *J Nutr*, 2000. **130**(10): p. 2434–43.
83. PETRIK, M.B., MCENTEE, M.F., CHIU, C.H., and WHELAN, J., Antagonism of arachidonic acid is linked to the antitumorigenic effect of dietary eicosapentaenoic acid in $Apc^{(Min/+)}$ mice. *J Nutr*, 2000. **130**(5): p. 1153–8.
84. PAULSEN, J.E., ELVSAAS, I.K., STEFFENSEN, I.L., and ALEXANDER, J., A fish oil derived concentrate enriched in eicosapentaenoic and docosahexaenoic acid as ethyl ester suppresses the formation and growth of intestinal polyps in the Min mouse. *Carcinogenesis*, 1997. **18**(10): p. 1905–10.
85. WHELAN, J., PETRIK, M.B., MCENTEE, M.F., and OBUKOWICZ, M.G., Dietary EPA reduces tumor load in $Apc^{Min/+}$ mice by altering arachidonic acid metabolism, but conjugated linoleic acid, gamma- and alpha-linolenic acids have no effect. *Adv Exp Med Biol*, 2002. **507**: p. 579–84.
86. ROYNETTE, C.E., CALDER, P.C., DUPERTUIS, Y.M., and PICHARD, C., *n*-3 Polyunsaturated fatty acids and colon cancer prevention. *Clin Nutr*, 2004. **23**(2): p. 139–51.
87. RAO, C.V., SIMI, B., WYNN, T.T., GARR, K., and REDDY, B.S., Modulating effect of amount and types of dietary fat on colonic mucosal phospholipase A2, phosphatidylinositol-specific phospholipase C activities, and cyclooxygenase metabolite formation during different stages of colon tumor promotion in male F344 rats. *Cancer Res*, 1996. **56**(3): p. 532–7.
88. SINGH, J., HAMID, R., and REDDY, B.S., Dietary fat and colon cancer: modulation of cyclooxygenase-2 by types and amount of dietary fat during the postinitiation stage of colon carcinogenesis. *Cancer Res*, 1997. **57**(16): p. 3465–70.
89. COLLETT, E.D., DAVIDSON, L.A., FAN, Y.Y., LUPTON, J.R., and CHAPKIN, R.S., *n*-6 and *n*-3 polyunsaturated fatty acids differentially modulate oncogenic *Ras* activation in colonocytes. *Am J Physiol Cell Physiol*, 2001. **280**(5): p. C1066–75.

90. VANAMALA, J., GLAGOLENKO, A., YANG, P., CARROLL, R.J., MURPHY, M.E., NEWMAN, R.A., FORD, J.R., BRABY, L.A., CHAPKIN, R.S., TURNER, N.D., and LUPTON, J.R., Dietary fish oil and pectin enhance colonocyte apoptosis in part through suppression of *PPAR*^{delta}*/PGE2* and elevation of *PGE3*. *Carcinogenesis*, 2008. **29**(4): p. 790–6.
91. DAVIDSON, L.A., NGUYEN, D.V., HOKANSON, R.M., CALLAWAY, E.S., ISETT, R.B., TURNER, N.D., DOUGHERTY, E.R., WANG, N., LUPTON, J.R., CARROLL, R.J., and CHAPKIN, R.S., Chemopreventive *n*-3 polyunsaturated fatty acids reprogram genetic signatures during colon cancer initiation and progression in the rat. *Cancer Res*, 2004. **64**(18): p. 6797–804.
92. ONOGI, N., OKUNO, M., KOMAKI, C., MORIWAKI, H., KAWAMORI, T., TANAKA, T., MORI, H., and MUTO, Y., Suppressing effect of perilla oil on azoxymethane-induced foci of colonic aberrant crypts in rats. *Carcinogenesis*, 1996. **17**(6): p. 1291–6.
93. NARISAWA, T., FUKAURA, Y., YAZAWA, K., ISHIKAWA, C., ISODA, Y., and NISHIZAWA, Y., Colon cancer prevention with a small amount of dietary perilla oil high in alpha-linolenic acid in an animal model. *Cancer*, 1994. **73**(8): p. 2069–75.
94. NARISAWA, T., TAKAHASHI, M., KOTANAGI, H., KUSAKA, H., YAMAZAKI, Y., KOYAMA, H., FUKAURA, Y., NISHIZAWA, Y., KOTSUGAI, M., ISODA, Y., *et al.*, Inhibitory effect of dietary perilla oil rich in the *n*-3 polyunsaturated fatty acid alpha-linolenic acid on colon carcinogenesis in rats. *Jpn J Cancer Res*, 1991. **82**(10): p. 1089–96.
95. HIROSE, M., MASUDA, A., ITO, N., KAMANO, K., and OKUYAMA, H., Effects of dietary perilla oil, soybean oil and safflower oil on 7,12-dimethylbenz[a]anthracene (DMBA) and 1,2-dimethyl-hydrazine (DMH)-induced mammary gland and colon carcinogenesis in female SD rats. *Carcinogenesis*, 1990. **11**(5): p. 731–5.
96. WILLIAMS, D., VERGHESE, M., WALKER, L.T., BOATENG, J., SHACKELFORD, L., and CHAWAN, C.B., Flax seed oil and flax seed meal reduce the formation of aberrant crypt foci (ACF) in azoxymethane-induced colon cancer in Fisher 344 male rats. *Food Chem Toxicol*, 2007. **45**(1): p. 153–9.
97. DWIVEDI, C., NATARAJAN, K., and MATTHEES, D.P., Chemopreventive effects of dietary flaxseed oil on colon tumor development. *Nutr Cancer*, 2005. **51**(1): p. 52–8.
98. OIKARINEN, S.I., PAJARI, A.M., SALMINEN, I., HEINONEN, S.M., ADLERCREUTZ, H., and MUTANEN, M., Effects of a flaxseed mixture and plant oils rich in alpha-linolenic acid on the adenoma formation in multiple intestinal neoplasia (*Min*) mice. *Br J Nutr*, 2005. **94**(4): p. 510–18.
99. LEE, K.W., LEE, H.J., CHO, H.Y., and KIM, Y.J., Role of the conjugated linoleic acid in the prevention of cancer. *Crit Rev Food Sci Nutr*, 2005. **45**(2): p. 135–44.
100. LIEW, C., SCHUT, H.A., CHIN, S.F., PARIZA, M.W., and DASHWOOD, R.H., Protection of conjugated linoleic acids against 2-amino-3-methylimidazo[4,5-f]quinoline-induced colon carcinogenesis in the F344 rat: a study of inhibitory mechanisms. *Carcinogenesis*, 1995. **16**(12): p. 3037–43.
101. PARK, H.S., RYU, J.H., HA, Y.L., and PARK, J.H., Dietary conjugated linoleic acid (CLA) induces apoptosis of colonic mucosa in 1,2-dimethylhydrazine-treated rats: a possible mechanism of the anticarcinogenic effect by CLA. *Br J Nutr*, 2001. **86**(5): p. 549–55.
102. YANG, H., STUART, G.R., GLICKMAN, B.W., and DE BOER, J.G., Modulation of 2-amino-1-methyl-6-phenylimidazo[4,5-b]pyridine-induced mutation in the cecum and colon of big blue rats by conjugated linoleic acid and 1,2-dithiole-3-thione. *Nutr Cancer*, 2001. **39**(2): p. 259–66.
103. EALEY, K.N., EL-SOHEMY, A., and ARCHER, M.C., Conjugated linoleic acid does not inhibit development of aberrant crypt foci in colons of male Sprague–Dawley rats. *Nutr Cancer*, 2001. **41**(1–2): p. 104–6.

104. YASUI, Y., SUZUKI, R., KOHNO, H., MIYAMOTO, S., BEPPU, F., HOSOKAWA, M., MIYASHITA, K., and TANAKA, T., 9*Trans*, 11*trans* conjugated linoleic acid inhibits the development of azoxymethane-induced colonic aberrant crypt foci in rats. *Nutr Cancer*, 2007. **59**(1): p. 82–91.
105. KOHNO, H., SUZUKI, R., NOGUCHI, R., HOSOKAWA, M., MIYASHITA, K., and TANAKA, T., Dietary conjugated linolenic acid inhibits azoxymethane-induced colonic aberrant crypt foci in rats. *Jpn J Cancer Res*, 2002. **93**(2): p. 133–42.
106. SUZUKI, R., NOGUCHI, R., OTA, T., ABE, M., MIYASHITA, K., and KAWADA, T., Cytotoxic effect of conjugated trienoic fatty acids on mouse tumor and human monocytic leukemia cells. *Lipids*, 2001. **36**(5): p. 477–82.
107. KOHNO, H., YASUI, Y., SUZUKI, R., HOSOKAWA, M., MIYASHITA, K., and TANAKA, T., Dietary seed oil rich in conjugated linolenic acid from bitter melon inhibits azoxymethane-induced rat colon carcinogenesis through elevation of colonic *PPAR*^{gamma} expression and alteration of lipid composition. *Int J Cancer*, 2004. **110**(6): p. 896–901.
108. KOHNO, H., SUZUKI, R., YASUI, Y., HOSOKAWA, M., MIYASHITA, K., and TANAKA, T., Pomegranate seed oil rich in conjugated linolenic acid suppresses chemically induced colon carcinogenesis in rats. *Cancer Sci*, 2004. **95**(6): p. 481–6.
109. SUZUKI, R., YASUI, Y., KOHNO, H., MIYAMOTO, S., HOSOKAWA, M., MIYASHITA, K., and TANAKA, T., Catalpa seed oil rich in 9*t*, 11*t*, 13*c*-conjugated linolenic acid suppresses the development of colonic aberrant crypt foci induced by azoxymethane in rats. *Oncol Rep*, 2006. **16**(5): p. 989–96.
110. TAN, K.Y. and SEOW-CHOEN, F., Fiber and colorectal diseases: separating fact from fiction. *World J Gastroenterol*, 2007. **13**(31): p. 4161–7.
111. POOL-ZOBEL, B.L., Inulin-type fructans and reduction in colon cancer risk: review of experimental and human data. *Br J Nutr*, 2005. **93** Suppl 1: p. S73–90.
112. LE LEU, R.K., BROWN, I.L., HU, Y., ESTERMAN, A., and YOUNG, G.P., Suppression of azoxymethane-induced colon cancer development in rats by dietary resistant starch. *Cancer Biol Ther*, 2007. **6**(10): p. 1621–6.
113. VAN LOO, J., COUSSEMENT, P., DE LEENHEER, L., HOEBREGS, H., and SMITS, G., On the presence of inulin and oligofructose as natural ingredients in the western diet. *Crit Rev Food Sci Nutr*, 1995. **35**(6): p. 525–52.
114. SCHNEEMAN, B.O., Fiber, inulin and oligofructose: similarities and differences. *J Nutr*, 1999. **129**(7 Suppl): p. 1424S–7S.
115. ELLEGARD, L., ANDERSSON, H., and BOSAEUS, I., Inulin and oligofructose do not influence the absorption of cholesterol, or the excretion of cholesterol, Ca, Mg, Zn, Fe, or bile acids but increases energy excretion in ileostomy subjects. *Eur J Clin Nutr*, 1997. **51**(1): p. 1–5.
116. REDDY, B.S., HAMID, R., and RAO, C.V., Effect of dietary oligofructose and inulin on colonic preneoplastic aberrant crypt foci inhibition. *Carcinogenesis*, 1997. **18**(7): p. 1371–4.
117. POULSEN, M., MOLCK, A.M., and JACOBSEN, B.L., Different effects of short- and long-chained fructans on large intestinal physiology and carcinogen-induced aberrant crypt foci in rats. *Nutr Cancer*, 2002. **42**(2): p. 194–205.
118. JACOBSEN, H., POULSEN, M., DRAGSTED, L.O., RAVN-HAREN, G., MEYER, O., and LINDECRONA, R.H., Carbohydrate digestibility predicts colon carcinogenesis in azoxymethane-treated rats. *Nutr Cancer*, 2006. **55**(2): p. 163–70.
119. RAO, C.V., CHOU, D., SIMI, B., KU, H., and REDDY, B.S., Prevention of colonic aberrant crypt foci and modulation of large bowel microbial activity by dietary coffee fiber, inulin and pectin. *Carcinogenesis*, 1998. **19**(10): p. 1815–19.
120. BOLOGNANI, F., RUMNEY, C.J., POOL-ZOBEL, B.L., and ROWLAND, I.R., Effect of lactobacilli, bifidobacteria and inulin on the formation of aberrant crypt foci in rats. *Eur J Nutr*, 2001. **40**(6): p. 293–300.

121. ROWLAND, I.R., RUMNEY, C.J., COUTTS, J.T., and LIEVENSE, L.C., Effect of Bifidobacterium longum and inulin on gut bacterial metabolism and carcinogen-induced aberrant crypt foci in rats. *Carcinogenesis*, 1998. **19**(2): p. 281–5.
122. FEMIA, A.P., LUCERI, C., DOLARA, P., GIANNINI, A., BIGGERI, A., SALVADORI, M., CLUNE, Y., COLLINS, K.J., PAGLIERANI, M., and CADERNI, G., Antitumorigenic activity of the prebiotic inulin enriched with oligofructose in combination with the probiotics *Lactobacillus rhamnosus* and *Bifidobacterium lactis* on azoxymethane-induced colon carcinogenesis in rats. *Carcinogenesis*, 2002. **23**(11): p. 1953–60.
123. VERGHESE, M., RAO, D.R., CHAWAN, C.B., WILLIAMS, L.L., and SHACKELFORD, L., Dietary inulin suppresses azoxymethane-induced aberrant crypt foci and colon tumors at the promotion stage in young Fisher 344 rats. *J Nutr*, 2002. **132**(9): p. 2809–13.
124. VERGHESE, M., RAO, D.R., CHAWAN, C.B., and SHACKELFORD, L., Dietary inulin suppresses azoxymethane-induced preneoplastic aberrant crypt foci in mature Fisher 344 rats. *J Nutr*, 2002. **132**(9): p. 2804–8.
125. MISIKANGAS, M., PAJARI, A.M., PAIVARINTA, E., and MUTANEN, M., Promotion of adenoma growth by dietary inulin is associated with increase in cyclin D1 and decrease in adhesion proteins in *Min*/+ mice mucosa. *J Nutr Biochem*, 2005. **16**(7): p. 402–9.
126. ENGLYST, H.N., KINGMAN, S.M., and CUMMINGS, J.H., Classification and measurement of nutritionally important starch fractions. *Eur J Clin Nutr*, 1992. **46** Suppl 2: p. S33–50.
127. THORUP, I., MEYER, O., and KRISTIANSEN, E., Effect of potato starch, cornstarch and sucrose on aberrant crypt foci in rats exposed to azoxymethane. *Anticancer Res*, 1995. **15**(5B): p. 2101–5.
128. CASSAND, P., MAZIERE, S., CHAMP, M., MEFLAH, K., BORNET, F., and NARBONNE, J.F., Effects of resistant starch- and vitamin A-supplemented diets on the promotion of precursor lesions of colon cancer in rats. *Nutr Cancer*, 1997. **27**(1): p. 53–9.
129. MAZIERE, S., MEFLAH, K., TAVAN, E., CHAMP, M., NARBONNE, J.F., and CASSAND, P., Effect of resistant starch and/or fat-soluble vitamins A and E on the initiation stage of aberrant crypts in rat colon. *Nutr Cancer*, 1998. **31**(3): p. 168–77.
130. LIU, R. and XU, G., Effects of resistant starch on colonic preneoplastic aberrant crypt foci in rats. *Food Chem Toxicol*, 2008. **46**(8): p. 2672–9.
131. FERGUSON, L.R., ZHU, S., and KESTELL, P., Contrasting effects of non-starch polysaccharide and resistant starch-based diets on the disposition and excretion of the food carcinogen, 2-amino-3-methylimidazo[4,5-f]quinoline (IQ), in a rat model. *Food Chem Toxicol*, 2003. **41**(6): p. 785–92.
132. BAUER-MARINOVIC, M., FLORIAN, S., MULLER-SCHMEHL, K., GLATT, H., and JACOBASCH, G., Dietary resistant starch type 3 prevents tumor induction by 1,2-dimethylhydrazine and alters proliferation, apoptosis and dedifferentiation in rat colon. *Carcinogenesis*, 2006. **27**(9): p. 1849–59.
133. LE LEU, R.K., BROWN, I.L., HU, Y., MORITA, T., ESTERMAN, A., and YOUNG, G.P., Effect of dietary resistant starch and protein on colonic fermentation and intestinal tumourigenesis in rats. *Carcinogenesis*, 2007. **28**(2): p. 240–5.
134. SAKAMOTO, J., NAKAJI, S., SUGAWARA, K., IWANE, S., and MUNAKATA, A., Comparison of resistant starch with cellulose diet on 1,2-dimethylhydrazine-induced colonic carcinogenesis in rats. *Gastroenterology*, 1996. **110**(1): p. 116–20.
135. PIERRE, F., PERRIN, P., CHAMP, M., BORNET, F., MEFLAH, K., and MENANTEAU, J., Short-chain fructo-oligosaccharides reduce the occurrence of colon tumors and develop gut-associated lymphoid tissue in Min mice. *Cancer Res*, 1997. **57**(2): p. 225–8.
136. YOUNG, G.P., MCINTYRE, A., ALBERT, V., FOLINO, M., MUIR, J.G., and GIBSON, P.R., Wheat bran suppresses potato starch – potentiated colorectal tumorigenesis at

the aberrant crypt stage in a rat model. *Gastroenterology*, 1996. **110**(2): p. 508–14.
137. WILLIAMSON, S.L., KARTHEUSER, A., COAKER, J., KOOSHKGHAZI, M.D., FODDE, R., BURN, J., and MATHERS, J.C., Intestinal tumorigenesis in the Apc1638N mouse treated with aspirin and resistant starch for up to 5 months. *Carcinogenesis*, 1999. **20**(5): p. 805–10.
138. LUPTON, J.R. and TURNER, N.D., Potential protective mechanisms of wheat bran fiber. *Am J Med*, 1999. **106**(1A): p. 24S–27S.
139. GAZZANIGA, J.M. and LUPTON, J.R., Dilution effect of dietary fiber sources – an *invivo* study in the rat. *Nut Res*, 1987. **7**(12): p. 1261–8.
140. LUPTON, J.R. and MEACHER, M.M., Radiographic analysis of the effect of dietary-fibers on rat colonic transit-time. *Am J Physiol*, 1988. **255**(5): p. G633–9.
141. KESTELL, P., ZHAO, L., ZHU, S., HARRIS, P.J., and FERGUSON, L.R., Studies on the mechanism of cancer protection by wheat bran: effects on the absorption, metabolism and excretion of the food carcinogen 2-amino-3-methylimidazo[4,5-f]quinoline (IQ). *Carcinogenesis*, 1999. **20**(12): p. 2253–60.
142. HU, Y., MARTIN, J., LE LEU, R., and YOUNG, G.P., The colonic response to genotoxic carcinogens in the rat: regulation by dietary fibre. *Carcinogenesis*, 2002. **23**(7): p. 1131–7.
143. REDDY, B.S., MORI, H., and NICOLAIS, M., Effect of dietary wheat bran and dehydrated citrus fiber on azoxymethane-induced intestinal carcinogenesis in Fischer-344 rats. *J Nat Cancer Inst*, 1981. **66**(3): p. 553–7.
144. WATANABE, K., REDDY, B.S., WEISBURGER, J.H., and KRITCHEVSKY, D., Effect of dietary alfalfa, pectin, and wheat bran on azoxymethane-induced or methylnitrosourea-induced colon carcinogenesis in F344 rats. *J Nat Cancer Inst*, 1979. **63**(1): p. 141–5.
145. BARNES, D.S., CLAPP, N.K., SCOTT, D.A., OBERST, D.L., and BERRY, S.G., Effects of wheat, rice, corn, and soybean bran on 1,2-dimethylhydrazine-induced large bowel tumorigenesis in F344 rats. *Nutr Cancer*, 1983. **5**(1): p. 1–9.
146. ALABASTER, O., TANG, Z., and SHIVAPURKAR, N., Inhibition by wheat bran cereals of the development of aberrant crypt foci and colon tumours. *Food Chem Toxicol*, 1997. **35**(5): p. 517–22.
147. ALABASTER, O., TANG, Z.C., FROST, A., and SHIVAPURKAR, N., Potential synergism between wheat bran and psyllium: enhanced inhibition of colon cancer. *Cancer Lett*, 1993. **75**(1): p. 53–8.
148. ALABASTER, O., TANG, Z., FROST, A., and SHIVAPURKAR, N., Effect of beta-carotene and wheat bran fiber on colonic aberrant crypt and tumor formation in rats exposed to azoxymethane and high dietary fat. *Carcinogenesis*, 1995. **16**(1): p. 127–32.
149. YANG, C.S. and WANG, Z.Y., Tea and cancer. *J Natl Cancer Inst*, 1993. **85**(13): p. 1038–49.
150. YANG, C.S., MALIAKAL, P., and MENG, X., Inhibition of carcinogenesis by tea. *Annu Rev Pharmacol Toxicol*, 2002. **42**: p. 25–54.
151. CHUNG, F.L., SCHWARTZ, J., HERZOG, C.R., and YANG, Y.M., Tea and cancer prevention: studies in animals and humans. *J Nutr*, 2003. **133**(10): p. 3268S–74S.
152. CRESPY, V. and WILLIAMSON, G., A review of the health effects of green tea catechins in *in vivo* animal models. *J Nutr*, 2004. **134**(12 Suppl): p. 3431S–40S.
153. KHAN, N., AFAQ, F., SALEEM, M., AHMAD, N., and MUKHTAR, H., Targeting multiple signaling pathways by green tea polyphenol (–)-epigallocatechin-3-gallate. *Cancer Res*, 2006. **66**(5): p. 2500–5.
154. KIM, S., LEE, M.J., HONG, J., LI, C., SMITH, T.J., YANG, G.Y., SERIL, D.N., and YANG, C.S., Plasma and tissue levels of tea catechins in rats and mice during chronic consumption of green tea polyphenols. *Nutr Cancer*, 2000. **37**(1): p. 41–8.

155. LAMBERT, J.D., LEE, M.J., LU, H., MENG, X., HONG, J.J., SERIL, D.N., STURGILL, M.G., and YANG, C.S., Epigallocatechin-3-gallate is absorbed but extensively glucuronidated following oral administration to mice. *J Nutr*, 2003. **133**(12): p. 4172–7.
156. BLOT, W.J., CHOW, W.H., and MCLAUGHLIN, J.K., Tea and cancer: a review of the epidemiological evidence. *Eur J Cancer Prev*, 1996. **5**(6): p. 425–38.
157. KOHLMEIER, L., WETERINGS, K.G., STECK, S., and KOK, F.J., Tea and cancer prevention: an evaluation of the epidemiologic literature. *Nutr Cancer*, 1997. **27**(1): p. 1–13.
158. BUSHMAN, J.L., Green tea and cancer in humans: a review of the literature. *Nutr Cancer*, 1998. **31**(3): p. 151–9.
159. LAMBERT, J.D. and YANG, C.S., Mechanisms of cancer prevention by tea constituents. *J Nutr*, 2003. **133**(10): p. 3262S–7S.
160. SUN, C.L., YUAN, J.M., KOH, W.P., and YU, M.C., Green tea, black tea and colorectal cancer risk: a meta-analysis of epidemiologic studies. *Carcinogenesis*, 2006. **27**(7): p. 1301–9.
161. YANG, G., SHU, X.O., LI, H., CHOW, W.H., JI, B.T., ZHANG, X., GAO, Y.T., and ZHENG, W., Prospective cohort study of green tea consumption and colorectal cancer risk in women. *Cancer Epidemiol Biomarkers Prev*, 2007. **16**(6): p. 1219–23.
162. YUAN, J.M., GAO, Y.T., YANG, C.S., and YU, M.C., Urinary biomarkers of tea polyphenols and risk of colorectal cancer in the Shanghai Cohort Study. *Int J Cancer*, 2007. **120**(6): p. 1344–50.
163. TAKAYAMA, T., KATSUKI, S., TAKAHASHI, Y., OHI, M., NOJIRI, S., SAKAMAKI, S., KATO, J., KOGAWA, K., MIYAKE, H., and NIITSU, Y., Aberrant crypt foci of the colon as precursors of adenoma and cancer. *N Engl J Med*, 1998. **339**(18): p. 1277–84.
164. ADLER, D.G., GOSTOUT, C.J., SORBI, D., BURGART, L.J., WANG, L., and HARMSEN, W.S., Endoscopic identification and quantification of aberrant crypt foci in the human colon. *Gastrointest Endosc*, 2002. **56**(5): p. 657–62.
165. YIN, P., ZHAO, J., CHENG, S., ZHU, Q., LIU, Z., and ZHENGGUO, L., Experimental studies of the inhibitory effects of green tea catechin on mice large intestinal cancers induced by 1,2-dimethylhydrazine. *Cancer Lett*, 1994. **79**(1): p. 33–8.
166. SUGANUMA, M., OHKURA, Y., OKABE, S., and FUJIKI, H., Combination cancer chemoprevention with green tea extract and sulindac shown in intestinal tumor formation in Min mice. *J Cancer Res Clin Oncol*, 2001. **127**(1): p. 69–72.
167. ORNER, G.A., DASHWOOD, W.M., BLUM, C.A., DIAZ, G.D., LI, Q., and DASHWOOD, R.H., Suppression of tumorigenesis in the *Apc(min)* mouse: down-regulation of beta-catenin signaling by a combination of tea plus sulindac. *Carcinogenesis*, 2003. **24**(2): p. 263–7.
168. JU, J., HONG, J., ZHOU, J.N., PAN, Z., BOSE, M., LIAO, J., YANG, G.Y., LIU, Y.Y., HOU, Z., LIN, Y., MA, J., SHIH, W.J., *et al.*, Inhibition of intestinal tumorigenesis in $Apc^{(min/+)}$ mice by (−)-epigallocatechin-3-gallate, the major catechin in green tea. *Cancer Res*, 2005. **65**(22): p. 10623–31.
169. JU, J., LIU, Y., HONG, J., HUANG, M.T., CONNEY, A.H., and YANG, C.S., Effects of green tea and high-fat diet on arachidonic acid metabolism and aberrant crypt foci formation in an azoxymethane-induced colon carcinogenesis mouse model. *Nutr Cancer*, 2003. **46**(2): p. 172–8.
170. HAO, X., SUN, Y., YANG, C.S., BOSE, M., LAMBERT, J.D., JU, J., LU, G., LEE, M.J., PARK, S., HUSAIN, A., and WANG, S., Inhibition of intestinal tumorigenesis in $Apc^{(min/+)}$ mice by green tea polyphenols (polyphenon E) and individual catechins. *Nutr Cancer*, 2007. **59**(1): p. 62–9.
171. KIM, M., HAGIWARA, N., SMITH, S.J., YAMAMOTO, T., YAMANE, T., and TAKAHASHI, T., Preventive effect of green tea polyphenols on colon carcinogenesis, in *Food Phytochemicals in Cancer Prevention*, M.-T. Huang, Osaswa, T., Ho, C.-T., and Rosen, R.T., Editors. 1994, ACS Symposium Series 546. p. 51–5.

172. XU, M., BAILEY, A.C., HERNAEZ, J.F., TAOKA, C.R., SCHUT, H.A., and DASHWOOD, R.H., Protection by green tea, black tea, and indole-3-carbinol against 2- amino-3-methylimidazo[4,5-f]quinoline-induced DNA adducts and colonic aberrant crypts in the F344 rat. *Carcinogenesis*, 1996. **17**(7): p. 1429–34.
173. CHALLA, A., RAO, D.R., and REDDY, B.S., Interactive suppression of aberrant crypt foci induced by azoxymethane in rat colon by phytic acid and green tea. *Carcinogenesis*, 1997. **18**(10): p. 2023–6.
174. HIROSE, M., YAMAGUCHI, T., MIZOGUCHI, Y., AKAGI, K., FUTAKUCHI, M., and SHIRAI, T., Lack of inhibitory effects of green tea catechins in 1,2-dimetylhydrazine-induced rat intestinal carcinogenesis model: comparison of the different formulations, administration routes and doses. *Cancer Lett*, 2002. **188**(1–2): p. 163–70.
175. HIROSE, M., HOSHIYA, T., MIZOGUCHI, Y., NAKAMURA, A., AKAGI, K., and SHIRAI, T., Green tea catechins enhance tumor development in the colon without effects in the lung or thyroid after pretreatment with 1,2-dimethylhydrazine or 2,2′-dihydroxy-di-*n*-propylnitrosamine in male F344 rats. *Cancer Lett*, 2001. **168**(1): p. 23–9.
176. WEISBURGER, J.H., RIVENSON, A., ALIAGA, C., REINHARDT, J., KELLOFF, G.J., BOONE, C.W., STEELE, V.E., BALENTINE, D.A., PITTMAN, B., and ZANG, E., Effect of tea extracts, polyphenols, and epigallocatechin gallate on azoxymethane-induced colon cancer. *Proc Soc Exp Biol Med*, 1998. **217**(1): p. 104–8.
177. CADERNI, G., DE FILIPPO, C., LUCERI, C., SALVADORI, M., GIANNINI, A., BIGGERI, A., REMY, S., CHEYNIER, V., and DOLARA, P., Effects of black tea, green tea and wine extracts on intestinal carcinogenesis induced by azoxymethane in F344 rats. *Carcinogenesis*, 2000. **21**(11): p. 1965–9.

16

Using stable isotopes to determine mineral bioavailability of functional foods

S. A. Abrams, Baylor College of Medicine and Texas Children's Hospital, USA

Abstract: Mineral stable isotopes allow for the direct assessment of mineral absorption in all population groups. The most widely used in human nutrition are calcium, magnesium, zinc and iron. These can be used to demonstrate the effects of interventions, including the use of functional foods, on mineral absorption both from an individual meal and from whole diets. Methodologies are safe, practical and well tolerated, even by small children.

Key words: calcium absorption, iron, zinc, stable isotopes, mineral metabolism.

16.1 Introduction

16.1.1 What are mineral stable isotopes and which minerals can be studied?

Mineral stable isotopes are naturally occurring, non-radioactive forms of minerals in which the lower abundance atomic mass fractions have been enriched so that they may be used to trace the metabolism of the native compounds. By enriching what are usually rare isotopes, followed by administration of small amounts of these enriched isotopes to human or animal subjects, the rate at which these minerals enter the body or are distributed and excreted can be determined. In nutritional research, by far the most commonly studied minerals are calcium, iron, zinc and magnesium. Some research has been done with copper and selenium. Key additional minerals, most notably phosphorus, do not have any naturally occurring low abundance isotopes and thus cannot be studied using stable isotope techniques. The use of mineral stable isotopes has largely, but not completely, replaced the use of radioactive isotopes in human nutrition research (Abrams, 1999).

16.1.2 How are mineral stable isotopes produced, obtained and tested for safety?

Stable isotopes are usually obtained as the metal, oxide, carbonate or chloride forms. Enriched isotopes are produced by a number of methods described elsewhere (Yergey and Yergey, 1997; Abrams, 1999). Currently, virtually all of the mineral stable isotopes are produced either via the calutron facilities in Russia (calcium and magnesium) or via European gas centrifugation facilities (iron and zinc). The isotopes need to be converted into a soluble form, usually the aqueous chloride or sulfate prior to administration. All chemicals used in isotope preparation and sample preparation must be high purity to avoid any trace contaminants. The soluble isotope is diluted to the desired concentration, or further preparation is conducted if necessary, depending on the mineral and the form in which it is to be administered. If the isotope is to be administered intravenously, the solutions need to be sterile-filtered, packaged into vials and tested for sterility and pyrogenicity before human or animal use. This is usually done by a licensed pharmacy experienced in these procedures. Unfortunately, in the United States there are few such pharmacies and this can be an issue in obtaining isotopes prepared for human use. As with all medications, stable isotopes must be prepared and administered in accordance with accepted pharmaceutical standards. There is no intrinsic risk to the isotopes as they are naturally occurring and as currently provided by reputable dealers, are free of contamination and can usually be provided at the desired enrichment.

Mineral stable isotopes are not usually purchased directly from the manufacturers. Instead they are purchased from reputable isotope sales companies. In the past, inappropriate sales and distributions of inadequately tested materials were common problems. However, at the present time, this is not a substantial problem and with appropriate diligence, there should be no concern about the availability or safety of purchased mineral isotopes. Typical isotopes used are listed in Table 16.1. With the exception of ^{46}Ca, isotopes are usually purchased at >80% purity, often >95%. This decreases problems with using multiple isotopes of the same mineral as there is little cross-over of isotope. A unique exception is ^{46}Ca with a natural abundance of 0.003%. This isotope is usually purchased at 5–10% purity, although a maximum of about 30% has been reached. This is not problematic as extremely small doses of ^{46}Ca are used in studies.

16.1.3 What are the approximate costs of mineral stable isotopes and how are they analyzed?

The costs of a mineral stable isotope study depend on the mineral being studied, the type of study being done (absorption or absorption and kinetic turnover rate study), the size of the subjects and their age. In the case

Table 16.1 Mineral stable isotopes frequently used in nutritional research

Isotope	Natural abundance (%)	Typical dose in adults (absorption)
^{42}Ca	0.65	1–2 mg intravenously
^{44}Ca	2.08	10–15 mg by mouth
^{57}Fe	2.14	6–8 mg by mouth
^{58}Fe	0.29	3 mg by mouth
^{25}Mg	10.0	15–20 mg intravenously
^{26}Mg	11.0	25–30 mg by mouth
^{67}Zn	4.1	2–4 mg by mouth
^{70}Zn	0.6	0.4–0.5 mg intravenously

Typical doses are based on dual tracer studies involving adults and children over 12 years of age. Other isotopes may be chosen and dosing depends on physiological conditions, expected absorption and analytical methodology/precision.

of calcium, for example, the largest isotope doses must be used on adolescents due to their high rates of bone turnover. For iron, as the tracer is primarily distributed into red blood cells, the whole body quantity of which is body weight dependent, it is usually less expensive to study small children than adults. Studies in which it is expected that absorption will be low due to dietary inhibitors or subject characteristics would need a greater dose. Ultimately, it is the precision of the measurement equipment being used for each isotope that determines how much the isotopes need to be enriched in the body fluid sample to be measured and thus what dosing is needed.

Analytical techniques for isotope analysis for minerals are very different from those for organic substances or other elements such as oxygen and nitrogen (e.g. deuterium). Briefly, most analysis are currently undertaken using either thermal ionization mass spectrometry or inductively coupled plasma mass spectrometry. These techniques are specialized and generally available only at a small number of institutions, as discussed below.

However, with these caveats in mind, it is not uncommon for the isotope costs for a single measurement of calcium, iron or zinc absorption to be between $100 and $200/subject. Magnesium measurements can be about twice this expensive. The cost of analysis is dependent on the mineral, the type of equipment used, the precision needed and the general operating characteristics of the laboratory. Costs typically range from $50 to $200 for a sample analysis in laboratories that process a large number of nutritional samples. Some laboratories may change considerably more for small sample volumes or high-precision measurements.

16.2 Methodological issues in using stable isotopes to study human nutrition

The methodologies used in mineral stable isotope studies are primarily mineral specific, rather than food specific. By this it is meant that very similar methods are used to evaluate the effects of diet and dietary interventions using stable isotopes regardless of the food or meal matrix in which the mineral of interest is found (Tables 16.2 and 16.3). What is different in how the research is conducted is which minerals are being evaluated. Calcium, magnesium, zinc and iron methodologies will be considered below.

16.2.1 Calcium

There are six naturally occurring stable isotopes of calcium. Choice of isotopes and dosing levels depends greatly on the type of study being conducted (i.e. absorption or kinetic), the likely level of mineral absorption and the type and precision of analytical technique being used (Abrams, 1999). The method used for most current studies for calcium (and magnesium and zinc) is the dual-tracer method. In this method, one isotope (e.g. ^{44}Ca) is given by mouth while a second enriched isotope (e.g. ^{42}Ca) is given intravenously. The relative enrichment of the oral versus the intravenous (IV)

Table 16.2 Minerals and preferred collection methods

Mineral	Dosing method	Collection method
Calcium	IV and oral	24–48 hour urine
Zinc	IV and oral	Spot urine 72–96 hours
Magnesium	IV and oral	Complete 72 hour urine
Iron	Oral	Red blood cells 14 days

Table 16.3 Guidelines for obtaining and preparing isotopes

Purchasing
- Experienced dealer
- Provision of complete tracking of isotopes from source
- Certified analysis
- Pricing based on volume and enrichment

Testing and preparation
- Certification by dealer
- Compounding by licensed pharmacist
- Sterility and pyrogenicity testing as needed
- Testing of final compounds for total mineral and isotopic enrichment

tracer in an appropriate body fluid is a measure of the absorption over 50 years ago (Bronner and Harris, 1956).

Early in the morning of the study, subjects are instructed to empty their bladders, and are given breakfast. Toward the end of the meal, the subjects are given an isotope of calcium that has been premixed (and allowed to equilibrate in the refrigerator for 12–24 h) with milk or juice. After breakfast, a different calcium isotope is administered intravenously over 2–3 min (Abrams *et al.*, 1997).

After administration of the tracers, a complete 24 h urine collection is carried out. The relative fraction of the oral vs. the IV tracer dose in this 24 h urine pool is determined and represents the fraction of the oral tracer dose that was absorbed. Spot determinations of urine or serum isotope levels of the tracers may also be used. However, for calcium, this method may not be as accurate as that determined from complete 24 h collections (Yergey *et al.*, 1994). Calcium is extracted from the urine sample via oxalate precipitation. For magnesium, iron and zinc, ion exchange columns are needed. Published methods are available for each of these minerals. In general, it is best to have the sample preparation done at the laboratory performing the mass spectrometric analysis.

In studies in adults, it may be more convenient to obtain a single timed blood sample rather than a 24 h urine collection. In this variation of the method described above, the oral isotope is given about 2 h before the IV isotope. Then a single blood sample is obtained usually 3–4 hours after the IV dose. The relative enrichment of the oral versus the IV tracer in the blood is used to calculate absorption. In theory, this method may be slightly less accurate than the urine method due to variable rates of absorption of the oral tracer. However, in practical terms, they appear to give very similar results and either method may be used in research studies (Abrams, unpublished observations). When used for clinical purposes on an individual patient, the dual-tracer method with 24 h urine collection would remain the gold standard at this time.

In studies in adults, some have used only a single oral tracer and estimated the IV results using height and weight of the subject (Heaney *et al.*, 2002). In general, this approach is less preferred than the dual tracer approach, especially for clinical use or smaller research studies. The IV tracer is a relatively small part of the overall study cost and is safely administered without difficulty in adults. Studies using only an oral tracer are likely to give accurate answers in relatively large sample groups of adults, but more reliance can be given to those conducted using both an oral and an IV tracer.

An important variation in this methodology was necessary for studies of prebiotics and calcium absorption. It was observed from some studies that a benefit was seen in some cases and not in others (Griffin and Abrams, 2005). A key feature of studies that did not show a benefit was that the 24 h urine method had been used. Since prebiotics primarily increases calcium absorption by increasing calcium absorption in the colon, using a 24 h urine collection may be inadequate to identify this effect. Instead, collecting all urine for a total of 36–48 h after dosing may be needed to evaluate factors which affect calcium absorption by the colon. Therefore, when evaluating dietary factors which may alter the site of calcium absorption, a 48 h urine collection should be performed rather than a 24 h collection to be certain of capturing this effect (Abrams *et al.*, 2007).

16.2.2 Magnesium

There are only three naturally occurring isotopes of magnesium, none of which is a true low-abundance one. This means that higher doses must be used than for other minerals and the relative cost is greater, as is the analytical challenge. Nonetheless, magnesium stable isotope studies are quite feasible and have been used in the evaluation of prebiotics (Holloway *et al.*, 2007).

The methods used in studies of magnesium absorption are extremely similar to those used for calcium with one important difference. That difference, identified in early studies, is that magnesium absorption is a slow process and collection of urine for a full 72 h after ingestion of the oral isotope is needed to measure absorption. Therefore, in studies of magnesium absorption it is necessary to collect urine for 3 days after dosing (Abrams *et al.*, 1997; Abrams 2003). This is challenging for many people due to work and schooling issues. The reliability of a 3-day urine collection may be less as well. Nonetheless, this method has been successfully used in studies involving both children and adults.

16.2.3 Zinc

There are five naturally occurring stable isotopes of zinc. Two are widely used in clinical studies (^{67}Zn and ^{70}Zn) and a third (^{68}Zn) can be used in some situations. Assessment of zinc isotopes in blood and urine is one of the more readily performed mineral stable isotope analysis by mass spectrometry. Recognition of the crucial role of zinc in promoting health has led to zinc becoming one of the most widely studied minerals in nutritional sciences at this time. Isotope-based studies have often evaluated factors such as the interaction of zinc and iron on the absorption of these minerals. Extremely few studies have evaluated the effects of food or diet on zinc absorption in humans. It is very likely, however, given the high frequency of zinc deficiency and the need to provide more enhanced methods of zinc delivery, that this type of research will increase.

Methodologically, there are two important issues differentiating zinc from calcium and magnesium research studies. The first is that it generally is not necessary to collect a complete 24–72 h urine after dosing of the isotopes. A spot urine sample, collected at least 72 h after dosing, is usually adequate. This spot method is much more reliable for zinc than for calcium or magnesium which simplifies the clinical protocols (Friel *et al.*, 1992; Griffin *et al.*, 2004).

A second, more difficult issue is related to determining what information is obtained from isotopic zinc absorption studies based on the regulation of zinc absorption. This requires consideration of what is actually meant by the term 'absorption'. Absorption, as calculated based on the difference between enteral intake and fecal excretion of a nutrient, consists of two components. The first is the quantity of material that is absorbed from the diet and enters the bloodstream via the gastrointestinal tract. This is referred to as 'true' dietary absorption. The other is the total difference between the amount of a nutrient in the diet and the amount that is recovered in the stool. This difference is referred to as 'net' absorption. These two 'absorptions' are different because some of what is excreted in the stool does not come from a particular meal that is traced, but from secretion of nutrients into the gastrointestinal tract (Abrams *et al.*, 1991). This additional loss of a nutrient is not measured by dual tracer studies in which urine or blood are collected as described above.

For some nutrients, this additional nutrient loss, called 'endogenous secretion', is not a major factor in the regulation of the nutrient and can either be ignored as it is very small (e.g. magnesium) or estimated for other purposes based on dietary intake (e.g. calcium) (Abrams *et al.*, 1991). Zinc, however, is unique in that nutrient regulation is significantly related to endogenous secretion and failure to measure this may not provide a complete picture of the effects of diet on zinc homeostasis (Griffin *et al.*, 2004).

If the research question being asked is specific to the bioavailability of the source of zinc and its solubility and dietary absorption, then the dual-tracer method with urinary assessment of absorption will provide the desired answer. If, however, the dietary change considered may affect gut function and the research question is to evaluate these effects, then endogenous secretion needs to be measured. For example, if one is comparing the absorption of zinc oxide and zinc gluconate in a food source, then the dual tracer method with urinary excretion measurement of absorption will distinguish between the absorption of these two zinc sources. If, however, one is looking at whether prebiotics or probiotics beneficially affect the gastrointestinal tract in people with inflammatory bowel disease and thus lead to less zinc wasting, then the urinary method will not be adequate for that assessment of absorption.

It is possible to directly measure the rate of endogenous secretion of minerals with tracers and thus answer these questions. Unfortunately, this is most accurately done with fecal collections. Fecal collections are difficult and cumbersome to obtain, process and analyze, but would be needed for some types of zinc-related research. Further details are provided elsewhere related to this issue (Abrams, 1999; Griffin *et al.*, 2004).

16.2.4 Iron

Iron presents different issues in measuring dietary bioavailability. There are four naturally occurring iron stable isotopes. The lowest-abundance isotopes, ^{58}Fe and ^{57}Fe, are most commonly used in human nutrition research. Iron stable isotopes are usually converted to ferrous sulfate prior to oral administration. Because dosing of iron stable isotopes is dependent on enriching the circulating body iron pool, the dose administered is usually dependent on the subject's weight, and increases in proportion to weight and hemoglobin concentration (Abrams *et al.*, 1994).

The methods for iron isotope studies are somewhat different from those for the other minerals. In general, the incorporation of a dietary iron dose into the red blood cells (RBC) is measured by collecting a single blood sample, usually 14 days after an oral dose and determining the isotopic enrichment relative to the total body circulating iron. This requires measuring hemoglobin concentration and estimating blood volume. In healthy children after the first year of life, about 80–90% of absorbed iron will appear in the red blood cells by 14 days. However, in special circumstances, including children with anemia associated with inflammatory diseases and infants, this percentage may be much lower. The actual percentage of absorbed iron that can be found in red blood cells can be measured by giving an iron stable isotope intravenously and determining the incorporation of this isotope into red blood cells 14 days later (Ames *et al.*, 1999). However, this method may not accurately reflect dietary iron handling and its use is limited because of safety concerns related to infusing iron intravenously.

For practical purposes, an intravenous tracer of iron is rarely administered. Commonly, however, one dose of iron isotope is administered orally with a meal or the form of iron being investigated and a second dose of a different isotope administered after an overnight fast with ascorbic acid. This second dose is referred to as a 'reference dose' and its absorption reflects the patient's iron status. Red blood cell incorporation of this dose is usually well correlated with serum ferritin or other iron status markers (Abrams *et al.*, 1994; Abrams, 1999).

Because the use of ^{57}Fe in larger children (>about 40 kg) or adults generally requires a dose of at least 6–8 mg, it is often given split over 2 days so that the total dose on any given day does not represent too large a proportion of usually daily iron intake. In most studies, a maximum of 4 mg of iron is given as the isotope in a 24 h period. Similar concerns are not as great for the other minerals as oral isotope doses are usually <10% of typical daily intake.

16.3 Study example: enhancement of calcium absorption by prebiotics in adolescents

Several studies have evaluated the use of stable isotopes to assess the effects of prebiotics on calcium absorption. We conducted a study using both calcium absorption and bone mineralization as outcomes. This study and its findings, especially methodological issues, will be considered in this section as an example of how the stable isotopic methodologies described in this chapter are used to evaluate functional foods (Abrams *et al.*, 2005).

16.3.1 Study design

We conducted a study using healthy young adolescents in which we randomized 100 subjects in a double-blinded fashion, stratified by gender to one of two carbohydrate supplement groups; either 8 g/day oligosaccharides of an inulin-type fructan, or maltodextrin placebo. Subjects mixed the carbohydrate supplement with calcium-fortified orange juice and drank it with breakfast daily for 12 months. After 8 weeks of receiving the carbohydrate supplement, subjects returned for a repeat calcium absorption study. Twelve months after the initial baseline study, they returned for a follow-up visit in which measurements of calcium absorption and bone mineralization were performed.

Subjects received a breakfast that contained approximately one-third of their daily intake of calcium (including the tracer-containing juice). Toward the end of breakfast, subjects were given 20 μg of ^{46}Ca which had been mixed with 240 mL of calcium-fortified orange juice. After breakfast, ^{42}Ca (1.2 mg) was infused over 2 min via a heparin lock catheter. Beginning with breakfast, a complete 48 h urine collection was obtained. Calcium absorption was calculated from the relative recovery of the oral and the intravenous tracer during the 48 h study period.

Two methodological issues can be commented upon. The first is the decision to give the calcium stable isotope once during the day with breakfast. An alternative approach would have been to determine the usual distribution of calcium in each subject's diet and then distribute the isotope proportionally between those multiple meals. Using multiple isotope doses may more accurately reflect the isotope distribution during a day. However, even that cannot completely reflect the distribution of calcium in the daily diet and each time that the isotope is mixed with food leads to potential dosing errors and inaccuracies. In general, we prefer to limit to one dose for each study and find this to provide adequate information about calcium absorption over the course of a day.

The second issue is the choice of material to which to add the tracer. It is important to be consistent in doing studies in individuals and therefore most groups have used fixed meals to which the tracer is added. However, for studies in subjects that have very low or very high usual calcium intakes, this can be problematic. For example, if a subject has a usual calcium intake of <500 mg/day and does not drink milk or calcium-fortified beverages, then it can be very difficult to accurately assess their usual calcium absorption using a fixed meal single-dose approach. That is because most of their daily calcium may be associated with vegetables or other non-dairy calcium sources for which the extrinsically administered isotopes, especially when given with only one meal, do not accurately reflect usual absorption (Heaney *et al.*, 1990, 2000).

16.4 Results from this study

After adjustment for ethnicity, gender, *Fok1* genotype, calcium intake at each visit and Tanner stage at enrolment, the effect of the prebiotic on fractional absorption of calcium was significant ($p = 0.02$) (Abrams *et al.*, 2005).

We further evaluated the results for calcium absorption at 8 weeks and 1 year relative to the baseline absorption values. These results demonstrated significantly greater calcium absorption at 8 weeks (difference 8.5 ± 1.6%, $p < 0.001$) and 1 year (difference 5.9 ± 2.8%, $p = 0.04$) for prebiotic subjects compared with control subjects. Similarly, both whole body bone mineral content (BMC) and whole body bone mineral density (BMD) were increased at one year in those receiving the prebiotic. For whole body BMC, the increase in BMC was 245 ± 11 g/year vs 210 ± 10 g/year for the control ($p = 0.03$). For whole body (areal) BMD, the increment was 0.047 ± 0.004 g/cm^2/year for the prebiotic group versus 0.032 ± 0.004 g/cm^2/year for the control group ($p = 0.01$).

An important methodological point related to these studies is the feasibility of performing repeat studies on the same individuals. Limitations to this can come in several areas. First, is the concern that isotope from the previous study will still be in the urine or blood at the time of the subsequent study limiting the ability to repeat studies. This is a complex issue, but this problem is dependent on the isotopes and the turnover rate of the minerals. For calcium, we have found that a time period of 2 weeks between studies readily allows for a repeat study. In adults, but not generally in children (because of slow bone turnover in adults), a baseline sample would be needed before a second study spaced apart by less than about 6 weeks. Using this baseline sample, we can correct for the small amount of 'residual isotope' in present at baseline. For zinc and magnesium, a similar approach can be taken, although experience is more limited with the time needed between studies.

The most important issues related to this are for studies of iron. Unlike the other minerals which are deposited in tissues or excreted, iron, once absorbed, remains in a relatively fixed pool of RBCs. Once dosed, it is possible to measure residual iron isotope in a sample of RBCs years after initial dosing. Furthermore, although most absorption and incorporation occurs within 14 days after dosing, in infants this can take longer and the levels do not stay constant. These issues can be managed by measuring the baseline levels of isotopes in the blood between studies but we tend to be cautious about multiple iron studies in small children and avoid them when possible.

16.5 Sources of further information and advice

16.5.1 Finding laboratories to perform mineral mass spectrometry analyses

Mineral stable isotope analyses are commonly performed either in specialized nutrition laboratories experienced in these analyses. In the United States there are about eight to ten such laboratories routinely performing these analyses. Most or all of these groups will perform 'outside' analyses for nutrition investigators, but their capacity to do so is often limited. Some may be able to only analyze one mineral such as zinc, whereas others will do all of the minerals described here.

An alternative source for mineral mass spectrometric analysis is a geology laboratory that performs these analyses. Many of these laboratories routinely perform analyses of lead and other minerals not of nutritional interest. However, a large number of laboratories in geology research have the technical capacity to measure iron, zinc, calcium and magnesium. Although this can be a useful approach to obtaining sample analysis, it can also be problematic because geology laboratories often have little, if any, experience in handling and processing biological samples. Also, they may perform only a small number of analyses daily, consistent with geological research needs. High-volume sample output as is needed in nutrition research may be difficult or impossible for these laboratories. Finally, non-nutritional laboratories may not provide much insight into interpreting the results of these studies and dealing with the specialized methodological issues described in this chapter.

For these reasons, we recommend that consultation be obtained with a researcher experienced in performing and interpreting results in planning a study. Even if the analysis is to be performed by a geology laboratory, this can be helpful to everyone, including the geologists.

16.5.2 Sources of purchasing the isotopes

Commercial isotope distributors are available for consultation and obtaining mineral isotopes. A few guidelines for working with distributors can be recommended. First, any distributor must provide complete information on the original source of the isotopes, their composition and any contamination. They should also be able to fully identify the pathway by which the isotopes were obtained. They should be prepared to have a sample tested if desired by an independent laboratory to assure the composition.

Once purchased, it is mandatory that end-users have batches of isotopes tested independently before human administration. This should be done in a laboratory experienced at these analyses.

16.5.3 Sample size for human studies

An important issue for researchers interested in this field is to identify the number of research subjects needed for participation. This number depends on the mineral, the variability in the expected results and whether a cross-over or a cross-sectional study is planned. With these key variables in mind, it is not uncommon for cross-over studies in which two conditions for absorption of the same mineral (e.g. iron) are being assessed to have adequate sample size with approximately 20–30 subjects. Studies involving calcium, zinc and magnesium may have slightly larger sample sizes. It is generally not appropriate to conduct studies with fewer than about 18–20 subjects in each group as variability in absorption is too great to have adequate power to identify a result.

16.6 Future trends

Three areas specifically relevant to functional foods will be considered. The first is the use of multi-mineral studies to evaluate the benefits of these products. Mineral stable isotope studies can readily be combined among minerals. It is not difficult to assess the nutritional effects of a dietary intervention or calcium, magnesium, iron and zinc simultaneously. The most important problems with such combined studies are dietary regulation and the actual administration of isotopes. It can be difficult to provide a fixed diet for 10 days to 2 weeks in which contents of all of the minerals are constant or relatively so. Also, it is not common to mix zinc or iron isotopes in a calcium-containing beverage. This requires some planning and consideration of the types of questions being asked before deciding how to give each isotope. It may be necessary to separate the meals or even the days in which the oral isotopes of different minerals are given in order to standardize the usual conditions for administration of each.

A related future trend is the intrinsic labeling of food products or meals with stable isotopes. This can be especially important for calcium. The solubility of the isotope and the way it is provided can affect the measured absorption. In some cases, there may be substantial error in providing an external tracer if a particular food effect is being studied (Heaney *et al.*, 2000). Intrinsic labeling refers to preparing the form of the mineral and sometimes the food with the desired chemical form of the isotope being evaluated (Weaver *et al.*, 1992). This can also be technically challenging but may be necessary for some studies.

The third topic is the performance of these studies in developing countries. It is increasingly recognized that functional foods may have key benefits for at-risk populations in developing countries. Specific benefits to the use of these products, such as increased iron and zinc absorption could be important from a public health perspective. However, as whole diets are very different in these settings, it is mandatory that hypothesized benefits be tested in the populations at risk and using their usual diet. Remarkably, this is not difficult to accomplish. We have conducted or consulted in dozens of such studies. As an example (Avalos Mishaan *et al.*, 2004), we evaluated the effects of a novel micronutrient-fortified beverage on iron and zinc absorption in schoolchildren in a low-income urban area of Lima, Peru. We were able to utilize local resources to conduct the studies and collect samples, and then we sent the samples to the United States for analysis.

16.7 Summary and conclusions

Direct assessment of mineral absorption is possible in all population groups. Using stable isotopes, the effects of functional foods on the absorption of calcium, iron, zinc and magnesium can be identified. Therefore, it is not necessary to make assumptions about these effects, without supporting absorption data. Methodologies vary for each mineral, but are generally minimally invasive and well tolerated by children of all ages and adults. The availability of these methods may be used to support specific health benefits from functional foods and enhance their acceptance by individuals.

16.8 References

ABRAMS S A (1999), 'Using stable isotopes to assess mineral absorption and utilization by children', *Am J Clin Nutr*, **70** (6), 955–964.

ABRAMS S A (2003), 'Stable isotope studies of mineral metabolism: calcium, magnesium, and iron', In: Abrams SA, Wong WW (eds): *Stable Isotopes in Nutrition*. Wallingford, CABI, 35–60.

ABRAMS S A, SIDBURY J B, MUENZER A, ESTEBAN N V, VIEIRA N E and YERGEY A L (1991), 'Stable isotopic measurement of endogenous fecal calcium excretion in children', *J Pediatr Gastroenterol Nutr*, **12** (4), 469–473.

ABRAMS S A, WEN J, O'BRIEN K O, STUFF J E and LIANG L K (1994), 'Application of magnetic sector thermal ionization mass spectrometry to studies of erythrocyte iron incorporation in small children', *Biol Mass Spectromet*, **23** (12), 771–775.

ABRAMS S A, GRUSAK M A, STUFF J and O'BRIEN K O (1997), 'Calcium and magnesium balance in 9–14-y-old children', *Am J Clin Nutr*, **66** (5), 1172–1177.

ABRAMS S A, GRIFFIN I J, HAWTHORNE K M, LIANG L, GUNN S K, DARLINGTON G and ELLIS K J (2005), 'A combination of prebiotic short- and long-chain inulin-type fructans enhances calcium absorption and bone mineralization in young adolescents', *Am J Clin Nutr*, **82** (2), 471–476.

ABRAMS S A, HAWTHORNE K M, ALIU O, HICKS P D, CHEN Z and GRIFFIN I J (2007), 'An inulin-type fructan enhances calcium absorption primarily via an effect on colonic absorption in humans', *J Nutr*, **137** (10), 2208–2212.

AMES S K, GORHAM B M and ABRAMS S A (1999), 'Effects of high vs low calcium intake on calcium absorption and red blood cell iron incorporation by small children', *Am J Clin Nutr*, **70** (1), 44–48.

AVALOS MISHAAN A M, ZAVALETA N, GRIFFIN I J, HILMERS D C, HAWTHORNE K M and ABRAMS S A (2004), 'Bioavailability of iron and zinc from a multiple micronutrient-fortified beverage', *J Pediatr*, **145** (1), 26–31.

BRONNER F and HARRIS R S (1956), 'Absorption and metabolism of calcium in human beings, studied with calcium45', *Ann N Y Acad Sci*, **64** (3), 314–325.

FRIEL J L, NAAKE V L, MILLER L V, FENNESSEY P V and HAMBRIDGE K M (1992), 'The analysis of stable isotopes in urine to determine the fractional absorption of zinc', *Am J Clin Nutr*, **55** (2), 473–477.

GRIFFIN I J and ABRAMS S A (2005), 'Methodological issues in assessing calcium absorption in humans: relevance to study the effects of inulin-type fructans', *Br J Nutr*, **93** (suppl 1), S105–S110.

GRIFFIN I J, HICKS P M D, LIANG L K and ABRAMS S A (2004), 'Metabolic adaptations to low zinc intakes in premenarcheal girls', *Am J Clin Nutr*, **80** (2), 385–390.

HEANEY R P, WEAVER C M and FITZSIMMONS M L (1990), 'Influence of calcium load on absorption fraction', *J Bone Miner Res*, **5** (11), 1135–1138.

HEANEY R P, DOWELL M S, RAFFERTY K and BIERMAN J (2000), 'Bioavailability of the calcium in fortified soy imitation milk, with some observations on method', *Am J Clin Nutr*, **71** (5), 1166–1169.

HEANEY R P, DOWELL M S and WOLF R L (2002), 'Estimation of true calcium absorption in men', *Clin Chem*, **48** (5), 786–788.

HOLLOWAY L, MOYNIHAN S, ABRAMS S A, KENT K, HSU A R and FRIEDLANDER A L (2007), 'Effects of oligofructose-enriched inulin on intestinal absorption of calcium and magnesium and bone turnover markers in postmenopausal women', *Brit Nutr J*, **97** (2), 365–372.

WEAVER C M, HEANEY R P, MARTIN B R and FITZSIMMONS M L (1992), 'Extrinsic vs. intrinsic labeling of the calcium in whole-wheat flour', *Am J Clin Nutr*, **55** (2), 452–454.

YERGEY A L and YERGEY A K (1997), 'Preparative scale mass spectrometry: a brief history of the calutron', *J Am Soc Mass Spectrom*, **8** (9), 943–953.

YERGEY A L, ABRAMS S A, VIEIRA N E, ALDROUBI A, MARINI J and SIDBURY J B (1994), 'Determination of fractional absorption of dietary calcium in humans', *J Nutr*, **124** (5), 674–682.

Part III

Implications

17

Optimising the flavour of low-fat foods

S. Bayarri and E. Costell, Instituto de Agroquímica y Tecnología de Alimentos, CSIC, Spain

Abstract: The elimination or reduction of fat in foods modifies its composition and structure and also the expected interactions among components, giving rise in most cases to perceptible changes in flavour. To optimise the flavour of low-fat foods, a multidisciplinary approach is necessary. This chapter will deal with the more relevant aspects of the mechanisms involved in the release and perception of flavour as well as with the role of fat in flavour perception and with some strategies for replacing fat in formulation of low-fat foods.

Key words: low-fat foods, flavour release, flavour perception, perceptual interactions, fat replacers.

17.1 Introduction

Low-fat foods are an interesting option for consumers interested in reducing the risks of suffering certain illnesses derived from the ingestion of saturated fatty acids or cholesterol or simply interested in maintaining an adequate body weight and a healthy physical condition. In addition, consumers look for healthy foods showing adequate sensory characteristics or even similar to those of the corresponding conventional product (Verbeke, 2006). Consumer acceptance of functional food is far from being unconditional. Functional benefits may provide added value to consumers but cannot outweigh the sensory properties of foods (Siró *et al.*, 2008). The success of a functional or healthy food will depend on whether it responds to consumer needs and on the degree of satisfaction that it is able to provide (Heldman, 2004; Urala and Lähtennmäki, 2004).

The elimination or reduction of fat in a certain foodstuff evidently modifies its composition and structure and also the expected interactions among components, giving rise in most cases to clearly perceptible changes in colour, flavour and/or texture. These changes may influence the final acceptance of the product by the consumer. Lowering the fat contained in a food product will decrease its known whitening effect, for example: reducing the fat content, milk is perceived as less white (Phillips *et al.*, 1995), vanilla ice cream is perceived as more yellow (Guinard *et al.*, 1997) and dark chocolate gets darker (Afoakwa *et al.*, 2008). The effect of fat reduction on food flavour is more complex. It depends mainly on the volatility of volatile compounds and on the hydrophobicity of both volatile and non-volatile compounds. Fat influences the qualitative, quantitative and temporal flavour profile of foods. In general, a decrease in fat content results in an increase in flavour strength, a decrease in flavour persistence and in a change in flavour character (de Roos, 1997). Moreover, although most taste compounds do not dissolve in fats, when fat content is lowered, the salty, sweet, sour and umami tastes weaken, while the bitter taste becomes enhanced (Metcalf and Vickers, 2002). Fat is an important contributor to texture in different types of foods. Thickness of liquid foods (Villegas and Costell, 2007), consistency of semisolids (Guven *et al.*, 2005; Tárrega and Costell, 2006) firmness of solids (Kavas *et al.*, 2004) and other textural attributes, such as creaminess, smoothness or fattiness, depend on fat content. Besides the direct influence of fat on colour, texture and flavour, the effect of the physiological and cognitive interactions among them also modify the sensations perceived by the consumer.

Flavour is considered to be the key factor for the acceptance of low-fat or non-fat foods, but its measurement and control present serious problems. The first question is: what is flavour? There is no universally accepted definition. Some authors identify flavour with the volatiles content, owing to the unquestionable influence of their presence and concentration. Others consider flavour to be the global sensation produced on humans during consumption of the particular foodstuff. More often accepted and used is to consider flavour as the combination of the sensations perceived simultaneously by the senses of taste and olfaction. Both of them are chemical senses, e.g. they respond to stimuli that are essentially molecules capable of activating the different receptors located in the sensitive cells in the mouth and nose (Durán and Costell, 1999). It is evident that the origin of such a sensation is linked to the presence in the food of those components capable of stimulating the senses of taste and smell when in certain concentrations, but flavour is not the result of the sum of both volatile and non-volatile compounds of a food. Flavour perception is the result of a complex process that involve different physicochemical, physiological and psychological phenomena (Overbosch *et al.*, 1991; Taylor 2002; Taylor and Roberts, 2004).

A very important drawback found when optimising the flavour of low-fat foods is that, for complex matrices, the establishment of relationships between the chemical stimuli and the physiological reaction of humans, and between the latter and the perception experienced by people upon consuming food, is not an easy task. It is necessary to combine information on different factors: concentration of both volatile and non-volatile stimuli, structure and other physical characteristics of the food matrix, physicochemical mechanisms governing release of tasting and odouring compounds, modification of product during oral food processing, sensory techniques to ascertain how flavour is perceived and how this perception affects the final acceptance of the product under study. This is why it is very difficult to make predictions as to the possible perceptible differences between products differing in composition and/or structure as a result of changes in formulation or processing.

Even more difficult will be to predict the degree of acceptance by the consumer. Regarding this last point, it must be considered that, when consumers eat food, their responses are not only based on the sensory characteristics of the product but are also related to other factors, such as the previous information acquired by the consumers about the product, their past experience, and their attitudes and beliefs (Aaron *et al.*, 1994; Zandstra *et al.*, 2001). The consumer's response to foods depends on the interaction of several factors that are different in nature (Jaeguer, 2006). In addition to the characteristics of the food itself and the sensations the consumer experiences on eating it, there are other influential factors, such as the opinion each consumer has on the nutritional characteristics or on the composition of the product, its safety and even its trade name or its price. All these factors can influence their choice at the moment of purchase and modify the degree of pleasure they experience when consuming it. This fact is of particular importance in the acceptance or rejection of some types of foods, like functional or 'healthy' foods, including low-fat foods, which the consumer sees as a possible alternative to conventional foods (Tuorila *et al.*, 1994; Wilcock *et al.*, 2004).

The design, measurement and control of food flavour present serious problems. To optimise the flavour of low-fat foods, a multidisciplinary approach is necessary. This chapter will deal with the more relevant aspects of the mechanisms involved in the release and perception of flavour as well as with the role of fat in flavour perception and with some strategies for replacing fat in formulation of low-fat foods.

17.2 Flavour perception

As stated by Keats *et al.* (2004), 'The flavour of the food/beverage is the result of complex stimulus–response interactions between a food matrix and human sensory, perceptual and cognitive processes.' The flavour perception process begins when the flavouring and odouring molecules are released from the food matrix and travel to either the taste or the smell receptors, located in the mouth and nose, respectively. The non-volatile compounds are transported in the saliva to the in-mouth taste receptors, while the volatile ones are carried through in the air to the odour receptors located in the nose. Then a process of transduction of the signals detected by the corresponding receptors through to the brain occurs, where a person's flavour perception is generated.

17.2.1 Release of chemical stimuli out of the food matrix

The first phase of the flavour perception process is related to the release of the chemical stimuli out of the food matrix. It is well known that the characteristics and structure of the matrix and the chemical interactions among the ingredients exert a decisive influence on the effective concentration of the chemical stimuli and on their rate of transport to the receptors. Release of tasting and odouring substances basically depends on their nature, concentration and characteristics, on the possible interactions among them, on the physicochemical and structural properties of the food matrix and finally on the interactions between stimuli and matrix (Taylor and Roberts, 2004). From a practical point of view, the more viscous a fluid food or the harder a solid food is, the less flavour is perceived on eating (Clark, 2002; Boland *et al.*, 2006). However, flavour release patterns as a function of viscosity and texture modifications are still not completely understood (Hollowood *et al.*, 2002; de Roos, 2003).

Regarding the perception of basic tastes (sweetness, bitterness, saltiness, sourness and umami), it is generally accepted that the extent of taste suppression when viscosity or texture increases may be attributed to the delay or the partial inhibition of the transport of the taste stimulus within the food matrix and from the matrix itself to the taste receptors. This process may be partially governed by the rate of diffusion of the stimulus within the food, by the rheological behaviour of the system and, in some cases, by binding of taste compounds with other food components (Durán and Costell, 1999). Cook *et al.* (2003) pointed out that, when adding thickeners to liquid model systems, there are implications for both taste intensity and taste profile. These authors observed that viscous solutions of hydroxypropylmethyl cellulose suppressed perception of both sweet and salt qualities, but had no significant effect on both acidity and bitterness. In solid foods, taste perceived was clearly related with some textural characteristics such as breaking strain, elasticity or cohesiveness (Clark, 2002). Bayarri *et al.* (2003), working with gelled systems sweetened with different types and concentrations of sweeteners, observed that, besides sweetener concentration, the main factors determining gel sweetness were related to the mechanical properties of gels and particularly to the amount of deformation required to break the network and to its resistance to deformation. In this case, the influence of the sweetener's diffusion constant on sweetness of the studied gel systems was negligible. This fact can be due, as stated by Morris (1995), to the fact that diffusion of small molecules through polymer networks to the surface of the gel is slow and it can be neglected as a significant factor in taste suppression.

Most of the studies in flavour release have focused on the release of odorants. Abundant information can be found in the literature on the partition coefficients of different volatiles in different matrices, obtained by analysis of headspace, generally by gas chromatography–mass spectrometry (GC-MS) with static or dynamic techniques (Cayot *et al.*, 2000; Arvisent *et al.*, 2002a, b; Seuvre *et al.*, 2004). Dynamic methods better simulate flavour release in the mouth, but only static measurements allow a determination of thermodynamic and kinetic parameters with a good precision (Juteau *et al.*, 2004). The theoretical bases of the transport phenomena governing the release of chemical stimuli out of the food matrix, such as phase partition, mass transport and diffusion, are well defined. The methods used to monitor diffusion and mass transport of volatile compounds have been recently described by Cayot *et al.* (2008). Unfortunately, this information is not directly related to the flavour perceived sensorially on consumption of actual foods. In the first place, most data have been obtained in model systems for some individual volatile compounds without contemplating the effect on flavour of the possible interactions among the different volatiles. Secondly, in these experiences the conditions are far from those that occur in the oral cavity on eating foods. Additionally, as commented by Brossard *et al.* (2002), measuring odorant concentration in the air does not ensure a reliable prediction of odour intensity, as sensory perception in humans is much more sensitive to the surroundings and context than are instruments. Several theoretical models have been proposed to predict the effect of the food matrix characteristics on stimuli delivery, but none of them is totally validated (Taylor, 2002). Basic knowledge of the effects of the different factors involved in the release of stimuli from the food matrix is needed to understand the first phase of the flavour perception process, related to the transport of chemical stimuli out of the food matrix.

17.2.2 Release of chemical stimuli into the mouth

During oral food processing, starting from the first bite, the food is transformed from its initial shape and size to a form suitable for swallowing (Chen, 2009) and chemical stimuli are released into the mouth and transferred to the taste and smell receptors. However, the study of these processes in the actual mouth conditions during mastication is far more complex. The food surface area in contact with saliva and the concentration of both volatile and non-volatile stimuli present in the aqueous and air phases undergo continuous changes mainly due to the continuous movements of the mouth components during mastication and deglutition (Engelen and Van der Bilt, 2008; Chen 2009). Rabe *et al.* (2004) studied the influences of shear rate, air-flow, in-mouth headspace volume, synthetic saliva and human epithelial cells on the initial dynamic flavour release from liquids. They concluded that three main factors: shearing/mastication forces, head-space volume and volumetric air-flow rate, were of significant importance for initial dynamic flavour release. Recently, Trelea *et al.* (2008) have proposed a mechanistic mathematical model for aroma release in the oro-pharynx to the nasal cavity during eating of semiliquid foods. The authors considered that this approach constitutes a first step towards accurate prediction of volatile concentration in the nasal cavity of humans consuming flavoured foods. This type of study gets even more complicated, especially in the case of solid foods, owing to the individual differences in respiration rates, in salivation and in mastication patterns (Buettner and Schieberle, 2000; van Ruth and Buhr, 2003). All these factors affect the breakdown of the food matrix and the transport of the stimuli to the receptors.

In the past few years several new techniques have been developed to evaluate aroma release *in vivo* at the nose or at the mouth (Taylor *et al.*, 2000). Some of these techniques are: measurement of the concentration of volatiles exhaled through the nose and subsequent analysis by GC-MS (Denker *et al.*, 2006) and the direct measurement of these volatiles with spectrometric methods such as atmospheric pressure chemical ionisation (APCI-MS) (Taylor and Linforth, 2003; Lethuaut *et al.*, 2004; González-Tomás *et al.*, 2007) or proton transfer reaction (PTR-MS) (Mestres *et al.*, 2005, 2006; Van Ruth *et al.*, 2006; Gallardo-Escamilla *et al.*, 2007). With these techniques the evolution of the concentration of volatiles carried by the respired air during consumption of a certain food can be analysed. They provide information closer to the evolution of the concentration of volatiles released during food consumption and consequently a better knowledge of the odour stimuli reaching the nose receptors. Interpretation of the information obtained with the above-mentioned techniques presents the problems associated with the use of persons as measuring instruments, e.g. the unavoidable individual variability in the volatiles exhaled in the mouth or in the nose. This variability originates mainly due to differences in respiration and mastication rates and in the deglutition movements. Attempts have been made to overcome this problem by using mechanical devices to mimic the processes occurring in mouth during eating such as model mouths (van Ruth and Roozen, 2000; Rabe *et al.*, 2002, 2004; Ghosh *et al.*, 2008) or the chewing simulator recently developed by Salles *et al.* (2007) that reproduces most of the functions of the human mouth during mastication. Besides the recognised influence of the stimuli perceived retronasally, other factors such as the odour stimuli perceived ortonasally or the taste and trigeminal stimuli perceived in mouth have to be taken into consideration when the flavour of foods is studied.

17.2.3 Flavour sensation and perception

The third phase of flavour perception begins when the signals from peripherals receptors are conveyed to the central nervous system, to specific regions of the brain. During food consumption, the brain receives different sensory inputs (visual, olfactory, gustatory, tactile. trigeminal, sound) and the information from physiologically distinct sensory modalities is integrated in the final flavour perception (Prescott, 2004). Delwiche (2004) have reviewed how all these sensations interact, both at the perceptual and at the physical level, and discussed the resulting impact that each one of them has on flavour rating. Each perceived sensation responds not only to a certain sensory input but also to the other inputs perceived simultaneously. Though all these inputs influence flavour perception, through physical or perceptual interactions, the interaction between taste and odour is so strong that they jointly make the flavour perceived. When either the taste or the odour compound of a highly familiar odour–taste pair is presented in isolation, it may elicit weak ratings of the missing component (Delwiche, 2004). For example, odours that are normally presented together with sweet tastes in mouth, such as vanilla, are commonly described as 'sweet' odours. This perception does not result from any direct physiological effect of such odours on taste receptors, rather it reflects a central neural process which appears to be based upon simultaneous associations between taste and smell. This type of learning effect has also been observed for sour and bitter tastants, resulting in odours that come to smell 'sour' and 'bitter', respectively (Sundqvist *et al.*, 2006).

A distinctive characteristic of odour–taste integration is that, for enhancement effects to occur, the odour and taste components need to be perceptually congruent (Small and Prescott, 2005). In studies using functional magnetic resonance imaging (fMRI), Rolls (2005) showed where interactions between taste and odour stimuli in the human brain take place to implement flavour. He commented on data obtained in a previous work (de Araujo *et al.*, 2003) in which two taste stimuli (sucrose and monosodium glutamate) and two odour stimuli (strawberry and methional) were delivered unimodally or in different combinations. The results obtained in this work revealed that, while some brain areas respond to either taste or retronasal olfactory stimuli, other brain areas respond to both. Rolls (2005) concluded that these results provide evidence on the neural substrate for the convergence of taste and olfactory stimuli to produce flavour. In addition, flavour perception is highly dependent on both the subject's past experience with specific odour–taste combinations (the origin of congruence) and on the cognitive factors that determine whether the flavour elements are combined or not (Prescott, 2004). In this line, other aspects about consumer response to food flavour must be considered. The increase in flavour acceptability due to the habitual consumption of food (Stein *et al.*, 2003; Luckow *et al.*, 2005) or the effect of confirmation or not of consumers' expectations about flavour can lead to either repeated consumption or rejection of a product (Kähkönen *et al.*, 1999).

In a simplified manner, consumer response to food flavour is mainly defined by: (1) a cognitive component, coming from knowledge and opinions about a product; (2) an affective component, responsible for positive or negative feelings towards a product; and (3) a behavioural component, involving intentions or actions, defining how willing a consumer is to do something in certain situations. The cognitive component is related to the information that a person has about an object, the affective component summarises the general feelings of a person about a product and the behavioural component relative to an action reflects the intentions of a person about his/her future behaviour (Barrios and Costell, 2004).

17.3 The role of fat in flavour perception

Fat content has a strong influence on the mechanisms involved in the release and perception of flavour in two ways: directly, it has a significant effect on the release of chemical stimuli from the food matrix and into the mouth and indirectly, due to its influence on the product texture. Fat also influences flavour perception, through perceptual interactions. Moreover, fat plays an important role in the consumer hedonic responses to foods. In summary, elimination or reduction of fat in a food product produces changes in the different phases of flavour perception.

17.3.1 Influence of fat on release of chemical stimuli out of the food matrix

Fat plays an important role as a solvent for lypophilic flavour compounds. These compounds concentrate in the lipid phase of foods, which greatly reduces their partitioning into the air or the aqueous phase. Fat content mainly affects the release of both tasting and odouring lypophilic compounds out of the food matrix. Generally, flavour release decreases with increasing lipid level in the food matrix, with the exception of hydrophilic compounds showing partition coefficients ($\log P$) values near or below zero (Bayarri *et al.*, 2007).

Most of the studies about the influence of fat on the release of chemical stimuli have focused on volatile compounds and little has been reported about the influence of fat content on taste compounds. Most taste compounds, except some bitter tastants, are water soluble and, in theory, their release from the matrix should not be affected by changes in fat content. Metcalf and Wickers (2002) studied the effect of fat on the intensity of sweet, salty, sour, bitter and umami tastes in oil–water emulsions with different fat contents. They found that increasing fat content suppressed bitterness and had no effect on any of the other taste compounds. The suppression of bitter taste is due to the hydrophobic nature of quinine, the bitter stimulus used in this work. When comparing the tastes of the different stimuli, either diluted with oil or with water, the authors also observed a decrease in bitterness but an increase in the intensity of the other basic tastes. They concluded that, when removing fat from a food, the product can be perceived as more bitter and with lower intensity in the other tastes.

This modification of the taste profile can lower the acceptability of low-fat products since consumers, as a general rule, dislike bitter taste and like the other tastes. The results obtained in model systems, such as those described above, are useful for clarifying the effects of fat on taste, but do not allow prediction of the extent of the changes in perceived flavour due to reduction of fat content in more complex food matrices.

Changes in the microstructure and/or the rheological properties of a food product due to altering its fat content may also influence the release of taste compounds. Increasing fat content may increase the concentration of tastants in the aqueous phase and favour their release, increasing the taste intensity perceived. This effect can get masked or outweighed by the contrary effect that the higher viscosity of fatty foods exert on the release of taste stimuli. Samil *et al.* (1991/92) found that the reduction of fat in cheese increased bitterness and decreased saltiness. The first effect can be explained by the hydrophobic character of the bitter compound. When the fat level was reduced, the bitter tastant concentration in the aqueous phase of the cheese matrix increased and the saltiness decreased, which can be attributed to the reduced concentration of salt in the aqueous phase. Malone *et al.* (2003b) investigated the relationship between fat content of iso-viscous oil–water emulsions and salty taste perception. Using a constant salt concentration, they found that saltiness increased with oil content, which can be due to the increase in salt concentration in the aqueous phase which ranged from 0.5% in the absence of oil to 1.25% in the 60% oil emulsion. In contrast, Bayarri *et al.* (2007) working with model oil–water emulsions with different oil contents and with the same viscosity in the mouth, observed that samples containing the highest oil content were perceived as significantly less sweet. In this case the effect on sweetness can be due to the different resistance to deformation of the emulsions, which may affect the release of sucrose.

The distribution of the aroma compounds within a food depends on their affinity for each of the different phases of the product. In products containing aqueous and lipid phases, a flavour compound distributes over three phases: fat, water and air. The oil-to-water partition coefficient indicates the distribution of each flavour component in both phases. The higher the value of this coefficient, the more lypophilic or hydrophobic is the flavour compound (de Roos, 1997). Contrary to what happens with the chemical stimuli of taste, most aroma compounds are lypophilic. In general, reduction of fat content results in higher aroma release out of the food matrix. The extent of this effect depends mainly on the hydrophobic nature of each volatile compound (Miettinen *et al.*, 2002; Van Ruth *et al.*, 2002; Weel *et al.*, 2004; Gonzalez-Tomas *et al.*, 2007). In model oil-in-water emulsions, Bayarri *et al.* (2006) observed that, when fat content was increased, the decrease in headspace concentration of some volatile compounds was different. The headspace concentrations were reduced by factors that ranged from 37 (ethyl hexanoate) to 2 (*cis*-3-hexenol-1-ol) and the variations observed were consistent with the hydrophobicity of the volatile compounds (partition coefficients for ethyl hexanoate and for *cis*-3-hexenol-1-ol, were 2.83 and 1.61, respectively). The information obtained in this type of study is important in understanding the effect of fat on flavour release, but, as commented above, the information obtained does not always relate well to the release profile observed during consumption of a product (Doyen *et al.*, 2001). The different effect of fat content reduction on release of the different volatiles determining the odour of a certain foodstuff generally alters its aroma balance. The original equilibrium will be disturbed when the fat content is changed. Hyvónen *et al.* (2003), on studying the flavour of samples of strawberry ice creams with different types and contents of fat, showed that intensity of aroma and flavour were significantly greater in fat-free samples than in fat-containing ice creams. However, flavour was perceived as a typical and strawberry aroma was regarded as less typical in fat-free and low-fat samples.

17.3.2 Influence of fat on release of chemical stimuli into the mouth

As commented above, it is hypothesised that the taste stimuli and the volatile compounds have different release mechanisms in mouth. It can then be expected that fat content will affect each type of stimulus differently. In the case of the volatile compounds, the key release mechanism is partition at the air–thin liquid film interface in the mouth; for the taste stimuli, the main mechanism is mass transfer across the saliva layer, which depends on the ability of the sample and saliva layers to mix. The retention effect of oil on aroma release is smaller under *in vivo* conditions than under static headspace conditions. A plausible explanation is that release of aroma compounds in mouth occurs from thin liquid layers and in this situation the reservoir of the fat phase is not so important as in the bulk phase (Bayarri *et al.*, 2007).

Weel *et al.* (2004) showed clear differences in the intensity of ethyl hexanoate aroma evaluated ortonasally and retronasally in emulsions containing different oil contents (from 0 to 1.0%). They studied the effect of emulsion properties on release of four esters with different hydrophobicities under *in vivo* and static headspace conditions. The aims of this work were to investigate why the effect of oil content on *in vivo* aroma release or on flavour perception was smaller than expected from equilibrium headspace studies. They showed that, with increasing oil content and with a higher hydrophobicity of the aroma compound, a stronger decrease in aroma release was detected. For hydrophobic compounds the concentration in the oil phase is much higher than in the aqueous phase. When oil content is increased, the aroma concentration in the oil phase decreases as a result of dilution, and consequently the concentration in the water phase decreases as a result of partitioning. Thus, a smaller concentration gradient between the emulsion and air is produced. This effect was stronger under static headspace conditions than under *in vivo* conditions and was also stronger at orthonasal than at retronasal evaluation. The authors concluded that orthonasal evaluation was performed by sniffing, the conditions of this process being similar to those of headspace analysis, governed by the partition coefficient.

Retronasal perception and *in vivo* release of aroma compounds occur upon exhalation after swallowing: the aroma compounds release from the thin layer in the throat and reach the olfactory epithelium aroma intensity. In these conditions a large gradient in aroma concentration exists between the thin liquid film in the throat and the relatively large air mass that flows along it. The physiological premises for retronasal aroma perception have not been fully elucidated. Buettner *et al.* (2002) studied the transfer of odorants from the oral to the nasal cavity during food consumption by observation of the swallowing process using both videofluoroscopic and real-time MRI techniques. The results revealed a direct link between dynamic retronasal aroma perception and intermittent openings of velum–tongue and velum–pharynx connections during the eating process.

Lipids in contact with the tongue and palate can also influence flavour perception. In studies on foods emulsions, to assess the effect of oil mouthcoatings on the perception of tastes, it was found that oil tended to have a suppressive effect because fat mouthcoatings may physically interfere with tastant access to the taste receptors (Valentova and Pokorny, 1998; Malone *et al.*, 2003a). According to Silletti *et al.* (2007), electrostatic interactions of saliva with food components can be one of the mechanisms that drives the deposition of compounds on oral surfaces. Recently, Pivk *et al.* (2008) investigated the influence of oil volume, after being processed in mouth, on the deposition of lipids on the tongue and palate. They concluded that the lipids were only weakly retained in the oral surfaces, but that the lipid deposition, especially on the tongue, was related to sensory perception.

In the case of solid foods, the effect of oral processing on the release of chemical stimuli into the mouth is very important (Linforth *et al.*, 2005). The amounts of odorants being released from foods directly depend on the duration of mastication and the release rates of each single odorant. The flavour profile changes significantly with increasing duration of mastication (Buettner and Schieeberle, 2000). Tárrega *et al.* (2008) studied aroma release and chewing activity during eating different model cheeses with the same flavourings content. Differences in chewing behaviour explained most of the variability in aroma release among subjects. The authors showed a strong interaction between cheese characteristics and composition and chewing behaviour on aroma release during cheese consumption. The texture of the product influenced the chewing pattern and both influenced aroma release. Thus, when the increase in texture leads to an increase in chewing activity, the negative effect the structure has on aroma release can be counteracted and even inversed. When the change in texture due to composition or processing conditions does not result in a great change in the chewing activity, aroma release will be dependent exclusively on the food matrix composition.

In summary, fat can influence the release of chemical stimuli into the mouth during oral processing of foods in several ways: (a) forming a barrier between the taste stimuli and taste receptors; (b) increasing the concentration of water-soluble compounds in the aqueous phase; (c) changing the viscosities of liquid and semisolid foods; (d) decreasing the dilution of the product by saliva during mastication; and (e) changing the firmness or texture of solid foods. For each type of food matrix, the relative influence of each one of these effects on flavour release will depend not only on the physicochemical characteristics and composition of the matrix but also on the differences in respiration and mastication rates and on the deglution movements of the different consumers. Deeper knowledge on the modifications the foods undergo during their stay in the mouth is needed to understand to what extent reduction or elimination of fat will affect the release of chemical stimuli from the matrix and their transport to the receptors.

17.3.3 Fat perception

When optimising the flavour of low-fat products, the objective should not simply be reduced to duplicating that of full-fat products. In this type of food the sensory inputs initiated by the perception of fat play an important role in product acceptability by consumers. Reduction or elimination of this component, besides directly affecting the processes of flavour release and perception, modify the signals received by the brain on consuming the particular food and may partially determine its acceptance or rejection. Fat perception is firstly associated with some texture attributes (viscosity, consistency, creaminess, smoothness), though no single textural attribute can be associated only with fat content. Although fat perception probably relies upon texture, the textural cues themselves and the way they are detected are probably multimodal (Sundqvist *et al.*, 2006).

Results obtained by de Araujo and Rolls (2004), on investigating the representation of oral texture and fat in the human brain using event-related fMRI, seem to confirm this idea. They found activation of a brain region by oral viscosity stimuli, this activation being proportional to the log of the viscosity of the oral stimuli. They also found activation of another brain region that was activated by both viscosity and fat. A third brain region was activated by oral fat independently of viscosity. This third region was also activated by sucrose taste and is a strong candidate for a brain region activated by the hedonic properties of fat. These results start to reveal a brain mechanism that may be important in perception of both food texture and oral fat. This information may help to understand some of the conclusions previously obtained by other authors about the relations between fat perception and food acceptability. Drewnowski and Schwartz in 1990 commented that, although many subjects are unable to accurately assess the fat content of foods, hedonic ratings are surprisingly sensitive to stimulus fat content.

The relation between fat perception and acceptability has increased the general interest for the possibility of enhancing the fattiness sensation by manipulating the flavour content of a food. Yackinous and Guinard (2000) investigated the effects of fat and aroma on the sensory impression of fat in four different foods (mashed potatoes, vanilla pudding, chocolate drink and potato chips). Flavour content significantly enhanced the perception of fattiness for two of the four foods: mashed potatoes and potato chips. Comparing the fattiness rating obtained first without and then with nose clips, they observed that the nose clips significantly reduced the fattiness ratings for all products, thus indicating that the aroma components of fat-based food can influence fat perception. With a similar approach, Sundqvist *et al.* (2006) investigated whether odours could acquire all or any fat-like properties in four milk types prepared with two concentrations of fat and two concentrations of sucrose. They concluded that odours can indeed acquire the perceived fatty properties of foods they are associated with. These results suggest that the type of cross-modal learning effect related to flavour is probably not restricted to odour and tastes but may extend into other sensory domains.

17.4 Strategies for replacing fat and implications for flavour

In order to solve the problems associated with the influence of reduction or elimination of fat in foods on their flavour, several strategies have been launched. The most frequent action is the use of ingredients capable of compensating or reducing the effects on texture of the total or partial reduction in fat content. Another strategy, applicable to food emulsions, consists of modifying the matrix structure in order to improve the release of the aroma compounds.

17.4.1 Fat replacers

Fat replacers have facilitated the development of both low-fat and fat-free foods that emulate the flavour and texture of full-fat foods, but with fewer calories and less fat and/or cholesterol. In most cases the main objective of the inclusion of these ingredients in the formulation of a new food is, besides its effect on its nutritional properties, the compensation of the defects in texture derived from the reduction or elimination of the fat content. There are several types of fat replacers for substituting fat in the formulation of different types of foods (Sandrou and Arvanitoyanis, 2000). According to their chemical composition and properties, they can be classified into two large groups: fat substitutes and fat mimetics.

The first group includes compounds showing physical properties similar to fat, such as fatty acids esterified with carbohydrates, alkyl glycosides, and polyols (Akoh, 1995). Olestra and Salatrim are the most famous commercial products and are manufactured either by chemical reaction between sugars and fatty acids or by modification of triglycerides. In general, they are considered to have the organoleptic and thermal properties of fat but they can neither be hydrolysed by gastric or pancreatic lipase nor be absorbed in the gastrointestinal tract. Some of the fat substitutes are heat stable at both cooking and frying temperatures. Some of them have a legally restricted use because of the possibility of production of some adverse physiological effects such as loose stools or the inhibition of absorption of fat-soluble vitamins (Bimal and Zhang, 2006).

The second group, fat mimetics, is formed by ingredients that imitate one or several functions typical of fat and related to the physical properties or with the sensory characteristics of the food product. They consist mainly of proteins, carbohydrates or a mixture of them. In each case, the choice of the ingredient to be used for the partial or total substitution of fat first depends on the characteristics of the initial food and on the functions that each fat mimetic can develop in the new formulation (Sandrou and Arvanitoyannis, 2000). For example, in cooking or salad oils the fat mimetics of proteinic nature are preferred, while for meat and poultry products those based on carbohydrates are recommended (Archer *et al.*, 2004; Cáceres *et al.*, 2004; Hsu and Sun, 2006). In dairy products the selection depends on the composition and characteristics of the specific item. Either those of proteinic origin, those based on carbohydrates or a mixture of both can be used.

Initially the use of proteinic ingredients to replace fat in food emulsions was considered an interesting option because of their emulsifying and stabilising capacities. They enabled some of the texture defects occasioned by the lack of fat to be solved and in addition they enriched the food nutritional value. The major limitation of these ingredients, especially those containing proteins from milk whey or soya, is that they not only reduce the perceptible intensity of desired flavours but can also give some off-flavours to the food. Although most proteins do not contribute to the emulsion flavour in a direct manner they can interact with some volatile compounds and give rise to unbalanced or even unacceptable sensory profiles. Proteins can combine with some volatiles and hinder or delay flavour release (Overbosch *et al.* 1991). When proteins replace the fat content in product formulation, both the structure and composition of the product undergo a dramatic change. The dominant component, the protein, interacts with volatile compounds in a different way from that of fat. The food–air partition coefficients of the substances responsible for flavour, especially of the lipophilic ones, get altered, the flavour release process is modified and the final food flavour can experience an important change.

Most of the available information on interactions between proteins and volatile compounds comes from studies carried out in very simple model systems (aqueous solutions of one or two proteins with one or two volatile compounds) using different instrumental techniques (gas and liquid chromatography, infrared spectroscopy, nuclear magnetic resonance, etc.) with not always coincident results (Kühn *et al.*, 2006). This type of information may be useful to demonstrate the occurrence of molecular interactions between proteins and volatiles, but it does not represent the phenomena taking place in more complex matrices and does not permit prediction of the volatiles release from an actual food matrix or of the way the released volatiles get transported to the nose to stimulate the odour receptors. On designing low-fat foods, with protein fat mimetics, the volatiles content needed to produce a certain flavour intensity will have to be increased in many cases. Moreover, in the case of intending to obtain a specific flavour, the proportion of the different volatile compound established for full-fat foods must be modified to compensate not only for the lack of fat but also for the effects of the above-discussed protein–volatiles interactions.

Several ingredients of different composition and characteristics are included under the denomination of fat substitutes of the carbohydrate type: cellulose, dextrins, maltodextrins, gums, fibres, modified starch, etc. Their main function in the formulation of low-fat foods is related with their capacity to hold water, reduce syneresis or act as thickeners, gellifying agents or stabilizers, and consequently they become one of the best options when intending to compensate for the texture changes originated from the partial or total reduction in the product fat content (Setser and Racette, 1992). The properties of these fat replacers result from the association of water with the structure of carbohydrate particles which bind water in such a way as to provide a sensation similar to that of fat in the oral cavity (Sandrou and Arvanitoyanis, 2000). In the past few years the interest for this type of ingredients, such as cellulose, gums or pectic substances, has grown because, besides their physicochemical properties, they also show health-friendly characteristics, since some of them function as dietetic fibres and others, like inulin, are also of prebiotic character (Tárrega and Costell, 2006; Warrand, 2006). Using this type of ingredient it is possible, though not always easy, to match the rheological behaviour of some low-fat dairy products with that of the full-fat counterpart. This does not guarantee matching the sensorially perceived texture. Some textural attributes, creaminess, fattiness or smoothness, of high incidence on the final product acceptance of some low-fat dairy foods, mainly depend on the food microstructure, on some surface properties and on certain crossed interactions between texture attributes and some flavours (Frost *et al.*, 2001; De Wijk *et al.*, 2003; Weenen *et al.*, 2005).

The major problem in the use of these fat substitutes is, as in the case of proteins, the control of flavour. The available information on the possible interactions between carbohydrates and the volatile compounds is rather poor, compared with that on protein–volatile interactions. Most of it deals with interactions between volatiles and starch (Cayot *et al.*, 2000; Arvisent *et al.*, 2002a,b). In general, the changes in flavour produced in formulated foods by the use of fat mimetics of the carbohydrate type, with the exception of starch, is qualitatively similar to that due to the simple reduction of fat content, since most of them do not exert any specific affinity for the volatile substances. In this case the decrease in the rate of release of volatiles from the food matrix is almost exclusively due to the increase in texture (Rega *et al.*, 2002).

At present, different combinations of protein, starches and hydrocolloids have been suggested to have synergistic effects for lowering fat and retaining textural characteristics of the products. Combinations of various fat replacers can have an important potential in the development of low-fat foods with greater acceptability.

17.4.2 Structured emulsions

It has been shown that the structure of the food matrix can affect the aroma release and perception in oil-in-water and in water-in-oil emulsions (Charles *et al.*, 2000). Structure differences can change the affinity of the volatile compounds for the food matrix by modifying the nature and the number of binding sites that are available to the odour compounds (Druaux and Voilley, 1997), though not all the available information on the structure–release relationship is in agreement. Van Ruth *et al.* (2002) analysed the influence of oil-in-water emulsion composition and structure on aroma retention for 20 volatile compounds. They observed that emulsions with larger particles showed increased aroma retention, which was independent of the lipid fraction and of the polarity of the aroma compounds. In contrast, Weel *et al.* (2004), on studying the effect of oil content and droplet size distributions of dilute oil-in-water emulsions on release of four esters with different hydrophobicities, concluded that the effect of droplet size distribution on aroma release strongly depends on the hydrophobicity of the aroma compound. They suggested that, by modulating the oil droplet size distribution, a large change in aroma release might be accomplished without changing the emulsion oil content.

With this approach, Malone *et al.* (2003b) proposed the design of specific food microstructures to control aroma release. They developed a gelled microstructured emulsion with the objective of reducing the rate of lypophilic aroma release in low-fat products. In this type of microstructure the oil droplets are enveloped in a gel phase, creating a static diffusion layer around the oil droplets that can reduce the rate of aroma release. In this work a microstructured emulsion consisting of 3% sunflower oil entrapped in gelatine–gum arabic gel particles was dispersed in a continuous xanthan solution and the aroma release was evaluated and compared with that of a control emulsion. Microstructured emulsions suppress the release of lypophilic molecules, such as ethyl hexanoate, but have no effect on hydrophylic aromas such as butanone. Results obtained showed that the microstructured emulsions can be effective in balancing the flavour profile in low-fat products without producing a significant change in the product's texture.

On the same line and based on the applications of the self-assembly structures used in the pharmaceutical industry as delivery systems for active compounds such as enzymes, hormones or drugs, Phan *et al.* (2008) investigated the possibility of the application of such self-assembly emulsions in low-fat and free-fat products. Temporal release and retention of aroma compounds in an emulsified water solution, where unsaturated monoglycerides are added to the oil, and in a conventional oil-in-water emulsion, were studied by different instrumental methods. The results showed that the instrumental aroma release profile of the 5% lipid structured emulsion was close to that obtained for the oil-in-water emulsion containing 10% lipid. Under static conditions, the 5% lipid structured emulsion retained more of the most lypophilic compounds than its counterpart non-structured emulsion. The authors concluded that this work shows the potential applications of structured emulsions to improve aroma in low-fat products. The latter two proposals deal with changes in the instrumental aroma profile on modifying the emulsion structure. Their actual usefulness is conditioned to the possible sensorially perceived changes and to their consequences on flavour perception.

17.5 Acknowledgements

To Fondo Social Europeo for financing the contract of author S. Bayarri in the program I3P from CSIC, to MEC of Spain for financial support (Project AGL2007-63444) and to Prof. Luis Durán for his invaluable contribution.

17.6 References

AARON JI, MELA DJ, EVANS RE (1994). The influences of attitudes, beliefs and label information on perceptions of reduced-fat spread. *Appetite* **22**: 25–37.

AFOAKWA EO, PATERSON A, FOWLER M, VIEIRA J (2008). Particle size distribution and compositional effects on textural properties and appearance of dark chocolates. *J. Food Eng.* **87**: 181–190.

AKOH CC (1995). Lipid-based fat substitutes. *Crit. Rev. Food Sci. Nutr.* **35**: 405–430.

ARCHER BJ, JOHNSON SK, DEVEREUX HM, BAXTER AL (2004). Effect of fat replacement by inulin or lupin-kernel fibre on sausage patty acceptability, post-meal perceptions of satiety and food intake in men. *Br. J. Nutr.* **91**: 591–599.

ARVISENET G, LE BAIL P, VOILLEY A, CAYOT N (2002a) Influence of physicochemical interactions between amylose and aroma compounds on the retention of aroma in food-like matrices. *J. Agric. Food Chem.* **50**: 7088–7093.

ARVISENET G, VOILLEY A, CAYOT N (2002b). Retention of aroma compounds in starch matrices: competitions between aroma compounds toward amylose and amylopectin. *J. Agric. Food Chem.* **50**: 7345–7349.

BARRIOS EX, COSTELL E (2004). Use of methods of research into consumers' opinions and attitudes in food research. *Food Sci. Technol. Int.* **10**: 359–371.

BAYARRI S, DURÁN L, COSTELL, E (2003). Compression resistance, sweetener's diffusion and sweetness of hydrocolloids gels. *Int. Dairy J.* **13**: 643–653.

BAYARRI S, TAYLOR AJ, HORT J (2006). The role of fat in flavor perception: Effect of partition and viscosity in model emulsions. *J. Agric. Food Chem.* **54**: 8862–8868.

BAYARRI S, SMITH T, HOLLOWOOD T, HORT J (2007). The role of rheological behaviour in flavour perception in model oil/water emulsions. *Eur. Food Res. Technol.* **226**: 161–168.

BIMAL C, ZHANG GN (2006). A solution to food fat?. *Food Rev. Int.* **22**: 245–258.

BOLAND AB, DELAHUNTY CM, VAN RUTH SM (2006). Influence of the texture of gelatine gels and pectin gels on strawberry flavour release and perception. *Food Chem.* **96**: 452–460.

BROSSARD C, ROUSSEAU F, DUMONT JP (2002). Oil-water partition coefficient of odorants: reliable index for smell but deceptive for odor rating. *Food Qual. Pref.* **13**: 65–72.

BUETTNER A, SCHIEBERLE P (2000). Influence of mastication on the concentrations of aroma volatiles–some aspects of flavour release and flavour perception. *Food Chem.* **71**: 347–354.

BUETTNER A, BEER A, HANNIG C, SETTLES M, SCHIEBERLE P (2002). Physiological and analytical studies on flavour perception dynamics as induced by the eating and swallowing process. *Food Qual. Pref.* **13**: 497–504.

CÁCERES E, GARCIA ML, TORO J, SELGAS MD (2004). The effect of fructooligosaccharides on the sensory characteristics of cooked sausages. *Meat Sci.* **68**: 87–96.

CAYOT N, TAISANT C, ARVISENET G, MEUNIER JM, VOILLEY A (2000). Flavouring ratios and partition coefficients for isoamyl acetate in various starch-based food matrices. *Sci. Alim.* **20**: 561–574.

CAYOT N, DURY-BRUN C, KARBOWIAK T, SAVARY G, VOILLEY A (2008). Measurement of transport phenomena of volatile compounds: a review. *Food Res. Int.* **41**: 349–362.

CHARLES M, ROSSELIN V, BECK L, SAUVAGEOT F, GUICHARD E (2000). Flavor release from salad dressings. Sensory and physicochemical approaches in relation with structure. *J. Agric. Food Chem.* **48**: 1810–1816.

CHEN J (2009). Food oral processing. A review. *Food Hyd.* **23**: 1–25.

CLARK R (2002). Influence of hydrocolloids on flavour release and sensory-instrumental correlations. In PA Williams, GO Phillips, *Gums and Stabilisers for the Food Industry* (Vol. 11) (pp. 217–225). Cambridge: The Royal Society of Chemistry.

COOK DJ, HOLLOWOOD TA, LINFORTH RST, TAYLOR AJ (2003). Oral shear stress predicts flavour perception in viscous solutions. *Chem. Sens.* **28**: 11–23.

DELWICHE J (2004). The impact of perceptual interactions on perceived flavour. *Food Qual. Pref.* **15**: 137–142.

DE ARAUJO IET, ROLLS ET (2004). Representation in the human brain of food texture and oral fat. *J. Neurosci.* **24**: 3086–3093.

DE ARAUJO IET, ROLLS ET, KRINGELBACH L, MCGLONE F, PHILLIPS N (2003). Taste-olfactory convergence, and the representation of the pleasantness of flavour in the human brain. *Eur. J. Neurosci.* **18**: 2374–2390.

DE ROOS KB (2003). Effect of texture and microstructure on flavour retention and release. *Int. Dairy. J.* **13**: 593–605.

DE ROOS KB (1997). How lipids influence food flavour. *Food Tech.* **51**: 60–62.

DE WIJK RA, VAN GEMERT LJ, TERPSTRA MEJ, WILKINSON CL (2003). Texture of semi-solids; sensory and instrumental measurements on vanilla custard desserts. *Food Qual. Pref.* **14**: 305–307.

DENKER M, PARAT-WILHELMS M, DRICHELT G, PAUCKE J, LUGER A, BORCHERDING K, HOFFMANN W, STEINHART H (2006). Investigation of the retronasal flavour release during the consumption of coffee with additions of milk constituents by oral breath sampling. *Food Chem.* **98**: 201–218.

DOYEN K, CAREY M, LINFORTH RST, MARIN M, TAYLOR AJ (2001). Volatile release from an emulsion: headspace and in-mouth studies. *J. Agric. Food Chem.* **49**: 804–810.

DREWNOWSKI A, SCHWARTZ M (1990). Invisible fats: sensory assessment of sugar/fat mixtures. *Appetite* **14**: 203–217.

DRUAUX C, VOILLEY A (1997). Effect of food composition and microstructure on volatile flavour release. *Trends Food Sci. Tech.* **8**: 364–368.

DURÁN L, COSTELL E (1999). Perception of taste: physiochemical and psychophysical aspects. *Food Sci. Tech. Int.* **5**: 17–24.

ENGELEN L, VAN DER BILT A (2008). Oral physiology and texture perception of semisolids. *J. Food Text.* **39**: 83–113.

FROST MB, DIJKSTERHUIS GY, MARTENS M (2001). Sensory perception in off milk. *Food Qual. Pref.* **12**: 327–336.

GALLARDO-ESCAMILLA FJ, KELLY AL, DELAHUNTY CM (2007). Mouthfeel and flavour of fermented whey with added hydrocolloids. *Int. Dairy J.* **17**: 308–315.

GHOSH S, PETERSON DG, COUPLand JN (2008). Temporal aroma release profile of solid and liquid droplet emulsions. *Food Biophys.* **3**: 335–343.

GONZÁLEZ-TOMÁS L, BAYARRI S, TAYLOR AJ, COSTELL E (2007). Flavour release and perception from model dairy custards. *Food Res. Int.* **40**: 520–528.

GUINARD JX, ZOUMAS-MORSE C, MORI B, UATONI B, PANYAM D, KILARA A (1997). Sugar and fat effects on sensory properties of ice cream. *J. Food Sci.* **62**: 1087–1094.

GUVEN M, YASAR K, KARACA OB, HAYALOGLYU AA (2005). The effect of inulin as a fat replacer on the quality of set-type low-fat yogurt manufacture. *Int. J. Dairy Tech.* **58**: 180–184.

HELDMAN DR (2004). Identifying food science and technology research needs. *Food Technol.* **58**: 32–34.

HOLLOWOOD TA, LINFORTH RST, TAYLOR AJ (2002). The effect of viscosity on the perception of flavour. *Chem. Sens.* **27**: 583–591.

HSU SY, SUN LY (2006). Comparisons on 10 non-meat protein fat substitutes for low-fat kung-wans. *J. Food Eng.* **78**: 47–53.

HYVÖNEN L, LINNA M, TUORILA H, DIJKSTERHUIST G (2003). Perception of meeting and flavor release of ice cream containing different types and contents of fat. *J. Dairy Sci.* **86**: 1130–1138.

JAEGER SR (2006). Non-sensory factors in sensory science research. *Food Qual. Pref.* **17**: 132–144.

JUTEAU A, CAYOT N, CHABANET C, DOUBLIER JL, GUICHARD E (2004). Flavour release from polysaccharide gels: different approaches for the determination of kinetic parameters. *Trends Food Sci. Technol.* **15**: 394–402.

KÄHKÖNEN P, HAKANPÄÄ P, TUORILA H (1999). The effect of information related to fat content and taste on consumer responses to a reduced-fat frankfurter and a reduced-fat chocolate bar. *J. Sensory Stud.* **14**: 35–46.

KAVAS G, OYSUN G, KINIC O, UYSAL H (2004). Effect of some fat replacers on chemical, physical and sensory attributes of low-fat white pickled cheese. *Food Chem.* **88**: 381–388.

KEATS SJ, DALTON PH, BRESLIN PAS (2004). Flavor interactions at the sensory level. In AJ Taylor and DD Roberts, *Flavor Perception* (pp. 228–249). Oxford. Blackwell Publ. Ltd.

KÜHN J, CONSIDINE T, SINGH H (2006). Interactions of milk proteins and volatile flavour compounds: implications in the development of protein foods. *J. Food Sci.* **71** (5): R72–R82.

LETHUAUT L, WEEL KGC, BOELRIJK AEM, BROSSARD CD (2004). Flavor perception and aroma release from model dairy desserts. *J. Agric. Food Chem.* **52**: 3478–3485.

LINFORTH RST, BLISSET A, TAYLOR AJ (2005). Differences in the effect of bolus weight on flavour release into the breath between low-fat and high-fat products. *J. Agric. Food Chem.* **53**: 7217–7221.

LUCKOW T, SHEEHAN V, DELAHUNTY C, FITZGERALD G (2005). Determining the odor and flavor characteristics of probiotic, health-promoting ingredients and the effects of repeated exposure on consumer acceptance. *J. Food Sci.* **70**: S53–S59.

MALONE ME, APPELQVIST IAM, NORTON IT (2003a). Oral behaviour of food hydrocolloids. Part 1. Lubrication and deposition considerations. *Food Hyd.* **17**: 763–773.

MALONE ME, APPELQVIST IAM, NORTON IT (2003b). Oral behaviour of food hydrocolloids. Part 2. Taste and aroma release. *Food Hyd.* **17**: 775–784.

MESTRES M, MORAN N, JORDAN A, BUETTNER A (2005). Aroma release and retronasal perception during and after consumption of flavored whey protein gels with different textures. 1. *In vivo* release analysis. *J. Agric. Food Chem.* **53**: 403–409.

MESTRES M, KIEFFER R, BUETTNER A (2006). Release and perception of ethyl butanoate during and after consumption of whey protein gels: relation between textural and physiological parameters. *J. Agric. Food Chem.* **54**: 1814–1821.

METCALF KL, VICKERS ZM (2002). Taste intensities of oil-in-water emulsions with varying fat content. *J. Sen. Stud.* **17**: 379–390.

MIETTINEN SM, TOURILA H, PIIRONEN V, VEHKALATHI K, HYVÖNEN L (2002). Effect of emulsion characteriastics on the release of aroma as detected by sensory evaluation, static headspace gas chromatografy and electronic nose. *J. Agric. Food Chem.* **50**: 4232–4239.

MORRIS ER (1995). Polysaccharide rheology and in-mouth perception. In AM Stephen, *Food Polysaccharides and their Applications* (pp. 517–546). New York: Marcel Dekker, Inc.

OVERBOSCH P, AFTEROF WGM, HARING PGM (1991). Flavor release in the mouth. *Food Rev. Int.* **7**: 137–184.

PHAN VA, LIAO YC, ANTILLE N, SAGALOWICZ L, ROBERT F, GODINOT N (2008). Delayed compound release properties of self-assembly structures in emulsions. *J. Agric. Food Chem.* **56**: 1027–1077.

PHILLIPS LG, MCGIFF ML, BARBANO DM, LAWLESS HT (1995). The influence of fat on the sensory properties, viscosity and color of low-fat milk. *J. Dairy Sci.* **78**: 1258–1266.

PIVK U, GODINOT N, KELLER C, ANTILLE N, JUILLERAT MA, RASPOR P (2008). Lipid deposition on the tongue after oral processing of medium-chain triglycerides and impact on the perception of mouthfeel. *J. Agric. Food Chem.* **56**: 1058–1064.

PRESCOTT J (2004). Psyological processes in flavour perception. In AJ Taylor and DD Roberts, *Flavor Perception* (pp. 256–274). Oxford. Blackwell Publ. Ltd.

RABE S, BANAVARA DS, KRINGS U, BERGER RG (2002). Computerized apparatus for measuring dynamic flavour release from liquid food matrices. *J. Agric. Food Chem.* **50**: 6440–6447.

RABE S, LINFORTH RST, KRINGS U, TAYLOR AJ, BERGER RG (2004). Volatile release from liquids: a comparison of *in-vivo* APCI-MS, in mouth headspace trapping and *in vitro* mouth model data. *Chen. Senses* **29**: 163–173.

REGA B, GUICHARD E, VOILLEY A (2002). Flavour release from pectin gels: effects of texture, molecular interactions and aroma compounds diffusion. *Sciences Aliment.* **22**: 235–248.

ROLLS E (2005). Taste, olfactory and food texture processing in the brain, and the control of food intake. *Physiol. Behavior.* **85**: 45–56.

SALLES C, TARREGA A, MIELLE P, MARATRAY J, GORRIA P, LIABOEUF J, LIODENOT JJ (2007). Development of a chewing simulator for food breakdown and the analysis of *in vitro* flavor compound release in a mouth enviroment. *J. Food Eng.* **82**: 189–198.

SAMIL S, WYETH L, KILCAST D (1991/92). Flavour release and perception in reduced-fat foods. *Food Qual. Pref.* **3**: 51–60.
SANDROU DK, ARVANITOYANNIS IS (2000). Low fat/calorie foods: current state and perspectives. *Crit. Rev. Food Sci. Nutr.* **40**: 427–447.
SETSER CS, RACETTE WL (1992). Macromolecule replacers in food-products. *Crit. Rev. Food Sci. Nutr.* **32**: 275–297.
SEUVRE AM, DIAZ MDLA, CAYOT P, VOILLEY A (2004). Influence of the composition and the structure of different media on the release of aroma compounds. *Lait.* **84**: 305–316.
SILLETTI E, VINGERHOEDS M, NORDE W, VAN AKEN G (2007). The role of electrostatics in saliva-induced emulsion flocculation. *Food Hyd.* **21**: 596–606.
SIRÓ I, KÀPOLNA E, KÀPOLNA B, LUGASI A (2008). Functional food. Product development, marketing and consumer acceptance. A review. *Appetite.* **51**: 456–457.
SMALL DM, PRESCOTT J (2005). Odor/taste integration and the perception of flavour. *Exp. Brain Res.* **166**: 345–357.
STEIN LJ, NAGAI H, NAKAGAWA M, BEAUCHAMP GK (2003). Effects of repeated exposure and health-related information on hedonic evaluation and acceptance of a bitter beverage. *Appetite* **40**: 119–129.
SUNDQVIST NC, STEVENSON RJ, BISHOP IRJ (2006). Can odours acquire fat-like properties? *Appetite* **47**: 91–99.
TÁRREGA A, COSTELL E (2006). Effect of inulin addition on rheological and sensory properties of fat-free starch-based dairy desserts. *Int. Dairy J.* **16**: 1104–1112.
TÁRREGA A, YVEN C, SEMON E, SALLES C (2008). Aroma release and chewing activity during eating different model cheeses. *Int. Dairy J.* **18**: 849–857.
TAYLOR AJ (2002). Release and transport of flavors *in vivo*: physicochemical, physiological, and perceptual considerations. *Comp. Rev. Food Sci. Food Saf.* **1**: 45–57.
TAYLOR AJ, LINFORTH RST (2003). Direct mass spectrometry of complex volatile and non-volatile flavour mixtures. *Int. J. Mass Spectrometry* **223**: 179–191.
TAYLOR AJ, ROBERTS DD (2004). *Flavor Perception.* Oxford. Blackwell Publ. Ltd.
TAYLOR AJ, LINFORTH RST, HARVEY BA, Y BLAKE A (2000). Atmospheric pressure chemical ionisation mass spe ctrometry for *in vivo* analysis of volatile flavour release. *Food Chem.* **71**: 327–338.
TRELEA IC, ATLAN S, DÉLÉRIS I, SAINT-EVE A, MARIN M, SOUCHON I (2008). Mechanistic mathematical model for *in vivo* aroma release during eating of semiliquid foods. *Chem. Sens.* **33**: 181–192.
TUORILA H, CARDELLO AV, LESHER L (1994). Antecedents and consequences of expectations related to fat-free and regular-fat foods. *Appetite* **23**: 247–263.
URALA N, LÄHTENNMÄKI L (2004). Attitudes behind consumers' willingness to use functional foods. *Food Qual. Prefer.* **15**: 793–803.
VALENTOVA H, POKORNY J (1998). Effect of edible oils and oil emulsions on the perception of basic tastes. *Nahrung* **42**: 406–408.
VAN RUTH SM, FLORIS V, FAYOUX S (2006). Characterisation of the volatile profiles of infant formulas by proton transfer reaction-mass spectrometry and gas chromatography-mass spectrometry. *Food Chem.* **98**: 343–350.
VAN RUTH SM, BUHR K (2003). Influence of saliva on temporal volatile flavour release from red bell peppers determined by proton transfer reaction–mass spectrometry. *Eur. Food Res. Technol.* **216**: 220–223.
VAN RUTH SM, KING C, GIANNOULI P (2002). Influence of lipid fraction, emulsifier fraction and mean particle diameter of oil-in water emulsions on the release of 20 aroma compounds. *J. Agric. Food Chem.* **50**: 2365–2371.
VAN RUTH SM, ROOZEN JP (2002). Influence of mastication and saliva on aroma release in a model mouth system. *Food Chem.* **71**: 339–345.

VERBEKE W (2006). Functional foods: consumer willingness to compromise on taste for health? *Food Qual. Prefer.* **17**: 126–131.

VILLEGAS B, COSTELL E (2007). Flow behaviour of inulin-milk beverages. Influence of inulin average chain length and of milk fat content. *Int. Dairy J.* **17**: 776–781.

WEENEN H, JELLEMA RH, DE WIJK RA (2005). Sensory sub-attributes of creamy mouthfeel in commercial mayonnaises, custard desserts and sauces. *Food Qual. Pref.* **16**: 163–170.

WARRAND J (2006). Healthy polysaccharides. The next chapter in food products. *Food Tech. Biotech.* **44**: 355–370.

WEEL KGC, BOELRIJK AEM, BURGER JJ, JACOBS MA, GRUPPEN H, VORAGEN AGJ, SMIT G (2004). Effect of emulsion properties on release of esters under headspace, *in vivo* and artificial throat conditions in relation to sensory intensity. *J. Agric. Food Chem.* **52**: 6572–6577.

WILCOCK A, PUN M, KHANONA J (2004). Consumer attitudes, knowledge and behaviour: a review of food safety issues. *Trends Food Sci. Tech.* **15**: 56–66.

YACKINOUS C, GUINARD JX (2000). Flavor manipulation can enhance the impression of fat in some foods. *J. Food Sci.* **65**: 909–914.

ZANDSTRA EH, DE GRAAF C, VAN STAVEREN WA (2001). Influence of health and taste attitudes on the consumption of low- and high-fat foods. *Food Qual. Pref.* **12**: 75–82.

18

Design of foods for the optimal delivery of basic tastes

G. J. van den Oever, J. Busch, E. van der Linden, G. Smit and N. J. Zuidam, Unilever Research and Development, The Netherlands

Abstract: This chapter focuses on the perception of basic tastes of food products. Firstly, an overview of the sensation of tastants by receptors upon oral intake of food and how food is broken down within the mouth is described. Secondly, the effects of food structural product parameters on taste perception are reviewed, followed by the influence of other senses on taste perception (cross-modal interactions). Then, we show how all these effects on taste perception can be understood and quantified in one model, which we are currently using in our research and product design. Finally, the future effects of health demands and technological progress in other fields on taste research are discussed.

Key words: flavour, cross-modal interactions, perception, microstructure, modelling.

18.1 Introduction

All the five classical senses (vision, audition, taste, smell and touch) play a role during eating and food perception. Other senses such as temperature and pain, and receptors in the gastrointestinal tract (e.g. to signal satiety) may also contribute. This chapter focuses on the perception of basic tastes of food products, i.e. salt, sour, sweet, bitter and umami. Such knowledge is important to enable the design of food products with less salt, sugar and fat. Public health organisations (such as the World Health Organization (WHO) and the British Government's Food Standards Agency) have recommended reductions from the current sodium chloride intake of 9–12 g/day to 5–6 g/day (World Health Organization, 2007), which would help to reduce blood pressure and subsequently incidences of strokes and ischaemic heart disease. More and more people suffer from being overweight, and therefore there is a need to eat less sugar and fat (World Health

Organization, 2004). However, reduction of salt, sugar and fat levels has a tremendous impact on taste and also aroma perception. Furthermore, more and more food products contain functional ingredients which often impart off-tastes (e.g. polyphenols, carotenoids, peptides). Therefore, design of good-tasting products is needed.

In this chapter we will firstly describe how food can be sensed by taste receptors upon oral intake and how the food is broken down within the mouth. Secondly, the effects of food structural product parameters on taste perception are discussed, followed by the influence of other senses on taste perception (cross-modal interactions). Then, we show how all these effects on taste perception can be understood and quantified in one model, as we are currently using in research and product design. Finally, the future effects of health demands and technological progress in other fields on taste research will be discussed.

18.2 Oral factors

18.2.1 Taste receptor activation and sensation

By definition, tastes are perceived by taste receptor cells located inside taste buds, the gustatory papillae that are located on the tongue, in the palate and the back of the throat (Tareilus, 2000; Chandrashekar *et al.*, 2006). Taste receptors are either ion channels (salt, sour) or G-protein coupled receptors (sweet, bitter, umami). Recent studies have revealed that, contrary to popular belief, there is no tongue 'map': responsiveness to the five basic modalities is present in all areas of the tongue in each taste bud (Chandrashekar *et al.*, 2006). Each taste pore connects the interior of the taste bud with the oral cavity and is 5–12 μm in diameter (Arvidson, 1976). It has been suggested that the taste pore contains fluids that are derived from the salivary glands and perhaps from cells in the taste buds (Brouwer and Wiersma, 1980). Some studies have shown that the chemical composition of the taste pore fluid (although not completely elucidated) is different from that of saliva, implying that saliva may not come into immediate contact with the taste receptors. The mucous substance in saliva (mucin glycoproteins) forms a viscous type of gel, which firmly binds to the oral mucosa and is not easily removed by rinsing with at least water (McMillan, 1980). Thus, it is thought that saliva provides a fluid layer, which lies over the top of the taste pore as well as the surface of the oral epithelium. Changes in the quantity and quality of saliva can affect taste sensitivity during the initial processes of taste stimulation.

A tastant can be sensed by receptors only once it is fully hydrated and transferred by saliva and taste pore fluids to the receptor. The perception of taste (T) is a function of the taste threshold and the activation of taste receptors by tastants which can be quantified by, amongst others, Stevens' power law (Stevens, 1975):

$$T = k(C - C^{\#})^{S} \qquad [18.1]$$

where k is a constant, $C^{\#}$ is the concentration of tastant, C^{*} is the threshold concentration and S is a constant (also called the Stevens value) indicating how fast the taste intensity rises with the tastant concentration. It should be noted that psychophysical curves for single taste stimuli can already be complex, particularly for bitter compounds, as signal transduction occurs via different bitter receptors (Chandrashekar *et al.*, 2006). For example, the relationships between concentration, detection threshold, and supra-threshold intensity were investigated for caffeine, quinine and *n*-propyl-6-thiourea (PROP). This study revealed a significant correlation between PROP threshold and supra-threshold intensity, but no such correlation was found for caffeine, highlighting the complex underlying mechanisms that are not yet fully understood (Keast and Roper, 2007). The taste intensity of salt (sodium ion) is affected by its counter-ion. The saltiness perception in the presence of large anions such as gluconate, glutamate or acetate is reduced compared with the saltiness in the presence of small anions, such as chloride or sulphate (Van der Klaauw and Smith, 1995). This can be explained by a flux of the anions via a paracellular pathway, needed to depolarise the taste receptor cells.

Sourness is elicited by acids, which donate/release hydrogen ions into the aqueous phase. The perceived acidity is dependent on the pH when using strong acids, but is determined by both the pH and the amount of undissociated hydrogen ions in the case of weak organic acids. The combined effect of the latter two, also in the case of mixtures of acids, can be determined by measurement of the product titratable acidity, TA (Da Conceicao Neta *et al.*, 2007). TA is used in equation 18.1 as a measure for the tastant concentration C driving sourness.

18.2.2 Oral processing

When food is eaten, it is subject to temperature changes, mechanical deformation, dilution with saliva and enzymatic breakdown induced by salivary enzymes (Van Aken *et al.*, 2007). The kinetics at which tastants reach receptors will influence taste perception. Oral factors occurring during mastication, which can influence these kinetics, may include:

- the breakdown of food into smaller units (pieces, lumps) from which the tastants migrate into the saliva-based phase which reaches the receptors;
- dilution of the aqueous phase by saliva;
- the viscosity of this saliva-based phase;
- other saliva effects, such as composition, amount, flow and interactions with tastants (Stokes and Davies, 2007);
- coating of the oral mucosa by an oily layer reducing mass transport of tastants to the receptors.

18.3 Effects of food structures on tastes

18.3.1 Effect of viscosity

In general, a large increase in viscosity of food products results in a decrease of taste perception. This might be caused by a combination of different mechanisms:

1. Food products with a higher viscosity or gel strength will be broken down slower in the oral cavity than ones with a low viscosity. Therefore, relatively large amounts of taste molecules might not be available for perception. Bayarrri *et al.* (2007b) determined the temporal perception of sweetness for sweetened κ-carrageenan and gellan gum gelled systems with different mechanical properties. The authors demonstrated that the maximum sweetness intensity in these systems was closely related to the amount of deformation required to break the hydrocolloid network and to the resistance to deformation. The resistance to rupture influenced the variation in the rate of intensity decrease. Although gellan gels were harder and more rigid, the sweetness intensities were higher than that of κ-carrageenan gels. This was explained by the fact that gellan gels were more brittle and thus easier to breakdown in the mouth (Bayarri *et al.*, 2007b). The same authors also demonstrated that, in hard κ-carrageenan and gellan gum gels of 20% sucrose, the sucrose had a significant contribution to the compression resistance in these gels, also indirectly influencing the texture of the gels (Bayarri *et al.*, 2007b).
2. Recently, it has been argued that the reduction in taste perception of liquid food is not fundamentally related to viscosity, but to a reduction in the efficiency of mixing between the liquid food and saliva (Ferry *et al.*, 2006a,b). This mixing determines the amount of tastants that reach the receptors. It is influenced by the type of thickener. Ferry *et al.* showed that granular structures like unmodified wheat starch and modified (cross-linked) waxy maize starch mix more efficiently with saliva than random-coil polymers like native waxy maize starch and especially hydroxypropyl methylcellulose (HPMC), since the latter polymers have entanglements between their chains. Such an entanglement might especially happen when the concentration of random-coil biopolymers exceeds the so-called coil-overlap concentration (C^*), at which the hydrocolloid chains begin to overlap in solution (Baines and Morris, 1987; Cook *et al.*, 2002; Hollowood *et al.*, 2002). This overlap reduces the molecular movements of the biopolymers and results in a sharp increase in viscosity. The efficiency of mixing hypothesis could explain why HPMC had a larger decreasing effect on saltiness than starch, and the waxy maize starch a lower saltiness perception than the modified one and wheat starch (Ferry *et al.*, 2006a). A decrease in saltiness by HPMC above its C^* was found before by Cook *et al.* (2002), who also reported decreased sweetness perceptions of sucrose and aspar-

tame, fructose and neohesperidin dihydrochalcone. The same was also found for the sweetness of sucrose and asparatame with guar gum and λ-carrageenan. However, no effect of increasing HPMC above its C* could be found on the acidity of citric acid and on the bitterness of quinine hydrochloride at the concentrations used (Cook *et al.*, 2002). In the mouths of individuals with high amylase activity the granular structures of wheat and modified waxy maize starch can be disrupted in seconds, which results in decreased mixing capabilities with saliva and therefore lower saltiness scores (Ferry *et al.*, 2006b). So for starch systems the higher the amylase activity of an individual, the lower the saltiness perception. Amylase activity will also reduce starch viscosity (Ferry *et al.*, 2004), so here a decrease in viscosity is not associated with an increase in taste perception.

3. The structure of the matrix (network of entangled hydrocolloids or three-dimensional network) can affect the diffusivity and mass transfer coefficients of taste compounds. Kokini has shown that the diffusion constant of sucrose decreased when the thickness (viscosity) of tomato juices was increased by addition of tomato solids, which corresponded with a decrease in sweetness perception (Kokini, 1982). Bayarri *et al.* (2001) demonstrated that the diffusion constant of sucrose at 37 °C was significantly higher in soft κ-carrageenan gels than in hard κ-carrageenan gels and (soft and hard) gellan gum gels. However, this did not correlate with taste intensity (see above).
4. Panellists can adapt their mastication process depending on the food texture, which in turn is likely to affect flavour release (Wilson and Brown, 1997). Sweetened and flavoured gelatin samples with increasing hydrocolloid concentrations were sensorially evaluated during normal mastication. Increased mechanical strength and melting point of the samples resulted in longer chewing times and lower intensity and more prolonged flavour perception. The authors could show that the temporal pattern of flavour perception was closely linked with mastication patterns for each subject, although large individual differences were observed. Similar conclusions were drawn from a study on sweet chewy confectionery products (Blissett *et al.*, 2006).
5. Increased viscosity will increase the texture perception, and this can have a decreased, cross-modal effect on taste perception (see Section 18.4.4).

In practice, it is hard to discriminate between the different mechanisms mentioned above. One should keep in mind that large changes in viscosity are required to control taste perception, and that, in practice, this is an ineffective way for the design of food products, since viscosity is often set to meet other consumer demands (Malone *et al.*, 2003; Pripp *et al.*, 2004).

18.3.2 Effect of biopolymers

Biopolymers may affect taste perception in several ways:

- The use of biopolymers may decrease the efficiency of mixing of a liquid or gelled food with saliva, which in general decreases the taste perception (see above).
- The thickener may have a taste effect itself.
- Biopolymers may bind taste molecules, which result in decreased perceptions. For example, sodium ions can bind to oppositely charged biopolymers. Rosett *et al.* (1994, 1996) found that saltiness in chicken broths was suppressed by the use of 0.3% (w/w) xanthan gum. This was explained by ^{23}Na nuclear magnetic resonance (NMR) spectroscopy, which showed ionic binding of sodium ions to xanthan. Binding of sapid components to biopolymers might also be used to decrease off-tastes of healthy ingredients; e.g. tea and olive oil phenolics were less bitter in the presence of proteins (Haslam, 1998; Pripp *et al.*, 2004). Katsuragi *et al.* (1995) found that bitter tastes could be masked by lipoproteins. They suggested binding of the hydrophobic region to the receptor membrane, but an alternative mechanism could be complexation of the bitter molecules with the lipoproteins.

18.3.3 Effect of lipids and emulsions

The majority of flavour studies in emulsion-based foods have been focused on aroma release, and some studies on addition of lipids to emulsion-based food products indicate that lipids may also alter taste perception by the following mechanisms:

- Lipids may influence the partitioning between the food, saliva and the taste receptors, e.g. by changing the concentration of tastants in the aqueous phase of the food product as the lipid content is altered. The reduction of fat in cheese led to an increase in bitterness and astringency and a reduction in saltiness (Shamil *et al.*, 1991). Increased bitterness and astringency were assumed to arise from hydrophobic ingredients, whose concentration increased in the aqueous phase of the food product when the fat level was reduced. Conversely, the decrease in salt intensity when the fat level was reduced was proposed to be due to the reduced concentration of salt in the aqueous phase of the food product. A decrease in fat content of mayonnaise led to a decrease in sour taste owing to the reduced concentration of the acid in the aqueous phase of the food product (Wendin *et al.*, 1999).
- Changes in the rate of regeneration of interfacial surfaces required for release of sapid compounds into the surrounding media. For example, reduction of fat in cheese also increases its hardness and therefore slows its oral break-up (Shamil *et al.*, 1991).

- Oral mouth coating may also limit the access or binding of taste molecules to receptors. Lynch and co-workers (1993) found that all taste modalities were affected, albeit by a small amount, and that coconut oil had a more suppressive effect than sunflower oil. They proposed that mouth coating by fats physically interferes with tastant access to the taste receptors. Valentova and Pokorny (1998) found that the intensity of sweet, bitter and astringent compounds were reduced by prior consumption of oil, but acidic and salty tastes were not affected.

Yamamoto and Nakabayashi (1999) concluded from their work on effects of increasing oil phase volume on salt perception in o/w emulsions that taste intensity will be influenced by a combination of an increased concentration of salt in the aqueous phase and a suppressed contact of salt with taste receptors. This was confirmed by Malone *et al.* (2003), who showed that, as the fat content was increased for emulsion-based products that were kept at constant salt concentration, the perceived saltiness increased due to the associated increase in the salt concentration in the aqueous phase (see Fig. 18.1). However, when the salt concentration on aqueous phase was kept constant, the saltiness decreased with increasing fat content (see Fig. 18.1), suggesting that perceived saltiness is non-linearly dependent on a combination of salt concentration and aqueous phase volume. Based on these results, a psychophysical model was developed that related taste intensity not only to salt concentration (see equation 18.1) but also to the phase volume of fat (Appelqvist *et al.*, 2007):

$$T = k[C]_{\mathrm{p}}^{S}(1-\phi_{\mathrm{fat}})^{-S}\{1-\exp[-q(1-\phi_{\mathrm{fat}})]\} \qquad [18.2]$$

where C_{p} is the concentration of tastant in the whole product, ϕ_{fat} is the fat phase volume (= 1 − ϕ_{aqueous}) and q is a constant.

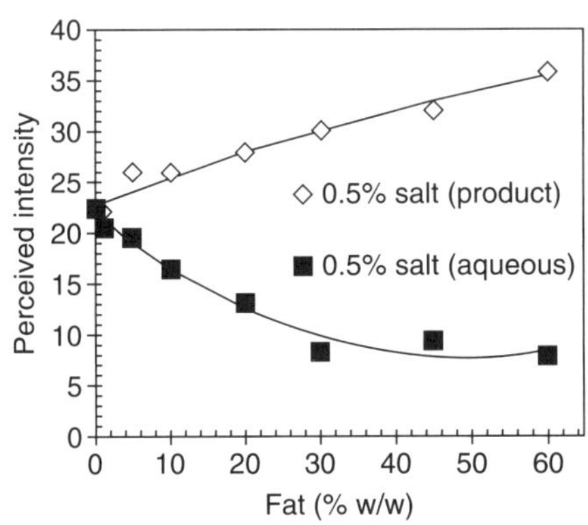

Fig. 18.1 Effect of oil phase volume in o/w emulsions on salty taste perception for constant sodium chloride concentration in product or in aqueous phase. Reprinted from Malone *et al.* (2003), with permission from Elsevier.

Some food products have their aqueous phase dispersed in a fat continuum as w/o emulsions, e.g. most spreads containing 40% or more fat. One of the key requirements for a good spread is phase inversion during breakdown in the mouth, thereby releasing, for example, salt. Both the aqueous phase and the organisation of the shell/crystalline fat structure around the water droplet affect the phase inversion process. Margarines that do not invert in the mouth are often perceived as waxy and with very little taste. In principle, stable w/o emulsions that do not invert well in the mouth should be able to trap, for example, bitter, hydrophilic molecules (such as peptides) in the water phase without being perceived.

18.3.4 Effect of encapsulates

Taste molecules that are entrapped within microparticles and which do not release during oral processing are not perceived. Malone *et al.* (2003) also studied the acid perception of citric acid in w/o/w duplex emulsions with fixed oil contents of 30% (w/w). The results are shown in Fig. 18.2. Citric acid was located in both the internal and external water phase. As more aqueous product was incorporated (from 0 to 50%, w/w), the perceived sourness decreased. The acid inside the duplex emulsions could not be perceived, and the taste perception was dependent on the volume of the external aqueous phase.

Molecular inclusion of sapid compounds in cyclodextrins might reduce undesired taste (Szente and Szejtli, 2004, and references therein), especially

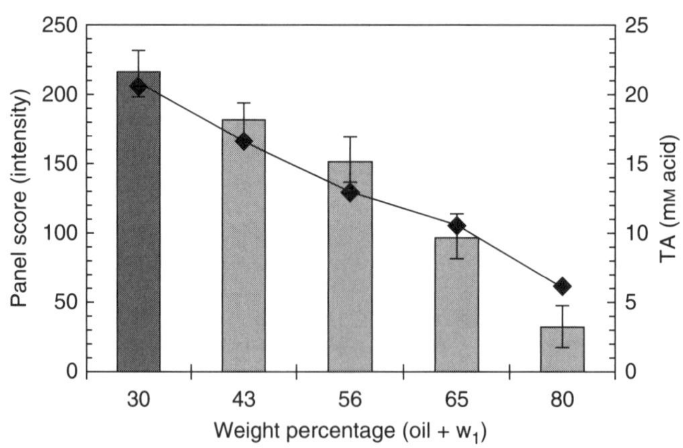

Fig. 18.2 Effect of the internal water volume within of $w_1/o/w_2$ duplex emulsions on the perception of citric acid. The oil content was fixed at 30% (w/w). The left column (darkly shaded) is an o/w emulsion, and the other, lightly shaded columns are duplex emulsions. On consumption, the sourness of the external aqueous phase w_2 could be perceived, in contrast to the internal aqueous phase w_1. Reprinted from Malone *et al.* (2003), with permission from Elsevier.

when the conditions are optimal for complexation (i.e. cold temperature and excess of cyclodextrin). For example, the bitter taste of milk casein hydrolysate, ginseng extract, grapefruit and mandarin juices could be eliminated by addition of β-cyclodextrin. Gel beads (e.g. composed of calcium alginate) with acids will normally leak all their contents during eating, unless they are quite large (>1 mm; unpublished Unilever data). Therefore, such beads are not very useful in practice to reduce sourness. Other encapsulates used to mask health ingredients with off-taste might be fluid bed coated ones (Desai and Park, 2005).

18.4 Effects of cross-modal interactions on tastes

Several authors have reviewed the impact of flavour interactions at the sensory level (Keast *et al.*, 2004b; Delwiche, 2004; Tournier *et al.*, 2007). It is generally accepted that different types of interactions can be distinguished: chemical interactions occurring in the food matrix, peripheral physiological interactions, mechanical/structural interactions during mastication, which can all be categorised as physicochemical interactions, and cognitive interactions (Keast *et al*, 2004b). The following part will primarily deal with perceptual interactions relevant for taste perception, but physicochemical aspects will also be discussed. The perceptual interactions of temperature, sound and trigeminal stimuli will not be discussed here, since their impact is relatively small, their occurance low, and the underlying mechanisms not very clear. Please see the reviews above for more information on this. Here, we will consider taste–taste, aroma–taste, colour–taste and texture–taste interactions, respectively.

18.4.1 Taste–taste interactions

When mixing two or more tastants, as is the case in most food and beverage products, perceptual interactions occur that follow complex sets of rules that are not well understood (Keast and Breslin, 2002). The number of papers that have investigated specific binary or ternary taste–taste interactions is vast. A review of these studies by Keast and Breslin (2002) revealed many contradictions in the literature. This can be attributed to individual variations in taste sensitivities, different experimental approaches used and the specific tastants studied. For example, bitter compounds are known to activate different taste receptors and this can affect the resulting interactions and perception accordingly (Chandrashekar *et al.*, 2006).

As indicated above, different interactions may take place concerning taste–taste interactions. Chemical interactions may occur between tastants, e.g. between an acid and a base. Oral physiological interactions can occur between a tastant in a mixture and taste receptor or taste transduction mechanism of the other tastant. The bitter masking effect of sodium salts on many bitter compounds is of this nature, as was demonstrated by Kroeze and Bartoshuk (1985) in split tongue experiments. Bitterness suppression occurred only when the sodium salt and the bitter stimulus were applied to the same tongue half. This demonstrated the peripheral nature of the interaction: the two lateral halves of the tongue are neurologically independent and perceptual integration of tastants applied to the two halves separately can only occur in the brain (Kroeze and Bartoshuk 1985). Keast *et al.* (2001, 2004a) demonstrated later on that sodium salts can mask the bitterness of most bitter compounds, but not those of $MgSO_4$ and tetralone. Very recently, the inhibition of the sweet transduction pathway by a bitter tastant was demonstrated. Quinine and its stereoisomer quinidine, but not denatonium benzoate, were shown to inhibit TRPM5, a cation channel involved in sweet taste transduction (Talavera *et al.*, 2007). It has also been shown that serotonin and ATP play a role in cell-to-cell signalling and sensory output in the gustatory end organs (Roper, 2006). This has initiated speculations on the potential impact on perception of cell–cell communication (synaptic processing in taste buds), e.g. with respect to bitterness masking.

Lastly, cognitive effects can occur when different tastants are present in a mixture. Mixture suppression is a typical example of cognitive effects: when two or more taste stimuli (above threshold) are mixed, the intensity is less than the sum of the individual taste intensities (Pangborn, 1960). Here again, split tongue experiments proved to be a powerful method, that was used to demonstrate this time that suppression (e.g. of sweet and bitter stimuli) has a central cognitive origin rather than a peripheral one (Kroeze and Bartoshuk, 1985). Keast and Breslin (2002) used the sigmoidally shaped concentration–intensity psychophysical curve to explain common effects of taste–taste interactions. They divided the curve into three different phases: an expansion phase at low concentration/intensity, a linear phase at medium concentration/intensity and a compressive phase at high concentration/intensity, the latter being due to the oral peripheral effect of saturation of the receptors. Keast and Breslin used this distinction to order the reported (cognitive) effects of binary taste–taste interactions. This approach helped to summarise effects and identify some general trends, which are often different for the different phases of the psychophysical curve. For example, mixtures of bitter and sweet stimuli are variably affected at low intensity/concentration, but mixtures at medium and high intensity/concentration are mutually suppressive. Bitterness, on the other hand, is suppressed by saltiness, while salty taste is not affected by bitterness, mostly at all three phases. Keast and Breslin defined some (more or less) general rules for binary taste–taste interactions of different taste qualities. At low intensity/concentration enhancement is reported more often, at moderate intensity/concentration a mix of enhancement, suppression and linear interaction is observed, while at high intensity/concentration suppression is most common.

When more than two compounds are mixed, resulting interactions become even more complex. The following example, reported by Breslin and Beauchamp (1997), illustrates how peripheral and central cognitive effects can interact in a mixture of sodium acetate, sucrose and urea. They showed that addition of sodium to a bitter–sweet mixture suppressed the bitterness (peripheral effect), while sweetness was enhanced owing to release from the cognitive suppression of the lower bitterness.

18.4.2 Aroma–taste interactions

There are numerous pieces of evidence now on the interactions between aroma and taste (Noble, 1996), but the focus of the work has been primarily on the influence of aroma on taste perception. Some compounds elicit taste and odour attributes, for example acetic acid, which may be interpreted as leading to aroma–taste interactions (Delwiche, 2004). However, in most cases stimuli operate in one modality. Strong evidence for the occurrence of aroma–taste interactions was provided by Dalton *et al.*, who demonstrated that the combination of subthreshold orthonasal concentrations of an odorant (benzaldehyde) and a subthreshold tastant (sodium saccharin) is perceived as the result of cross-modal summation (Dalton *et al.*, 2000). These findings have recently been extended with neuroimaging studies, that also highlighted the importance of the right timing of the delivery of odour and taste stimuli for taste–aroma integration (Pfeiffer *et al.*, 2005; Marciani *et al.*, 2006). Furthermore, headspace measurements of aroma concentrations in the nose space have excluded physicochemical interaction at the release level (Davidson *et al.*, 1999), thus confirming the role of cognition in aroma–taste interactions.

The importance of congruency between odour–taste pairs has been highlighted. Many examples of enhancement by congruent pairs have been reported, especially for sweetness. Examples are strawberry and sweetness (Frank *et al.*, 1993; Schifferstein and Verlegh, 1996) and vanilla and sweetness (Sakai *et al.*, 2001). Absence of enhancement is seen for incongruent pairs, e.g. for ham flavour and sweetness (Schifferstein and Verlegh, 1996) and soy flavour and sweetness (Djordjevic *et al.*, 2004). Recently, we have shown in our own laboratory that beef aroma can be used to increase perceived saltiness in a beef bouillon (Dötsch *et al.*, 2009).

The extent of taste or aroma enhancement is largely dependent on the evaluation strategy of the assessor. The synthetic approach of consumers favours aroma–taste interactions, while an analytical approach focusing on the components of a sample (typically used by trained panellists) can abolish cross-modal interactions (Bingham *et al.*, 1990; Prescott, 1999; Hort and Hollowood, 2004; Prescott *et al.*, 2004). This indicates that cross-modal interactions are to a large extent based on learned associations rather than 'hard-wired'. This also explains why aroma–taste interactions can be experienced to a different extent amongst different cultures of people (Sauvageot *et al.*, 2000).

In conclusion, both psychophysical and neuroimaging findings have provided evidence that aroma and taste can interact perceptually, while it is also generally recognised that the observed effects are highly dependent on factors such as congruency and sensory methodology.

18.4.3 Colour–taste interactions

Several studies have shown that colour can greatly impact the ability of subjects to identify food and beverages (Delwiche, 2004). These studies indicate that the impact of colour is largest for strong colour–flavour associations. For example, Morrot *et al.* (2001) have reported that, when white wine was coloured red, individuals tended to describe the wine with more red wine terms instead of using white wine descriptors, as was done for the uncoloured wines. For colour–odour pairs (but not for taste–odour pairs) Zellner and Kautz (1990) found that solutions were rated as having more intense odours in the presence of colour cues but not without, regardless of the colour–odour appropriateness. However, the impact of a particular colour on a certain taste is inconsistent across studies (see Delwiche, 2004, for an overview). Several studies have shown that taste and/or flavour intensity increase as the colour intensity increases (e.g. DuBose *et al.*, 1980; Johnson *et al.*, 1982). It seems likely that some association exists between colour intensity and flavour intensities. Clydesdale (1993) has argued that the effect of colour on perception seems to result from learned associations rather than inherent psychophysical characteristics because the effects of colour often do not follow Stevens' power law.

18.4.4 Texture–taste interactions

Texture–taste interactions might have two primary origins: (1) a physical effect in the mouth (see Section 18.3) and (2) a perceptual interaction effect, i.e. via touch. In this section perceptual data, which can be the result of physicochemical effects and perceptual interactions, are discussed, as well as the current status in the literature on cross-modal texture-taste interactions.

An increase in perceived texture has been found to decrease taste perception. For example, gel hardness (rupture) and gel rigidity (deformability) correlated negatively with sweetness perception of sucrose and aspartame (Bayarri *et al.*, 2007a,b). The sweetness also depended on the nature of the gels; although gellan gels were harder and more rigid, the sweetness intensities were higher than for κ-carrageenan gels. This could be explained by the fact that the gellan gels were more brittle and thus easier to break down in the mouth (see also Section 18.3.1).

The type of thickener has a limited effect on the perceived thickness of a sample. HPMC and native waxy maize starch (amylopectin) gave a similar thickness (Ferry *et al.*, 2006a), although the latter is rapidly degraded by in mouth amylase. Unmodified wheat starch and modified (cross-linked) waxy maize starch were perceived slightly lower in thickness at high viscosities, most likely because of their granular structure. Granular structures are also regarded as having a more pleasant mouthfeel (rather than perceived viscosity) compared with waxy maize or HPMC (Ferry *et al.*, 2006b).

Several measures have been described in the literature to correlate perceived thickness or viscosity with instrumental measurements (Van Vliet, 2002). For example, perceptual data have often been linked to the viscosity measured at a shear rate of 50 s^{-1}, which was taken as an 'average' shear rate for the one in the mouth. However, Malone *et al.* (2003) proposed that higher shear rates (up to 1000 s^{-1}) may be more relevant. The shear rate in the oral cavity is not a constant and is hard to define.

Perceptual data has also been correlated with the so-called Kokini oral shear stress (Ejejalde and Kokini, 1992; Cook *et al.*, 2004; Ferry *et al.*, 2006a), which is based on a 'parallel-plate' model for the mouth (i.e. upper surface of the tongue and the palate) and can be defined as the rate at which a sample thins under increasing rates of shear. Van Vliet (2002) and Ferry *et al.* (2006a), however, argued that shear viscosity and Kokini oral shear stress are only loosely connected to taste and aroma perception. Elongation flows and therefore extensional viscosities are more likely to correlate with mouthfeel and taste perception. Unfortunately, these are more difficult to measure. Furthermore, turbulence may occur for low-viscosity liquids at high shear rates in the mouth, resulting in effective higher evaluated viscosities (Van Vliet, 2002).

Functional magnetic resonance imaging (fMRI) studies have shown that texture, taste and aroma stimuli converge in the same cortical areas in the brain (Cerf-Ducastel *et al.*, 2001; de Araujo and Rolls, 2004; Rolls, 2005), giving a likely explanation for the possibility of texture–aroma and texture–taste interactions. Most studies concerning texture–flavour interactions have dealt with texture–aroma interactions rather than texture–taste interactions. Aroma can be delivered and measured separately from texture and taste (Heilmann and Hummel, 2004; Hummel *et al.*, 2005), which is not possible with the taste modality. As a consequence, perceptual texture–aroma interactions can be studied more easily. Weel *et al.* (2002) attributed the lower-flavour intensity of whey protein gels of increasing hardness to perceptual texture–aroma interactions rather than to physicochemical effects, as the in-nose aroma concentration was the same for all gels. Visschers *et al.* (2006) and Bult *et al.* (2007) have also reported evidence of perceptual texture–aroma interactions. Some of the underlying principles and effects observed for texture–aroma interactions may also be valid for texture–taste ones.

18.5 Integrated sensory response modelling

As shown in Sections 18.3 and 18.4, taste is not only directly linked to the concentration of tastants, but many other parameters influence taste as well.

For product design, of course, it is essential to know which of these parameters influence the taste perception of real, complete products and to which extent. Integrated sensory response modelling (ISRM) has been developed to test hypotheses in this area and to translate theoretical insights into quantitative design rules (Van den Oever, 2003, 2005). The ISRM approach has been applied to cereal products (Van den Oever, 2003) and to spreads on bread (Van den Oever, 2005) and here we show this approach for a study on the taste of mayonnaises and pourable dressings as an example to quantify the relative impact of drivers of taste.

Within Unilever a large taste study was performed with 76 mayonnaises and 192 pourable dressings (including ketchup), focusing on three of the five basic tastes. A range of hypotheses was identified, which resulted both in a list of physical and chemical properties and in a number of psychophysical model shapes (expressed in mathematical equations), which could best represent the relationships tested. The chemical properties generally relate to the composition of the food products, and the physical properties relate to composition, processing and storage factors. This initial step in ISRM generally results in a long list of physical and chemical properties which each represent a hypothesis on a theoretical effect on the sensory attribute under study. Many of these hypotheses will relate to the theory given in Sections 18.3 and 18.4. Each of these hypotheses (identified by product properties) represents an element of theory, a mechanism, and ISRM helps to reveal which element of theory, which mechanism, appears to be relevant for the sensory attribute of a given product under study and which mechanism apparently has no added value in that study. This also may help to identify the mechanisms through which technological solutions for taste problems of a given product might be feasible (or not) and also to what extent the problem could be affected through a given mechanism (definition of the operational window).

In order to preselect chemical and physical properties for entering in a final, integrating model, the statistical significance of each parameter in its relationship with the sensory attribute should be determined. Partial least squares (PLS) analysis with noise addition is a useful tool for this (Centner and Massart, 1996). We extended this technique with an internal cross-validation test and a comparison between parameters based on their correlation coefficient. Only those parameters are selected for a final model which have a high statistical significance and are independent of each other (have relatively low mutual correlation coefficients). This also promotes the selection of truly different mechanisms for the final, integrating multivariate model.

The ISRM model is given by the following equation:

$$T = I + P * E \qquad [18.3]$$

in which T is the taste perception, I is the intercept, P is the proportionality constant and E is the integrated effect of tastants, microstructures, oral processing and interactions (of the hypotheses explained above). I and P are factors determined by the operational scale used by the sensory panel. Mathematical descriptions (submodels) of E for the mayonnaises and pourable dressings tested were combined into one coherent, logically built model consisting of the following, interconnected sub-equations:

$$E_{\text{sour}} = (O * B_{\text{sour}} * \text{TA}_{\text{sour}})^{S\text{sour}} + d * (O * B_{\text{sweet}} * \text{Sug}_{\text{aq}})^{S\text{sweet}} + e * (O * B_{\text{salt}} * \text{Salt}_{\text{aq}})^{S\text{salt}} \quad [18.4]$$

$$E_{\text{sweet}} = (O * B_{\text{sweet}} * \text{Sug}_{\text{sweet}})^{S\text{sweet}} + i * (O * B_{\text{sour}} * \text{TA}_{\text{aq}})^{S\text{sour}} + j * (O * B_{\text{salt}} * \text{Salt}_{\text{aq}})^{S\text{sal}} \quad [18.5]$$

$$E_{\text{salt}} = (O * B_{\text{salt}} * \text{Salt}_{\text{salt}})^{S\text{salt}} + n * (O * B_{\text{sour}} * \text{TA}_{\text{aq}})^{S\text{sour}} + o * (O * B_{\text{sweet}} * \text{Sug}_{\text{aq}})^{S\text{sweet}} \quad [18.6]$$

$$O = 1 - \exp\left[\frac{-q * (100 - \%\ \text{oil})/100 - r}{D_{32}\text{oil}}\right] \quad [18.7]$$

$$B_{\text{sour}} = \exp[f\,(f\text{vis} * \text{viscosity} + fc\text{strain} * \text{crit. strain} + f\text{amylase} * A_{400/50}) \quad [18.8]$$

$$B_{\text{sweet}} = (B_{\text{sour}})^{b\text{sweet}} * \exp[s * \text{crit. stress}] \quad [18.9]$$

$$B_{\text{salt}} = (B_{\text{sour}})^{b\text{salt}} * \exp[t * A_{400/50}] \quad [18.10]$$

$$\text{TA}_{\text{sour}} = \text{TA} * \left(\frac{1 + a * \text{Sug} + b * \text{Salt} + c * \text{Sug} * \text{Salt}}{100 - \%\ \text{oil}}\right) \quad [18.11]$$

$$\text{Sug}_{\text{sweet}} = \text{Sug} * \left(\frac{1 + f * \text{TA} + g * \text{Salt} + h * \text{TA} * \text{Salt}}{100 - \%\ \text{oil}}\right) \quad [18.12]$$

$$\text{Salt}_{\text{salt}} = \text{Salt} * \left(\frac{1 + k * \text{TA} + l * \text{Sug} + m * \text{TA} * \text{Sug}}{100 - \%\ \text{oil}}\right) \quad [18.13]$$

$$\text{TA}_{\text{aq}} = \frac{\text{TA}}{100 - \%\ \text{oil}} \quad [18.14]$$

$$\text{Sug}_{\text{aq}} = \frac{\text{Sug}}{100 - \%\ \text{oil}} \quad [18.15]$$

$$\text{Salt}_{\text{aq}} = \frac{\text{Salt}}{100 - \%\ \text{oil}} \quad [18.16]$$

$$\text{TA} = \text{Titratable acidity (expressed in equivalent acetic acid in mol/l)} \quad [18.17]$$

$$\text{Sug} = \text{equivalent sucrose in mol/l} = (10/342.3) * (\%\ \text{sucrose} + f\text{fruc} * \%\ \text{fructose} + f\text{malt} * \%\ \text{maltose} + f\text{gluc} * \%\ \text{glucose} + f\text{lact} * \%\ \text{lactose} + \Sigma f\text{sw.}\ \%\ \text{sweetener}) \quad [18.18]$$

$$\text{Salt} = [\text{Na in mol/l}] + fK * [K \text{ in mol/l}] \qquad [18.19]$$

in which O is the effect of oil level and droplet size (D_{32}oil) on the 'openness' of the structure, the accessibility of the receptors, B is the breakup effect as result of rheological properties, S is the Stevens' value, $A_{400/50}$ the amylase effect, a–m = constants quantifying the different tastant-tastant interactions, and *f*fruc, fK, etc. are constants quantifying the relative taste effect of the parameter.

Equations 18.4–18.6 indicate that E is an effect of openness, break-up effects, aqueous tastant perception, and their interactions. This is an extension of Stevens' law (equation 18.1). The openness (equation 18.7) is derived from equation 18.2, which indicates the oil hindrance effect of taste receptors by oil and in which we also took into account a possible oil droplet size effect. The break-up effect as a result of oral processing is expressed in equations 18.8–18.10, and related to viscosity parameters and amylase activity. The viscosity was measured at a shear rate of 50 s^{-1}. Here we tested the hypothesis that the viscosity measured at 50 s^{-1} already represented the integration of all viscosity-related effects (including a cognitive interactions with thickness perception) and that the theory and complexity given by the Kokini oral shear stress (see Section 18.4.4) does not provide additional value in this context. The critical strain and stress were obtained from the point in an oscillatory strain sweep (measuring elastic and viscous modulus at 1 Hz as a function of deformation strain), where the elastic and viscous modulus had the same value. The amylase effect ($A_{400/50}$) was the ratio of the flow resistance after and before amylase (see legend of Fig. 18.7 for more information on this). Please note that we found that the break-up effects for sour tastants were different from the ones for sweet and salt. The break-up effects as defined in our study also include the cognitive texture–taste interactions, which may not have the same effects for the three tastes investigated. The tastant concentration which influences sour, sweetness and saltiness is expressed in equations 18.17–18.19. Equations 18.14–18.16 indicate how these concentrations in the aqueous phase are increased by the addition of oil to the product. Finally, equations 18.11–18.13 express the cross-modal tastant effects, corrected by the enhancement of the aqueous phase concentration of the tastants by addition of oil. The theory on taste–taste interaction (Section 18.4.1), which distinguishes oral, peripheral interactions and cognitive, central interactions lead us into two mathematical shapes (submodels) of testing the taste–taste interactions: (a) an effect which involves a multiplication of two concentrations (e.g. the effect of sugar on sourness is proportional both to the sugar and acid level: equations 18.11–18.13) and (b) an effect which is only given by the concentration of the interacting tastant (e.g. here the effect of sugar on sourness is the same at all acid levels and only proportional to sugar level; equations 18.4–18.6).

In the final stage of ISRM, the above model was tested against available data applying advanced mathematical modelling and validation techniques.

Quality criteria applied to reduce the model into the state which could be accepted, included:

- model fit: lowest mean model fit error;
- statistical significance model coefficients;
- cross-validation fit: mean prediction error;
- stability of coefficients in cross-validation;
- maximum simplicity (lowest number of parameters);
- akaike index: penalty for overfitting;
- f-test: statistical significance of more complexity;
- predictability of independent sensory measurements;
- fit with insights from other sources.

ISRM could model the saltiness, sweetness and sourness of mayonnaises and pourable dressings very well (remaining model error approached the sensory measurement error). As an example, Fig. 18.3 gives the result for saltiness of mayonnaises. This final model also identified five 'building blocks' from the initial inventory which, together, dominate and explain measured variation in each of the three taste modalities in the products tested:

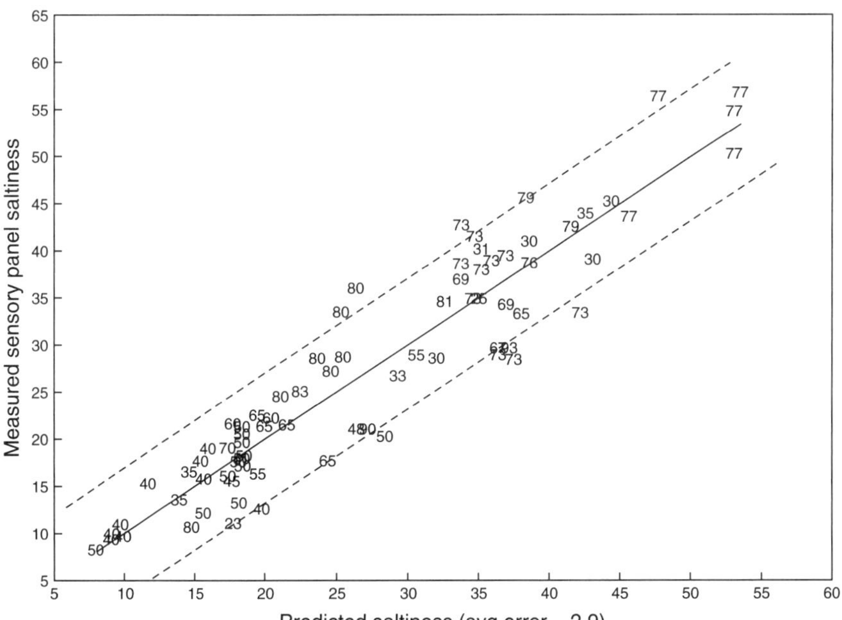

Fig. 18.3 ISRM model for the saltiness of mayonnaises as a function of acid/sugar/salt/oil level plus viscosity, critical strain and amylase thinning. The non-broken line in this figure is fitted to equation 18.3, and the two outer lines indicate the 95% confidence interval.

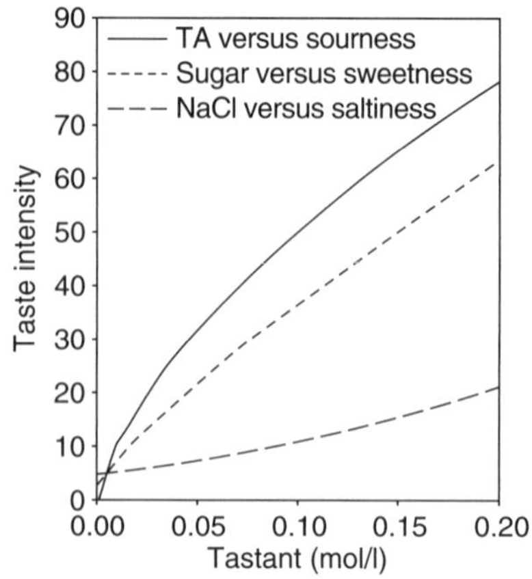

Fig. 18.4 ISRM-identified effect of molar tastant concentration on relative taste intensity of dressings.

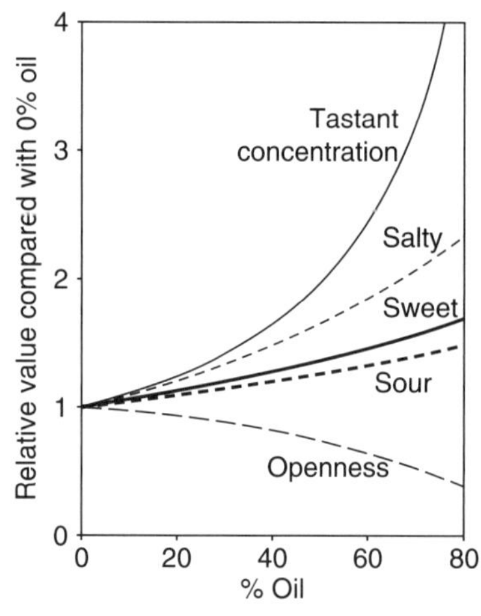

Fig. 18.5 ISRM-identified effect of oil phase volume on accessibility of taste receptors (openness), relative tastant concentration on water phase and on relative intensities of sourness, sweetness and saltiness.

1. *Effects of main tastants* (sugar on sweetness, salts on saltiness, etc.: Fig. 18.4). The Stevens' values quantified were within the ranges reported in literature (Meiselman *et al.*, 1972).

2. *Effects of oil volume fraction* (Fig. 18.5). The presence of oil limits the accessibility of taste receptors (openness) for tastants, and the relative tastant concentration in water and thus the taste perception increased upon addition of oil.

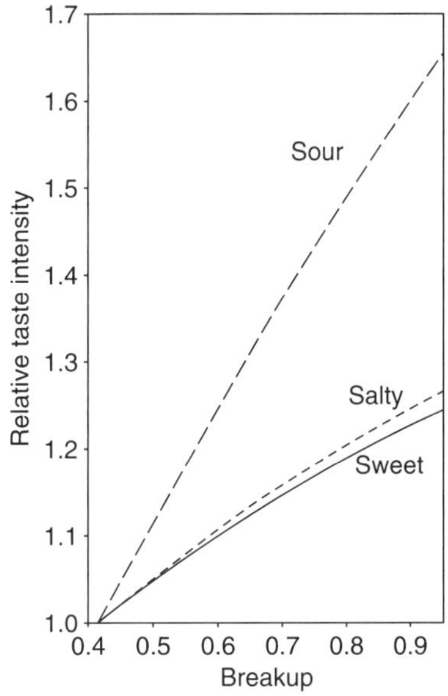

Fig. 18.6 ISRM-identified effect of rheological parameters modelling oral break-up and tastant release of mayonnaises and pourable dressings. Cognitive, texture–taste interactions are probably also taken into account indirectly here.

3. *Effects related to product break-up* (different for each taste: Fig. 18.6). The product break-up is calculated with equations 18.8–18.10, which describe how food products are broken down into smaller pieces in the oral cavity (see Section 18.2) and thereby making tastants available for interacting with the taste receptors. As written before, we found that the break-up effects for sour tastants were different from the ones for sweet and salt. Equations 18.8–18.10 do not describe cross-modal texture–taste effects directly, although we believe they are taken into account by these equations indirectly. If necessary and available in the future, the ISRM approach may take this into account by use of other sub-equations. It is possible that differences in the cross-modal effects are responsible for the different break-up effects found.
4. *Additional rheological effects of amylase breakdown.* These are shown in Fig. 18.7 as a function of the viscosity ratio after and before the addition of amylase. As expected (see Section 18.3.1) reduction in viscosity by amylase breakdown of starch (leading to lower values of the viscosity ratio in Fig. 18.7) resulted in an increase of sweetness and sourness. Surprisingly, this was not found for saltiness. Saltiness increased with decreasing amylase-induced product thinning of the products tested. At the moment, we cannot explain this.

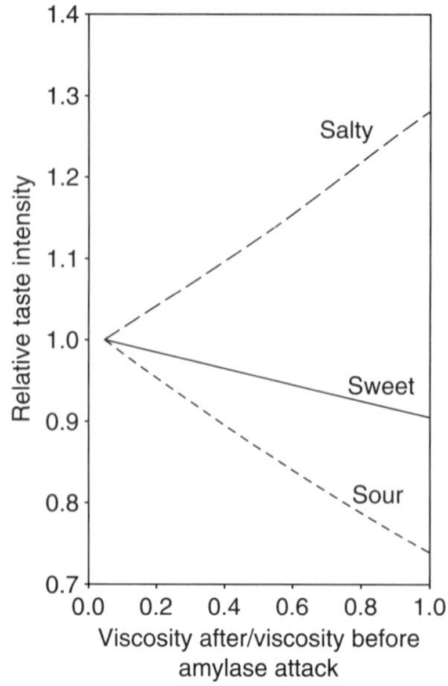

Fig. 18.7 ISRM-identified effect of amylase-induced product breakdown as a function of viscosity before and 400 s after amylase addition on sourness, sweetness and saltiness of mayonnaises and pourable dressings. An amount of 20 grams of each sample was measured within a C-VOR Rheometer from Bohlin Instruments at $1000\,s^{-1}$ and 32 °C. 0.25% of 1 ml fungal amylase solution was added to each sample. A higher value means a smaller amylase effect (and is inversely proportional to starch level).

5. *Cross-modal effects of tastants plus interactions.* As an example, these are shown for reduced oil mayonnaise in Fig. 18.8:
   - Sourness increased with increasing salt level and decreased with increasing sugar level, both independent of acid level (d and e in equation 18.4 were significantly different from zero; a, b and c in equation 18.11 were not).
   - Sweetness decreased with increasing salt level and decreased with increasing acid level, both effects increasing with sugar level (i in equation 18.5 and f, g and h in equation 18.12 were significantly different from zero, j in equation 18.5 was not).
   - Saltiness appeared to decrease with increasing sugar level, proportional to salt level, and to increase with increasing acid level (an effect decreasing with increasing salt level: n in equation 18.6 and k, l and m in equation 18.13 were significantly different from zero, o in equation 18.6 was not). Figure 18.8 also shows that the effect of salt reduction on saltiness can be compensated by sugar reduction and the effect of sugar reduction on sweetness can be compensated by salt reduction.

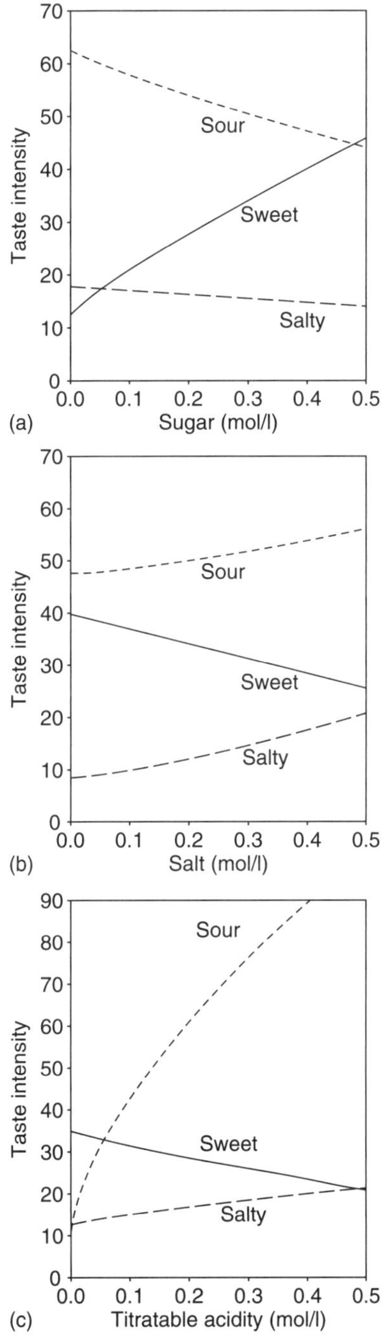

Fig. 18.8 ISRM-identified cross-modal effects of molar concentrations of (a) sugar, (b) salt and (c) titratable activity on sour, sweet and salty intensities of reduced oil mayonnaise.

The following hypotheses were supported by our ISRM analysis:

- The integrating structure of product properties determining basic tastes is the same for mayonnaises (spoonable) and pourable dressings and for tomato ketchup.
- Amylase induced product thinning increases sourness and sweetness (see Fig. 18.7).
- Effects of microstructure and oil level are different for different taste modalities (see Fig. 18.3–18.7).
- Aroma variations used in the pourables tested have negligible effects on basic tastes. Products from a wide varieties of dressings (mayonnaises, pourable dressings and even ketchup) could be used in our current ISRM model, without taking into account possible aroma–taste interactions. This result does not exclude that aroma–taste interactions may occur with other aroma variations and other products, as has been reported before (see Section 18.4.2).

The following hypotheses could not be confirmed by our analysis:

- On a molar basis, potassium ions contribute less to taste effects than sodium ions. We were interested in the molar saltiness of potassium ions versus sodium ones in order to compare these values with possible activation values of salt receptors if they might come available.
- Amylase-induced product thinning increases saltiness. The opposite was found (see Fig. 18.7), which cannot bc cxplaincd at this moment.
- Larger oil droplet sizes increase taste perception. We found no effect of oil droplet size in our studies (r in equation 18.7 was not significantly different from zero).

The novel ISRM approach presented here can be easily extended with other sub-equations to test other hypotheses as explained in Sections 18.3 and 18.4 or new ones in the future. Using this approach, we have acquired a better scientific understanding and quantification of tastants, aromas and food structures, and their interactions within real food products. Effects studied in isolation with aqueous (thickened) model solutions were not always relevant for fully formulated products.

The insights obtained by ISRM are actionable in several ways: the potential scope of different technological solutions for taste challenges follows directly from the relative impact of the building block on which each solution acts upon. We have also tested over 20 commercial sourness maskers and sucrose replacers in our ISRM approach (data not shown). We had to conclude that sourness maskers operate only through known sweetness effects of sugars within these samples. The relative sweetness value of sucrose replacers were within ranges given in the literature.

Further, ISRM allows us to predict basic tastes, and predictive models for all basic tastes are now via advanced IT tools available to Unilever product developers worldwide to speed up product development, also allowing the design of better-tasting low salt, low sugar and low-fat products, evaluating novel flavour maskers or enhancers, and/or cost-saving by reduction of fat.

18.6 Future trends

As discussed in the introduction and shown in the other parts of this chapter, the lowering of fat, sugar and salt levels in food products for health reasons has a large impact on flavour perception. Fortunately, as documented in this chapter, the directly linked taste attributes of sweetness and saltiness can also be influenced by other product properties than sugar or salt level, respectively. Still, closing the sensory gap caused by sugar or salt reduction often appears to be not straightforward and easy in product design. Such a reduction influences interdependently all five tastes and other sensory attributes in different ways. The ISRM approach developed within Unilever quantifies these interdependent influences and allows us to speed up product development, design healthy and better tasting low-fat, low-salt and low-sugar products, evaluate novel flavour maskers or enhancers, and/or allow cost-saving by reduction of fat.

In the future, this kind of approach will be further optimised by using advanced mathematical methods and by applying new insights to the mathematical models developed. Advanced mathematical methods could be the Full Information Maximum Likelihood method (Csiszar and Matus, 2008) and the MARS technique (Friedman, 1991). New insights might be obtained by the design of novel food structures, identification of healthy and cost-effective tastant replacers, use of taste receptor and neurophysiological studies in relation to taste (Marciani *et al.*, 2006), use of improved *in vitro* mouth models to determine tastant release from foods upon mastication (e.g. Salles *et al.*, 2007), multivariate psychophysics, role of genetics to determine whether or not human preference for taste is partly genetically determined, perception and preference of taste of the children, teenagers, adults and elderly (e.g. Zandstra and De Graaf, 1998; Mojet *et al.*, 2001, 2004), consumer studies, etc. Temporal delivery of stimuli is also thought to be highly important for the actual perception (e.g. Buettner *et al.*, 2008), as was demonstrated for example by Baek *et al.* (1999) and Linforth *et al.* (2007) who correlated the rate of aroma change in nose to perception. Recently, we have demonstrated the impact of tastant (salt) delivery profile on perception (Busch *et al.*, 2009). These pieces of evidence suggest the relevance of contrast in perception, which is in line with the general view on receptors as contrast detectors (Alberts *et al.*, 1994). Post-ingestive effects of tastants might be another factor to consider. For example, De Araujo *et al.* (2008) found that mice lacking sweetness perception still preferred water with sucrose over water with sucralose, although the sweetness was the same. This was attributed to the fact that sucrose intake induced dopamine release in the ventral striatum of the sweet-blind mice, which is associated with the receipt of palatable rewards.

18.7 References

ALBERTS B, BRAY D, LEWIS J, RAFF M, ROBERTS K and WATSON J D (1994), 'Cell signalling', in Alberts B, Bray D, Lewis J, Raff M, Roberts K and Watson J D, *Molecular Biology of the Cell*, New York, Garland Publishing Inc., 721–785.

APPELQVIST I A M, GOLDING M, VREEKER R and ZUIDAM N J (2007), 'Emulsions as delivery systems in Foods', in Lakkis J M, *Encapsulation and Controlled Release: Technologies in Food systems*, Ames, Blackwell Publishing, 41–81.

ARVIDSON K (1976), 'Scanning electron-microscopy of fungiform papillae on tongue of man and monkey', *Acta Oto-laryngol*, **81**(5–6), 496–502.

BAEK I, LINFORTH RST, BLAKE A, *et al.* (1999), 'Sensory perception is related to the rate of change of volatile concentration in-nose during eating of model gels', *Chem. Senses*, **24**(2), 155–160.

BAINES Z V and MORRIS E R (1987), 'Flavour/taste perception in thickened systems: the effect of guar gum above and below *c**', *Food Hydrocolloids*, **1**(3), 197–205.

BAYARRI S, RIVAS I, COSTELL E and DURÁN L (2001), 'Diffusion of sucrose and aspartame in kappa-carrageenan and gellan gum gels', *Food Hydrocolloids*, **15**, 67–73.

BAYARRI S, IZQUIERDO L and COSTELL E (2007a), 'Sweetening power of aspartame in hydrocolloids gels: influence of texture', *Food Hydrocolloids*, **21**, 1265–1274.

BAYARRI S, RIVAS I, IZQUIERDO L and COSTELL E (2007b), 'Influence of texture on the temporal perception of sweetness of gelled systems', *Food Res. Int.*, **40**, 900–908.

BINGHAM, A F, BIRCH G G, DE GRAAF C, BEHAN J M and PERRING K D (1990), 'Sensory studies with sucrose–maltol mixtures', *Chem. Senses*, **15**(4), 447–456.

BLISSETT A, HORT J and TAYLOR A J (2006), 'Influence of chewing and swallowing behavior on volatile release in two confectionery systems', *J. Texture Studies*, **37**, 476–496.

BRESLIN P A and BEAUCHAMP G K (1997), 'Salt enhances flavour by suppressing bitterness', *Nature*, **387**, 563.

BROUWER J N and WIERSMA A (1980), 'Stimulus-induced appearance of proteinaceous material in the taste pore', in Starre van der H, ed. *Olfaction and Taste*, London, IRL Press, 179–182.

BUETTNER A, OTTO S, BEER A *et al.* (2008), 'Dynamics of retronasal aroma perception during consumption: cross-linking on-line breath analysis with medico-analytical tools to elucidate a complex process', *Food Chem.*, **108**(4), 1234–1246.

BULT J H F, DE WIJK R A and HUMMEL T (2007), 'Investigation on multimodal sensory integration: texture, taste, and othro- and retronasal olfactory stimuli in concert', *Neurosci. Lett.*, **411**(1), 6–10.

BUSCH J L H C, TOURNIER C, KNOOP J E, KOOYMAN G, and SMIT G. (2009), 'Temporal contrast of salt delivery in mouth increases salt perception', *Chem. Senses*, **34**, 341–348.

CENTNER V and MASSART D-L (1996), 'Elimination of uninformative variables for multivariate calibration', *Anal. Chem.*, **68**, 3851–3858.

CERF-DUCASTEL B, VAN DE MOORTELE P-F, MACLEOD P, LE BIHAN D and FAURION A (2001), 'Interaction of gustatory and lingual somatosensory perceptions at the cortical level in the human: a functional magnetic resonance imaging study', *Chem. Senses*, **26**, 371–383.

CHANDRASHEKAR J, HOON M A, RYBA N J P and ZUKER C S (2006), 'The receptors and cells for mammalian taste', *Nature*, **444**(16), 288–294.

CLYDESDALE F M (1993), 'Color as a factor in food choice', *Crit. Rev. Food Sci. Nutr.*, **33**(1), 83–101.

COOK D J, HOLLOWOOD T A, LINFORTH R S T and TAYLOR A J (2002), 'Perception of taste intensity in solutions of random-coil polysaccharides above and below *c**', *Food Qual. Pref.*, **13**, 473–480.

COOK D J, HOLLOWOOD T A, PETTELOT E and TAYLOR A J (2004), '*Effects of Viscosity on Flavor Perception: A Multimodal Approach*', *ACS Symposium Series*, Washington, DC, American Chemical Society, 240–253.

CSISZAR I and MATUS F (2008), 'Generalized maximum likelihood estimates for exponential families', *Prob. Theory Related Fields*, **141**, 213–246.

DA CONCEICAO NETA E R, JOHANNINGSMEIER S D and MCFEETERS R F (2007), 'The chemistry and physiology of sour taste – a review', *J. Food Sci.*, **72**(2), R33–R38.

DALTON P, DOOLITTLE N, NAGATA H and BRESLIN P A S (2000), 'The merging of the senses: integration of subthreshold taste and smell', *Nat. Neurosci.*, **3**, 431–432.

DAVIDSON J M, LINFORTH R S, HOLLOWOOD T A and TAYLOR A J (1999), 'Effect of sucrose on the perceived flavor intensity of chewing gum', *J. Agric. Food Chem.*, **47**, 4336–4340.

DE ARAUJO I E and ROLLS E T (2004), 'Representation in the human brain of food texture and oral fat', *J. Neurosci.*, **24**(12), 3086–3093.

DE ARAUJO I E, OLIVIERA-MAIA A J, SOTNIKOVA T D, GAINETDINOV R R, CARON M G, NICOLELIS M A L and SIMON S A (2008), 'Food reward in the absence of taste receptor signaling', *Neuron* **57**, 930–941.

DELWICHE J (2004), 'The impact of perceptual interactions on perceived flavor', *Food Qual. Pref.*, **15**, 137–146.

DESAI K G H and PARK H J (2005), 'Recent developments in microencapsulation of food ingredients', *Drying Technol.*, **23**, 1361–1394.

DJORDJEVIC J, ZATORRE R J and JONES-GOTMAN M (2004), 'Odor-induced changes in taste perception', *Exp. Brain Res.*, **159**, 405–408.

DÖTSCH M, BUSCH J L H C, BATENBURG A M, LIEM G, TAREILUS E, MUELLER R and MEIJER G (2009), 'Strategies to reduce sodium consumption; a food industry perspective', *Crit. Rev. Food Sci. Nutr.*, in press.

DUBOSE C N, CARDELLO A V and MALLER O (1980), 'Effects of colorants and flavorants on identification, perceived flavor intensity, and hedonic quality of fruit-flavored beverages and cake', *J. Food Sci.*, **45**, 1393–1399.

ELEJALDE C C and KOKINI J L (1992), 'The psychophysics of pouring, spreading and in-mouth viscosity', *J. Texture Studies*, **23**(3), 315–336.

FERRY A L, HORT J, MITCHELL J R, COOK D J, LAGARRIGUE S and VALLES PAMIES B (2004), 'Effect of amylase activity on starch paste viscosity and its implications for flavor perception', *J. Texture Studies*, **35**, 511–524.

FERRY A L, HORT J, MITCHELL J R, COOK D J, LAGARRIGUE S and VALLES PAMIES B (2006a), 'Viscosity and flavour perception: why is starch different from hydrocolloids', *Food Hydrocolloids*, **20**, 855–862.

FERRY A L, MITCHELL J R, HORT J, HILL S E, TAYLOR A J, LAGARRIGUE S and VALLES PAMIES B (2006b), 'In-mouth amylase activity can reduce perception of saltiness in starch-thickened foods', *J. Agric. Food Chem.*, **54**, 8869–8873.

FRANK R A, VAN DER KLAAUW N J and SCHIFFERSTEIN H N (1993), 'Both perceptual and conceptual factors influence taste-odor and taste-taste interactions', *Percept. Psychophys.*, **54**, 343–354.

FRIEDMAN J H (1991), 'Multivariate adaptive regression splines', *Annals Statistics*, **1**(19), 1–141.

HASLAM E (1998), *Practical Polyphenols – From Structure to Molecular Recognition and Physiological Action*, Cambridge: CambridgeUniversity Press.

HEILMANN S and HUMMEL T A (2004), 'New method for comparing orthonasal and retronasal olfaction', *Behav. Neurosci.*, **118**, 412–419.

HOLLOWOOD T A, LINFORTH R S T and TAYLOR A J (2002), 'The effect of viscosity on the perception of flavour', *Chem. Senses*, **27**, 583–591.

HORT J and HOLLOWOOD T A (2004), 'Controlled continuous flow delivery system for investigating taste–aroma interactions', *J. Agric. Food Chem.*, **52**, 4834–4843.

HUMMEL T, HEILMANN S, LANDIS, B N, REDEN J, FRASNELLI J, SMALL D M and GERBER J (2005), 'Perceptual differences between chemical stimuli presented through the ortho- or retronasal route', *Flav. Fragr. J.*, **21**, 42–47.

JOHNSON D L, DZENDOLET E, DAMON R, SAWYER M and CLYDESDALE F M (1982), 'Psychophysical relationships between perceived sweetness and colour in cherry-flavoured beverages', *J. Food Prot.*, **45**(7), 601–606.

KATSURAGI Y, SUGIURA Y, LEE C, OTSUJI K and KURIHARA K (1995) Selective inhibition of bitter taste of various drugs by lipoprotein, *Pharm. Res.*, **12**(5), 658–662

KEAST R S J and BRESLIN P A S (2002), 'An overview of binary taste–taste interactions', *Food Qual. Pref.*, **14**, 111–124.

KEAST R S J and ROPER J (2007), 'Complex relationship among chemical concentration, detection threshold, and suprathreshold intensity of bitter compounds', *Chem. Senses*, **32**, 245–253.

KEAST R S J, BRESLIN P A S and BEAUCHAMP G K (2001), 'Suppression of bitterness using sodium salts', *Chimia*, **55**, 441–447.

KEAST R S J, CANTY T M and BRESLIN P A S (2004a), 'The influence of sodium salts on binary mixtures of bitter-tasting compounds', *Chem. Senses*, **29**, 431–439.

KEAST R S J, DALTON P H, and BRESLIN P A S (2004b), 'Flavor interactions at the sensory level', in Taylor A J and Roberts D D, *Flavor Perception*, Ames, Blackwell Publishing, 228–295.

KOKINI J L, BISTANY K, POOLE M *et al.* (1982), 'Use of mass-transfer theory to predict viscosity–sweetness interactions of fructose and sucrose solutions containing tomato solids', *J. Texture Studies*, **13**(2), 187–200.

KROEZE J H and BARTOSHUK L M (1985), 'Bitterness suppression as revealed by split-tongue taste stimulation in humans', *Physiol. Behav.*, **35**, 779–783.

LINFORTH R S T, PEARSON K S K and TAYLOR A J (2007), '*In vivo* flavor release from gelatin–sucrose gels containing droplets of flavor compounds', *J. Agric. Food Chem.*, **55**, 7859–7863.

LYNCH J, LIU J-H, MELA D J and MACFIE H (1993), 'A time–intensity study of the effect of oil mouthcoatings on taste perception', *Chem. Senses*, **18**, 121–129.

MALONE, M E, APPELQVIST I A M and NORTON I T (2003), 'Oral behaviour of food hydrocolloids and emulsions. Part 2. Taste and aroma release', *Food Hydrocolloids*, **17**, 775–784.

MARCIANI L, PFEIFFER J C, HORT J, HEAD K, BUSH D, TAYLOR A J, SPILLER R C, FRANCIS S and GOWLAND P A (2006), 'Improved methods for fMRI studies of combined taste and aroma stimuli', *J. Neurosci. Methods*, **158**, 186–194.

MCMILLAN M D (1980), 'Transmission and scanning electron microscope studies on the surface coat of the oral mucosa in the rat', *J. Periodontal Res.*, **15**(3), 288–296.

MEISELMAN H L, BOSE H E and NYKVIST W F (1972), 'Magnitude production and magnitude estimation of taste intensity', *Perception Psychophys.*, **12**, 2B, 249.

MOJET J, CHRIST-HAZELHOF E and HEIDEMA J (2001), 'Taste perception with age: generic or specific losses in threshold sensitivity to the five basic tastes?', *Chem. Senses*, **26**, 845–860.

MOJET J, CHRIST-HAZELHOF E and HEIDEMA J (2004), 'Effect of concentration on taste–taste interactions in foods for elderly and young subjects', *Chem. Senses*, **26**, 845–860.

MORROT G, BROCHET F and DUBOURDIEU D (2001), 'The color of odors', *Brain Language*, **79**, 309–320.

NOBLE A C (1996), 'Taste–aroma interactions', *Trends Food Sci. Technol.*, **7**(12), 439–444.

PANGBORN R M (1960), 'Taste interrelationships', *Food Res.*, **25**, 245–256.

PFEIFFER J C, HOLLOWOOD, T A, HORT J and TAYLOR A J (2005), 'Temporal synchrony and integration of sub-threshold taste and smell signals', *Chem. Senses*, **30**, 539–545.

PRESCOTT J (1999), 'Flavour as a psychological construct: implications for perceiving and measuring the sensory qualities of foods', *Food Qual. Pref.*, **10**, 349–356.

PRESCOTT J, JOHNSTONE V and FRANCIS J (2004), 'Odor–taste interactions: effects of attentional strategies during exposure', *Chem. Senses*, **29**, 331–340.

PRIPP A H, BUSCH J and VREEKER R (2004), 'Effect of viscosity, sodium caseinate and oil on bitterness perception of olive oil phenolics', *Food Qual. Pref.*, **15**, 375–382.

ROLLS E T (2005), 'Taste, olfactory, and food texture processing in the brain, and the control of food intake', *Physiol. Behavi.*, **85**(1), 45–56.

ROPER S D (2006), 'Signaling in the chemosensory systems', *Cell. Mol. Life Sci.*, **63**, 1494–1500.

ROSETT T, SHIRLEY L, KLEIN B P and SCHMIDT S J (1994), 'Na+ binding as measured by 23Na nuclear magnetic resonance spectroscopy influences the perception of saltiness in gum solutions', *J. Food Sci.*, **59**, 206–210.

ROSETT T R, KENDREGAN S L, GAO Y, SCHMIDT S J and KLEIN B P (1996), 'Thickening agents effects on sodium binding and other taste qualities of soup systems', *J. Food Sci.*, **61**, 1099–1104.

SAKAI N, KOBAYAKAWA T, GOTOW N, SAITO S and IMADA S (2001), 'Enhancement of sweetness ratings of aspartame by a vanilla odor presented either by orthonasal or retronasal routes', *Percept. Motor Skills*, **92**, 1002–1008.

SALLES C, TARREGA A, MIELLE P, MARATRAY J, GORRIA P, LIABOEUF J and LIODENOT J J (2007), 'Development of a chewing simulator for food breakdown and the analysis of *in vitro* flavor compound release in a mouth environment', *J. Food Eng.*, **82**, 189–198.

SAUVAGEOT F, NGUYEN H D and VALENTIN D (2000), 'Les mots évoquent – ils des saveur? Une comparaison entre étudiants de France, du Vietnam et des U.S.A', *Sci. Aliments*, **20**, 491–522.

SCHIFFERSTEIN H N and VERLEGH P W (1996), 'The role of congruency and pleasantness in odor-induced taste enhancement', *Acta Psychol.*, **94**, 87–105.

SHAMIL S, WYETH L J and KILCAST D (1991), 'Flavour release and perception in reduced fat foods', *Food Qual. Pref.*, **3**(1), 51–60.

STEVENS S S (1975), *Psychophysics: Introduction to its Perceptual, Neural and Social Prospects*, Wiley, New York.

STOKES J R and DAVIES G A (2007), 'Viscoelasticity of human whole saliva collected after acid and mechanical stimulation', *Biorheology*, **44**, 141–160.

SZENTE L and SZEJTLI J (2004), 'Cyclodextrins as food ingrdients', *Trends Food Sci. Technol.*, **15**, 137–142.

TALAVERA K, YASUMATSU K, YOSHIDA R, MARGOLSKEE, R F, VOETS T, NINOMIYA Y and NILIUS B (2007), 'The taste transduction channel TRPM5 is a locus for bitter–sweet taste interactions', *FASEB J.*, **22**, 1–13.

TAREILUS E (2000), 'The taste of salt', Unilever Research Prize 1999, Unilever Research Vlaardingen, 14–17.

TOURNIER C, SULMONT-ROSSÉ and GUICHARD E (2007), 'Flavour perception: aroma, taste and texture interactions', *Food,* **1**(2), 246–257.

VALENTOVA H and POKORNY J (1998), 'Effect of edible oils and oil emulsions on the perception of basic tastes', *Nahrung*, **42**(6), 406–408.

VAN AKEN G A, VINGERHOEDS M H and DE HOOG E H A (2007), 'Food colloids under oral conditions', *Curr. Opin. Colloid Interface Sci.*, **12**, 251–262.

VAN DEN OEVER G J (2003), 'Integrated sensory response (ISR) modeling: a new methodology to understand and predict sensory attributes in terms of physical properties', *Cereal Chem.*, **80**(4), 409–418.

VAN DEN OEVER G J (2005), 'Fat reduction in foods: microstructure control of oral texture, taste and aroma in reduced oil systems', in: *Food Lipids: Chemistry, Flavor and Texture*, F. Shahidi and H. Weenen, *ACS Symposium Series*, vol. 920(14), Washington, DC, American chemical society, 171–189.

VAN DER KLAAUW N J and SMITH D V (1995), 'Taste quality profiles for fiftheen organic and inorganic salt', *Physiol. Behav.*, **58**(2), 295–306.

VAN VLIET T (2002), 'On the relation between texture perception and fundamental mechanical parameters for liquids and time dependent solids', *Food Qual. Pref.*, **13**(4), 227–236.

VISSCHERS R W, JACOBS M A, FRASNELLI J, HUMMEL T, BURGERING M and BOELRIJK A E M (2006), 'Cross-modality of texture and aroma perception is independent of orthonasal or retronasal stimulation', *J. Agric. Food Chem.*, **54** (15), 5509–5515.

WEEL K G C, BOELRIJK E M, ALTING A C, VAN MIL P J J M, BURGER J J, GRUPPEN H, VORAGEN A G J and SMIT G (2002), 'Flavour release and perception of flavoured whey protein gels: perception is determined by texture rather than by release', *J. Agric. Food Chem.*, **50**, 5149–5155.

WENDIN K, ELLEKJAER M R and SOLHEIM R (1999), 'Fat content and homogenization effects of flavour and texture of mayonnaise with added aroma', *Food Sci. Technol. Lebensmittel Wissenschaft and Technologie*, **32**, 377–383.

WILSON C E and BROWN W E (1997), 'Influence of food matrix structure and oral breakdown during mastication on temporal perception of flavor', *J. Sensory Studies*, **12**(1), 69–86.

WORLD HEALTH ORGANIZATION (2004), 'Global strategy on diet, physical activity, and health', *World Health Assembly (WHA57.17)* held on 22 May 2004.

WORLD HEALTH ORGANIZATION (2007), *Reducing Salt Intake in Populations*, Report of a WHO Forum and Technical Meeting, WHO Document Production Services, Geneva.

YAMAMOTO Y and NAKABAYASHI M (1999), 'Enhancing effect of an oil phase on the sensory intensity of salt taste of NaCl in oil/water emulsions', *J. Food Texture Stud.*, **30**, 581–590.

ZELLNER D A and KAUTZ M A (1990), 'Color affects perceived odor intensity', *J. Exp. Psychol.: Human Percept. Perform.*, **16**(2), 391–397.

ZANDSTRA E H and DE GRAAF C (1998), 'Sensory perception and pleasantness of orange beverages from childhood to old age', *Food Qual. Pref.*, **9**, 5–12.

19

Oral processing and perception of food emulsions: the relevance for fat reduction in food

G. A. van Aken and E. H. A. de Hoog, TI Food and Nutrition, The Netherlands and NIZO Food Research, The Netherlands; and M. H. Vingerhoeds, TI Food and Nutrition, The Netherlands and Wageningen University and Research Centre, The Netherlands

Abstract: The textural sensory functionality of emulsion droplets in foods is largely due to their effect on the rheological behaviour (such as viscosity and fracture behaviour), and importantly also to their effects on friction between the oral surfaces and on lubrication of the food bolus. Crucial in this is that much of this functionality is dependent on structural changes in the food emulsions that occur upon processing in the mouth. This chapter gives an overview of the main topics relevant for understanding the role of fat in the textural sensory perception of food emulsions, and discusses strategies to compensate for the sensory loss that accompanies fat reduction.

Key words: texture of food emulsion, sensory perception, fat perception, creaminess, fat reduction, fat content in food, oral processing.

19.1 Introduction

Emulsion droplets strongly affect the sensory perception of food material not only by their role in the overall rheological behaviour, but also by their interaction with the oral environment. One of the consequences is that a full understanding of the sensory properties of a food emulsion can be obtained only by including the way the structure is changed upon processing in the mouth. Another consequence is that it is possible to gain control of the sensory efficacy of emulsified fat in food products by making specific engineering choices.

This chapter is mainly based on our pioneering study on the role of oral processing on the perception of food emulsions at TI Food and Nutrition (previously named Wageningen Centre for Food Sciences; WCFS),

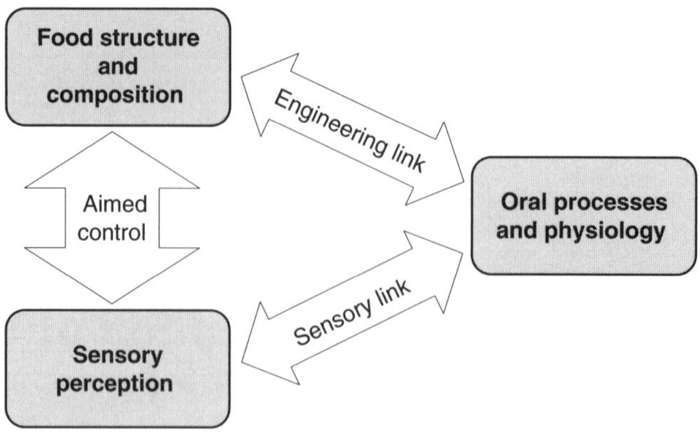

Fig. 19.1 Diagram sketching the role of knowledge on oral processes and physiology for achieving the aimed sensory control by modification of food structure and composition.

motivated by previous studies focusing on oral processing of mainly solid food systems (Hutchings and Lillford, 1988; Lucas *et al.*, 2002), and sensory studies on mayonnaise and custards (De Wijk *et al.*, 2003). The overall objective of this chapter is to present mechanistic understanding of factors and processes determining emulsion-related sensory attributes relevant for the oral perception of compound food systems and the way this knowledge can be used to engineer these systems with respect to sensory quality. Control of sensory perception of a food emulsion can be obtained by modifying the structure and composition of the emulsions. However, in-mouth sensory perception of a food system depends on the structure, composition and behaviour of the food system during processing in the mouth rather than before it is taken in the mouth. Therefore, the aimed sensory control can only be obtained by taking into account the physiology of the mouth and the way the food system is processed in the mouth. This is illustrated in Fig. 19.1.

This chapter is organised as follows. Section 19.2 starts with a general description of the interaction of foods with the oral environment, focusing mainly on tactile sensations. The special role of emulsion droplets is highlighted in more detail in the next subsections. Using the mechanistic understanding described in Section 19.2, Section 19.3 discusses a number of 'engineering' control variables that affect the efficacy by which reduced fat food products can impart a full fat 'creamy' taste. To conclude, some future trends on the role of fat in food products are discussed in Section 19.4.

19.2 Behaviour and perception of emulsions in the oral environment

19.2.1 Mastication and sensing of food in the mouth

The oral cavity forms the first chamber of the digestive tract, where food is mechanically broken up into smaller pieces and mixed with saliva, forming a slippery bolus that can safely pass through the pharynx and oesophagus to the stomach (Hutchings and Lillford, 1988). An important function of the mouth as the portal to the digestive tract is the control of the quality and safety of food by the various sensory receptors. Examples of these receptors are the taste buds on the tongue, the flavour receptors located in the nose and the pressure, stress and heat sensors located in the oral tissues.

This sensing occurs during the whole process of mastication. For solid or semi-solid foods aspects of the temperature and fracture behaviour are sensed during the 'first bite' stage, followed by the 'masticatory' stage, during which the product is processed into a swallowable food bolus, consisting of particles of the broken down food material stuck together by saliva (Brandt *et al.*, 1963; Lucas *et al.*, 2002). This stage is very important for perception. The brittleness of solid products will determine how fast the product is broken up by grinding between the teeth or squeezing between tongue and palate into sufficiently small particles. The temperature of the food material will gradually adapt to the mouth temperature, which can induce important structural changes such as the melting of fat crystals and gelatine gels. Volatile flavours (aromas) are partially dissolved in the saliva and released in the air, reaching the nose retro-nasally (Van Ruth and Roozen, 2000; Malone *et al.*, 2003). Non-volatile flavours (tastants) are dissolved in saliva and then reach the taste buds in the tongue. The rheological properties of the food material are monitored during mastication by both the ease of spontaneous flow through the mouth and the tongue pressure needed to make it flow. Finally, the tongue is rubbed against remaining food particles, palate and teeth. This provides tribological information on the smoothness of the food bolus, the presence, size and shape of small 'gritty' particles in the bolus, and the degree of lubrication of the oral surfaces (Engelen *et al.*, 2005). In the 'swallowing stage' the ease of swallowing gives information about the overall fluidity of the product, and in the final stage, after swallowing, the mouth is cleaned by saliva and tongue movements, and the persistence of food remnants and adsorbed layers on the oral surfaces are sensed (Brandt *et al.*, 1963).

Since the in-mouth sensory quality of a food product is determined by the set of aspects sensed during oral processing, detailed knowledge of the way food products interact with the oral environment is needed for a full understanding and control of this quality. Upon consumption, food emulsions come into contact with saliva. Saliva is a complex heterogeneous biological fluid, composed of proteins, electrolytes, small organic compounds and water (Zalewska *et al.*, 2000; Humphrey and Williamson, 2001; Van Nieuw Amerongen *et al.*, 2004). Proteins include α-amylase, serum albumin, immunoglobulins (sIgA), cystatins, lysozyme, histatins, a group of proline-rich proteins (PRP) and highly glycosylated salivary mucins (MUC5B and MUC7). Salivary mucins belong to a family of molecules composed of disulphide-linked, negatively charged protein monomers containing heavily glycosylated domains, interspersed with less glycosylated ones. These glycoproteins, especially MUC5B, are responsible for the typical viscoelastic behaviour of saliva. The amount and composition of human saliva are affected by many factors, such as the flow rate, time of the day, type and size of the gland, duration and type of the stimulus, diet, drugs, age and sex. For a review on saliva properties, we refer to a recent review of Schipper and co-workers (2007).

Saliva is produced in and secreted by three pairs of major salivary glands, i.e. parotid glands (PAR; ear), submandibular glands (SM), and sublingual glands (SL; under the tongue), and numerous minor ones present in the mucosa (epithelial surface plus adherent mucous layer) of the tongue (von Ebner glands), cheeks, lips and palate (PAL). The glands differ in the type of secretion they produce, which is determined by the ratio of serous to mucous cells. Serous cells (PAR, SM, PAL, lingual) secrete a watery fluid, essentially devoid of mucin; this secretion is strongly activated by stimuli. Mucous cells (SM, SL, labial, PAL, lingual) produce a very mucin-rich secretion, which is viscous and more or less elastic; this secretion continues during resting. The mucin concentration in whole saliva is about 200 μg/ml (ranging from 30 to >500 μg/ml, depending on the stimulus), i.e. 10–25% of all saliva proteins (Fox *et al.*, 1985). Saliva components, like mucins, are known to be able to interact with themselves and a range of other components. These components include, amongst others, proteins, surfactants, bacteria, lipids and tannins. In this way a complex three-dimensional structure is formed (Glantz *et al.*, 1989; Glantz, 1997).

The epithelial surfaces of tongue and palate consist of stratified squalors epithelium (Keeton and McFadden, 1967). Like in skin epidermis, the epithelium is constantly renewing, with dead cells flaking-off from the top layer. The epithelial surfaces are normally covered by a mucous layer with a mean thickness of 50–100 μm (Wolff and Kleinberg, 1998), largely formed by the interaction with saliva, which retains the surface moist and protects the underlying tissue. The gel properties of this layer are attributed to entanglements of mainly the MUC5B mucin (Glantz *et al.*, 1996; Glantz, 1997; Wickström *et al.*, 1998), mediated by hydrophobic interaction (Bromberg and Barr, 2000), carbohydrate–carbohydrate interactions and calcium-mediated crosslinks (Raynal *et al.*, 2003).

The upper (dorsal) surface of the tongue is covered by papillae, which contain the taste buds (Keeton and McFadden, 1967). The most abundant type of papilla is the papillae filiformis (Leonhardt, 1971). These papillae do not contain taste buds or secretory cells. They cover almost the whole tongue surface and give the tongue its roughness, thus allowing food handling (Kessel and Kardon, 1979), and they also contain the mechanoreceptors which are involved in the sense of touch on the surface of the tongue. Trulsson and co-workers have measured the sensitivity and spatial distribution of three main types of mechanoreceptors (Trulsson and Essick, 1997).

Oral tactile sensations of food systems depend on the forces sensed by the mechanoreceptors in the mouth. Several publications related fracturing of food gels and diminution of the gel particle size (Hutchings and Lillford,

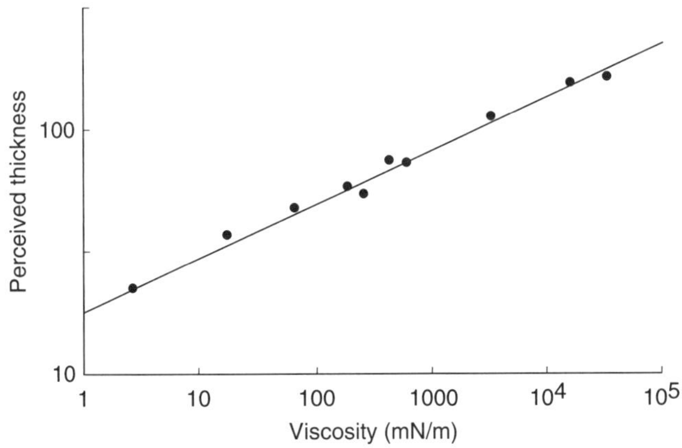

Fig. 19.2 Perceived thickness as a function of viscosity of Newtonian solutions. Best fit through the data points: perceived thickness = 81(viscosity (mN/m))$^{0.22}$. Adapted from Cutler *et al.* (1983).

1988; Lucas *et al.*, 2002) and viscous flow of food liquids (Shama and Sherman, 1973; Cutler *et al.*, 1983; Morris, 1995) to perceived hardness, thickness and creaminess. As an example, Cutler *et al.* (1983) showed for a broad range of Newtonian fluids (mainly solutions of small carbohydrates) that an increase in rated thickness is related to an increase in viscosity (Fig. 19.2).

Generally, whether emulsified fat or oil is present or not, food systems are described by the same set of panel-defined sensory attributes. In general, it turns out to be very difficult to obtain a complete match of the sensory attributes between systems that do contain fat or oil and those that do not. In other words, even though emulsified fat or oil can be replaced by other compounds to restore the intensity of each individual fat-related attribute, a complete match of the whole profile of tactile attributes is not obtained.

For an emulsion without thickener, an increase in the oil content leads to an increase in rated thickness and creaminess (Akhtar *et al.*, 2005; Vingerhoeds *et al.*, 2008). However, this increase is not proportional between the two attributes; initially the rated creaminess increases more than the rated thickness (Fig. 19.3), based on systems given in Table 19.1. Only if the fat content of the emulsion is higher than a certain minimum value (in the order of a percent, but probably dependent on the system), the rated creaminess is roughly proportional to the rated thickness (rising branch in Fig. 19.3). At zero fat, the thickness ratings increased with the viscosity (which varies in these systems by a variation in protein and starch content), but the creaminess ratings remained constant at low value (horizontal branch in Fig. 19.3). An interesting exception in Fig. 19.3 is the case of skimmed milk (number 13), which contains almost no fat but nevertheless scores among the samples on the rising branch. The reason for this is not clear, but

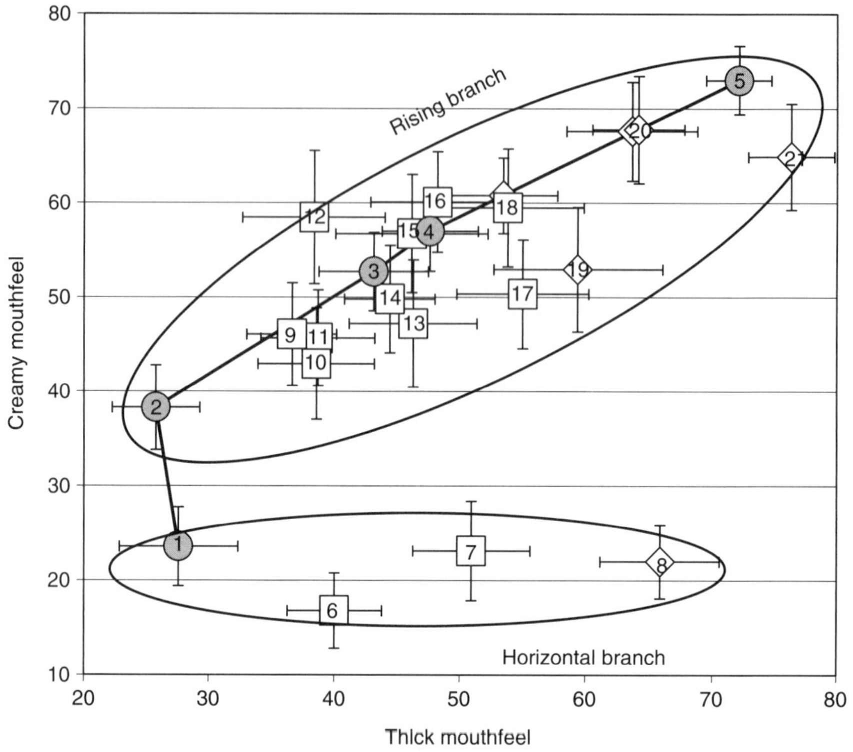

Fig. 19.3 Plot of averaged panel scores of creamy mouthfeel versus thick mouthfeel for liquid emulsions with variable fat content. The systems ranged in viscosity between 1 and 10 mPa s by variation in fat content (0–40%) and thickener (starch), variation in protein content and the use of various emulsifiers (see Table 19.1). The products were evaluated in three separate panel tests, indicated with different symbols (○, □, ◇).

it might be due to a specific interaction with saliva (van Aken *et al.*, 2005), possibly caused by the presence of casein micelles, or to the typical milk-flavour which is associated with creaminess. Fat-free systems thickened by starch score low in creaminess (Fig. 19.3; number 8), possibly because starch is quickly hydrolysed by salivary amylase, in this way quickly losing its thickening capacity close to the tongue surface.

Akhtar *et al.* (2005, 2006) showed that the addition of a thickener increases the viscosity, which leads to higher ratings in perceived thickness. The fat content was shown to have an additional small, but significant, effect on both thickness and creaminess. We confirmed this result in a study where the oil content was varied (0–40%) in the presence of a constant concentration of the thickener (van Aken *et al.*, to be published). In agreement with the studies of Akhtar and co-workers, it turned out that the presence of a thickener enhances both the thick and creamy mouthfeel at any fat content

Table 19.1 Composition of experimental systems for sensory analysis shown in Fig. 19.3. Experimental data taken from Vingerhoeds *et al.* (2008) and Van Aken *et al.* (2005)

Sample	Sunflower oil content (wt%)	Emulsifier	Thickener
1	0	1 wt% WPI	
2	5	1 wt% WPI	
3	10	1 wt% WPI	
4	20	1 wt% WPI	
5	40	1 wt% WPI	
6	0	5 wt% WPI	
7	0	5 wt% Na caseinate	
8	0	1 wt% WPI	4.5 wt% waxy maize
9	10	Stearoyl lactylate	
10	10	1 wt% Na caseinate	
11	10	1 wt% WPI	
12	10	1 wt% lecithin	
13	0	Skimmed milk	
14	10	Skimmed milk	
15	10	5 wt% WPI	
16	10	1 wt% monoglyceride	
17	10	1 wt% sucrose ester	
18a	10	5 wt% Na caseinate	
18b	10	1 wt% WPI	4 wt% rice starch
19	10	1 wt% WPI	4 wt% potato starch
20a	10	1 wt% WPI	5% moderately cross-linked waxy maize (wt% corn starch)
20b	10	1 wt% WPI	4 wt% waxy maize, strongly cross-linked
21	10	1 wt% WPI	4.5 wt% pregelatinised waxy maize starch

and that the rated creamy mouthfeel and especially creamy afterfeel always appeared somewhat increased for higher fat content. From the foregoing, it is apparent that emulsion droplets add a specific tactile sensory effect to liquid systems, which cannot be ascribed directly to the viscosity increase by the presence of emulsion droplets.

In the following sections, we will give our explanation for this tactile sensory effect of emulsions on the basis of the specific interaction of emulsions in the oral environment. To do so, we will give a general treatment of the way emulsion droplets affect the way the food material is processed in the mouth, how this affects the properties of the food bolus and the interaction with the oral surfaces, and how this relates to the tactile perception of mouthfeel and afterfeel. Because a gelled system is transformed by mastication into a semi-liquid bolus, which in a way resembles a viscous liquid emulsion taken directly into the mouth, we start by describing the effect of mastication on the structure of food gels containing emulsion droplets and how this is perceived in the mouth. Subsequently, we will describe the way liquid emulsions are processed and perceived in the mouth.

19.2.2 Role of emulsion droplet in the tactile perception of emulsion-filled gels

The fracture properties of a gel determine the perceived firmness and brittleness of the gel. The first-bite sensory attributes relate to the fracture properties of the gel, which is predominantly dependent on the gelling agent. The presence of emulsion droplets in a gelled matrix affects the first fracture events in a system-dependent way, leading to variations in 'first bite' sensory ratings (Sala *et al.*, 2007a, 2008).

Before the product is swallowed, gels are broken up by mastication to form a bolus of small gel particles bound together by saliva (Hutchings and Lillford, 1988; Lucas *et al.*, 2002). The presence of emulsion droplets in gelled matrices disturbs the structure of these matrices in such a way that the fracture properties are altered, and this affects 'masticatory' attributes, like hardness and brittleness. For a wide range of gel properties and droplet–matrix interactions, obtained by selection of model systems, the behaviour of the gels until first fracture (relevant for first bite perception, notably the firmness of the gel) could be described on the basis of a number of basic physical processes: (a) viscoelastic behaviour of the gel matrix; (b) stress concentration around the droplets; (c) viscous flow of the matrix; (d) friction between structural elements (droplets and matrix segments); (e) unzipping of physical bonds between the matrix elements; and (f) bulking effect by the droplets (Sala, 2007; Sala *et al.*, 2009).

Of perhaps larger importance is the subsequent diminution of the gel particles by multiple fracturing forming a viscous bolus of gel particles of variable size determined by the emulsion droplet content, size and binding to the matrix. If the droplets are not bound to the matrix, they are released from the fracture planes into the solution (saliva) (Sala *et al.*, 2007b). If the droplets are bound to the matrix, they are retained in the gel particles (Sala *et al.*, 2007b). The gel particles in the masticated gel also become slightly smaller, increasing both the bolus viscosity and the rated spreadibility and creaminess of the gel (Chojnicka *et al.*, 2008). Although this process is also a fracturing process, it is related to brittleness rather than hardness, and the precise relation with first fracture behaviour is not completely clear yet. The presence of emulsified fat was, however, shown to reduce the friction between rubber surfaces, which related to an increased perceived smoothness and creaminess of the gels (Chojnicka *et al.*, 2008).

The masticated food bolus can be viewed as a viscous liquid emulsion, and the explanation for the perceived tactile perception for these liquid systems, as given in the next section, may give an explanation for the perceived creaminess and smoothness of the masticated bolus of gelled emul-

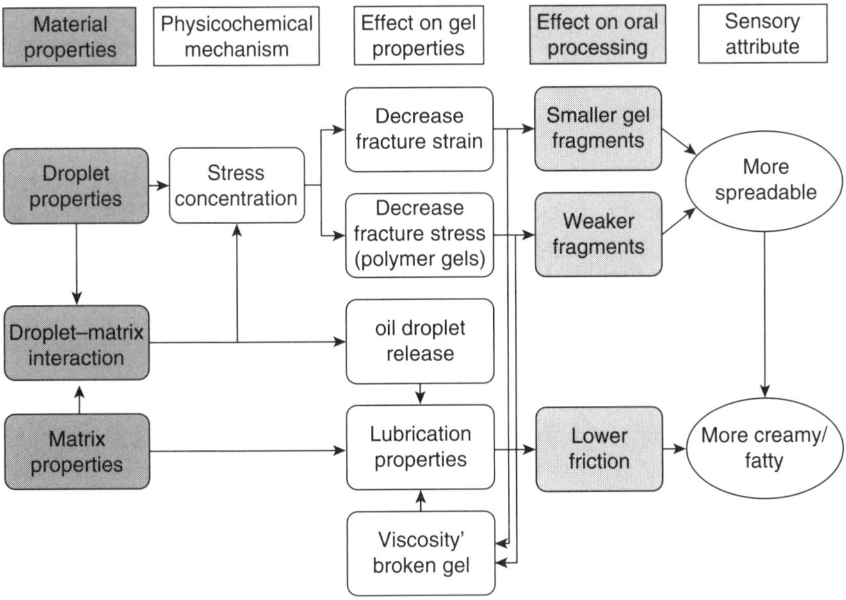

Fig. 19.4 Relations between gel properties and sensory attributes (after Sala, 2007).

sions. Figure 19.4 gives a schematic overview of the proposed mechanism and its consequence on perception as described by Sala (2007).

19.2.3 Role of emulsion droplet in the tactile perception of liquid emulsions

For liquid emulsions, three main specific properties of the emulsion droplets in the mouth are important. Firstly, the interaction with saliva leads to droplet flocculation, which increases the viscosity of previously unflocculated emulsion droplets. Secondly, the emulsion droplets appear to interact with the epithelial surfaces by being retained in the adherent mucous layer and by depositing fat onto the tongue surface, which reduces the boundary lubrication. Thirdly, there is some indication that fat in the oral cavity can be detected by chemoreceptors in the tongue as a taste attribute, which might be interpreted by the brain as a textural attribute as well. The combination of these three factors likely forms the key in understanding and controlling the sensory role of fat in food emulsions. These factors are discussed in more detail in the next sections.

Interaction with saliva

Saliva induces flocculation in thin liquid emulsions (Vingerhoeds *et al.*, 2005; Silletti *et al.*, 2007a,c). The effect is very general and seems to occur with all food grade emulsifiers. Saliva-induced flocculation considerably increases the viscosity of the emulsion–saliva mixture, measurable *in vitro* (Silletti *et al.*, 2008) or in the spit-out (Vingerhoeds *et al.*, 2009), and leads to the formation of a viscous layer consisting of flocculated droplets and salivary components adhering to the tongue surface before it is rinsed off by saliva (Dresselhuis, 2008; Dresselhuis *et al.*, 2008a). As saliva is predominantly present at the oral surfaces when the emulsion is taken into the mouth, flocculation immediately occurs at these surfaces, which is also the locus of the mechanoreceptors. As a consequence, the mechanoreceptors 'experience' a higher viscosity than the viscosity of the bulk of the food emulsion, which is still hardly mixed with saliva. This viscous coating may also explain the often reported sensation of a 'soft coating' or 'velvety coating' related to liquid emulsions.

The flocculation is caused by a range of interaction forces between the droplets, including depletion, van der Waals, electrostatic and molecular bridging interactions between the adsorbed layers on the emulsion droplets and salivary proteins and peptides. Saliva-related parameters, such as the salivary protein concentration in the mixture and the use of stimulated versus unstimulated saliva largely affect flocculation. Silletti and co-workers (Silletti, 2008; Silletti *et al.*, submitted for publication) carried out a biochemical study to identify the salivary components that interact with emulsions. Focus was on β-lactoglobulin- and lysozyme-stabilised emulsions at neutral pH, which reversibly and irreversibly flocculated with saliva, respectively. With the reversibility of flocculation, we point to the reversibility upon dilution with water or upon shear. A large number of salivary proteins and peptides in the molecular mass (M_r) range between 0.8 and 100 kDa and the salivary mucins MUC5B and MUC7 (M_r > 200 kDa) were found to be associated with the emulsion droplets. The emulsifying protein at the oil–water interface determines which salivary components associate with the droplets in the flocs. Lastly, the influence of the reversibility of saliva-induced flocculation on sensory perception was studied (Vingerhoeds *et al.*, 2009). Emulsions stabilised by whey protein isolate (WPI, mostly consisting of β-lactoglobulin) show reversible flocculation, which causes an increase in the viscosity of the saliva–emulsion mixture up to one order of magnitude compared with the emulsion itself and whole saliva. These were perceived as creamy. Instead, lysozyme-stabilised emulsions, which showed irreversible flocculation and a very high viscosity of the emulsion–saliva mixture (Silletti *et al.*, 2007b), were perceived as dry, rough and astringent, probably because the lubricating salivary proteins are depleted from the saliva. Moreover, small precipitates of lysozyme and salivary proteins are formed, which might be sensed as gritty particles. Interestingly, thickening of the lysozyme emulsions with guar gum restored lubrication and resulted in similar perceived creaminess as in case of thickened WPI emulsions, possibly because the guar gum restores the lubrication either by adhesion to the tongue surface or because the increased viscosity favours hydrodynamic lubrication. In addition, guar gum may interact with lysozyme, resulting in

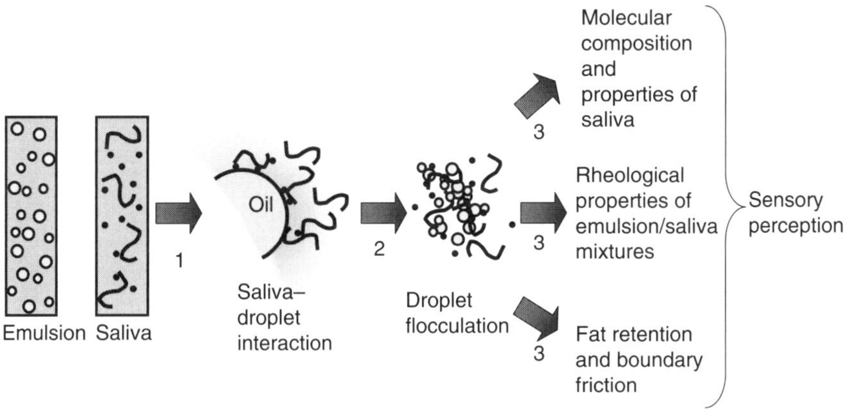

Fig. 19.5 Schematic representation of the different steps occurring upon mixing emulsions with saliva. Adsorption of salivary proteins and peptides to the oil–water interface of emulsion droplets (step 1), followed by floc formation with characteristic structural features (step 2), are key factors influencing sensory perception. As a consequence of floc formation, changes in saliva properties, rheological properties of emulsion/saliva mixtures, and changes in friction and lubrication in the mouth determine differences in perception of low-viscosity emulsions (after Silletti, 2008).

adsorption to the droplet surfaces and the formation of lysozyme–guar complexes, which both may result in reduced perceived astringency. Figure 19.5 gives a schematic overview of the proposed mechanism for saliva-induced emulsion flocculation and its consequence on perception.

Interaction with oral surfaces

Oil originating from the emulsions was found to be retained at the tongue surface, either in the form of emulsion droplets in a viscous adherent layer at the tongue surface and entrapped between the papillae, or in the form of an adherent spread oil layer or oil lenses at the surface (Dresselhuis, 2008; Dresselhuis *et al.*, 2008a,c). This retention seems to be related to the stability of an emulsion towards coalescence and was found to increase on decreasing the emulsion stability towards coalescence, either by varying the composition of the adsorbed layer on the emulsion droplets (Dresselhuis *et al.*, 2008b) or by partial coalescence (Benjamins *et al.*, 2009). For reversibly flocculated emulsions, this leads to increased ratings of fat-related tactile sensory attributes such as thickness, fattiness and creaminess and decreased friction-related sensory attributes such as roughness, dryness and astringency (Dresselhuis *et al.*, 2008a,b). It appeared that the sensory effect due to the increased sensitivity towards coalescence was not caused by the formation of large droplets, as very large droplets are not perceived as more creamy than small droplets (unpublished results), and therefore should be related to the way these coalescence-sensitive droplets interact with the tongue. It was indeed demonstrated by *in vitro* measurements that factors that increase the sensitivity towards coalescence also lead to a reduction in friction of rubber surfaces and to an increase in fat spreading on glass surfaces (Dresselhuis *et al.*, 2008c). In addition to this, since the emulsions that are more sensitive to coalescence are more strongly retained at the tongue surface, this coating forms a reservoir of fat that can be deposited as an adsorbed layer on the tongue surface, affecting the afterfeel of the emulsions.

Emulsions stabilised by positively charged lysozymes, which flocculate irreversibly with saliva, also show a stronger retention on the tongue surface than negatively charged WPI emulsions (Vingerhoeds *et al.*, 2009), but this leads to dry, rough and astringent sensations. The main difference with the reversibly flocculating emulsions is the strong interaction with salivary proteins such as mucins, thereby negatively affecting lubrication.

Motivated by the finding that fat deposition onto the tongue surface increases the sensory efficacy of the fat, the possible role of the formation of a hydrodynamic lubricating layer by the viscous oil was investigated. It turned out that a 20-fold variation in the oil viscosity has only a minor effect on instrumental friction and perception (Dresselhuis *et al.*, 2007; van Aken *et al.*, to be published). This suggests that fat deposition changes perception mainly in another way, e.g. by adsorption and hydrophobisation of the tongue surface, reducing boundary lubrication. This reduced boundary friction probably leads to the more smooth mouthfeel described by sensory panels in relation to emulsions. Figure 19.6 gives a schematic overview of the type of interactions of emulsion droplets with saliva and the oral surfaces.

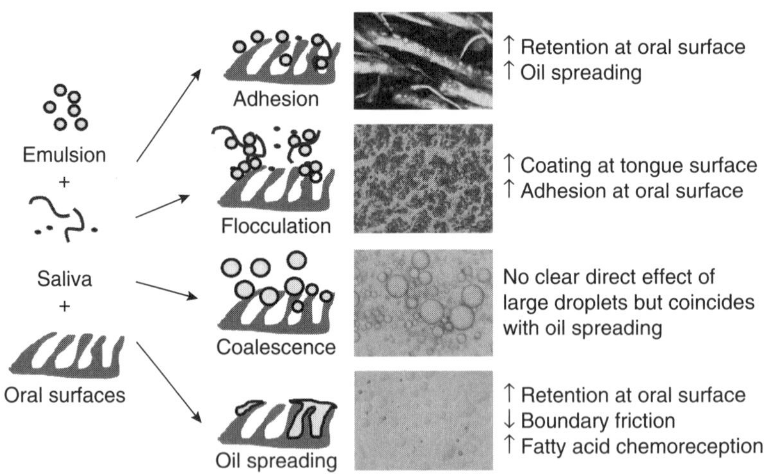

Fig. 19.6 Interaction of emulsions with oral surfaces in the presence of saliva: schematic representation of the mechanisms, microscope images of the processes and the effects of these mechanisms. Top microscope image: emulsion droplets in contact with pig's tongue papillae; second image: *in vitro* saliva-induced flocculation of emulsion droplets; third image: large emulsion droplets in expectorated emulsion formed by in-mouth coalescence; bottom image: spread emulsion droplets on glass surface.

Chemo-perception of fats

An increase in the unsaturation of the oil resulted in a small but statistically significant increase in the scoring of a number of fat-related taste attributes, such as taste intensity, oil taste and cream taste (de Hoog *et al.*, submitted for publication). In this study the degree of unsaturation of the oil was defined as the average number of double C—C bonds per fatty acid residue, averaged over all triglyceride species in the oil (ranging from olive oil (~0.9) to fish oil (~2.15). It should be noted that this correlation was found only for fresh oils with low peroxide numbers and purified by steam distillation, and panel members wearing nose clips to avoid aroma cues from the oil as much as possible. If these precautions were not taken, the very strong and specific flavours of the different oils overcast the much smaller effect related to unsaturation. This result suggests that fat is, to some extent, also perceived by a chemoreceptor that is somewhat dependent on the unsaturation of the fat.

Several studies reported in literature suggest that fat chemoreceptors might contribute to liking and taste-induced satiation by fat. For example, it has been demonstrated in isolated taste cells from rats that *cis*-polyunsaturated fatty acids are able to inhibit the delayed rectifying K+ (DRK) channels, which are involved in the transduction pathway of taste stimuli (Gilbertson, 1998; Gilbertson and Kim, 2002). Furthermore, the fatty acid transporter CD36 is located in the lingual gustatory papillae of rats and is involved in the detection of long chain fatty acids in the oral cavity (Fukuwatari *et al.*, 1997; Laugerette *et al.*, 2005). Whether analogous fat chemoreception also occurs in humans and whether it influences the gustatory system and the food intake behaviour is still under investigation. Nevertheless, experimental evidence is growing that oral lipid detection also occurs in humans, eliciting cephalic phase responses rather than a clear taste reported by a sensory panel. These cephalic phase responses include the release of gastric lipase, pancreatic digestive enzymes, mobilisation of lipid from prior meals stored in the intestine, pancreatic endocrine secretion (Mattes, 2005). Although it cannot be excluded that the oral lipid detection occurs through textural aspects of dispersed fat discussed in the previous sections, it is thought that this occurs at least partially through chemoreceptors in the mouth. Although further studies are clearly needed on this subject, our observation that the degree of unsaturation of the fat leads to a small but significant sensory effect does suggest that chemoreception of fatty acids in humans indeed occurs, and can also lead to a small but significant sensory effect.

19.3 Creating food emulsions with improved texture and mouthfeel

The implication of the research findings summarised in Section 19.2 is that a restoration of the tactile sensory loss in reduced fat products can be obtained by restoring the specific interactions of the emulsified fat with the mouth. Because of the various possible interactions of food materials with the oral environment, sensorially compensating a reduction in fat content will set different requirements for different food systems. When excluding the contribution of fat to flavour perception, the main targets should be on (1) the rheological properties (viscosity) of the food bolus, (2) the formation of a viscous coating at the tongue surface, (3) a reduction of boundary lubrication of the tongue against palate, and (4) the use of specific lipids or fatty acids that provoke a stimulation of the fat receptors in the tongue.

In the following we discuss some possibilities to reach each of these targets. We note, however, that it will be highly dependent on the structure of the specific product or product group.

19.3.1 Rheological properties (viscosity) of the food bolus

An increase in the viscosity of the liquid food product generally leads to higher ratings of the creaminess of the food product. Especially at higher fat contents, the presence of emulsion droplets can considerably increase the viscosity of the food product. This, for example, explains the higher perceived thickness of full cream (40% fat) compared with milk (3.5% fat). A reduction in the fat content therefore leads to a thinner product, which is for this reason rated as less creamy. This is often compensated for by adding polysaccharide thickeners or starches. Although this approach has proven its value for relatively thick food products, there are some possible drawbacks. Especially for thin liquid products, such as milk or ice cream after it has melted in the mouth, the addition of a thickener will also increase the perceived thickness of the food product, which might be undesirable. Moreover, a higher thickener content can change the perceived mouthfeel towards more sliminess.

Another option is to use foam bubbles to replace the filler properties of emulsion droplets. Examples of existing food systems that already incorporate this feature are whipped cream and ice cream. The most important parameters for sensory perception of fat-free model foams appear to be the overall fluidity of the foam and the amount of air that is released during oral processing (Minor *et al.*, 2009). The more gas is retained in the foam, the creamier the foam is rated, likely because of similar reasons as emulsion droplets increase the creaminess of a gel. Instead, high gas release leads to high 'airy' scorings. This gas release was shown to be modulated by the following parameters (unpublished results):

- The amount of gas bubbles (overrun).
- The size of the gas bubbles.
- The fluidity of the matrix (ranging between 'brittle gel' and 'viscous fluid'). Gelled matrices stabilise the foam bubbles against disproportionation and coalescence in rest, but fast release of gas is obtained during

oral processing. For fluid matrices, gas release during oral processing is much slower, but since the matrix does not stabilise against disproportionation, special precaution must be taken to stabilise the bubbles 'on the shelf'.

19.3.2 Formation of a viscous coating at the tongue surface

Especially for thin liquid food emulsions, the formation of a viscous coating right at the tongue surface by saliva-induced droplet flocculation is probably sensed as a soft coating, which adds to the perceived creaminess of the product. Moreover, since such a coating can persist for some time, it may add to the creamy afterfeel of these thin food emulsions. For reduced-fat emulsions, the approach can be to use emulsifiers that lead to binding of the emulsion droplets to the tongue surface, which seems to be related to a higher propensity for in-mouth coalescence (Dresselhuis *et al.*, 2008a) and the electrical charge of the emulsifier. Another approach is to add small and preferably soft particles that reversibly flocculate in interaction with saliva. Fat replacers such as inulin or aggregated proteins may already serve this function. It has been suggested that milk proteins can interact with saliva to form a slimy viscous structure at the tongue surface (van Aken *et al.*, 2005). This would suggest the possibility of forming a tongue coating by using food components that form a viscous structure with salivary proteins to compensate for a reduction of the fat content.

19.3.3 Reduction of boundary lubrication of the tongue against palate

An important effect of the emulsion droplets seems to originate from a reduction in friction forces in the boundary regime of lubrication. Since it can be argued that this reduction is predominantly due to a reduction in surface adhesion forces between the mucosal surfaces of tongue and palate (and in the case of food gels between gel particles and the oral mucosa of tongue and palate), caused by a deposited layer of fat at the mucosal surfaces (Dresselhuis *et al.*, 2008a,c), focus should be on a reduction of these adhesive forces. To compensate for a reduction in fat content, one approach could be to improving the lubricating effect of the remaining fat droplets. This can be done by improving the retention of emulsion droplets at the tongue surface by the formation of a viscous emulsion–saliva coating, improving the targeted deposition of a fatty layer at the tongue surface, or by using added ingredients that are also or better able to adhere to the surface and reduce boundary lubrication (possibly a surfactant such as a monoglyceride, a lecithin or an adsorbing polysaccharide or mucin).

An example of the approach of increasing the sensitivity to coalescence in the mouth, is the use of hydrophobised starch as the emulsifier. This emulsifier is quickly broken down by salivary amylase, leading to fast and extensive coalescence in the mouth, resulting in high creaminess ratings

(Dresselhuis *et al.*, 2008a,b). Also the presence of fat crystals in the droplets can increase the sensory efficacy of the dispersed fat, probable through the effect on emulsion viscosity by partial coalescence, and probable also increase deposition of the fat to the tongue surface in a mechanism related to partial coalescence (Benjamins *et al.*, 2009). In this way the steepness of the melting curve and melting point (clear point) of the fat, together with the use of monoglycerides (and probably other surfactants), give important control variables to increase the perceived thickness and creaminess of the emulsion (Benjamins *et al.*, 2009). It was found that a protein-stabilised emulsion of non-crystalline fat (sunflower oil) was rated creamier by the addition of monoglyceride to the oil phase (Benjamins *et al.*, 2009). This might be due to imparted stability of the emulsion due to displacement of the adsorbed protein by the monoglyceride. However, because there was no indication for an increase in coalescence in the spat-out emulsion, the effect may also be due to a decreased adhesion of the mucosal surfaces by adsorption of the monoglyceride.

Another possibility is to use the sensitivity of emulsion droplets to spread at bubble surfaces. The general mechanisms for this effect were studied by Hotrum *et al.* (2002, 2003) in a study on emulsion whipping. It was demonstrated as part of the study by Benjamins *et al.* (2009) on the role of partial coalescence on fat perception, that introduction of air bubbles in the emulsion in the mouth leads to oil spreading at the bubble surfaces, which in turn increases sensory efficacy of the dispersed fats.

For gelled emulsions, both aspects (formation of a viscous coating and reduction of boundary lubrication) are also important, with the difference that first a food bolus must be formed by multiple fracturing. These observations strongly suggest that diminished creaminess of gelled systems with reduced fat content can be improved by adapting the gel structure. Possibilities would be (1) to improve the masticatory breakdown into smaller gel particles (which occurs for smaller droplets that are bound to the matrix), which increases the viscosity of the bolus and possibly also reduces the perceived grittiness, (2) to increase the viscosity of the resulting food bolus by other means, such as the addition of thickeners, (3) to restore the lubricating effect of the fat in the gel by other lubricants, which could be thickeners, surfactants or perhaps mucins, and (4) to compensate for the reduction in fat-related taste attributes (see below). Furthermore, if the droplets are unbound to the matrix, the release of droplets to the saliva might be used to increase the release of fat-soluble flavours (not investigated).

19.3.4 The use of specific lipids or fatty acids that provoke a stimulation of the fat receptors in the tongue

The finding by de Hoog and co-workers (submitted for publication) that fat-related taste attributes (intensity, oil, cream) are perceived slightly more strongly for more unsaturated triglycerides suggests that a reduction in fat content can, in part, be compensated by using more unsaturated fats. It should, however, be noted that the effect is rather small and can easily be overcast by off-flavours related to oxidation products of the more unsaturated oils. Therefore, it is unlikely that this effect can be used to fortify the creamy mouthfeel and afterfeel of mildly flavoured products such as milk. On the other hand, the principle might work for products that are so strongly flavoured that off-flavours from the unsaturated fats are easily masked.

19.4 Future trends

The recent development to include oral processing into the mechanistic picture of in-mouth sensory perception appears to give important new understanding and tools to control the sensorial properties of food systems. For food emulsions, our studies have shown that the specific role of fat in tactile perception is related not only to an effect on the rheological properties of the food material before it is taken into the mouth, but especially also in the way the emulsion droplets change the fracturing of a gelled or solid food material, react to the ambient temperature in the mouth and interact with saliva and the tongue surface. Our studies underlined the role of fat retention on the tongue surface, mediated by saliva-induced droplet flocculation, and points to sensitivity to coalescence and the formation of a spread fatty layer at the tongue surface as the main controllable key effects of emulsified fat on sensory perception.

Future developments are foreseen in two directions, namely towards application in food products and towards fundamental studies. Towards application, for example in the development of reduced fat products with unabated sensory quality, further studies are needed to identify which of the fat-specific effects are prevalent in perception. This will be highly dependent on the type of food product (e.g. liquid, thickened or gelled; acidified or not; aerated or not; high or low in fat content). For example, in thin liquid emulsions an enhanced retention on the tongue seems to be related to the sensitivity towards coalescence, but this is probably not so relevant for thickened or gelled emulsions. The low pH in acidified emulsions will affect the behaviour of saliva and probably also the ability of saliva to induce droplet flocculation. In aerated emulsions, such as whipped cream, the emulsion droplets are already highly coalesced at the bubble surfaces and this will probably affect the interaction with the tongue surface.

Towards fundamental studies, more understanding is needed on how the fat-specific mechanisms affect sensory perception. A more detailed description of the location of the emulsion droplets on the oral surfaces on a smaller length scale, and a better understanding of how the retained emulsion droplets are perceived as described by the sensory attributes scored by a panel test are needed. Furthermore, under the conditions operative in the mouth, the presence of emulsion droplets and the deposited fatty layer at the tongue surface will depend on a dynamic competition between one hand droplet aggregation and coalescence delivering fat to the tongue surface and on the other hand the removal of this layer by emulsification by saliva and shear forces.

19.5 Sources of further information and advice

A general introduction on in-mouth behaviour of food systems and how these can be established by physical and sensory studies is given by van Aken (2007). A review on the oral processing of solid food materials is given by Hutchins and Lillford (1988), and detailed studies of food bolus formation is given by Lucas and co-workers (2002). A review on oral physiology and texture perception of semi-solid foods is given by Engelen and van der Bilt (2008). Mastication of semi-solid food gels leads to a variable release of water in the mouth and a variable size of the gel particles, which is described in a study by van den Berg and co-workers (2007a,b). An introduction and references on the role of tribology on texture perception in fat-containing semi-solids can be found in a publication by Chojnicka and co-workers (2008). An overview of the oral processing of food emulsions is given by van Aken and co-workers (2007). More fundamental studies on tribology of soft surfaces and the role of saliva are described by Bongaerts and co-workers (2007a,b).

19.6 References

AKHTAR M, STENZEL J, MURRAY B S & DICKINSON E (2005) 'Factors affecting the perception of creaminess of oil-in-water emulsions', *Food Hydrocolloids*, **19**, 521–526.

AKHTAR M, MURRAY B S & DICKINSON E (2006) 'Perception of creaminess of model oil-in-water dairy emulsions: influence of the shear-thinning nature of a viscosity-controlling hydrocolloid', *Food Hydrocolloids*, **20**, 839–847.

BENJAMINS J, VINGERHOEDS M H, ZOET F, DE HOOG E H A & VAN AKEN G A (2009) 'Partial coalescence as a tool to control sensory perception of emulsions', *Food Hydrocolloids*, **23**(1), 102–115.

BONGAERTS J, ROSSETTI D & STOKES J (2007a) 'The lubricating properties of human whole saliva', *Tribology Letters*, **27**, 277–287.

BONGAERTS J H H, FOURTOUNI K & STOKES J R (2007b) 'Soft-tribology: lubrication in a compliant PDMS-PDMS contact', *Tribology International*, **40**, 1531–1542.

BRANDT M A, SKINNER E Z & COLEMAN J A (1963) 'Texture profile method', *J. Food Sci.*, **28**, 404–409.

BROMBERG L & BARR D (2000) 'Self-association of mucin', *Biomacromolecules*, **1**, 325–334.

CHOJNICKA A, SALA G, DE KRUIF C G & VAN DE VELDE F (2008) 'The interactions between oil droplets and gel matrix affect the lubrication properties of sheared emulsion-filled gels', *Food Hydrocolloids*, **23**, 1038–1046.

CUTLER A N, MORRIS E R & TAYLOR L J (1983) 'Oral perception of viscosity in fluid foods and model systems', *J. Texture Studies*, **14**, 337–395.

DE HOOG E H A, VINGERHOEDS M H, DE WIJK R A & VAN AKEN G A (submitted for publication) 'Taste perception of fat: the effect of variation in the degree of unsaturation of fatty acids in emulsified dietary triglycerides'.

DE WIJK R A, PRINZ J F & ENGELEN L (2003) 'The role of intra-oral manipulation in the perception of sensory attributes', *Appetite*, **40**, 1–7.

DRESSELHUIS D M (2008) *The Fate of Fat: Tribology, Adhesion, and Fat Perception of Food Emulsions*. Ph D thesis Wageningen, The Netherlands, Wageningen University.

DRESSELHUIS D M, KLOK H J, COHEN STUART M A, DE VRIES R J & VAN AKEN G A (2007) 'Tribology of o/w emulsions under mouth-like conditions: determinants of friction', *Food Biophysics*, **2**, 158–171.

DRESSELHUIS D M, COHEN STUART M A, VAN AKEN G A, SCHIPPER R G & DE HOOG E H A (2008a) 'Fat retention at the tongue and the role of saliva: adhesion and spreading of 'protein-poor' versus 'protein-rich' emulsions', *J. Coll. Interface Sci.*, **321**, 21–29.

DRESSELHUIS D M, DE HOOG E H A, COHEN STUART M A, VINGERHOEDS M H & VAN AKEN G A (2008b) 'The occurrence of in-mouth coalescence of emulsion droplets in relation to perception of fat', *Food Hydrocolloids*, **22**, 1170–1183.

DRESSELHUIS D M, VAN AKEN G A, DE HOOG E H A & COHEN STUART M A (2008c) 'Direct observation of adhesion and spreading of emulsion droplets at solid surfaces', *Soft Matter*, **4**, 1079–1085.

ENGELEN L & VAN DER BILT A (2008) 'Oral physiology and texture perception of semisolids', *J. Texture Studies*, **39**, 83–113.

ENGELEN L, DE WIJK R A, VAN DER BILT A, PRINZ J F, JANSSEN A M & BOSMAN F (2005) 'Relating particles and texture perception', *Physiology & Behavior*, **86**, 111–117.

FOX P C, BODNER L, TABAK L A & LEVINE M J (1985) 'Quantitation of total human salivary mucins', *J. Dental Res.*, **64**, 327, Abstract 1376.

FUKUWATARI T, KAWADA T, TSURUTA M, HIRAOKA T, IWANAGA T, SUGIMOTO E & FUSHIKI T (1997) 'Expression of hte putative membrane fatty acid transporter (FAT) in taste buds of the circumvallate papillae in rats', *FEBS Lett.*, **414**, 461–464.

GILBERTSON T A (1998) 'Gustatory mechanisms for the detection of fat', *Curr. Opin. Neurobiol.*, **8**, 447–452.

GILBERTSON T A & KIM I (2002) 'Chemoreception of fat', *Chemistry of Taste: Mechanisms, Behaviors, and Mimics.* ACS Symposium Series vol. 825. Washington, DC, ACS, 180–191.

GLANTZ P O (1997) 'Interfacial phenomena in the oral cavity', *Colloids Surfaces A: Physicochem. Eng. Aspects*, **123–124**, 657–670.

GLANTZ P O, NATIELLA J R, VAUGHAN C D, MEYER A E & BAIER R E (1989) 'Structural studies of human saliva', *Acta Odontol. Scand.*, **47**, 17–24.

GLANTZ P O, BAIER R E & CHRISTERSSON C E (1996) 'Biochemical and physiological considerations for modeling biofilms in the oral cavity: a review', *Dental Mater.*, **12**, 208–214.

HOTRUM N E, VAN VLIET T, COHEN STUART M A & VAN AKEN G A (2002) 'Monitoring entering and spreading of emulsion droplets at an expanding air/water interface: a novel technique', *J. Colloid Interface Sci.*, **247**, 125–131.

HOTRUM N E, COHEN STUART M A, VAN VLIET T & VAN AKEN G A (2003) 'Entering and spreading of protein stabilized emulsion droplets at the expanding air/water interface', in Dickinson, E & Van Vliet, T, *Food Colloids, Biopolymers and Materials.* Cambridge, The Royal Society of Chemistry, 192–199.

HUMPHREY S P & WILLIAMSON R T (2001) 'A review of saliva: normal composition, flow and function', *J. Prosthetic Dentistry*, **85**, 162–169.

HUTCHINGS J B & LILLFORD P J (1988) 'The perception of food texture – the philosophy of the breakdown path', *J. Texture Stud.*, **19**, 103–115.

KEETON W T & MCFADDEN C H (1967) *Elements of Biological Science*, New York, W.W. Norton & Company.

KESSEL R G & KARDON R H (1979) *Tissues and Organs, A Text Atlas of Scanning Electron Microscopy*, San Francisco, W.H. Freeman and Company.

LAUGERETTE F, PASSILLY-DEGRACE P, PATRIS B, NIOT I, FEBBRAIO M, MONTMAYEUR J-P & BESNARD P (2005) 'CD36 involvement in orosensory detection of dietary lipids, spontaneous fat preference, and digestive secretions', *J. Clin. Invest.*, **115**, 3177–3184.

LEONHARDT H (1971) *Histologie und Zytologie des Menschen*, Stuttgart, Georg Thieme Verlag.

LUCAS P W, PRINZ J F, AGRAWAL K R & BRUCE I C (2002) 'Food physics and oral physiology', *Food Qual. Pref.*, **13**, 203–213.

MALONE M E, APPELQVIST I A M & NORTON I T (2003) 'Oral behaviour of food hydrocolloids and emulsions. Part 2. Taste and aroma release', *Food Hydrocolloids*, **17**, 775–784.

MATTES R D (2005) 'Fat taste and lipid metabolism in humans', *Physiol. Behavi.*, **86**, 691–697.

MINOR M, VINGERHOEDS M H, ZOET F D, DE WIJK R A & VAN AKEN G A (2009) 'Preparation and sensory perception of fat-free foams – effect of matrix properties and level of aeration', *Int. J. Food Sci. Technol.* **44**, 735–747.

MORRIS E R (1995) 'Polysaccharide rheology and in-mouth perception', in Stephen, A M, *Food Polysaccharides and their Applications.* New York, Marcel Dekker, Inc., 517–546.

RAYNAL B D E, HARDINGHAM T E, SHEEHAN J K & THORNTON D J (2003) 'Calcium-dependent protein interactions in MUC5B provide reversible crosslinks in salivary mucus', *J. Biol. Chem.*, **278**, 28703–28710.

SALA G (2007) *Food Gels Filled with Emulsion Droplets. Linking Large Deformation Properties to Sensory Perception.* Ph D thesis Wageningen, The Netherlands, Wageningen University.

SALA G, VAN AKEN G A, COHEN STUART M A & VAN DE VELDE F (2007a) 'Effect of droplet–matrix interactions on large deformation properties of emulsion-filled gels', *J. Texture Studies*, **38**, 511–535.

SALA G, VAN DE VELDE F, COHEN STUART M A & VAN AKEN G A (2007b) 'Oil droplet release from emulsion-filled gels in relation to sensory perception', *Food Hydrocolloids*, **21**, 977–985.

SALA G, DE WIJK R A, VAN DE VELDE F & VAN AKEN G A (2008) 'Matrix properties affect the sensory perception of emulsion-filled gels', *Food Hydrocolloids*, **22**, 353–363.

SALA G, VAN VLIET T, COHEN STUART M A, VAN AKEN G A & VAN DE VELDE F (accepted for publication) 'Deformation and fracture of emulsion-filled gels. 1 Effect of oil volume fraction and deformation speed', *Food Hydrocolloids*.

SCHIPPER R G, SILLETTI E & VINGERHOEDS M H (2007) 'Saliva as research material: biochemical, physicochemical and practical aspects', *Arch. Oral Biol.*, **52**, 1114–1135.

SHAMA F & SHERMAN P (1973) 'Identification of stimuli controlling the sensory evaluation of viscosity, II Oral methods', *J. Texture Studies*, **4**, 111–118.

SILLETTI E (2008) *When Emulsions Meet Saliva. A Physical–Chemical, Biochemical and Sensory Study*. Ph D thesis Wageningen, The Netherlands, Wageningen University.

SILLETTI E, VINGERHOEDS M H, NORDE W & VAN AKEN G A (2007a) 'Saliva-induced emulsion flocculation: The role of droplet charge', in Dickinson, E & Leser, M, *Food Colloids: Self-assembly and Material Science.* Cambridge, UK, Royal Society of Chemistry, 463–472.

SILLETTI E, VINGERHOEDS M H, NORDE W & VAN AKEN G A (2007b) 'Complex formation in mixtures of lysozyme-stabilized emulsions and human saliva', *J. Colloid Interface Sci.*, **313**, 485–493.

SILLETTI E, VINGERHOEDS M H, NORDE W & VAN AKEN G A (2007c) 'The role of electrostatics in saliva-induced emulsion flocculation', *Food Hydrocolloids*, **21**, 596–606.

SILLETTI E, VINGERHOEDS M H, VAN AKEN G A & NORDE W (2008) 'Rheological behaviour of food emulsions mixed with saliva: effect of oil content, salivary protein content and saliva type', *Food Biophys.*, **3**, 318–328.

SILLETTI E, VITORINO R, DE GROOT J, VINGERHOEDS M H & AMADO F (submitted for publication) 'Analysis and identification of salivary peptides interacting with beta-lactoglobulin and lysozyme stabilized emulsions by SELDI-TOF-MS and RP-HPLC coupled to MS-TOF-TOF'.

TRULSSON M & ESSICK G K (1997) 'Low-threshold mechanoreceptive afferents in the human lingual nerve', *J. Neurophys.*, **77**, 737–748.

VAN AKEN G A (2007) 'Relating food microstructure to sensory quality', in McClements, D J, *Understanding and Controlling the Microstructure of Complex Foods.* Abington, Cambridge, UK, Woodhead Publishing, 449–482.

VAN AKEN G A, VINGERHOEDS M H & DE HOOG E H A (2005) 'Colloidal behaviour of food emulsions under oral conditions', in Dickinson, E, *Food Colloids 2004: Interactions, Microstructure and Processing.* Cambridge, The Royal Society of Chemistry, 356–366.

VAN AKEN G A, VINGERHOEDS M H & DE HOOG E H A (2007) 'Food colloids under oral conditions', *Curr. Opin. Colloid Interface Sci.*, **12**, 251–262.

VAN AKEN G A, VINGERHOEDS M H & DE WIJK R A (to be published) 'The role of the viscosity of the oil and continuous phase in the sensory perception of emulsions'.

VAN DEN BERG L, VAN VLIET T, VAN DER LINDEN E, VAN BOEKEL M A J S & VAN DE VELDE F (2007a) 'Breakdown properties and sensory perception of whey proteins/polysaccharide mixed gels as a function of microstructure', *Food Hydrocolloids*, **21**, 961–976.

VAN DEN BERG L, VAN VLIET T, VAN DER LINDEN E, VAN BOEKEL M A J S & VAN DE VELDE F (2007b) 'Serum release: the hidden quality in fracturing composites', *Food Hydrocolloids*, **21**, 420–432.

VAN NIEUW AMERONGEN A, VEERMAN E C I & VISSINK A (2004) *Speeksel, Speekselklieren en Mondgezondheid*, Houten, Bohn Stafleu Van Loghum.

VAN RUTH S M & ROOZEN J P (2000) 'Influence of mastication and saliva on aroma release in a model mouth system', *Food Chem.*, **71**, 339–345.

VINGERHOEDS M H, BLIJDENSTEIN T B J, ZOET F D & VAN AKEN G A (2005) 'Emulsion flocculation induced by saliva and mucin', *Food Hydrocolloids*, **19**, 915–922.

VINGERHOEDS M H, DE WIJK R A, ZOET F D, NIXDORF R R & VAN AKEN G A (2008) 'How emulsion composition and structure affect sensory perception of low viscosity model emulsions', *Food Hydrocolloids*, **22**, 631–646.

VINGERHOEDS M H, SILLETTI E, DE GROOT J, SCHIPPER R & VAN AKEN G A (2009) 'Relating the effect of saliva-induced emulsion flocculation on rheological properties and adherence to the tongue surface with sensory perception', *Food Hydrocolloids*, **23**, 773–785.

WICKSTRÖM C, DAVIES J R, ERIKSEN G V, VEERMAN E C I & CARLSTEDT I (1998) 'MUC5B is a major gel-forming, oligomeric mucin from human salivary gland, respiratory tract and endocervix: identification of glycoforms and C-terminal cleavage', *Biochem. J.*, **334**, 685–693.

WOLFF M & KLEINBERG I (1998) 'Oral mucosal wetness in hypo- and normosalivators', *Arch. Oral Biol.*, **43**, 445–462.

ZALEWSKA A, ZWIERZ K, ZÓLKOWSKI K & GINDZIENSKI A (2000) 'Structure and biosynthesis of human salivary mucins', *Acta Biochim. Polonica*, **47**, 1067–1079.

20

Controlling lipid bioavailability using emulsion-based delivery systems

D. J. McClements and E. A. Decker, University of Massachusetts, USA

Abstract: This chapter focuses on the development of emulsion-based delivery systems for controlling the bioavailability of lipophilic components, such as triacylglycerols, cholesterol, oil-soluble vitamins and nutraceuticals. The major physicochemical and physiological processes that occur in the mouth, stomach and small intestine that are relevant to understanding how lipid droplets behave in the human gastrointestinal tract are briefly reviewed. The concept of lipid bioavailability and how it is influenced by the molecular properties of food lipids is then discussed. Finally, a number of emulsion-based delivery systems that can potentially be used to control the bioavailability of lipids are presented, including conventional emulsions, solid lipid nanoparticles, multiple emulsions, multilayer emulsions, and filled hydrogel particles. The preparation, properties and potential applications of each of these systems is discussed.

Key words: digestion, lipids, emulsions, delivery systems, bioavailability.

20.1 Introduction

Humans ingest a variety of different types of lipid that play important roles in the human diet, e.g., triacylglycerols, cholesterol, oil-soluble vitamins, antioxidants, and nutraceuticals (Decker and McClements, 2007). Triacylglycerols are a major source of energy and provide essential fatty acids that cannot be synthesized by the human body. Oil-soluble vitamins, such as vitamins A, D, E, and K, help maintain the proper functioning of the human body. Lipid-soluble bioactive components, such as ω-3 fatty acids, phytosterols, and carotenoids, are believed to promote health and prevent diseases such as heart disease, diabetes and cancer (Decker and McClements, 2007). On the other hand, consumption of certain types of lipids can have an adverse impact on human health. Over-consumption of saturated fatty acids, *trans*-fatty acids and cholesterol has been linked to increased incidences of heart disease, obesity, diabetes, and cancer.

The bioavailability of lipids varies widely depending on their molecular characteristics and the nature of the food matrix that they are consumed with (Wildman and Kelley, 2007b). In healthy humans, the digestion and absorption of triacylglycerols is normally highly efficient with >95% of the lipids that are ingested being absorbed (Patton *et al.*, 1985). Nevertheless, some human diseases greatly decrease the bioavailability of triacylglycerols by inhibiting either their digestion or absorption, such as short gut, cystic fibrosis, and other pancreas deficiencies (Bauer *et al.*, 2005; Fave *et al.*, 2004; Pafumi *et al.*, 2002). Individuals with these diseases have problems obtaining sufficient calories or essential lipid-soluble nutrients from their diets, which can lead to severe health problems. In these cases, it would be beneficial to increase the bioavailability of lipids by increasing the efficiency of lipid digestion and/or absorption. It would also be beneficial to increase the bioavailability of those highly hydrophobic components that have been shown to be helpful to health but that typically have poor absorption characteristics, such as β-carotene, lutein and lycopene (Wright *et al.*, 2008; Faulks and Southon, 2001; Wildman and Kelley, 2007a). On the other hand, triacylglycerols have a high caloric density and their over-consumption can result in obesity. In addition, high intake of saturated fatty acids, *trans*-fatty acids or cholesterol could also be deleterious since these lipids are associated with increased risk of cardiovascular disease. It may therefore be beneficial to decrease the bioavailability of these lipid components to avoid their deleterious impact on human health.

Finally, there is a considerable interest in developing structured delivery systems to encapsulate, protect and release lipophilic food components (Aguilera, 2006; Sanguansri and Augustin, 2006). These structured delivery systems may be designed for one purpose (e.g., improving the chemical or physical stability of an encapsulated component during storage), but they may have unexpected side effects on the nutritional performance of a food (e.g., altered bioavailability). It is therefore important to understand how food structure impacts lipid bioavailability so as to avoid any potentially adverse impacts. This knowledge could also be used to design structured delivery systems to control the release of lipid components within specific regions of the human digestive tract, e.g., mouth, stomach, small intestine, large intestine, or colon.

The purpose of this chapter is to show how emulsion-based delivery systems can be designed to alter the bioavailability of encapsulated lipids. The same delivery systems may also be used to incorporate lipids into different food matrices or to protect lipids during storage and transport (McClements *et al.*, 2007). We begin the chapter by briefly discussing the most important physicochemical and physiological processes that occur as lipids pass through the human digestive tract, since this knowledge is essential for understanding how emulsion-based delivery systems can be designed to alter lipid bioavailability. We then discuss the meaning of the term *bioavailability* in the context of the digestion and absorption of lipids. Finally, we outline some of the emulsion-based technologies that could potentially be used to alter lipid bioavailability, giving examples of previous studies where possible.

20.2 Lipid ingestion, digestion and absorption

A brief overview of the basic physicochemical and physiological processes that occur as ingested emulsified lipids pass through the mouth, stomach, and small intestine is given in this section (Carey *et al.*, 1983; Fave *et al.*, 2004; Pafumi *et al.*, 2002; Porter *et al.*, 2007; Tso, 2000).

20.2.1 Mouth

Initially, we will assume that a human ingests a food containing a lipid phase within an emulsion-based delivery system, i.e., lipid droplets dispersed within an aqueous medium. The composition, structure and properties of the ingested food change appreciably within the human mouth due to the complex physiochemical, physiological, and biochemical processes occurring during mastication (Sanz and Luyten, 2006a, b, 2007; Van Aken, 2007). The food will be mixed with saliva, it may change its pH, ionic strength, and temperature, it may be acted on by various digestive enzymes, it will interact with the biological surfaces of the tongue and mouth, it will be subjected to a complex fluid flow profile, and it may be broken down into smaller pieces by chewing (Blijdenstein *et al.*, 2004; de Hoog *et al.*, 2006; Gwartney *et al.*, 2004; Malone *et al.*, 2003a, b; Silletti *et al.*, 2007; Vingerhoeds *et al.*, 2005). The nature and extent of the changes of the lipid phase within the food will depend on the initial characteristics of the lipid phase (e.g., composition, physical state, polarity), the initial structure of the lipid droplets (e.g., size, polydispersity, interfacial composition, surrounding matrix), and various other factors (e.g., food temperature, serving size, ingredient interactions, saliva type, and output). There is currently limited knowledge of the physicochemical and structural changes that occur when different types of fatty foods are consumed. Nevertheless, much progress has been made for emulsion-based systems within recent years (Malone *et al.*, 2003a, b; Van Aken, 2007; Vingerhoeds *et al.*, 2005).

An important factor that influences the mastication of emulsified foods is their mixing with saliva after ingestion. Typically, human saliva is at pH 5.5 to 6.1 during fasting, and at pH 7 to 8 after stimulation by food ingestion (Kalantzi *et al.*, 2006). Saliva is secreted at a rate of about 0.3 to 0.7 ml per minute, with a total saliva output of 500 to 1500 mL per day (Vingerhoeds *et al.*, 2005). It contains water (~99%), minerals (<1%), and proteins (0.1–0.2%). The protein fraction is compositionally complex containing many different types of molecule, including enzymes, immunoglobulins, antibacterial proteins, proline-rich proteins, and glycosylated proteins (mucins) (Amado *et al.*, 2005; Vitorino *et al.*, 2004a, b). Recent research has shown that mucins are able to induce droplet aggregation in emulsified products, which has been attributed to depletion and/or bridging mechanisms (Silletti *et al.*, 2007; Vingerhoeds *et al.*, 2005).

The material that is swallowed after ingestion and mastication of a food is referred to as the 'bolus' (Tso, 2000). Typically, swallowing takes a few seconds to complete, and involves integrated movements of the tongue, pharynx, esophagus, and stomach (Weisbrodt, 2001c). The structural organization of the lipids within the bolus depends on their initial structure and properties within the ingested food, the duration and intensity of mastication, and the physiological characteristics of the individual consuming the food.

20.2.2 Stomach

After the bolus is swallowed, it passes down the esophagus and into the stomach (Fig. 20.1), where it is mixed with acidic digestive juices containing gastric enzymes, minerals and surface active compounds, and is subjected to a complex flow/force profile due to the stomach's contractions (Weisbrodt, 2001a, b). Typically, the pH of the fasting human stomach is within the range 1 to 3, and the ionic strength is around 100 mM (Ekmekcioglu, 2002; Kalantzi *et al.*, 2006; Lindahl *et al.*, 1997). The pH and ionic composition of the stomach change considerably after a food is ingested,

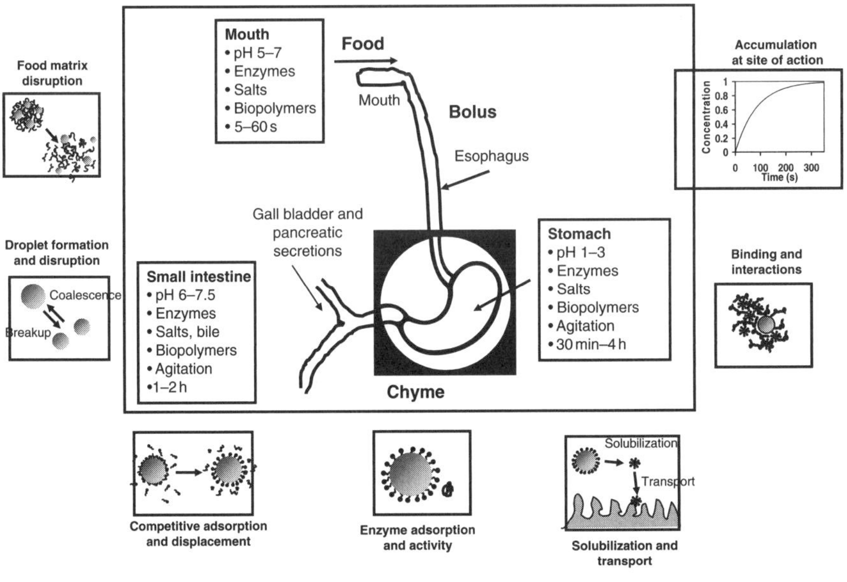

Fig. 20.1 Highly schematic diagram of the human digestive system and the various processes occurring during lipid digestion and absorption.

by an amount that depends on the quantity and nature of the ingested food, and there may be large person-to-person variations (Kalantzi *et al.*, 2006). Typically, there is an appreciable increase in the pH of the stomach contents after ingestion of a food, followed by a gradual decrease to around pH 2 over the next hour or so. The time taken for the stomach to return to pH 2 depends on the initial pH, buffering capacity, composition, and quantity of food ingested (Kalantzi *et al.*, 2006). After ingestion of a meal, there is usually an appreciable increase in the ionic strength of the stomach contents due to the additional ions and other solutes arising from the food, with the increase depending on the type and quantity of food consumed (Kalantzi *et al.*, 2006).

The stomach goes through a variety of contractive motions to mix the ingested food components with the digestive juices, break down any large fragments within the food, and transport partially digested material into the small intestine (Schulze, 2006; Schwizer *et al.*, 2003; Shafik *et al.*, 2007; Weisbrodt, 2001a, b). After being ingested, a food component may remain in the stomach for a period ranging from a few minutes to a few hours depending on its quantity, physical state, structure, and location. Typically, the amount of food remaining in the stomach after ingestion decreases by about 50% in 30 to 90 minutes, with liquid components being emptied more rapidly than solid components (Weisbrodt, 2001a, b).

The size of the lipid droplets within the bolus depends on the original size of the lipid droplets within the ingested food, as well as any changes brought about during passage through the mouth and esophagus. A number of studies have shown that the lipid droplet size may increase, decrease or remain the same as emulsified lipids passes through the stomach depending on the initial droplet size and interfacial composition (Bauer *et al.*, 2005; Fave *et al.*, 2004). A study using phospholipid-stabilized lipid droplets has shown that the final mean droplet diameter in the human stomach was between 10 and 20 μm, irrespective of the initial droplet size (Armand *et al.*, 1997, 1999; Bauer *et al.*, 2005; Fave *et al.*, 2004). When the initial lipid droplets were larger than this size, they tended to be broken down in the stomach, but when they were smaller they tended to coalesce. Presumably, a steady-state situation was reached where the rate of droplet disruption was balanced by the rate of droplet coalescence. On the other hand, studies using milk protein-stabilized lipid droplets showed that the droplets remained small throughout the digestion process, presumably because the proteins protected the droplets from droplet coalescence within the stomach (Armand *et al.*, 1996b; Michalski *et al.*, 2005).

There may also be considerable variations in the properties of the interfacial layers surrounding the lipid droplets in the bolus depending on the type of emulsifier(s) originally present in the food, as well as the possible adsorption of any surface active components to the droplet surfaces during mastication or transfer to the stomach (Kalantzi *et al.*, 2006). The properties of the interfacial coating surrounding lipid droplets will affect the ability of lipase to adsorb to the droplet surfaces and interact with the emulsified lipids. It may be possible to create interfacial coatings around lipid droplets in emulsion-based delivery systems that are more or less susceptible to displacement by surface active substances, which may prove to be a useful means of controlling lipid digestibility (see later).

The composition of the lipid phase that enters the stomach depends on the type of oils and fats used in the preparation of the delivery system. The lipid phase may consist primarily of a particular type of lipid (e.g., triacylglycerols) or it may consist of a minor lipid component (e.g., carotenoid) dispersed within a carrier lipid (e.g., triacylglycerols). The composition of the lipid phase may be altered within the stomach due to the activity of gastric lipases, which are typically present at levels of around 0.5 to 1 μM. Human gastric lipase is a highly glycosylated globular protein with a molecular weight of about 50 kDa (Armand, 2007; Bauer *et al.*, 2005; Mukherjee, 2003) and an isoelectric point around pH 7 (Miled *et al.*, 2005). Gastric lipase binds to the surface of lipid droplets within the stomach, where it hydrolyzes the conversion of surface triacylglycerols (TAG) into diacylglycerols (DAG), monoacylglycerols (MAG), and free fatty acids (FFA) (Armand, 2007; Jurado *et al.*, 2006; Whitcomb and Lowe, 2007). Gastric lipases preferentially hydrolyse the sn-3 ester bond of TAGs, resulting in the formation of sn-1,2 DAGs, although it also has some activity for the sn-1 ester bond (Mu and Hoy, 2004). As a result of lipase activity, there is a change in the composition of the lipid phase within the droplets (Bauer *et al.*, 2005; Pafumi *et al.*, 2002). Lipid hydrolysis usually stops when about 10–30% of the fatty acids have been released from the TAGs, which corresponds to a surface load of about 120–170 $\mu mol/m^2$ of fatty acids at the oil–water interface (Fave *et al.*, 2004). Hence, the digestion of TAGs in the stomach is usually greater for smaller droplets (with a larger surface area), than for larger droplets (with a lower surface area). The limited amount of lipid hydrolysis that occurs in the human stomach is important for individuals whose pancreatic lipase system functions improperly, e.g., patients with cystic fibrosis or other pancreatic disorders (Fave *et al.*, 2004). In addition, the lipid hydrolysis that occurs in the stomach may enhance subsequent lipid digestion in normal humans by promoting lipid droplet disruption, increasing solubilization of digestion products, stimulating hormone release, increasing the binding of co-lipase, and increasing the activity of pancreatic lipase in the small intestine (Bauer *et al.*, 2005; Mu and Hoy, 2004).

Foods are compositionally and structurally complex materials that normally contain a wide variety of different components, including sugars, salts, proteins, polysaccharides, lipids, vitamins, etc. Potentially, some of these components could interfere with lipid digestion within the stomach, e.g., by interfering with droplet breakdown/coalescence, by altering interfacial composition, or by influencing lipase activity. For example, some studies have shown that hydrocolloids can retard the breakdown of lipid droplets in the stomach, which has been attributed to their ability to greatly increase the viscosity of the stomach contents (Pasquier *et al.*, 1996; Lairon, 1997a, b). On the other hand, other studies using rats have shown that soluble fibers have little influence on the droplet size (FilleryTravis *et al.*, 1997).

20.2.3 Small intestine

The partially digested food that leaves the stomach and enters the small intestine is usually referred to as 'chyme' (Fig. 20.1). The emulsified lipids within the chyme are transferred from the stomach to the duodenum where they are mixed with sodium bicarbonate, bile salts, phospholipids and enzymes secreted by the liver, pancreas, and gall bladder (Tso, 2000). The composition of the lipids within the droplets at this stage will depend on the nature of the original oil phase, and any changes that occurred as it passed through the mouth and stomach (e.g., due to hydrolysis by gastric lipase). If the ingested lipid was a typical food oil, then the lipid phase entering the small intestine would typically consist of a mixture of TAG, DAG, MAG, FFA, cholesterol, carotenoids, and fat-soluble vitamins. These components would be distributed between the hydrophobic core and amphiphilic shell of the lipid droplets depending on their polarities and surface activities (Bauer *et al.*, 2005; Fave *et al.*, 2004). The sodium bicarbonate secreted into the small intestine causes the pH to increase from highly acidic (pH 1 to 3) in the stomach to around neutral (pH 5.8–6.5) in the duodenum, where the pancreatic enzymes work most efficiently (Bauer *et al.*, 2005). Nevertheless, studies with human subjects have shown that there may be large variations in both stomach and duodenum pH (Kalantzi *et al.*, 2006). The bile salts and phospholipids originating from the liver (via the gall bladder) are surface active and can facilitate emulsification of the lipids by adsorbing to the droplet surfaces (Tso, 2000). They may also displace some of the original surface active substances from the lipid droplet surfaces, thereby altering the access of the lipase/co-lipase complex to the lipids (see below). Lipid hydrolysis continues within the duodenum through the actions of lipases and other enzymes originating from the pancreas (Armand, 2007; Mukherjee, 2003). Pancreatic lipase bound to the surface of the lipid droplets will convert TAGs into DAGs, MAGs, and FFAs (Armand, 2007; Mukherjee, 2003). Cholesterol esterase converts cholesteryl ester to free cholesterol (which is the only form absorbed), as well as hydrolyzing various other types of lipid esters, such as acylglycerols, phospholglycerides, and esters of vitamins A and D (Tso, 2000). Lipids and lipid digestion products (e.g., FFAs, MAGs, cholesterol, phospholipids, and fat-soluble vitamins) are transported from the surface of the lipid droplets to the intestinal mucosa via mixed micelles and vesicles, where they are absorbed (Van Aken, 2007).

In the fasted state, the ionic strength of the small intestine has been reported to be about 140 mM (Lindahl *et al.*, 1997). After ingestion of food, there is usually an appreciable increase in the ionic strength due to the additional ions arising from the food. Over time, the ionic strength will then progressively decrease back to the value of the fasting state (Kalantzi *et al.*, 2006). The type and concentration of ions present are particularly important because they influence the magnitude and range of any electrostatic interactions in the system. For example, multivalent cations (such as Ca^{2+} and Mg^{2+}) may promote precipitation of bile salts and long chain saturated fatty acids in the small intestine, thereby decreasing their absorption (Karupaiah and Sundram, 2007; Read, 2004; Vaskonen, 2003).

The type and concentrations of surface active substances surrounding the lipid droplets may change considerably when they enter the small intestine, owing to the secretion of the bile salts and phospholipids, but also due to the presence of digestion products, such as MAGs, FFAs, lysophospholipids, peptides, and oligosaccharides (Bauer *et al.*, 2005). In the fasted state the bile salt concentration in the duodenum has been reported to be around 4.3 to 6.4 mM, while after ingestion of a meal it increases to around 5 to 15 mM (Kalantzi *et al.*, 2006). Many of these substances may compete with the surface active molecules already present at the lipid droplet surfaces, which may lead to an appreciable change in the type of molecules present at the lipid–water interface. The interfacial composition is therefore likely to change during lipid digestion, and will depend on changes in the relative concentrations and surface activities of the various amphiphilic components secreted by the body or arising from the food (originally present or produced during digestion) (Kalantzi *et al.*, 2006). If may therefore be possible to design emulsion-based delivery systems with interfacial coatings that are more or less susceptible to displacement by other surface active substances in the small intestine, thereby altering their susceptibility to lipase digestion (see below).

Typically, the lipid droplets present within the duodenum after ingestion of a fatty food have diameters that range between about 1 and 50 μm (Armand *et al.*, 1996a). Pancreatic lipase adsorbs to the surface of the emulsified lipids, usually as a complex with co-lipase and possibly bile salts (Bauer *et al.*, 2005). It then rapidly breaks down TAGs and DAGs to FFAs and MAGs (sn-2 position). It preferentially attacks fatty acids in the sn-1 and sn-3 positions, and has little specificity for fatty acid chain length (Mu and Hoy, 2004). The extent of binding of pancreatic lipase to the droplet surfaces depends on the 'quality' of the interface, although this term is not yet fully understood (Bauer *et al.*, 2005). It is likely to depend on the electrical charge of the interface, since this will affect any electrostatic interactions between the enzyme complex and the surface. In addition, there may be competitive adsorption processes occurring between the enzyme complex, bile salts, phospholipids, digestion products, and other surface active substances for the droplet surfaces, which could interfere with the binding of the lipase to the droplet surfaces. The pH optimum of pancreatic lipase is around pH 8.5, but it also operates well at pH 6.5. A co-enzyme known as 'co-lipase' is required for the optimum activity of lipase. It has been proposed that this co-enzyme forms a stoichiometric complex with lipase that adsorbs to the oil–water interface and brings the lipase into close contact with the lipid substrate. Co-lipase is a polypeptide with a molecular weight of about 10 kDa, which has a hydrophobic side that is believed to bind to the oil–water interface, and a hydrophilic side that is believed to bind the lipase. Co-lipase is secreted from the pancreas as pro-co-lipase, and then is converted into its active form when trypsin cleaves off a peptide called enterostatin. This peptide is believed to be a hormone that regulates satiety, reduces fat intake, and inhibits pancreatic secretion (Bauer *et al.*, 2005).

The presence of bile salts may either promote or inhibit the activity of pancreatic lipase depending on their concentration (Bauer *et al.*, 2005; Lowe, 2002). At relatively low concentrations, they tend to promote lipase activity, which can mainly be attributed to their ability to solubilize lipid digestion products and remove them from the oil–water interface, e.g., sn-2 MAGs and FFAs. If these products were not removed from the droplet surfaces, then the fatty acids might accumulate at the oil–water interface, thereby preventing the lipase from adsorbing and getting access to the TAGs and DAGs within the droplets. In addition, if the lipid digestion products were not removed from the site of enzyme activity, then the conversion of TAGs to MAGs and FFAs would be inhibited by the high local concentration of reaction products. On the other hand, relatively high bile salt concentrations may inhibit the ability of lipase to digest emulsified lipids. This effect can be attributed to the ability of the bile salts to compete for the oil–water interface with the lipase, thereby preventing it from coming into close proximity to the lipid substrate (Gargouri *et al.*, 1983). One of the key roles of the bile salts is to form micelles that solubilize and transport the lipid digestion products from the lipid droplet surfaces to the intestinal membrane where they are absorbed. It is therefore important that the bile salt concentration exceeds the critical micelle concentration (CMC), which is usually around 1 to 2 mM (Bauer *et al.*, 2005). In practice, the bile salt concentrations in the small intestine are above the CMC: ~6–15 mM in the duodenum (being higher after consumption of a meal); ~10 mM in the ileum; <4 mM in the ileum (where the bile salts are reabsorbed by the body).

Important insights into the physicochemical and structural mechanisms of lipid digestion in the small intestine have been obtained using light microscopy (Patton and Carey, 1979; Patton *et al.*, 1985), electron microscopy (Fatouros *et al.*, 2007a), and X-ray scattering (Fatouros *et al.*, 2007b). These studies have shown that digestion of emulsified lipids by pancreatic lipase takes place by a sequence of steps involving the formation of different phases. A liquid crystalline or crystalline phase is observed around the lipid droplet surfaces within the first few minutes of lipolysis, which gets thicker over time. Eventually, any undigested oil within the interior of the droplet may be expelled as a smaller oil droplet, leaving the liquid crystalline or crystalline phase behind. These latter phases are presumably formed due to the high local concentration of surface active lipids (FFA and MAG) at the droplet surfaces. The liquid crystalline phase tends to form at low calcium concentrations, whereas the crystalline phase forms at high calcium concentrations (due to fatty acid calcium soap formation). Nevertheless, in the presence of sufficiently high concentrations of bile salt micelles the lipid reaction products are solubilized and therefore the liquid crystalline phases may not be observed. The amount of bile salt micelles required to solubilize the reaction products depends on their solubilization capacity – once the available micelles have been saturated with digestion products, then liquid crystalline phases may be observed. It should be noted that a variety of different liquid crystalline phases have been observed depending on the nature of the original lipid, solution composition and digestion time (Patton and Carey, 1979; Patton *et al.*, 1985). Microscopy studies in our laboratory using an *in vitro* digestion model have shown that extensive droplet coalescence may occur during the digestion of emulsified lipids by lipase, which depends on the nature of the emulsifier present at the droplet surfaces (Mun *et al.*, 2007).

Potentially, the digestion and absorption of lipids in the small intestine can be affected by many different physicochemical processes. The rate of digestion will depend on the size of the emulsion droplets in the small intestine, since this influences the amount of lipid surface area exposed to the lipase. The droplet size is likely to depend on the physical organization of the lipid in the original emulsion-based delivery system, as well as the disruptive processes experienced by the lipids in the mouth, throat, and stomach. In addition, the breakdown and coalescence of the lipid droplets will depend on the composition of the droplet surfaces and the rheological properties of the surrounding medium. There may also be food components that can interact or influence the properties of the enzyme, co-enzyme, bile salts or lipid droplets. For example, it has been proposed that dietary fibers can affect lipid digestion or absorption in the small intestine through a variety of physicochemical mechanisms, e.g., increase in aqueous phase viscosity, alteration of droplet disruption or coalescence kinetics, binding of bile salts, phospholipids or enzymes, etc. (Lairon, 1997a, b; Lairon *et al.*, 2007; Mun and *et al.*, 2005).

20.2.4 Post-absorption events

Once lipid digestion products have been incorporated into micelles and vesicles and transported across the 'unstirred layer', they are absorbed by the intestinal enterocyte cells (Bauer *et al.*, 2005; Bermudez *et al.*, 2004; Fave *et al.*, 2004). Their subsequent transport to the systemic circulation depends on their chemical structure. Small chain ($<C_8$) and medium chain (C_8 to C_{12}) fatty acids tend to pass directly through the enterocyte cells and enter the portal vein where they are transported into the systemic system via the liver. On the other hand, long chain ($\geq C_{14}$) fatty acids tend to be reassembled into triacylglycerols in the enterocyte cells, packed into lipoproteins, and then transported into the systemic circulation via the lymph system, i.e.,

they do not pass through the liver first (Mu and Hoy, 2004). Different kinds of lipoproteins are formed that vary in their composition and structural organization, with the two most common being chylomicrons (CM) and very low density lipoproteins (VLDL). The type of lipoprotein that dominates depends mainly on the type and amount of fat consumed in the diet. VLDL tends to be preferentially produced during fasting, whereas CM tends to be produced after the consumption of a fatty meal.

20.2.5 Summary of key events

The above discussion has highlighted the complex series of processes that an emulsion-based delivery system will experience as it passes through the mouth, stomach, and small intestine. An improved understanding of these processes should lead to the design of emulsion-based delivery systems that can control the bioavailability of lipids. We highlight some of the key processes below that need to be considered when designing such a delivery system:

- *pH.* There are considerable variations in the pH of the aqueous phase surrounding lipid droplets as they pass through the digestive tract: mouth (pH ≈ 7); stomach (pH ≈ 2); small intestine (pH ≈ 7). These variations may cause changes in the electrical charge on the lipid droplet surfaces, as well as causing alterations in the properties and interactions of other charged species (such as enzymes, proteins, amino acids, ionic polysaccharides, and lipids).
- *Ionic composition.* There may be considerable variations in the type and concentration of ions surrounding the lipid droplets, which may impact the electrostatic interactions in the system. For example, long chain FFAs may be precipitated in the presence of calcium ions, thereby reducing their absorption. On the other hand, the complexation of long chain fatty acids with calcium ions increases the rate and efficiency of triacylglycerol digestion by removing free fatty acid digestion products away from the lipid droplet surfaces.
- *Surface active components.* There are a variety of endogeneous (e.g., proteins, phospholipids and bile salts), exogeneous (e.g., surfactants, proteins), and internally generated (e.g., lipid digestion products) surface active substances present within the aqueous phase surrounding the lipid droplets. These substances compete with the surface active substances already present at the oil–water interface, potentially leading to changes in interfacial composition and properties.
- *Enzyme activity.* There are various kinds of enzymes in the mouth, stomach, and small intestine that can digest food components, such as lipids (lipases), proteins (proteases), and starch (amylases). The ability of these enzymes to interact with the specific substrates will determine the digestibility of the various ingested food components.
- *Temperature.* There may be a large change in temperature from the initial food to the human body, which may cause changes in the physical

state, conformation or interactions of specific components that impact digestibility, e.g., melting of fats.
- *Flow/force profile.* The encapsulated lipids may be exposed to various kinds of forces and flow profiles during their passage through the human body. These processes will mix the various components together, as well as potentially breaking down various structures (lipid droplets, protein particles, hydrogel matrices, etc.).

Knowledge of how emulsion-based delivery systems behave under these different conditions may be used to design foods that either increase, decrease, or control lipid bioavailability.

20.3 Lipid bioavailability

It is informative to consider the meaning of the term 'bioavailability' in the context of lipid digestion and absorption. Prior to ingesting, a food contains definite concentrations of specific lipid components, which can be defined in terms of the grams of lipid per gram of food. As the lipids pass through the digestive tract some of them are chemically modified prior to absorption (e.g., hydrolysis of triacylglycerols, diacylglycerols, or cholesterol esters), so that the absorbed species is different from the one originally present in the food. It is therefore important to be aware of any potential chemical changes that occur to a lipid, the rate at which these changes occur, and the factors that impact them, since this will affect the subsequent digestion and absorption of the lipid (Verhagen *et al.*, 2004).

The term *bioavailability* has been defined as the fraction of an ingested component that eventually ends up in the systemic circulation (Versantvoort *et al.*, 2004). The bioavailability (F) of a particular component can be divided into a number of physicochemical contributions (Versantvoort *et al.*, 2004):

- *Bioaccessibility* – the fraction of the component that is released from the food matrix into the juices of the gastrointestinal tract (F_B).
- *Transport* – the fraction of the released component that is transported across the intestinal epithelium and into the enterocyte cells (F_T).
- *Metabolism* – the fraction of the component that passes through the liver without being metabolized (F_M) – if the lipid is absorbed via the portal vein.

Hence the fraction of the ingested component that eventually reaches the systemic circulation is given by $F = F_B \times F_T \times F_M$. The value of the F_M term depends on the pathway that the lipid takes after it enters the enterocyte cells. Small and medium chain fatty acids tend to pass directly through the enterocyte cells and enter the portal vein where they are transported into the systemic system via the liver. In this case, the value of F_M depends on whether the lipid components are metabolized during this first pass through the liver. On the other hand, long chain fatty acids tend to be reassembled into triacylglycerols in the enterocytes, then packed into lipoproteins (see

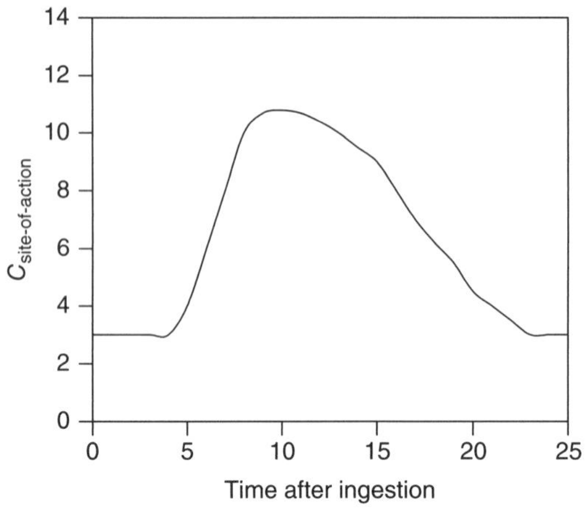

Fig. 20.2 Highly schematic representation of the change in the concentration of a lipophilic component at a particular tissue over time after ingestion of a food.

below), and then transported into the systemic circulation via the lymph system, i.e., they do not pass through the liver first. In this case, F_M should equal one, since these lipids will not be metabolized within the liver. After the component reaches the systemic circulation it may be distributed between different tissues, where it may be stored, utilized, or excreted (Verhagen *et al.*, 2004). The relative rates of these various processes will determine the time-dependence of the concentration of the lipid and its metabolites at specific locations within the body. The concentration–time profile of a specific lipid component at a particular site of action will determine its beneficial or adverse affects on human health and wellness. Consequently, it may be important to measure the concentration of a lipid component at a particular location in order to establish its efficacy (Verhagen *et al.*, 2004).

The time-dependence of the concentration of a lipid component at a specific site of action in the human body after ingestion of a food often looks something like Fig. 20.2. There is usually a lag period between ingestion of a food and the first appearance of the lipid component within the tissue of interest. The duration of this lag period depends on the time taken for the lipid component to be released from the food matrix, and then digested, absorbed, and transported to the site where the sample was collected. The overall shape of the curve depends on where the concentration of the component is measured (e.g., blood, liver, muscle, adipose tissue, feces), as well as the relative rates of release, digestion, absorption, transport, utilization, and excretion of the component.

By analogy to pharmaceuticals, there may be a range of concentrations where the optimum efficacy of a bioactive component is demonstrated. If the concentration is too high, the component may have adverse effects or be toxic, but if it is too low it may be ineffective. It is therefore important to establish the dose dependence of specific bioactive components, and to ensure that they are delivered to the required site of action within the optimum concentration range. The aim of a food scientist should therefore be to formulate an emulsion-based delivery system so that the concentration of specific bioactive components falls within this desirable range.

When considering factors that can impact the bioavailability of food components, it is also important to distinguish between their influence on the *rate* and *extent* of lipid digestion or absorption. Some factors may affect the rate at which a lipid component is digested or absorbed, without affecting the final amount, whereas others may affect the final amount of material that is digested or absorbed. If a food component spends sufficient time within the gastrointestinal (GI) tract, then the rate of digestion and absorption may be less important than their total extent. For example, a lipid in the solid state may be digested more slowly than one in the liquid state, but the food may spend sufficient time within the GI tract for all the lipid phase to be digested anyway. On the other hand, if the rate of digestion or absorption can be slowed down sufficiently, it may reduce the bioavailability of the component.

20.4 Impact of lipid type and concentration on bioavailability

Before discussing the impact of the structural properties of emulsion-based delivery systems on lipid bioavailability, it is useful to discuss the general effects of lipid type and concentration on bioavailability. There are large variations in the chemical structure of lipid molecules that have a pronounced impact on their bioavailability (McClements and Decker, 2007). Triacylglycerols typically have a high bioavailability, with over 95% of the ingested lipids being absorbed, which can be attributed to their ability to be broken down by lipase into digestion products (MAGs and FFAs) that can be incorporated into colloidal carrier structures within the GI tract (Patton *et al.*, 1985). On the other hand, highly hydrophobic bioactive components often have poor bioavailability owing to difficulties associated with releasing them from food matrices and incorporating them within colloidal carrier structures, e.g., β-carotene, lutein and lycopene (Faulks and Southon, 2001; Wildman and Kelley, 2007a; Wright *et al.*, 2008).

The digestion of triacylglycerols depends on their molecular structure, i.e., the type and position of the fatty acid chains on the glycerol backbone (Bauer *et al.*, 2005; Fave *et al.*, 2004). The rate of fatty acid release from TAGs during lipolysis is faster for short and medium chain FAs than for long chain FAs, and is faster for FAs at the sn-1 and sn-3 positions than in the sn-2 position, since pancreatic lipase has high specificity for sn-1 and sn-3. In addition, the rate of absorption of FAs in the sn-2 position is usually higher than that in the sn-1 or sn-3 positions, because MAGs are absorbed more rapidly than FFAs. Long chain saturated FFAs in particular are poorly absorbed because they tend to form insoluble soaps in the small intestine due to their high melting points and the strong electrostatic attraction between the anionic fatty acids and cationic multivalent mineral ions, such as calcium and magnesium (Karupaiah and Sundram, 2007). The low bioavailability of long chain saturated fats such as stearic and palmitic acid results in certain fats having less than 9 kcal/g. For instance, tristearin has been estimated to have only 3 kcal/g when fed to young rats (Ranhotra *et al.*, 1998). Food lipids vary in the location of fatty acids at different positions on the triacylglycerol. For example, tropical oils such as cocoa butter, coconut and palm oil have large amounts of long chain saturated fatty acids at sn-1 and sn-3, while bovine and human milk fat have saturated fatty acids primarily at sn-2 (Decker, 1996; Karupaiah and Sundram, 2007). These differences could be partially attributed to the biological role of the fat in the case of bovine milk fat since the purpose of milk fat is to deliver calories to the calf and thus maximal bioavailability of long chain saturated fatty acids is desirable. Interesterification of tropical oils increases the amount of long chain saturated fatty acid at the sn-2 position and increases fatty acid absorption (Karupaiah and Sundram, 2007). The stereospecific location of fatty acids can also impact atherosclerosis with inter-esterified peanut oil (less saturated at sn-1 and sn-3) being less atherogenic than native peanut oil (Kritchevsky *et al.*, 1975). Dietary calcium concentrations can also impact fatty acid bioavailability (Karupaiah and Sundram, 2007; Lorenzen *et al.*, 2007; Scholz-Ahrens and Schrezenmeir, 2006). Denke and co-workers found that 2200 mg calcium/day increased human excretion of saturated fatty acids and decreased total and LDL plasma cholesterol concentrations (Denke *et al.*, 1993). The fact that the absorption of long chain saturated fatty acids can be influenced by their stereospecific location led to the development of low-calorie food lipids. These products included Salatrim and Caprenin which have relatively high concentrations of stearic acid or behenic acid (22:0) at the sn-1 and sn-3 positions, respectively, thus decreasing the absorption and thus the caloric contribution of the saturated fatty acids. These structured fats have an estimated 5–7 kcal/g (Finley *et al.*, 1994; Hayes *et al.*, 1994; Klemann *et al.*, 1994; Ranhotra *et al.*, 1998).

It should also be noted that the type of TAGs in a lipid may also influence the digestion and absorption processes indirectly, through their influence on the tendency for droplets to be broken up or to coalesce in the mouth, stomach and small intestine (Fave *et al.*, 2004). In particular, the TAG type, and the presence of surface active lipids (such as FFAs, phospholipids, MAGs, and DAGs) may alter the size of the lipid droplets in the stomach or small intestine, which will alter the efficiency of lipid digestion. The TAG composition will also influence the solid fat content of the lipid phase, which may influence their digestibility and absorption (see later). In addition, if there is a high concentration of surface active lipids present, these may displace the TAGs from the droplets surfaces, and thereby reduce the rate of digestion by altering the droplet interfacial composition (Bauer *et al.*, 2005; Fave *et al.*, 2004).

The type and amount of TAGs ingested also affect lipid digestion and absorption. Research in the pharmaceutical area has shown that the bioavailability of highly hydrophobic drugs can be greatly increased by ingesting them with a triacylglycerol carrier lipid (Porter *et al.*, 2007). The origin of this enhanced bioavailability has been attributed to a number of different effects of the carrier lipid on digestion and absorption:

- *Increased solubilization capacity*: the solubilization of a hydrophobic bioactive component within the colloidal carrier structures present within the small intestine (micelles and vesicles) is greatly increased in the presence of a carrier lipid. Firstly, this increase in solubilization power can be attributed to the enhanced secretion of bile salts and phospholipids that occurs when lipids are co-ingested. Secondly, the lipid digestion products (fatty acids and monoacylglycerols) themselves can be incorporated into micelles and vesicles and increase their solubilization capacity. The extent of the increase in solubilization power in the presence of lipids has been found to depend on lipid type, particularly the chain length of the fatty acids. Long chain ($\geq C_{14}$) fatty acids have been found to be more effective than medium chain (C_8 to C_{12}) or short chain ($\leq C_6$) fatty acids at increasing the solubilization power of the colloidal structures within the small intestine, although this may depend somewhat on the type of bioactive component solubilized (Porter *et al.*, 2007).
- *Transport pathway.* The ingestion of a highly hydrophobic bioactive component with a triacylglycerol carrier lipid may also increase its bioactivity by influencing the transport pathway within the enterocyte cells. After absorption of a bioactive lipid into the enterocyte cells it may be transported to the systemic circulation by either the portal vein (where it passes through the liver) or the intestinal lymphatic system (thereby avoiding first-pass through the liver). The transport pathway taken depends on the chain length of the fatty acids that are ingested. Small and medium chain fatty acids tend to be absorbed via the portal vein, whereas long chain fatty acids tend to be absorbed via the lymphatic system. In addition, monounsaturated and polyunsaturated fatty acids tend to be more readily absorbed via the lymph system than saturated fatty acids. When a highly hydrophobic bioactive component is ingested with a triacylglycerol carrier lipid that contains long chain fatty acids, then it may be incorporated within the hydrophobic core of lipoproteins formed within the enterocyte cells, thereby favoring its transport via the lymph system. If a bioactive component is metabolized within the liver, then it may be more favorable to direct its transport through the lymph system to avoid its degradation.

- *Enterocyte absorption.* There is some evidence that carrier lipids and bioactive components may interact with transport pathways into and across the enterocyte cells, e.g., altering the performance of cell membrane transporters or lipid-binding proteins (Porter *et al.*, 2007). Nevertheless, the importance of these mechanisms is still not clearly understood and research is ongoing.

20.5 Emulsion-based delivery systems

Many different kinds of delivery system have been developed to encapsulate lipophilic functional agents, including simple solutions, association colloids (micelles, microemulsions, vesicles), emulsions, biopolymer matrices, powders, etc. Each kind of delivery system has its own advantages and disadvantages for encapsulation, protection, and delivery of functional agents, as well as in its cost, regulatory status, ease of use, biodegradability, biocompatibility, etc. In this chapter, we focus on emulsion-based delivery systems since these systems offer the food industry a particularly convenient means of encapsulating, protecting, and releasing lipids. They can be fabricated entirely from food-grade components using relatively simple processing operations. There structural properties, such as droplet size, droplet concentration, and interfacial properties, can be controlled in a rational and systematic fashion. They can be conveniently incorporated into many food products in either a wet (emulsion) or dry (powder) form without adversely affecting their properties, e.g., beverages, dressings, deserts, sauces, dips, soups, batters, spreads, meat products, and baked goods.

Bioactive lipids differ widely in their molecular properties (e.g., molecular weights, structures, functional groups, polarities and charge), which lead to differences in their physicochemical and physiological properties (e.g., solubility, physical state, rheology, optical properties, chemical stability, surface activity, and bioactivity). Consequently, delivery systems often have to be designed to address the specific molecular, physicochemical, and physiological concerns that are unique to each bioactive lipid.

20.5.1 Desirable characteristics of delivery systems

There are a number of characteristics that an edible delivery system must have if it is going to be suitable for utilization by the food and other industries. Some of the most important attributes are listed below:

- *Food grade*: the delivery system must be fabricated entirely from permitted food ingredients using processing operations that have regulatory approval. Some of the most common food-grade ingredients that can be used to assemble emulsion-based delivery systems are listed in Table 20.1.

Table 20.1 Major food-grade components that can be used to construct emulsion-based delivery systems

Name	Important characteristics	Examples
Lipids	Polarity Physical state Chemical stability	• *Animal fats*: beef, pork, chicken • *Fish oils*: cod liver, menhedan, salmon, tuna • *Plant oils*: palm, coconut, sunflower, safflower, corn, flax seed, soybean • *Flavor oils*: lemon, orange
Surfactants	Solubility (HLB) Charge Molecular geometry Surface load Surface activity	• *Non-ionic*: Tween, Span • *Anionic*: SLS, DATEM, CITREM • *Cationic*: Lauric arginate • *Zwitterionic*: lecithin
Biopolymers	Molar mass Conformation Charge Hydrophobicity Flexibility Transition temperature	• *Globular proteins*: whey, soy, egg • *Flexible proteins*: casein, gelatin • *Non-ionic polysaccharides*: starch, dextran, agar, galactomannans, cellulose • *Anionic polysaccharides*: alginate, pectin, xanthan, carrageenan, gellan, gum Arabic • *Cationic polysaccharides*: chitosan

HLB: hydrophile – lipophile balance.

- *Economic production*: the delivery system should be capable of being economically and consistently manufactured from inexpensive ingredients.
- *Protection against chemical degradation*: the delivery system may have to protect an encapsulated bioactive lipid against some form of chemical degradation during storage, e.g., oxidation, hydrolysis.
- *Loading capacity and retention*: a delivery system should be capable of encapsulating a relatively large amount of bioactive lipid per unit mass of carrier material, and should efficiently retain the encapsulated component until it needs to be delivered.
- *Delivery mechanism*: the delivery system may have to be designed so that it releases the bioactive lipid at a particular site of action, at a controlled rate or in response to a specific environmental stimulus (e.g., pH, ionic strength, enzyme activity, or temperature).
- *Food matrix compatibility*: the delivery system should be compatible with the surrounding food or beverage matrix, i.e., it should not adversely affect the appearance, texture, flavor, or stability of the final product.
- *Bioavailability/bioactivity*: a delivery system should enhance (or at least not adversely affect) the bioavailability/bioactivity of the encapsulated component.

20.5.2 Preparation and properties of emulsion-based delivery systems

A brief overview of the major kinds of delivery systems that can be assembled from food grade components using emulsion technology is given in this section. We limit the scope of this overview to emulsion-based delivery systems with aqueous-based continuous phases, as well as to delivery systems based on emulsions (which are thermodynamically unstable), rather than on microemulsions (which are thermodynamically stable).

Prior to creating an emulsion-based delivery system, it is important to consider how the oil phase will be prepared and handled. Many liquid oils can be used directly to prepare an emulsion, e.g., olive, fish, corn, or soybean oils. Lipids that are partially or fully solid at ambient temperatures may have to be melted prior to emulsion preparation to avoid fouling of homogenizers, e.g., lard, palm or coconut oils. If a minor lipid component is to be delivered (e.g., a vitamin, antioxidant or nutraceutical), then it may first have to be dispersed within a *carrier oil* (such as corn, soybean, or olive oils) prior to homogenization. If a minor lipid component is crystalline (e.g., phytosterols or carotenoids), then it may be necessary to ensure that it is used at a level below its saturation concentration in the carrier oil, or to warm the lipid phase prior to homogenization to melt any crystals present. If the lipid is susceptible to chemical degradation (e.g., ω-3 fatty acids, conjugated linoleic acid (CLA), and carotenoids), then it may be necessary to carefully control preparation conditions to avoid exposure to factors that increase the degradation rate (e.g., high temperatures, oxygen, light or transition metals).

Conventional emulsions

Structure: Conventional oil-in-water (O/W) emulsions consist of lipid droplets dispersed in an aqueous continuous phase, with the lipid core being surrounded by a thin interfacial layer consisting of emulsifier molecules (Fig. 20.3) (Dickinson, 1992; Friberg *et al.*, 2004; McClements, 2005a). The

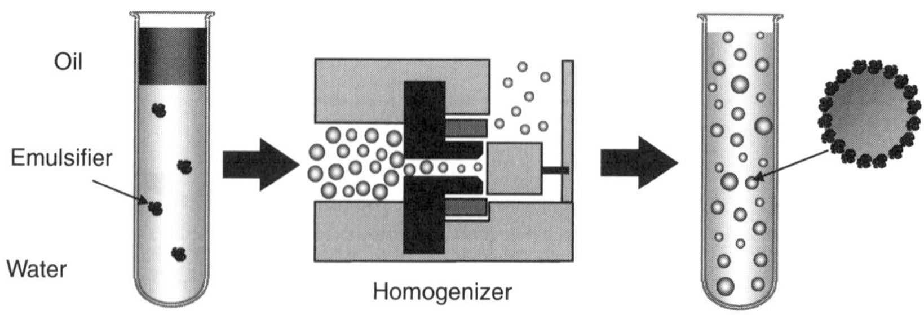

Fig. 20.3 Schematic representation of the formation of conventional oil-in-water emulsions. These emulsions are formed by homogenizing oil and aqueous phases together in the presence of a water-soluble emulsifier.

particle size distribution and concentration of the lipid droplets in O/W emulsions can be controlled, as can the nature of the emulsifier used to stabilize the system. Typically, O/W emulsions are prepared with lipid droplets having diameters in the range of 0.1 to 100 μm, although it is possible to prepare emulsions with larger or smaller droplets for specific applications. The thickness, packing, and charge of the interfacial layer can be controlled by selecting different kinds of food grade emulsifiers, e.g., surfactants, phospholipids, proteins, or polysaccharides. Typically, the thickness of the interfacial layer lies somewhere within the range of 1 to 50 nm and can be controlled by selection of different emulsifiers. The charge on the interfacial layer can be made positive, negative or neutral by selection of cationic, anionic, or non-ionic food grade emulsifiers.

Preparation: conventionally, O/W emulsions are prepared by homogenizing an oil phase and an aqueous phase together in the presence of a water-soluble emulsifier (Fig. 20.3). A variety of different kinds of homogenizers are available, including high-shear mixers, high-pressure homogenizers, colloid mills, ultrasonic homogenizers, and membrane homogenizers (McClements, 2005a; Walstra, 1993, 2003). The choice of a particular kind of homogenizer and of the operating conditions used depend on the characteristics of the materials being homogenized (e.g., viscosity, interfacial tension, shear sensitivity) and of the required final properties of the emulsion (e.g., droplet concentration, droplet size, viscosity). For example, the size of the droplets in an O/W emulsion produced by a high-pressure homogenizer can be decreased by increasing the homogenizer pressure or the number of passes of the emulsion through the device (Kanafusa *et al.*, 2007).

Potential methods of controlling lipid bioavailability: in principle, there are a number of ways that emulsion-based delivery systems produced from conventional oil-in-water emulsions could be designed to control lipid bioavailability:

- *Control of droplet size.* Lipid hydrolysis occurs when lipases adsorb to lipid droplet surfaces, i.e., it is a surface mediated reaction. The specific surface area of the lipids in an oil-in-water emulsion is given by the following expression: $A_N = 6\phi/d_{32}$, where, A_N is the surface area of lipids exposed to the aqueous phase per unit volume of emulsion, d_{32} is the surface-weighted mean diameter, and ϕ is the disperse phase volume fraction. Consequently, the rate of hydrolysis should be inversely proportional to the mean droplet diameter. *In vitro* experiments of lipase catalyzed digestion of emulsified lipids have shown that the rate of lipid hydrolysis does increase with decreasing droplet size (Armand *et al.*, 1992; Borel *et al.*, 1994). In principle, it is therefore possible to control the rate of lipid digestion by controlling the initial lipid droplet size in an emulsion-based delivery system – the smaller the droplets, the faster lipid digestion. Nevertheless, *in vivo* studies where oil-in-water emulsions were injected directly into the stomach (rather than being consumed) have shown that the overall extent of lipid hydrolysis is unaffected by the initial size of the lipid droplets (0.7 versus 10 μm) (Armand *et al.*, 1999). One of the reasons for the differences between *in vitro* and *in vivo* experiments is that the size of the lipid droplets often changes considerably after ingestion due to the various processes discussed earlier, e.g., droplet coalescence and disruption (Bauer *et al.*, 2005; Fave *et al.*, 2004). In addition, differences in the initial rate of lipid digestion may be unimportant over the relatively long timescales that foods remain in the human digestive tract (hours), since all the lipids may eventually be digested.

- *Interfacial composition.* For lipid hydrolysis to occur, it is necessary for lipases to adsorb to the surfaces of lipid droplets. The propensity for lipase to adsorb to a lipid droplet surface depends on the nature of the surface (Reis *et al.*, 2006; Sonesson *et al.*, 2006). The initial composition and characteristics of the droplet surfaces can be controlled by selection of appropriate emulsifiers and processing operations. In principle, it should therefore be possible to control the interactions between lipase and lipid droplet surfaces. Indeed, a number of *in vitro* studies of the digestibility of lipid droplets have shown that the rate and extent of lipid digestion depend on emulsifier type (Mun *et al.*, 2006, 2007). A recent *in vitro* study in our laboratory on the impact of emulsifier type on the digestion of emulsified lipids showed that the rate and extent of fatty acid release was higher for protein-coated droplets (casein or whey protein) than for surfactant-coated droplets (Tween or lecithin) (Fig. 20.4). Nevertheless, it should be stressed that the interfacial properties of lipid droplets normally change appreciably after a food is ingested because of displacement by other surface active substances and/or because the original emulsifier molecules are digested by enzymes (Sonesson *et al.*, 2006, 2007). Consequently, the surface properties of the lipid droplets in the stomach and small intestine could be dominated by the presence of endogenous surface active substances, rather than by the surface active substances initially present at the droplet surfaces in the food. If one wanted to increase the bioavailability of an encapsulated lipid component, then one may want to ensure that the lipase can adsorb to the droplet surfaces. In this case, one would want to use an emulsifier that is either digested or that is displaced from the droplet surfaces within the digestive tract. Conversely, if one wished to decrease the bioavailability of an encapsulated lipid component, then one may want to ensure that the lipase cannot adsorb to the droplet surfaces and access the lipids. In this case, one would want to use an emulsifier that remains intact around the lipid droplets (i.e., it is neither digested nor displaced) and that is impermeable to enzyme diffusion.
- *Physical state.* The physical state of the lipids in oil-in-water emulsions can be controlled by appropriate selection of lipid type (e.g., solid

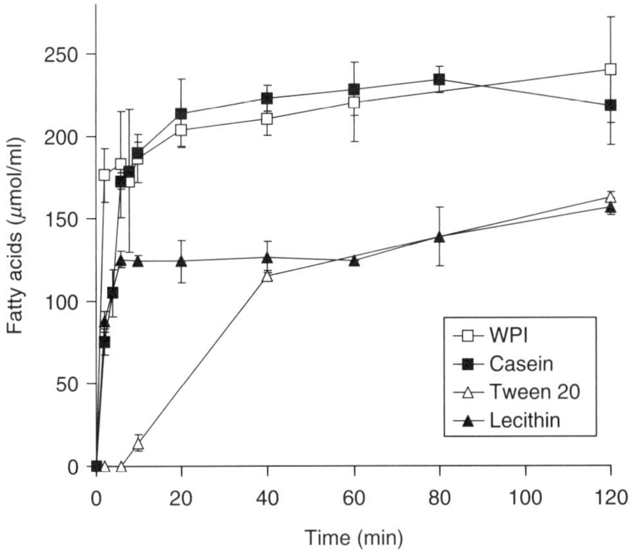

Fig. 20.4 Influence of emulsifier type on the *in vitro* digestibility of emulsified corn oil.

fat content versus temperature profile) and thermal history (e.g., temperature–time profile). It is possible to prepare emulsions with completely liquid droplets, completely solid droplets, or a mixture of solid and liquid within the droplets (Bunjes *et al.*, 2003; Ghosh *et al.*, 2006; McClements *et al.*, 1990). Emulsions containing fully or partially crystallized lipid droplets are sometimes referred to as *solid lipid nanoparticles* (SLN), and may be utilized to encapsulate, protect, and deliver functional lipid components (Bummer, 2004; Muller and Keck, 2004; Muller *et al.*, 2000). Potentially, the crystallinity of the lipid phase may alter the ability of enzymes to digest the emulsified lipids (i.e., to convert the triacylglycerols to free fatty acids, diacyglycerols and monoacyglycerols) or to alter the absorption of the digestion products (e.g., solubilization and transport in mixed micelles). *In vitro* and *in vivo* studies have shown that encapsulated lipophilic molecules are released from SLN, which would suggest that the solidified lipids are still digested and the encapsulated lipophilic components are still bioavailable (Olbrich *et al.*, 2002a, b).

Nevertheless, the release rate of lipophilic molecules from emulsified lipids during digestion depends on the crystallinity and structural organization of the lipid phase. For example, it has been shown that the release rate of a lipophilic drug decreased with increasing crystallinity of the lipid droplets (Olbrich *et al.*, 2002b). A recent study in our laboratory has shown that solid tripalmitin particles are digested at a slower rate than liquid tripalmitin droplets by lipase (Fig. 20.5). Consequently, it may be possible to control the bioavailability of lipids by changing the physi-

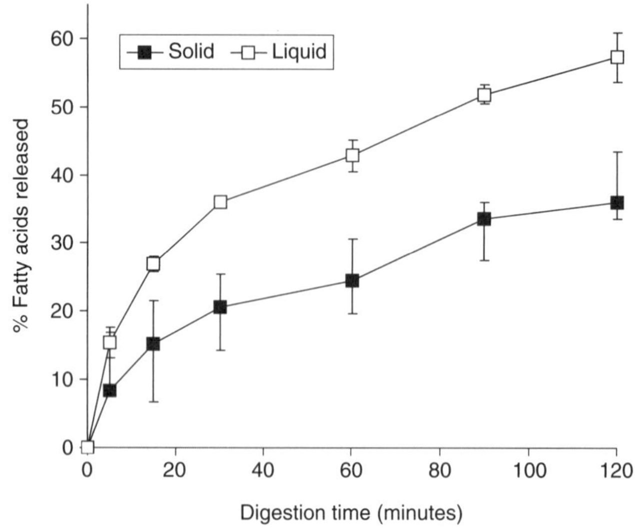

Fig. 20.5 Influence of lipid physical state (completely solid versus completely liquid) on the *in vitro* digestibility of emulsified tripalmitin.

cal state of the lipid droplets – the greater the solid fat content, the slower lipid digestion. As mentioned earlier the physical state of the lipids may also alter the absorption of lipid digestion products via mixed micelles and vesicles. For example, long chain fatty acids have been shown to form insoluble soaps in the presence of multivalent cations (such as Ca^{2+} and Mg^{2+}), thereby retarding their absorption (Read, 2004; Vaskonen, 2003).

In principle, careful design of lipid droplet size, surface properties and physical state may be used to control lipid digestibility and absorption, although more research is certainly needed in this area to understand how these systems behave within animals and humans.

Multiple emulsions

Structure: multiple emulsions of the water-in-oil-in-water (W/O/W) type consist of small water droplets contained within larger oil droplets, which are themselves dispersed in an aqueous continuous phase (Garti, 1997a, b; Garti and Benichou, 2004; Garti and Bisperink, 1998) (Fig. 20.6). Water-in-oil-in-water emulsions are more accurately designated as $W_1/O/W_2$ emulsions, where W_1 is the inner water phase and W_2 is outer water phase, since these two aqueous phases usually have different compositions. There are two different interfacial regions in this type of emulsion: the W_1–O layer surrounding the inner water droplets, and the O–W_2 layer surrounding the oil droplets. Consequently, two different types of emulsifier are usually needed to stabilize W/O/W emulsions: an oil-soluble emulsifier for the inner

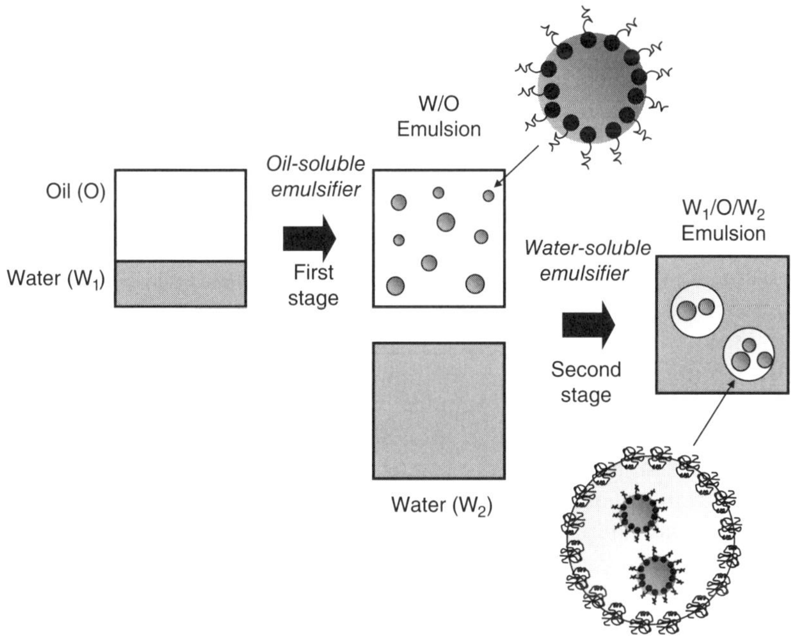

Fig. 20.6 Schematic representation of the formation of a multiple water-in-oil-in-water (W/O/W) emulsion. First, a W/O emulsion is formed by homogenizing an oil and aqueous phase together in the presence of an oil-soluble emulsifier. Second, a W/O/W emulsion is formed by homogenizing the W/O emulsion with an aqueous phase containing a water-soluble emulsifier.

water droplets and a water-soluble emulsifier for the oil droplets (Fig. 20.6). In this system, it is possible to control the particle size distribution and concentration of both the inner water droplets and the oil droplets, as well as the interfacial characteristics of the W_1–O and O–W_2 layers surrounding the various types of droplet (e.g., thickness, charge, permeability, chemical reactivity, and environmental responsiveness).

Preparation: multiple emulsions of this kind are normally produced using a two-step procedure (Fig. 20.6): (1) a W_1/O emulsion is produced by homogenizing water, oil, and an oil-soluble emulsifier together; (2) a $W_1/O/W_2$ emulsion is then produced by homogenizing the W_1/O emulsion with an aqueous solution containing a water-soluble emulsifier. Similar kinds of homogenizers can be used to produce $W_1/O/W_2$ emulsions as to produce O/W emulsions, e.g., high shear mixers, high pressure homogenizers, colloid mills, ultrasonic homogenizers, and membrane homogenizers (McClements, 2005b). Nevertheless, the homogenization conditions used in the second stage are often less intense than those used in the first stage, so as to avoid disruption or expulsion of the W_1 droplets within the oil phase. The size of the water droplets in the W_1/O emulsion can be controlled by varying emulsifier type, emulsifier concentration, and homogenization conditions (e.g., energy intensity and duration) in the first stage. Similarly, the size of the oil droplets in the final $W_1/O/W_2$ emulsion can be controlled by varying emulsifier type, emulsifier concentration, and homogenization conditions in the second stage. The concentration of water droplets in the W_1/O emulsion can be controlled by using a different ratio of W_1 to oil phase in the first homogenization step, whereas the concentration of W_1/O droplets in the final $W_1/O/W_2$ emulsion can be controlled by using a different ratio of W_1/O emulsion to W_2 phase in the second homogenization step. Consequently, one has great scope for creating structured delivery systems with different compositions and microstructures based on multiple emulsions.

Bioactive components can potentially be located in a number of different molecular and physical environments within a $W_1/O/W_2$ emulsion. Hydrophilic components can be incorporated into the inner water phase by dispersing them in the W_1 phase prior to the first homogenization step, or in the outer water phase by dispersing them in the W_2 phase after the second homogenization step. Lipophilic components can be incorporated into the oil droplets by dispersing them in the oil phase either before or after the first homogenization step. Surface active components could be located at either the W_1/O or O/W_2 interfaces depending on when they were incorporated during the emulsion preparation procedure.

Potential methods of controlling lipid bioavailability: the bioavailability of lipids in W/O/W emulsions may be controlled using the same approaches used for O/W emulsions, e.g., controlling lipid droplet size, interfacial properties, or lipid physical state (see above). The main advantage of using W/O/W emulsions is to deliver hydrophilic bioactive components that would normally be degraded within the highly acidic environment of the stomach. For example, W/O/W emulsions could be designed to deliver hydrophililc bioactive components (such as peptides, proteins, or minerals) to the small or large intestine, while protecting them from degradation within the stomach. The hydrophililc bioactive component would be encapsulated within the inner water phase (W_1), while the oil phase would be designed to be digested primarily in the small or large intestine. Only after the lipid phase was digested would the hydrophilic bioactive component be released. Previous studies have shown that various hydrophilic components can be encapsulated within W/O/W emulsions, including vitamin B (Fechner *et al.*, 2007; Kukizaki and Goto, 2007; Owusu *et al.*, 1992), immunoglobulins (Chen *et al.*, 1999; Lee *et al.*, 2004), insulin (Cournarie *et al.*, 2004), proteins (Su *et al.*, 2006), and amino acids (Owusu *et al.*, 1992; Weiss *et al.*, 2005). Nevertheless, there are few examples of *in vitro* or *in vivo* studies of lipid digestibility in these systems.

Multilayer emulsions

Structure: multilayer oil-in-water (M-O/W) emulsions consist of small lipid droplets dispersed in an aqueous medium, with each lipid droplet being

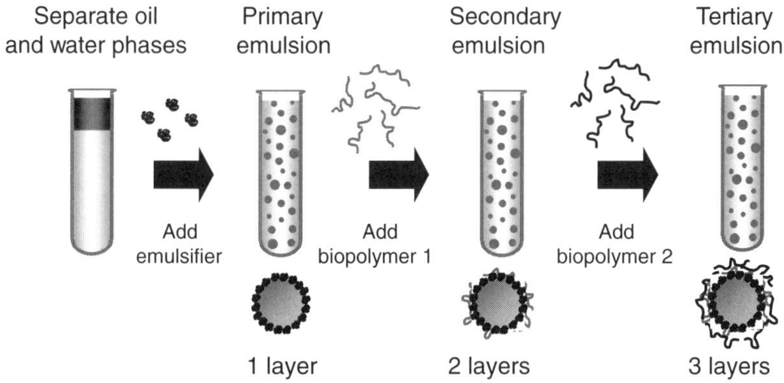

Fig. 20.7 Schematic representation of the formation of multilayer oil-in-water emulsions. An O/W emulsion is formed by homogenizing oil and aqueous phases together in the presence of a water-soluble ionic emulsifier. Multilayer coatings are then formed around the lipid droplets by adding oppositely charged polyelectrolytes.

surrounded by a nano-laminated coating consisting of layers of emulsifier and/or biopolymer molecules (Fig. 20.7). The particle size distribution and concentration of the oil droplets in M-O/W can be controlled, as can the characteristics of the interfacial layer surrounding the droplets, e.g., composition, thickness, charge, permeability, and environmental responsiveness.

Preparation: the method used to form multilayer emulsions is shown schematically in Fig. 20.7 (McClements, 2005b). Initially, an oil-in-water emulsion is prepared by homogenizing an oil and aqueous phase together in the presence of an ionized water-soluble emulsifier. The resulting 'primary' emulsion consists of electrically charged lipid droplets dispersed within an aqueous medium. An oppositely charged polyelectrolyte is then added to the system so that it adsorbs to the droplet surfaces and produces a 'secondary' emulsion consisting of lipid droplets coated by a two-layer emulsifier–polyelectrolyte interface. This procedure can be repeated a number of times to form lipid droplets coated by nano-laminated interfaces containing three or more layers.

One of the major advantages of using multilayer emulsions as delivery systems is that the properties of the interfacial layer surrounding the oil droplets can be carefully controlled, e.g., composition, structure, charge, thickness, permeability, rheology, and environmental responsiveness (Decher and Schlenoff, 2003). This can be achieved by careful control of system composition and preparation conditions during the production of the multilayer emulsions, e.g., emulsifier type and concentration, polyelectrolyte type and concentration, pH, ionic strength, order of ingredient

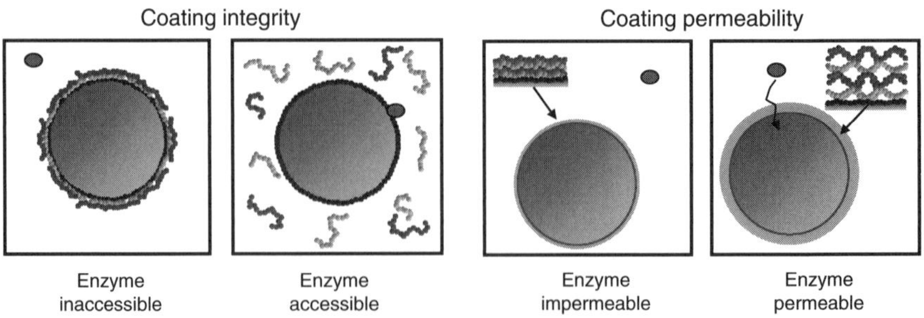

Fig. 20.8 The integrity and permeability of a nano-laminated coatings determine the ability of digestive enzymes to access encapsulated lipids.

addition, mixing conditions, and post-mixing conditions (Guzey and McClements, 2006). In principle, the ability to systematically control interfacial properties in a rational manner enables one to control the bioavailability of encapsulated lipids.

Potential methods of controlling lipid bioavailability: In principle, the bioactivity of an encapsulated lipid could be controlled using multilayer emulsions (Fig. 20.8):

- *Coating integrity.* If a lipid droplet is surrounded by a coating of material that prevents the enzymes from reaching the encapsulated lipids, then the lipid phase may not be digested and bioactive components released. The *integrity* of a nano-laminated coating may be greatly altered during the passage of an encapsulated lipid through the GI tract due to changes in pH, ionic strength, levels of surface active components, and enzyme activities (McClements, 2005a). Surface active components may displace biopolymer layers through a competitive adsorption process. Changes in pH and ionic strength may cause biopolymer layers to become detached by weakening electrostatic interactions. Enzymes such as proteases or amylases may degrade certain biopolymer layers. The bioavailability of encapsulated lipids may therefore be controlled by controlling the responsiveness of a coating's integrity to different biological fluids (e.g., saliva, or gastric or pancreatic juices).
- *Coating permeability.* Even if the nano-laminated coating remains around the lipid droplets within the GI tract, the digestibility of the encapsulated lipids will depend on the ability of the digestive enzymes to penetrate through the layers and access the lipid phase (Angelatos *et al.*, 2007). The *permeability* of a nano-laminated coating will depend on its pore size, as well as specific interactions between the enzyme molecules and biopolymers in successive layers. Previous studies have shown that the permeability of nano-laminated coatings formed by the layer by layer (LbL) method depends strongly on ionic strength and pH because they are held together by electrostatic interactions. For example,

when the solution pH or ionic strength is changed so that the electrostatic interactions between the polymer layers are weakened, a coating may swell considerably, thereby increasing its permeability to small molecules (Rubner, 2003; Schlenoff, 2003). It is therefore possible to 'tune' the permeability of coatings by careful control of biopolymer type and assembly conditions (Angelatos *et al.*, 2007). Consequently, it may be possible to control the bioavailability of an encapsulated lipid by controlling the responsiveness of a coating's permeability to different biological fluids (e.g., saliva, or gastric or pancreatic juices).

Research in non-food applications means that there is currently a fairly good understanding of the major factors that influence the formation of nano-laminated coatings around colloidal particles (Decher and Schlenoff, 2003). These studies have shown that the thickness and properties of the interfacial membranes formed around colloidal particles depend on: the electrical charge density, flexibility and molecular weight of the polymer; the concentration, ζ-potential and radius of the colloidal particles; and the pH, ionic strength, and temperature of the aqueous phase surrounding the particles (Schoeler *et al.*, 2002, 2003). Nevertheless, research is still needed within the food industry to establish: (i) how nano-laminated coatings with different integrities and permeabilities can be produced using food grade ingredients; (ii) how these coatings respond to the conditions found within the human GI tract; and (iii) how this information can be used to design delivery systems that can be used to control the bioavailability of lipophilic food components.

Our research group has carried out preliminary experiments to study the impact of nano-laminated coatings on the digestibility of encapsulated lipids (Mun *et al.*, 2006; Park and Pariza, 2007). Initially, we examined the influence of coating properties on the *in vitro* digestion of encapsulated lipids by pancreatic lipase. The electrostatic layer-by-layer deposition technique was used to prepare corn oil-in-water emulsions (3 wt% oil) that contained droplets coated by (i) lecithin, (ii) lecithin–chitosan, or (iii) lecithin–chitosan–pectin. Pancreatic lipase and/or bile extract were added to each emulsion and the FFA released due to digestion were measured. In the presence of bile extract, the amount of fatty acids released was much lower in the emulsions containing droplets coated by lecithin–chitosan (38 ± 16 μmol ml^{-1}) than those containing droplets coated by lecithin (250 ± 70 μmol ml^{-1}) or lecithin–chitosan–pectin (274 ± 80 μmol ml^{-1}) (Fig. 20.9).

We postulated that lipase activity was reduced in the lecithin–chitosan emulsion due to the formation of a relatively thick cationic layer around each droplet, as well as the formation of large flocs, which restricted the access of the pancreatic lipase to the lipids within the droplets. The observation that a lecithin–chitosan–pectin coating did not inhibit lipase activity was attributed to desorption of a chitosan/pectin complex from the lipid droplet surfaces, thereby enabling the digestive enzymes to access the lipid

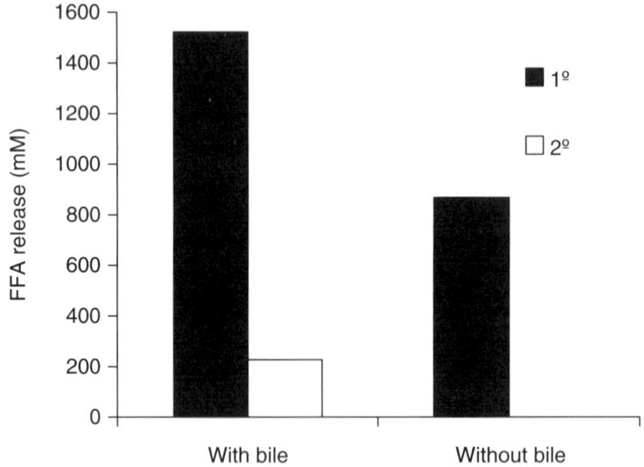

Fig. 20.9 Evidence of the potential ability of nano-laminated coatings to alter the *in vitro* digestibility of lipids encapsulated. Lipid droplets coated by lecithin–pectin layers (2°) showed less digestion than those coated by a lecithin layer (1°).

surfaces. This study highlighted the potential for nano-laminated coatings to be used to modulate the bioavailability of encapsulated lipids.

An animal feeding study was then used to investigate the influence of nano-laminated coatings on the *in vivo* digestibility of encapsulated lipids (Park *et al.*, 2007). The electrostatic layer-by-layer deposition technique was used to prepare soybean oil-in-water emulsions that contained lipid droplets coated by either lecithin or by lecithin–chitosan. Mice were divided into four groups and fed treatment diets for 4 weeks; atherogenic diets supplemented with (A) non-emulsified fat, without chitosan (control); (B) non-emulsified fat, with chitosan; (C) emulsified fat, without chitosan; or, (D) emulsified fat encapsulated by chitosan. We found no significant differences in fecal fat contents between all treatment groups, with total fat absorption being greater than 90% in all treatments. These results therefore suggested that encapsulation of lipids by a single layer of chitosan *did not* inhibit their *in vivo* digestibility, even though our earlier study indicated that a chitosan coating did inhibit their *in vitro* digestibility (Mun *et al.*, 2006).

The most likely reason for the different behavior of chitosan-encapsulated lipids within *in vitro* and *in vivo* digestion models is that the *in vitro* model used did not accurately simulate the complex physicochemical and physiological processes occurring within an animal's digestive system. In particular, we hypothesize that the chitosan coating may have become detached from the lipid droplet surfaces during passage of the lipids through the mouse GI tract, which enabled the digestive enzymes to access the lipid surfaces. The difference between the *in vitro* and *in vivo*

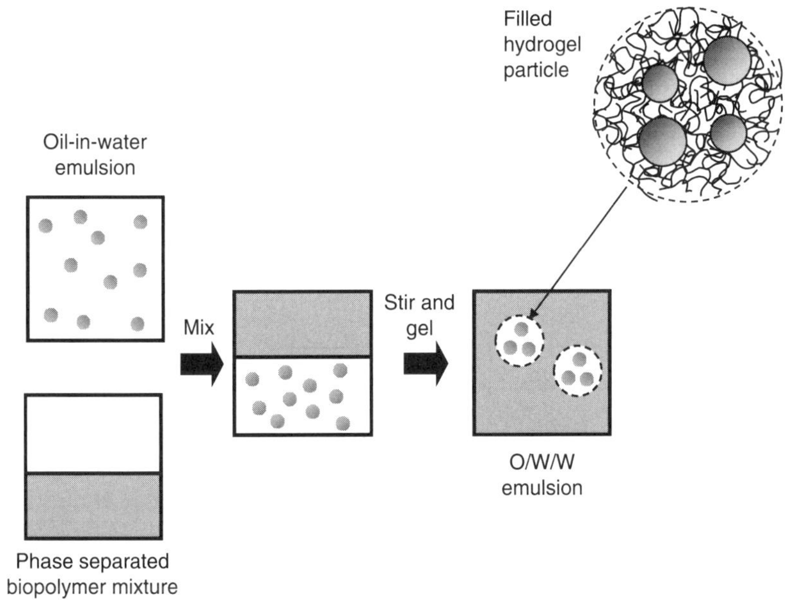

Fig. 20.10 Schematic representation of production of an oil-in-water-in-water (O/W/W) emulsion from a two-phase system consisting of two aqueous phases and an O/W emulsion.

models noted in these studies highlights the *critical* importance of verifying the results of mechanistic studies in a laboratory with animal feeding studies.

Filled hydrogel particles

Structure: filled hydrogel particles consist of lipid droplets (O) dispersed within hydrogel particles (W_1) that are themselves dispersed within an aqueous medium (W_2) (Fig. 20.10). This kind of delivery system can be thought of as a type of oil-in-water-in-water ($O/W_1/W_2$) emulsion. The particle size distribution, concentration, and spatial location of the lipid droplets within the hydrogel particles can be varied, as well as the properties of the hydrogel particles themselves, e.g., their particle size, electrical charge, permeability, and sensitivity to environmental conditions.

Preparation: filled hydrogel particles can be fabricated using a variety of approaches (Chen *et al.*, 2006; Norton and Frith, 2001; Pich and Adler, 2007; Zhang *et al.*, 2007), and the most important ones relevant to the food industry are summarized below. Most of these methods involve initially preparing an oil-in-water emulsion by homogenizing an oil and aqueous phase together in the presence of a water-soluble emulsifier. The size, concentration, and charge of the lipid droplets in these emulsions can be controlled by selecting an appropriate emulsifier (type and concentration) and appropriate homogenization procedure (homogenizer type and operating conditions). A filled hydrogel particle can then be created by combining the O/W emulsion with an appropriate biopolymer solution and then adjusting the conditions to promote hydrogel particle formation and stabilization (Fig. 20.10). Some of the most important methods for forming filled hydrogel particles are outlined below:

- *Phase separation and gelation of single component biopolymer solutions.* Under certain conditions biopolymer molecules dispersed within an aqueous solution can be made to associate and form a separate hydrogel phase by adjusting the solvent 'quality', e.g., by changing dielectric constant, temperature, pH, or ionic strength (Chen *et al.*, 2006). This process is usually referred to as *simple coacervation* and can be used to form filled hydrogel particles. For example, the lipid droplets could be mixed with the biopolymer solution prior to adjusting the solvent quality. The solvent quality could then be adjusted to promote the formation of small hydrogel particles that trap the lipid droplets within them. If necessary, the solution conditions could then be adjusted to promote gelation of the biopolymer molecules within the hydrogel droplets. In this case, it is important to ensure that the biopolymer concentration is not too high, or else gelation of the whole system may occur.
- *Injection and gelation of single component biopolymer solutions.* Many biopolymers are capable of forming gels when the solution or environmental conditions are altered in a specific manner, e.g., heating, cooling, mineral addition, pH adjustment, or enzyme treatment. Small hydrogel particles can be formed by starting off with a solution of biopolymers that is liquid, and then dispersing it (e.g., by injecting, spraying, atomizing, or extruding) into another phase that promotes biopolymer gelation (Senuma *et al.*, 2000; Zhang *et al.*, 2007). The size of the particles produced can be controlled by varying the injection conditions, e.g., injection flow rates, pore sizes or stirring conditions (Zhang *et al.*, 2007). This process can be adapted to form filled hydrogel particles (Zhang *et al.*, 2006). The lipid droplets are mixed with the biopolymer solution prior to gelation, and the resulting mixture is then injected into another liquid that promotes rapid biopolymer gelation so that a hydrogel matrix is formed around the lipid droplets.
- *Gelation of single biopolymer solutions within double emulsions.* In this approach, an oil-in-water-in-oil (O/W/O) emulsion is formed by homogenizing an O/W emulsion with an (outer) oil phase containing a lipophilic emulsifier (Cho *et al.*, 2003; Ribeiro *et al.*, 1999). The (inner) oil phase of the O/W emulsion contains the lipophilic component that is to be encapsulated, while the water phase contains a biopolymer that is capable gelling. After the O/W/O emulsion has been produced the gelation of the biopolymer is induced, e.g., enzymatically, chemically, or thermally (Cho *et al.*, 2003; Hwang *et al.*, 2005; Ribeiro *et al.*, 1999). The oil phase is then removed from the O/W/O emulsion by centrifuging or

filtering to collect the W/O droplets, followed by washing with an organic solvent, and then drying to remove any excess external oil. Alternatively, the O/W/O emulsion can be formed by homogenizing a O/W emulsion with an organic solvent that acts as the outer oil phase, which can then be removed by evaporation (Freitas *et al.*, 2005). Finally, the filled hydrogel particles are collected and can be used directly or dispersed in water. The size and properties of the internal oil droplets can be controlled by varying the composition (e.g., emulsifier type and concentration) and homogenization conditions (e.g., duration and intensity) used to produce the initial O/W emulsion, whereas the size and properties of the hydrogel particles can be controlled by varying the composition and homogenization conditions used to produce the O/W/O emulsion.

- *Aggregative separation and gelation of mixed biopolymer solution.* If an aqueous solution contains two biopolymers that have a sufficiently strong attractive force between them (Fig. 20.6), then it will separate into two phases: a phase that is rich in both biopolymers and a phase that is depleted in both biopolymers (Burgess, 1990; Cooper *et al.*, 2005; de Kruif *et al.*, 2004; Renard *et al.*, 2002; Weinbreck *et al.*, 2003). The major driving force for this type of phase separation is usually an electrostatic attraction between oppositely charged biopolymers, e.g., an anionic polysaccharide and a cationic protein. The biopolymer-rich phase may either be a *coacervate* or a *precipitate* depending on the strength of the electrostatic attraction and the charge densities of the two biopolymers (Cooper *et al.*, 2005). Nevertheless, coacervates are usually more suitable for use as delivery systems because they tend to form particles with more well-defined properties (size and charge) and they have better stability to aggregation and sedimentation. Small coacervate droplets tend to be formed when a mixed biopolymer solution is adjusted to conditions where complex coacervation is favored (Cooper *et al.*, 2005). These coacervate droplets are usually susceptible to coalescence, and may dissociate when either the pH or ionic strength of the solution is adjusted. Consequently, it may be necessary to stabilize them so that one or both of the biopolymers forms a gel, e.g., by heating, cooling, mineral addition, or enzyme treatment. In this case, filled hydrogel particles could be created by mixing an O/W emulsion with a mixed biopolymer solution before inducing complex coacervation. After coacervation is induced, the coacervate phase forms around the oil droplets and traps them within the coacervate particles. Alternatively, the O/W emulsion could be mixed with a preformed coacervate phase and then the filled coacervate phase could be injected into or blended with an aqueous solution.
- *Segregative separation and gelation of mixed biopolymer solution.* If an aqueous solution contains two biopolymers (A and B) that have a sufficiently strong repulsive force between them, then it may separate into two phases (Benichou *et al.*, 2002; Norton and Frith, 2001; Schmitt *et al.*,

1998; Tolstoguzov, 2002, 2003). One of the phases is rich in biopolymer A and depleted in biopolymer B, whereas the other phase is rich in biopolymer B and depleted in biopolymer A. Typically, the driving force for this kind of phase separation is steric exclusion or electrostatic repulsion. When the solution conditions are adjusted so that segregative separation is promoted in a mixed biopolymer solution, the system often initially forms droplets of one phase dispersed in a continuous medium of the other phase. This kind of system is often referred to as a water-in-water (W/W) emulsion. As with coacervates, the water droplets formed due to segregative separation are often unstable to coalescence and gravitational separation and so it may be necessary to stabilize them by adjusting the solution or environmental conditions so that one or both of the water phases gels, e.g., by heating, cooling, mineral addition, or enzyme treatment. In this case, filled hydrogel particles could be formed by mixing the O/W emulsion with the mixed biopolymer solution prior to inducing segregative phase separation, or by mixing the O/W emulsion with the biopolymer phase that will become the dispersed phase of the W/W emulsion and then incorporating this into the biopolymer phase that will become the continuous phase (e.g., by mixing, injecting, or spraying).

- *Spray drying*. Spray drying can also be used to form filled hydrogel particles (Gibbs *et al.*, 1999; Madene *et al.*, 2006). Initially, an oil-in-water emulsion is produced by homogenizing an oil phase and an aqueous phase together in the presence of a hydrophilic emulsifier. A substance that will form the hydrogel matrix within the particles in the final powder is then added to the emulsion, e.g., protein or polysaccharide. The emulsion and biopolymer mixture is then used as the feed material to a spray dryer. The emulsion is pumped through a nozzle that disperses it into fluid particles. These particles consist of a number of small lipid droplets trapped inside a larger water particle. The particles are mixed with a hot drying medium (usually air), which causes most of the water inside them to evaporate, leaving solid particles consisting of lipid droplets embedded within a biopolymer matrix. When these particles are hydrated, the biopolymer molecules may simply dissolve and release the lipid droplets. Nevertheless, if the biopolymer molecules are physically or chemically cross-linked within the powder particles, then it is possible to retain a hydrogel matrix around the lipid droplets after hydration.

Filled hydrogel particles with different microstructures and functional properties can be created by varying the type of biopolymers used (e.g., charge sign and density, molecular weight, flexibility, hydrophobicity), the solution composition (e.g., pH, ionic strength), the mixing conditions (e.g., order of addition, stirring speed, homogenization pressure), and environmental conditions (e.g., temperature). The precise methods used will depend on the particular approach used to form the filled hydrogel particles. Thus,

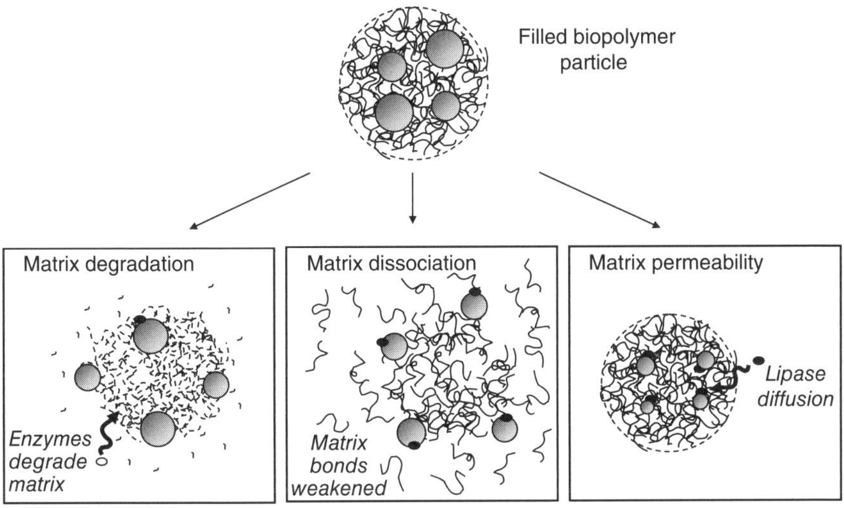

Fig. 20.11 Possible mechanisms impacting the ability of digestive enzymes accessing encapsulated lipids.

it is possible to prepare filled hydrogel particles that have different sizes, electrical charges, permeability, loading capacity, release properties, and stabilities to environmental conditions.

Potential methods of controlling lipid bioavailability: in addition to the approaches described for conventional emulsions, the bioactivity of encapsulated lipids could be controlled using filled hydrogel particles in various other ways. The biopolymer matrix that surrounds the lipid droplets could be designed to respond to specific conditions within the GI tract (Fig. 20.11):

- *Matrix dissociation.* The biopolymer matrix may dissociate within the GI tract and release the encapsulated lipid droplets if the bonds holding the biopolymer molecules are weakened. For example, electrostatic interactions may be weakened when the pH or ionic strength is altered to change the sign or magnitude of the charge on biopolymer molecules. Once the lipid droplets are released then the lipase molecules can access them.
- *Matrix digestion.* The biopolymer matrix may disintegrate within the GI tract and release the encapsulated lipid droplets if the biopolymer molecules themselves are digested. Some types of biopolymer molecule are indigestible within the GI tract, such as dietary fibers and resistant starch, and therefore matrices fabricated from these molecules should remain intact and prevent lipid release. This type of system could be used to decrease the bioavailability of the encapsulated lipids, e.g., by decreasing the rate or extent of lipid digestion. On the other hand, other types of biopolymer molecules are digestible, such as proteins and starch,

and so they may be broken down within the GI tract and release the encapsulated lipids. This type of system should not adversely impact the bioavailability of the encapsulated lipids.

- *Matrix permeability.* The permeability of the biopolymer matrix will determine which types of molecule can diffuse through it, and the rate at which they can diffuse. If the matrix is completely impermeable to enzyme molecules, then it may restrict lipid digestion by preventing the lipase molecules from reaching the lipid droplet surfaces. On the other hand, if the matrix is completely permeable to the enzyme molecules, then the lipid droplets may be digested even though the biopolymer matrix stays intact. The permeability of a matrix may change with environmental conditions such as pH or ionic strength due to swelling or shrinking of the hydrogel particles (Kashyap *et al.*, 2005; Lin and Metters, 2006; Renard *et al.*, 2002). Thus, it may be possible to design a system that is impermeable to enzyme penetration under one set of conditions (e.g., within the stomach) but permeable under another set of conditions (e.g., in the small or large intestine).

In principle, it is possible to control the release and digestion of lipids by surrounding them by hydrogel matrices that alter the interaction between digestive enzymes and encapsulated lipids. It is possible to design hydrogel matrices that only break down or change permeability in response to particular stimuli within the GI tract, e.g., pH, ionic strength, or enzyme activity. This kind of system could be designed to protect and release an encapsulated component at a particular site-of-action. The potential of filled hydrogel particles for controlled release of bioactive substances has recently been demonstrated using *in vitro* digestion models (Chen and Subirade, 2007; Chen *et al.*, 2006). It has been shown that the rate and extent of digestion or dissociation of biopolymer matrices can be controlled by changing its composition, cross-linking or particle size. Nevertheless, more research is required to identify suitable food grade methods of preparing biopolymer matrices with controlled digestibility.

20.5.3 Applications

As mentioned earlier, delivery systems are usually designed to carry out a variety of different functions in addition to controlling lipid bioactivity, e.g., protection of the encapsulated lipids against chemical degradation during storage, convenient means of delivery, and compatibility with food matrices. A variety of different kinds of lipids can be encapsulated within emulsion-based delivery systems. The encapsulated lipid may be a macroscopic phase that comprises the entirety of the droplets, such as fish, flax, algae, corn, soybean, palm, coconut, or olive oils (Chee *et al.*, 2005, 2007; Lee *et al.*, 2005, 2006a,b; McClements and Decker, 2000; Sharma, 2005). A delivery system may be designed to ensure that the encapsulated lipids are fully digested and released, e.g., for oils containing beneficial bioactive fatty acids (such as ω-3 or CLA) or for humans with diseases that impair lipid digestion and absorption. For example, one could use a conventional emulsion that contains lipid droplets that are easily digested. On the other hand, the delivery system could be designed to decrease the bioavailability of the lipid phase if it contains components that are detrimental to health when overconsumed, e.g., saturated or *trans*-fatty acids. In this case, one might design an indigestible coating or matrix around the lipid droplets to prevent the lipase from getting to the lipid droplets. The encapsulated lipid could also be a minor component that is dispersed within a carrier oil, e.g., carotenoids, phytosterols or oil-soluble vitamins (Ribeiro *et al.*, 2003, 2006; Tyssandier *et al.*, 2001, 2003). In these cases, it is important to ensure that the delivery system increases or does not adversely affect the bioactivity of the encapsulated bioactive component.

20.6 Future trends

A wide variety of emulsion-based delivery systems has been developed for the encapsulation of bioactive lipids, each with its own advantages and disadvantages. This chapter has provided an overview of the major types of emulsion-based delivery system that are available, and has highlighted some of the advantages and disadvantages of each one. Conventional oil-in-water emulsions are currently the most widely used method of encapsulating bioactive lipids, but they are often susceptible to breakdown over time or when they are exposed to certain environmental stresses during production, transport, storage, or utilization. In addition, they have limited ability to encapsulate, protect, and deliver certain types of bioactive lipids. Consequently, there is a need for certain applications to have alternative types of delivery systems. Other types of lipid-based delivery systems, such as multiple emulsions, multilayer emulsions, filled hydrogel particles, and solid lipid particle emulsions, have certain advantages over conventional emulsions, but they are often more complicated to prepare and are sometimes more unstable. It is likely that additional approaches will be developed for controlling lipid digestibility based on emulsion technology in the future. In particular, the authors see particular merit in combining two or more existing technologies to create composite systems, such as multiple emulsions with multilayer coatings.

20.7 Sources of further information and advice

Research into the rational design of structures to control the bioavailability of lipophilic components is rapidly growing, especially in the pharmaceutical industry where there is a need to increase the bioavailability of highly hydrophobic drugs. Much of the research carried out in the pharmaceutical industry can be directly translated into the design of functional foods. For example, there have been a number of excellent reviews on novel colloidal strategies for controlling the bioavailability of hydrophobic drugs recently (Ansari *et al.*, 2008; Kesisoglou *et al.*, 2007; Narang *et al.*, 2007; Porter and Charman, 2001; Porter *et al.*, 2007). There are also many excellent books on drug delivery that can serve as a basis for the design of functional foods. The authors would therefore strongly recommend that food scientists search the physical chemistry, colloid science, and pharmaceutical literature to identify effective approaches for controlling the bioavailability of lipophilic food components.

20.8 Acknowledgements

This material is based upon work supported by the Cooperative State Research, Extension, Education Service, United State Department of Agriculture, Massachusetts Agricultural Experiment Station (Project No. 831) and an United States Department of Agriculture, CREES, NRI Grant (Award Numbers 2005-01357 2008-02191 and 2008-01368).

20.9 References

AGUILERA JM. 2006. Food microstructure affects the bioavailability of several nutrients. *J Food Sci* **72**(2):R21–R32.

AMADO FML, VITORINO RMP, DOMINGUES P, LOBO MJC & DUARTE JAR. 2005. Analysis of the human saliva proteome. *Expert Rev Proteomics* **2**(4):521–539.

ANGELATOS AS, JOHNSTON APR, WANG YJ & CARUSO F. 2007. Probing the permeability of polyelectrolyte multilayer capsules via a molecular beacon approach. *Langmuir* **23**(8):4554–4562.

ANSARI MJ, KOHLI K & DIXIT N. 2008. Microemulsions as potential drug delivery systems: a review. *PDA J Pharm Sci Technol* **62**(1):66–79.

ARMAND M. 2007. Lipases and lipolysis in the human digestive tract: where do we stand? *Current Opin Clin Nutr Metabolic Care* **10**(2):156–164.

ARMAND M, BOREL P, YTHIER P, DUTOT G, MELIN C, SENFT M, LAFONT H & LAIRON D. 1992. Effects of droplet size, triacylglycerol composition, and calcium on the hydrolysis of complex emulsions by pancreatic lipase – an *in vitro* study. *J Nutr Biochem* **3**(7):333–341.

ARMAND M, BOREL P, PASQUIER B, DUBOIS C, SENFT M, ANDRE M, PEYROT J, SALDUCCI J & LAIRON D. 1996a. Physicochemical characteristics of emulsions during fat digestion in human stomach and duodenum. *Am J Physiol-Gastrointestinal Liver Physiol* **34**(1):G172–G183.

ARMAND M, HAMOSH M, MEHTA NR, ANGELUS PA, PHILPOTT JR, HENDERSON TR, DWYER NK, LAIRON D & HAMOSH P. 1996b. Effect of human milk or formula on gastric function and fat digestion in the premature infant. *Pediatr Res* **40**(3):429–437.

ARMAND M, PASQUIER B, BOREL P, ANDRE M, SENFT M, PEYROT J, SALDUCCI J & LAIRON D. 1997. Emulsion and absorption of lipids: the importance of physicochemical properties. *Ocl-Oleagineux Corps Gras Lipides* **4**(3):178–185.

ARMAND M, PASQUIER B, ANDRE M, BOREL P, SENFT M, PEYROT J, SALDUCCI J, PORTUGAL H, JAUSSAN V & LAIRON D. 1999. Digestion and absorption of 2 fat emulsions with different droplet sizes in the human digestive tract. *Am J Clin Nutr* **70**(6):1096–1106.

BAUER E, JAKOB S & MOSENTHIN R. 2005. Principles of physiology of lipid digestion. *Asian-Australasian J Animal Sci* **18**(2):282–295.

BENICHOU A, ASERIN A & GARTI N. 2002. Protein–polysaccharide interactions for stabilization of food emulsions. *J Disper Sci Technol* **23**(1–3):93–123.

BERMUDEZ B, PACHECO YM, LOPEZ S, ABIA R & MURIANA FJG. 2004. Digestion and absorption of olive oil. *Grasas y Aceites* **55**(1):1–10.

BLIJDENSTEIN TBJ, VAN DER LINDEN E, VAN VLIET T & VAN AKEN GA. 2004. Scaling behavior of delayed demixing, rheology, and microstructure of emulsions flocculated by depletion and bridging. *Langmuir* **20**(26):11321–11328.

BOREL P, ARMAND M, YTHIER P, DUTOT G, MELIN C, SENFT M, LAFONT H & LAIRON D. 1994. Hydrolysis of emulsions with different triglycerides and droplet sizes by gastric lipase *in-vitro* – effect on pancreatic lipase activity. *J Nutr Biochem* **5**(3):124–133.

BUMMER PM. 2004. Physical chemical considerations of lipid-based oral drug delivery – solid lipid nanoparticles. *Crit Rev Therapeutic Drug Carrier Systems* **21**(1):1–19.

BUNJES H, KOCH MHJ & WESTESEN K. 2003. Influence of emulsifiers on the crystallization of solid lipid nanoparticles. *J Pharmaceut Sci* **92**(7):1509–1520.

BURGESS DJ. 1990. Practical analysis of complex coacervate systems. *J Colloid Interface Sci* **140**(1):227–238.

CAREY MC, SMALL DM & BLISS CM. 1983. Lipid digestion and absorption. *Annu Rev Physiol* **45**:651–677.

CHEE CP, GALLAHER JJ, DJORDJEVIC D, FARAJI H, MCCLEMENTS DJ, DECKER EA, HOLLENDER R, PETERSON DG, ROBERTS RF & COUPLAND JN. 2005. Chemical and sensory analysis of strawberry flavoured yogurt supplemented with an algae oil emulsion. *J Dairy Res* **72**(3):311–316.

CHEE CP, DJORDJEVIC D, FARAJI H, DECKER EA, HOLLENDER R, MCCLEMENTS DJ, PETERSON DG, ROBERTS RF & COUPLAND JN. 2007. Sensory properties of vanilla and strawberry flavored ice cream supplemented with omega-3 fatty acids. *Milchwissenschaft* **62**(1):66–69.

CHEN CC, TU YY & CHANG HM. 1999. Efficiency and protective effect of encapsulation of milk immunoglobulin G in multiple emulsion. *J Agric Food Chem* **47**(2): 407–410.

CHEN LY & SUBIRADE M. 2007. Effect of preparation conditions on the nutrient release properties of alginate–whey protein granular mincrospheres. *Eur J Pharm Biopharm* **65**(3):354–362.

CHEN LY, REMONDETTO GE & SUBIRADE M. 2006. Food protein-based materials as nutraceutical delivery systems. *Trends Food Sci Tech* **17**(5):272–283.

CHO YH, SHIM HK & PARK J. 2003. Encapsulation of fish oil by an enzymatic gelation process using transglutaminase cross-linked proteins. *J Food Sci* **68**(9):2717–2723.

COOPER CL, DUBIN PL, KAYITMAZER AB & TURKSEN S. 2005. Polyelectrolyte–protein complexes. *Curr Opin Colloid Interface Sci* **10**(1–2):52–78.

COURNARIE F, SAVELLI MP, ROSILIO W, BRETEZ F, VAUTHIER C, GROSSIORD JL & SEILLER M. 2004. Insulin-loaded W/O/W multiple emulsions: comparison of the performances of systems prepared with medium-chain-triglycerides and fish oil. *Eur J Pharm Biopharm* **58**(3):477–482.

DE HOOG EHA, PRINZ JF, HUNTJENS L, DRESSELHUIS DM & VAN AKEN GA. 2006. Lubrication of oral surfaces by food emulsions: the importance of surface characteristics. *J Food Sci* **71**(7):E337–E341.

DE KRUIF CG, WEINBRECK F & DE VRIES R. 2004. Complex coacervation of proteins and anionic polysaccharides. *Curr Opin Colloid Interface Sci* **9**(5):340–349.

DECHER G & SCHLENOFF JB. 2003. *Multilayer Thin Films: Sequential Assembly of Nanocomposite Materials*. Weinheim: Wiley-VCH.

DECKER EA. 1996. The role of stereospecific saturated fatty acid position on lipid nutrition. *Nutr Rev* **54**:108–110.

DECKER EA & MCCLEMENTS DJ. 2007. Lipids. In: Damodarin, S., Parkin, K. & Fennema, O. R., editors. *Food Chemistry*, 4th edition. New York: Marcel Dekker.

DENKE MA, FOX MM & SCHULTE MC. 1993. Short-term dietary calcium fortification increases fecal saturated fat-content and reduces serum-lipids in men. *J Nutr* **123**(6):1047–1053.

DICKINSON E. 1992. *Introduction to Food Colloids*. Cambridge, UK: Royal Society of Chemistry.

EKMEKCIOGLU C. 2002. A physiological approach for preparing and conducting intestinal bioavailability studies using experimental systems. *Food Chem* **76**(2):225–230.

FATOUROS DG, BERGENSTAHL B & MULLERTZ A. 2007a. Morphological observations on a lipid-based drug delivery system during *in vitro* digestion. *Europ J Pharmaceut Sci* **31**(2):85–94.

FATOUROS DG, DEEN GR, ARLETH L, BERGENSTAHL B, NIELSEN FS, PEDERSEN JS & MULLERTZ A. 2007b. Structural development of self nano emulsifying drug delivery systems (SNEDDS) during *in vitro* lipid digestion monitored by small-angle X-ray scattering. *Pharmaceut Res* **24**(10):1844–1853.

FAULKS RM & SOUTHON S. 2001. Carotenoids, metabolism and disease. In: Wildman, R. E. C., editor. *Handbook of Nutraceuticals and Functional Foods*, 1st edition. Boco Raton, FL: CRC Press. p. 143.

FAVE G, COSTE TC & ARMAND M. 2004. Physicochemical properties of lipids: new strategies to manage fatty acid bioavailability. *Cell Molec Biol* **50**(7):815–831.

FECHNER A, KNOTH A, SCHERZE I & MUSCHIOLIK G. 2007. Stability and release properties of double-emulsions stabilised by caseinate–dextran conjugates. *Food Hydrocolloids* **21**(5–6):943–952.

FILLERYTRAVIS AJ, GEE JM, WALDRON KW, ROBINS MM & JOHNSON IT. 1997. Soluble non-starch polysaccharides derived from complex food matrices do not increase average lipid droplet size during gastric lipid emulsification in rats. *J Nutr* **127**(11):2246–2252.

FINLEY JW, LEVEILLE GA, DIXON RM, WALCHAK CG, SOURBY JC, SMITH RE, FRANCIS KD & OTTERBURN MS. 1994. Clinical-assessment of Salatrim, a reduced-calorie triacylglycerol. *J Agric Food Chem* **42**(2):581–596.

FREITAS S, MERKLE HP & GANDER B. 2005. Microencapsulation by solvent extraction/evaporation: reviewing the state of the art of microsphere preparation process technology. *J Controlled Release* **102**(2):313–332.

FRIBERG S, LARSSON K & SJOBLOM J. 2004. *Food Emulsions*, 4th edition. New York: Marcel Dekker.

GARGOURI Y, JULIEN R, BOIS AG, VERGER R & SARDA L. 1983. Studies on the detergent inhibition of pancreatic lipase activity. *J Lipid Res* **24**(10):1336–1342.

GARTI N. 1997a. Double emulsions – scope, limitations and new achievements. *Colloid Surface A* **123**:233–246.

GARTI N. 1997b. Progress in stabilization and transport phenomena of double emulsions in food applications. *Food Sci Technol – Lebensmittel-Wissenschaft & Technologie* **30**(3):222–235.

GARTI N & BENICHOU A. 2004. Recent developments in double emulsions for food applications. In: Friberg, S. E., Larsson, K. & Sjoblom, J., editors. *Food emulsions*. 4th edition. New York: Marcel Dekker.

GARTI N & BISPERINK C. 1998. Double emulsions: progress and applications. *Curr Opin Colloid Interface Sci* **3**(6):657–667.

GHOSH S, PETERSON DG & COUPLAND JN. 2006. Effects of droplet crystallization and melting on the aroma release properties of a model oil-in-water emulsion. *J Agric Food Chem* **54**(5):1829–1837.

GIBBS BF, KERMASHA S, ALLI I & MULLIGAN CN. 1999. Encapsulation in the food industry: a review. *Int J Food Sci Nutr* **50**(3):213–224.

GUZEY D & MCCLEMENTS DJ. 2006. Formation, stability and properties of multilayer emulsions for application in the food industry. *Adv Colloid Interface* **128**:227–248.

GWARTNEY EA, LARICK DK & FOEGEDING EA. 2004. Sensory texture and mechanical properties of stranded and particulate whey protein emulsion gels. *J Food Sci* **69**(9):S333–S339.

HAYES JR, PENCE DH, SCHEINBACH S, DAMELIA RP, KLEMANN LP, WILSON NH & FINLEY JW. 1994. Review of triacylglycerol digestion, absorption, and metabolism with respect to salatrim triacylglycerols. *J Agric Food Chem* **42**(2):474–483.

HWANG YJ, OH C & OH SG. 2005. Controlled release of retinol from silica particles prepared in O/W/O emulsion: the effects of surfactants and polymers. *J Controlled Release* **106**(3):339–349.

JURADO E, CAMACHO F, LUZON G, FERNANDEZ-SERRANO M & GARCIA-ROMAN M. 2006. Kinetic model for the enzymatic hydrolysis of tributyrin in O/W emulsions. *Chem Eng Sci* **61**(15):5010–5020.

KALANTZI L, GOUMAS K, KALIORAS V, ABRAHAMSSON B, DRESSMAN JB & REPPAS C. 2006. Characterization of the human upper gastrointestinal contents under conditions simulating bioavailability/bioequivalence studies. *Pharmaceut Res* **23**(1):165–176.

KANAFUSA S, CHU BS & NAKAJIMA M. 2007. Factors affecting droplet size of sodium caseinate-stabilized O/W emulsions containing beta-carotene. *Europ J Lipid Sci Technol* **109**(10):1038–1041.

KARUPAIAH T & SUNDRAM K. 2007. Effects of stereospecific positioning of fatty acids in triacylglycerol structures in native and randomized fats: a review of their nutritional implications. *Nutr Metabolism* **4**(16):1–17.

KASHYAP N, KUMAR N & KUMAR M. 2005. Hydrogels for pharmaceutical and biomedical applications. *Crit Rev Therapeutic Drug Carrier Systems* **22**(2):107–149.

KESISOGLOU F, PANMAI S & WU YH. 2007. Application of nanoparticles in oral delivery of immediate release formulations. *Current Nanosci* **3**(2):183–190.

KLEMANN LP, FINLEY JW & LEVEILLE GA. 1994. Estimation of the absorption-coefficient of stearic-acid in Salatrim fats. *J Agric Food Chem* **42**(2):484–488.

KRITCHEVSKY D, TEPPER SA, VESSELINOVITCH D *et al.* 1975. Atherogenic semipurified, cholesterol-free diets – effect of peanut oil. *Federation Proc* **34**(3):235.

KUKIZAKI M & GOTO M. 2007. Preparation and evaluation of uniformly sized solid lipid microcapsules using membrane emulsification. *Colloid Surface A* **293**(1–3):87–94.

LAIRON D. 1997a. *Dietary Fiber in Health and Disease*. New York: Plenum Press.

LAIRON D. 1997b. Soluble fibers and dietary lipids. *Adv Exp Med Biol* **427**:99–108.

LAIRON D, PLAY B & JOURDHEUIL-RAHMANI D. 2007. Digestible and indigestible carbohydrates: interactions with postprandial lipid metabolism. *J Nutr Biochem* **18**(4):217–227.

LEE JJ, PARK IB, CHO YH, HUH CS, BAEK YJ & PARK J. 2004. Whey protein-based IgY microcapsules prepared by multiple emulsification and heat gelation. *Food Sci Biotechnol* **13**(4):494–497.

LEE S, DECKER EA, FAUSTMAN C & MANCINI RA. 2005. The effects of antioxidant combinations on color and lipid oxidation in *n*-3 oil fortified ground beef patties. *Meat Sci* **70**(4):683–689.

LEE S, FAUSTMAN C, DJORDJEVIC D, FARAJI H & DECKER EA. 2006a. Effect of antioxidants on stabilization of meat products fortified with *n*-3 fatty acids. *Meat Sci* **72**(1):18–24.

LEE S, HERNANDEZ P, DJORDJEVIC D, FARAJI H, HOLLENDER R, FAUSTMAN C & DECKER EA. 2006b. Effect of antioxidants and cooking on stability of *n*-3 fatty acids in fortified meat products. *J Food Sci* **71**(3):C233–C238.

LIN CC & METTERS AT. 2006. Hydrogels in controlled release formulations: network design and mathematical modeling. *Adv Drug Deliver Rev* **58**(12–13):1379–1408.

LINDAHL A, UNGELL AL, KNUTSON L & LENNERNAS H. 1997. Characterization of fluids from the stomach and proximal jejunum in men and women. *Pharmaceut Res* **14**(4):497–502.

LORENZEN JK, NIELSEN S, HOLST JJ, TETENS I, REHFELD JF & ASTRUP A. 2007. Effect of dairy calcium or supplementary calcium intake on postprandial fat metabolism, appetite, and subsequent energy intake. *Am J Clin Nutr* **85**(3):678–687.

LOWE M. 2002. The triglyceride lipases of the pancreas. *J Lipid Res* **43**(12):2007–2016.

MADENE A, JACQUOT M, SCHER J & DESOBRY S. 2006. Flavour encapsulation and controlled release – a review. *Int J Food Sci Tech* **41**(1):1–21.

MALONE ME, APPELQVIST IAM & NORTON IT. 2003a. Oral behaviour of food hydrocolloids and emulsions. Part 1. Lubrication and deposition considerations. *Food Hydrocolloids* **17**(6):763–773.

MALONE ME, APPELQVIST IAM & NORTON IT. 2003b. Oral behaviour of food hydrocolloids and emulsions. Part 2. Taste and aroma release. *Food Hydrocolloids* **17**(6):775–784.

MCCLEMENTS DJ. 2005a. *Food Emulsions: Principles, Practice, and Techniques*, 2nd edition. Boca Raton, FL: CRC Press.

MCCLEMENTS DJ. 2005b. Theoretical analysis of factors affecting the formation and stability of multilayered colloidal dispersions. *Langmuir* **21**(21):9777–9785.

MCCLEMENTS DJ & DECKER EA. 2000. Lipid oxidation in oil-in-water emulsions: impact of molecular environment on chemical reactions in heterogeneous food systems. *J Food Sci* **65**(8):1270–1282.

MCCLEMENTS DJ & DECKER EA. 2007. Lipids. In: Damodaran, S., Parkin, K. L. & Fennema, O. R., editors. *Food Chemistry*. 4th edition. Boca Raton, FL: CRC Press. p. 155–216.

MCCLEMENTS DJ, DICKINSON E & POVEY MJW. 1990. Crystallization in hydrocarbon-in-water emulsions containing a mixture of solid and liquid droplets. *Chem Phys Lett* **172**(6):449–452.

MCCLEMENTS DJ, DECKER EA & WEISS J. 2007. Emulsion-based delivery systems for lipophilioc bioactive components. *J Food Sci* **72**(8):R109–R124.

MICHALSKI MC, BRIARD V, DESAGE M & GELOEN A. 2005. The dispersion state of milk fat influences triglyceride metabolism in the rat – A (CO2)-C-13 breath test study. *Europ J Nutr* **44**(7):436–444.

MILED N, RIVIERE M, CAVALIER JF, BUONO G, BERTI L & VERGER R. 2005. Discrimination between closed and open forms of lipases using electrophoretic techniques. *Analyt Biochem* **338**(2):171–178.

MU HL & HOY CE. 2004. The digestion of dietary triacylglycerols. *Prog Lipid Res* **43**(2):105–133.

MUKHERJEE M. 2003. Human digestive and metabolic lipases – a brief review. *J Molecular Catalysis B – Enzymatic* **22**(5–6):369–376.

MULLER RH & KECK CM. 2004. Challenges and solutions for the delivery of biotech drugs – a review of drug nanocrystal technology and lipid nanoparticles. *J Biotechnol* **113**(1–3):151–170.

MULLER RH, MADER K & GOHLA S. 2000. Solid lipid nanoparticles (SLN) for controlled drug delivery – a review of the state of the art. *Eur J Pharm Biopharm* **50**(1): 161–177.

MUN S, DECKER EA & MCCLEMENTS DJ. 2005. Influence of droplet characteristics on the formation of oil-in-water emulsions stabilized by surfactant–chitosan layers. *Langmuir* **21**(14):6228–6234.

MUN S, DECKER EA, PARK Y, WEISS J & MCCLEMENTS DJ. 2006. Influence of interfacial composition on *in vitro* digestibility of emulsified lipids: potential mechanism for chitosan's ability to inhibit fat digestion. *Food Biophys* **1**(1):21–29.

MUN S, DECKER EA & MCCLEMENTS DJ. 2007. Influence of emulsifier type on *in vitro* digestibility of lipid droplets by pancreatic lipase. *Food Res Int* **40**(6):770–781.

NARANG AS, DELMARRE D & GAO D. 2007. Stable drug encapsulation in micelles and microemulsions. *Int J Pharmac* **345**:9–25.

NORTON IT & FRITH WJ. 2001. Microstructure design in mixed biopolymer composites. *Food Hydrocolloids* **15**(4–6):543–553.

OLBRICH C, KAYSER O & MULLER RH. 2002a. Enzymatic degradation of Dynasan 114 SLN – effect of surfactants and particle size. *J Nanoparticle Res* **4**(1–2):121–129.

OLBRICH C, KAYSER O & MULLER RH. 2002b. Lipase degradation of Dynasan 114 and 116 solid lipid nanoparticles (SLN) – effect of surfactants, storage time and crystallinity. *Int J Pharmaceutics* **237**(1–2):119–128.

OWUSU RK, ZHU QH & DICKINSON E. 1992. Controlled release of L-tryptophan and vitamin-b2 from model water oil-water multiple emulsions. *Food Hydrocolloids* **6**(5):443–453.

PAFUMI Y, LAIRON D, DE LA PORTE PL, JUHEL C, STORCH J, HAMOSH M & ARMAND M. 2002. Mechanisms of inhibition of triacylglycerol hydrolysis by human gastric lipase. *J Biol Chem* **277**(31):28070–28079.

PARK GY, MUN S, PARK Y, RHEE S, DECKER EA, WEISS J, MCCLEMENTS DJ & PARK Y. 2007. Influence of encapsulation of emulsified lipids with chitosan on their *in vivo* digestibility. *Food Chem* **104**(2):761–767.

PARK Y & PARIZA MW. 2007. Mechanisms of body fat modulation by conjugated linoleic acid (CLA). *Food Res Int* **40**(3):311–323.

PASQUIER B, ARMAND M, CASTELAIN C, GUILLON F, BOREL P, LAFONT H & LAIRON D. 1996. Emulsification and lipolysis of triacylglycerols are altered by viscous soluble dietary fibres in acidic gastric medium *in vitro*. *Biochem J* **314**:269–275.

PATTON JS & CAREY MC. 1979. Watching fat digestion. *Science* **204**(4389):145–148.

PATTON JS, VETTER RD, HAMOSH M, BORGSTROM B, LINDSTROM M & CAREY MC. 1985. The light-microscopy of triglyceride digestion. *Food Microstructure* **4**(1):29–41.

PICH AZ & ADLER HJP. 2007. Composite aqueous microgels: an overview of recent advances in synthesis, characterization and application. *Polymer Int* **56**(3): 291–307.

PORTER CJH & CHARMAN WN. 2001. *In vitro* assessment of oral lipid based formulations. *Advanced Drug Delivery Rev* **50**:S127–S147.

PORTER CJH, TREVASKIS NL & CHARMAN WN. 2007. Lipids and lipid-based formulations: optimizing the oral delivery of lipophilic drugs. *Nature Rev Drug Discovery* **6**(3): 231–248.

RANHOTRA GS, GELROTH JA & LEINEN SD. 1998. Energy value of a fat high in stearic acid. *J Food Sci* **63**(2):363–365.

READ I. 2004. Effects of calcium supplementation on circulating lipids – potential pharmacoeconomic implications. *Drugs Aging* **21**(1):7–17

REIS P, HOLMBERG K, DEBECHE T, FOLMER B, FAUCONNOT L & WATZKE H. 2006. Lipase-catalyzed reactions at different surfaces. *Langmuir* **22**(19):8169–8177.

RENARD D, ROBERT P, LAVENANT L, MELCION D, POPINEAU Y, GUEGUEN J, DUCLAIROIR C, NAKACHE E, SANCHEZ C & SCHMITT C. 2002. Biopolymeric colloidal carriers for encapsulation or controlled release applications. *Int J Pharmaceutics* **242**(1–2): 163–166.

RIBEIRO AJ, NEUFELD RJ, ARNAUD P & CHAUMEIL JC. 1999. Microencapsulation of lipophilic drugs in chitosan-coated alginate microspheres. *Int J Pharmaceutics* **187**(1):115–123.

RIBEIRO HS, AX K & SCHUBERT H. 2003. Stability of lycopene emulsions in food systems. *J Food Sci* **68**(9):2730–2734.

RIBEIRO HS, GUERRERO JMM, BRIVIBA K, RECHKEMMER G, SCHUCHMANN HP & SCHUBERT H. 2006. Cellular uptake of carotenoid-loaded oil-in-water emulsions in colon carcinoma cells *in vitro*. *J Agric Food Chem* **54**(25):9366–9369.

RUBNER MF. 2003. pH-controlled fabrication of polyelectrolyte multilayers: Assembly and applications. In: Decher, G. & Schlenoff, J. B., editors. *Multilayer Thin Films: Sequential Assembly of Nanocomposite Materials.* Weinheim: Wiley-VCH. p. 133–154.

SANGUANSRI P & AUGUSTIN MA. 2006. Nanoscale materials development – a food industry perspective. *Trends Food Sci Tech* **17**(10):547–556.

SANZ T & LUYTEN H. 2006a. Effect of thickening agent in the *in vitro* mouth, stomach and intestine release of tyrosol from enriched custards. *Food Hydrocolloids* **20**(5):703–711.

SANZ T & LUYTEN H. 2006b. Release, partitioning and stability of isoflavones from enriched custards during mouth, stomach and intestine *in vitro* simulations. *Food Hydrocolloids* **20**(6):892–900.

SANZ T & LUYTEN H. 2007. *In vitro* evaluation of genistein bioaccessibility from enriched custards. *Food Hydrocolloids* **21**(2):203–211.

SCHLENOFF JB. 2003. Charge balance and transport in polyelectrolyte multilayers. In: Decher, G. & Schlenoff, J. B., editors. *Multilayer Thin Films: Sequential Assembly of Nanocomposite Materials.* Weinheim: Wiley-VCH. p. 99–132.

SCHMITT C, SANCHEZ C, DESOBRY-BANON S & HARDY J. 1998. Structure and technofunctional properties of protein-polysaccharide complexes: a review. *Crit Rev Food Sci* **38**(8):689–753.

SCHOELER B, KUMARASWAMY G & CARUSO F. 2002. Investigation of the influence of polyelectrolyte charge density on the growth of multilayer thin films prepared by the layer-by-layer technique. *Macromolecules* **35**:889–897.

SCHOELER B, POPTOSCHEV E & CARUSO F. 2003. Growth of multilayer films of fixed and variable charge density polyelectrolytes: effect of mutual charge and secondary interactions. *Macromolecules* **36**(14):5258–5264.

SCHOLZ-AHRENS KE & SCHREZENMEIR J. 2006. Milk minerals and the metabolic syndrome. *Int Dairy J* **16**(11):1399–1407.

SCHULZE K. 2006. Imaging and modelling of digestion in the stomach and the duodenum. *Neurogastroenterology Motility* **18**(3):172–183.

SCHWIZER W, FOX M & STEINGOTTER A. 2003. Non-invasive investigation of gastrointestinal functions with magnetic resonance imaging: towards an 'ideal' investigation of gastrointestinal function. *Gut* **52**:34–39.

SENUMA Y, LOWE C, ZWEIFEL Y, HILBORN JG & MARISON I. 2000. Alginate hydrogel microspheres and microcapsules prepared by spinning disk atomization. *Biotechnol Bioeng* **67**(5):616–622.

SHAFIK A, EL SIBAI O, SHAFIK AA & SHAFIK IA. 2007. Mechanism of gastric emptying through the pyloric sphincter: a human study. *Med Sci Monitor* **13**(1): CR24–CR29.

SHARMA R. 2005. Market trends and opportunities for functional dairy beverages. *Aust J Dairy Technol* **60**(2):195–198.

SILLETTI E, VINGERHOEDS MH, NORDE W & VAN AKEN GA. 2007. The role of electrostatics in saliva-induced emulsion flocculation. *Food Hydrocolloid* **21**(4):596–606.

SONESSON AW, ELOFSSON UM, BRISMAR H & CALLISEN TH. 2006. Adsorption and mobility of a lipase at a hydrophobic surface in the presence of surfactants. *Langmuir* **22**(13):5810–5817.

SONESSON AW, BRISMAR H, CALLISEN TH & ELOFSSON UM. 2007. Mobility of *Thermomyces lanuginosus* lipase on a trimyristin substrate surface. *Langmuir* **23**(5): 2706–2713.

SU JH, FLANAGAN J, HEMAR Y & SINGH H. 2006. Synergistic effects of polyglycerol ester of polyricinoleic acid and sodium caseinate on the stabilisation of water–oil–water emulsions. *Food Hydrocolloids* **20**(2–3):261–268.

TOLSTOGUZOV V. 2002. Thermodynamic aspects of biopolymer functionality in biological systems, foods, and beverages. *Crit Rev Biotechnol* **22**(2):89–174.

TOLSTOGUZOV V. 2003. Some thermodynamic considerations in food formulation. *Food Hydrocolloids* **17**(1):1–23.

TSO P. 2000. Overview of digestion and absorption. In: Crissinger, K. D. & Stipanuk, M. H., editors. *Biochemical and Physiological Aspects of Human Nutrition.* Philadelphia, PA: W.B. Saunders Company. p. 75–90.

TYSSANDIER V, LYAN B & BOREL P. 2001. Main factors governing the transfer of carotenoids from emulsion lipid droplets to micelles. *Biochim Biophys Acta Molec Cell Biol Lipids* **1533**(3):285–292.

TYSSANDIER V, REBOUL E, DUMAS JF, BOUGTELOUP-DEMANGE C, ARMAND M, MARCAND J, SALLAS M & BOREL P. 2003. Processing of vegetable-borne carotenoids in the human stomach and duodenum. *Am J Physiol Gastrointestinal Liver Physiol* **284**(6):G913–G923.

VAN AKEN GA. 2007. Relating food microstructure to sensory quality. In: McClements, D. J., editor. *Understanding and Controlling the Microstructure of Complex Foods.* Boca Raton, FL: CRC Press. p. 449–482.

VASKONEN T. 2003. Dietary minerals and modification of cardiovascular risk factors. *J Nutr Biochem* **14**(9):492–506.

VERHAGEN H, COOLEN S, DUCHATEAU G, HAMER M, KYLE J & RECHNER A. 2004. Assessment of the efficacy of functional food ingredients-introducing the concept 'kinetics of biomarkers'. *Mutation Res – Fundamental Molec Mechanisms Mutagenesis* **551**(1–2):65–78.

VERSANTVOORT CHM, VAN DE KAMP E & ROMPELBERG CJM. 2004. *Development and Applicability of an* in vitro *Digestion Model in Assessing the Bioaccessibility of Contaminants from Food.* Bilthoven: Inspectorate of Health Inspection. p. 1–87.

VINGERHOEDS MH, BLIJDENSTEIN TBJ, ZOET FD & VAN AKEN GA. 2005. Emulsion flocculation induced by saliva and mucin. *Food Hydrocolloids* **19**(5):915–922.

VITORINO R, LOBO MJC, DUARTE JAR, FERRER-CORREIA AJ, DOMINGUES PM & AMADO FML. 2004a. Analysis of salivary peptides using HPLC-electrospray mass spectrometry. *Biomed Chromatogr* **18**(8):570–575.

VITORINO R, LOBO MJC, FERRER-CORREIRA AJ, DUBIN JR, TOMER KB, DOMINGUES PM & AMADO FML. 2004b. Identification of human whole saliva protein components using proteomics. *Proteomics* **4**(4):1109–1115.

WALSTRA P. 1993. Principles of emulsion formation. *Chem Eng Sci* **48**:333.

WALSTRA P. 2003. *Physical Chemistry of Foods.* New York: Marcel Decker.

WEINBRECK F, DE VRIES R, SCHROOYEN P & DE KRUIF CG. 2003. Complex coacervation of whey proteins and gum arabic. *Biomacromolecules* **4**(2):293–303.

WEISBRODT NW. 2001a. Gastric emptying. In: Johnson, L. R., editor. *Gastrointestinal Physiology*, 6th edition. St. Louis, MI: Mosby. p. 37–45.

WEISBRODT NW. 2001b. Motility of the small intestine. In: Johnson, L. R., editor. *Gastrointestinal Physiology*, 6th edition. St. Louis, MI: Mosby. p. 47–56.

WEISBRODT NW. 2001c. Swallowing. In: Johnson, L. R., editor. *Gastrointestinal Physiology*, 6th edition. St. Louis, MI: Mosby. p. 27–35.

WEISS J, SCHERZE I & MUSCHIOLIK G. 2005. Polysaccharide gel with multiple emulsion. *Food Hydrocolloids* **19**(3):605–615.
WHITCOMB DC & LOWE ME. 2007. Human pancreatic digestive enzymes. *Dig Dis Sci* **52**(1):1–17.
WILDMAN REC & KELLEY M. 2007a. Lycopene: Food sources, properties and health. In: Wildman, R. E. C., editor. *Handbook of Nutraceuticals and Functional Foods*, 2nd edition. Boco Raton, FL: CRC Press. p. 55–72.
WILDMAN REC & KELLEY M. 2007b. Nutraceuticals and functional foods. In: Wildman, R. E. C., editor. *Handbook of Nutraceuticals and Functional Foods*, 2nd edition. Boco Raton, FL: CRC Press. p. 1–22.
WRIGHT AJ, PIETRANGELO C & MACNAUGHTON A. 2008. Influence of simulated upper intestinal parameters on the efficiency of beta carotene micellarisation using an *in vitro* model of digestion. *Food Chemi* **107**(3):1253–1260.
ZHANG FJ, CHENG GX, GAO Z & LI CP. 2006. Preparation of porous calcium alginate membranes/microspheres via an emulsion templating method. *Macromolecular Mater Eng* **291**(5):485–492.
ZHANG H, TUMARKIN E, SULLAN RMA, WALKER GC & KUMACHEVA E. 2007. Exploring microfluidic routes to microgels of biological polymers. *Macromolecular Rapid Commun* **28**(5):527–538.

21

Controlling the delivery of glucose in foods

G. Zhang, Jiangnan University, China; Z. Ao and B.R. Hamaker, Purdue University, USA

Abstract: Glucose is the principal biological fuel for the body, and it has been classified into rapidly available glucose (RAG) and slowly available glucose (SAG) based on glycemic carbohydrate digestion rate that is related to human health. This chapter first reviews the concept of glycemic index (GI), and the digestion and nutritional classification of glycemic carbohydrates. The structural properties, slow digestion mechanism, and the biological functions of slowly digestible carbohydrates (SDC), mainly slowly digestible starch (SDS), are then discussed. Finally, potential formulation and testing of low-GI foods, using SDCs to control the glucose delivery, are described for the purpose of improving human health.

Key words: slowly digestible carbohydrate (SDC), slowly digestible starch (SDS), slowly available glucose (SVG), glycemic carbohydrate, glycemic index (GI).

21.1 Introduction

According to the Dietary Guidelines for Americans 2005 (USDA, 2005), dietary carbohydrates should provide 45–65% of total caloric intake, indicating their important role in human health. However, the calories provided by a specific carbohydrate component cannot be accurately assessed based on its quantity alone due to variations of the rate and extent of its digestion and glucose absorption (Jenkins *et al.*, 1981; Englyst *et al.*, 2003). Thus, the concept of glycemic index (GI) reflecting these variations was proposed by Jenkins *et al.* (1981) in which the GI is the percentage of the area under the glycemic response curve (AUC) of a test food compared to a reference sample (glucose or white bread) with the same amount (50 g) of available carbohydrate. High GI (GI > 70), low GI (GI < 55), and intermediate GI foods are categorized according to the measured GI values (Brand *et al.*, 1991). Although the GI of a food is determined by *in vivo* testing involving both food and human factors, the digestion property of the carbohydrate component is the ultimate determinant of the food's GI value (Wolever *et al.*, 2006). Since the proposition of the GI concept, there have been extensive clinical and nutritional investigations on dietary carbohydrates, particularly the potential health benefits of low-GI foods (Wolever, 2003). Related to this, a comprehensive GI table for different foods has been published (Foster-Powell *et al.*, 2002).

Starch is one of the most important glycemic carbohydrate components in foods as it is supplied by traditional staple food materials such as cereals, roots and tubers, and the myriad of products made from them. Categorized similarly as GI, starch is classified into rapidly digestible starch (RDS), slowly digestible starch (SDS), and resistant starch (RS) based on the *in vitro* Englyst assay (Englyst *et al.*, 1992). RDS is rapidly digested and absorbed in the duodenum and proximal regions of the small intestine, and it is correlated to the GI values of the sample. RS is not digested in the upper gastrointestinal tract, while SDS is the digested portion between RDS and RS, and is thought to be digested along the whole small intestine. Concerning glucose delivery, RDS provides a rapid and high level of glucose delivery (high GI), RS theoretically does not provide glucose (GI = 0), and SDS provides a slow and prolonged glucose delivery (low GI). Non-starch carbohydrates can also be categorized in a similar manner as rapid digesting (including most glycemic monosaccharides and disaccharides), intermediate digesting (such as isomaltulose), as well as non-digestible carbohydrates (dietary fiber). Thus, common terms of rapidly digestible carbohydrate (RDC), slowly digestible carbohydrate (SDC), and dietary fiber will be used to describe glucose delivery control. Regarding controlled delivery of glucose to the body, SDCs, including SDS and other types of slowly digestible carbohydrates, will be related in this chapter to their structural property, slow digestion mechanism, and function in low-GI food formulations.

21.2 Glucose delivery and health effects

Glucose, the major molecule from glycemic carbohydrate digestion, is the principal biological fuel for the body, and particularly for the central nervous system. Its level in the blood is tightly controlled by complex regulatory systems. Although some glucose can be synthesized from TCA, or citric acid, cycle intermediates, glycemic carbohydrates in foods are the major source of glucose, and its release from carbohydrate digestion in the digestive system is the starting point of the glucose homeostasis regulatory cascade. Control of glucose delivery in foods is determined mostly by food structure and the physicochemical properties of the carbohydrate components in foods.

The rate and extent of glucose production from carbohydrate digestion reflect the physiological property of a specific carbohydrate component. RDC is rapidly digested and absorbed in the duodenum and proximal regions of the small intestine, leading to a rapid elevation of blood glucose and, when in large amount, usually a subsequent episode of hypoglycemia. This large fluctuation in blood glucose generates high stress on the regulatory system of glucose homeostasis (Ludwig, 2002) that can lead to cell, tissue, and organ damages under a long-term stress (Brownlee, 2001). Dietary fiber is not digested in the upper gastrointestinal tract, but short chain fatty acids (SCFA), resulting from its fermentation in the colon, provide additional energy to the body. A high proportion of butyrate during RS fermentation is well recognized to be beneficial to colonic health (Topping and Clifton, 2001). The classification, development, and physiological consequences of RS have been extensively reviewed (Annison and Topping, 1994; Champ, 2004; Higgins, 2004; Sajilata *et al.*, 2006). SDC, the intermediate fraction between RDC and dietary fiber, is digested slowly throughout the entire small intestine to provide sustained glucose release, and this digestion property is consistent with the fundamental basis of low-GI foods: providing low initial glycemia and subsequently a slow and prolonged release of glucose, which indicates the beneficial effect to health of SDC. Overall, different digestion rates and different locations of glucose production do have different physiological consequences related to health.

Commonly consumed foods, which contain highly refined carbohydrates, often have a high value of GI and glycemic load (GL, GI × amount). The high postprandial glycemic response elicited by highly refined carbohydrates usually leads to a concomitant high level of plasma insulin, which is the major hormone to control and maintain postprandial blood glucose levels. High insulin level promotes glucose absorption and fat synthesis, and long-term consumption of high-GL foods has a high tendency to result in weight gain for people with susceptible genetic backgrounds (Livesey, 2005), as well as insensitivity to insulin. Both obesity and insulin-insensitivity are related to chronic metabolic diseases such as type 2 diabetes, cardiovascular disease, and possibly cancer (Ludwig, 2002). Chronic high levels of plasma insulin were also shown to be related to a reduced lifespan and unhealthy aging (Taguchi *et al.*, 2007), which has a common biological link to cancer (Finkel *et al.*, 2007). Additionally, a high GL food may produce oxidative stress (Hu *et al.*, 2006) that is a causative factor for many diseases. Thus, controlling the rate and location of glucose delivery as part of nutrient homeostasis is an important consideration for health.

With the above noted, there is still no good consensus within the scientific and industrial communities on the value of glycemic response, or GI, on health. The basic structures, mechanisms, and outcomes of low glycemic response from food carbohydrates need further study. Moreover, an intermediate rate and prolonged glucose delivery provided by foods or food ingredients is still not well understood. It is this aspect of glycemic carbohydrate that will be the focus of this chapter, that being foods with controlled glucose delivery. It is possible that a full spectrum of glucose delivery ingredients and foods could be realized utilizing different proportions of RDC, SDC, and dietary fibers.

21.3 The carbohydrate digestion process and human enzyme properties

Starch, as the main glycemic carbohydrate in foods, is a pure glucose polymer composed of essentially linear amylose and highly branched amylopectin macromolecules. The starch component in foods is digested in the gastrointestinal tract by the amylolytic α-amylases from saliva and pancreas, and the brush border glucogenic enzymes of maltase–glucoamylase and sucrase–isomaltase (Swallow *et al.*, 2001; Nichols *et al.*, 2003). These enzymes belong to the family of α-glucosidases. After food is consumed, the starch component is first digested by α-amylase to α-limit dextrins and oligosaccharides that are then cleaved by the brush border enzymes into glucose, and absorbed by the sodium–glucose cotransporter (SGLT-1) anchored at the luminal surface of enterocytes (Pencek *et al.*, 2002). Any factors affecting enzyme activity (quantity, different isoforms, inhibitors) and the susceptibility of substrate to hydrolytic enzymes will influence starch digestion and its nutritional property (Tester *et al.*, 2004). Amorphous or completely dispersed starches are highly susceptible to enzyme action; but starches that are physically entrapped, B-type raw starch granules, retrograded amylose, and some that are chemically modified are resistant to digestion. Starches may have an intermediate slow digestion pattern if either some degree of physical structure is retained during food processing or structural aspects dictate slow kinetics of digestion.

Most processed starchy foods have low to medium moisture contents, thus their digestion is basically a solid–liquid two-phase reaction, and the enzyme (particularly α-amylase) needs first to diffuse into the hydrated solid food matrix, bind to the substrate, and then cleave the glycosidic linkages of the starch molecules (Leloup *et al.*, 2004). Human α-amylase has five subsites for binding the starch substrate and cleavage of the α-1,4 glycosidic linkages (Brayer *et al.*, 2000) using a multiple attack mechanism (Mazur and Nakatani, 1993). Factors affecting the binding of α-amylase to substrates (e.g. substrate inhibition by the hydrolysis products maltose and maltotriose; Seigner *et al.*, 1985) will slow down the enzyme reaction. Brush border glucogenic enzymes cleave both α-1,4 and α-1,6 glycosidic bonds. Generally α-1,6 glycosidic bonds are more difficult to be cleaved compared with α-1,4 bonds (Kerr *et al.*, 1951), therefore, more α-1,6 bonds will slow the starch digestion (Ao *et al.*, 2007). Pancreatic α-amylase is the more dominant enzyme in digestion of starch (Englyst *et al.*, 1992), though the brush border enzymes (maltase-glucoamylase and sucrase-isomaltase) also play an important role with their glucogenic, or glucose-generating, property. Recent reports (Quezada-Calvillo *et al.*, 2007, 2008) showed that certain luminal α-amylase degradation products such as maltotriose, maltotetraose, and maltopentose inhibit the action of maltase-glucoamylase that is important for glucose production.

During the passage of foods in the gastrointestinal tract, there are other factors that affect food digestion and absorption including gastric emptying, enzyme inhibitors, and viscosity in the digestive tract (affecting enzyme accessibility to substrate and the absorption of glucose). It is possible that these can be used to generate a slow digestion effect.

21.3.1 Human α-amylase

The salivary and pancreatic α-amylases (EC 3.2.1.1), which are α-1,4 endo-glucosidases, are the initial and important enzymes in carbohydrate digestion. After starch or other glucans are slightly digested by the salivary amylase in the mouth, more extensive hydrolysis occurs by the action of pancreatic α-amylase. Compared with porcine pancreatic α-amylase, which is often used in starch analysis, human pancreatic α-amylase has 83% similarity in gene sequence (Ferey-Roux *et al.*, 1998).

Substantial efforts have been made to elucidate the catalytic mechanism of pancreatic α-amylase. α-Amylase is efficient in hydrolyzing large molecules as evidenced by a decrease in apparent K_m (more affinity to substrate) with the increasing of glucose units in the substrate (David, 1982). For the oligosaccharides, the action patterns are concentration dependent. Thus, different substrate concentration would leads to changes in α-limit dextrins that will influence the subsequent enzyme reactions (Robyt and French, 1970).

21.3.2 Brush border enzyme function in glucose production

Since glucose is only a minor product of the α-amylase digestion of large glycemic carbohydrate molecules, the products of α-limit dextrins and small linear oligomers from α-amylase digestion need further hydrolysis to become glucose monomers before absorption. Mucosal maltase-glucoamylase (MGAM, EC 3.2.1.20 and 3.2.1.3, encoded by the gene MGAM, located on chromosome 7q34) and sucrase-isomaltase (SI, EC 3.2.1.48 and 3.2.1.10, encoded by the gene SI, located on chromosome 3q26) (Nichols *et al.*, 1998 and 2003) are the enzymes for this final step. Both enzymes belong to the glucohydrolyase Family 31, and their proteins show 60% amino acid sequence homology. Human MGAM and SI each have two subunits with five distinct protein domains: an N-terminal cytoplasmic tail domain (26 amino acids), a transmembrane domain (anchoring domain, 21 amino acids), an *O*-glycosylated stalk domain (52 amino acids), and two similar catalytic domains (MGAM N-terminal subunit, NtMGAM; MGAM C-terminal subunit, CtMGAM; SI N-terminal subunit, NtSI; SI C-terminal subunit, CtSI; each ~900 residues) (Fig. 21.1) (Nichols *et al.*, 1998, 2003; Rossi *et al.*, 2006; Sim *et al.*, 2008). MGAM and SI are anchored to the brush border epithelial cells of the small intestine. Each of the enzymes has two subunits with complete conservation of the catalytic residues. NtMGAM and NtSI are found near the cell membrane.

Both MGAM and SI display α-1,4 exo-glucosidic activity from the non-reducing ends of linear chains of glucose oligomers and polymers to release

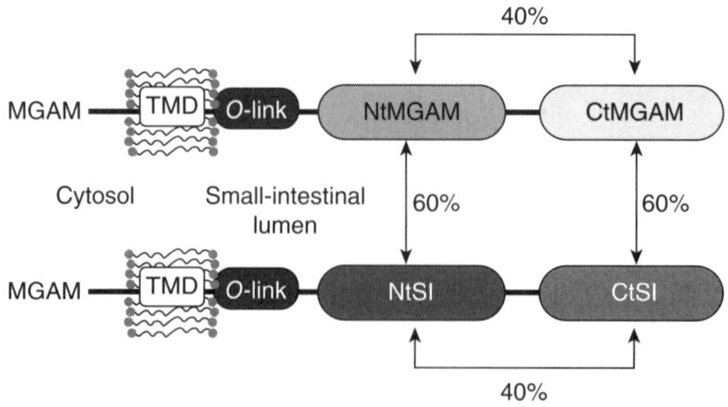

Fig. 21.1 A linear representation of the protein organization of the MGAM and SI complexes. The percentage of sequence identities between the catalytic subunits is indicated. (From: Sim *et al.*, 2008.)

glucose monomers. The hydrolytic action on branched α-1,6 linkages shown by SI (NtSI, isomaltase activity) is complementary to the hydrolytic activity to α-1,4 linkages by MGAM and SI with certain degree of substrate overlaps. The CtSI catalytic subunit also displays specific activity on α-1,2 linkage of sucrose. NtMGAM and CtMGAM, with 40% identity, have different substrate specificities, although both domains contain maltase and glucoamylase activities. The crystal structure of the N-terminal subunit of human MGAM has been resolved (Sim *et al.*, 2008), and recent research also showed that, at low oligomer concentrations, MGAM was ten times more active than SI, but at high concentrations MGAM experienced substrate inhibition while SI was not affected (Quezada-Calvillo *et al.*, 2007). Of particular note, maltotriose, maltotetraose, and maltopentose displayed a substrate inhibitory 'brake' effect on MGAM activity (Quezada-Calvillo *et al.*, 2008). The results suggested that the CtMGAM has a greater catalytic efficiency due to a higher affinity for glucan substrates and larger number of binding configurations to its active site. Sequence study also indicates that CtMGAM has higher affinity to substrates with longer chains (Sim *et al.*, 2008). Thus, CtMGAM is mainly responsible for the MGAM peptide's 'glucoamylase' activity and is the location of the substrate inhibitory brake (Quezada-Calvillo *et al.*, 2008).

21.4 Structural basis and mechanism of slowly digestible carbohydrate

Slowly digestible starch is the major SDC in processed foods. SDS itself is a method-oriented concept without specification on structural requirements of starch materials, making it difficult to be fabricated based simply on its definition. Consequently, an understanding of the fundamental structure and mechanism of SDS is essential for SDS product development. From the current available data, there are two fundamental mechanisms for SDS from the point of view of the starch itself: (1) physical structures that decrease enzyme accessibility and (2) chemical structures limiting the rate of enzyme action. Additionally, other factors such as decrease in gastric emptying, increase in viscosity inside the gastrointestinal tract, use of enzyme inhibitors, and interaction with other food components will possibly lead to a slow digestion property that is of physiological nature.

21.4.1 Physical structures for slowly digestible starch

Physical structures leading to SDS character are often found in processed foods, such as pasta in which the starch component is protected by other food components such as protein. The raw starch granule is perhaps the best representative of a SDS material caused by a physical structure. Starch granules have a unique semi-crystalline supramolecular structure with concentric layers of amorphous and crystalline regions radiating from the hilum. Amylopectin is the major molecule that forms the semi-crystalline regions showing A, B, or C types of X-ray diffraction patterns depending on its fine structure, namely, the non-random arrangement and length of each linear chain in the molecule (Thompson, 2000). The major intrinsic factors affecting raw starch digestibility include the supramolecular structure (packing of crystallites inside starch granule), ratio of amylose and amylopectin, amylopectin fine structure, and surface characteristics of starch granules (Oates, 1997). Investigators (Jane *et al.*, 1997; Planchot *et al.*, 1997; Gérard *et al.*, 2001) showed that B-type starches are resistant to enzyme digestion while A-type starches are slowly digestible. Most raw cereal starches have a high proportion of SDS material as measured by the *in vitro* Englyst test, and human testing of normal corn starch (A-type) confirms a slow and prolonged postprandial glucose release profile (Seal *et al.*, 2003). A good understanding of the slow digestion mechanism of raw cereal starch, as described below, provides a theoretical basis for fabricating SDS materials using appropriate physical structures.

Cereals have A-type starches in which the crystalline regions and amorphous regions are arranged concentrically, and there are channels, ranging in amount, that connect the central hilum region to the surface of the starch granules (Fig. 21.2). When starch granules are incubated with amylolytic enzymes, the enzymes migrate inside the starch granules through the channels (Fannon *et al.*, 1992) and initiate hydrolysis leading to an inside-out pattern of digestion (Benmoussa *et al.*, 2004). Although the amorphous regions have been generally thought to be easily digested (Gallant *et al.*, 1992), owing to the fact that they are not dense compared with the crystalline regions that are packed with dense double helices, Zhang *et al.* (2006a) observed no change of crystallinity before and after digestion, indicating

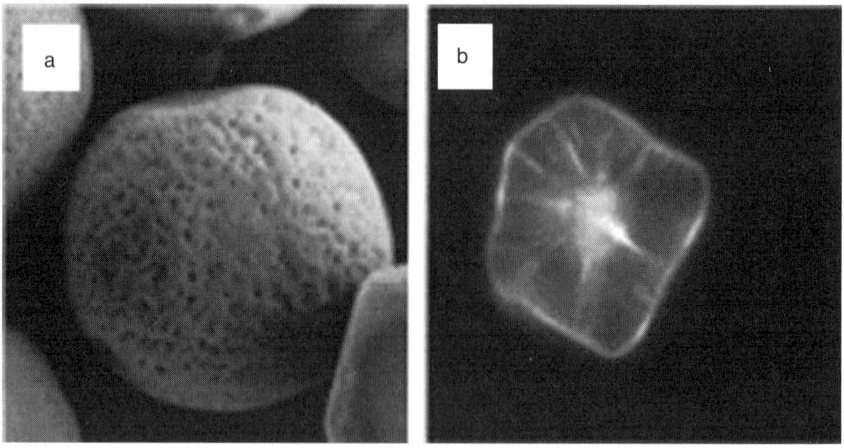

Fig. 21.2 Cereal starch granule surface pore (a, SEM) and the interior channel and cavity revealed using aqueous solution of merbromin (b, micrograph). (From Huber and BeMiller 1997.)

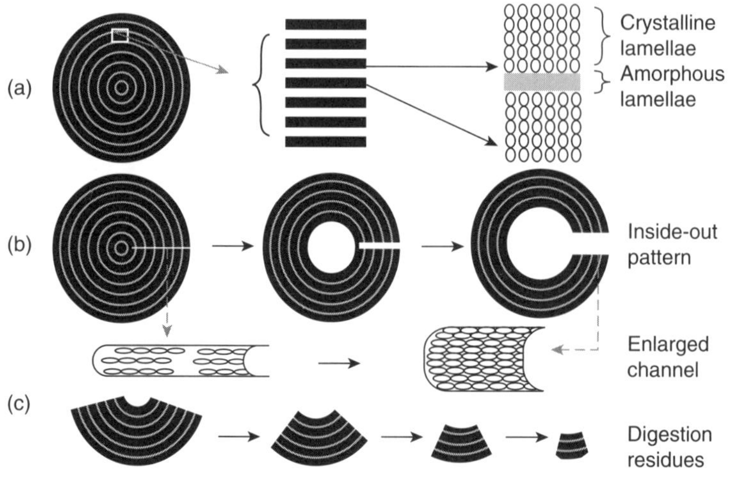

Fig. 21.3 Schematic representation of a dynamic side-by-side digestion mechanism and resulted static inside-out digestion pattern. (From: Zhang *et al.*, 2006a.)

that the amorphous region and crystalline region are digested simultaneously. A side-by-side and even digestion mechanism starts from the channels (Fig. 21.3), and is likely the mechanism leading to the simultaneous digestion of crystalline and amorphous regions. This digestion process produces the generally accepted inside-out digestion pattern. The side-by-side digestion mechanism is probably caused by the tight linkage between adjacent amorphous and crystalline layers so that the two regions remain together throughout the digestion process. Although other starches, such as potato and banana, also have concentrically arranged amorphous and crystalline regions, they are resistant to digestion owing to their B-type crystallites and absence of channels (Zhang *et al.*, 2006a,b).

Starch granules have a nicely packed physical structure without the involvement of covalent bonds between each compartment of the structure. A-type raw cereal starches are slowly digested with >50% SDS by the Englyst test and moreover, cereal starch granules are almost pure SDS material from the digestion kinetics perspective. This is because SDS, as measured by the Englyst assay at 120 min, can be digested further, if longer digestion time is permitted. Thus, a supramolecular structure composed of layer-by-layer crystalline (A-type) and amorphous regions is the structural basis for the slow digestion property of native cereal starches, and one might speculate that similar structures could be fabricated in food products or ingredients for a slow digestion effect.

Food matrices with physical structures that induce slow digestion can be found in pasta and spaghetti in which a network of protein limits the accessibility of amylolytic enzymes to the starch component (Fardet *et al.*, 1998). Similarly, a polymer structure that entraps starch into microspheres generates a slowly digestible starch with digestion proceeding from the peripheral to interior regions (Fig. 21.4) (Venkatachalam *et al.*, 2006). This latter example lends starch a slowly digestible character with a prolonged release of glucose when tested *in vivo* (Fig. 21.5).

21.4.2 Molecular structures for slowly digestible starch

When starch is used in food preparations, starch gelatinization, or the process of disrupting starch crystalline structure with heat and moisture, usually results in a decrease or loss of the slow digestion property of native cereal starches (Zhang *et al.*, 2006a). Depending on the moisture content of the final food, gelatinized starch may disperse in a liquid suspension, form a thick paste, or exist as swollen granules in a partial or complete amorphous state. For the liquid and paste gelatinized starch forms, the granular or supramolecular structures within the starch granule are almost completely lost, and the molecular structure of starch likely becomes the only determinant for its functionality regarding food and nutritional properties. Since starch is composed of essentially linear amylose consisting mostly of α-1,4 linked D-glucopyranosyl units and highly branched amylopectin in which α-1,4 linked linear chains are interconnected by α-1,6 glycosidic linkages, the structure of molecularly dispersed starch mainly depends on the ratio of amylose to amylopectin and the fine structure of amylopectin, namely its chain length distribution and branching pattern.

Starch retrogradation, which is the reassociation of amylose and amylopectin molecules to form double helices and possible crystalline structures, is another important process that occurs during food storage, particularly

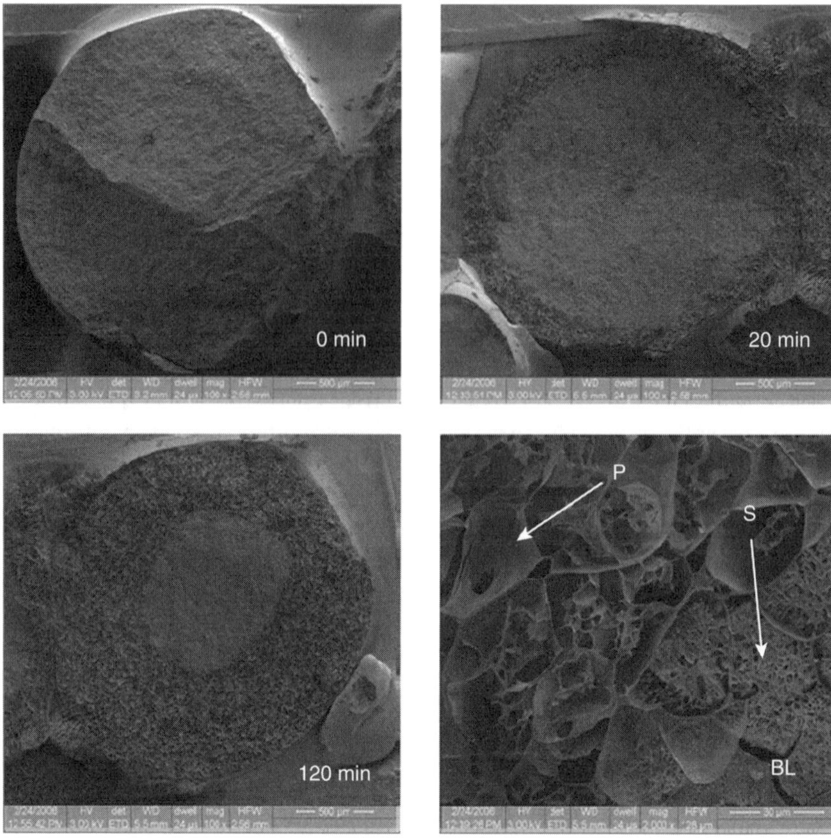

Fig. 21.4 With the Englyst test of cooker starch-entrappel alginate-based microspheres lower right panel micrograph is an enlargement of the boundary layer (BL) between digested and undigested matrix showing the polymer (P) and starch (S). (From Venkatachalam *et al.*, 2006.)

at low temperatures, but at a sufficiently high temperature to surpass its glass transition temperature (T_g). Researchers (Farhat *et al.*, 2001; Okuda *et al.*, 2006) have shown that starch retrogradation decreases starch's susceptibility to enzyme hydrolysis. The high RS nutritional property of starches with a high ratio of amylose to amylopectin is mostly related to the retrogradation of amylose (Haralampu, 2000). Related to this, retrogradation of partially debranched amylopectin after isoamylase treatment has been used to make SDS (Shi *et al.*, 2003; Shin *et al.*, 2004).

Other methods to make SDS have been to modify chemically the molecular structure of starch molecules including 1-octenyl succinic anhydride (OSA) modified starch (Han and BeMiller, 2007; He *et al.*, 2008) and enzyme modified starch with high density of α-1,6 linkages (Backer and

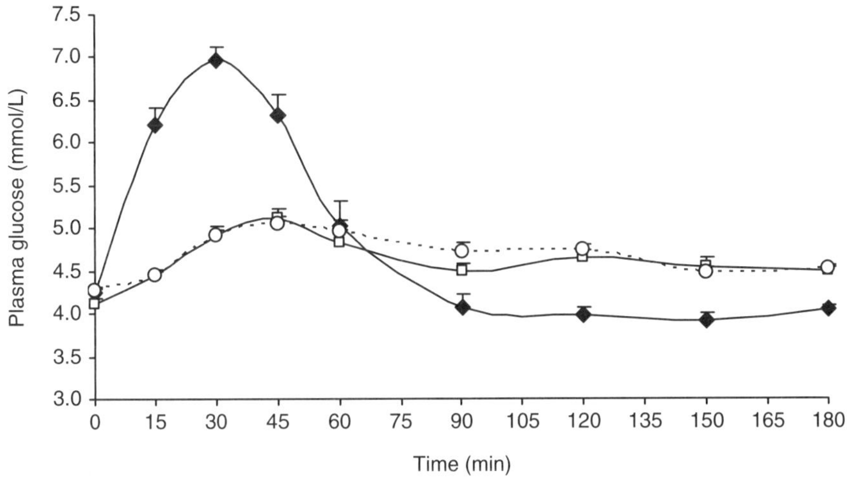

Fig. 21.5 Postprandial plasma glucose concentrations (mean ± SEM) in healthy subjects after consumption of 50 g of glucose (♦), 50 g starch equivalent microsphere test diet 1 (□) and test diet 2 (○), respectively. (From Venkatachalam *et al.*, 2006.)

Saniez, 2005; Ao *et al.*, 2007). These studies show that the molecular structure of starch molecules is a key for SDS production.

Our investigation (Zhang *et al.*, 2008a,b) using a variety of genetic maize mutants revealed a parabolic relationship between SDS content and the weight ratio of amylopectin short chains (degree of polymerization (DP) < 13) to long chains (DP ≥ 13), showing that amylopectins with either higher amount of short chains or long chains have comparably high content of SDS (Fig. 21.6). Further study of the mechanism of the parabolic relationship showed that there are two different mechanisms leading to the slow digestion of gelatinized starches. For those with more amylopectin long chains, starch retrogradation shows a bell-shaped pattern of SDS content with retrogradation time (Fig. 21.7), indicating the imperfect crystallites formed in retrogradation are associated with the slow digestion property. On the other hand, the molecular structure itself, or the branch pattern, is associated with the slow digestion property of samples with more short chains (with high branch density). An extreme example of molecular structure-dependent SDS is high molecular pullulan with an amylase-resistant linkage pattern in which the basic structure unit of maltotriose or maltotetraose is linked through α-1,6 glycosidic linkages (Wolf *et al.*, 2003). Amylose, as another component of starch, is mainly associated with RS formed through retrogradation during food storage. Therefore, amylopectin is the major component of SDS, and an optimum molecular structure of amylopectin required for SDS might be realized through chemical, physical, enzymatic, and genetic modifications; however, clinical studies would ultimately be required to show their physiological significance.

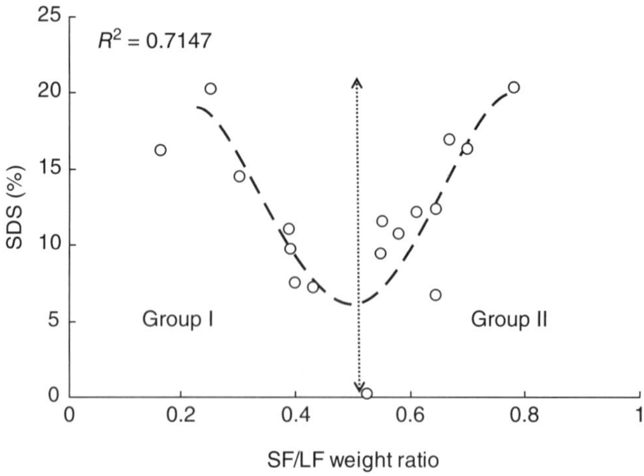

Fig. 21.6 The parabolic relationship between SDS percentage and the weight ratio of short chain (SF) to long chain fraction (LF); Groups I and II signing two structural paths for gaining a slowly digesting starch property. (From: Zhang *et al.*, 2008a.)

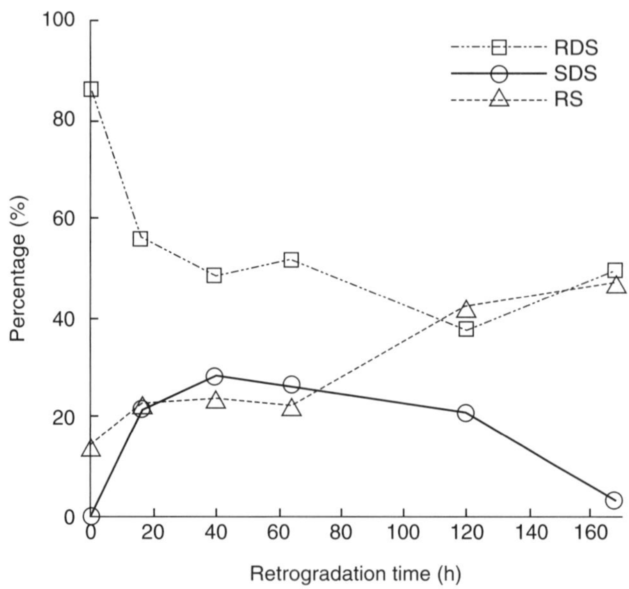

Fig. 21.7 The bell-shaped SDS content with the retrogradation time for starch mutant *AeWx* with high portion of longer chains. (From: Zhang *et al.*, 2008b.)

21.4.3 Physiological mechanisms for slowly digestible starch

Although the molecular structure of starch is the basis for starch granule supramolecular structure and the structures formed after starch gelatinization/retrogradation that impact digestion rate, there are extrinsic factors that need to be considered when the food is consumed. These include the effect of chewing, gastric emptying rate, transit time in the small intestine, as well as the properties of digestive enzymes discussed above. SDS of a physiological nature can be generated if these factors are modified to slow down the digestion of starch, or more broadly glycemic carbohydrates with a slow and prolonged glycemic response profile. Gastric emptying rate, viscosity of the food in the digestive tract, and enzyme inhibitors are reviewed below from the available literature related to physiology-oriented SDS.

The presence of organic acids or acid salts, such as those produced during sourdough fermentation or added during the baked food preparation, influences glycemic and insulinemic responses (Liljeberg and Björck, 1996, 1998; Liljeberg *et al.*, 1995). For example, consumption of sourdough bread (with lactic acid produced during fermentation) or breads with added Ca-lactate, or Na-propionate, significantly reduced glycemic and insulinemic indexes as compared with whole meal bread in the absence of these acids (Liljeberg *et al.*, 1995). Intake of bread with a high concentration of Na-propionate not only lowered postprandial blood glucose and insulin responses, but also significantly prolonged the duration of satiety compared with other breads. *In vitro* digestion, however, showed significant decrease in the rate of amylase digestion only in bread containing lactic acid. The authors concluded that the effect of acid salts such as sodium propionate on metabolic responses and satiety was due to delayed gastric emptying (Liljeberg and Björck, 1996). Similar effects were observed upon addition of vinegar to a starchy meal (Liljeberg and Björck, 1998). Thus, there is a potential of using fermentative processes, or practices that incorporate organic acids, to improve the nutritional features of carbohydrates needs.

A decreased gastric emptying rate and improvement of glucose tolerance is also seen in the 'second meal effect' caused by fermentation of dietary fibers (e.g. RS, soluble fibers) in the colon. The so-called 'second meal effect' was first described by Jenkins *et al.* (1982) and Wolever *et al.* (1988), whereby a low GI food improves the glycemic response in the second meal, as was later demonstrated due to an elevated amount of RS (Björck *et al.*, 2000). Brighenti *et al.* (2006) showed that the fermentation of dietary fibers has the potential to regulate postprandial glycemic response by decreasing gastric emptying rate. A similar finding showed that RS addition to food improves the sensitivity of insulin to clear glucose in the muscle, and causes a higher uptake of SCFAs by adipose tissues (Robertson *et al.*, 2005). Studies on the physiological function of SCFAs revealed that they induce the secretion of the incretin hormones GLP-1 and polypeptide YY (PYY) to reduce the motility of the gastrointestinal tract and stomach (Massimino *et al.*, 1998; Cuche *et al.*, 2000). Therefore, SCFAs produced during colonic fermentation behave as a negative feedback signal to decrease gastric emptying rate and the motility of other parts of gastrointestinal tract.

The viscosity effect of water-soluble dietary fibers has been shown to induce a slow digestion and absorption of carbohydrates with lowered postprandial glycemic and insulinemic responses (Jenkins *et al.*, 1976, 1977). Guar gum, psyllium, β-glucan, arabinoxylan, and others effectively flatten glycemic response, and their effects were still maintained when they were incorporated in food products (Yokayama *et al.*, 1997; Jenkins *et al.*, 2002). The mechanism of these soluble fibers on glycemic response is generally considered to result from the viscosity effect (Wood *et al.*, 1990) leading to a reduced rate of gastric emptying, decreased accessibility of hydrolytic enzymes to its substrates (Leclère *et al.*, 1994; Slavin, 2005), and/or slowed diffusion rate of digested carbohydrates (i.e. α-limit dextrins and oligosaccharides) towards the small intestine surface for glucogenesis and absorption (Briani *et al.*, 1987).

Inhibitors of human α-glucosidases can also be used to moderate carbohydrate digestion and its associated insulin response. Acarbose, an oligosaccharide formed by strains of the genus *Actinoplanes*, functions as an inhibitor of both α-amylase and the mucosal α-glucosidases (mainly maltase-glucoamylase) (Hiele *et al.*, 1992). It has been effective in the treatment of diabetes as it slows digestion of starch (Chiasson *et al.*, 1994; Conniff *et al.*, 1994) and is used in some countries to treat diabetes. Starch blockers, purified amylase inhibitors from great northern beans (phaseolamin), have also shown promise in providing good glucose homeostasis (Boivin *et al.*, 1988) and are marketed as dietary supplements (Phase 2 Starch Neutralizer™, Udani *et al.*, 2004). Unlike these blockers, which need to be ingested in large quantities (4–6 g per meal) to show significant effect, trestatin (a mixture of complex oligosaccharides produced microbiologically) has been proven to be a potent inhibitor (3–6 mg per 75 g starch) of pancreatic α-amylase in several *in vitro* and *in vivo* studies (Golay *et al.*, 1991). Glycemic and insulinemic responses in healthy and diabetic volunteers were moderated after consumption of breads containing trestatin added during processing without serious gastrointestinal side effects. Phenolic compounds extracted from some plants (such as green tea), with an anti-oxidation property, also inhibit the enzyme activity and the absorption of carbohydrate resulting in a low glycemic response (Konishi *et al.*, 2006). Although the use of enzyme inhibitors has shown promise, further studies are needed to evaluate the efficacy of these inhibitors after addition to starch-based processed foods, the dose–response relationship, and more importantly long-term tolerance and side effects of such inhibitors.

21.4.4 Non-starch slowly digestible carbohydrates

Other types of SDCs, although not SDS, that are completely determined by their chemical structure include isomaltulose, trehalulose (also called

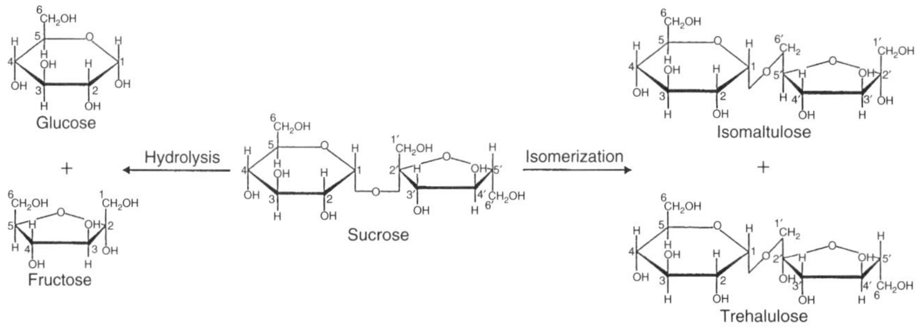

Fig. 21.8 Sucrose isomerization catalyzed by isomaltulose synthase. (From: Zhang *et al.*, 2003.)

trehalose), and sucromalt. Isomaltulose and trehalulose are made from sucrose using isomaltulose synthase (*Pal*I), also known as sucrose isomerase (EC 5.4.99.11) with the product α-D-glucosylpyranosyl-1,6-D-fructofuranose termed isomaltulose, and α-D-glucosylpyranosyl-1,1-D-fructofuranose termed trehalulose (Zhang *et al.*, 2003, Fig. 21.8). Sucromalt is composed of fructose and an oligosaccharide of alternan that has an alternating sequence of α-1,3 and α-1,6 linked D-glucopyranosyl units. It is produced by enzyme alternansucrase (EC 2.4.1.140) using sucrose as the substrate (Argüello-Morales *et al.*, 2001). These carbohydrates have unique glycosidic bonds that are different from starch molecules, and are completely digested and absorbed at a slower rate, leading to a blunted glycemic response and insulinemic response (Grysman *et al.*, 2007). Owing to their special molecular structures, they can be applied to a variety food products to provide a slow release of energy and blunted glycemic response.

21.5 Formulating low-glycemic index foods

From the above discussion, a potentially wide range of health benefits is possible from SDC in the diet and implies an importance to exploring ways to produce SDC for human health, that is particularly relevant considering the scarcity of SDC in common food products (Björck *et al.*, 2000). A better understanding of the slow digestion mechanism of carbohydrate also provides the basis for exploring approaches to generate SDC. Application-oriented approaches to make low-GI food using SDC include: (1) SDC ingredients where carbohydrate molecular structure is the foundation for its slow digestion and (2) SDC where the food matrix is the slow digestion mechanism.

21.5.1 Slowly digestible carbohydrate ingredient

Thermal processing, which causes starch gelatinization (in the presence of water), is essential to food quality and safety. Because of the loss of SDS property in thermally processed starchy foods, it is the molecular structures of starch molecules of these foods that hold more potential in achieving a slow digestion property. In this respect, chemical, enzymatic, and genetic methods can be applied to produce an appropriate starch structure that is slowly digestible. We have shown previously that a molecular structure with multiple short chains and a high degree of branch density in a certain distribution pattern will slow down the enzyme reaction, and this is one of the goals of amylopectin structure modification for enhancement of SDS. *In vivo* studies are still necessary to determine physiological effect of these altered starches.

For chemical modification, functional groups can be added to the chains of starch molecules to make the starch with desired structural characteristics from the viewpoint of enzyme digestion. Most chemical modifications (oxidation, acetylation, cross-linking, and etherification), however, make starch resistant to digestion (Wolf *et al.*, 1999). Recently, a slowly digestible starch, as defined by the *in vitro* Englyst test, was designed by Han and BeMiller (2007) using octenyl succinic anhydride (OSA) esterfication. A previous study showed an attenuated *in vivo* glycemic response of OSA-modified starch compared with the unmodified starch (Wolf *et al.*, 2001). The OSA-modified starch molecules were later shown to be an uncompetitive inhibitor that slows enzyme digestion (He *et al.*, 2008). The potential to produce a real SDS through chemical modification is worth further investigation.

Enzymatic modification is another method to change the molecular structure (chain length and branch pattern) of amylopectin molecules. The most commonly used enzyme approaches include α-amylase to remove some of the RDS fraction, β-amylase to shorten the branched chains (relatively increased the branch density), branching enzymes to add more branches into the amylopectin to further increase the branch density, and transglucosidase to add glucose or maltose through α-1,6 linkages (Hamaker and Han, 2006; Ao *et al.*, 2007). A highly branched soluble glucose polymer was produced by Backer and Saniez (2005) utilizing a series of enzymes including α-amylase, β-amylase, amyloglucosidase, α-transglucosidase, and branching enzymes.

Genetic modification can be considered as the extension of the enzyme modification of starch molecular structures through changing the activities of starch biosynthetic enzymes including starch synthases, branching enzymes, and debranching enzyme. A coordinated action of different enzymes would be needed to produce SDS. Although there are no identified SDS products using this approach, this is an area with good potential for future development.

The chemical structure-determined SDC can be directly added into food as slow digestion carbohydrate, especially in beverages. SDS, on the other hand, would be suitable as texture-forming ingredients.

21.5.2 Slowly digestible carbohydrate generation in a food matrix

Food processing technologies provide another good opportunity to make SDC by controlling the extent of starch gelatinization, and interactions between starch and other food components. Lowering the degree of starch gelatinization and partially retaining the A-type crystalline structure of related starches may be one effective way to increase the content of SDC in food products. Most of the common cereal food processing technologies use high moisture content, high temperature, and shear force that completely gelatinize starches and make them highly susceptible to enzyme digestion (Le Francois, 1989; Bravo *et al.*, 1998). However, some low-GI foods such as biscuits, with a low moisture content, have a lower extent of starch gelatinization and higher content of SDC because of the remaining partially intact starch granules (Englyst *et al.*, 2003). Most legume foods cooked in the whole grain form also have a high content of SDC, because of the entrapment of starch granules in the cell wall (Englyst *et al.*, 1996). Hydrothermal treatment can be used to increase the thermal stability of starch granules through an increase of crystallite perfection, alteration of crystalline packing from B or C to A type, and increased interaction of molecules within amorphous and crystalline regions (see review of Jacobs and Delcour, 1998). Shin *et al.* (2005) reported that hydrothermal treatment of sweet potato converted its C-type structure to A-type, and the SDS of the treated granule increased 200% compared with native starch granules.

Interactions between starch and non-starch food components that lead to production of new chemical or physical structures are another way to decrease the starch digestibility. The complex formed between amylose and monoglycerides during food preparation has been recognized to have a lower digestibility (Holm *et al.*, 1983; Seneviratne and Biliaderis, 1991; Murray *et al.*, 1998). Use of longer saturated monoglycerides causes a greater resistance to digestion (Eliasson and Krog, 1985). Using an *in vivo* animal model (dog), an amylose–lipid complex-containing diet slightly lowered serum glucose and insulin more than a maltodextrin-containing control diet (Patil *et al.*, 1998). A network of protein limiting the accessibility of amylolytic enzymes to the starch component, such as in pasta and spaghetti (Fardet *et al.*, 1998), is another example with physical structures that induce slow digestion of starch. For molecular structure-induced SDC with a chemical entity, conjugated starch with protein or amino acids made through the Maillard reaction is an example that reduced digestibility (Yang *et al.*, 1998). However, the potential side effects caused by consumption of these glycated products need to be considered since diet-derived glycation end products are a major contributor to the body's pool of advanced glycation end products (AGE) (Uribarri *et al.*, 2005), which are associated with pathogenesis in various diseases (Vlassara *et al.*, 2002).

Theoretically speaking, a molecular structure that is naturally slowly digestible and has good functionality is the ideal approach to make a thermally stable SDC to seamlessly combine functional and nutritional properties. SDC related to its physical structure is normally associated with a dense food matrix, whereas SDC obtained from a physiological mechanism needs introduction of other ingredients (e.g. enzyme inhibitors) that can lead to a slow digestion of starch materials.

21.6 Testing the glycemic index of foods

Glycemic index (GI) was developed to systematically classify dietary carbohydrates based on its glycemic response after consumption (Wolever *et al.*, 1991). To provide an accurate and comparative value of GI, a defined methodology must be used to reflect differences in dietary carbohydrates in food, and to fulfill the criteria of consistency of the GI value, application to individual and to mixed diets, as well as to demonstrate clinically significant therapeutic improvements by practical dietary changes. Since the measurement of the GI involves both the food and human factors, there are many considerations in its testing, including the number of testers, the number of replicates in the experiment, blood sampling time interval, sampling duration, the food portion size, the reference food, and requirements for the conditions of measurement. This is necessary to minimize the influence of human factors (individual differences) and reflect the true quality of dietary carbohydrates that is related to glucose absorption rate as controlled by insulin, the counter-regulation response, and affected by insulin resistance.

Currently, the defined method of GI measurement is to use 50 g available carbohydrate portion size consumed by 10–12 healthy subjects after overnight fasting, with blood sampling conducted at 0, 15, 30, 45, 60, 90 and 120 min from the start of eating, and using a reference food of glucose or white bread. The area under the glycemic (AUG) response curve from 0–120 min is calculated (only the positive portion), and the GI value is the ratio of test food to reference food multiplied by 100. Three replications are performed. Outliers of the individual subjects are decided based on GI > 2SD (standard deviation) from the mean. The human factors affecting the glycemic response include age, sex, body fitness, glucose tolerance status, and the fasting blood glucose on the day of test. Although outliers can be removed from the final calculation, a standard control of the subjects is necessary to give an accurate GI value of the test foods. The calculation of the AUC has been automated using a computer program.

Some food issues also need to be considered for the accuracy of GI measurement in addition to the factors mentioned above. One is the accurate measurement of the available carbohydrate content (not the total carbohydrate content in the food) using enzymatic methods (such as in the Englyst method RDS + SDS = available carbohydrate) since the measured GI value of the food is usually negatively related to the content of the resistant starch or dietary fibers (Björck *et al.*, 2000) (which should not be the case). Another point is the composition of food containing insulinotropic proteins, such as whey protein from milk, that will falsely make the GI value smaller. These food issues are one of the reasons for variations of food GI values. Although a true low-GI food should contain a high portion of SDC as the available carbohydrate providing a slow and prolonged release of glucose, attention must be paid to the measurement of GI values for various foods.

21.7 Future trends

A relatively good understanding of SDC concerning its structure and mechanism has been achieved through a series of investigations on its physical, chemical, and physiological aspects. One can at least speculate, and go on to test hypotheses experimentally, as to further SDC food or ingredient products that can be made. Although there remains some controversy about the GI concept and its use, there is good reason to further pursue SDC as one of the carbohydrates for true low-GI foods. Moreover, study of well-defined SDC foods or components can be used to elucidate some of these inconsistencies.

However, there still exist many challenges to transform this knowledge into real food products. Many of the claimed 'slowly digestible starch' products in patents do not have a high content of practically utilizable SDC, and raw cereal starch made by nature is still the SDC model used in many physiological studies. Future research on SDC needs to focus on novel technologies to make SDC, developing *in vivo* methods to evaluate the qualities of different SDC materials, and further understanding of the physiological consequences of SDC including satiety, cognitive performance, physical performance, energy metabolism, and metabolic diseases. The physiological relationship between SDC and different dietary fibers, and their colonic effect, also need to be investigated to have a complete picture of glycemic carbohydrate nutrition to better control of glucose delivery through foods.

21.8 References

ANNISON G. and TOPPING D.L. (1994). Nutritional role of resistant starch: chemical structure vs physiological function. *Annu. Rev. Nutr.* **14**:297–320.

AO Z., SIMSEK S., ZHANG G., VENKATACHALAM M., REUHS B., and HAMAKER B.R. (2007). Starch with slow digestion property produced by altering branch density, chain length and crystalline structure. *J. Agric. Food. Chem.* **55**:4540–4547.

ARGÜELLO-MORALES M.A. REMAUD-SIMEON M., WILLEMOT R., VIGNON M.R., and MONSAN P. (2001). Novel oligosaccharides synthesized from sucrose donor and cellobiose acceptor by alternansucrase. *Carbohydr. Res.* **331**:403–411.

BACKER D. and SANIEZ M.H. (2005). Soluble highly branched glucose polymers and their method of production. Patent, US 2005/0142167A1.

BENMOUSSA M., SUHENDRA B., ABOUBACAR A., and HAMAKER B.R. (2004). Distinctive sorghum starch granule morphologies appear to improve raw starch digestibility. *Starch/Stärke* **58**:92–99.

BJÖRCK I., LILJEBERG H., and OSTMAN E., (2000). Low glycaemic-index foods. *Br. J. Nutr.* **83**:S149–155.

BOIVIN M., FLOURIE B., RIZZA R.A., GO V.L.W., and DIMAGNO E.P. (1988). Gastrointestinal and metabolic effects of amylase inhibition in diabetics. *Gastroenterology* **94**:387–394.

BRAND J.C., COLAGIURI S., CROSSMAN S., ALLEN A., ROBERTS D.C., and TRUSWELL A.S. (1991). Low-glycemic index foods improve long-term glycemic control in NIDDM. *Diabetes Care* **14**:95–101.

BRAVO L., ENGLYST H.N., and HUDSON J.H. (1998). Nutritional evaluation of carbohydrates in Spanish diet: non-starch polysaccharides and *in vitro* starch digestibility of breads and breakfast products. *Food Res. Int.* **31**:129–135.

BRAYER G.D., SIDHU G., MAURUS R., RYDBERG E.H., BRAUN C., WANG Y., NGUYEN N., OVERALL C.M., and WITHERS S.G. (2000). Subsite mapping of the human pancreatic α-amylase active site through structural, kinetic, and mutagenesis techniques. *Biochemistry* **39**:4778–4791.

BRIANI G., BRUTTOMESSO D., BILARDO G., GIORATO C., DUNER E., IORI E., SGNAOLIN E., PEDRINI P., and TIENGO A. (1987). Guar-enriched pasta and guar gum in the dietary treatment of type II diabetes. *Phytother Res.* **1**:177–179.

BRIGHENTI F., BENINI L., RIO D.D., CASIRAGHI C., PELLAGRINI N., SCAZZINA F., JENKINS D.J., and VANTINI I. (2006). Colonic fermentation of indigestible carbohydrate contributes to the second-meal effect. *Am. J. Clin. Nutr.* **83**:817–822.

BROWNLEE M. (2001). Biochemistry and molecular cell biology of diabetic complications. *Nature* **414**:813–820.

CHAMP M. (2004). Physiological aspects of resistant starch and *in vivo* measurement. *J. AOAC Int.* **87**:749–755.

CHIASSON J.L., JOSSE R.G., HUNT J.A., PALMASON C., RODGER N.W., ROSS S.A., RYAN E.A., TAN M.H., and WOLEVER T.M. (1994). The efficacy of acarbose in the treatment of patients with non-insulin-dependent diabetes mellitus. A multicenter controlled clinical trial. *Ann. Intern. Med.* **121**:928–935.

CONNIFF R.F., SHAPIRO J.A., and SEATON T.B. (1994). Long-term efficacy and safety of acarbose in the treatment of obese subjects with non-insulin-dependent diabetes mellitus. *Arch. Intern. Med.* **154**:2442–2448.

CUCHE G., CUBER J.C., and MALBERT C.H. (2000). Ileal short-chain fatty acids inhibit gastric motility by a humoral pathway. 1. *Am. J. Physiol. Gastrointest. Liver Physiol.* **279**:G925–930.

DAVID H. (1982). Hydrolysis by human alpha-amylase of *p*-nitrophenyloligosaccharides containing four to seven glucose Units. *Clin. Chem.* **28**:1485–1489.

ELIASSON A.C. and KROG N. (1985). Physical properties of amylose monoglyceride complexes *J. Cereal Sci.* **3**:239–248.

ENGLYST H.N., KINGMAN S.M., and CUMMINGS J.H. (1992). Classification and measurement of nutritionally important starch fractions. *Eur. J. Clin. Nutr.* **46**:S33–S50.

ENGLYST H.N., KINGMAN S.M., HUDSON G., and CUMMINGS J.H. (1996). Measurement of resistant starch *in vitro* and *in vivo*. *Br. J. Nutr.* **75**:749–755.

ENGLYST K.N., VINOY S., ENGLYST H.N., and LANG V. (2003). Glycaemic index of cereal products explained by their rapidly and slowly available glucose. *Br. J. Nutr.* **89**:329–339.

FANNON J.E., HAUBER R.J., and BEMILLER J.N. (1992). Surface pores of starch granules. *Cereal Chem.* **69**:284–288.

FARDET A., HOEBLER C., BALDWINT P.M., BOUCHET B., GALLANT D.J., and BARRY J.L. (1998). Involvement of the protein network in the *in vitro* degradation of starch from spaghetti and lasagne: a microscopic and enzymatic study. *J. Cereal Sci.* **27**:133–145.

FARHAT I.A., PROTZMANN J., BECKER A., VALLES-PAMIES B., NEALE R., and HILL S.E. (2001). Effect of the extent of conversion and retrogradation on the digestibility of potato starch. *Starch/Stärke* **53**:431–436.

FEREY-ROUX G., PERRIER J., FOREST E., MARCHIS-MOUREN G., PUIGSERVER A., and SANTIMONE M. (1998). The human pancreatic α-amylase isoforms: isolation structural studies and kinetics of inhibition by acarbose. *Biochim. Biophys. Acta* **1388**:10–20.

FINKEL T., SERRANO M., and BLASCO M.A. (2007). The common biology of cancer and ageing. *Nature* **448**:767–774.

FOSTER-POWELL K., HOLT S.H., and BRAND-MILLER J.C. (2002). International table of glycemic index and glycemic load values'. *Am. J. Clin. Nutr*. 76 5–56.

GALLANT D.J., BOUCHET B., BULÉON A., and PEREZ S. (1992). Physical characteristics of starch granules and susceptibility to enzymatic degradation. *Europ. J. Clin. Nutr.* **46**:S3–16.

GÉRARD C., COLONNA P., BULÉON A., and PLANCHOT V. (2001). Amylolysis of maize mutant starches. *J. Sci. Food Agric.* **81**:1281–1287.

GOLAY A., SCHNEIDER H., TEMLER E., and FELBER J.P. (1991). Effect of trestatin, an amylase inhibitor, incorporated into bread, on glycemic responses in normal and diabetic patients. *Am. J. Clin. Nutr*. **53**:61–65.

GRYSMAN A., CARLSON T., and WOLEVER T.M.S. (2007). Effect of sucromalt on postprandial response in human subjects. *Eur. J. Clin. Nutr.* **62**:1364–1371.

HAMAKER B.R. and HAN X. (2006). Slowly digestible starch. US Patent 20060257977.

HAN J. and BEMILLER J.N. (2007). Preparation and physical characteristics of slowly digesting modified food starches. *Carbohydr. Polym*. **67**:366–374.

HARALAMPU S.G. (2000). Resistant starch – a review of the physical properties and biological impact of RS3. *Carbohydr. Polym.* **41**:285–292.

HE J., LIU J., and ZHANG G. (2008). Slowly digestible waxy maize starch prepared by octenyl succinic anhydride esterification and heat-moisture treatment: glycemic response and mechanism. *Biomacromolecules* **9**:175–184.

HIELE M., GHOOS Y., RUTGEERTS P., and VANTRAPPEN G. (1992). Effects of acarbose on starch hydrolysis. Study in healthy subjects, ileostomy patients, and *in vitro*. *Dig Dis Sci*. **37**:1057–1064.

HIGGINS J.A. (2004). Resistant starch: metabolic effects and potential health benefits. *J. AOAC Int.* **87**:761–768.

HOLM J., BJÖRCK I., OSTROWSKA S., ELIASSON A.C., ASP N.G., LARSSON K., and LUNDQUIST I. (1983). Digestibility of amylose–lipid complexes *in vitro* and *in vivo*. *Starch/Stärke*, **35**:294–297.

HU Y., BLOCK G., NORKUS E.P., MORROW J.D., DIETRICH M., and HUDES M. (2006). Relations of glycemic index and glycemic load with plasma oxidative stress markers. *Am. J. Clin. Nutr.* **84**:70–76.

HUBER K.C. and BEMILLER J.N. (1997). Visualization of channels and cavities of corn and sorghum starches. *Cereal Chem.* **74**:537–541.

JACOBS H. and DELCOUR J.A. (1998). Hydrothermal modifications of granular starch with retention of the granular structure – a review. *J. Agric. Food Chem.* **46**:2895–2905.

JANE J.-L., WONG K.S., and MCPHERSON A.E. (1997). Branch structure difference in starches of A- and B-type X-ray patterns revealed by their naegeli dextrin. *Carbohydr. Res.* **300**:219–227.

JENKINS A.L., JENKINS D.J.A., ZDRAVKOVIC U., WURSCH O., and VUKSAN V. (2002). Depression of the glycemic index by high levels of β-glucan fiber in two functional foods tested in type 2 diabetes. *Eur. J. Clin. Nutr.* **56**:622–628.

JENKINS D.J.A., LEEDS A.R., GASSUL M.A., WOLEVER T.M.S., GOFF D.V., ALBERTI K.G.M.M., and HOCKADAY T.D.R. (1976). Unabsorbable carbohydrates and diabetes. Decreased post-prandial hyperglycemia. *Lancet* **2**:172–174.

JENKINS D.J.A., LEEDS R., GASSUL M.A., COCHET R., and ALBERTI K.G.M.M. (1977). Decrease in post-prandial insulin and glucose concentrations by guar and pectin. *Ann. Intern. Med.* **86**:20–23.

JENKINS D.J.A., KENDALL C.W.C., AUGUSTIN L.S.A., FRANSESCHI S., HAMAIDI M., MARCHIE A., WOLEVER T.M.S., and TAYLOR R.H. (1981). Glycemic index of foods: a physiological basis for carbohydrate exchange. *Am. J. Clin. Nutr.* **34**:362–366.

JENKINS D.J., WOLEVER T.M., and TAYLOR R.H. (1982). Slow release dietary carbohydrate improves second meal tolerance. *Am. J. Clin. Nutr.* **35**:1339–1346.

JENKINS D.J.A., KENDALL C.W.C., AUGUSTIN L.S.A., FRANSESCHI S., HAMAIDI M., MARCHIE A., and AXELSEN M. (2002). Glycemic index: overview of implications in health and disease. *Am. J. Clin. Nutr.* **76**:266S–273S.

KERR R.W., CLEVELAND F.C., and KATZBECK W.J. (1951). The action of amylo-glucosidase on amylose and amylopectin. *J. Am. Chem. Soc.* **73**:3916–3921.

KONISHI Y., AITANI M., YAMAGUCHI H., ARIMURA T., OKADA T., and MURAI H. (2006). Method of treating diabetes and obesity using carbohydrate absorption inhibitors. US Patent 20060024396.

LECLÈRE C.L., CHAMP M., BOILLOT J., GUILLE G., LECANNU G., MOLIS C., BORNET F., KREMPF M., DELORT-LAVAL J., and GALMICHE J.-P. (1994). Role of viscous guar gums in lowering the glycemic response after a solid meal. *Am. J. Clin. Nutr.* **59**:914–921.

LE FRANCOIS P. (1989). *In vitro* availability of starch in cereal products. *J. Sci. Food Agric.* **49**:499–501.

LELOUP V.M., COLONNA P., and RING S.G. (2004). α-Amylase adsorption on starch crystallites. *Biotech. Bioeng.* **38**:127–134.

LILJEBERG H.G. and BJÖRCK I.M. (1996). Delayed gastric emptying rate as a potential mechanism for lowered glycaemia after eating sourdough bread: studies in humans and rats using test products with added organic acids or an organic salt. *Am. J. Clin. Nutr.* **64**:886–893.

LILJEBERG H. and BJÖRCK I. (1998). Delayed gastric emptying rate may explain improved glycaemia in healthy subjects to a starchy meal with added vinegar. *Eur. J. Clin. Nutr.* **52**:368–371.

LILJEBERG H.G., LONNER C.H., and BJÖRCK I.M. (1995). Sourdough fermentation or addition of organic acids or corresponding salts to bread improves nutritional properties of starch in healthy humans. *J. Nutr.* **125**:1503–1511.

LIVESEY G. (2005). Low-glycemic diets and health: implications for obesity. *Proc. Nutr. Soc.* **64**:105–113.

LUDWIG D.S. (2002). The glycemic index physiological mechanism relating to obesity, diabetes, and cardiovascular disease. *J. Am. Med. Assoc.* **287**:2414–2423.

MASSIMINO S.P., MCBURNEY M.I., FIELD C.J., THOMPSON A.B.R., KEELAN M., HAYEK M.G., and SUNVOID G.D. (1998). Fermentable dietary fiber increases GLP-1 secretion and improves glucose homeostasis despite increased intestinal glucose transport capacity in healthy dogs. *J. Nutr.* **128**:1786–1793.

MAZUR A.K. and NAKATANI H. (1993). Multiple attack mechanism in the porcine pancreatic alpha-amylase hydrolysis of amylose and amylopectin. *Arch. Biochem. Biophys.* **306**:29–38.

MURRAY S., PATIL A., FAHEY G., MERCHEN N., WOLF B., LAI S.-C., and GAREB K. (1998). Apparent digestibility of a debranched amylopectin-lipid complex and resistant starch incorporated into enteral formulas fed to ileal-cannulated dogs. *J. Nutr.* **128**:2032–2035.

NICHOLS B.L., ELDERING J., AVERY S., HAHN D., QUARONI A., and STERCHI E. (1998). Human small intestinal maltase-glucoamylase cdna cloning: homology to sucrase-isoamylase. *J. Biol. Chem.* **273**:3076–3081.

NICHOLS B.L., AVERY S.E., SEN P., SWALLOW D.M., HAHN D., and STERCHI E.E. (2003). The maltase-glucoamylase gene: common ancestry to sucrase-isomaltase with complementary starch digestion activities. *Proc. Natl. Acad. Sci.* **100**:1432–1437.

OATES C.G. (1997). Towards an understanding of starch granule structure and hydrolysis. *Trends Food Sci. Tech.* **8**:375–382.

OKUDA M., ARAMAKI I., KOSEKI T., INOUCHI N., and HASHIZUME K. (2006). Structural and retrogradation properties of rice endosperm starch affect enzyme digestibility of steamed milled-rice grains used in sake production. *Cereal Chem.* **83**:143–151.

PATIL A.R., MURRAY S.M., FAHEY G.C., MERCHEN N.R., WOLF B.W., LAI C., and GARLEB K.A. (1998). Apparent digestibility and glycemic responses to a debranched amylopectin–lipid complex and resistant starch incorporated into enteral formulas fed to dogs cannulated in the ileum. *FASEB J.* **12**, A210 (abs.).

PENCEK R.R., KOYAMA Y., LACY D.B., JAMES F.D., FUEGER P.T., JABBOUR K., WILLIAM P.E., and WASSERMAN D.H. (2002). Transporter-mediated absorption is the primary route of entry and is required for passive absorption of intestinal glucose into the blood of conscious dogs. *J. Nutr.* **132**:1929–1934.

PLANCHOT V., COLONNA P., and BULÉON A. (1997). Enzymatic hydrolysis of α-glucan crystallites. *Carbohydr. Res.* **298**:319–326.

QUEZADA-CALVILLO R., ROBAYO-TORRES C.C., AO Z., HAMAKER B.R., QUARONI A., BRAYER G.D., STERCHI E.E., BAKER S.S., and NICHOLS B.L. (2007). Luminal substrate 'brake' on mucosal maltase-glucoamylase activity regulates total rate of starch digestion to glucose. *J. Ped. Gastr. Nutr.* **45**:32–43.

QUEZADA-CALVILLO R., SIM L., AO Z., HAMAKER B.R., QUARONI A., BRAYER G.D., STERCHI E.E., ROBAYO-TORRES C.C., ROSE D.R., and NICHOLS B.L. (2008). Localization of luminal starch substrate 'brake' on maltase-glucoamylase activity within the glucoamylase subunit. *J. Nutr.* **138**:685–692.

ROBERTSON M.D., BICKERTON A.S., DENNIS A.L., VIDAL H., and FRAYN K.N. (2005). Insulin-sensitizing effects of dietary resistant starch and effects on skeletal muscle and adipose tissue metabolism. *Am. J. Clin. Nutr.* **82**:559–567.

ROBYT J.F. and FRENCH D. (1970). The action pattern of porcine pancreatic α-amylase in relationship to the substrate binding site of the enzyme. *J. Biol. Chem.* **245**:3917–3927.

ROSSI E.J., SIM L., KUNTZ D.A., HAHN D., JOHNSTON B.D., GHAVAMI A., SZCZEPINA M.G., KUMAR N.S., STERCHI E.E., NICHOLS B.L., PINTO B.M., and ROSE D.R. (2006). Inhibition of recombinant human maltase glucoamylase by salacinol and derivatives. *FEBS J.* **273**:2673–2683.

SAJILATA M.G., SHINGHAL R.S., and KULKARNI P.K. (2006). Resistant starch – a review. *Comp. Rev. Food Sci. Food Safety.* **5**:1–17.

SEAL C.J., DALY M.E., THOMAS L.C., BAL W., BIRKETT A.M., JEFFCOAT R., and MATHERS J.C. (2003). Postprandial carbohydrate metabolism in healthy subjects and those with type 2 diabetes fed starches with slow and rapid hydrolysis rates determined *in vitro*. *Br. J. Nutr.* **90**:853–864.

SEIGNER C., PRODANOV E., and MARCHIS-MOUREN G. (1985). On porcine pancreatic α-amylase action: kinetic evidence for the binding of two maltooligosaccharide molecules (maltose, maltotriose and *o*-nitrophenylmaltoside) by inhibition study. *Eur. J. Biochem.* **148**:161–168.

SENEVIRATNE H.D. and BILIADERIS C.G. (1991). Action of α-amylases on amylose–lipid complex superstructures. *J. Cereal Sci.* **13**:129–143.

SIM L., QUEZADA-CALVILLO R., STERCHI E.E., NICHOLS B.L., and ROSE D.R. (2008). Human intestinal maltase–glucoamylase: crystal structure of the N-terminal catalytic subunit and basis of inhibition and substrate specificity. *J. Mol. Biol.* **375**:782–792.

SHI Y.C., CUI X., BIRKETT A.M., and THATCHER M.G. (2003). Slowly digestible starch products. US Patent Application 20030219520, 20030215562.

SHIN S.I., CHOI H.J., CHUNG K.M., HAMAKER B.R., PARK K.H., and MOON T.W. (2004). Slowly digestible starch from debranched waxy sorghum starch: preparation and properties. *Cereal Chem.* **81**:404–408.

SHIN S.I., KIM H.J., HA H.J., LEE S.H., and MOON T.W. (2005). Effect of hydrothermal treatment on formation and structural characteristics of slowly digestible non-pasted granular sweet potato starch. *Starch/Stärke* **57**:421–430.

SLAVIN J.L. (2005). Dietary fiber and body weight. *Nutrition* **21**:411–418.

SWALLOW D.M., POULTER M., and HOLLOX E.J. (2001). Intolerance to lactose and other dietary sugars. *Drug Meta. Dispo.* **29**:513–516.

TAGUCHI A., WARTSCHOW L.M., and WHITE M.F. (2007). Brain IRS2 signaling coordinates life span and nutrient homeostasis. *Science* **317**:369–372.

TESTER R.F., KARKALAS J., and QI X. (2004). Starch structure and digestibility enzyme-substrate relationship. *Worlds Poultry Sci. J.* **60**:186–195.

THOMPSON D.B. (2000). On the non-random nature of amylopectin branching. *Carbohydr. Polym.* **43**:223–239.

TOPPING D.L. and CLIFTON P.M. (2001). Short-chain fatty acids and human colonic function: roles of resistant starch and nonstarch polysaccharides. *Physiol. Rev.* **81**:1032–1054.

UDANI J., HARDY M., and MADSEN D. (2004). Blocking carbohydrate absorption and weight loss: a clinical trial using Phase 2 brand proprietary fractionated white bean extract. *Alter. Med. Rev.* **9**:63–69.

URIBARRI J., CAI W., SANDU O., PEPPA M., GOLDBERG T., and VLASSARA H. (2005). Diet-derived advanced glycation end products are major contributors to the body's AGE pool and induce inflammation in healthy subjects. *Ann. N.Y. Acad. Sci.* **1043**:461–466.

USDA (2005). *U.S. Department of Health and Human Services and U.S. Department of Agriculture. Dietary Guidelines for Americans.* 6th edition, Washington, DC: U.S. Government Printing Office, January 2005.

VLASSARA H., CAI W., and CRANDALL J. (2002). Inflammatory mediators are induced by dietary glycotoxins: a major risk factor for diabetic angiopathy. *Proc. Natl. Acad. Sci. USA.* **99**:15596–15601.

VENKATACHALAM M., ZHANG G., and HAMAKER B.R. (2006). Use of polymer encapsulated starches as a novel method to make low glycemic foods. World Grain Summit: Foods and Beverages (AACC International), Abstract P-285, Sept.17–20, San Francisco, CA.

WOLEVER T.M. (2003). Carbohydrate and the regulation of blood glucose and metabolism. *Nutr. Rev.* **61**:S40–S48.

WOLEVER T.M., JENKINS D.J., OCANA A.M., RAO V.A., and COLLIER G.R. (1988). Secondmeal effect: low-glycemic-index foods eaten at dinner improve subsequent breakfast glycemic response. *Am. J. Clin. Nutr.* **48**:1041–1047.

WOLEVER T.M.S., JENKINS D.J.A., JENKINS A.L., and JOSSE R.G. (1991). The glycemic index: methodology and clinical implications. *Am. J. Clin. Nutr.* **54**:846–854.

WOLEVER T.M., YANG M., ZENG X.Y., ATKINSON F., and BRAND-MILLER J.C. (2006). Food glycemic index, as given in glycemic index tables, is a significant determinant of glycemic responses elicited by composite breakfast meals. *Am. J. Clin. Nutr.* **83**:1306–1312.

WOLF B.W., BAUER L.L., and FAHEY G.C. (1999). Effects of chemical modification on *in vitro* rate and extent of food starch digestion: an attempt to discover a slowly digested starch. *J. Agric. Food Chem.* **47**:4178–4183.

WOLF B.W., WOLEVER T.M.S., BOLOGNESI C., ZINKER B.A., GARLEB K.A., and FIRKINS J.L. (2001). Glycemic response to a food starch esterified by 1-octenyl succinic anhydride in humans. *J. Agric. Food chem.* **49**:2674–2678.

WOLF B.W., GARLEB K.A., CHOE Y.S., HUMPHREY P.M., and MAKI K.C. (2003). Pullulan is a slowly digestible carbohydrate in humans. *J. Nutr.* **133**:1051–1055.

WOOD P.J., BRAATEN J.T., FRASER W.S., RIEDEL D., and POSTE L.M. (1990). Comparisons of viscous properties of oat and guar gum and the effects of these and oat bran on glycemic index. *J. Agric. Food Chem.* **38**:753–757.

YANG W., HATTORI M., KAWAGUCHI T., and TAKAHASHI K. (1998). Properties of starches conjugated with lysine and poly(lysine) by the Maillard reaction. *J. Agric. Food Chem.* **46**:442–445.

YOKOYAMA W.H., HUDSON C.A., KNUCKLES B.E., CHIU M.M., SAYRE R.N., and TURNLAND J.R. (1997). Effect of barley β-glucan in durum wheat pasta on human glycemic response. *Cereal Chem.* **74**:293–296.

ZHANG D., LI N., LOK S.-M., ZHANG L.-H., and SWAMINATHAN K. (2003). Isomaltulose synthase (*Pal*I) of *Klebsiella* sp. LX3, crystal structure and implication of mechanism. *J. Biol. Chem.* **278**:35428–35434.

ZHANG G., AO Z., and HAMAKER B.R. (2006a). Slow digestion property of native cereal starches. *Biomacromolecules* **7**:3252–3258.

ZHANG G., VENKATACHALAM M., and HAMAKER B.R. (2006b). Structural basis for the slow digestion property of native cereal starch. *Biomacromolecules* **7**:3259–3266.

ZHANG G., AO Z., and HAMAKER B.R. (2008a). Nutritional property of endosperm starches from maize mutants: a parabolic relationship between slowly digestible starch and amylopectin fine structure. *J. Agric. Food Chem.* **56**:4686–4694.

ZHANG G., SOFYAN M., and HAMAKER B.R. (2008b). Slowly digestible state of starch: mechanism of slow digestion property of gelatinized maize starch. *J. Agric. Food Chem.* **56**:4695–4702.

22

Protein micro/nanoparticles for controlled nutraceutical delivery in functional foods

L. Chen, University of Alberta, Canada

Abstract: As a vital macronutrient in food, proteins possess unique functional properties and excellent biodegradability, which enable them to be generally regarded as safe materials for encapsulation of nutraceutical compounds. This chapter focuses on the current knowledge and techniques for development of food protein-based micro/nanoparticles of desirable structures at precisely controlled sizes for target release of nutracetuical compounds at the site of absorption. Their potential applications in functional foods are illustrated.

Key words: food proteins, micro/nanoparticles, nutraceutical delivery, functional foods.

22.1 Introduction

Growing interest in the enormous potential of microencapsulation has been recently triggered by the emergence of nutraceutical compounds. These are the active ingredients in functional foods which convey health benefits, for example, unsaturated fatty acids, antioxidants, probiotics and bioactive peptides (Wildman, 2001). The incorporation of nutraceutical compounds into food systems can provide a simple way to improve public health and/or reduce the risk of disease (Elliott and Ong, 2002). However, many of these compounds remain unavailable by oral administration, owing to instability under the conditions encountered during food processing (e.g. high temperature, exposure to oxygen and light) or in the gastrointestinal tract (e.g. low pH, digestive enzymes, presence of other nutrients) (Bell, 2001), and low permeability and/or solubility within the gut. Micro/nano-encapsulation systems can be used to overcome these limitations. Formulations for intelligent, modulated and selective delivery of drugs to specific areas in the body in order to maximize drug action and minimize side effects in the biomedical and pharmaceutical sectors have been successfully developed (Langer and Peppas, 2003; Peppas *et al.*, 2000). However, these formulations often cannot be used in food applications due to limitations imposed by the requirement: (1) to use materials generally recognized as safe (GRAS); (2) not to affect food sensory qualities (Champagne and Fustier, 2007; Chen *et al.*, 2006) and (3) the requirement for low-cost additives in the final foodstuff considering that the profit margins in the food industry are much more stringent than in pharmaceutical industries (Gouin, 2004). Therefore, design and development of novel encapsulation systems to maintain the active molecular form of nutraceutical compounds during processing and storage and to deliver this form effectively to the physiological target are important challenges for food scientists and the industry.

The type and physicochemical properties of the wall material used for encapsulation are the most critical aspects that govern the functionality of these systems (Gharsallaoui *et al.*, 2007). Food proteins as wall materials to encapsulate nutraceutical compounds are receiving growing scientific and industrial interest. Food proteins are GRAS materials with abundant natural sources and are widely used in formulated foods because they have high nutritional value and are degradable by digestive enzymes. The bioactive peptides generated from food protein degradation may exert a number of physiological effects *in vivo* on the gastrointestinal, cardiovascular, endocrine, immune and nervous systems. The functional properties of food proteins have been extensively described in the scientific literature (Bryant and McClements, 1998; Clark, 1998; Dickinson, 2003; Walstra, 2003). Documented physicochemical characteristics of food proteins indicate that these biopolymers offer unique potential in developing microcapsules for controlled release in food applications (Lee and Rosenberg, 2000a). During the past two decades, various kinds of micro/nanoparticles based on animal proteins (gelatin, casein and whey protein) and plant proteins (soy protein, zein and wheat gliadin) have been developed, as illustrated in Table 22.1. Examples of nutraceuticals that have been incorporated in the core are minerals, vitamins, unsaturated fatty acids, antioxidants and probiotic microorganisms.

This chapter will focus on the current knowledge and techniques for development of protein-based matrices and their potential applications for controlled delivery of nutraceutical compounds in functional foods. Micro/nanoparticles will be emphasized since only smaller particles can be incorporated into most foods, including solid and semi-solid products, without changing their sensory qualities (Augustin, 2003). More importantly, by decreasing the matrix size from micrometers to nanometers, new protein vehicles with improved delivery properties can be developed.

22.2 Advantages of protein matrices for controlled delivery

In recent years, the concept of controlled release of the encapsulated ingredient at the right place and at the right time has become more and more of

Table 22.1 Food protein micro/nanoparticles incorporating nutraceuticals

Protein	Encapsulated ingredient	Particle size	Reference
Whey protein	Retinol	1–2 mm	Beaulieu *et al.* (2002)
	Unsaturated fatty acids	μm range	Jimenez *et al.* (2004)
	Riboflavin	3–10 μm	Chen and Subirade (2006, 2007a)
	Probiotics	3 μm–3 mm	Picot and Lacroix (2003, 2004) Reid *et al.* (2005), Anal and Singh (2007)
	Avocado oil	2–4 μm	Bae and Lee (2008)
Soy protein	Retinol	150 μm	Chen and Subirade (2008b)
	Riboflavin	10 μm	
	Fish oil	30–280 μm	Cho *et al.* (2003), Gan *et al.* (2008)
Caseinate	Fish oil	20–50 μm	Augustin *et al.* (2006), Kagami *et al.* (2003)
Gelatin	Immunoglobulin	μm range	Cho *et al.* (2005)
	Lycopene	2–15 μm	Chiu *et al.*, (2007), Shu *et al.* (2006)
Gliadin, hordein, zein	Unsaturated fatty acids	μm range	Iwami *et al.* (1987)
Gliadin	Tocopherol	900 nm	Duclairoir *et al.* (2003)

interest (Desai and Park, 2005). Controlled release of the encapsulated nutraceuticals can broaden their applications in various food formulations, improve their effectiveness and ensure optimal dosage. The excellent functional properties of food proteins allow controlled release properties to be achieved by formulating to obtain the desired micro/nanoparticle structure or by precisely controlling the particle size (Usha and Gustavo, 1995).

22.2.1 Gelling and film forming capacity

Gel forming capacities are essential for development of delivery formulations. Gel forming involves self aggregation of protein molecules into a three-dimensional network (Aguilera, 1995; Twomey *et al.*, 1997) via weak physical bonds (hydrophobic effects, van der Waals, hydrogen bonding) and covalent interactions (Ziegler and Foegeding, 1990) owing to the diverse functional groups (carboxyl, amino, aromatic and sulfate side chains) on protein molecular chains. This process can be triggered by heating, drying, acidification and addition of calcium/iron or crosslinking agents. Since these intermolecular interactions are generally sensitive to the physicochemical conditions of the medium, modulating the pH, temperature, ionic strength and protein concentration can result in a large variety of ordered structures, which may lead to matrices of various desirable structures for different applications. In general, matrices prepared from food proteins are excellent oxygen barriers (Lee and Rosenberg, 2000b). Traditionally, heating has been applied to prepare food protein gels; however, thermal treatment has limited their applicability to formulations containing heat-sensitive ingredients. Recently, cold gelation provides an alternative gel development method for globular proteins such as whey and soy proteins (Barbut and Foegeding, 1993; Maltais *et al.*, 2005). This method requires a heating step during which food proteins are denatured and polymerized into soluble aggregates, followed by a cooling step and subsequent addition of salt or acid, which results in the formation of a network of soluble aggregates. The ability to form cold set gels opens interesting opportunities for food proteins as carriers of heat-sensitive bioactive compounds. The gel allows protection of nutraceuticals in protein networks and the ability to release them in a controlled way under different conditions.

Food proteins can form films on the surface of target core ingredients upon drying. The film-forming process involves intermolecular S—S bonding, hydrogen bonding and hydrophobic interactions (Guilbert *et al.*, 2002; Padua and Wang, 2002; Krochta, 2002; Park *et al.*, 2002; Chen and Subirade, 2008a). Food proteins can also form complex films with other polymers in solution. They form complex films with polysaccharides on the surface of emulsified droplets generally at pH values lower than the isoelectric point of the protein (De Kruif *et al.*, 2004; Turgeon *et al.*, 2003). The association is based on the formation of a complex between the positively charged protein and the negatively charged polysaccharide. Levy and co-workers also demonstrated that whey protein could form a complex film with alginate at alkaline pH owing to the formation of amide bonds between these two polymers (Levy and Edwards-Levy, 1996). Depending on their composition and properties, some complex films showed reinforced water barrier capacity. The ability to form complex films provides another way to entrap nutraceutical compounds at ambient temperature.

22.2.2 Emulsifying properties

Food proteins often have emulsifying properties because of their amphiphilic nature. The flexible molecular chains on proteins can rapidly adsorb to the emulsion interface, where they self-aggregate and form continuous and homogeneous coatings around oil droplets to prevent flocculation and coalescence (Dickinson and Chen, 1999; Dickinson *et al.*, 1996; Jost *et al.*, 1986, 1989; Lefèvre and Subirade, 2003; McClements *et al.*, 1993; Phillips *et al.*, 1994). The ability to bridge oil/water interfaces suggests that protein coatings can efficiently entrap lipophilic nutraceuticals for incorporation into functional foods (Beaulieu *et al.*, 2002; Leung *et al.*, 2005). Most polysaccharides used in encapsulation applications, such as starches and gums, do not share this characteristic. Virtually any ingredient can be incorporated into and be protected by food protein matrices whether hydrophilic, lipophilic or even microorganisms. Lipophilic compounds are generally incorporated into a protein matrix by a two-step process. The nutraceutical of interest is dissolved in a lipid carrier and emulsified with an aqueous dispersion of protein that functions as an emulsifier and a wall material. Solidification of the protein around the lipid droplets follows. Hydrophilic and other ingredients such as probiotic microorganisms can be dissolved or dispersed into protein solutions directly and then be encapsulated in protein microparticles by various protein drying or gelation techniques.

22.2.3 Nutraceutical binding

A food protein matrix is not an inert system. Food proteins have strong binding affinity to a number of nutraceuticals via hydrogen bonding and hydrophobic and ionic interactions (De Wolf and Brett, 2000; Pérez and Calvo, 1995; Wang *et al.*, 1997). The milk protein β-lactoglobulin (β-lg) has been the object of extensive research because of its well-defined structure and wide applications in the food industry. Although the binding mechanism is still not entirely clear, current research suggests that the most probable binding site for unsaturated fatty acids and retinol is in the hydrophobic pocket of β-lg. In addition to this primary binding site, β-lg is thought to contain weaker secondary binding sites that are also capable of undergoing interactions with hydrophobic molecules (Dufour and Haertlé 1990; O'Neill and Kinsella 1988; Robillard and Wishnia 1972; Spector and Fletcher, 1970). Other milk proteins such as α-lactalbumin and bovine serum albumin bind various types of compounds as well (Futterman and Heller, 1972; Morrisett *et al.*, 1975; Pérez *et al.*, 1989; Spector, 1975). The type of binding between a protein and a nutraceutical compound depends on their molecular characteristics, and thus there is no universal mechanism for these bindings. This favorable binding property allows increased loading efficiency of nutraceuticals in protein gel and film networks, especially those with low solubility, and protection of these compounds during food processing and storage.

22.2.4 Active side chains for modification

The active side chains (carboxyl, amino and sulfate side chains) on food protein molecules allow the possibility of physical, chemical and enzymatic modifications to develop new or improved properties (Means and Feeney, 1998). The most frequently used modification is crosslinking to reinforce the protein matrix. This process usually involves aldehyde derivatives such as formaldehyde and glutaraldehyde, which must be used carefully according to the local legislation (Chen and Subirade, 2008a). Safety concerns of chemical crosslinking renders enzymatic crosslinkers a possible alternative approach for food applications. For instance, a process involving a transglutaminase enzyme as a crosslinking agent for protein wall materials induced a hardened shell of coacervate around the targeted nutraceutical compounds. This effect was achieved by catalyzing the formation of a covalent bond between a free amine group (e.g. lysine) and the gamma-carboxamide group of glutamine (Cho *et al.*, 2003; Gan *et al.*, 2008). Bonds formed by transglutaminase exhibit high resistance to proteolytic degradation.

The advantageous functional properties of food proteins mentioned above allow adaptation of existing techniques or the development of new technology to produce micro/nanoparticles of various formulations at precisely controlled sizes ranging from several millimeters to nanometers. Particle size plays a very important role in regulating the rate of degradation of the polymer matrix as well as the rate of release, uptake and distribution of the nutraceutical compound. The ability to control the particle size improves the possibility for controlled release at a specific absorption site to maximize health benefits and minimize side effects. The following section describes current techniques for development of protein-based micro/nanoparticles and a variety of formulations prepared for food applications.

22.3 Formation of food protein micro/nanoparticles

22.3.1 Techniques

Food protein-based micro/nanoparticles have found wide and rapidly increasing applications in the food industry and a great variety of processes have been developed so far. Common techniques to produce micro/nanoparticles include spray drying, coacervation, extrusion and emulsification–gelation. The selection of the microencapsulation process is governed by the physicochemical properties of the core materials (i.e. nutraceutical compounds), the coating materials (i.e. protein) and the intended applications of the food ingredients.

Spray-drying

Spray-drying is a unit operation by which a liquid product is atomized in a current of hot gas to instantaneously obtain a powder. It is the most widely applied technique in the food industry. The merits of the process have ensured its widespread use; these include availability of the equipment, low processing costs, a wide choice of carrier solids, good stability of the finished product and the possibility of large-scale production in continuous mode (Baisier and Reineccius, 1989; Gharsallaoui *et al.*, 2007). Materials suitable for microencapsulation by spray drying should have high solubility, low viscosity in concentrated solution, and exhibit good emulsification, film-formation and drying properties. However, suitable coating materials which also have GRAS status are relatively limited. In spite of the extensive application of carbohydrates such as starches and maltodextrins in microencapsulation of food ingredients, wall materials that are based on these compounds have poor interfacial properties and often must be chemically modified in order to improve their surface activity (Young *et al.*, 1993).

In contrast, proteins manifest good functional properties that allow them to be viable coating materials for microencapsulation by spray-drying. During the past decades, properties of food protein microparticles prepared by spray-drying methods have been investigated extensively. Typical protein wall materials include sodium caseinate, whey proteins, soy proteins and gelatin (Baranauskiene *et al.*, 2006; Kagami *et al.*, 2003; Keogh *et al.*, 2001; Sheu and Rosenberg, 1998). The initial liquid feeding the sprayer can be a protein solution, emulsion or suspension. Depending on the starting feed material and operating conditions, spray-drying produces protein microparticles of 1–50 μm. Among proteins, whey protein and casein have been shown to be excellent coating materials. They have been successfully formulated into microparticles incorporating anhydrous milk fat, conjugated linoleic acid, avocado oil and probiotic microorganisms (Bae and Lee, 2008; Jimenez *et al.*, 2004; Keogh and O'Kennedy, 1999; Moreau and Rosenberg, 1996; Picot and Lacroix, 2003; Young *et al.*, 1993). Hydrolysed starches (glucose, lactose, corn syrup solids and maltodextrin) are generally added as a secondary wall material to improve the drying properties of the sprayed droplets by enhancing the formation of a dry crust around the droplets and increasing the oxidative stability of the encapsulated ingredients by reducing oxygen permeability of the wall (Kagami *et al.*, 2003; Sheu and Rosenberg, 1995).

Coacervation

The concept of coacervation is the phase separation of one or more hydrocolloids from the initial solution and the subsequent deposition of the newly formed coacervate phase around the active ingredient suspended or emulsified in the same reaction media. A coacervation process can be 'simple' or 'complex'. Complex coacervation is based on the formation of a coacervate between oppositely charged polymers, usually proteins and polysaccharides as mentioned in Section 21.2. If the required conditions are met, the polysaccharide and the protein form a complex, which may form a film around the target material that needs to be encapsulated. Complexes of food protein (gelatin, albumin, β-lactoglobulin, casein, legumin) with polysaccharide (acacia gum, pectin, gellan gum, xanthan gum, alginate, carrageenan and carboxymethyl cellulose) have been developed into various microcapsulations (Kim *et al.*, 1996; De Kruif *et al.*, 2004; Weinbreck *et al.*, 2004). The core ingredients include fish oil and various flavor compounds. Complex coacervation generates particles with sizes ranging from 1 to 200 μm. Factors that influence compatibility and the formation of the complex are the protein/polysaccharide ratio, pH, ionic strength and the nature of the polymers (molecular weight, net charge, ternary structure and flexibility of chains) (Benichou *et al.*, 2002).

Simple coacervation results from the removal of the solvent from a single colloid dispersed in solution by addition of chemical compounds which have a greater affinity for the solvent than the colloid. This causes the colloid chains to come closer together and form the coacervate. This phenomenon provides a convenient approach to prepare protein nanoparticles by pouring protein solutions into desolvating agents. For example, gelatin, albumin, and whey protein nanoparticles were successfully prepared using alcohol and acetone as desolvating agents, respectively; while gliadin and zein nanoparticles (100 nm) were prepared by pouring their alcoholic solution into a saline buffer (Arnedo *et al.*, 2002; Gunasekaran *et al.*, 2007; Liu *et al.*, 2005; Mauguet *et al.*, 2002; Muthuselvi and Dhathathreyan, 2006; Weber *et al.*, 2000). Sub-microparticles have also been prepared by a salting-out coacervation process by adding a salt such as sodium sulfate to a protein solution (Mauguet *et al.*, 2002). It has been shown that precise control of the nanoparticle size was realized by carefully modulating the parameters affecting the thermal aggregation process such as the amount of added desolvating or salting-out agent (Weber *et al.*, 2000). The need of further crosslinking steps to produce water-insoluble coatings for hydrophilic proteins may leave hydrophobic proteins such as zein and gliadin more advantageous for preparing nanoparticles by simple coacervation methods.

Extrusion

Extrusion is a relatively low-temperature microencapsulation method. It involves forcing protein droplets containing the fixing agent into a gel-forming solution through a micro-size nozzle. The coating material hardens on contact with the liquids, forming an encapsulating matrix to entrap the core material. In this method, microparticle size is easily controlled by adjusting the nozzle diameter. The smallest particles produced in this way are about 1 mm in diameter. This method is thought to be less detrimental to bioactive compounds and allows them to be completely surrounded by the protein wall material to provide a good barrier.

One typical example is the preparation of gelatin microspheres by forcing the heated gelatin solution into chilled liquid paraffin (Di Silvio *et al.*, 1994; Franz *et al.*, 1998). Cooling of the dispersion resulted in the formation of beads of 1–2 mm, which were subsequently crosslinked to form microspheres insoluble at 37 °C. More recently, whey protein micro-beads (1–2 mm) were developed by an extrusion method consisting of dropping a whey protein/oil emulsion into a $CaCl_2$ solution (Beaulieu *et al.*, 2002). This method is based on the Ca^{2+} induced gelation of pre-denatured whey protein. Higher $CaCl_2$ concentrations resulted in accelerated gelation kinetics, which led to rapid entrapment and stabilization of the emulsion droplets by the protein network and a more regular shape. Properties such as swelling, elasticity, deformability and resistance at fracture depend on pH and preparation conditions. One of the drawbacks of extrusion is the formation of rather large particles, which limits the use of extruded encapsulated nutraceuticals in applications where mouthfeel is important. However, it has been shown recently that the calcium concentration can be judiciously controlled to obtain desired particle sizes in the μm to mm range (Lavoie *et al.*, 2005).

Emulsification–gelation

Emulsification–gelation is another method frequently used to prepare protein microparticles. This method involves a process to stabilize emulsions of oil droplets in aqueous protein solution (O/W) or aqueous protein droplets in oil phase (W/O), followed by gelification of the protein by heating, chemical or enzymatic crosslinking (Cho *et al.*, 2003; Gan *et al.*, 2008; Heelan and Corrigan, 1998). The particle size varies from several micrometers to 500 μm. The advantages of this technique are its feasibility for large-scale production and its ability to produce microparticles with a wide range of diameters by controlling the emulsion size. However, concerns about the heating process for formulations containing heat-sensitive ingredients, and the safety of chemical crosslinking, have limited the application of this technique.

Enzymatically induced protein gelation using transglutaminase may be a promising technique for the formation of micro/nanoparticle nutraceutical delivery systems. Emulsification/internal cold gelation is another safe method that may be feasible to prepare food protein microparticles on a large scale for food applications (Chen and Subirade, 2007a; Chen *et al.*, 2006). The method is based on the release of calcium ions from an acid-soluble calcium salt in emulsified pre-denatured protein solution. This is achieved by acidification with an oil-soluble acid, which partitions to the dispersed aqueous phase, releasing soluble calcium and initiating gelation. Using this technique, whey and soy protein microspheres have been successfully developed at ambient temperature. By modulating emulsification conditions, the particle size can be controlled from 30 to 500 μm in diameter. This method may open interesting opportunities for the use of food proteins as carriers of sensitive nutraceutical compounds in functional foods.

Comparison of methods

The techniques presented above have their specific advantages and disadvantages and their use will depend on the intended product use. In spite of the merits of the spray-drying technique as mentioned above, one disadvantage is the elevated temperature. High temperatures and the presence of oxygen may lead to an increased oxidation of core ingredient. Nutraceutical stability can be increased by lowering the outlet air temperature; however, sufficient temperature is required to achieve complete and satisfactory drying of the feed suspensions. In order to overcome this problem, freeze-drying has been used to prepare protein microencapsulations at low temperature. However, the particles had a very porous structure and addition of antioxidants to the core ingredients was necessary to achieve an adequate shelf-life (Heinzelmann *et al.*, 2000). The complex coacervation

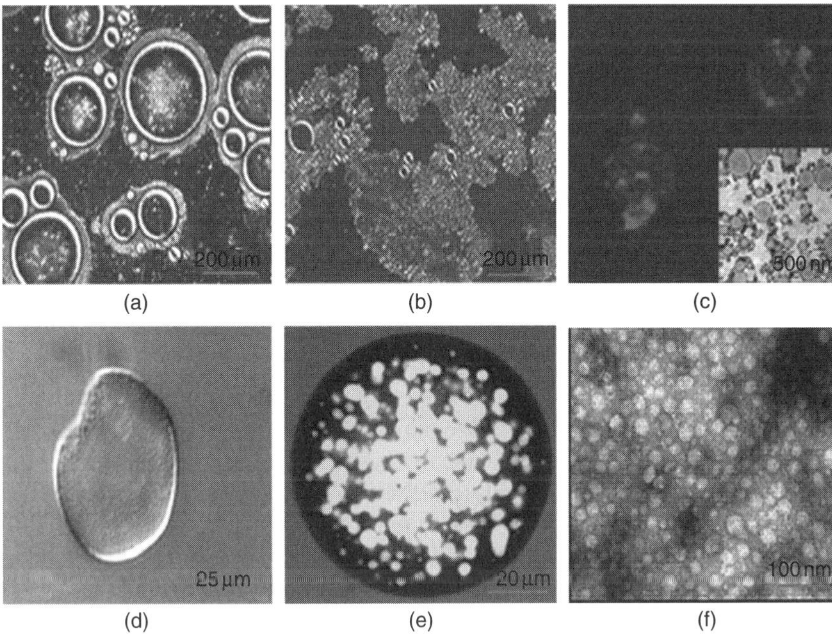

Fig. 22.1 Food protein-based micro/nanoparticle formulations for controlled nutraceutical delivery.

process of microencapsulation has several drawbacks, including a need for constant attention and the adjustment of stirring conditions, solution viscosity, pH and temperature. The process also often produces significant amount of agglomerated microcapsules. In the emulsification–gelation method, large amounts of oil are needed for extraction and for washing. Extrusion allows narrower size distributions in the final product. However, scale-up of this technique presents a challenge. Thus, there is a continuing need for improved methods of preparation of protein microparticles.

22.3.2 Formulation examples

Various food protein-based micro/nanoparticles have been developed, as illustrated in Fig. 22.1. Figure 22.1(a) depicts a typical protein-based microparticle prepared by complex coacervation of whey protein and gum arabic (Weinbreck *et al.*, 2004). From microscopic observations, large droplets (100–250 µm) were individually surrounded by a thin coacervate layer, whereas small droplets were encapsulated in a matrix of coacervate as shown. The encapsulation of large droplets requires the aggregation and the partial coalescence of a great amount of coacervate droplets. On the other hand, for encapsulation of small droplets, entrapment of the substance in one coacervate droplet is more likely to occur and requires less rearrangement than wetting and spreading, which involves a change of shape of the coacervate.

Figure 22.1(b) shows oil globules encapsulated in soy protein microparticles of 150 μm prepared by extrusion in a gelation bath containing $CaCl_2$ (Chen and Subirade, 2008b). The photomicrographs show uniform and homogeneous distribution of oil globules stabilized by a layer of soy protein aggregates in the gel networks. During the emulsification step, thermally pre-denatured soy proteins, acting as emulsifiers, rapidly adsorbed to the surface of the oil droplets. In the presence of calcium, the protein aggregated to create a stabilizing coating that protected the fine droplets against coalescence and provided physical stability to the emulsion. Increasing the $CaCl_2$ concentration led to a thicker protein aggregate layer, which should have ensured a more stable internal structure. In this work, retinal was incorporated inside as a model core material. In principle, any lipid or lipid-soluble nutraceuticals could be incorporated in these emulsion microparticles. In addition, the oil droplets stabilized in soy protein matrices have sizes of 200 nm. This submicron size may result in interesting properties, such as enhanced absorption in the small intestine leading to improved bioavailability compared to the traditional fish oil capsules available in the market.

Figure 22.1(c) shows the slightly granular aspect of the internal gel (50 μm), surrounded by a continuous, dense and rather thin membrane of protein–alginate composite covalently bound by a transacylation reaction (Levy and Edwards-Levy, 1996). The reaction involves the formation of amide bonds between protein and alginate, producing a membrane on the bead surface, which resists gastric pH and pepsin activity. This means that encapsulation in membrane-coated gel beads could be used to protect nutraceuticals during their transit through the gastrointestinal tract.

Figure 22.1(d) presents a fluorescent micrograph of alginate–whey protein granular microspheres prepared by an emulsification/internal cold gelation method (Chen and Subirade, 2005). The distribution of the whey protein microparticles, with diameters ranging from 3 to 10 μm, is homogeneous within the alginate matrix. Riboflavin crystals were homogeneously distributed in the whey protein microparticles, as revealed by optical microscopy. The advantage of this specific structure is that, in simulated gastric fluid (SGF), the alginate coating remained in a shrunken state due to conversion of sodium alginate to insoluble alginic acid, which acted as a barrier to whey protein microparticle degradation by pepsin, thereby retarding riboflavin release. When transferred to simulated intestinal fluid (SIF), the alginate matrix eroded, liberating the whey protein microparticles, which were then digested by pancreatin, followed by complete release of the riboflavin. This research has thus provided novel protein-based microparticles suitable as oral delivery vehicles for nutraceutical compounds.

Nanotechniques are a relatively new area of research. Owing to their subcellular size, nanoparticles offer a promising means of improving the bioavailability of nutraceutical compounds, especially poorly soluble substances such as functional lipids (e.g. carotenoids and phytosterols), natural antioxidants and numerous other compounds that are widely used as active ingredients in various food products. Nanoencapsulation can dramatically prolong compound residence time in the gastrointestinal tract by decreasing the influence of intestinal clearance mechanisms and increasing the surface available to interact with the biological support (Arbós *et al.*, 2002; Kawashim, 2001; Peppas, 1995). Nanoparticles can also penetrate deeply into tissues through fine capillaries, cross the epithelial lining fenestration (e.g. in the liver) and are generally taken up efficiently by cells (Desai *et al.*, 1996, 1997; Lamprecht *et al.*, 2004; Schäfer *et al.*, 1992), thus allowing efficient delivery of active compounds to target sites in the body.

Figure 22.1(e) demonstrates β-lactoglobulin (βlg) coated chitosan nanoparticles (around 100 nm), obtained by cold ionic gelation of chitosan and βlg mixtures (Chen and Subirade, 2005). Native βlg coated nanoparticles exhibited the desirable property of retarding molecule release into the gastric environment to some extent. A pepsin degradation assay revealed that the coating resists acid and pepsin, which may be attributed to the hydrophobic amino acids of native βlg being hidden inside its calyx-like globular structure, given that pepsin preferentially attacks peptide bonds involving hydrophobic aromatic amino acids. Under simulated intestinal conditions, the coatings were degraded by pancreatin. Owing to its muco-adhesive nature, the chitosan core should then adhere to the intestinal wall to facilitate the absorption of the nutraceutical compound. This study suggests that βlg, especially in its native configuration, is an interesting candidate for coating nanoparticles to protect carried nutrients from exposure to gastric fluids.

Recently, monodisperse suspensions of 40 nm whey protein nanospheres were prepared by modulating the parameters affecting the thermal aggregation process in the presence of the calcium (Leclerc *et al.*, 2005). The aggregation mechanism was investigated and the electrostatic interactions between protein and calcium, hydrophobic interactions between proteins, and the consolidation of the structure by intermolecular disulfide bonds were revealed to be involved in the nanosphere formation.

As demonstrated above, the excellent functional properties of food proteins allow them to be formulated into various structures from micro- to nano-size, alone or in combination with other natural polymers, providing opportunity to improve the stability of encapsulated nutraceuticals and release them in a controlled way at the site of action for food applications.

22.4 Protein structure, physical and biological behavior in gastrointestinal tract

A rational design of controlled release systems based on food proteins requires an understanding of their physical and biological behavior in the gastrointestinal tract in relation to protein molecular structures. Among the factors that modulate the release properties of protein matrices, swelling, degradation and bioadhesion play major roles.

22.4.1 Swelling

As amphoteric polyelectrolytes containing both cationic and anionic fixed charges, hydrophilic protein matrices show typical polyampholyte hydrogel characteristics, exhibiting swellability (volume change) in response to external conditions such as pH and ionic strength (Chen *et al.*, 2004). The swelling behavior of whey and soy protein microparticles was investigated at different pH conditions including simulated gastric (pH 1.9) and intestinal buffer (pH 7.5), as well as protein isoelectric point (pI). The pH of the medium has a significant effect on the degree of swelling of these microspheres. Swelling was at a minimum near the pI, and increased with pH decreasing to 1.2 or increasing to 7.4, suggesting that swelling behavior is mainly governed by the net charge of the protein molecules. Near the pI, the numbers of NH_3^+ and COO^- groups on the protein molecular chains are equal. Intraionic attraction between opposite charges seldom results in a residual ionic group. In the simulated gastric buffer, protein molecular chains are positively charged owing to protonated amino groups, while in the simulated intestinal buffer, protein molecular chains are negatively charged due to unprotonated carboxyl groups. Strong electrostatic repulsion among positive/negative charges at the surface of the gel microstructure allows water diffusion into the protein network (Chen and Subirade, 2007b). Whey protein microparticles formed by cold gelation are more swollen at intestinal pH than at gastric pH, because the amine groups in the hydrogel are fewer than the carboxyl groups and hence greater electrostatic repulsive forces (between COO^- groups) at pH 7.4 allow water to infiltrate the interchain spaces more easily.

pH-responsive polymeric networks have been extensively used for the development of controlled release formulations for oral administration. Highly swollen microparticles at pH 7.4 are favorable for nutraceutical release in the small intestine (Beaulieu *et al.*, 2002). In contrast, microspheres prepared by hydrophobic proteins such as zein and gliadin are generally not sensitive to pH changes and swell little in gastrointestinal buffers due to the hydrophobic characteristics of the network surface, which forms a strong barrier to prevent permeation of the gut fluids. Although research is still under way, these microparticles show promising abilities to carry nutraceuticals that are sensitive to stomach conditions with the presence of pepsin and low pH (Chen and Subirade, 2007b). The examples above demonstrate that swelling behavior of food protein microparticles in the gastrointestinal tact can be modulated by controlling the balance of free NH_3^+ and COO^- groups on the protein molecular chains and controlling the network surface hydrophobicity to design formulations for small intestine target release.

22.4.2 Degradation

Food proteins are digested by many different enzymes in the gastrointestinal tract. Pepsins are located in the stomach and trypsin, chymotrypsin and carboxypeptidases from the pancreas are located in the small intestinal lumen (Carino and Mathiowitz, 1999). Breakdown of the polymer matrix plays an important role in regulating core release. Therefore, development of protein micro/nanoparticles with controlled degradation, and, consequently, desirable release profiles of nutraceutical compounds to mimic their administration schedules, present a great challenge. The number of susceptible peptide bonds is likely important in determining the rate and extent of degradation. In the stomach, pepsin preferentially attacks peptide bonds involving hydrophobic aromatic amino acids (Chen and Subirade, 2005). β-Lactoglobulin apparently remains mostly intact after it passes through the stomach because of its globular structure with hydrophobic amino acids located in the internal core of its calyx-like structure and hydrophilic amino acids at the surface (Morr and Ha, 1993). Recent research demonstrated that denatured β-lactoglobulin can also prevent degradation by pepsin to some extent when adsorbed onto a hydrophobic surface (oil globules) in an end- on orientation with the hydrophilic charged groups located on the outside of the protein in contact with the gut fluids (Beaulieu *et al.*, 2002).

Accordingly, gastroresistant protein microparticles were prepared with oil droplets entrapped inside a whey protein matrix. Notably, these particles exhibited resistance to pepsin, but were completely degraded by pancreatin, leading to total release of the core compounds. Another example is the whey protein granules distributed in alginate microspheres as shown in Fig. 22.1(d), which showed a significant delay of degradation in the simulated stomach conditions in the presence of the pepsin. This delay can be attributed to two mechanisms. The first one is protection by the shrunken alginate matrix in stomach conditions, which created a barrier to penetration by the enzyme. The second one may be due to whey protein conformations in the special alginate/protein matrix–granule structures. In this structure, whey protein tends to form spherical structures with the hydrophobic side chains buried in the core of the sphere and the hydrophilic side chains facing the alginate matrix. Since pepsin preferentially attacks peptide bonds involving hydrophobic aromatic amino acids, these protein granules presented a less vulnerable substrate, resulting in slower degradation. As mentioned in Section 22.3.2, protein–alginate composite also produces a membrane on the protein microparticle surface, which resists gastric pH and pepsin activity to enable protection of nutraceuticals during their transit through the gastrointestinal tract.

These examples suggest that the degradation of protein-based micro/nanoparticles may be modulated by designing different protein conformations and/or complex formulations with other natural polymers to preserve gastric-sensitive bioactive molecules until delivery in the intestine, where they can be absorbed through the intestinal walls. Other factors such as particle size and network density can also significantly affect the degradation of the matrix of protein micro/nanoparticles. Larger particles are generally degraded slowly and over longer time periods due to smaller surface area/volume ratios.

Development of submicron particles in the range of several μm to nm may bring interesting new properties; however, these particles may suffer from quick degradation in the gut and lose their ability to protect the nutraceuticals incorporated inside. This problem may be overcome by cross-linking to develop a denser protein matrix which protects against proteolytic degradation by preventing the enzymes from penetrating into the particles.

22.4.3 Bioadhesion

Bioadhesion is classically defined in pharmaceutical science as the ability of a material to adhere to a biological substrate with the objective of improving the therapeutic efficiency of drugs by increasing the residence time at the site of activity or absorption (Park and Robinson, 1984; Peppas and Buri, 1985). The use of nanoparticles is of interest for bioadhesion purposes because these dosage forms have a large specific surface, which is indicative of a high interactive potential with biological surfaces. Traditionally, the bioadhesive properties of natural or synthetic polymers have principally been explained by hydrogen bonding, van der Waals, hydrophobic or ionic interactions. Owing to the abundant functional groups on food protein molecular chains, nanoparticles based on food proteins have a high chance of adhering to the gastrointestinal surface by developing various interactions with gut mucosa.

Arangoa *et al.* (2001) evaluated the bioadhesive activity of gliadin nanoparticles in rat small and large intestinal mucosa. The amount of adsorbed nanoparticles was estimated to be around 8 and 4 g/m in the small and large intestine, respectively. However, no significant differences in the extent of interaction were found among duodenum, jejunum and ileum. This high capacity of non-specific interactions with the mucosa may be explained by gliadin composition, which is rich in neutral and lipophilic residues that can promote hydrogen bonding and hydrophobic interactions with the small intestinal mucosa. In addition, by conjugating with lectin, a category of bioadhesive glycoproteins, the same nanoparticles showed 2 g/m absorbed nanoparticles in the small intestine and greater than 4 g/m in the caecum and distal colon, indicating a greater specificity for colonic mucosa (Ezpeleta *et al.*, 1999). This work demonstrated the high potential to develop food protein bioadhesive nanoformulations to improve bioavailability of nutraceuticals by prolonging the formulation residence time or increasing the nutrient absorption via reduction of the diffusion pathway or direct uptake of the nanoparticle carrier. The adhesive specificity of the food protein nanoparticles can also be improved by surface modifications. Nevertheless, food protein nanoformulation development is still in its infancy and it seems that other proteins have rarely been investigated as potential mucoadhesives.

22.4.4 Controlled release

The mechanisms of core compound release from a polymer matrix can be categorized into three main processes or systems (Arifin *et al.*, 2006): (1) diffusion from the non-degraded polymer (diffusion-controlled system); (2) enhanced drug diffusion due to polymer swelling (swelling-controlled system); (3) release by polymer degradation and erosion (erosion-controlled system). The release mechanism from protein micro/nanoparticles varies depending on the physicochemical properties of the protein matrix and the core nutraceutical compounds.

Rosenberg and co-workers (Lee and Rosenberg, 1999, 2000a; Satpathy and Rosenberg, 2003) systematically investigated hydrophilic core ingredient release from crosslinked whey protein microparticles and revealed that the release mechanism could be contributed to diffusion, matrix swelling or a combination of both. Figure 22.2(a) depicts that the release profile of core ingredient with limited water solubility can be divided into two linear segments that differ in their slope and a non-linear segment representing the final stages of core release (Satpathy and Rosenberg, 2003). The first linear segment represented the events during the time that was needed for swelling of the dry microparticles in the dissolution medium and involved release of 1–6% of the core. In this process, the protein matrix changed to a gel state upon interaction with the penetrant. The protein molecular chains in the gel state, being more mobile than those in the dry state, allow the active agent to diffuse out of the matrix more rapidly. The second linear segment represented the diffusion-governed events after the wall matrices have become fully hydrated and involved release of 85–97% of the core. Following hydration and swelling of the wall matrices, the core release fitted the Higuchi model. In all cases, a non-linear segment, where the Higuchi model was no longer valid, followed the two linear segments of the release profile. This segment represented the effects of the dissolution medium filling empty core domains via the diffusion mechanism that governed core release. At a comparable core load, the release rate of water soluble core ingredients was significantly quicker, indicating that the core ingredient solubility has a significant effect on the release. Within 1 h, almost 80% of the core ingredient was released from all the microparticles, regardless of the size and crosslinking degree (Lee and Rosenberg, 1999, 2000a). Conversely, the release rate of core materials with limited solubility was greatly influenced by a combined effect of particle size and crosslinking conditions. Complete core release from large (>700 μm), medium (500–700 μm) and small (<500 μm) microcapsules ranged from 28.6 to 81.2 h, from 16.8 to 28.6 h and from 7.2 to 15.9 h, respectively. The quicker release for small

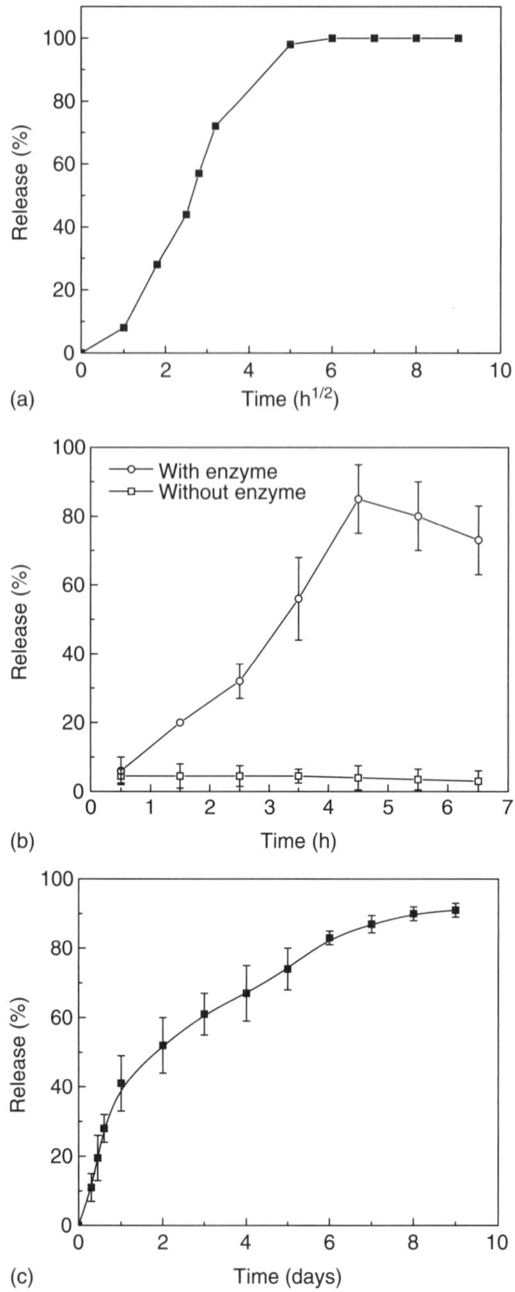

Fig. 22.2 (a) Higuchi plots depicting limited water-soluble core release from whey microcapsules (>700 μm). (b) Release of retinol from beads in the presence and in the absence of digestive enzyme. (c) *In vitro* release profile of IVM as a function of time from zein microspheres in PBS, pH 7.4, 37 °C.

particles can be attributed to their large surface area-to-volume ratio, which facilitated core ingredient diffusion. At a given particle size, higher crosslinking density resulted in a significantly slower core release rate, indicating crosslinking slowed down the rate of diffusion through the wall matrix.

In contrast, whey protein microparticles incorporating lipophilic nutrients did not show obvious core ingredient release in the gastrointestinal tract in the absence of digestive enzymes. Figure 22.2(b) demonstrates that the release of retinol from whey protein emulsion beads (1 mm) in solution is weak and only 5–10% of the incorporated retinol is released even after 6.5 h. However, in the presence of pancreatic enzymes, a progressive release of retinol from beads was observed. The release of retinol from whey protein beads was 75–95% in about 4.5 h. At the same time, a degradation assay confirmed the particle degradation in pancreatic media as observed by microscope. After 6 h, the particles were completely destroyed, leaving only lipid globules in the solution (Beaulieu *et al.*, 2002). This research suggests that lipophilic nutrient release from whey protein formulations is mainly due to the biodegradation of the protein shell matrices. The same release mechanism was observed for soy protein microparticles of 100 μm incorporating lipophilic vitamins according to our recent experimental data. Compared with protein beads of 1 mm, microparticles of 100 μm underwent a much more rapid degradation process. The protein matrix disappeared within 1–2 hours of the test in the simulated gastrointestinal tract, resulting in a quick retinol release. Thus, particle size is an important factor in the release of lipophilic ingredients from whey/soy protein formulations as well. However, in this case, the increased surface area-to-volume ratio promotes enzymatic attack instead of core diffusion.

The above examples showed release properties of hydrophilic protein formulations. Hydrophobic proteins, such as zein and gliadin, are another important category of food proteins that are candidates in developing delivery formulations (Liu *et al.*, 2005). Figure 22.2(c) showed the release of ivermectin (IVM) (water-soluble) from zein nanoparticles during the 9-day test. A biphasic release profile for IVM was observed. At the initial stage, the burst effect is attributed to the core ingredient entrapped near the surface of the microspheres, and this was followed by a very slow release stage. After 1 day, about 40% of the entrapped IVM was released, but the release rate tapered off in the subsequent 'slower' phase. About 90% of the entrapped IVM was released after 9 days. The slowing of the release rate probably represents the long diffusion route of IVM that was entrapped deeper in the zein matrix. Compared with whey protein matrices, the release rate of a hydrophilic ingredient was significantly lower from zein microparticles, suggesting that hydrophobicity of the protein material used for formulation plays a very important role in regulating core ingredient release rate. Hydrophilic protein networks such as whey and soy protein swell in the gastrointestinal tract owing to the abundance of polar amino acids, rendering the matrix more permeable to the release media. In the swollen network, when the nutraceutical is in an aqueous environment, its water solubility becomes an important consideration and compounds with appreciable water solubility will rapidly leach out. The significantly slower release rate of core ingredients from zein microparticles can be attributed to the hydrophobic nature of zein which contains many non-polar amino acids. Therefore, microparticles prepared from it have a highly hydrophobic surface which prevents penetration of the aqueous buffer, resulting in slower diffusion of the nutraceutical into the release medium. Microparticles formed by hydrophilic proteins alone have difficulty in achieving sustained release of hydrophilic nutrients, especially those in submicron formulations. When these systems absorb water and swell, core ingredients rapidly diffuse out. For a comparable size range, hydrophobic systems have the advantage of facilitating sustained drug release.

The examples above indicate that controlled release of nutraceuticals from food protein micro/nanoparticles relies on tailoring protein formulation structures with desirable release, medium permeation and enzymatic degradation properties. This can be achieved by careful design of proper formulation, particle size and crosslinking density. Thus, a systematic understanding of the relationship of food protein micro/nanoparticle structures and nutraceutical release properties presents a challenge for food scientists, which is essential for the development of efficient delivery systems and novel functional foods.

22.5 Food applications

22.5.1 Unsaturated fatty acids

There is a growing demand for polyunsaturated fatty acids (PUFA), particularly long chain omega-3 fatty acids, to be incorporated into foods because of their many health benefits relating to coronary heart disease, inflammatory and immune disorders, early childhood development and psychiatric disorders (De Deckere *et al.*, 1998). One of the major hurdles associated with the delivery of oils high in PUFA into food is the susceptibility of these oils to oxidative deterioration and the development of undesirable rancid odor and taste.

Microencapsulation provides a convenient approach to protect oils high in PUFA and make them more stable during processing and storage. This protection relies on the oxygen permeability of the wall matrix. Materials with pores small enough to exclude or resist the permeation of oxygen are favorable as a choice of microencapsulation (Kärger and Ruthven, 1992). Among food proteins, whey proteins have been shown to be good encapsulating materials for protecting omega-3 fatty acid against oxidation owing to their good oxygen barrier properties. Conjugated linoleic acid (CLA) as the free acid was microencapsulated using whey protein concentrate (WPC) as a wall material by Jimenez *et al.* (2004), involving an emulsification process followed by spray-drying. The stability of the microcapsules was affected by water activity and storage temperature. Microcapsules stored at water activity of 0.743 and 0.727 at 35 and 45 °C had very good stability against oxidation for at least 60 days. Augustin *et al.* (2006) proposed the use of Maillard reaction products (MRPs) obtained by the reaction at high temperature between protein and carbohydrate to encapsulate fish oil. The MRPs greatly reduced the susceptibility of the fish oil to oxidation at 35 °C for four weeks, compared with non-encapsulated spray dried samples in ordinary shell material (Augustin *et al.*, 2006). The prolamin powder systems also demonstrated interesting antioxidant effects against lipid deterioration (Iwami *et al.*, 1987; Kawase *et al.*, 1998). Experimental results revealed that gliadin, hordein and zein could inhibit the autoxidation of ethyl esters of linoleic, linolenic and arachidonic acids, i.e. with two to four unsaturated bonds. The antioxidative effect of the prolamins did not extend to PUFA with five or more unsaturated bonds. Only hordein effectively inhibited the oxidation of eicosapentaenoic acid ethyl ester from autoxidation in the powder system for 7 days. None of the prolamins completely inhibited the autoxidation of docosahexaenoic acid ethyl ester. A special spiral supersecondary structure and the ability of the whole molecule to take on a rod conformation may explain the good antioxidant properties of hordein, which forms a pocket to protect unsaturated fatty acid against oxidation.

22.5.2 Carotenoids

Carotenoids play an important potential role in human health by acting as biological antioxidants, protecting cells and tissues from the damaging effects of free radicals and singlet oxygen. However, because of the presence of unsaturated bonds in molecular structure, they are susceptible to oxidants, light and heat, and can easily deteriorate when exposed to such factors (Lee and Chen, 2002). Therefore, they generally need protection against damage in microcapsules. Lycopene is one kind of carotenoid found in ripe tomato, watermelon and pink grapefruit, giving these foods a characteristic red pigmentation. A great number of literature reports suggest that supplementation of food rich in lycopene is associated with a decreased risk of cardiovascular diseases and cancer (Clinton, 1998; Rao and Agarwal, 1999), and such foods are now desired by the public.

Lycopene has been successfully microencapsulated by spray-drying using a wall system consisting of gelatin and sucrose (Shu *et al.*, 2006). The storage stability of the microencapsulated lycopene was enhanced significantly compared with the free powders. After four weeks, 90% of the encapsulated lycopene still remained in its active form, while the lycopene in free powder was almost completely destroyed. This excellent protection capacity may be due to the ability of gelatin-based wall materials to effectively avoid the damage from oxygen and light during storage.

Chiu *et al.* (2007) further investigated the release profile of lycopene incorporated in gelatin/poly (γ-glutamic acid) (γ-PGA) microparticles of 39 μm. Fast release of lycopene in the powder occurred at pH 5.5 and 7.0, while no lycopene was released at pH 2.0 and 3.5, indicating that a low pH makes the core material difficult to release. This difficulty is likely due to the formation of a tight structure through an electrostatic interaction between gelatin and γ-PGA. In addition, the carboxyl groups of γ-PGA remain un-ionized at pH 2.0, and a tight α-helix structure would make γ-PGA less soluble in water. However, following a rise in pH, the α-helix structure can be extended to form a linear and more hydrophilic polyanionic structure, accounting for the fast release of lycopene from the encapsulated powder at high pH (5.5 and 7.0). From a physiological point of view, lycopene microcapsules could remain intact when passing through the stomach (pH 2.0–3.5), but would undergo fast release in the intestinal system (pH 5.5–7.0). These characteristics would enhance the bioavailability of lycopene by oral administration.

22.5.3 Microorganisms

Probiotics, defined as 'living microorganisms which, upon ingestion in certain numbers, exert health benefits beyond inherent general nutrition' (Guarner and Schaafsma, 1998) have become increasingly popular during the past decade. In most cases, bacteria must be viable at high concentrations when reaching the gut in order to confer the health benefits to the host. However, the survival of probiotics in food systems is often low under the harsh conditions of acidity and bile concentration commonly encountered in the gastrointestinal tract of humans (Berrada *et al.*, 1991; Lankaputhra & Shah, 1995). Moreover, many technological processes and storage conditions are detrimental to the viability of probiotics (Anal & Singh, 2007). Thus, there is interest in developing novel encapsulation systems that would improve the survival of probiotics during the processing and storage of functional foods as well as in gastrointestinal conditions.

Entrapping probiotic bacteria in whey protein beads (3 mm) crosslinked by Ca^{2+} was achieved by extrusion of the cell/protein mixture in a $CaCl_2$ solution. Scanning electron microscopy of beads before freeze-drying showed a tight protein network containing encapsulated *Lactobacillus rhamnosus* cells homogeneously distributed throughout the matrix. A study of the viability of microentrapped cells in a dynamic gastrointestinal model showed that the protein matrix provided protection against acidic conditions in the stomach after 90 min, as well as against bile after 30, 60 and 90 min in the duodenum. These results suggest that the whey protein beads can protect the cells against adverse conditions of the gastrointestinal system (Reid *et al.*, 2005). *Bifidobacterium breve* and *Bifidobacterium longum* were also encapsulated as freeze-dried powders or fresh cultures in whey protein microparticles (3–75 μm) produced by emulsion and/or spray-drying (Picot and Lacroix, 2004). Dispersion of fresh cells in a heat-treated whey protein suspension followed by spray-drying was the least destructive immobilization technique tested, with a survival rate of 25.7% and 1.4% for *Bifidobacterium breve* and *Bifidobacterium longum*, respectively. Viable counts of *Bifidobacterium breve* cells entrapped in whey protein microcapsules were significantly higher than those of free cells after 28 days in yoghurt stored at 4 °C (+2.6 log cycles), and after sequential exposure to simulated gastric and intestinal juices (+2.7 log cycles). In contrast, no protective effect of encapsulation was observed with *Bifidobacterium longum*.

Reid *et al.* (2007) investigated the effect of whey protein microencapsulation on the viability of *Lactobacillus rhamnosus* during the production and storage of biscuits, frozen fruit and vegetable juice. The results demonstrated that whey protein microencapsulation can be useful in protecting cells during a short heat treatment. Although this encapsulation delayed mortality of cells, possibly by limiting their rehydration, water activity in biscuits was too high to allow stable viability during storage at room temperature in the presence of oxygen. In addition, the encapsulated cells could be added to vegetable juice since they maintained high viability after a two-week storage period. These findings demonstrated that the immobilization of probiotic cultures in whey protein-based microcapsules can increase cell survival when subjected to extreme conditions, making this approach potentially useful for delivery of viable bacteria to the gastrointestinal tract of humans via fermented dairy and other food products. However, the particle-forming steps such as calcium gelation and spray-drying still need to be optimized, in order to limit the mortality of the cells. In addition, the probiotic strain chosen for microencapsulation should be taken into consideration for functional food development.

22.5.4 Immunoglobulin

There has been considerable interest in recent years in using orally administered immunoglobulins as a means of providing immunization. However, during oral administration, immunoglobulins are subject to denaturation at gastric pH levels and digestion by pepsin in the human stomach, resulting in reduced antibody activities. To preserve the therapeutic potential of immunoglobulins, consideration of the stability of immunoglobulin during storage and processing and upon ingestion is important (Chen *et al.*, 1999). Emulsification-heat gelation was used for preparation of whey protein–based microcapsules containing immunoglobulin in yolk IgY (Cho *et al.*, 2005). The residual activity of IgY during the emulsion preparation and the effects of microencapsulation on IgY stability under harsh conditions were investigated. Microencapsulated IgY showed remarkable stability against both pepsin and acid owing to the good barrier properties of whey protein, which prevented contact between IgY and the artificial gastric juice and pepsin solution.

Thermal treatment, including pasteurization, sterilization, evaporation concentration and spray-drying, are often performed during food processing. Thus, effects of thermal processing and storage conditions on the residual activity of microencapsulated IgY have been investigated for application in food industry. The residual activity of IgY after heating at 70 °C remained stable. Thus, microencapsulated IgY can be used for sterile processes in food processing. The residual activity of IgY was monitored over a four-week period under different storage temperatures. There was no difference in the residual activity of microencapsulated IgY at 4, 25 and 37 °C. In addition, microencapsulated IgY showed good storage stability under different temperatures for four weeks of storage and was superior to non-encapsulated IgY under similar conditions.

22.6 Conclusion and future trends

Food proteins are promising new GRAS materials for food applications owing to their excellent functional properties and their acceptability as naturally occurring food components, which are degradable by digestive enzymes. This chapter has described the potential of engineering food proteins into various formulations at micro/nano-scale for stabilization of nutraceuticals and releasing them in a controlled fashion to a targeted site. The aim of making these formulations is to develop novel functional foods that can effectively and efficiently deliver beneficial nutrients in their active form. To date, most systems that have been investigated consist of one nutraceutical compound. Functional food systems are much more complex, consisting of mixtures of nutraceutical components. Thus, further research on these complex systems is becoming increasingly important. Another area that is likely to see intense research activity in the future is enhancing the absorption and bioavailability of nutraceuticals. Food protein nanoparticles are a promising technology that can increase the apparent solubility of the active ingredient, prolong the retention time in the small intestine, or even be directly uptaken by the mucosa cells. Formation of nanoparticles can be achieved by self-assembly of the proteins into tailored nanostructures with desirable properties and high surface area. Finally, rational design of food protein micro/nanoparticles as nutraceutical delivery systems relies on a fundamental understanding of the relationship between the structures of food protein formulations and their functional properties. Further experiments are required to understand protein–protein and protein–nutrient interactions at the molecular level, their impact on microscopic features of the resulting micro/nanoparticles, and their capacity to stabilize and target release nutraceuticals. Successful development of versatile protein-based encapsulation systems will lead to greater application in the food industry.

22.7 Acknowledgement

This work was funded by Alberta Crop Industry Development Fund Inc. (ACIDF) and Alberta Barley Commission.

22.8 References

AGUILERA JM (1995), 'Gelation of whey proteins' *Food Tech.*, **49**, 83–89.

ANAL AK, SINGH H (2007), 'Recent advances in microencapsulation of probiotics for industrial applications and targeted delivery' *Trends Food Sci. Technol.*, **18**, 240–251.

ARANGOA MA, CAMPANERO MA, RENEDO MJ, PONCHEL G, IRACHE JM (2001), 'Gliadin nanoparticles as carriers for the oral administration of lipophilic drugs. Relationships between bioadhesion and pharmacokinetics' *Pharm. Res.*, **18**, 1521–1527.

ARBÓS P, ARANGOA MA, CAMPANERO MA, IRACHE JM (2002), 'Quantification of the bioadhesive properties of protein-coated PVM/MA nanoparticles' *Int. J. Pharm.*, **242**, 129–136.

ARIFIN DY, LEE LY, WANG CH (2006), 'Mathematical modeling and simulation of drug release from microspheres: implications to drug delivery systems' *Adv. Drug Deliv. Rev.*, **58**, 1274–1325.

ARNEDO A, ESPUELAS S, IRACHE JM (2002), 'Albumin nanoparticles as carriers for a phosphodiester oligonucleotide' *Int. J. Pharm.*, **244**, 59–72.

AUGUSTIN MA (2003), 'The role of microencapsulation in the development of functional dairy foods' *Aust. J. Dairy Tech.*, **58**(2), 156–160.

AUGUSTIN MA, SANGUANSRI L, BODE O (2006), 'Maillard reaction products as encapsulants for fish oil powders' *J. Food Sci.*, **71**, 25–32.

BAE EK, LEE SJ (2008), 'Microencapsulation of avocado oil by spray drying using whey protein and maltodextrin' *J. Microencapsul.*, **6**, 1–12.

BAISIER W, REINECCIUS GA (1989), 'Spray drying of food flavors. V: factors influencing shelf-life of encapsulated orange peel oil' *Perfum. Flavor*, **14**, 48–50, 52–43.

BARANAUSKIENE R, VENSKUTONIS PR, DEWETTINCK K, VERHE R (2006), 'Properties of oregano (*Origanum vulgare* L.), citronella (*Cymbopogon nardus* G.) and marjoram (*Majorana hortensis* L.) flavors encapsulated into milk protein-based matrices' *Food Res. Int.*, **39**, 413–425.

BARBUT S, FOEGEDING EA (1993), 'Ca^{2+}-induced gelation of pre-heated whey protein isolate' *J. Food Sci.*, **58**, 867–871.

BEAULIEU L, SAVOIE L, PAQUIN P, SUBIRADE M (2002), 'Elaboration and characterization of whey protein beads by an emulsification/cold gelation process: application for the protection of retinol' *Biomacromolecules*, **3**, 2239–2248.

BELL LN (2001), 'Stability testing of nutraceuticals and functional foods' *Handbook of Nutraceuticals and Functional Foods*, Wildman REC, ed (pp. 501–516). New York: CRC Press.

BENICHOU A, ASERIN A, GARTI N (2002), 'Protein–polysaccharide interactions for stabilization of food emulsions' *Disp. Sci. Tech.*, **23**, 93–123.

BERRADA N, LEMELAND JF, LAROCHE G, THOUVENOT P, PIAIA M (1991), '*Bifidobacterium* from fermented milks: survival during gastric transit' *J. Dairy Sci.*, **74**, 409–413.

BRYANT CM, MCCLEMENTS DJ (1998), 'Molecular basis of protein functionality with special consideration of cold-set gels derived from heat-denatured whey' *Trends Food Sci. Technol.*, **9**, 143–151.

CARINO GP, MATHIOWITZ E (1999), 'Oral insulin delivery' *Adv. Drug Deliv. Rev.*, **35**, 249–257.

CHAMPAGNE CP, FUSTIER P (2007), 'Microencapsulation for the improved delivery of bioactive compounds into foods' *Curr. Opin. Biotechnol.*, **18**, 184–190.

CHEN CC, TU YY, CHANG HM (1999), 'Efficiency and protective effect of encapsulation of milk immunoglobulin G in multiple emulsion' *J. Agric. Food Chem.*, **47**, 407–410.

CHEN L, SUBIRADE M (2005), 'Chitosan/β-lactoglobulin coreshell nanoparticles as nutraceutical carriers' *Biomaterials*, **26**, 6041–6953.

CHEN L, SUBIRADE M (2006), 'Alginate–whey protein granular microspheres as oral delivery vehicles for bioactive compounds' *Biomaterials*, **27**, 4646–4654.

CHEN L, SUBIRADE M (2007a), 'Effect of preparation conditions on the nutrient release properties of alginate/whey protein granular microspheres' *Eur. J. Pharm. Biopharm.*, **65**, 354–362.

CHEN L, SUBIRADE M (2007b), 'Microspheres based on soy, zein protein as oral delivery vehicles I. Microsphere fabrication, characterization and dissolution properties' 34th conference in Controlled Release Society, 7–14 July, California, USA.

CHEN L, SUBIRADE M (2008), 'Kinetics of the breakdown of cross-linked soy protein films for drug delivery' *Biomaterials*, **29**, 3750–3756.

CHEN L, SUBIRADE M (2009), 'Calcium crosslinked soy microspheres for nutraceutical delivery carriers' *American Chemistry Society Symposium series*, in press.

CHEN L, TIAN Z, DU Y (2004), 'Synthesis and pH sensitivity of carboxymethyl chitosan based polyampholyte hydrogels for protein carrier matrices' *Biomaterials*, **25**, 3725–3732.

CHEN L, REMONDETTO G, SUBIRADE M (2006), 'Food protein-based materials as nutraceutical delivery systems' *Trends Food Sci. Technol.*, **17**, 272–283.

CHIU YT, CHIU CP, CHIEN JT, HO GH, YANG J, CHEN BH (2007), 'Encapsulation of lycopene extract from tomato pulp waste with gelatin and poly(γ-glutamic acid) as carrier' *J. Agric. Food Chem.*, **55**, 5123–5130.

CHO YH, SHIM HK, PARK J (2003), 'Encapsulation of fish oil by an enzymatic gelation process using transglutaminase cross-linked proteins' *J. Food Sci.*, **68**, 2717–2723.

CHO YH, LEE JJ, PARK IB, HUH CS, BAEK YJ, PARK JY (2005), 'Protective effect of microencapsulation consisting of multiple emulsification and heat gelation processes on immunoglobulin in yolk' *J. Food Sci.*, **70**, 148–151.

CLARK AH (1998), 'Gelation of globular proteins' *Functional Properties of Food Macromolecules*, Hill SE, Leward DA, Mitchell JR, eds. Gaithersburg, MD: Aspen.

CLINTON SK (1998), 'Lycopene: chemistry, biology, and implications for human health and disease' *Nutr. Rev.*, **56**, 35–51.

DECKERE EAM, KORVER O, VERSCHUREN PM, KATAN MB (1998), 'Health aspects of fish and n-3 polyunsaturated fatty acids from plant and marine origin' *Eur. J. Clin. Nutr.*, **52**, 749–753.

DE KRUIF CG, WEINBRECKA F, VRIES R (2004), 'Complex coacervation of proteins and anionic polysaccharides' *Curr. Opin. Colloid Interface Sci.*, **9**, 340–349.

DE WOLF FA, BRETT GM (2000), 'Ligand-binding proteins: their potential for application in systems for controlled delivery and uptake of ligands' *Pharm. Rev.*, **52**, 207–236.

DESAI KGH, PARK HJ (2005), 'Recent developments in microencapsulation of food ingredients' *Drying Tech*, **23**, 1361–1394.

DESAI MP, LABHASETWAR V, AMIDON GL, LEVY RJ (1996), 'Gastrointestinal uptake of biodegradable microparticles: effect of particle size' *Pharm. Res.*, **13**, 1838–1845.

DESAI MP, LABHASETWAR V, WALTER E, LEVY RJ, AMIDON GL (1997), 'The mechanism of uptake of biodegradable microparticles in Caco-2 cells is size dependent' *Pharm. Res.*, **14**, 1568–1573.

DICKINSON E (2003), 'Colloidal aggregation: Mechanism and implications' *Food Colloids, Biopolymers and Materials*, Dickinson E, Vlie T van, eds. (pp. 68–83). Cambridge: Royal Society of Chemistry.

DICKINSON E, CHEN J (1999), 'Heat-set whey protein emulsion gels: role of active and inactive filler particles' *J. Dispersion Sci. Tech.*, **20**, 197–213.

DICKINSON E, HONG S T, YAMAMOTO Y (1996), 'Rheology of heat-set emulsion gels containing β-lactoglobulin and small-molecule surfactants' *Netherlands Milk Dairy J.*, **50**, 199–207.

DI SILVIO L, GURAV N, KAYSER MV, BRADEN M, DOWNES S (1994), 'Biodegradable microspheres: a new delivery system for growth hormone' *Biomaterials*, **15**, 931–936.

DUCLAIROIR C, ORECCHIONI AM, DEPRAETERE P, OSTERSTOCK F, NAKACHE E (2003), 'Evaluation of gliadin nanoparticles as drug delivery systems: a study of three different drugs, *Int. J. Pharm.*, **2003**, 133–144.

DUFOUR E, HAERTLÉ T (1990), 'Binding affinities of β-ionone and related flavor compounds to β-lactoglobulin: effects of chemical modifications' *J. Agric. Food Chem.*, **38**, 1691–1695.

ELLIOTT R, ONG TJ (2002), 'Science, medicine, and the future nutritional genomics' *British Medical J.*, **324**, 1438–1442.

EZPELETA I, ARANGOA MA, IRACHE JM, STAINMESSE S, CHABENAT C, POPINEAU Y, ORECCHIONI AM (1999), 'Preparation of *Ulex europaeus* lectin–gliadin nanoparticle conjugates and their interaction with gastrointestinal mucus' *Int. J. Pharm.*, **191**, 25–32.

FRANZ J, POKOROVA D, HAMPL J, DITTRICH M (1998), 'Adjuvant efficacy of gelatine particles and microparticles' *Int. J. Pharm*, **168**, 153–161.

FUTTERMAN S, HELLER J (1972), 'The enhancement of fluorescence and the decreased susceptibility to enzymatic oxidation of retinol complexed with bovine serum albumin, β-lactoglobulin, and the retinol-binding protein of human plasma' *J. Biol. Chem.*, **247**, 5168–5172.

GAN CY, CHENG LH, EASA AM (2008), 'Evaluation of microbial transglutaminase and ribose cross-linked soy protein isolate-based microcapsules containing fish oil' *Innovat. Food Sci. Emerg. Technol.*, **9**, 563–569.

GHARSALLAOUI A, ROUDAUT G, CHAMBIN O, VOILLEY A, SAUREL R (2007), 'Applications of spray-drying in microencapsulation of food ingredients: an overview' *Food Res. Int*, **40**, 1107–1121.

GOUIN S (2004), 'Microencapsulation: industrial appraisal of existing technologies and trends' *Trends Food Sci. Technol.*, **15**, 330–347.

GUARNER F, SCHAAFSMA GJ (1998), 'Probiotics' *Int. J. Food Microbiology*, **39**, 237–238.

GUILBERT S, GONTARD N, MOREL MH, CHALIER P, MICARD V, REDL A (2002), 'Formation and properties of wheat gluten films and coatings' *Protein-based Films and Coatings*, Gennadios A, ed. (pp. 1–42). Boca Raton, FL: CRC Press.

GUNASEKARAN S, KO S, XIAO L (2007), 'Use of whey proteins for encapsulation and controlled delivery applications' *J. Food Eng.*, **83**, 31–40.

HEELAN BA, CORRIGAN OI (1998), 'Preparation and evaluation of microspheres prepared from whey protein isolate' *J. Microencapsul.*, **15**, 93–105.

HEINZELMANN K, FRANKE K, JENSEN B, HAAHR AM (2000), 'Protection of fish oil from oxidation by microencapsulation using freeze-drying techniques' *Eur. J. Lipid Sci. Technol.*, **102**, 114–121.

IWAMI K, HATTORI M, NAKATANI S, IBUKI F (1987), 'Spray-dried gliadin powders inclusive of linoleic acid (microcapsules): their preservability, digestibility and application to bread making' *Agric. Biol. Chem.*, **51**, 3301–3307.

JIMENEZ M, GARC HS, BERISTAIN CI (2004), 'Spray-drying microencapsulation and oxidative stability of conjugated linoleic acid' *Eur. Food Res. Technol.*, **219**, 588–592.

JOST R, BAECHLER R, MASSON G (1986), 'Heat gelation of oil-in-water emulsions stabilized by whey protein' *J. Food Sci.*, **51**, 440–444.

JOST R, DANNENBERG F, ROSSET J (1989), 'Heat-set gels based on oil/water emulsions: an application of whey protein functionality' *Food Microstructure*, **8**, 23–28.

KAGAMI Y, SUGIMURA S, FUJISHIMA N, MATSUDA K, KOMETANI T, MATSUMURA Y (2003), 'Oxidative stability, structure, and physical characteristics of microcapsules formed by spray drying of fish oil with protein and dextrin wall materials' *J. Food Sci.*, **7**, 2248–2255.

KÄRGER J, RUTHVEN DM (1992), *Diffusion in Zeolites and other Microporous Solids*, (pp. 1–20), New York: Wiley-Interscience.

KAWASE S, MATSUMURA Y, MURAKAMI H, MORI T (1998), 'Comparison of antioxidative activity among three types of prolamin subunits' *J. Cereal Sci.*, **28**, 33–41.

KAWASHIM Y (2001), 'Nanoparticulate systems for improved drug delivery' *Adv. Drug Delivery Rev.*, **47**, 1–2.

KEOGH MK, O'KENNEDY BT (1999), 'Milk fat microencapsulation using whey proteins' *Int. Dairy J.*, **9**, 657–663.

KEOGH MK, O'KENNEDY BT, KELLY J, AUTY MA, KELLY PM, FUREBY A, HAAHR AM (2001), 'Stability to oxidation of spray-dried fish oil powder microencapsulated using milk ingredients' *J. Food Sci.*, **66**, 217–224.

KIM YD, MORR CV, SCHENZ TW (1996), 'Microencapsulation properties of gum arabic and several food proteins: liquid orange oil emulsion particles' *J. Agric. Food Chem.*, **44**, 1308–1313.

KROCHTA JM (2002), 'Proteins as raw materials for films and coatings: definitions, current status, and opportunities' *Protein-based Films and Coatings*, Gennadios A, eds. (pp. 1–42). Boca Raton, FL: CRC Press.

LAMPRECHT A, SAUMET JL, ROUX J, BENOIT JP (2004), 'Lipid nanocarriers as drug delivery system for ibuprofen in pain treatment' *Int. J. Pharm.*, **278**, 407–414.

LANGER R, PEPPAS NA (2003), 'Advances in biomaterials, drug delivery, and bionanotechnology' *AIChE J*, **49**, 2990–3006.

LANKAPUTHRA WEV, SHAH NP (1995), 'Survival of *Lactobacillus acidophilus* and *Bifidobacterium* spp. in the presence of acid and bile salts' *Cultured Dairy Products J.*, **30**, 2–7.

LAVOIE C, REMONDETTO GE, ANGERS P, SUBIRADE M (2005), 'Encapsulation of omega-3 fatty acids in a protein matrix: characterization and protective effect study' in XIIth International Workshop on Bioencapsulation, Kingston, 24–26 June.

LECLERC PL, REMONDETTO GE, RAMASSAMY C, SUBIRADE M (2005), 'Whey protein nanospheres as drug carriers for oral administration' In XIIth International Workshop on Bioencapsulation, Kingston, 24–26 June.

LEE MT, CHEN BH (2002), 'Stability of lycopene during heating and illumination in a model system' *Food Chem.*, **78**, 425–432.

LEE SJ, ROSENBERG M (1999), 'Preparation and properties of glutaraldehyde cross-linked whey protein-based microcapsules containing theophylline' *J. Control. Release*, **61**, 123–136.

LEE SJ, ROSENBERG M (2000a), 'Microencapsulation of theophylline in whey proteins: effects of core-to-wall ratio' *Int. J. Pharm.*, **205**, 147–158.

LEE SJ, ROSENBERG M (2000b), 'Whey protein-based microcapsules prepared by double emulsification and heat gelation' *Lebensmittel-Wissenschaft and Technologic,* **33**, 80–88.

LEFEAVRE T, SUBIRADE M (2003), 'Formation of intermolecular β-sheet structures: a phenomenon relevant to protein film structure at oil/water interfaces of emulsions' *J. Colloid Interface Sci.*, **263**, 59–67.

LEUNG SLV, REMONDETTO GE, SUBIRADE M (2005), 'Controlled release of α-tocopherol from cold-set β-lactoglobulin emulsion gels' in XIIth International Workshop on Bioencapsulation, Kingston, 24–26 June, 87–89.

LEVY MC, EDWARDS-LEVY F (1996), 'Coating alginate beads with cross-linked biopolymers: A novel method based on a transacylation reaction' *J. Microencapsul.*, **13**, 169–183.

LIU X, SUN Q, WANG H, ZHANG L, WAN J (2005), 'Microspheres of corn protein, zein, for an ivermectin drug delivery system' *Biomaterials*, **26**, 109–115.

MALTAIS A, REMONDETTO GE, GONZALES R, SUBIRADE M (2005), 'Formation of soy protein isolate cold-set gels: protein and salt effects' *J. Food Sci.*, **70**, 67–73.

MAUGUET MC, LEGRAND J, BRUJES L, CARNELLE G, LARRE C, POPINEAU Y (2002), 'Gliadin matrices for microencapsulation processes by simple coacervation method' *J. Microencapsul.*, **19**, 377–384.

MCCLEMENTS D J, MONAHAN F J, KINSELLA J E (1993), 'Effect of emulsion droplets on the rheology of whey protein isolate gels' *J. Texture Stud.*, **24**, 411–422.

MEANS GE, FEENEY RE (1998), 'Chemical modifications of proteins: a review' *J. Food Biochem.*, **22**, 399–426.

MOREAU DL, ROSENBERG M (1996), 'Oxidative stability of anhydrous milkfat microencapsulated in whey proteins' *J. Food Sci.*, **61**, 39–43.

MORR CV, HA EYW (1993) 'Whey protein concentrates and isolates: processing and functional properties' *Food Sci. Nutr.*, **33**, 431–476.

MORRISETT JD, POWNALL HJ, GOTTO AMG (1975), 'Bovine serum albumin: study of the fatty acid and steroid binding sites using spin-labelled lipids' *J. Biol. Chem.*, **250**, 2487–2494.

MUTHUSELVI L, DHATHATHREYAN A (2006), 'Simple coacervates of zein to encapsulate gioxin' *Colloids Surf. B: Biointerfaces*, **51**, 39–43.

O'NEILL T, KINSELLA JE (1988), 'Effect of heat treatment and modification on conformation and flavor binding by β-lactoglobulin' *J. Food Sci.*, **53**, 906–909.

PADUA GW, WANG Q (2002), 'Formation and properties of corn zein films and coatings' *Protein-based Films and Coatings*, Gennadios A, eds. (pp. 1–42). Boca Raton, FL: CRC Press.

PARK K, ROBINSON JR (1984), 'Bioadhesive polymers as platforms for oral-controlled drug delivery: method to study bioadhesion' *Int. J. Pharm.*, **19**, 107–127.

PARK SK, HETTIARACHCHY NS, JU ZY, GENNADIOS A (2002), 'Formation and properties of soy protein films and coatings' *Protein-based Films and Coatings*, Gennadios A, eds. (pp. 1–42). Boca Raton, FL: CRC Press.

PEPPAS LB (1995), 'Recent advances on the use of biodegradable microparticles and nanoparticles in controlled drug delivery' *Int. J. Pharm.*, **116**, 1–9.

PEPPAS NA, BURI PA (1985), 'Surface, interfacial and molecular aspects of polymer bioadhesion on soft tissues' *J. Control. Release*, **2**, 257–275.

PEPPAS NA, BURES R, LEOBANDUNG W, ICHIKAWA H (2000), 'Hydrogels in pharmaceutical formulations' *Europ. J. Pharm. Biopharm*, **50**, 27–46.

PEREZ MD, CALVO M (1995), 'Interaction of β-lactoglobulin with retinol and fatty acids and its role as a possible biological function for this protein: a review' *J. Dairy Sci.*, **78**, 918–988.

PEREZ MD, DIAZ DE VILLEGAS MC, SANCHEZ L, ARANDA P, ENA JM, CALVO M (1989), 'Interaction of fatty acids with β-lactoglobulin and albumin from ruminant milk' *J. Biochem.*, **106**, 1094–1097.

PHILLIPS LG, WHITEHEAD DM, KINSELLA JE (1994), *Structure–Function Properties of Food Proteins*, San Diego, CA: Academic Press.

PICOT A, LACROIX C (2003), 'Production of multiphase water-insoluble microcapsules for cell microencapsulation using an emulsification/spray-drying technology' *J. Food Sci.*, **68**, 2693–2700.

PICOT A, LACROIX C (2004), 'Encapsulation of bifidobacteria in whey protein-based microcapsules and survival in simulated gastrointestinal conditions and in yoghurt' *Int. Dairy J.*, **14**, 505–515.

RAO AV, AGARWAL S (1999), 'Role of lycopene as antioxidant carotenoid in the prevention of chronic diseases: a review' *Nutr. Res.*, **19**, 305–323.

REID AA, VUILLEMARD JC, BRITTEN M, ARCAND Y, FARNWORTH E, CHAMPAGNE CP (2005), 'Microentrapment of probiotic bacteria in a Ca^{2+}-induced whey protein gel and effects on their viability in a dynamic gastro-intestinal model' *J. Microencapsul.*, **22**, 603–619.

REID AA, CHAMPAGNE CP, GARDNER N, FUSTIER P, VUILLEMARD JC (2007), 'Survival in food systems of *Lactobacillus rhamnosus* R011 microentrapped in whey protein gel particles' *J. Food Sci.*, **72**, 31–37.

ROBILLARD KA, WISHNIA A (1972), 'Aromatic hydrophobes and β-lactoglobulin A. Thermodynamics of binding' *Biochemistry*, **11**, 3835–3840.

SATPATHY G, ROSENBERG M (2003), 'Encapsulation of chlorothiazide in whey proteins: effects of wall-to-core ratio and cross-linking conditions on microcapsule properties and drug release' *J. Microencapsul.*, **20**, 227–245.

SCHÄFER V, VON BRIESEN H, ANDREESEN R, STEFFAN AM, ROYER C, TROSTER S (1992), 'Phagocytosis of nanoparticles by human immunodeficiency virus (HIV)-infected macrophages: a possibility for antiviral drug targeting' *Pharm. Res.*, **9**, 541–546.

SHEU TY, ROSENBERG M (1995), 'Microencapsulation by spray drying ethyl caprylate in whey protein and carbohydrate wall systems' *J. Food Sci.*, **60**, 98–103.

SHEU TY, ROSENBERG M (1998), 'Microstructure of microcapsules consisting of whey proteins and carbohydrates' *J. Food Sci.*, **63**, 491–494.

SHU B, YU W, ZHAO Y, LIU X (2006), 'Study on microencapsulation of lycopene by spray-drying' *J. Food Eng.*, **76**, 664–669.

SPECTOR AA (1975), 'Fatty acid binding to plasma albumin' *J. Lipid Res.*, **16**, 165–179.

SPECTOR AA, FLETCHER JE (1970), 'Binding of long-chain fatty acids to β-lactoglobulin' *Lipids*, **5**, 403–411.

TURGEON SL, BEAULIEU M, SCHMITT C, SANCHEZ C (2003), 'Protein–polysaccharide interactions: phase-ordering kinetics, thermodynamic and structural aspects' *Curr. Opin. Colloid Interface Sci.*, **8**, 401–414.

TWOMEY M, KEOGH MK, MEHRA R, O'KENNEDY (1997), 'Gel characteristics of β-lactoglobulin, whey protein concentrate and whey protein isolate' *J. Texture Studies*, **28**, 387–403.

USHA RP, GUSTAVO VBG (1995), 'Fundamental aspects of controlled release in foods' *Trends. Food Sci. Technol.*, **61**, 397–406.

WALSTRA P (2003), 'Studying food colloids: past, present and future' *Food Colloids, Biopolymers and Materials,* Dickinson E, Vlie T van, eds. (pp. 68–83). Cambridge: Royal Society of Chemistry.

WANG Q, ALLEN JC, SWAISGOOD HE (1997), 'Binding of vitamin D and cholesterol to β-lactoglobulin' *J. Dairy Sci.*, **80**, 1054–1059.

WEBER C, COESTER C, KREUTER J, LANGER K (2000), 'Desolvation process and surface characterisation of protein nanoparticles' *Int. J. Pharm.*, **194**, 91–102.

WEINBRECK F, MINOR M, DE KRUIF CG (2004), 'Microencapsulation of oils using whey protein/gum arabic coacervates' *J. Microencapsul.*, **21**, 667–679.

WILDMAN REC, ED (2001), *Handbook of Nutraceuticals and Functional Foods*. New York: CRC Press.

YOUNG SL, SARDA X, ROSENBERG M (1993), 'Microencapsulating properties of whey proteins. 2. Combination of whey proteins with carbohydrates' *J. Dairy Sci.*, **76**, 2878–2885.

ZIEGLER GR, FOEGEDING EA (1990), 'The gelation of proteins' *Adv. Food Nutr. Res.*, **34**, 203–298.

23

Self-assembling structures in the gastrointestinal tract

T. J. Foster, University of Nottingham, UK; and I. T. Norton, University of Birmingham, UK

Abstract: This chapter introduces the concept of microstructure self-assembly during the digestive process. It extends the thinking of food microstructure, moving on from its creation, by design, and how it is deconstructed upon consumption. New thinking is introduced, highlighting how microstructure conceptualisation might throw fresh light on how food is ultimately digested and taken up by the body. It begins to bridge the gap between the structure of food as consumed and the importance of food structures in the gastrointestinal tract, for optimal uptake of nutrients and how they respond to and even influence physiological processes. To introduce such thoughts, the effects of physiological triggers (e.g. enzyme action, pH and temperature jumps, dilution/concentration and how food interacts with bodily surfaces and fluids) are considered and reviewed as to how they might affect the fat and water structures that make up food microstructure. The impact on the incorporation of these concepts into food products, as well as how they fit with future food trends is also discussed.

Key words: self-assembly, biopolymers, microstructure, emulsions, viscosity, gelation, digestion, satiety, food products.

23.1 Introduction

The area of self-assembling structures in the gastrointestinal tract (GI) is of hot scientific interest, in which the students of food science are coming face to face with biophysicists, human physiologists, gastroenterologists, physicists and pharmacists as it emerges as a key approach for the future design of food functionality. In the past the focus has been on the production and stability of food structures, with the requirement for optimising (often at lowest cost) the process and ingredient usage. This was possible as scientists and technologists developed a keen understanding of the unit operations in a process line, the specific ingredient structure/functionality and how the two interacted. This control enabled the food manufacturers of today to develop products which are safe to consumers, are enjoyable to eat, convenient to prepare and cheap. A few examples of this have been ingredient flexibility allowing manufactures to switch between ingredients as the need arose from cost or availability to the use of microstructure design for, for example, fat reduction or removal of gelatine, while still maintaining acceptable delivery of tastants and aromas for a pleasurable eating experience (Malone and Appelqvist, 2003). In a recent article Norton *et al.* (2006a) outlined the product/process integration in food manufacture, highlighting the future need to be able to better understand and predict the digestion and subsequent metabolism of structured foods. We therefore move from a position of thinking about how food microstructure is created, to thinking about how foods are broken down and reassembled within the body, how they pass through and impact on the GI tract, and how quickly they release nutrients. The unit operations in this human 'process' are not movable, but the way in which food is broken down can influence which parts of the 'process' different food formats see. The link then starts to be made between how food is constructed and, during consumption and digestion, deconstructed. In this chapter we extend this thinking by reviewing and discussing how microstructures and microstructure understanding can be used to construct materials inside humans as a response to the physiological triggers imposed by the GI tract and how these might be optimised in the future so that the food manufacturer can use the understanding to provide design rules for functional food creation. To enable this to be achieved, a new way of thinking about the food that we eat needs to begin. We need to consider how the effects of enzyme digestion, pH and temperature jumps, dilution/concentration and the interaction with bodily surfaces and fluids impact on the microstructure and functionality of food. However, it is pertinent to emphasise that food has a complex multiphase structure often comprising water, fat and air. These structures are typically not in thermodynamic equilibrium and are stabilised in their kinetically trapped form by the use of water soluble ingredients, surface active components and via crystallisation/gelation of either the fat or water phase (Norton *et al.*, 2006a; Ubbink and Mezzenga, 2006; Mezzenga, 2007). The water phase often exists in a multiphase state in its own right, as the ingredients used are often incompatible and form their own separate phases. We will explore the relevance of how these phases are arranged in relation to how they behave when consumed.

In recent years there have been a number of initial studies in this area with the workers extolling the virtues of using realistic simulations of oral, gastric and intestinal fluid environments. A limited number of groups now have models for various parts of the human digestive system. Workers in IFR and TNO have models for the stomach while recently a mechanical model of the intestine has been constructed and initial studies of how food behaves under peristaltic flow investigated by the chemical engineering department at the University of Birmingham. Challenges still exist in simulating these environments in both a chemical and physical sense (Minekus *et al.*, 1995; Janssen *et al.*, 2007; Wickham *et al.*, 2007). As these techniques develop, they will allow researchers to rapidly test their new microstructures in realistic conditions before they progress to test the effects in large scale nutritional trials or with consumers.

When we turn our attention to the food itself, a number of investigations have been carried out. Dietary fibres have been compared in simulated human gastric and small intestinal digesta (Dikeman *et al.*, 2006) and linked to their role in controlling blood glucose and lipid digestion. Riccardi *et al.* (2003) investigated the role of food structure on digestion rates and showed that the microstructure can have significant effects. Kim *et al.* (2004) studied the physical properties of rice, in determining the accessibility of starch to digestion and how it impacts on glycaemic index.

The structure of food not only affects the way that the individual receives nutrients: it has been shown that there can be a significant effect on the release of other molecules as well. Moreno (2007) discusses the effect of food structure on food allergenicity, indicating that the food matrix has a critical impact on allergen release. Sanz and Luyten (2007) used custard with varying microstructure and composition (fat content and thickener type) to investigate the bioaccessibility of soy agylocone, genistein. In the future it is likely that structures will be used to control the timescale and location of release of a wide range of micronutrients and therapeutic ingredients.

Following from the effects of food microstructure, the properties of the individual components have been shown to influence their digestibility. Moreno *et al.* (2004) and Koppelman *et al.* (2005) show the structure of protein and its resistance to digestion has also been linked to the body's immune response. Kumagai *et al.* (2006) have shown that the nutritive value of proteins from rice can be improved when prepared by alkaline extraction. This process changes the structural properties of the protein bodies, making them swollen and fragile, therefore allowing enzymes more access and improving their digestibility. Hernandez-Ledesma *et al.* (2004) have shown that biologically active peptides can be produced in simulated gastrointestinal digestion of milk. Other studies have shown that such peptide systems can be the source of self-assembling structures (Nowak *et al.*, 2002; Adams *et al.*, 2007), producing strong gels with novel microstructures (Ipsen *et al.*, 2001). The gelation of pure caseins (Dickinson and Krishna, 2001) and monomeric peptide fractions of whey (Veerman *et al.*, 2003) indicates that, while proteins might be broken down during digestion, the products of digestion might then have the ability to form extended three-dimensional structures. Indeed, such self-assembled structures might be induced by lipid/water interfaces as they concentrate the peptides at the interface so that they can aggregate together (Egan *et al.*, 2006). Semo *et al.* (2007) have also shown that reassembled casein micelles can be used as encapsulation vehicles to deliver health actives.

A more recent development has been to design structures in such a way as to respond in predetermined ways to different environments in the different parts of the GI tract. This can be achieved by designing particles that are tuned to different parts of the digestive tract, for instance through controlled layer-by-layer deposition. Antipov and Sukhorukov (2004) indicate through clever design that the capsules made in this way can be sensitive to shifts in pH, ionic strength or solvent, leading to changes in their permeability properties. Such capsules can then be used for delivery at different sites of the GI tract, depending on local physiological conditions. Additionally, they point out that such capsules can be envisaged as micro-reactors or crystallisation compartments, which would allow control of self-assembling structures as a function of the GI tract environment. In a similar vein Guzey and McClements (2006) take the concept of multilayering to interfaces typically found in food products, e.g. those in emulsions. They indicate that the stability/structuring potential of the dispersed phase of the emulsion can be controlled, depending on the layering and outer surface design. Furthermore, they also suggest that the outer surface of the multilayered structure can be induced to detach as a result of changes in pH, ionic strength or temperature, again indicating the opportunity for controlled/triggered release of the contents of the dispersed phase. They are, however, cautious about the cost-effective use of this technology. As we mentioned earlier, this may require a redesign of how 'functional' foods are applied and marketed in the future, which could give this technology an opportunity for delivery of highly active and desirable molecules to control some of the chronic diseases associated with food and diet. Thus the potential of the technology could be in the area of targeted and controlled release.

Targeting can be seen as creating a structure that interacts with specific parts of the GI tract (Remunan-Lopez *et al.*, 1998). Their work focused on design of bilayered devices for buccal drug delivery containing chitosan and ethylcellulose, where adhesion and the physical properties to cope with erosion and controlled diffusion are introduced as combinatory factors in defining the overall delivery profile. The self-assembly nature of this approach is therefore the structuring of the imbibed material with natural body services and has also been utilised for controlled aroma delivery (Malone *et al.*, 2003). Harding (2003, 2006) has focused on the potential to extend such delivery opportunities to the rest of the GI tract. This work and that of Bansil and Turner (2006) start to provide some good understanding of the state of the mucins lining the surfaces in the body, and how best food might mix and interact with such surfaces. Indeed, this is similar to the approach that has recently been taken by Janssen *et al.* (2007) for understanding the breakdown of food in the mouth.

There are three major structuring agents in foods, and so far we have touched on proteins and mentioned carbohydrates (this will be expanded upon in the next section). The third material that needs careful consideration is fats and the issues around their self-assembly possibilities. Fats are used to impart structure in wet (emulsion-based) and dry foods typically through their propensity to crystallise. They also are key constituents in foods due to their impact on the overall flavour delivery of foods, as they are sinks for lipophilic aroma volatiles (Malone and Appelqvist, 2003). Fat is digested in the small intestine and is broken down by lipase to release free fatty acids from the mono-, di- or triglyceride starting material. The digestion of fats from the bulk or from emulsion droplets needs to be considered as a surface effect. Thus as the surface area increases, the rate of digestion will increase. Bile salts are used in this process to disrupt interfacial layers and make the fats more accessible for digestion.

One way that fat structuring could be used for self-structuring inside people and for subsequent delivery of actives is to produce and use liquid crystalline phases. Heertje *et al.* (1998) described the structures that could be formed using monoglycerides, from lamellar liquid crystal phases to α-gel and coagel phases. More recently, these self-assembling structures have been studied, with the proposal made that such structures can be used as micro-reactors for flavour formation (Raemy *et al.*, 2005). Leser *et al.* (2006) and Sagalowicz *et al.* (2006) extend this to using such devises for solubilisation of poorly water-soluble ingredients and controlled release. van Amelsvoort *et al.* (2005) have utilised such technology to improve the bioavailability of lipophilic physiologically active ingredients. We believe that this is an interesting self-assembly problem, owing to the complexity of fat digestion; the mix of fat, fat digestion products and water. Additionally the introduction by the body of bile salts and bile acids complicate the situation further, with the self-assembly of dietary mixed micelles. Amar-Yuli and Garthi (2005) have attempted to unravel some of this complexity by studying the effect of introducing fats of differing chain length to a mesophase structure, looking at the effect on the phase diagram. The situation is obviously more complicated in the digestion of 'real' food systems, as fat, protein and carbohydrates will be present together and will all be undergoing the digestion process at different rates and in different locations in the GI tract, where some or all of the self-assembly mechanisms outlined above might be taking place. In addition to these sorts of structures, an interesting area for consideration is mixed polysaccharide–surfactant systems; with Grant *et al.* (2006) showing that self-assembly can be induced in these mixtures.

The way fats are emulsified into droplets and the surfactants used can also impact dramatically on their digestion (Marciani *et al.*, 2003; Bialek *et al.*, 2006). If the emulsion is designed to be sensitive to the pH of the stomach, then coarsening of the fat droplets or total phase separation of the fat can be induced. As mentioned earlier, the rate of digestion is dependent on surface area so such changes will impact on the digestive process. However, if the emulsion is designed in such a way as to rearrange structurally in the GI tract, then aggregated self-structured systems may well be produced, thus impacting on both the rheological properties of the stomach and the digestion rates. In addition, if the aqueous phase self-structures on consumption and traps acid-resistant oil droplets that were designed into the food product, slow release of energy over extended periods of time may well be possible.

As discussed earlier, the digestive mechanisms could well be dictated by the physical stability of the food structure in question. Such complexity in this area has ignited fresh impetus in the field of food science and nutrition which undoubtedly will lead to a range of healthy but indulgent products in the future, with potentially dramatic impact on the health of the consumer.

23.2 Self-structuring liquid products

The thought of liquid products obviously brings into focus the ever-expanding drinks market. However, it would be a remission if the other categories of liquid products are not included in this discussion, i.e. soups, sauces and other condiments. Very few of such products are high in fat, or indeed fat continuous. Therefore, the attention should be on products that are high in water content, and in some cases water continuous emulsions. The water phase in such products often contains protein and/or carbohydrates, which serve to thicken and stabilise the water phase and emulsify the fat phase if present. These sorts of products are normally based on mixtures of two or more biopolymers. The usual consequence of mixing carbohydrates and proteins is to form complex phase separated structures, which can be tuned for specific structural functionality (Foster, 2007). The food products will have initially been formulated to be stable, as liquid products for the optimal consumption quality related to the product in question, i.e. a milky drink full of 'body' or a soup that is nicely thickened and not too watery. But what happens to the structure upon ingestion as the product is subjected to a number of 'body-process' environments, involving shear, enzyme attack, a pH jump (eventually to pH 2 in the stomach – depending on mixing rate, and then to pH ~7 in the small intestine), a dilution via inclusion of saliva, gastric juices and bile, and depending on the temperature of the product, a temperature jump to the body temperature of 37 °C. All of these effects will be discussed now.

23.2.1 pH jump

A number of proteins and polysaccharides are known to be pH sensitive and aggregate as the overall charge on the polymer approaches zero. The structures that are formed not only depend upon the final pH but also on the rate of pH change (pH jump). For proteins the structures and rate of pH change have been investigated by a number of groups Heertje *et al.*, 1985; Roefs *et al.*, 1985; Fox and Mulvihill, 1990; Kuipers *et al.*, 2005. Many of the food grade proteins will aggregate at stomach pHs and form particulate gels. However, any manipulation of the three-dimensional structure will be difficult for the proteins alone as the aggregation is very rapid and the proteins are trying to dewater, thus resulting in highly compact structures. One potential way of overcoming these problems, however, might be to have the protein at the oil–water interface of an emulsion droplet. As the protein aggregates and dewaters with the pH jump, it will cause the oil droplets to form an extended three-dimensional network.

A number of polysaccharides are pH sensitive and can form acid gels. The best known examples are the alginates and pectins, which have been investigated by a number of different groups (Capel *et al.*, 2006; Draget *et al.*, 2006; Strom *et al.*, 2007). The gel network for each is dependent upon the rate of pH change and on the molecular fine structure of the polysaccharide. For alginate, the guluronic acid to mannuronic acid ratio and distribution of the sugars affect the rate of gel formation as well as the final gel properties. The degree of esterification (DE) of the galacturonic acid sugars and the DE distribution and blockiness have been shown to be important in pectin gelation. Hoad *et al.* (2004) compared alginates of different guluronic acid content in a model milk drink and followed intragastric gelation using state-of-the-art magnetic resonance imaging (MRI) techniques. Norton *et al.* (2006b) showed, by controlling the acidification of alginates, that acid gels could be produced under conditions experienced in the stomach. From this they postulated that, in the presence of shear forces in the stomach, a string-like gel is formed rather than a homogeneous three-dimensional gel. This might be expected when considering the way that the alginate drink enters the stomach and the acid gel forms in the gently mixed environment of the stomach. These structures are probably governed by the same effects as had previously been shown to be relevant for the formation of fluid gels (Norton *et al.*, 1999). From comparisons with non-gelling galactomannan, Hoad concluded that the gelling of the alginates was important in the control of satiety (this will be discussed in detail in the next section).

An area which has not really been investigated for a self-structuring and nutritional control viewpoint is mixed biopolymer systems. Schorsch *et al.* (1999) established that mixtures of milk protein and galactomannans are incompatible and create two phases, whose relative volumes are determined by the concentrations of polysaccharide and protein. Foster *et al.* (1996) showed that the properties of gelling phase separated systems are still determined by the relative phase volumes of the two discrete phases, but that the overall microstructure and material properties are controlled by the gelation process of one or both of the biopolymer phases. The ability to kinetically trap different microstructures in mixed biopolymer systems is likely to have significant effects on the self-assembled structures that can be produced (Fig. 23.1). It is unclear whether the galactomannan system in the Hoad study was phase separated, and more to the point, whether the alginate–milk mixtures were compatible or not, and whether this has any

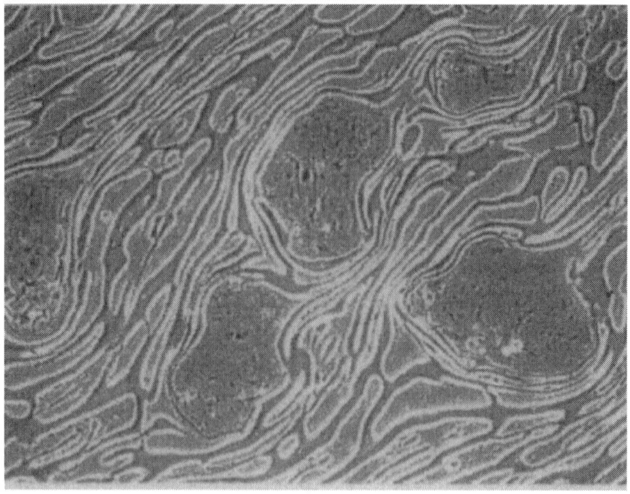

Fig. 23.1 An example of a phase separated biopolymer mixture, in which one of the biopolymers is gelling. The large particle of LBG gel is approximately 100 μm in diameter.

bearing on the intragastric properties of such systems. All these need to be fully investigated before real conclusions can be drawn.

As has been discussed, the gelation kinetics for self-assembling biopolymer systems is key to the sorts of structures that can be formed and, indeed, if the whole stomach contents or only part of the stomach content are gelled on ingestion. The kinetics of gelation of single biopolymers can be controlled by selecting or engineering the required molecular structure; however, if mixed acid-sensitive biopolymers, or a single acid-sensitive biopolymer in combination with a non-acid-sensitive biopolymer, are used, then we can envisage a selection based not only on the molecular structure of both biopolymers but also on the phase volumes and phase continuity of the polymers. These aspects will be more fully discussed later.

Another area of interest in considering pH jumps is the effect that this might have on charge of the biopolymer and thus its effect on the water holding capacity. Butler *et al.* (2006) have used this to control the swelling of biopolymer hydrogel particles containing chitosan and bovine serum albumin in order to enhance gastric retention or for controlled release in gastric conditions.

23.2.2 Dilution

Having just introduced the concept of creating structure upon entering the stomach, it seems strange to introduce the concept of the effects of dilution. However, as Foster *et al.* (2001), Cassin *et al.* (2000) and more recently Ferry *et al.* (2006) have shown, dilution can aid effective dispersion of liquids.

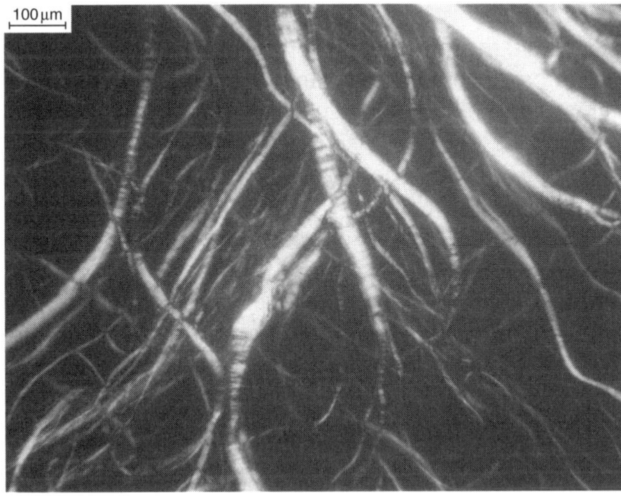

Fig. 23.2 A phase separated xanthan 'strand' in a much lower molecular weight polyelectrolyte continuous phase. Scale bar is 100 μm.

Liquids can be structured via particle–particle interaction or via soluble polymeric coils. Particles disperse more effectively than polymer thickened solutions and indeed, Marciani *et al.* (2001a) showed that solutions viscosified with random coil polymers do not disperse well in the stomach.

Two pieces of work that show structure creation upon dilution are those from Ryan *et al.* (2000) and Boyd *et al.* (2004). Both utilise the concept of phase separation, where the more viscous phase is the dispersed phase. Upon dilution or enzyme degradation of the continuous phase, a high viscosity 'self-assembled' structure is created as a result of phase inversion. In both cases the high molecular weight, high-viscosity polymer is mixed with a much lower molecular weight polymer (Fig. 23.2). If the more viscous polymer also was able to gel under gastric conditions, then this would be a second wave of self-assembly that could be possible.

23.2.3 Temperature-induced structuring

An environmental change that might be used to cause self-structuring on ingestion of food is temperature. However, the number of systems that can be used to cause structuring on increasing the temperature to 37 °C is small. Some work has been carried out by Tomlin *et al.* (1993) who first showed that a room temperature solution of ethylhydroxyethylcellulose could be induced to gel on increasing the temperature to 37 °C. This 'liquid fibre' (LF) was shown to gel in the stomach of humans and rats and dramatically delay gastric emptying times (Tomlin, 1995). However, the composition also contained a surfactant molecule (sodium dodecyl sulphate (SDS)), which is not allowed in food products. The concept of using a phase separated surfactant and biopolymer mixture might be useful in the future. Spyropoulos *et al.* (2008a,b) have reported on the mechanism of phase separation of such mixtures and shown how it relates to phase separated biopolymer mixtures. Such ideas will guide the future activities using food grade surfactants as these sorts of systems could potentially be optimised by selection of the biopolymer and the emulsifier phase to give self-structuring in the GI tract.

23.2.4 Emulsions

The properties of water continuous emulsions are determined by both the materials that are dispersed in the aqueous phase and the nature of the interaction of the dispersed fat phase. Two types of emulsions are possible and need consideration. These are either bulk emulsions which are kinetically trapped, or micro-emulsions which are in thermodynamic equilibrium. Bulk emulsions can be controlled to change structure by modification of the interfacial layer as a response to the environment, e.g. the surfactant packing at the interface can be modified as the pH is changed in the case of proteins emulsifiers. An important consideration with bulk emulsions is the size of the oil droplets. Until recently, droplet sizes were limited to be in the micron scale. However, just recently, Henry *et al.* (2008) have published the first results on production and stabilisation of food grade nanoemulsions. Such small droplets are potentially highly important when trying to self-structure systems. For bulk emulsions the interactions of the oil droplets are controlled by the interfacial layer, the molecular size and charge of the surfactant, the way the emulsion has been made and often the rheological nature of the fat phase itself, i.e. the amount of solid fat in the droplet. As micro-emulsions are thermodynamically stable, then the dilution process on ingestion might be used to control and manipulate structures. However, the problem currently is that most of the emulsifiers used for micro-emulsions are not food grade and they have to be used at such high concentrations that they have side issues such as bitterness and off-tastes.

Control of product performance by interfacial design has been known in the food industry for many years and is used to impart the desired textural properties to mayonnaise, salad dressings, dairy creams, non-dairy creams, whipping creams and acidified milk products. Milk proteins, small molecular weight emulsifiers and, in some cases, surface active polysaccharides have been used individually or in combination to control emulsion stability/instability (Campbell *et al.*, 1996; Buffet and Foster, 2003). The question is how can the emulsion behaviour and the nature of the interfacial layer be used to cause self-structuring when a food product experiences the environment of the human GI tract? Marciani *et al.* (2003, 2006, 2007) have shown, using MRI, that the stability of an emulsion to acidic conditions can vary the extent of gastric emptying. Emulsions that were unstable to the acidic gastric environment were seen to 'break' and cream in the

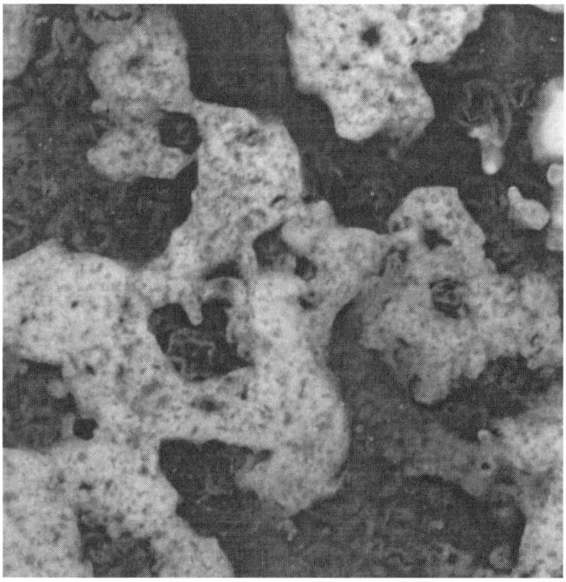

Fig. 23.3 An example of a bicontinuous fat and biopolymer structured water phase microstructure. Image width is 50 μm.

stomach, whereas those that were stable were emptied from the stomach as intact emulsion droplets. Similar results were seen by Bialek *et al.* (2006). However, as mentioned earlier, the rate of digestion of fat is dependent upon the amount of interface and on the way the interface is constructed. It is well known that solid fat is digested more slowly than are liquid oils. Thus we predict that, if an emulsion has a solid fat shell at body temperatures, then the rate of digestion of the inner core liquid oil will be slowed. In addition, if the interfacial layer is designed to cause aggregation of the droplets after ingestion of the food, then it seems likely to us that these sorts of self-assembled structures could be used to supplement self-structuring from the aqueous components (Fig. 23.3).

23.3 Effects on satiety

All of the self-assembling structures discussed above have been shown to affect satiety and are therefore worthy of consideration by the food industry in the need to address the increased prevalence of obesity in today's society.

23.3.1 Viscosity and gelation

Ryan *et al.* (2000) describe their glucomannan compositions lowering blood glucose and cholesterol, whose therapeutic mechanisms are thought to have their effects in increased viscosity and decreased uptake as a function of intestinal diffusion. Recent work by Bakalis *et al.* (2007), using a model of the human intestine, has shown how viscosity increases using guar solutions can impact on flow of material in the GI tract and how this can impact on digestion and uptake of other nutritional components.

Hoad *et al.* (2004) investigated the effects of viscous and intragastric gel-forming drink formats on satiety. They studied gastric emptying, gastric volume, the sense of fullness and feeling of hunger. They compared high and low guluronic acid content alginates (high G and low G, respectively), but also a viscous guar sample. The 'meals' containing the polysaccharides alginate or guar were four orders of magnitude more viscous than the control milk beverage. All four meals showed similar gastric emptying times, but the meals containing the polysaccharides all showed a significantly greater sense of fullness and the high G alginate decreased hunger. The more viscous samples of guar and high G alginate delayed the time for mean hunger values to return to the basal values by 60 and 75 minutes, respectively. The mechanism by which satiety is affected in this trial is therefore possibly a combination of viscosity and the effect of intragastric gelation. The idea that gelation has an effect was supported by the fact that the two alginate meals, when gelled in a controlled *in vitro* acidification regime, had a break force of 1.2 N for the high G alginate and 0.7 N for the lower G alginate. Previously, Marciani *et al.* (2001b), using gelled beads of agar of different firmness, indicated that the maximum force exerted by the gastric antrum was ~0.65 N, which was also shown to relate to feelings of fullness. Thus the gels produced via self-assembly inside the stomach had gel strengths above that required to get the feeling of fullness. Hoad's final hypothesis is that satiety can be affected by increasing the viscosity of a meal, but the opportunity presented by an intragastric gelling system distends the gastric antrum and the gel lumps transport nutrients to the small intestine. Evidently, there is much more scientific underpinning to be carried out to extend this fascinating finding.

Tomlin (1995) found that the so-called 'liquid fibre' (LF), body temperature gelling system delays gastric emptying times. When compared with the placebo, the mean time to the next meal was 67 minutes longer for the LF meal. These findings were mirrored by a decrease in hunger, increase in fullness and reduced food intake. While considering the delayed gastric emptying times and prolonged gastric distension, Tomlin also concluded that the gelling of LF delays nutrient release and nutrient–receptor interactions. It is not clear what functionality the SDS has in the formulation and how it relates to the effects on satiety. In this particular example it is likely that the surfactant improves the solubility of the ethylhydroxyethylcellulose, resulting in a more homogeneous system, which is mixed more evenly when the food enters the stomach. Thus, as the temperature is increased, the hydrophobic groups on the polymer interact to form an extended three-dimensional gel within the stomach. However, alternatively, the SDS could also play an important role in interactions with other surfactants that are naturally present in the human body or it could be encapsulating and 'emulsifying' nutrients. If this approach is to be used, however, alternative (food allowed) surfactants need to be found.

The examples given above for systems that increase the viscosity as temperature is increased via phase separation or phase inversion could provide satiety effects, induced for the same reasons as discussed above, i.e. increased gastric emptying times and/or delayed nutrient release.

23.3.2 Emulsions

The initial work carried out by Marciani *et al.* (2003, 2004, 2006, 2007) started to show how emulsion stability can impact on satiety. Model water continuous emulsions, with a 15% dispersed phase volume of olive oil were designed to either be stable or unstable in acidic conditions. Acid-tolerant emulsions were prepared using polyoxyethylene sorbitan monostearate (Tween 60), while acid-unstable emulsions were prepared using sorbitan monooleate (Span 80). *In vitro* studies at pH 2 showed that the acid-unstable emulsions 'broke', with droplet coalescence and rapid bulk phase separation into an oil layer. The acid-stable emulsion remained intact, with no change in droplet size distribution.

In vivo studies showed, however, that while the acid-unstable emulsion again separated, the acid-stable emulsion also formed a creamed layer. It was argued that creaming occurred due to charge screening in the stomach which reduced the repulsive forces between droplets. An important observation was that the cream layer of the acid-stable emulsion was formed much later than the broken oil layer of the acid-unstable emulsion. However, it is likely that the fat layer at the top of the stomach is re-emulsified with the natural emulsifiers present and the mechanical action of the stomach. This is a naturally occurring mechanism as enzymatic breakdown of the fats into fatty acids is an important step in digestion. As mentioned earlier, the rate of this process will be dependent on surface area, so there is a need to increase surface area for efficient digestion. Gastric emptying studies were undertaken using these two emulsions as the test meals (Marciani *et al.*, 2006, 2007). The acid-stable emulsion emptied more slowly and, as discussed above, led to prolonged gastric distension. It was shown that the acid-stable emulsion delivered small amounts of well-emulsified fat to the small intestine sooner than the unstable emulsion, and this occurred over a longer time period, showing increased indicators of improved satiety (fullness and hunger), and increased the release of cholecystokinin (CCK) and gall bladder contraction.

23.4 Incorporation into food products

The studies outlined in the previous sections begin to lay down design rules for in-body functionality of food stuffs, taking into account the environments that they have to survive/endure. The requirements, however, may not be compatible with current food formats owing to the unpalatability of the product offering. There are still many unanswered questions waiting to be investigated; the emulsion study uses one fat type and a couple of emulsifiers, indicating two ways in which the fat can be presented to the body for digestion. Following on from that model system discussed above, the next steps will probably develop understanding of fat type (chain length, degrees of saturation, molecular homogeneity solid/liquid ratio, encapsulation of liquid components inside droplets with crystalline shells designed to melt at specific temperatures), the interfacial layer (molecular design as well as interfacial layer thickness) and its ability to slow lipase activity, mixed emulsifier systems, droplet size and droplet size distribution, along with the design of complex microstructures, for instance, in which the oil droplet is encapsulated inside a gel bead which has been structured with the materials that in themselves self-structure. Recent work has shown the effectiveness of polyunsaturated fatty acids from Korean pine nuts to induce the release of high amounts of the appetite suppressing hormone CCK (Einerhand *et al.*, 2006), and some work has been carried out investigating the effects of very long chain ($>C_{18}$) versus long chain ($C_{12\text{-}18}$) triglycerides (Jonkers *et al.*, 2000) and the effect of emulsification (Ledeboer *et al.*, 1999).

The aqueous phase is often much more complicated in full food products than just a thickener/gelling agent. Hoad *et al.* (2004) and Tomlin (1995) have shown the opportunity of self-assembling in the body, but the complexity of food microstructures is not taken into account in their studies. The work of Ryan *et al.* (2000) and Boyd *et al.* (2004) begins to address the more complex nature of real foods. Their work points towards the redesign of foods for phase separated aqueous phases which can be designed to be palatable while having in-body functionality. For instance, Ryan *et al.* (2000) incorporated the action of α-amylase in the design of the functional microstructure. However, the action of pepsin and other gastric/intestinal enzymes must be considered in the construction of self-assembling/functionally active structures. An approach which could be of great potential here is the design of complex inclusions, using layer-by-layer techniques. Such structures could be designed to be stable in production and storage, and then be pleasant to eat before layers are removed in the rest of the GI tract to cause self-structuring and controlled release of bio-actives.

In the examples given so far the gelling agent and the emulsion droplet are the 'magic bullets' that have the functional effects of self-assembling systems. The area of functional foods has a tendency to focus on the 'magic bullet' and, depending on what it is, what its mode of action is, and where it needs to be delivered in the body, different mechanisms of incorporating it into various food formats can be envisaged.

23.4.1 Incorporation into current formats

A number of problems need to be overcome if self-assembling structures are to be incorporated into current food formats:

- Stopping the structuring from occurring before being consumed. The last thing a consumer wants is to open a can of meal replacement drink to find it has gelled.
- The addition of the self-assembling structure should be invisible to the consumer in terms of texture, taste and appearance, i.e. it has to have all the properties of the current product.

An approach that can be used to incorporate self-structuring systems into current products is one of encapsulation of the starting materials. This might best be illustrated by a couple of examples; there is a product, originally marketed as Olibra™, and now Fabuless™, which is an oil-in-water emulsion, containing small drops of palm oil and a galactolipid membrane, thought to delay the onset of digestion, thus imparting feelings of satiety via the 'ileal brake' mechanism (Burns *et al.*, 2000). Alternative encapsulates have been developed to serve a similar goal using natural oil bodies (Beindorff *et al.*, 2007) and complex coacervates (van Benthum *et al.*, 2004). Given that fabricated foods go through harsh process environments of shear, pressure and temperature, it is a valid question to ask whether such encapsulates would survive intact. If such systems are to be fully used throughout the food industry, they probably require a new process step of late-stage addition of the encapsulate carriers.

23.4.2 Redesigning current formats

Food microstructure can be designed by knowing how ingredients and processes interact (Norton and Foster, 2002; Norton *et al.*, 2006b; Foster, 2007). Therefore, depending on what is to be included in the product, a process sequence and/or ingredient mix can be formulated to serve the purpose required. Hill (2004) questions the use of unit operations in the production of certain products, introducing the thought of combining product and process design, i.e. only having the process steps and ingredient addition required at key points in the microstructure creation. This could potentially cause process complications, since different ingredients might be required to be added at different points in the process line. This complication in process flexibility would be outweighed if the product delivered the increased functionality of in-body self-assembly and thus impacted on the consumer in terms of real indulgence with healthy and nutritionally balanced foods. It is highly likely that such steps could lead to innovation in both process and ingredient.

23.4.3 New product design

The most likely way forward will be to design new products. The focus on designing new products specifically for self-assembly in the GI tract has a number of implications. The functionality could be in delivering ingredients to any part of the GI tract, to be absorbed by the body or designed to trigger the body's hormonal response to, for example, increase the feeling of satiety. The view should then be from the site of activity back up the GI tract to describe the requirements of the food product to provide what is required, when it is required, and to be stable until that point. This means that food structure design needs to consider the physiological triggers as discussed above. In doing so one might find that current food processing technologies are not precise enough to provide the accuracy of product requirements. Additionally, the current way we structure our foods could mean that not all of the designed functionality is expressed by the food format, in the location of the GI tract which it targeted. Again, there are indications of this route starting to happen. For instance, van Amelsvoort *et al.* (2005) attempted to deliver lipophilic physiologically active ingredients using mesophase structures in order to improve the delivery in the small intestine, and there are attempts to deliver bitter peptides to the stomach without oral perception using encapsulation, gel network entrapment and/or molecular chaperone interactions as the carrier/delivery mechanisms. The requirement for precise starting ingredient chemistry has implications on ingredient supply, utilising fractionation/separation technologies providing speciality/value-added status for ingredient suppliers. Process refinement may have to move from bulk structuring to precise particle creation and interactions, e.g. in the development of microfluidics (Stone and Kim, 2001).

23.5 Future trends

Norton and Foster (2002) published their ideas on how the world of hydrocolloids would change over the following decade. They suggested: the use of hydrocolloids from around the world, an increased use of biomaterials and natural sources of structuring for increased health perception, and an increased use of hydrocolloids in nutrition and nutrient control. Evidently, some of these ideas apply to this subject, but specifically we believe that this subject area will develop in the following three ways.

23.5.1 New ingredients/structures that meet the needs of self-assembling structures

If the full potential of self-assembling structures for foods is to be gained, it is highly likely that foods will be constructed in different ways in the future. This will be achieved using new processes and processing routes and the use of a whole range of different combinations of materials. This might be achieved through the particle assembly methodologies, or via compartmentation (Fig. 23.4) of specific ingredients or materials into structural elements that do not interact before they enter the required environmental conditions to trigger structural changes of the compartments, so that specific self-assembly only takes place at the site of action, and not before.

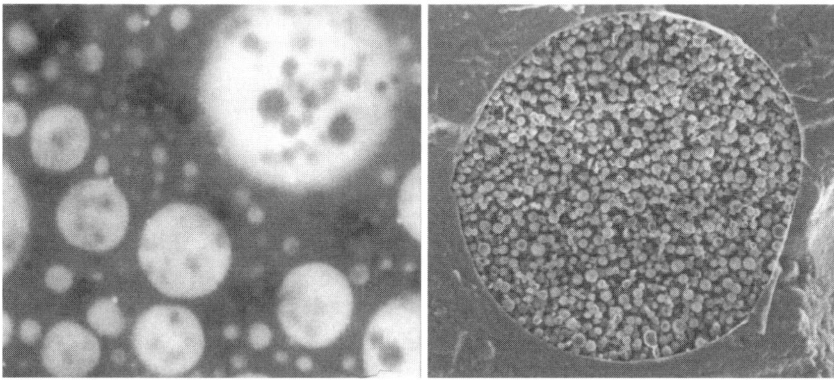

Fig. 23.4 Examples of complex compartmentalised structures of a water-in-water-in-water emulsion (left) and oil-in-water-in-oil emulsion (right). Image width is 50 μm in both cases.

Although the use of new ingredients is highly seductive, if they are to be used they will need to be cleared for use. This is likely to severely limit the number of new ingredients finding their way into the human food chain. Additionally, the use of plant cell structures or traditional therapeutic remedies will introduce new structuring options in the formulation of food products. An understanding of using such natural structures for controlled release and effects on satiety has already begun (Ellis *et al.*, 2004; Moorhead *et al.*, 2006).

23.5.2 The way in which the structures interact with the body

There will be much more emphasis placed on targeting sites of action, whether they are in the mouth, for controlled taste delivery or targeting sites of delivery/activity in other parts of the GI tract. Greater understanding of how food and food components interact with the body surfaces, controlling migration and delivery through the mucosal layers and membranes, as well as a better perspective of uptake mechanisms will be achieved. Furthermore, an appreciation for how food structures and their digestion products interact with one another and with the body fluids/secretions will aid the initial product design.

23.5.3 Mechanism of food consumption

The concepts outlined in this chapter address a change in emphasis on how food is manufactured and consumed. This change in emphasis has largely been in response to the need to control the onset of food-related chronic diseases, such as obesity, cardiovascular disease and diabetes. The role of such functional food is preventative, rather than curative (pharmaceutical industry). Such an idea is becoming much more prevalent in the food industry. A number of claims about the physiological benefits of specific food components are currently unsupported by strong scientific evidence, and so legislation is attempting to keep check of the claims made by food manufacturers for such products. The ultimate objective is to provide consumers with clearly understandable and scientifically supported health claims that can be used to make informed choices about dietary intake. This approach could be seen to be blurring the edges between the food and pharmaceutical industries, and in turn could determine how people choose to eat their food. An article by Boland (2006) indicates a shift to personalisation of foods at the point of sale, either for functional or sensory performance. Ultimately, people will eat the food that they can trust, be it cheap, authentic, functional or pleasurable, and we believe that providing a better understanding of how food behaves in the body will help enable that trust.

23.6 Sources of further information and advice

A good starting point for further information in this area is the European Technology Platform: Food For Life: http://etp.ciaa.be

Additionally, the conference series of: *Multi-scale Structures and Dynamics of Complex System*s and *Delivery of Functionality in Complex Food Systems*.

23.7 References

ADAMS DJ, HOLTZMANN K, SCHNEIDER C and BUTLER MJ (2007), 'Self-assembly of surfactant-like peptides', *Langmuir*, **23**, 12729–12736.

AMAR-YULI I and GARTHI N (2005), 'Transitions induced by solubilized fat into reverse hexagonal mesophases', *Colloids Surfaces B: Biointerfaces*, **43**, 72–82.

ANTIPOV AA and SUKHORUKOV GB (2004), 'Polyelectrolyte multilayer capsules as vehicles with tunable permeability', *Adv Colloids Interfaces*, **111**, 49–61.

BAKALIS S, THAKARAN A. NORTON IT and FRYER PJ (2007), *FASEB J*, **21**, 524.

BANSIL R and TURNER BS (2006), 'Mucin structure, aggregation, physiological functions and biomedical applications', *Curr Opinion Colloid Interface Sci*, **11**, 164–170.

BEINDORFF CM, LEMETTER CYG, MELNIKOV SM and WINTER I (2007), 'Food product, useful for treating or preventing overweight, and in weight-loss treatment, comprises oil bodies, where the oil bodies comprising lipid matrix surrounded by layer of phospholipids embedded with structural proteins', WO2007115899-A1.

BIALEK JM, MELNIKOV SM, WINTER I, GOLDING MD, DE GROOT PWN, KOPPERT RJ and PELAN EG (2006), 'Edible aqueous oil-in-water emulsion useful in food and beverages to treat or prevent obesity, comprises oil (having a saturated fatty acid), emulsifier (a protein) and water', WO2006053647-A1.

BOLAND M (2006), 'Perspective: mass customisation of food', *J Sci Food Agric*, **86**, 7–9.

BOYD MJ, MITCHELL JR, MELIA CD, JOLLIFFE IG and DETTMAR PW (2004), 'Thickenable compositions', WO2004096906-A1.

BUFFET G and FOSTER T (2003), 'Oil in water emulsion used as or part of food product, e.g. spreads, dressings, sauces, drinks and desserts, comprises surface active polymer and gelling polymer', WO2003053151-A1.

BURNS AA, LIVINGSTONE MBE, WELCH RW, DUNNE A, ROBSON PJ, LINDMARK L, REID CA, MULLANEY U and ROWLAND IR (2000), 'Short-term effects of yoghurt containing a novel fat emulsion on energy and macronutrient intakes in non-obese subjects', *Int J Obesity*, **24**, 1419–1425.

BUTLER MJ, CLARK AH and ADAMS S (2006), 'Swelling and mechanical properties of biopolymer hydrogels containing chitosan and bovine serum albumin', *Biomacromolecules*, **7**, 2961–2970.

CAMPBELL I, NORTON IT and MORLEY W (1996), 'Factors controlling the phase inversion of oil-in-water emulsions', *Neth Milk Dairy J*, **50**(2), 167–182.

CAPEL F, NICOLAI T, DURAND D, BOULENGUER P and LANGENDORFF V (2006), 'Calcium and acid induced gelation of (amidated) low methoxyl pectin', *Food Hydrocoll*, **20**(6), 901–907.

CASSIN G, APPELQVIST I, BOSSU N and NORTON IT (2000), 'Stress-induced alignment of fibres in a particulate matrix', *Colloid Polym Sci*, **278**, 783–788.

DICKINSON E and KRISHNA S (2001), 'Aggregation in a concentrated model protein system: a mesoscopic simulation of β-casein self-assembly', *Food Hydrocoll*, **15**, 107–115.

DIKEMAN CL, MURPHY MR and FAHEY GC (2006), 'Dietary fibers affect viscosity of solutions and simulated human gastric and small intestinal digesta', *J Nutr*, **136**(4), 913–919.

DRAGET KI, SKJAK-BRAEK G and STOKKE BT (2006), 'Similarities and differences between alginic acid gels and ionically crosslinked alginate gels', *Food Hydrocoll*, **20**(2–3), 170–175.

EGAN TJ, CHEN JY-J, DE VILLIERS KA, MABOTHA TE, NAIDOO KJ, NCOKAZI KK, LANGFORD SJ, MCNAUGHTON D, PANDIANCHERRI S and WOOD BR (2006), 'Haemozoin (β-haetmatin) biomineralisation occurs by self-assembly near the lipid/water interface', *FEBS Letts*, **580**, 5105–5110.

EINERHAND AW, PASMAN W, RUBINGH C, VAN DEN BERG R, O'SHEA M, GAMBELLI L and HENDRIKS H (2006), 'Korean pine nut fatty acids affect appetite sensations, plasma CCK and GLP1 in overweight subjects', *FASEB J*, **20**, A829.

ELLIS PR, KENDALL CWC, REN Y, PARKER C, PACY JF, WALDRON KW and JENKINS DJA (2004), 'Role of cell walls in the bioaccessibility of lipids in almond seeds', *Am J Clin Nutr*, **80**, 604–613.

FERRY AL, HORT J, MITCHELL JR, COOK DJ, LAGARRIGUE S and PAMIES BV (2006), 'Viscosity and flavour perception: why is starch different from hydrocolloids?', *Food Hydrocoll*, **20**(6), 855–862.

FOSTER T (2007), 'Structure design in the food industry', in Brockel U, Meier W and Wagner G, *Product design and engineering, Volume 2: Raw materials, Additives and Applications*, Weinheim, Wiley-VCH, 617–628.

FOSTER TJ, BROWN CRT and NORTON IT (1996), 'Phase inversion of water-in-water emulsions', in Williams PA, Phillips GO and Wedlock DJ, *Gums and Stabilisers for the Food Industry 8*, Oxford, IRL Press, 297–306.

FOSTER TJ, BROWN CRT, FRITH WJ and NORTON IT (2001), 'Textural and functional properties of fluid gels', in Berk Z, Leslie RB, Lillford PJ and Mizrahi S, *Water Science for Food, Health, Agriculture and Environment (ISOPOW 8)*, Lancaster, PA, Technomic Publishing Company, 87–96.

FOX PF and MULVIHILL DM (1990), 'Casein', in Harris P, *Food Gels*, London, Elsevier Applied Science, 121–174.

GRANT J, CHO J and ALLEN C (2006), 'Self-assembly and physiological and rheological properties of a polysaccharide–surfactant system formed from cationic biopolymer chitosan and nonionic sorbitan esters', *Langmuir*, **22**, 4327–4335.

GUZEY D and MCCLEMENTS J (2006), 'Formation, stability and properties of multilayer emulsions for application in the food industry', *Adv Colloid Interface Sci*, **128–130**, 227–248.

HARDING SE (2003), 'Mucoadhesive interactions', *Biochem Soc Trans*, **31**(5), 1036–1041.

HARDING SE (2006), 'Trends in mucoadhesive analysis', *Trends Food Sci Technol*, **17**, 255–262.

HEERTJE I, VISSER J and SMITS P (1985), 'Structure formation in acid milks gels', *Food Microstructure*, **4**(2), 267–277.

HEERTJE I, ROIJERS EC and HENDRICKX HACM (1998), 'Liquid crystalline phases in the structuring of food products', *Lebensm-Wiss u-Technol*, **31**, 387–396.

HERNANDEZ-LEDESMA B, AMIGO L, RAMOS M and RECIO I (2004), 'Application of high-performance liquid chromatography–tandem mass spectrometry to the identification of biologically active peptides produced by milk fermentation and simulated gastrointestinal digestion', *J Chromatography A*, **1049**, 107–114.

HENRY JV, FRITH WJ, FRYER PJ and NORTON IT (2008), 'Kinetically trapped food grade nano-emulsions', *Foods Food Ingredients J, Japan*, **213**, 192–196.

HILL M (2004), 'Product and process design for structured products', *AIChE J*, **47**, 1250–1254.

HOAD CL, RAYMENT P, SPILLER RC, MARCIANI L, DE CELIS ALONSO B, TRAYNOR C, MELA DJ, PETERS HP and GOWLAND PA (2004), '*In vivo* imaging of intragastric gelation and its effect on satiety in humans', *J Nutr*, **134**(9), 2293–2300.

IPSEN R, OTTE J and QVIST KB (2001), 'Molecular self-assembly of partially hydrolysed α-lactalbumin resulting in strong gels with a novel microstructure', *J Dairy Res*, **68**, 277–286.

JANSSEN AM, TERPSTRA MEJ, DE WIJK RA and PRINZ JF (2007), 'Relations between rheological properties, saliva-induced structure breakdown and sensory texture attributes of custards', *J Text Stud*, **38**, 42–69.

JONKERS IJAM, LEDEBOER M, STEENS J, SMELT AHM and MASCLEE AAM (2000), 'Effects of very long chain versus long chain triglycerides on gastrointestinal motility and hormone release in humans', *Digestive Diseases Sci*, **45**(9), 1719–1726.

KIM JC, KIM J-I, KONG B-W, KANG M-J, KIM M-J and CHA I-J (2004), 'Influence of the physical form of processed rice products on the enzymatic hydrolysis of rice starch *in vitro* and on the postprandial glucose and insulin responses in patients with type 2 diabetes mellitus', *Biosci, Biotechnol, Biochem*, **68**(9), 1831–1836.

KOPPELMAN SJ, NIEUWENHUIZEN WF, GASPARI M, KNIPPELS LM, PENNIKS AH, KNOL EF, HEFLE SL and DE JONGH HHJ (2005), 'Reversible dematuration of brazil nut albumin (Ber e1) and implication of structural destabilisation on digestion of pepsin', *J Agric Food Chem*, **53**, 123–131.

KUIPERS BJH, VAN KONINGSVELD GA, ALTING AC, DRIEHUS F, GRUPPEN H and VORAGEN AGJ (2005), 'Enzymatic hydrolysis as a means of expanding the cold gelation conditions of soy proteins', *J Agric Food Chem*, **53**(4), 1031–1038.

KUMAGAI T, KAWAMURA H, FUSE T, WATANABE T, SAITO Y, MASUMURA T, WATANABE R and KADOWARI M (2006), 'Production of rice protein by alkaline extraction improves its digestibility', *J Nutr Sci Vitaminol*, **52**, 467–472.

LEDEBOER M, MASCLEE AAM, BIEMOND I and LAMERS C (1999), 'Differences in cholecystokinin release and gallbladder contraction between emulsified and nonemulsified long-chain triglycerides', *J Parenter Enter Nutr*, **23**, 203–206.

LESER ME, SAGALOWICZ L, MICHEL M and WATZKE H (2006), 'Self-assembly of polar food lipids', *Adv Colloid Interface Sci*, **123–126**, 125–136.

MALONE ME and APPELQVIST IAM (2003), 'Gelled emulsion particles for the controlled release of lipophilic volatiles during eating', *J Cont Release*, **90**(2), 227–241.

MALONE ME, APPELQVIST IAM and NORTON IT (2003), 'Oral behaviour of food hydrocolloids and emulsions. Part 1. Lubrication and deposition considerations', *Food Hydrocoll*, **17**, 763–773.

MARCIANI L, GOWLAND PA, SPILLER RC, MANOJ P, MOORE RJ, YOUNG P and FILLERY-TRAVIS AJ (2001a), 'Effect of meal viscosity and nutrients on satiety, intragastric dilution, and emptying assessed by MRI', *Am J Physiol Gastrointest Liver Physiol*, **280**, G1227–G1233.

MARCIANI L, GOWLAND PA, FILLERY-TRAVIS A, MANOJ P, WRIGHT J, SMITH A, YOUNG P, MOORE R and SPILLER RC (2001b), 'Assessment of antral grinding of a model solid meal with echo-planar imaging', *Am J Physiol Gastrointest Liver Physiol*, **280**, G844–G849.

MARCIANI L, WICKHAM M, WRIGHT J, BUSH D, FAULKS R, FILLERY-TRAVIS A, GOWLAND P and SPILLER RC (2003), 'Magnetic resonance imaging (MRI) insights into how fat emulsion stability alters gastric emptying', *Gastroenterology*, **124**(4), A581.

MARCIANI L, WICKHAM M, HILLS BP, WRIGHT J, BUSH D, FAULKS R, FILLERY-TRAVIS A, SPILLER RC and GOWLAND PA (2004), 'Intragastric oil-in-water emulsion fat fraction measured using inversion recovery echo-planar magnetic resonance imaging', *J Food Sci*, **69**(6), E290.

MARCIANI L, WICKHAM MSJ, BUSH D, FAULKS R, WRIGHT J, FILLERY-TRAVIS A, SPILLER RC and GOWLAND PA (2006), 'Magnetic resonance imaging of the behaviour of oil-in-water emulsions in the gastric lumen of man', *Br J Nutr*, **95**, 331–339.

MARCIANI L, WICKHAM M, SINGH G, BUSH D, PICK B, COX E, FILLERY-TRAVIS A, FAULKS R, MARSDEN C, GOWLAND PA and SPILLER RC (2007), 'Enhancement of intragastric acid stability of a fat emulsion meal delays gastric emptying and increases cholecystokinin release and gallbladder contraction', *Am J Physiol Gastrointest Liver Physiol*, **292**, G1607–G1613.

MEZZENGA R (2007), 'Equilibrium and non-equilibrium structures in complex food systems', *Food Hydrocoll*, **21**, 674–682.

MINEKUS M, MARTEAU P, HAVENAAR R and HUISINTVELD JHJ (1995), 'A multicompartmental dynamic computer-controlled model simulating the stomach and small-intestine', *Alt Laboratory Animals*, **23**(2), 197–209.

MOORHEAD SA, WELCH RW, BARBARA M, LIVINGSTONE E, MCCOURT M, BURNS AA and DUNNE A (2006), 'The effects of the fibre content and physical structure of carrots on satiety and subsequent intakes when eaten as part of a mixed meal', *Br J Nutr*, **96**(3), 587–595.

MORENO FJ (2007), 'Gastrointestinal digestion of food allergens: effects on their allergenicity', *Biomed Pharmacotherapy*, **61**, 50–60.

MORENO FJ, MELLON FA, WICKHAM MSJ, BOTTRILL AR and MILLS ENC (2004), 'Stability of the major allergen brazil nut 2S albumin (Ber e1) to physiologically relevant *in vitro* gastrointestinal digestion', *FEBS J*, **272**, 341–352.

NORTON IT and FOSTER TJ (2002), 'Hydrocolloids in real food systems', in Williams PA and Phillips GO, *Gums and Stabilisers for the Food Industry 11*, Cambridge, RSC Special Publications, 187–200.

NORTON IT, JARVIS DA and FOSTER TJ (1999), 'A molecular model for the formation and properties of fluid gels', *Int J Biol Macromol*, **26**(4), 255–261.

NORTON I, FRYER P and MOORE S (2006a), 'Product/process integration in food manufacture: engineering sustained health', *AIChE J*, **52**(5), 1632–1640.

NORTON IT, FRITH WJ and ABLETT S (2006b), 'Fluid gels, mixed fluid gels and satiety', *Food Hydrocoll*, **20**, 229–239.

NOWAK AP, BREEDVELD V, PAKSTIS L, OZBAS B, PINE DJ, POCHAN D and DEMING TJ (2002), 'Rapidly recovering hydrogel scaffolds from self-assembling diblock copolypeptide amphiphiles', *Nature*, **417**, 424–428.

RAEMY A, NOUZILLE A, FROSSARD L, SAGALOWICZ L and LESER M (2005), 'Thermal behaviour of emulsifier–water systems studied by micro-DSC', *J Thermal Anal Calorimetry*, **80**, 439–443.

REMUNAN-LOPEZ C, PORTERO A, VILA-JATO JL and ALONSO MJ (1998), 'Design and evaluation of chitosan/ethylcellulose mucoadhesive bilayered devices for buccal drug delivery', *J Cont Release*, **55**, 143–152.

RICCARDI G, CLEMENTE G and GIACCO R (2003), 'Glycemic index of local foods and diets: the Mediterranean experience', *Nutr Revs*, **61**(5), S56–S60.

ROEFS SPFM, WALSTRA P, DALGLEISH DG and HORNE DS (1985), 'Preliminary note on the change in casein micelles caused by acidification', *Neth Milk Dairy J*, **39**, 119–122.

RYAN VJ, YUAN CR and CROSBY GA (2000), 'Methods for lowering viscosity of glucomannan compositions', WO0067592-A1.

SAGALOWICZ L, LESER ME, WATZKE HJ and MICHEL M (2006), 'Monoglyceride self-assembly structures as delivery vehicles', *Trends Food Sci Technol*, **17**, 204–214.

SANZ T and LUYTEN H (2007), '*In vitro* evaluation of genistein bioaccessibility from enriched custards', *Food Hydrocoll*, **21**, 203–211.

SCHORSCH C, JONES MG and NORTON IT (1999), 'Thermodynamic incompatibility and microstructure of milk protein/locust bean gum/sucrose systems', *Food Hydrocoll*, **13**(2), 89–99.

SEMO E, KESSELMAN E, DANINO D and LIVNEY YD (2007), 'Casein micelle as a natural nano-capsular vehicle for nutraceuticals', *Food Hydrocoll*, **21**, 936–942.

SPYROPOULOS S, DING P, FRITH WJ, NORTON IT, WOLF B and PACEK A (2008a), 'Interfacial tension in aqueous biopolymer–surfactant mixtures', *J Colloid Interface Sci*, **317**, 604–610.

SPYROPOULOS S, FRITH WJ, NORTON IT, WOLF B and PACEK AW (2008b), 'Sheared aqueous two-phase biopolymer-surfactant mixtures', *Food Hydrocoll*, **22**, 121–129.

STONE HA and KIM S (2001), 'Microfluidics: basic issues, applications and challenges', *AIChE J*, **47**, 1250–1254.

STROM A, RIBELLES P, LUNDIN LO, NORTON IT, MORRIS ER and WILLIAMS MAK (2007), 'Influence of pectin fine structure on the mechanical properties of calcium–pectin and acid–pectin gels', *Biomacromolecules*, **8**(9), 2668–2674.

TOMLIN J (1995), 'The effect of the gel-forming liquid fibre on feeding behaviour in man', *Br J Nutr*, **74**, 427–436.

TOMLIN J, BROWN N, ELLIS A, CARLSSON A, BOGENTOFT C and READ NW (1993), 'The effect of liquid fiber on gastric-emptying in the rat and humans and the distribution of small-intestinal contents in the rat', *Gut*, **34**(9), 1177–1181.

UBBINK J and MEZZENGA R (2006), 'Delivery of functionality in complex food systems: introduction', *Trends Food Sci Technol*, **17**, 194–195.

VAN AMELSVOORT JM, DUCHATEAU GS, MELNIKOV SM and WINTER I (2005), 'Water-continuous composition for food product, e.g. beverage, dressing, soup, sauce, dip, spread or filling, comprises lipophilic physiologically active ingredient in particular fat soluble nutrient', WO2006069619-A2.

VAN BENTHUM WA, DUCHATEAU GS and PETERS HP (2004), 'Food product e.g. for controlling body weight comprises a satiety agent encapsulated by cross-linked encapsulation material with a specified degree of cross-linking', WO2004105505-A1.

VEERMAN C, BAPTIST H, SAGIS LMC and VAN DER LINDEN E (2003), 'A new multistep Ca^{2+}-induced cold gelation process for β-lactoglobulin', *J Agric Food Chem*, **51**, 3880–3885.

WICKHAM MSJ, MANDALARI G, RICH GT, PICOUT DR, ELLIS PR and FAULKS R (2007), '*In vitro* and *in vivo* digestion studies of nutrients and phytochemicals from almond seeds', *Annals Nutr Metabolism*, **51**, 207.

24

Designing foods to induce satiation: a flavour perspective

R. M. A. J. Ruijschop, K. M. M. Burseg, T. T. Lambers and J. Overduin, NIZO Food Research, The Netherlands

Abstract: The epidemic of overweight and obesity is giving rise to the design of functional foods for durable suppression of appetite. Adopting a multidisciplinary approach that combines principles from the sensory science of flavours, gastrointestinal physiology, ingredient technology and texture design could bring the engineering of such food products within reach. In this chapter the special focus is on the possibility of using sensory triggers, particularly flavour, for inducing or increasing satiation. Different aspects influencing sensory satiation are first described. Secondly, opportunities to design food products that boost satiation by applying specific tools and technologies are discussed.

Key words: appetite, sensory perception, gastrointestinal behaviour, meal termination.

24.1 Introduction

24.1.1 A global need for sustained weight management

Worldwide, the prevalence of overweight and obesity, and associated co-morbidities, is increasing significantly. The World Health Organization (WHO) projects that by 2015, approximately 2.3 billion adults will be overweight and more than 700 million will be obese. The fundamental cause of obesity and overweight is an energy imbalance between calories consumed and calories expended. Global increases in overweight and obesity are attributable to a number of factors, including a global shift towards increased portion size and intake of energy-dense foods that are high in fat and sugar, but low in fibre, vitamins, minerals and other micronutrients. Added to this is a trend towards decreased physical activity associated with increasingly sedentary lifestyles (International Obesity Task Force, 2008).

To prevent energy imbalance by advising individuals to choose healthier diets with fewer calories, and to increase their level of exercise, has proven insufficient to deal with the epidemic. The human body exerts a strong defence against under-nutrition and weight loss, but applies a much weaker resistance to overconsumption and weight gain. This means that weight gain by overconsumption may occur despite the best efforts to prevent it (Blundell and King, 1996). Therefore, conventional weight management (dietary intervention, physical activity, behavioural therapy) often results in short-term successes only; sustained weight maintenance is difficult to achieve (Westerterp-Plantenga *et al.*, 2004). Hence, alternative weight reduction strategies might contribute to a solution. Various weight management approaches can be adopted with different modes of action, from boosting meal-induced thermogenesis and fat oxidation, inhibiting protein breakdown, and blocking intestinal fat absorption, to regulating mood (linked to food consumption), suppressing appetite and enhancing satiety.

24.1.2 Second generation of functional foods to address weight management

Multiple academic and industrial efforts are under way to find strategies to reduce overweight and obesity. For instance, in 2005 a large EC-funded project started called DiOGenes (an acronym for Diet, Obesity and Genes) whose main objective is to reduce overweight, obesity and its co-morbidities in Europe. This project is facilitated by an expanded knowledge base, which will generate the tools to optimise dietary intake with the aim of preventing weight (re)gain in different types of consumers (DiOGenes project, 2008). In recent years, the food industry has spearheaded a number of initiatives to reduce the fat, sugar and salt content of processed foods and portion sizes, without compromising on aroma, taste and mouthfeel. As an example, optimising the flavour release from low-fat products is an important topic in new product development. The release of aromas during food consumption can be measured and adjusted using atmospheric pressure chemical ionisation – mass spectrometry (APcI-MS) technology (Weel *et al.*, 2003). In Fig. 24.1 this is illustrated for yoghurt. The flavour release of an arbitrary (lipophilic) aroma compound is highly dependent on the amount of fat present in the food matrix as well as the type of fat. Lowering the fat content in yoghurt results in a striking increase of *in vivo* aroma release, while on the other hand, an alternative type of fat substantially decreases the aroma release from the yoghurt during actual consumption. Clearly, these three different food matrices affect the *in vivo* release of aroma volatiles and thus the final sensory perception of the food products. Typically, these types of studies are used to optimise the taste and aroma perception of reduced-fat food products.

While the development of this more classical generation of functional foods will continue, added functionalities, e.g. potency to induce satiety, are being increasingly explored. The ultimate aim in this case is to develop a good tasting low-fat food product that also induces an increased level of satiety, which will prevent consumers overeating.

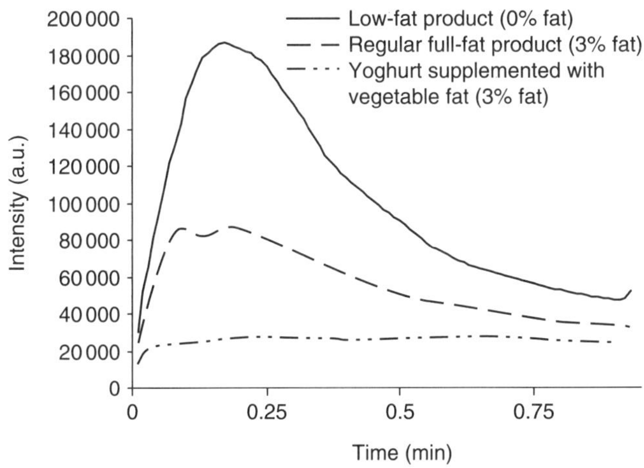

Fig. 24.1 Example of average *in vivo* flavour release curves of a lipophilic aroma compound of three yoghurts with different amounts and type of fat as measured with APcI-MS (adapted from van de Velde *et al.*, 2008).

24.1.3 Appetite control

The biological drive to eat can be linked with the satiating power or efficiency of food. Food brings about this effect by mediating certain processes that can be roughly classified as sensory, cognitive, post-ingestive and post-absorptive. The operation of these processes results from the activation by foods of physiological and biochemical mechanisms. Collectively, these processes have been referred to as the satiety cascade, consisting of processes related to satiation (intra-meal satiety) and satiety (inter-meal satiety) (Blundell and King, 1996; Blundell, 1999). Food-related stimuli can affect all phases of the satiety cascade. In Fig. 24.2 this 'satiety cascade' is depicted along with the meal intake cycle.

Satiation is associated with fullness and termination of food intake during meals. It develops during meal intake and ultimately brings the period of eating to an end. Satiation (intra-meal satiety), therefore, reduces hunger and limits the amount of energy consumed during a meal (Blundell *et al.*, 1996; Blundell and King, 1996). Satiety (inter-meal satiety), on the other hand, occurs after meal termination. It is the state of satiety that delays the onset of the next meal and may reduce food consumption at the next eating occasion (Blundell *et al.*, 1996). Satiation and satiety are distinct but interrelated factors that influence both the type and amount of food consumed.

Even before the food touches the mouth, physiological signals are generated by the sight and the smell of food. These events constitute the cephalic phase of appetite. Cephalic phase responses are generated throughout the gastrointestinal tract and one of their prime functions is to prepare the body

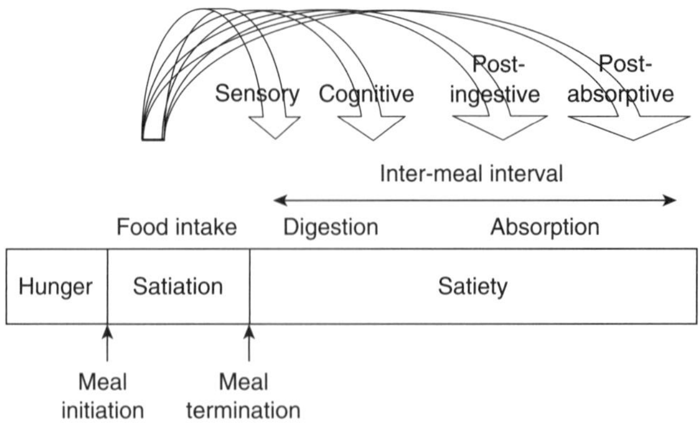

Fig. 24.2 Schematic overview of a food intake cycle and satiety cascade with related terminology (adapted from Blundell and King, 1996).

for effective food digestion. During and immediately after eating, afferent information exerts major control over appetite. Flavour and mouthfeel qualities of food give rise to hedonic responses via opioidergic and aminergic neural pathways. Food-induced gastrointestinal effects that decrease appetite include gastric distension, intestinal nutrient presence, hormone release and post-absorptive appearance of food metabolites in the circulation. These peripheral events lead to an activation of multiple pathways and networks within the central nervous system. Proteins, fats and carbohydrates generate different sets of physiological responses with different effects on the intensity and duration of satiety. Many studies have shown that proteins are the macronutrients that provide the most satiation per calorie, followed by carbohydrates and fats (de Castro, 1987; de Graaf *et al.*, 1992; Stubbs, 1995; Westerterp-Plantenga *et al.*, 1996). Not only the macronutrient composition of food, but also the overall energy density and food texture influence meal size and post-meal satiety (Blundell and King, 1996).

Currently, marketed functional food products that are claimed to suppress appetite are often combined with active ingredients that are aimed at later phases of the satiety cascade, e.g. the post-ingestive and post-absorptive stage. This chapter focuses on the possibility of using sensory triggers, particularly flavour, for inducing or increasing satiation. These sensory triggers take part in the early phases of the satiety cascade at the interface between satiation and satiety, and contribute to the process of meal termination.

24.2 Understanding of sensory satiation

24.2.1 Sensory modalities

Human perception of food aroma and texture during consumption is a complicated process in which taste, mouthfeel, vision, olfaction, the trigeminal system and even auditory signals contribute to the total appreciation of a food product (Sheperd, 1995; Meiselman, 1996). When food is processed in the mouth, it is subjected to changes in temperature, mechanical deformation and effects caused by saliva such as dilution and enzymatic breakdown of certain food ingredients such as starch (de Wijk and Prinz, 2005). Non-volatile compounds that are responsible for the basic tastes diffuse into the saliva and subsequently reach the gustatory receptors. Furthermore, during oral processing and after swallowing, volatile aroma compounds are released from the food matrix and are able to flow to the olfactory epithelium, where they interact with olfactory receptors. During food intake, the different senses interact in a non-linear way. Cross-modal phenomena, in which aroma influences the perception of the taste (and vice versa) of a food product, have been described (Stevenson *et al.*, 1999; Hort and Hollowood, 2004; Pfeiffer *et al.*, 2005). These interactions are most prominent for sweetness and congruent aromas like strawberry and include both synergistic and antagonistic effects. Additionally, perceived properties such as thickness and creaminess may be enhanced by congruent aromas (Bult *et al.*, 2007). Cross-modal interactions have, in particular, been reported for semi-solid gelled food systems such as yoghurt (Rolls, 2005; Hollowood *et al.*, 2002; Weel *et al.*, 2002; Cook *et al.*, 2003a,b; Lethuaut *et al.*, 2004; Saint-Eve *et al.*, 2004; Visschers *et al.*, 2006).

In the human brain the orbitofrontal cortex is an important site where representations of the various sensory properties of food converge. The orbitofrontal cortex is also the region where the short-term sensory-specific control of appetite and ingestion is regulated (Rolls, 2004). Sensory effects, generated by the sensory properties of food, are probably among the most important factors leading to satiation and meal termination (Sorensen *et al.*, 2003).

24.2.2 Sensory-specific satiation

Palatability of foods is positively related to the amount consumed (e.g. de Graaf *et al.*, 1999). As a food is eaten, its palatability declines and it becomes less likely that it will be eaten if other foods are also available. This phenomenon is called sensory-specific satiation, which refers to the decrease in pleasantness of a food after it is eaten compared with the decrease in pleasantness of foods that were tasted but not eaten to satiety. The decrease in liking is also associated with a lower intake of that particular food in a subsequent course. Sensory-specific satiation already occurs within 2 minutes after the start of consumption, when there has been little opportunity for digestion and absorption. Its magnitude does not seem to change over the next 20 minutes and it is specific for the sensory properties of food products. The duration of sensory-specific satiation is unknown. A number of studies show that drops in liking persist for more than one hour after consumption (Sorensen *et al.*, 2003). Sensory-specific satiation depends more on the sensory stimulation accompanying eating and less on absorptive events after consuming these foods (Rolls *et al.*, 1982; Hetherington *et al.*, 1989; Hetherington, 1996; Sorensen *et al.*, 2003; Snoek *et al.*, 2004). Factors that interrupt continued exposure, i.e. distractors introduced during a meal or variety in food and sensory properties, delay the development of (sensory-specific) satiation (Brunstrom and Mitchell, 2006; Hetherington *et al.*, 2006; Romer *et al.*, 2006; Harthoorn *et al.*, 2008). This implies that, when a food is eaten, introducing another food with different sensory properties slows the decline in desire to eat the food and increases meal size. Increasing the variety of sensorily distinct foods that are almost identical in composition can increase food and energy intake and alter energy balance in the short to medium term (Stubbs *et al.*, 2001).

Several studies have investigated which sensory properties of food are involved in sensory-specific satiation. Taste-, aroma-, texture- and appearance-specific satieties have been identified (Rolls *et al.*, 1982; de Graaf *et al.*, 1993; Hirsch and Gomez, 1995; Guinard and Brun, 1998; Mayer *et al.*, 1999; O'Doherty *et al.*, 2000; Maier *et al.*, 2007). Studies on the role of macronutrients and the energy content of the food in sensory-specific satiation have obtained equivocal results (Sorensen *et al.*, 2003).

24.2.3 Sensory perception and obesity

In general, obese subjects experience greater liking for foods than do non-obese subjects. In particular, they have a higher preference for sweet and high-fat foods (Bartoshuk *et al.*, 2006). Higher body mass index (BMI) is also associated with decreased perception of sweetness, which probably intensifies fat sensations via taste–taste interactions. Decreased intensity of one orosensory system is able to disinhibit another orosensory system.

Genetic variation may contribute to the defect in sweet taste in obese subjects (Bartoshuk *et al.*, 2006). In taste tests, individuals vary widely in their sensitivity to the bitter taste of phenylthiocarbamide (PTC) and chemical relatives such as 6-*n*-propylthiouracil (PROP), as reflected in PROP threshold levels and reported intensity ratings of supra-threshold PROP concentrations. The variation in PROP responses is presumed to have a genetic basis (inherited trait) that explains the classification of individuals into three groups: those that are insensitive (non-tasters; who appear to lack a receptor for the N—C=S group), moderately sensitive (tasters) and acutely sensitive (supertasters or PROP tasters) (Bartoshuk *et al.*, 1992). The number of taste buds is associated with the ability to taste PROP (Bartoshuk *et al.*, 1994). It has been reported that PROP tasters have greater sensitivity to a wide range of oral stimuli, including bitter tastes associated with fruits and vegetables, the textural sensations of fats and trigeminal irritation caused by chilli pepper and ethanol (e.g. Ko *et al.*, 2000; Prescott and Swain-Campbell, 2000; Prescott *et al.*, 2001).

An inverse association between PROP sensitivity and body weight is suggested by some, but not all, reported data. Lower weights among supertasters appear to result from less liking for high-sweet, high-fat foods (e.g. Duffy *et al.*, 2003). This relation is strongest in individuals who are normal-weight to mildly obese, and may be influenced by other factors including dietary restraint and disinhibition (Tepper and Ulrich, 2001; Lanier *et al.*, 2005; Bartoshuk *et al.*, 2006).

24.2.4 Cephalic phase responses, flavour learning and satiation

The term cephalic phase responses refers to physiological changes triggered by food- and meal-associated cues, such as the sight, smell and taste of foods and the usual location and timing of meals (Overduin and Jansen, 1997; Teff, 2000; Power and Schulkin, 2008). Several researchers (Robertson *et al.*, 2001; Arosio *et al.*, 2004) have used a 'modified sham-feeding' procedure to study these responses. Subjects are instructed to take a bite of food, keeping it in their mouths for several minutes, during which the food should be chewed but not swallowed. Thereafter, the food is expelled. Physiological responses observed during this procedure are increased salivation and flow of digestive gastric and pancreatic juices, a rise in plasma ghrelin and insulin levels, and a decrease in blood glucose (Broberg and Bernstein, 1989; Power and Schulkin, 2008). Rather than enhancing satiation or satiety, cephalic responses appear to reflect and favour appetitive and consummatory behaviours, i.e. they prime the body for smooth ingestion (salivation) and effective breakdown of food (digestive juices) and safeguard against perturbations of homeostasis (by limiting post-prandial hyperglycaemia). This raises the question whether cephalic phase physiological responses contribute significantly to satiation. The issue is currently unresolved. On the one hand, the gastrointestinally secreted peptides that are usually implicated in satiation and satiety (e.g. CCK, GLP-1, PYY) are not, or not consistently, stimulated cephalically. On the other hand, oro-sensory exposure to lipids or glucose stimulates the transfer of intestinally present triglycerides into the circulation (Mattes, 2002; Robertson *et al.*, 2003), and both of these responses could potentially contribute to satiation. One could speculate that, in the context of real meals, cephalic phase priming of food digestion and absorption could stimulate satiation by accelerated delivery of food's metabolites to the circulation. In addition, it should be noted that cephalic phase responses to aroma or sham-feeding may be biased towards appetitive responses, because the extent of retro-nasal perception of a potentially satiating aroma (Small *et al.*, 2005) may not be controlled for, as it would during normal meal intake. Cephalic phase responses are not entirely 'hard-wired', but amenable to learning experience. This is illustrated by arbitrary, non-food stimuli that may trigger them, e.g. the buzzer used by Russian physiologist Ivan Pavlov, to elicit conditioned salivation in his dogs, and the arbitrary time of the day at which pre-meal cephalic responses can be established (Woods *et al.*, 1977; Drazen *et al.*, 2006).

Importantly, alterations in flavour preference, food intake and presumably satiation can occur in the absence of cephalic phase responses following repeated exposure to flavour–food combinations (e.g. Crystal and Teff, 2006). The more general term flavour–nutrient learning applies to cases in which humans and animals alter their preference/food intake in response to experience with flavours that reliably signal caloric density or metabolic effects of a food (Mobini *et al.*, 2007). Although learned taste-aversion is a well-known example of flavour conditioning (Braveman and Bronstein, 1985), in many cases flavour–nutrient learning influences food preference and intake in ways that promote positive energy balance. For example, children readily learn to prefer food flavours paired with high caloric density of a food over those that predict fewer calories (Johnson *et al.*, 1991). These effects can also be macronutrient-specific, e.g. protein-specific hungers, provided that the previous meal was low in that macronutrient (e.g. Gibson *et al.*, 1995). This does not rule out the possibility that satiation or decreased preference for flavours signalling high nutrient density could be learned, especially during positive energy balance (Lucas and Sclafani, 1989; Gibson and Wardle, 2001; Sclafani and Acroff, 2004; Appleton *et al.*, 2006).

To summarise and conclude, the main cephalic phase physiological responses to food- and meal-related sensory stimuli seem to support appetite rather than satiation during sham feeding, although effects on satiation cannot be excluded during real feeding. Learned influences of flavour on food preference and intake can be appetitive or satiating, depending on the metabolic effects of food, and the energy state of the individual.

24.2.5 Satiation beyond the oro-nasal cavity: gastrointestinal mechanisms

Everyday expressions to describe hunger (empty stomach) and satiation (full stomach) suggest that the stomach is a prime source of satiation signals. Indeed, because of anatomical constraints, leading to rapid accumulation of ingested food in the stomach, this organ seems strategically well positioned to monitor caloric intake and signal short-term satiation.

How is satiation signalled by the stomach? Ingested food alters many stomach functions, causing, for example, receptive relaxation to accommodate the food bolus as well as increased motility and secretion of digestive juices that prime the food for intestinal absorption (Guyton and Hall, 2005). In humans, a correlation between stomach distension and satiation is evident in a number of cases. For example, diabetic patients with gastroparesis (impaired gastric emptying, leading to food retention in the stomach) experience early satiation as one of the major symptoms. Studies in healthy human subjects with a gastrically inserted inflatable bag have demonstrated an association between induced stomach distension and satiation. Interestingly, distension-induced satiation ratings were highest when nutrients had been concurrently infused into the small intestine (French and Cecil, 2001). This finding is in line with the limited and fleeting satiation resulting from ingestion of a considerable volume of non-caloric water. Long-term correlations of stomach functioning and body weight are probably limited in the general population. Obese and normal-weight subjects do not show clear differences in gastric emptying, gastric volume or gastric accommodation to food, although caloric intake by the obese is larger (Kim *et al.*, 2001; Park and Camilleri, 2005). Chronic attenuation of food intake and body weight by gastric banding surgery probably works via non-physiological mechanisms. In gastric banding surgery, a pouch is created near the oesophagal entrance to the stomach, leading to upper-gastric and oesophagal distension and back-up of food, which lowers the threshold for discomfort during meals (Schauer and Ikramuddin, 2001). In healthy individuals the stomach boundaries are elastic, so that meals are usually terminated before major distension has occurred. Thus, stomach wall tension is an important factor to control food intake.

Moving downstream from the stomach, nutrient presence in the small intestine may increase satiation acutely. Intestinal nutrients trigger a multitude of presumed satiation/satiety signals, including the release of gastrointestinal peptides such as CCK, GLP-1 and PYY (Chaudri *et al.*, 2006; Cummings and Overduin, 2007), and inhibition of the orexigenic stomach peptide, ghrelin (Overduin *et al.*, 2005, Foster-Schubert *et al.*, 2008). These peptides have widespread neural and hormonal effects that, combined with post-absorptive circulation of food metabolites, evoke satiation and maintain satiety. One of GLP-1's notable effects is its inhibition of gastric emptying by means of the so-called ileal brake, named after the area of the small intestine, the ileum, where GLP-1 is expressed most densely.

24.3 Design of tasty foods with enhanced satiation

24.3.1 Engineering sensory perception and gastrointestinal behaviour

With regard to the aforementioned need for a second generation of functional foods that may support weight management, a series of methods and technologies have been developed that assist in the development of food products that boost satiation. Both APcI-MS and olfactometry have proven to be of great importance in measuring as well as controlling aroma release and perception of foods and beverages.

Although originally developed for medical purposes, tailored olfactometer equipment is finding more and more application in (industrial) aroma research (Visschers *et al.*, 2006; Bult *et al.*, 2007; Ruijschop *et al.*, 2008), as it is able to deliver specific, well-defined aroma profiles consisting of a single or multiple aroma components. The ability to administer aroma stimuli to subjects separately from other stimuli from the food matrix (associated with other ingredients, textures and tastes) enables investigation of the relative importance of aroma stimuli for satiation. As described by Visschers *et al.* (2006), delivering food-related aroma stimuli to subjects via an olfactometer involves fine-tuning of many parameters, and delivery of aroma stimuli in a manner that reflects aroma release during food intake is a complex undertaking. The generally used approach is based on data from *in vivo* studies with real-time measurement of aroma release, using APcI-MS (Weel *et al.*, 2003; de Kok *et al.*, 2006). It has indeed been demonstrated that the aroma profile that is generated with the olfactometer closely resembles the concentration of volatiles in the oro-nasal cavity measured in individuals during ingestion of a specific food product. This enables the design of complete aroma release profiles that mimic those obtained by *in vivo* measurement during food consumption (Visschers *et al.*, 2006).

Another important tool in the engineering of enhanced satiating foods is the gustometer (or Dynataste system) – the taste equivalent of the olfactometer. The system includes a pumping device for controlled delivery of taste mixtures in a manner that resembles conditions during normal consumption (Hort and Hollowood, 2004; Bult *et al.*, 2007). Taste mixtures can be model solutions but also real food products (soups, milk, custard, etc.) that are pumped at specific flow rates and quantities into the mouth of the subject. This allows not only control of the total sample amount that is being consumed but also, when combined with an olfactometer, the delivery of any taste–aroma profile of interest. Besides sensory perception, other physical parameters during gastrointestinal passage such as meal viscosity, coagulation and emulsion stability control food intake. These food textural properties can be measured *in vitro* by *sim*ulation of *phy*siological *d*igestion (SIMPHYD). By combining simulation of *in vitro* digestion with in-line measurements of physical parameters the satiating potency of certain foods and food ingredients can be estimated. Overall, this provides a tool for engineering of the textural properties that contribute to satiation during gastrointestinal passage of food (ingredients).

24.3.2 Optimising flavour quality

When designing healthier foods, by reducing the fat, sugar and salt content or by including functional ingredients, it is important that aroma, taste and mouthfeel should never be compromised. Examples of functional ingredients are unsaturated fatty acids, flavonoids, minerals, prebiotics or soy protein (van Kleef *et al.*, 2005; Siro *et al.*, 2008). However, the application of these ingredients in foods and beverages has implications for the food flavour quality. Volatile off-flavour formation as a consequence of enzymatic and oxidative processes (e.g. in unsaturated fatty acids and soy protein; Reineccius, 1991; Leclercq *et al.*, 2007) or innate bitter taste qualities (e.g. of soy protein hydrolysates) have been reported (Seo *et al.*, 2008). As a consequence, different strategies and methods have been developed to mask both volatile and taste-related off-flavours. Volatile off-flavour perception can be masked by the addition of other volatiles that interact with the off-flavour at either receptor or perceptual level to either suppress or neutralise its perception (for aroma–aroma interactions see Oka *et al.*, 2004). Bitter taste perception can be masked by the addition of either other taste-masking compounds (taste–taste interaction (Ley *et al.*, 2005, 2006; Shah *et al.*, 2008) or volatiles (aroma–taste interaction). Unfortunately, there is no universal masking agent that solves either all volatile or all taste-related off-flavour problems. To facilitate the search for the right masking compound, several screening methods have been developed. The Olfactoscan®, for example, was developed to screen for both aroma–aroma interactions as well as aroma–taste interactions (Burseg and de Jong, 2008). So-called 'electronic tongues' are finding more and more application as screening devices for (bitter) taste-masking compounds (Legin *et al.*, 2004; Zheng and Keeney, 2006).

Also, the reduction of sugar and salt (NaCl) levels in foods and beverages has a negative impact on flavour quality. Different taste-enhancing strategies have been developed that include the addition of either sweet- or savoury-smelling aroma compounds (aroma–taste interaction; Dalton *et al.*, 2000; Hort and Hollowood, 2004; Pfeiffer *et al.*, 2006), the addition of non-volatile taste modifiers (Ottinger *et al.*, 2003; Soldo *et al.*, 2004), or the modification of food-texture properties to optimise the release and accessibility of the taste molecules to the receptors in the mouth (Cook *et al.*, 2003a; Burseg *et al.*, 2009).

24.3.3 Aroma as trigger for satiation

During the consumption of a meal, aroma molecules reach the olfactory epithelium retro-nasally (perceived as arising from the mouth). Activation of brain areas by a retro-nasally sensed food odour is associated with the perception of food and is hypothesised to contribute to satiation (Small *et al.*, 2005), i.e. sensory-related satiation.

The extent of sensory stimulation may be related to meal termination. There are indications that not all food types result in the same quality or quantity of retro-nasal aroma stimulation (Vickers and Holton, 1998). Additionally, interpersonal differences in retro-nasal aroma stimulation are of importance (Buettner *et al.*, 2002). These interpersonal differences are factors that are likely to escape control by the individual, such as saliva production, nasal anatomy, and oral processing habits (Brown *et al.*, 1996; Buettner *et al.*, 2001, 2002; Wright *et al.*, 2003; Pionnier *et al.*, 2004). It is hypothesised that difference in the extent of retro-nasal aroma stimulation is linked to interpersonal or food product differences in sensory satiation and food intake.

Using APcI-MS, *in vivo* in real-time retro-nasal aroma release was determined in 30 subjects consuming nine different food products that varied in physical structure (i.e. (semi)-liquid and solid food products) (Ruijschop

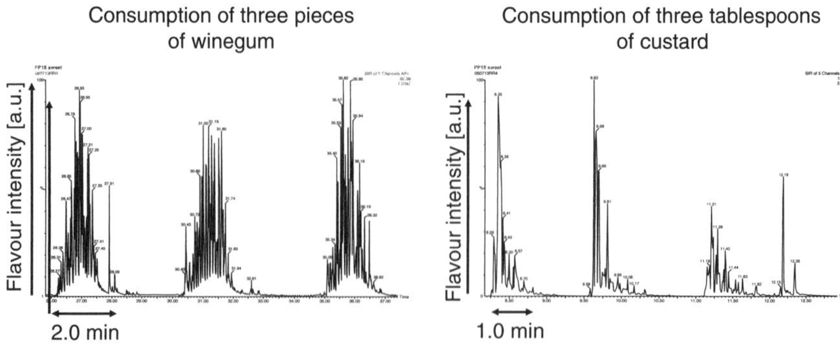

Fig. 24.3 Example of one subject, taken from Ruijschop *et al.* (2009d), illustrating the differences in the extent of retro-nasal aroma stimulation between (left) the consumption of three times one mouthful (on average 5 g per mouthful) of winegum candy ((soft) solid food) and (right) three times one mouthful (on average 19 g per tablespoon) of custard (liquid food), measured by *in vivo* APcI-MS technology (Weel *et al.*, 2003; Brauss *et al.*, 1999). As appears from the triplicate measurement, people are reproducible in the morphology and intensity of their aroma release profile (adapted from Ruijschop and Burgering, 2007; Ruijschop *et al.*, 2009a).

et al., 2009d). Absolute differences were observed between retro-nasal aroma release profiles of (semi)-liquid and solid food products, presumably due to differences in intensity and duration of oral processing (Fig. 24.3) (Ruijschop *et al.*, 2009d). The finding of differences in retro-nasal aroma release profiles associated with the type of food product consumed led us to study whether a beverage becomes more satiating when the retro-nasal aroma release profile coincides with the profile of a (soft) solid food (Ruijschop *et al.*, 2008). In a double-blind placebo-controlled randomised cross-over full factorial design, 27 healthy subjects were administered aroma profiles by a computer-controlled stimulator based on air-dilution olfactometry. Profile A reflected an aroma release profile typically observed during consumption of normal beverages. Profile B resembled that normally observed during consumption of (soft) solids. The quality of the aroma stimulus was strawberry, and it was administered in a retro-nasal fashion, while the subjects consumed a sweetened milk drink. Before, during and after sensory stimulation, appetite profile measurements were performed. A significant difference between perceived satiation during delivery of aroma release profiles A and B was observed (Fig. 24.4). Subjects felt significantly more satiated the longer the duration of the aroma stimulation ($F = 4.24$; $P = 0.04$). Despite these changes in perceived satiation, no impact was found on *ad libitum* amount consumed (Ruijschop *et al.*, 2008).

Figure 24.5 gives an overview of some of the main features that have been suggested to contribute to the extent of retro-nasal aroma stimulation and sensory satiation, from both the consumer and food product point of view. Sensitivity to (specific) aroma components and extent of *in vivo*

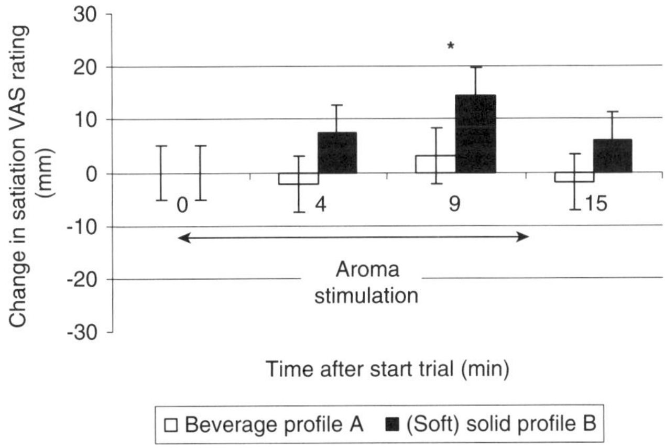

Fig. 24.4 Change in satiation visual analogue scale (VAS) rating after stimulation with aroma profile A vs. aroma profile B. Data are means with their standard errors represented by vertical bars. *Effect of *type* of aroma stimulation (profile A or B) on change in satiation VAS rating with $P < 0.05$ (Ruijschop *et al.*, 2008; adapted from Ruijschop and Burgering, 2007; Ruijschop *et al.*, 2009a).

retro-nasal aroma release (Ruijschop *et al.*, 2009d) are features that vary among individuals. In contrast, the physical structure of a food product and the oral processing it evokes (Ruijschop *et al.*, 2009d), the aroma quality (e.g. ingredient-related aroma cues; Ruijschop *et al.*, 2009b), the complexity (Ruijschop *et al.*, 2009c) and congruency in aroma and texture (Harthoorn *et al.*, 2008) are factors related more to food products with respect to the extent of retro-nasal aroma stimulation. Finally, bite size (Ruijschop *et al.*, 2009e) and eating speed have been suggested to be of importance for the extent of retro-nasal aroma stimulation, from both the subject and food product point of view. Tailoring these features may lead to a higher quality and/or quantity of sensory stimulation, which in turn may lead to enhanced feelings of satiation and ultimately contribute to a decrease in food intake.

24.3.4 Cross-modal sensory interactions as trigger for satiation

Besides aroma, taste and mouthfeel are other sensory modalities contributing to flavour perception that may interact, leading to cross-modal effects. The perceptual match of aroma with taste and mouthfeel is referred to as aroma–taste and aroma–texture congruency. Assuming that the total amount of exposure to a food's sensory properties determines the total decline in desire to eat, it is expected that an enhancement of sensory properties by a congruent aroma will further reduce the desire to eat, and boost satiation (Harthoorn *et al.*, 2008).

Viscosity is also an important physicochemical food property in sensory perception. Liquid foods appear to be less satiating than (soft) solid foods

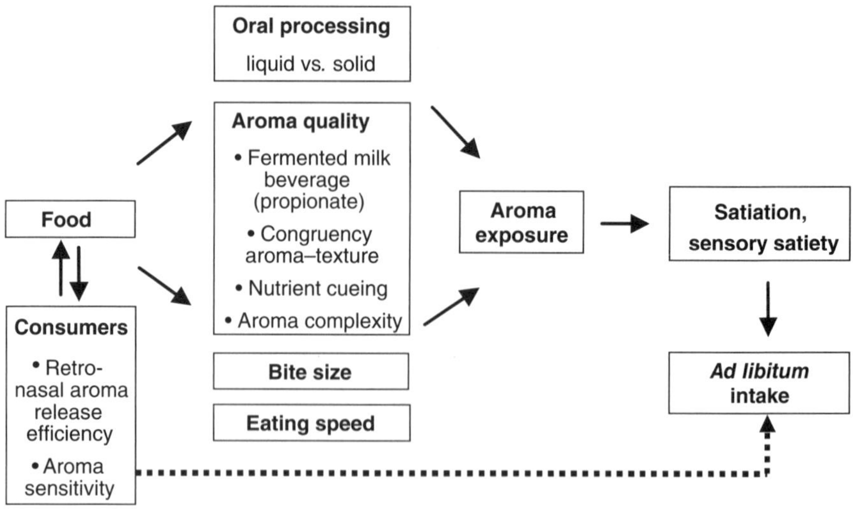

Fig. 24.5 Schematic representation of opportunities to engineer aroma-induced satiation, from both the consumer and food product points of view (adapted from Ruijschop *et al.*, 2009a).

(Mattes, 2005; Tsuchiya *et al.*, 2006). Zijlstra *et al.* (2008) demonstrated that food products different in viscosity, but similar in palatability, macronutrient composition and energy density evoke significant differences in intake. The caloric intake of the liquid was 14% higher than that of the semi-liquid and 30% higher than the semi-solid food product. This difference was partially explained by the higher eating rate for liquids. Maurao *et al.* (2007) also observed that food rheology exerts similar effects on food intake, independent of the nature of the energy source (protein, carbohydrate or fat). Caloric compensation for beverages is weaker than for solid food forms of comparable nutrient content. Thus, liquids pose a greater risk for promoting positive energy balance. Differences in structure and composition of the food and the oral processing it evokes may be (partly) responsible for this effect.

24.3.5 Gastrointestinal triggers for satiation

Meal-induced satiation signalling in the stomach is necessarily limited to a time-window of a few hours, i.e. the time it takes for the stomach to empty its food contents into the small intestine. Food design to enhance satiation and satiety based on stomach mechanisms can be aimed at controlled stomach retention and distension of the gastric wall. On the other hand, by delaying or enhancing gastric passage satiety signals occurring later than those in the stomach can be controlled. One way to achieve this is if the size of food particles is >2 mm (the diameter of the stomach exit when the pylorus is constricted), and sufficiently solid/viscous to resist immediate breakdown during antral grinding. These design principles were adopted by Hoad *et al.* (2004), who formulated beverages containing alginates, polymers that will form gel-like lumps in the acidic stomach, in the presence of calcium. Following ingestion by human subjects in this study, the alginate-containing beverages increased feelings of fullness (at defined gastric volumes) for up to 2 hours after ingestion, while suppressing hunger for up to 4 hours. The underlying mechanism probably involves slower gastric emptying due to solidification and increased antrum distension.

Another example is the principle of fast and slow proteins that differentially modulate food intake (Hall *et al.*, 2003). The underlying mechanism of slow proteins is reduced gastric passage, where these proteins precipitate and coagulate, resulting in a slower gastrointestinal passage. On the other hand, fast proteins remain soluble under gastric conditions, consequently are better accessible for proteases and reach the duodenum more rapidly to deliver their nutrients (amino acids) to the blood. This difference is seen in the whey and casein fractions of milk, which have different satiation profiles (Westerterp-Plantenga, 2003), owing partly to their different physicochemical properties. When in contact with stomach acid, casein molecules detach from milk micelles to form voluminous clumps, while whey proteins remain in solution.

In addition, the behaviour of emulsions under gastric conditions is directly related to feelings of fullness (Marciani *et al.*, 2008). An olive oil-in-water emulsion that remained stable under gastric conditions was identified to reduce gastric emptying and evoke increased fullness in comparison to its unstable equivalent.

In conclusion, these examples illustrate the interesting possibilities of altering, by technological modification, the behaviour of proteins and emulsions under stomach-like conditions. Such approaches could be used to enhance the satiating effects and efficacy of high-protein foods and emulsions that are developed for body-weight management.

24.3.6 Molecular gastronomy

In addition to the engineering of satiating food products, a reduction in portion size is also an important tool to prevent subjects from overeating. This would require focusing on food quality rather than on food quantity. Common experience indicates that subjects, when exposed to a more refined, higher-quality food product tend to consume less. For example, people will often gulp down large quantities of cheaper wines, but will more attentively sip smaller quantities of fine wines. The same holds true for having a meal in a fast-food restaurant compared with having dinner in an exclusive Michelin-star restaurant. To create food which is experienced as high in quality and exclusive, molecular gastronomy is emerging. Based on experimental and scientific cooking techniques, special combinations of foods are created to challenge the consumer by playing with their established culinary mindset and evoking surprise (e.g. This, 2006).

24.3.7 Examples of new food concepts based on sensory triggers

The application of flavours for induction of satiation seems promising and appealing. While active ingredients may induce satiety at later stages in the food intake cycle, sensory triggers operating during food ingestion have a consumer benefit that is immediately noticeable.

The results of the studies reviewed above are interesting for the development of foods containing triggers that induce or increase the feeling of satiation. For example, foods could be designed with an increase in aftertaste by lingering aroma, or with a long-chewable structure leading to substantially more oral processing and increased oral transit time and higher retro-nasal aroma release efficiency. These applications could evoke a higher quality or quantity of sensory stimulation, leading to enhanced feelings of satiation and, ultimately, decreased food intake. Enhancing the sensory stimulation of satiation influences consumers' motivational state. Perception of a food product as satiating yet low in caloric density could evoke feelings of well-being, especially in consumers who are conscious of their body weight.

24.4 Future trends

Because the epidemic of overweight and obesity, and associated co-morbidities, are forecast to increase in coming years, the demand for functional foods that prevent subjects from overeating will be high. As discussed before, control of caloric intake can be achieved via short-term (satiation) and longer-term (satiety and body weight) mechanisms. Flavour-induced satiation is expected to act primarily within meals, i.e. in the short term. In contrast, for induction of longer-lasting satiety, e.g. to suppress between-meal snacking behaviour, flavour-induced satiation is expected to be less effective. Food designs that enhance satiety often require inclusion of certain ingredients, and/or physicochemical adjustments of the food matrix to enhance or prolong nutrient availability. Useful approaches include the modification of ingredients (proteins or others) to induce gelling in the stomach for nutrient retention and stomach fill (Hoad *et al.*, 2004); altering the gastrointestinal transit times of slow proteins to increase their satiating power by shortening the time of nutrient delivery in blood; encapsulation of nutrients for slow release in the small intestine to stimulate satiety and inhibit gastric emptying (Gibson *et al.*, 2006; Gunasekaran *et al.*, 2007); and inclusion of pre- and probiotic ingredients for late-onset release and stimulation of hormone release from the colon (e.g. Delzenne *et al.*, 2005).

When designing functional foods for durable suppression of appetite, foods that combine induction of satiation and satiety would be the ultimate goal. Adopting a multidisciplinary approach that combines principles from the sensory science of flavours, gastrointestinal physiology, ingredient technology and texture design could bring the engineering of such food products within reach. Based on the aforementioned approaches it should be possible to engineer foods that not only are healthier, but at the same time reduce overall energy intake.

Also worth mentioning is that independently of the increasing prevalence of overweight and obesity, an increasing number of, for example, elderly individuals run a risk of suffering from malnutrition due to factors such as sensory impairments and frailty. Instead of engineering flavour-induced satiation, identical tools and technologies can be applied to engineer flavour-induced appetite in the design of clinical nutrition and nutrition for the frail elderly.

24.5 Acknowledgements

The work about aroma-induced satiation, referred to in Section 24.3.3, was carried out within DiOGenes. DiOGenes is the acronym of the project 'Diet, Obesity and Genes' supported by the European Community (Contract no. FOOD-CT-2005-513946). The Parties of the project are listed on the web site of the project: http://www.diogenes-eu.org/. In addition, special acknowledgement is made to the Dutch Dairy Organization for co-financing the research described in Section 24.3.3.

24.6 References

APPLETON, K M, GENTRY, R C, SHEPHERD, R (2006), 'Evidence of a role for conditioning in the development of liking for flavours in humans in everyday life', *Physiol Behav*, **87**, 478–486, doi: 10.1016/j.physbeh.2005.11.017.

AROSIO, M, RONCHI, C L, BECK-PECCOZ, P, GEBBIA, C, GIAVOLI, C, CAPPIELLO, V, CONTE, V, PERACCHI, M (2004), 'Effects of modified sham feeding on ghrelin levels in healthy human subjects', *J Clin Endocrinol Metab*, **89**, 5101–5104.

BARTOSHUK, L M, FAST, K, KARRER, T A, MARINO, S, PRICE, R A, REED, D A (1992), 'PROP supertasters and the perception of sweetness and bitterness', *Chem. Senses*, **17**, 594.

BARTOSHUK, L M, DUFFY, V B, MILLER, I J (1994), 'PTC/PROP tasting: anatomy, psychophysics, and sex effects', *Physiol Behav*, **56**, 1165–1171, doi: 10.1016/0031-9384(94)90361-1.

BARTOSHUK, L M, DUFFY, V B, HAYES J E, MOSKOWITZ, H R, SNYDER, D J (2006), 'Psychophysics of sweet and fat perception in obesity: problems, solutions and new perspectives', *Phil Trans R Soc B*, **361**, 1137–1148, doi: 10.1098/rstb.2006.1853.

BLUNDELL, J E (1999), 'The control of appetite: basic concepts and practical implications', *Schweiz Med Wochenschr*, **129**, 182–188.

BLUNDELL, J E, KING, N A (1996), 'Overconsumption as a cause of weight gain: behavioural-physiological interactions in the control of food intake (appetite)', in James P, Bouchard C and Bray G, eds., *The Origins and Consequences of Obesity*, Chichester, Wiley, 138–158.

BLUNDELL, J E, LAWTON, C L, COTTON, J R, MACDIARMID, J I (1996), 'Control of human appetite: implications for the intake of dietary fat', *Annu Rev Nutr*, **16**, 285–319, doi: 10.1146/annurev.nu.16.070196.001441.

BRAUSS, M S, BALDERS B, LINFORTH, R S T, AVISON, S, TAYLOR, A J (1999), 'Fat content, baking time, hydration and temperature affect flavour release from biscuits in model-mouth and real systems', *Flavour Fragr J*, **14**, 351–357, doi: 10.1002/(SICI)1099-1026(200001/02)15.

BRAVEMAN, N S, BRONSTEIN, P, eds. (1985), 'Experimental assessment and clinical applications of conditioned food aversion', *Ann NY Acad Sci*, **443**, 1–441.

BROBERG, D J, BERNSTEIN, I L (1989), 'Preabsorptive insulin release in bulimic women and chronic dieters', *Appetite*, **13**, 161–169, doi: 10.1016/0195-6663(89)90009-3.

BROWN, W E, DAUCHEL, C, WAKELING, I (1996), 'Influence of chewing efficiency on texture and flavour perceptions of food', *J Texture Stud*, **27**, 433–450.

BRUNSTROM, J M, MITCHELL, G L (2006), 'Effects of distraction on the development of satiety', *Br J Nutr*, **96**, 761–769, doi: 10.1079/BJN20061880.

BUETTNER, A, BEER, A, HANNING, C, SETTLES, M (2001), 'Observation of the swallowing process by application of videofluoroscopy and real-time magnetic resonance imaging-consequences for retro-nasal aroma stimulation', *Chem Senses*, **26**, 1211–1219.

BUETTNER, A, BEER, A, HANNING, C, SETTLES, M, SCHIEBERLE, P (2002), 'Physiological and analytical studies on flavor perception dynamics as induced by eating and swallowing process', *Food Qual Pref*, **13**, 497–504, doi: 10.1016/S0950-3293(02)00052-6.

BULT, J H F, DE WIJK, R A, HUMMEL, T (2007), 'Investigations on multimodal sensory integration: texture, taste, and ortho- and retronasal olfactory stimuli in concert', *Neurosci Lett*, **411**, 6–10, doi: 10.1016/j.neulet.2006.09.036.

BURSEG, K M M, DE JONG, C (2009), 'Olfactoscan: *in-vivo* screening for off-flavor solutions', in *Proceedings 12th Weurman Flavour Research Symposium*, Interlaken, *accepted for publication*.

BURSEG, K M M, HORT, J, MITCHELL, J R, TAYLOR, A J (2009), 'Flavor perception of biscuits and baked goods: biscuit composition, sweetness perception and texture', in *Abstracts of Papers of the American Chemical Society*, *in press*.

CHAUDHRI, O, SMALL, C, BLOOM, S (2006), 'Gastrointestinal hormones regulating appetite', *Philos Trans R Soc Lond B Biol Sci*, **36**, 1187–1209.

COOK, D J, HOLLOWOOD, T A, LINFORTH, R S, TAYLOR, A J (2003a), 'Oral shear stress predicts flavour perception in viscous solutions', *Chem Senses*, **28** (1), 11–23.

COOK, D J, LINFORTH, R S, TAYLOR, A J (2003b), 'Effects of hydrocolloid thickeners on the perception of savory flavors', *J Agric Food Chem*, **51**, 3067–3072, doi: 10.1021/jf0211581.

CRYSTAL, S R, TEFF, K L (2006), 'Tasting fat: cephalic phase hormonal responses and food intake in restrained and unrestrained eaters', *Physiol Behav*, **89**, 213–220, doi: 10.1016/j.physbeh.2006.06.013.

CUMMINGS, D E, OVERDUIN, J (2007), 'Gastrointestinal regulation of food intake', *J Clin Invest*, **117**, 13–23, doi: 10.1172/JCI30227.

DALTON, P, DOOLITTLE, N, NAGATA, H, BRESLIN, P A (2000), 'The merging of the senses: integration of subthreshold taste and smell', *Nat Neurosci*, **3**, 431–432, doi: 10.1002/1099-1026(200009/10)15.

DE CASTRO, J M (1987), 'Macronutrient relationships with meal patterns and mood in the spontaneous feeding behavior of humans', *Physiol Behav*, **39**, 561–569, doi: 10.1016/0031-9384(87)90154-5.

DE GRAAF, C, HULSHOF, T, WESTSTRATE, J A, JAS, P (1992), 'Short-term effects of different amounts of protein, fats, and carbohydrates on satiety', *Am J Clin Nutr*, **55**, 33–38.

DE GRAAF, C, SHREURS, A, BLAUW, Y H (1993), 'Short-term effects of different amounts of sweet and non-sweet carbohydrates on satiety and energy intake', *Physiol Behav*, **54**, 833–843, doi: 10.1016/0031-9384(93)90290-V.

DE GRAAF, C, DE JONG, L S, LAMBERS, A C (1999), 'Palatability affects satiation but not satiety', *Physiol Behav*, **66**, 681–688, doi: 10.1016/S0031-9384(98)00335-7.

DE KOK, P M T, BOELRIJK, A E M, DE JONG, C, BURGERING, M J M, JACOBS, M A (2006), 'MS-nose flavour release profile mimic using an olfactometer', in Bredie W and Petersen M A, eds., *Flavour Science, Recent Advances and Trends*, London, Elsevier, Developments in Food Science, vol. 43, 585–599.

DELZENNE, N M, CANI, P D, DAUBIOUL, C, NEYRINCK, A M (2005), 'Impact of inulin and oligofructose on gastrointestinal peptides', *Br J Nutr*, **93**, S157–S161, doi: 10.1079/BJN20041342.

DE WIJK, R A, PRINZ, J F (2005), 'The role of friction in perceived oral texture', *Food Qual Pref*, **16**, 121–123, doi: 10.1016/j.foodqual.2004.03.002.

DIOGENES PROJECT (2008), Retrieved 18 September 2008, from http://www.diogenes-eu.org.

DRAZEN, D L, VAHL, T P, D'ALESSIO, D A, SEELEY, R J, WOODS, S C (2006), 'Effects of a fixed meal pattern on ghrelin secretion: evidence for a learned response independent of nutrient status', *Endocrinology*, **147**, 23–30, doi: 10.1210/en.2005-0973.

DUFFY, V B, PETERSON, J M, DINEHART, M E, BARTOSHUK, L M (2003), 'Genetic and environmental variation in taste: associations with sweet intensity, preferences and intake', *Topics Clin Nutr*, **18**, 209–220.

FOSTER-SCHUBERT, K E, OVERDUIN, J, PRUDOM, C E, LIU, J, CALLAHAN, H S, GAYLINN, B D, THORNER, M O, CUMMINGS, D E (2008), 'Acyl and total ghrelin are suppressed strongly by ingested proteins, weakly by lipids, and biphasically by carbohydrates', *J Clin Endocrinol Metab*, **93**, 1971–1979.

FRENCH, S J, CECIL, J E (2001), 'Oral, gastric and intestinal influences on human feeding', *Physiol Behav*, **74**, 729–734, doi: 10.1016/S0031-9384(01)00617-5.

GIBSON, E L, WARDLE, J (2001), 'Effect of contingent hunger state on development of appetite for a novel fruit snack', *Appetite*, **37**, 91–101, doi: 10.1006/appe.2001.0420.

GIBSON, E L, WAINWRIGHT, C J, BOOTH, D A (1995), 'Disguised protein in lunch after low-protein breakfast conditions food-flavor preferences dependent on recent lack of protein intake', *Physiol Behav*, **58**, 363–371, doi: 10.1016/0031-9384(95)00068-T.

GIBSON, R S, PERLAS, L, HOTZ, C (2006), 'Improving the bioavailability of nutrients in plant foods at the household level', *Proc Nutr Soc*, **65**, 160–168, doi: 10.1079/PNS2006489.

GUINARD, J, BRUN, P (1998), 'Sensory-specific satiety: comparison of taste and texture effects', *Appetite*, **31**, 141–157, doi: 10.1006/appe.1998.0159.

GUNASEKARAN, S, KO, S, XIAO, L (2007), 'Use of whey proteins for encapsulation and controlled delivery applications', *J Food Eng*, **83**, 31–40, doi: 10.1016/j.jfoodeng.2006.11.001.

GUYTON, A C, HALL, J E (2005), *Textbook of Medical Physiology*, 11th ed., Philadelphia, Elsevier/Saunders.

HALL, W L, MILLWARD, D J, LONG, S J, MORGAN, L M (2003), 'Casein and whey exert different effects on plasma amino acid profiles, gastrointestinal hormone secretion and appetite', *Br J Nutr*, **89**, 239–248, doi: 10.1079/BJN2002760.

HARTHOORN, L F, RUIJSCHOP, R M A J, WEINBRECK, F, BURGERING, M J M, DE WIJK, R A, PONNE, C T, BULT, J H F (2008), 'Effects of aroma–texture congruency within dairy custard on satiation and food intake', *Food Qual Pref*, **19**, 644–650, doi: 10.1016/j.foodqual.2008.05.004.

HETHERINGTON, M M (1996), 'Sensory-specific satiety and its importance in meal termination', *Neurosci Biobehav Rev*, **20**, 113–117, doi: 10.1016/0149-7634(95)00048-J.

HETHERINGTON, M, ROLLS, B J, BURLEY, V J (1989), 'The time course of sensory-specific satiety', *Appetite*, **12**, 57–68, doi: 10.1016/0195-6663(89)90068-8.

HETHERINGTON, M M, FOSTER, R, NEWMAN, T, ANDERSON, A S, NORTON, G (2006), 'Understanding variety: tasting different foods delays satiation', *Physiol Behav*, **87**, 263–271, doi: 10.1016/j.physbeh.2005.10.012.

HIRSCH, A R, GOMEZ, R (1995), 'Weight reduction through inhalation of odorants', *J Neurol Orthop Med Surg*, **16**, 28–31.

HOAD, C L, RAYMENT, P, SPILLER, R C, MARCIANI, L, DE CELIS ALONSA, B, TRAYNOR, C, MELA, D J, PETERS, H P, GOWLAND, P A (2004), '*In vivo* imaging of intragastric gelation and its effect on satiety in humans', *J Nutr*, **134**, 2293–2300.

HOLLOWOOD, T A, LINFORTH, R S, TAYLOR, A J (2002), 'The effect of viscosity on the perception of flavour', *Chem Senses*, **27**, 583–591.

HORT, J, HOLLOWOOD, T A (2004), 'Controlled continuous flow delivery system for investigating taste–aroma interactions', *J Agric Food Chem*, **52**, 4834–4843, doi: 10.1021/jf049681y.

INTERNATIONAL OBESITY TASK FORCE (IOTF) (2008), retrieved 29 September 2008, from http://www.iotf.org.

JOHNSON, S L, MCPHEE, L, BIRCH, L L (1991), 'Conditioned preferences: young children prefer flavors associated with high dietary fat', *Physiol Behav*, **50**, 1245–1251, doi: 10.1016/0031-9384(91)90590-K.

KIM, D-Y, CAMILLERI, M, MURRAY J A, STEPHENS, D A, LEVINE, J A, BURTON, D D (2001), 'Is there a role for gastric accommodation and satiety in asymptomatic obese people?', *Obes Res*, **9**, 655–661.

KO, C W, HOFFMAN, H J, LUCCHINA, L A, SNYDER, D J, WEIFFENBACH, J M, BARTOSHUK, L M (2000), 'Differential perceptions of intensity for the four basic taste qualities in PROP supertasters versus nontasters', *Chem Senses*, **25,** 639–640.

LANIER, S, HUTCHINS, H, DUFFY, V B (2005), 'Taste and dietary predictors of central adiposity in adult females', *Chem Senses*, **30,** A34.

LECLERCQ, S, REINECCIUS, G A, MILO, C (2007), 'Effect of type of oil and addition of delta-tocopherol on model flavor compound stability during storage', *J Agric Food Chem*, **55**, 9189–9194, doi: 10.1021/jf071686i.

LEGIN, A, RUDNITSKAYA, A, CLAPHAM, D, SELEZNEV, B, LORD, K, VLASOV, Y (2004), 'Electronic tongue for pharmaceutical analytics: quantification of tastes and masking effects', *Anal Bioanal Chem*, **380**, 36–45, doi: 10.1007/s00216-004-2738-3.

LETHUAUT, L, WEEL, K G, BOELRIJK, A E, BROSSARD, C D (2004), 'Flavor perception and aroma release from model dairy desserts', *J Agric Food Chem*, **52**, 3478–3485, doi: 10.1021/jf035488c.

LEY, J P, KRAMMER, G, REINDERS, G, GATFIELD, I L, BERTRAM, H-J (2005), 'Evaluation of bitter masking flavanones from Herba Santa (*Eriodictyon californicum* (H. and A.) Torr., Hydrophyllaceae), *J Agric Food Chem*, **53**, 6061–6066, doi: 10.1021/jf0505170.

LEY, J P, BLINGS, M, PAETZ, S, KRAMMER, G E, BERTRAM, H J (2006), 'New bitter-masking compounds: hydroxylated benzoic acid amides of aromatic amines as structural analogues of homoeriodictyol', *J Agric Food Chem*, **54**, 8574–8579, doi: 10.1021/jf0617061.

LUCAS, F, SCLAFANI, A (1989), 'Flavor preferences conditioned by intragastric fat infusions in rats', *Physiol Behav*, **46**, 403–412, doi: 10.1016/0031-9384(89)90011-5.

MAIER, A, VICKERS, Z, JEFFREY INMAN, J (2007), 'Sensory-specific satiety, its crossovers, and subsequent choice of potato chip flavors', *Appetite*, **49**, 419–428, doi: 10.1016/j.appet.2007.02.006.

MARCIANI, L, FAULKS, R, WICKHAM, M S, BUSH, D, PICK, B, WRIGHT, J, COX, E F, FILLERY-TRAVIS, A, GOWLAND, P A, SPILLER, R C (2008), 'Effect of intragastric acid stability of fat emulsions on gastric emptying, plasma lipid profile and postprandial satiety', *Br J Nutr*, **5**, 1–10, doi: 10.1017/S0007114508039986.

MATTES, R D (2002), 'Oral fat exposure increases the first phase triacylglycerol concentration due to release of stored lipid in humans', *J Nutr*, **132**, 3656–3662.

MATTES, R (2005), 'Soup and satiety', *Physiol Behav*, **83**, 739–747, doi: 10.1016/j.physbeh.2004.09.021.

MAURAO, D M, BRESSAN, J, CAMPBELL, W W, MATTES R D (2007), 'Effects of food form on appetite and energy intake in lean and obese young adults', *Int J Obes*, **31**, 1688–1695, doi:10.1038/sj.ijo.0803667.

MAYER, S N, DAVIDSON, R S, HENSLEY, C B (1999), 'The role of specific olfactory stimulation in appetite suppression and weight loss', *J Adv Med*, **12**, 13–21.

MEISELMAN, H L (1996), 'The contextual basis for food acceptance, food choice and food intake: the food , the situation and the individual', in Meiselman, H L and MacFie, H J H, eds., *Food Choice, Acceptance and Consumption*, London, Blackie Academic & Professional, 239–263.

MOBINI, S, CHAMBERS, L C, YEOMANS, M R (2007), 'Effects of hunger state on flavour pleasantness conditioning at home: flavour-nutrient learning vs. flavour-flavour learning', *Appetite*, **48**, 20–28, doi: 10.1016/j.appet.2006.05.017.

O'DOHERTY, J, ROLLS, E T, FRANCIS, S, BOWTELL, R, MCGLONE, F, KOBAL, G, RENNER, B, AHNE, G (2000), 'Sensory-specific satiety related olfactory activation of the human orbitofrontal cortex', *Neuroreport*, **11**, 893–897.

OKA, Y, NAKAMURA, A, WATANABE, H, TOUHARA, K (2004), 'An odorant derivative as an antagonist for an olfactory receptor', *Chem Senses*, **29**, 815–822.

OTTINGER, H, SOLDO, T, HOFMANN, T (2003), 'Discovery and structure determination of a novel Maillard-derived sweetness enhancer by application of the comparative taste dilution analysis (cTDA)', *J Agric Food Chem*, **51**, 1035–1041, doi: 10.1021/jf020977i.

OVERDUIN, J, JANSEN, A (1997), 'Conditioned insulin and blood sugar responses in humans in relation to binge eating', *Physiol Behav*, **61**, 569–575, doi: 10.1016/S0031-9384(96)00504-5.

OVERDUIN, J, FRAYO, R S, GRILL, H J, KAPLAN, J M, CUMMINGS, D E (2005), 'Role of the duodenum and macronutrient type in ghrelin regulation', *Endocrinology*, **146**, 845–850, doi: 10.1210/en.2004-0609.

PARK, M, CAMILLERI, M (2005), 'Gastric motor and sensory functions in obesity', *Obes Res*, **13**, 491–500, doi: 10.1038/oby.2005.51.

PFEIFFER, J C, HOLLOWOOD, T A, HORT, J, TAYLOR, A J (2005), 'Temporal synchrony and integration of subthreshold taste and smell signals', *Chem Senses*, **30**, 539–545.

PFEIFFER, J C, HORT, J, HOLLOWOOD, T A, TAYLOR, A J (2006), 'Taste-aroma interactions in a ternary system: a model of fruitiness perception in sucrose/acid solutions', *Percept Psychophys*, **68**, 216–227.

PIONNIER, E, CHABANET, C, MIOCHE, L, LE QUERE, J L, SALLES, C (2004), '1. *In vivo* aroma release during eating of a model cheese: relationships with oral parameters', *J Agric Food Chem*, **52**, 557–564, doi: 10.1021/jf030544v.

POWER, M L, SCHULKIN, J (2008), 'Anticipatory physiological regulation in feeding biology: cephalic phase responses', *Appetite*, **50**, 194–206, doi: 10.1016/j.appet.2007.10.006.

PRESCOTT, J, SWAIN-CAMPBELL, N (2000), 'Responses to repeated oral irritation by capsaicin, cinnamaldehyde and ethanol in PROP tasters and nontasters', *Chem Senses*, **25**, 239–246, doi:10.1093/chemse/25.3.239.

PRESCOTT, J, JOHNSTONE, V, MUNRO, P (2001), 'Discriminability of fat content as a function of PROP sensitivity', *Chem Senses*, **26**, 800.

REINECCIUS, G A (1991), 'Off-flavors in foods', *Crit Rev Food Sci Nutr*, **29**, 381–402.

ROBERTSON, M D, JACKSON, K G, WILLIAMS, C M, FIELDING, B A, FRAYN, K N (2001), 'Prolonged effects of modified sham feeding on energy substrate mobilization', *Am J Clin Nutr*, **73**, 111–117.

ROBERTSON, M D, PARKES, M, WARREN, B F, FERGUSON, D J, JACKSON, K G, JEWELL, D P, FRAYN, K N (2003), 'Mobilisation of enterocyte fat stores by oral glucose in humans', *Gut*, **52**, 834–839.

ROLLS, E T (2004), 'Smell, taste, texture, and temperature multimodal representations in the brain, and their relevance to the control of appetite', *Nutr Rev*, **62** (11), S193–S204.

ROLLS, E T (2005), 'Taste, olfactory, and food texture processing in the brain, and the control of food intake', *Physiol Behav*, **85**, 45–56, doi: 10.1016/j.physbeh.2005.04.012.

ROLLS, B J, ROWE, E A, ROLLS, E T (1982), 'How sensory properties of food affect human feeding behaviour', *Physiol Behav*, **29**, 409–417, doi: 10.1016/0031-9384(82)90259-1.

ROMER, M, LEHRNER, J, VAN WYMELBEKE, V, JIANG, T, DEECKE, L, BRONDEL, L (2006), 'Does modification of olfacto-gustatory stimulation diminish sensory-specific satiety in humans?', *Physiol Behav*, **87**, 469–477, doi: 10.1016/j.physbeh.2005.11.015.

RUIJSCHOP, R M A J, BURGERING, M J M (2007), 'Aroma induced satiation. Possibilities to manage weight through aromas in food products', *Agro Food Industry Hi-tech*, **18**, 37–39.

RUIJSCHOP, R M A J, BOELRIJK, A E M, DE RU, J A, DE GRAAF, C, WESTERTERP-PLANTENGA, M S (2008), 'Effects of retro-nasal aroma release on satiation', *Br J Nutr*, **99**, 1140–1148, doi: 10.1017/S0007114507837482.

RUIJSCHOP, R M A J, BOELRIJK, A E M, BURGERING, M J M, DE GRAAF, C, WESTERTERP-PLANTENGA, M S (2009a), 'Novel approaches to induce satiation via aroma in foods', in *Proceedings 12th Weurman Flavour Research Symposium*, Interlaken, *accepted for publication.*

RUIJSCHOP, R M A J, BOELRIJK, A E M, BURGERING, M J M, DE GRAAF, C, WESTERTERP-PLANTENGA, M S (2009b), 'Effects of ingredient-related aroma cues on satiation and food intake', *submitted for publication.*

RUIJSCHOP, R M A J, BOELRIJK, A E M, BURGERING, M J M, DE GRAAF, C, WESTERTERP-PLANTENGA, M S (2009c), 'Acute effects of complexity in aroma composition on satiation and food intake', *submitted for publication.*

RUIJSCHOP, R M A J, BURGERING, M J M, JACOBS, M A, BOELRIJK, A E M (2009d), 'Retro-nasal aroma release depends on both subject and product differences: a link to food intake regulation?', *Chem Senses*, *accepted for publication.*

RUIJSCHOP, R M A J, ZIJLSTRA, N, BOELRIJK, A E M, BURGERING, M J M, DE GRAAF, C, WESTERTERP-PLANTENGA, M S (2009e), 'Effects of bite size and oral processing time on retro-nasal aroma release with a link to food intake regulation', *submitted for publication.*

SAINT-EVE, A, KORA-PACI, E, MARTIN, N (2004), 'Impact of flavour quality and complexity on the texture of low fat stirred yogurts assessed by three different sensory methods', *Food Qual Pref*, **15**, 655–668, doi: 10.1016/j.foodqual.2003.09.002.

SCHAUER, P R, IKRAMUDDIN, S (2001), 'Laparoscopic surgery for morbid obesity', *Surg Clinics North America*, **81**, 1145–1179.

SCLAFANI, A, ACKROFF, K (2004), 'The relationship between food reward and satiation revisited', *Physiol Behav*, **82**, 89–95, doi: 10.1016/j.physbeh.2004.04.045.

SEO, W H, LEE, H G, BAEK, H H (2008), 'Evaluation of bitterness in enzymatic hydrolysates of soy protein isolate by taste dilution analysis', *J Food Sci*, **73**, S41–S46, doi: 10.1111/j.1750-3841.2007.00610.x.

SHAH, P P, MASHRU, R C, RANE, Y M, THAKKAR, A (2008), 'Design and optimization of mefloquine hydrochloride microparticles for bitter taste masking', *AAPS PharmSciTech*, **9**, 377–389.

SHEPERD, R (1995), 'Psychological aspects of food choice', *Food Sci Technol Today*, **9**, 178–182.

SIRO, I, KAPOLNA, E, KAPOLNA, B, LUGASI, A (2008), 'Functional food. Product development, marketing and consumer acceptance – A review', *Appetite*, **51**, 456–467, doi: 10.1016/j.appet.2008.05.060.

SMALL, D M, GERBER, J C, MAK, Y E, HUMMEL, T (2005), 'Differential neural responses evoked by orthonasal versus retro-nasal odorant perception in humans', *Neuron*, **47**, 593–605, doi: 10.1016/j.neuron.2005.07.022.

SNOEK, H M, HUNTJENS, L, VAN GEMERT, L J, DE GRAAF, C, WEENEN, H (2004), 'Sensory-specific satiety in obese and normal-weight women', *Am J Clin Nutr*, **80**, 823–831.

SOLDO, T, FRANK, O, OTTINGER, H, HOFMANN, T (2004), 'Systematic studies of structure and physiological activity of alapyridaine. A novel food-born taste enhancer', *Mol Nutr Food Res*, **48**, 270–281.

SORENSEN, L B, MOLLER, P, FLINT, A, MARTENS, M, RABEN, A (2003), 'Effect on sensory perception of foods on appetite and food intake: a review of studies on humans', *Int J Obes Relat Metab Disord*, **27**, 1152–1166.

STEVENSON, R J, PRESCOTT, J, BOAKES, R A (1999), 'Confusing tastes and smells: how odours can influence the perception of sweet and sour tastes', *Chem Senses*, **24**, 627–635.

STUBBS, R J (1995), 'Macronutrient effects on appetite', *Int J Obes*, **19**, S11–S19.

STUBBS, R J, JOHNSTONE, A M, MAZLAN, N, MBAIWA, S E, FERRIS, S (2001), 'Effect of altering the variety of sensorially distinct foods, of the same macronutrient content, on food intake and body weight in men', *Eur J Clin Nutr*, **55**, 19–28, doi: 10.1038/sj.ejcn.1601117.

TEFF, K (2000), 'Nutritional implications of the cephalic-phase reflexes: endocrine responses', *Appetite*, **34**, 206–213, doi: 10.1006/appe.1999.0282.

TEPPER, B J, ULLRICH, N V (2001), 'Influence of genetic taste sensitivity to 6-n-propylthiouracil (PROP), dietary restraint and disinhibition on body mass index in middle-aged women', *Physiol Behav*, **75**, 305–312, doi:10.1016/S0031-9384(01)00664-3.

THIS, H (2006), 'Food for tomorrow? How the scientific discipline of molecular gastronomy could change the way we eat', *EMBO Rep*, **7** (11), 1062–1066.

TSUCHIYA, A, ALMIRON-ROIG, E, LLUCH, A, GUYONNET, D, DREWNOWSKI, A (2006), 'Higher satiety ratings following yoghurt consumption relative to fruit drink or dairy fruit drink', *J Am Diet Assoc*, **106**, 550–557, doi: 10.1016/j.jada.2006.01.004.

VAN DE VELDE, F, DE HOOG, E H A, RUIJSCHOP, R M A J (2008), 'Sensory perception of emulsions translating science into products', *Agro Food Industry Hi-tech*, **19** (3), 50–52.

VAN KLEEF, E, VAN TRIJP, H C, LUNING, P (2005), 'Functional foods: health claim-food product compatibility and the impact of health claim framing on consumer evaluation', *Appetite*, **44**, 299–308, doi: 10.1016/j.appet.2005.01.009.

VICKERS, Z, HOLTON, E A (1998), 'A comparison of taste test ratings, repeated consumption, and postconsumption ratings of different strengths of iced tea', *J Sensory Stud*, **13**, 199–212.

VISSCHERS, R W, JACOBS, M A, FRASNELLI, J, HUMMEL, T, BURGERING, M, BOELRIJK, A E M (2006), 'Cross-modality of texture and aroma perception is independent of orthonasal or retro-nasal stimulation', *J Agric Food Chem*, **54**, 5509–5515, doi: 10.1021/jf060533c.

WEEL, K G, BOELRIJK, A E, ALTING, A C, VAN MIL, P J, BURGER, J J, GRUPPEN, H, VORAGEN, A G, SMIT, G (2002), 'Flavor release and perception of flavored whey protein gels: perception is determined by texture rather than by release', *J Agric Food Chem*, **50**, 5149–5155, doi: 10.1021/jf0202786.

WEEL, K G C, BOELRIJK, A E M, BURGER, J J, GRUPPEN, H, VORAGEN, A G J, SMIT, G (2003), 'A protocol for measurement of *in vivo* aroma release from beverages', *J Food Sci*, **68**, 1123–1128, doi: 10.1002/ffj.1211.

WESTERTERP-PLANTENGA, M S (2003), 'The significance of protein in food intake and body weight regulation', *Curr Opin Clin Nutr Metab Care*, **6**, 635–638.

WESTERTERP-PLANTENGA, M S, PASMAN W J, YEDEMA M J W, WIJCKMANS-DUIJSENS, N E G (1996), 'Energy intake adaptation of food intake to extreme energy densities of food by obese and non-obese women', *Eur J Clin Nutr*, **50**, 401–407.

WESTERTERP-PLANTENGA, M S, LEJEUNE, M P G M, NIJS, I, VAN OOIJEN, M, KOVACS, E M R (2004), 'High protein intake sustains weight maintenance after body weight loss in humans', *Int J Obes Relat Metab Disord*, **28** (1), 57–64.

WOODS, S C, VASSELLI, J R, KAESTNER, E, SZAKMARY, G A, MILBURN, P, VITIELLO, M V (1977), 'Conditioned insulin secretion and meal feeding in rats', *J Comp Physiol Psychol*, **91**, 128–133.

WRIGHT, K M, SPRUNT, J, SMITH, A C, HILLS, B P (2003), 'Modeling flavor release from a chewed bolus in the mouth. Part 1. Mastication', *Int J Food Sci Technol*, **38**, 351–360.

ZHENG, J Y, KEENEY, M P (2006), 'Taste masking analysis in pharmaceutical formulation development using an electronic tongue', *Int J Pharm*, **310**, 118–124.

ZIJLSTRA, N, MARS, M, DE WIJK, R A, WESTERTERP-PLANTENGA, M S, DE GRAAF C (2008), 'The effect of viscosity on *ad libitum* food intake', *Int J Obes*, **32** (4), 676–683, doi: 10.1038/sj.ijo.080377.

25

Health food product composition, structure and bioavailability

G. S. M. J. E. Duchateau and W. Klaffke, Unilever Research and Development, The Netherlands

Abstract: As consumers become aware of the role functional foods can play in their personal health, the differentiating aspects of such functional foods need to be determined. One such aspect is the information provided on the bioavailability of the active ingredients responsible for functionality, which plays a role in marketing and the regulatory process. Regulators are starting to develop guidelines and criteria that take bioavailability into account. Although bioavailability is not a new term for foods, the many parameters which determine bioavailability in a food context are not understood in full. On one hand, bioavailability is controlled by the active ingredient itself, as determined by its physicochemical characteristics and the response of the human physiology upon exposure. Understanding the basic principles and physiology is, however, too simple an approach. On the other hand, for food-specific processing, the food matrix itself and the response of human physiology towards a food product and meal intake also play a role. They determine to a great extent the gastrointestinal milieu from which the active ingredient needs to be absorbed. This interplay of ingredient, matrix, gastrointestinal condition and body response, including post-absorption, has to be taken into account in determining bioavailability of a functional ingredient or in developing new functional food products. Thus the models that predict bioavailability based on physicochemical parameters should be used cautiously as other factors can be dominant. Within foods there is a need to expand these predictive models into the relevant chemical space. To test these predictions or food concepts, *in vitro* models are suitable as long as they reflect the actual intestinal conditions in the fasted or fed state. In this area considerable progress has been made, resulting in proper biorelevant models. One aspect, which is still little understood, is that of meal composition and meal conditions (e.g. is the active ingredient taken with the meal, or before or after) on bioavailability. No relevant standards have been agreed on experimental conditions, nor are all critical limits known for the physiology triggers and their inter- and intra-individual variations. To guide the functional foods researcher in this complex area, examples are given and a simple logic scheme is provided as a start in developing a bioavailability research strategy.

Key words: bioaccessibility, bioavailability, structure, functional foods.

25.1 Health foods: the role of bioavailability

25.1.1 The consumer

Consumers are showing an increased awareness towards their diet: recent surveys indicate a growing proportion of the public is well aware of the importance of a healthy diet for themselves and their families. A healthy diet is defined as consuming several servings per day of fruit and vegetables and maintaining a critical view of the daily consumption of (saturated) fat, sugar, and salt, i.e. as provided by the label information. Within this context, foods combining the three aspects of health, convenience and taste, have taken a strong and still growing market position. Consumers are interested in products which can reduce the risk of, for example, cardiovascular events, help avoid diet-related diseases, e.g. compromised 'digestive health', or help avoid nutritional deficiencies.[1] In response, regulatory bodies have set up, or are developing, guidelines or requirements to protect consumers against misleading health claims made on foods. As such, claims based about specific ingredients must be substantiated by tailored measurement or generally accepted scientific knowledge supporting availability regarding the ingredient concerned. Food product developers and producers must understand not only the mere composition of their products, but also the metabolic 'fate' of their product in order to determine the biological effects of its constituents on human physiology. This is true not only in the acute cases, but also in cases of potential long-term consumption.

25.1.2 Regulatory authorities

With the increased marketing of functional foods and the demand for healthy products as well as health-maintaining and risk-reducing diets, it has become apparent that none of the existing guidance and legal requirements of food or drugs would work for functional foods. Functional foods, although the term itself leaves quite some room for discussion (and we therefore prefer 'health food'), are neither simple foods nor pharmaceutical preparations. The definition given by the International Life Sciences Institute (ILSI) is: '...foods which provide a health benefit which goes beyond classical nutrition...'.[2] A regulatory framework for functional foods was developed, describing both the type of claims and how they should be substantiated. However, for any serious food manufacturer, the knowledge required even for a 'classical' fortified product needs to stretch beyond the fact that a given dose is added. Hence, a product can only be credibly advertised if the body can absorb it, to enable it to fully exert its intended physiological function – which should result in a quantifiable and testable outcome on body function or disease risk reduction.

Definitions and requirements for health claims based on functional foods were developed within the European Union (EU) by two subsequent projects: Functional Foods in Europe (FuFoSE) and Process for the Assessment of Scientific Support for Claims on Foods (PASSCLAIM).[3,4] As part of this thinking, it became obvious that the active ingredient on which the health claim of the functional food is based should indeed be bioavailable. As such, the draft guidance on Health Claims by the US Food and Drug Administration (FDA) (2007) refers to (bio)availability and the recent European legislation on health claims on foods (2006) discusses availability of the active ingredients to the body,[5] and with it – to some extent – the further systemic conversion of the active ingredients.

A thorough knowledge of bioavailability is also required for either expensive ingredients or cases where dose constraints are given by formulation or process. Furthermore, correcting poor bioavailability by increasing the dose per serving is limited by the recommended dietary allowance (RDA) values, since these do not differentiate between products with different bioavailability. Instead, they indicate a maximum level for the analytical content per serving.

In essence, optimizing bioavailability is also an ethical argument as it maximizes the use of resources, and the bought-in benefit for the consumer. Further to bioavailability data for the parent compound, additional detailed information on metabolism will reveal the nature of the molecule that reaches the target site, since the active species is not necessarily identical to the applied parent compound. Moreover, it might be a much better approach to formulate either the metabolite or a precursor that has a more favorable bioavailability.

Processing often has a double effect on the active: on the one hand, it might compromise the total level of active ingredient in the product due to heat or oxygen stress from the processing, but on the other hand, processing can render higher bioavailable actives. The latter is, for example, related to disintegration of plant cell structures or reducing crystal size or both with significant effects on the bioavailability of carotenoids.[6,7]

Along with the physiological value of an ingredient that is added, a thorough understanding of the physics and the chemistry of the ingredient is required. Hence, the manufacturer needs information on of the composition, the molecular identities and the complete uptake routes, metabolic processing and the kinetics of systemic circulation. Only then can the specific benefit be marketed in a believable and scientifically sound fashion. A fresh and revised view on nutritional parameters enhanced with knowledge that was gathered and developed in pharmacological sciences will thus yield better and stronger functional foods.

25.1.3 Bioavailability

Bioavailability refers to the amount of an ingested dose of a substance that reaches the systemic circulation. It is expressed as a fraction between 0 and 1 or as a percentage. The underlying assumption in the concept of bioavailability, particularly valid for functional food active ingredients, is that the active compound needs to circulate in the blood to allow entry into the target tissue somewhere else in the body. The bioavailability metric was developed in pharmacology to explain and understand differences in activity between drug compounds and between different formulations of the same active ingredient. Here it might be pointed out that sometimes the fraction absorbed is differentiated not only by the extent but also by the rate of absorption.[8]

In a further refinement of the definition, absolute bioavailability refers to the situation where an intravenous (IV) dose is used as the reference. Upon such IV dosing, the fraction entering the systemic circulation is by definition 100%. To calculate the bioavailability of the oral dose, plasma samples in both oral and IV situations are taken over a sufficient length of time to construct plasma concentration versus time curves. The Area Under the plasma concentration versus time Curve (AUC) from an oral dose relative to the AUC obtained after the IV dose is used to calculate the absolute bioavailability. Dose differences between the oral and IV dose need to be taken into account.

For functional food active ingredients, a similar approach can obviously not be taken, in that IV injections are often impossible to formulate or administer in a safe manner to volunteers. In such cases, a suitable reference can be defined, based on what is assumed the best bioavailable format for oral delivery. For example, an aqueous solution can be used as the reference in studying bioavailability from solid food formats. The bioavailability obtained in such experiments is defined as the relative bioavailability (as opposed to absolute bioavailability).

Four key subsequent processes, *a*bsorption from the gut, *d*istribution over the body, *m*etabolism and, finally, *e*xcretion shape the plasma concentration versus time curve. This step-wise description of the fate of an active ingredient is better known by the acronym 'ADME'. Product structure and composition can only influence the liberation step of the active ingredient in the gastrointestinal content, prior to actual gut-wall absorption. Influencing absorption itself and the subsequent processes is possible, but it requires chemical modification of the compound itself, a process that would change the food-like properties of the active ingredient and likely also the activity.

A consequence of this approach is that bioavailability and ADME properties are defined at the single, well-defined molecular species level. This is not so much a challenge for food active ingredients such as vitamins, minerals or single phytochemicals, but more so for compound classes to which certain effects are attributed, e.g. the definition of bioavailability or ADME of polyphenols. To get a better grip on this, it is necessary to describe as accurately as possible the chemical identity or, in case of mixtures, the composition, highlighting the key ingredient(s) with their concentration range limits. Having such a description also ensures constant quality over time. Suitable examples are the monographs as given in the Food Chemicals Codex.[9]

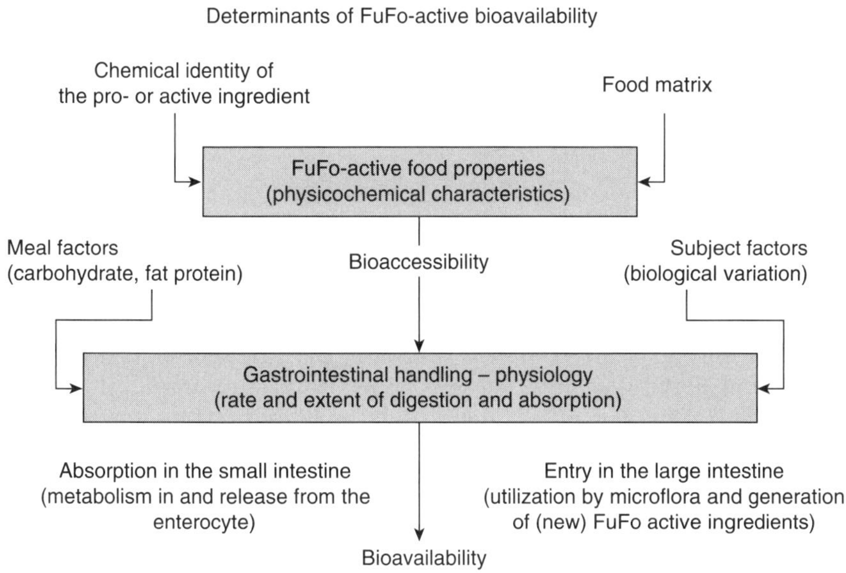

Fig. 25.1 General scheme of functional food (FuFo) active, food matrix and physiology interactions determining aspects of bioaccessibility and bioavailability.

Knowledge of the bioavailability, or proper experimental information, on all ADME parameters, is thus an important tool if not a prerequisite in communicating efficacy and mode of action of functional foods. This will result in product formulation criteria for the food active ingredient and, help in choosing a product format, and will furnish application information (dose, quantity, dietary information, RDA range limits). Bioavailability is not just a factor controlled by the active ingredient for which it is defined, but is the combined result of several aspects of the compound, the matrix from which it is delivered (the products), the content of the gastrointestinal (GI) tract as determined by, for example, meal eaten and the biology of the subject. These factors, and how they determine compound bioaccessibility and bioavailability are shown in Fig. 25.1. These factors will be discussed in subsequent sections.

As pointed out above, regulatory authorities, as well as consumers, will require a sound understanding of both the nutritional and pharmacological aspects of a functional product.

It is helpful to realize that all ingested compounds of any food are chemical entities, the chemical structure, including configuration and conformation, of which encodes the physiological effect. All factors together then define the relative position of the interacting groups with the target site. Ideally, one would like to be able to predict all of these at an atomic level, which is, however, a tedious process and not always needed. Molecular descriptors have been devised to characterize the permeation characteristics at a higher level of aggregation.

25.2 The role of physiology

To arrive within the systemic circulation, a compound has to pass several hurdles. First of all, the compound need to be released from the food matrix and go into solution in the volume-restricted, water-continuous GI content. Available areas in the human body for absorption of chemical entities are defined by (i) the surface areas and (ii) the respective physiological parameters (Table 25.1). The latter are obviously pH, transporter density (for active transport), gradients, energy supply (for active transport against gradients), efficacy of efflux transporters and transit times through the compartments.

The pH profile of the GI tract starts at about neutral in the mouth, dropping to low pH (1–2) in the stomach at the end of digestive phase. Immediately after the pylorus, pH increases to around 6 as result of the neutralizing bicarbonate from the pancreas. Along the small intestine, pH slowly increases to about 7.2 in the ileum. The pH in stomach and small intestine (SI) is logically highly dependent on whether they are in the fed or fasted state and the composition of the meal, especially the buffering capacity.[10] Colon pH is again lower, most likely as result of acid end products of bacterial fermentation[11] (see Fig. 25.2).

25.2.1 Intestinal milieu

Release and dissolution from the food matrix depend on the GI processes triggered by intake of food itself. Upon seeing, smelling and tasting of food, the GI system increases its motility, enzyme levels and fluid flows. Digestion starts with chewing and lingual enzyme effects, which are important, for example, flavour release and further triggering of physiological events such as increased GI motility and pancreatic and liver activity. The increased salivary flow contains amylases to aid food break-up within the oral cavity. In the gastric compartment, the presence of food triggers release of acid, mucus and lipolytic and proteolytic enzymes by the stomach wall. The low pH in the stomach breaks most protein-stabilized emulsions and alters the

Table 25.1 Intestinal surface areas and compartment pH

Stomach 3.5 m^2, pH 1–2
Duodenum 1.9 m^2, pH 4–5.5
Jejunum 184 m^2, pH 5.5–7
Ileum 276 m^2, pH 7–7.5
Colon 1.3 m^2, pH 7–7.5

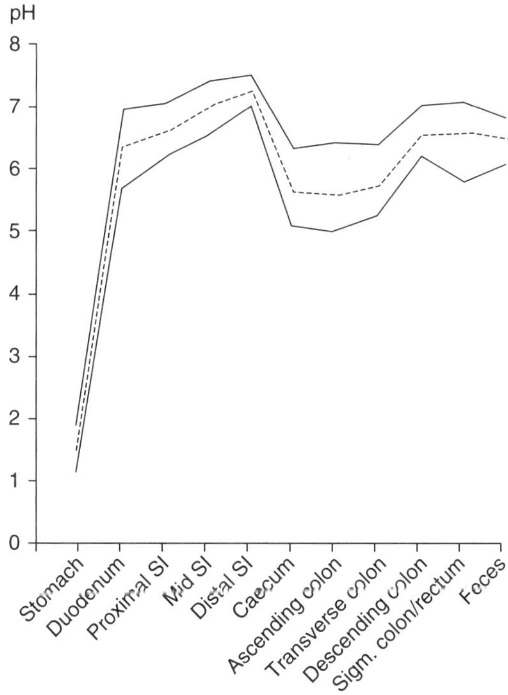

Fig. 25.2 Median and interquartile range of GI pH as measured with a radiotelemetry device. Figure taken from ref (11) with permission from the Danish Medical Bulletin.

tertiary structures of poly- and oligomeric structures (proteins and carbohydrates). The change of pH also changes the activities of the enzymes present, e.g. the enhanced activity of gastric lipase towards triglycerides at low pH.[12] The combined activity of enzymes and pH drives such small droplet emulsions into coalescence to form larger droplets. In contrast, large droplet size emulsions break up into smaller ones. Emulsification is further facilitated by the release of surface active products from triglyceride hydrolysis and small amounts of bile entering the gastric compartment from duodenal reflux.[13–15] The end result is an emulsion with droplet sizes in the range of 10–20 μm as it leaves the stomach.[16]

Further along in the small intestine, conditions change to a more neutral pH. A mix of pancreatic enzymes (proteases, lipases, amylases) is released from the pancreatic gland and bile is injected by the gall bladder, followed by a more continuous liver bile flow. Bile response from the gall bladder can be as high as a 70% release of its total volume of 20–30 mL, but depends on the amount of fat in the product or meal which serves as the main bile release trigger.[17–19]

For water-soluble compounds these GI conditions create an environment in which dissolving of active ingredients is defined by the compound's thermodynamic solubility. The assumption often made is that the aqueous volume present in the GI tract to dissolve the active ingredient is about 250 mL and small intestinal transit time is about 3–4 h.[20–24] The maximum dose or the dose held in a typical serving should dissolve and be absorbed within this volume and transit time-frame.[25] Dissolution data can easily be generated *in vitro* using simulated intestinal fluids for either the fasted or fed state.[15]

For lipophilic compounds, the situation is more complex. As these compounds are poorly soluble in water, micellization is required. Micellization takes place in the GI tract and relies on the presence of the bile acids, cholesterol, lecithin and the enzymatic hydrolysis products of triglycerides, such as free fatty acids and predominantly monoglycerides.[26] The transfer of the lipophilic compounds from the oil phase into the partially digested triglycerides and subsequently into vesicles and finally dietary mixed micelles has been studied in detail.[27–30] The strong solubilizing properties of the viscous isotropic phase formed out of the triglyceride digestion products remain intriguing.[31] The different (meso-)phases formed subsequently during the process of triglyceride digestion, e.g. from the pure oil to mono- and diglycerides, cubic and lamellar phase, and further dilution into the final aqueous micellar system show dramatic increases in solubilizing capacity towards poorly soluble lipophilic compounds. Solubility can increase by several orders of magnitude.[32–36]

25.2.2 Gut wall passage

Transport across the (small) intestinal wall can be via different mechanisms,[37] such as the following:

- *Passive*, Fickian, *diffusion*; concentration gradient driven and applicable for small, lipophilic molecules.
- *Carrier-mediated transport*; for small hydrophilic molecules. As a carrier protein is involved, this system is saturable. A further refinement can be made between the active, energy-dependent transport and passive carrier-mediated transport.
- *Endocytosis*: uptake of particles or large macromolecules. It also requires energy, is slow and limited in capacity.
- *Paracellular transport* across the tight junctions.

Opposing these mechanisms can be active, reverse transport from the intestinal cells back into the lumen or even from the circulation into the lumen. This is an important factor limiting bioavailability, as many natural compounds are substrates for these efflux transporters.

Transfer of the active into a genuine solution or into a micellized system is essential, as the epithelial cells can only absorb active ingredients from solutions. Once in a genuine solution or micellar state, the active ingredient has to pass the GI wall via entry into the cells lining the gut wall (epithelium). Inside these cells, the active ingredient might be metabolized, as the gut wall is a metabolically active tissue. Also, the compound might be recognized by the body as 'not essential' or even potentially harmful and be actively exported out of the epithelial cells back into the lumen of the gut.

Large particle uptake (pinocytosis) is possible, but the capacity is very limited and not physiologically relevant.[38] New nanoparticle technologies try to solve this, but the question remains, though, whether one would like to circumvent the selectivity of physiological uptake processes. Often, these processes have a feedback regulation and protective function. Circumventing normal uptake processes and their feedback loop via nanoparticle technology is thus subject to debate.[39–41]

25.2.3 Presystemic metabolism

The fraction of the dose delivered by the product or meal and which goes into solution is, in principle, available for uptake by the gut wall. This is also referred to as the bioaccessible part; the fraction of the dose which is theoretically available for absorption.[42] Presystemic metabolism, however, can still influence this theoretically available concentration. Examples for this are the breakdown of flavanol scaffolds or the deglycosylation of glycosidic structures by gut bacteria and the mucosal layer. This can have a large impact on the amount absorbed, the site where it is absorbed and whether activity is explained from the parent molecules or via the (fermentation) metabolites. For example, soy isoflavones, naturally present mostly as their glycosides, are not absorbed in significant amounts from the human small intestine, whereas the aglycones are absorbed.[43,44] The non-absorbed glycosides enter the colon and via colon fermentation even more active molecules (phyto-estrogens) can be formed.[45] The food chemistry thus determines the site of absorption as well as the possible fermentation fate (see Fig. 25.3). The ordering of factors involved in bioaccessibility and bioavailability are given in Fig. 25.4. The balance between either passive or active influx and efflux govern the intracellular concentrations.

Bioaccessibility, by and large, is defined by the dose that is dissolved during GI transit, more strictly the duodenal–jejunal part. Thus, it is aimed at complete and rapid dissolution of the given dose, in a reasonable amount of fluid matching with the small-intestinal content and volume. Typical transit times for the upper GI tract are 60 minutes in volumes of about 250 mL.

For the actual crossing of the gut wall of the total or nearly complete bioaccessible part of the dose, the effective permeation rate (P_{eff}) is the determining factor. A good relationship has been found between the human gut wall permeation rate P_{eff} and the actual fraction absorbed.[46,47] These two factors combined are used in what is called the Bio-pharmaceutical Classification System (BCS[48]). The use of this system allows prediction of human intestinal absorption based on these two factors. For functional food active

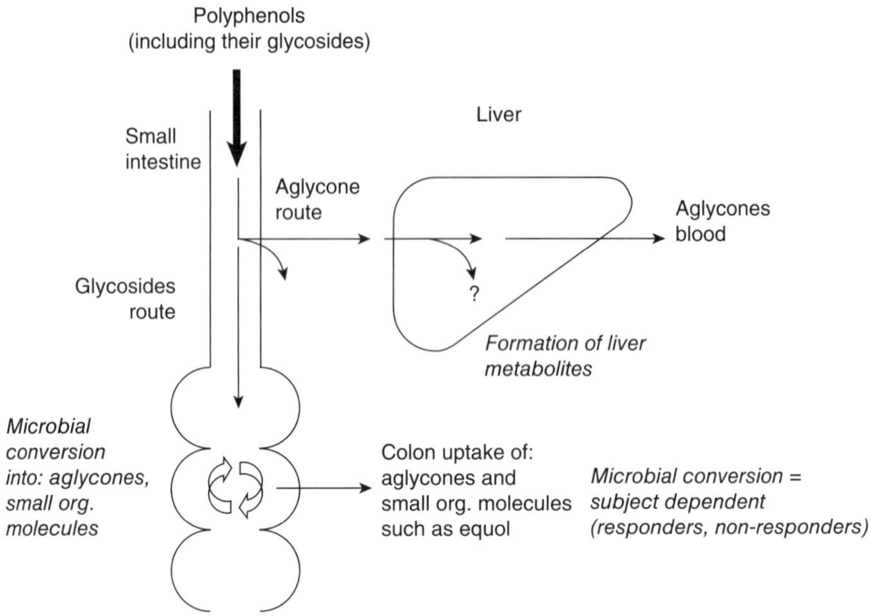

Fig. 25.3 Scheme of polyphenol uptake.

ingredients, the value of this approach could be that it will tell whether uptake is limited by the compound's physicochemical descriptors (e.g. via a limited or slow solubility) or by the actual transport rate, or a combination of the two. Both factors are measured with *in vitro* models, simplifying the approach. For the effective human permeation rate (P_{eff}), which is difficult to measure *in vivo* in humans, the alternative permeation rate across a cell line mimicking the small intestine can be used. It is important to validate or cross-correlate the results obtained in these models with actual data obtained in humans.[47,49]

25.2.4 Liver first-pass effect

The fraction of the dose which is indeed absorbed by the gut wall must not be confused with the bioavailable part. The mesenteric venous system draining from the gut flows first via the liver into the systemic circulation, and consequently, further metabolism might occur in the liver. This liver extraction immediately after absorption is referred to as the first-pass effect. Hence, the fraction absorbed (by the gut wall) is not necessarily the fraction bioavailable to the body. There could be a difference depending on the extent of liver first-pass metabolism, which again depends on the molecular structure of the circulating compound.

Food structure → Bioaccessibility → Bioavailability

Bioaccessibility:

- matrix release
- compound solubility
- gastrointestinal stability

Bioavailability:

- gut wall permeability
- metabolic stability
- excretion

Fig. 25.4 Factors involved in bioaccessibility and bioavailability.

The differentiation between uptake via the portal vein route or via the lymphatic pathway in the form of chylomicrons depends on the physicochemical properties ($\log P$) of the compound. For fatty acids this effect has been studied in more detail and the differentiation is at about carbon number (CN) of 12 (lauric acid). The calculated and experimental $\log P$ values of lauric acid are 5.00 and 4.60, respectively, hence a $\log P$ value of 5 is often used as a means of determing which route will be followed.[50]

So, fatty acids with a CN above 12 and highly lipophilic compounds will be transported into the lymph. However, to be micellized, not only do the compounds need to be lipophilic, but all the other building blocks needed to create the mixed micellar system should be present: free fatty acids, monoglycerides, phospholipids, bile acids, cholesterol. These building blocks are only available if enough substrate for triglyceride hydrolysis is present, as well as ample bile and enzymes. The presence of phospholipids from either bile or product is especially critical for chylomicron formation.[51] The trigger for this flow of micellar building blocks is the presence of free fatty acids released by lipases. Estimates for minimal intake amount of triglycerides to fully trigger GI motility, bile and pancreatic secretions are undefined, but range from as low as 2 g to above 25 g.[17,18]

As discussed in the two sections above, the final bioavailable fraction of the dose ingested, i.e. available for systemic circulation, is the end result of a step-wise reduction process. For optimal bioavailability, the reduction in any step should be as small as possible (Fig. 25.5). The initial steps are determined by physicochemical parameters of the active ingredient and food structure (bioaccessibility); subsequently biochemistry and physiology become more important.

25.3 Bioaccessibility parameters

According to the parameters as outlined in Figs 25.1 and 25.4, we can separate bioaccessibility from the overall bioavailability. In order to be bioaccessible, a hierarchy of various parameters can be set up as requirements:

- The molecular solubility, or simply whether or not the compound is soluble and how much of it can be dissolved in an equilibrium situation. As in all equilibria, the constant K is defined by the quotient of the

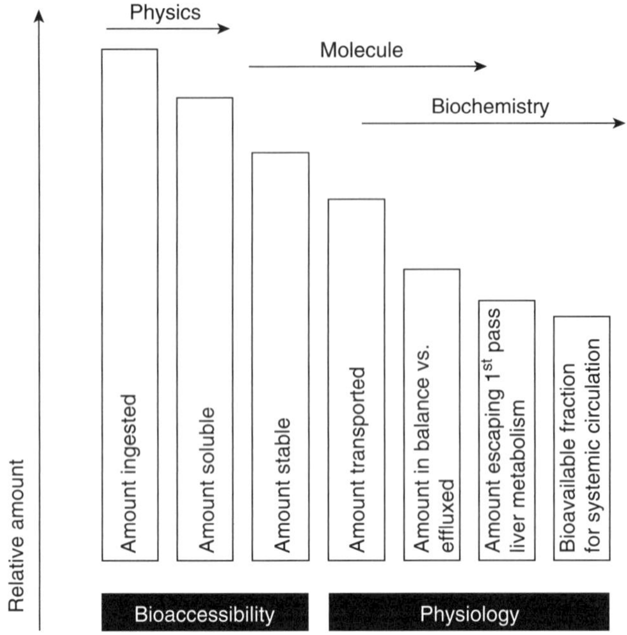

Fig. 25.5 Ordering of factors in bioaccessibility and bioavailability.

activities of the dissolved over the solid. The activity of the latter is set to 1 by definition, and hence K_S = [dissolved]. For ionic compounds, which will dissociate, the expression becomes the solubility product, $K_{SP} = [A^+][B^-]$.

- The temperature controls solubility as well as the molecular diffusion constant. In biological systems this effect, however, can be excluded as it is constant at 37 °C.
- Particle size plays a role in dissolution, since thermodynamic solubility only applies strictly for large monocrystals. Since additional surface energy mounts up, smaller crystals will dissolve more easily than larger ones. This can shift the thermodynamic equilibrium, since parameters such as surface tension of the solute particles will play a more dominant role.
- The situation of the thermodynamic equilibrium is statically influenced by parameters such as the free enthalpies of dissolution and crystallization (the crystal lattice energy that influences the thermodynamic solubility), but dynamic influence through the rate of dissolution also plays a role in living systems. Since the passage through the GI tract adds a spatial dimension to the time, a favorable equilibrium state obtained through slow solubilization rates can be as detrimental as a faster rate ending up in an unfavorable equilibrium.

- The final parameters to be mentioned here are molecular mass, polar surface area and ionizability. A given compound may well be soluble in aqueous media, but will be limited in permeation through lipid membranes. Either the compound lacks sufficient lipophilicity, is ionized, protonated or deprotonated at physiological pH, or is simply too large (molecular mass). Typically, these parameters are bundled into the 'rule-of-five' as derived from large drug molecule data sets.[52] All these parameters are also time dependent since, during passage, both pH and uptake processes may differ.

25.4 Release of the active ingredients from the food matrix

Probably the best studied group of food actives in this respect are carotenoids and lycopene, and interest is based on their antioxidant properties and, for some, also their role as pro-vitamin A. These compounds are present in relatively high concentrations in fruits (tomatoes) and vegetables (bell peppers, carrots, etc.), but are typically enclosed in the plant cell material and in the form of crystals. On top of that, carotenoids are poorly soluble, highly lipophilic compounds requiring uptake into micelles to allow gut wall crossing and transport into lymph.[42,53–55] The release from the food matrix depends heavily on the level of food processing and the presence of fat.

To assess the release from the matrix and the transfer to either the aqueous phase or the micellar phase, several systems are described. Critical here is that the fluids mimicking the GI content match with the *in vivo* situation. The presence of bile salts, lecithin, partial glycerides and cholesterol as well as enzymes strongly influences wetting and solubility properties. Suitable, biorelevant systems, which reflect recent knowledge on the actual GI content based on intubation studies are described in several papers.[14,15,56] Models to study the release range from simple stirred vessels known as dissolution models (Fig. 25.6), to complex systems such as the TNO Intestinal Model (TIM) model or the stomach model from Institute of Food Research (IFR).[57,58] More recently, it has been shown that the subtle grinding forces developed between food particles in different parts of the stomach are also important for release.[59,60] This is where food structure, physicochemical properties and physiology meet.

The dissolution system has been used to study release from carotenoids from encapsulates. Tiny encapsulates (100–300 μm) containing carotenoids are one way to include high levels of these strong coloring agents into a fat-continuous system such as a margarine. Without the use of the encapsulates, the matrix would be dark orange, versus a better situation with only a few tiny encapsulates, barely visible to the naked eye. In this application it was essential, prior to any human confirmation on the actual *in vivo* uptake, to test different encapsulate prototypes. To do so, the USP dissolution model was used and clearly demonstrated the impact of encapsulate matrix sensitivity for GI enzymes (Fig. 25.7).

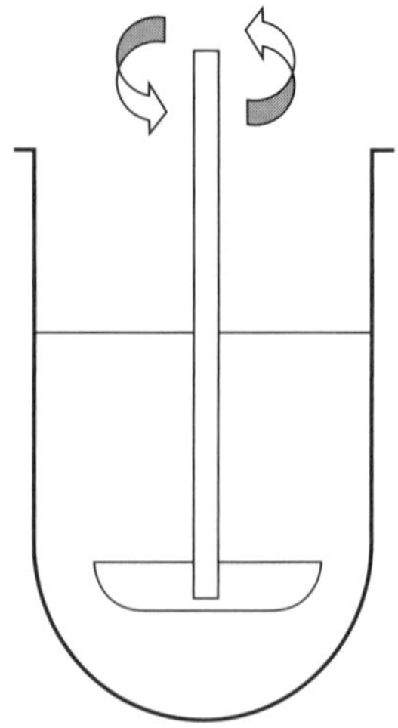

Fig. 25.6 USP dissolution apparatus, model 2 (paddle system). Typical conditions: 900 mL of simulated GI fluid, stirring at 50–100 rpm, 37°C, precisely described geometry of glass vessel and paddle and the paddle position from bottom.

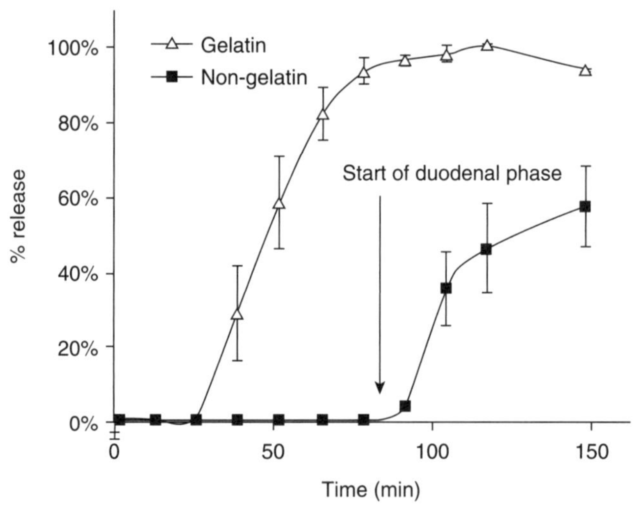

Fig. 25.7 Carotenoids release as tested in simulated GI conditions using the USP paddle apparatus for gelatin and non-gelatin (carbohydrate)-based encapsulates. Gelatin encapsulates disintegrate in the gastric phase, maximizing contact time with lipid, whereas a non-gelatin system only disintegrates in the small intestinal phase.

Iron deficiency is the most prevalent nutritional deficiency, affecting as much as 40% of the world's population.[61] Many food fortification programmes are ongoing to solve this. However, iron is a compound that is difficult to handle in this context as the different forms have quite different physicochemical behavior (solubility range, redox activity). The actual daily net amount needed to be taken up is quite small (1–2 mg/day), but food matrix effects can influence either product or uptake and the maneuvering space for dosing is small given the low RDA (in Europe, 14 mg for adults). Iron forms which can be used for food fortification or in supplements, range from simple reduced, but insoluble iron, to poorly soluble salts (e.g. iron fumarate) and fully soluble salts and complexes (iron sulfate, sodium–iron–EDTA (ethylenediaminetetraacetic acid). The bioavailability properties of these different forms can be classified in about the same order. At the same time, product stability and organoleptic properties in general seem to follow the reverse order.

For ample uptake into the small intestinal cells, the poorly soluble iron salts need to dissolve first in the acidic gastric environment, where they form a complex array of hydroxo complexes, depending on the local pH. For the poorly soluble and inexpensive reduced iron forms, the solubility rate in dilute acid is the main factor predicting *in vivo* effects.[62,63] In situations where gastric secretion is compromised, iron uptake from those poorly soluble salts is reported to be lower.[24] Choice of the iron fortificant is recommended by the WHO based on their solubility, but even within the same chemical form, *in vitro* differences might exist (Fig. 25.8).

As iron has strong redox properties, food systems with a high water concentration are notoriously different. Iron (as well as copper) promotes

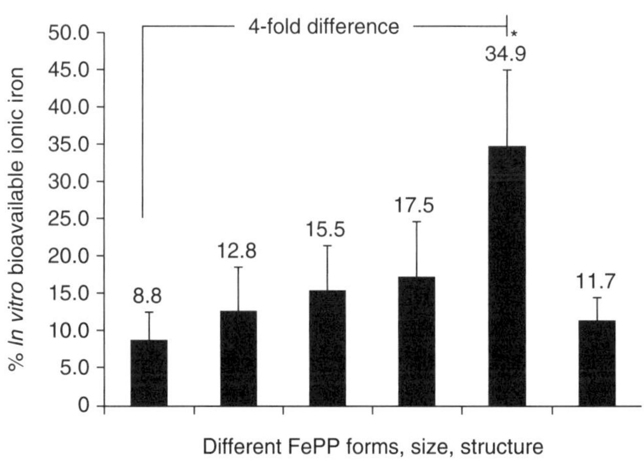

Fig. 25.8 Dialyzable iron as measured from a range of different iron pyrophosphate (FePP) commercial sources. A difference as wide as a factor of four can be seen.

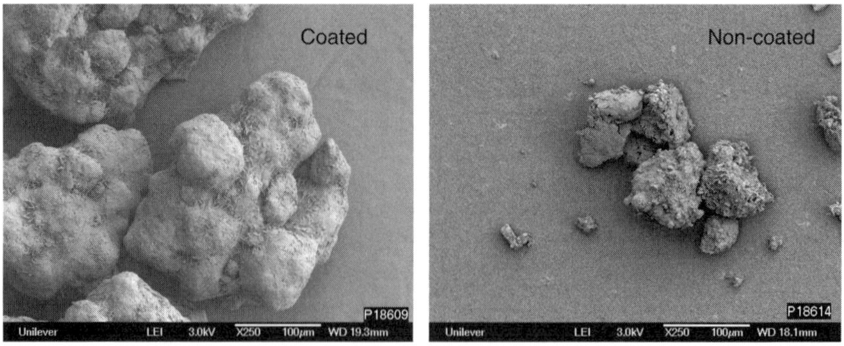

Fig. 25.9 Electron micrographs showing encapsulated and non-encapsulated ferro-fumarate.

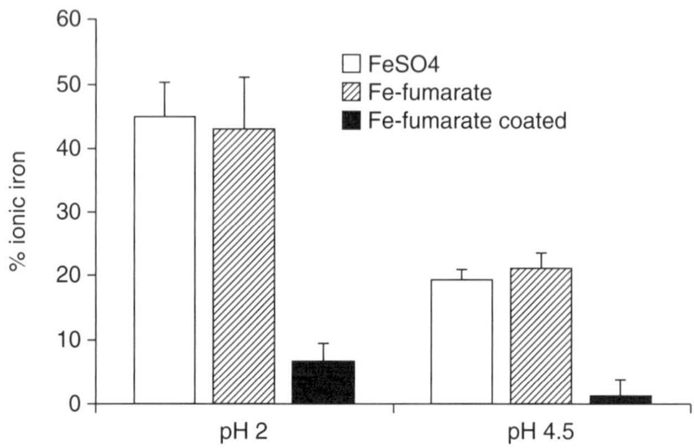

Fig. 25.10 Iron *in vitro* bioavailability measured as the dialyzable iron fraction for a fully water-soluble iron salt ($FeSO_4$), and a poorly soluble iron salt (Fe-fumarate), tested as such and with edible fat coating. Experiments ($n = 3$) were done at pH 2 and 4.5 to simulate the pH impact as seen in a compromised gastric function.

the oxidation process of unsaturated fatty acids. In such a system, use of less soluble or encapsulated iron forms can be a solution. Unilever has used iron-fumarate in various products for the Turkish and Indian markets with very acceptable organoleptics and stability profile. Use of soluble complexes such as EDTA is another option, but iron–sodium–EDTA is not generally accepted as food grade.

The release of iron from encapsulates, used for taste improvement of the poorly water-soluble iron form (fumarate), influenced the dialyzable fraction in an *in-vitro* model compared with the non-encapsulated form and iron sulfate (Figs 25.9 and 25.10). The pH sensitivity as shown in this case is of importance where stomach pH might be higher as normal (children, *Helicobacter pylori* infection[24]).

25.5 Physicochemical properties and bioavailability

In the pharmaceutical context, the lack of suitable bioavailability characteristics of new compounds contributes, together with toxicity problems, to the high attrition rate in developmental drugs. This has forced scientists to review the molecular properties, which can be linked to favorable human bioavailability and create rules based on this to use in early screening. Filters derived from this are so-called Lipinski or Veber (or other) rules; many refinements on these rules exist.[52,64] The key requirements are that:

- compounds need to dissolve within the time-frame of GI passage in a relatively small volume of water or simulated intestinal fluid (solubility *S*);
- the dose (*D*) should not exceed this *D*/*S* limit of about 250 mL;
- compounds need to match the Lipinski or Veber requirements with respect to molecular size, proton binding aspects and log *P*, to allow a high permeation rate across the intestinal wall;
- compounds should stay in solution, not degrade chemically or enzymatically, precipitate or form insoluble salts.

A thorough review of the molecular design rules for developmental drugs has been presented by Thomas *et al.*[65] Part of that set of rules is applicable to functional food active ingredients as well. In selecting or ranking compounds of interest, simple *in vitro* tests can be used to obtain this information. The actual solubility in systems mimicking the aqueous GI milieu can be assessed by methods that are standardized for temperature, shear, volume and composition. It is important that media used in these kind of tests reflect the GI fluid composition accurately to be reliable in their prediction of the *in vivo* situation.[15,56]

25.6 Gastrointestinal stability of the active ingredient

Besides the compound properties and the interaction with the cells lining the gut wall, direct chemical or enzymatic processing in the intestinal milieu can limit the bioaccessibility, simply because the amount of active ingredient is reduced due to chemical instability or enzymatic breakdown. Bioactive peptides have been proposed for several interesting functional food activities such as cholesterol lowering or blood pressure control. From a food perspective, peptides are very attractive as being common dietary components. For the functional effect, one may assume that a certain plasma concentration needs to be reached after intake. The human digestive system is designed to break down proteins and peptides very efficiently in the so-called proteolytic barrier, built from the luminal enzymes (gastric and small intestinal proteases) to finally even proteolytic enzymes in plasma. The likelihood of a reasonable peptide bioavailability is thus low and indeed experiments on the absolute bioavailability of particular tripeptides showed very low systemic exposure (~0.1%) with very rapid elimination half-lives in pigs.[66] It is unlikely that high plasma concentrations are reached after oral intake due to the efficient proteolytic barrier.

Interestingly, the enzyme activity present in the gut or gut wall can also be used to release the compound of interest from a precursor. This 'pro-drug' principle is used for vitamin-C-2-O-glycosides or -phosphates. These vitamin C derivatives are stable in product formulation, the redox reaction being blocked by derivatization of the functional groups involved in the process. After ingestion, vitamin C is released again from the C-2-O-derivative as it is hydrolyzed by the brush border enzyme α-glucosidase in the gut.[67]

25.7 Meal factors

25.7.1 Composition and structure of food matrix

Food intake triggers a number of physiological responses. However, the intensity of these responses depends on the macronutrient composition of the food. The emptying rate from the stomach is about 2–2.5 kcal/min as energy content is the main predictor of gastric emptying.[68,69] The composition also determines the buffer capacity and hence the pH changes in time upon gastric secretion. The time course of digestion and the transport rate from the gastric compartment to the small bowel depend on the energy density and viscosity.[68,70,71] In fact, gastric emptying is by no means a linear, homogeneous process and solids and liquids may empty at different rates;[72,73] even more so, fats and the aqueous phase may empty separately.[74] Gastric emptying, especially for liquid meals, follows a power equation, whereas for solid meals a time shift of about 30 minutes or more takes place.[72]

25.7.2 Meal and food format effects

As discussed earlier, for lipophilic compounds which rely on the presence of bile, pancreatic fluid, edible fats and GI motility to create, dissolve and transfer into the micellar space, a meal might be critical if the product is (too) low in calories from fat to act as an independent trigger. Examples of such food ingredients are the carotenoids and plant sterols (PS).

Factors influencing carotenoid bioaccessibility and bioavailability have been extensively studied. These factors range from processing of the plant material to finally the events in the GI tract. The range of factors have been captured in the acronym SLAMENGHI (Species, molecular Linkage, Amount, Matrix, Effectors of absorption and bioconversion, Nutrient status, Genetic factors, Host-related factors and Interactions). More recently, these acronym-captured factors were reviewed to detect gaps in knowledge in the area.[75] The known factors such as processing to release the carotenoids from the plant cellular matrix and the impact of fat have been reported and can be applied to most, though not all, carotenoids.[6] New insights in cellular active uptake and efflux mechanisms at the intestinal wall indicate that some of these processes are also valid for carotenoids. Here a gap in knowledge is identified.

The hypothesized micellar interaction of PS with cholesterol for intestinal uptake as the cholesterol lowering mechanism is indeed influenced by timing of the product and meal. Simultaneous consumption of a low-calorie drink containing a PS fatty acid ester (PSE) with a meal resulted in a larger effect on plasma cholesterol than separate consumption (9.1% low-density lipoprotein (LDL) lowering versus 6.0%).[76] A meta-analysis on all PSE and PS published studies indicated possible effects of food format and timing, but effects are not significant. There are few systematic studies in this area that focus on meal effects.[77]

25.7.3 Active-matrix (in-)compatibilities

In many cases the preferred consumer format is already defined for mundane reasons, such as similarity to the product already accepted in the marketplace, cost constraints, processing equipment constraints, minimal shelf-life, etc. As a result of this, freedom in optimizing active and matrix with respect to bioavailability no longer exists. In such situations, incompatibilities may occur, impacting release or bioavailability. On top of that, specific products, which are fine on their own with respect to bioaccessibility or bioavailability, will be used in a meal situation introducing compromising agents. Also, the opposite can be true and certain ingredients combined in a product or meal situation can promote the uptake of functional actives. Figure 25.11

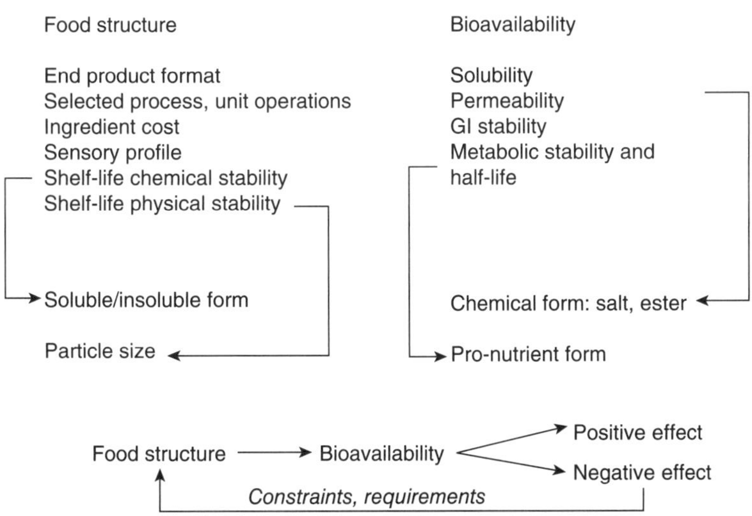

Fig. 25.11 Opposite nature of drives for food formulation and bioavailability.

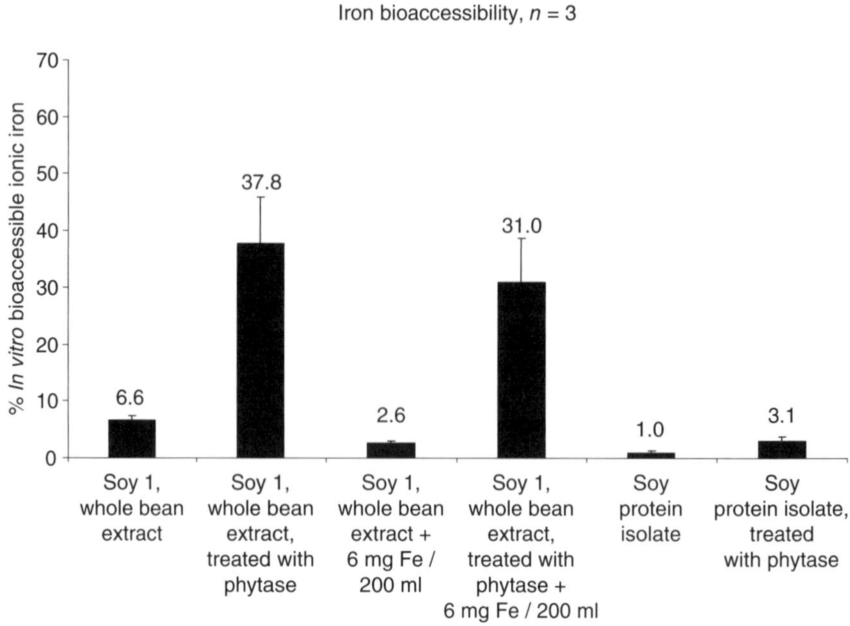

Fig. 25.12 Impact of phytase treatment on *in vitro* iron bioavailability. The test was performed in a USP dissolution II system, followed by a dialysis membrane step.

lists the often opposite nature of the drivers for food formulation and bioavailability. Some typical examples of such ingredient–food or meal matrix interactions are now given.

Iron–phytate interaction

One particular challenge is the low iron intake, typical for a vegetarian diet, with the high level of phytate from the vegetables. The strong phytate–iron interaction compromises bioaccessibility from the iron-fortified food product in a meal situation. The WHO has therefore recommended a decrease in the molar ratio of phytate–iron to below 1 or even 0.5 to ensure acceptable iron uptake.[61] The effect of, for example, phytases to improve this balance can be studied *in vitro* with a suitable model; see Fig. 25.12.[78] To a lesser extent, the same metal–ligand complexation mechanism plays a role for calcium and oxalate, although it is less critical, as calcium daily intake is much higher (hundreds of milligrams) than iron (tenths of milligrams). Also, oxalate intake is low.[79]

Iron–ascorbic acid interaction

This is an interesting example, as ascorbic acid has a double role here. The ionic form of iron, especially the Fe^{2+} form, forms a soluble metal–ligand complex with ascorbic acid with the proper dissociation constant. This prevents the iron from binding or complexing with, for example, proteins or polyphenols into non-absorbable complexes. At the same time, ascorbic acid is required to maintain the redox cycle by the intestinal cell surface enzyme ferri-reductase which converts Fe^{3+} to Fe^{2+}. The positive effect of ascorbic acid on iron bioavailability is well described and used in commercial products. The same positive effect on iron absorption via suitable solubilization in the form of a complex can be achieved via sodium–iron–EDTA. Although not allowed in most countries at the level required for that purpose, iron from sodium–iron–EDTA has a much better bioavailability than, for example, iron sulfate. Again, the complex formed has the right solubility and dissociation constant in the GI milieu to allow optimal uptake of iron by the intestinal iron transporter.[61]

Polyphenol–protein interaction

High polyphenol intake has been linked to a range of beneficial effects, most often explained via their antioxidant properties.[80] The oral bioavailability of most polyphenols is, however, dramatically low, about 10% or less and is the topic of many researchers (see the special issue of *Molecular Pharmaceutics*[81] and also Yang *et al.*[82]). The unfavorable physicochemical characteristics of these molecules in relation to bioavailability may be further compromised by the strong interaction with dietary proteins,[83,84] which can be to such a great extent that the attributed health effects are negated.[85]

Calcium salts and bioavailability

A high calcium intake during the period in which bone formation is still ongoing ensures a higher bone mass and might reduce the risk of fracture in later life. Calcium intake from the diet can be too low (calcium RDA is high, as high as 1300 mg/day for certain groups in the US recommendations) and calcium-containing food products or supplements can correct for this. For food use, calcium can be selected, from soluble to insoluble salts, including the oxide. The bioavailability of calcium from all these different chemical forms is close to 30%, despite huge differences in solubility. The overruling effect here is that the acidic stomach provides conditions that are favourable for dissociation into the ionic form.

25.8 'Practical guide'

With the many parameters involved in bioaccessibility and bioavailability, some guidance in the form of a number steps would be helpful. There is, however, no 'golden rule' which applies to all situations (i.e. active and format combination). However, if we appreciate that the compound as such needs to be bioavailable at an acceptable level, we can formulate some general requirements for the matrix. For water-soluble compounds, this is simpler than for lipophilic, poorly soluble compounds.

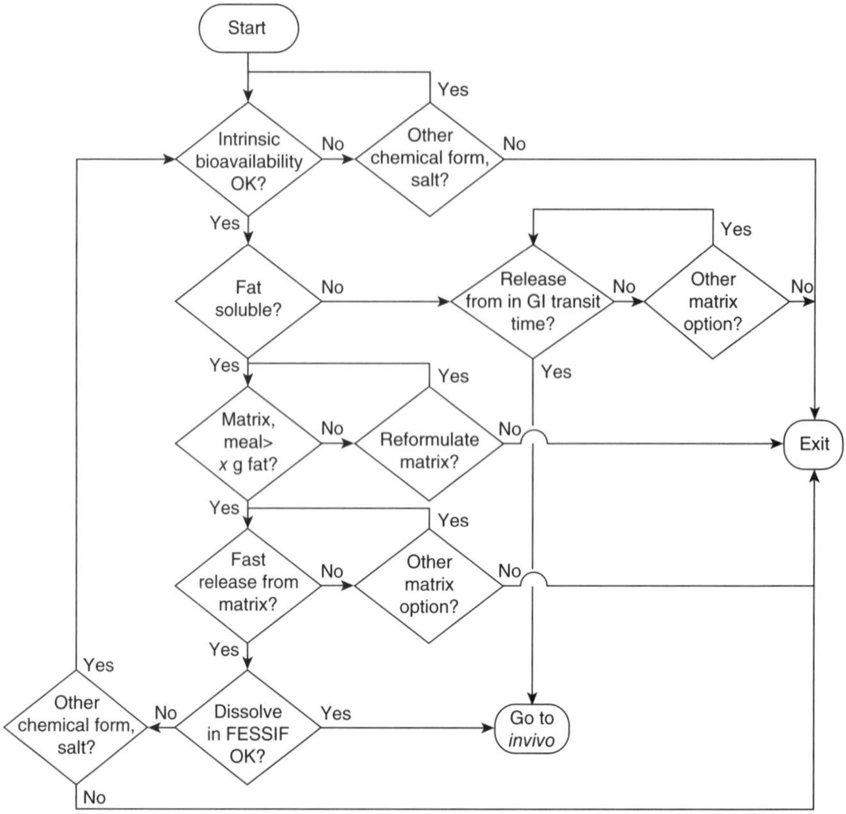

Fig. 25.13 Simplified flow diagram explaining steps and decision points to pass upon formulating an active ingredient into a food, while maintaining bioavailability (FESSIF = Fed State Simulated Intestinal Fluid[15]).

As a practical guide, the flow chart (see Fig. 25.13) outlines the principles for the improvement work that needs to be done. Here, factors such as intrinsic bioaccessibility (solubility, etc. see above), and liberation from the food matrix (mainly physical effects) of the compound(s) of interest are being studied and lead to a range of possible actions. Lastly, items such as palatability and stability throughout the intestinal passage need to be addressed.

When confronted with the task of formulating and including an active ingredient into a food, the first step will be to check the intrinsic bioavailability, as defined by solubility, p*K*, ionic form, etc. (discussed in Section 25.5 above). Hence, if that is not given, one needs to check for other routes to change the chemical form, by food grade chemical operations, such as esterification, oxidation, condensation with amines to yield Schiff bases, (chemo-enzymatic) phosphorylation or transformation into soluble ion-pairs. Should this route not yield any intrinsically bioavailable product, the room for manipulation is exhausted, and a search has to be made for alternative active ingredients or the case must be closed.

If the compound is lipophilic, but the solubility in a micellar system is sufficient, the question arises, whether the food product or the meal contains a fat amount that is below or above a critical threshold. There is no clear-cut limit here, but the fat amount required to trigger ample bile flow and GI motility is typically above 2–5 g. If there is ample fat, then the kinetics of release from such matrix is decisive; if the amount is below the critical concentration, either a reformulated matrix is needed or the route must be abandoned. The last hurdle for the accessibility issue is the solubility in fed-state (postprandial) intestinal fluid.

25.9 Conclusion

In developing and bringing functional foods to the market, a thorough knowledge of bioavailability is increasingly important, to substantiate the claim in order to achieve consumer acceptance or the regulatory approval. Food formulators must appreciate that bioavailability is built from several interdependent factors, ranging from the molecular properties of the active ingredient, to the food format and product structure itself, including its intended use, e.g. in the context of a meal or typical diet and the subsequent physiological responses of the GI tract upon ingestion. This complexity requires that the basic design rules can no longer be used, based on cost, taste, processing, shelf-life, etc. To design functional food formats which should show optimal bioavailability of the active ingredient, one also has to understand the processes taking place in the GI tract, such as luminal effects (dissolution, enzyme action), transport across the intestinal wall (role of permeation, impact of transporters and gut wall metabolism) to, ultimately, events after absorption (chylomicron uptake, metabolism). This new dimension in food design brings new challenges for the structures and compositions required as a simple analytical content claim no longer suffices.

For some active ingredients, such as water solubles, this is a simpler task and models and design rules keeping track of pH and solubility effects can easily be applied. More complex, though, is the design of food systems or food structures which ensure the proper bioavailability of poorly soluble, lipophilic functional compounds. Here, it is not only the food itself that should be taken into account to address the low solubility, but also the physiological response upon ingestion of the product either alone or as part of a meal.

Design rules and models to arrive at optimal bioavailability are available from, for example, the pharma area, but the large differences in the typical molecules and product formats that are common in food as opposed to pharma area result in a knowledge gap. In particular, this is true for the more lipophilic compounds and the minimal GI triggers required to allow sufficient solubilization and uptake. Further building on these rules and models in a structured way is required to improve the bioavailability of functional active ingredients from novel food structures.

25.10 Acknowledgements

Silvia Miret, Monique van de Burg and Serpil Tascioglu are kindly acknowledged for the information provided on the iron compounds. Our colleagues from the Food Structural Design department of Unilever R&D Vlaardingen are thanked for giving us insight in aspects of food formulation.

25.11 References

1. IFIC; *Consumer Attitudes Toward Functional Foods/Foods for Health*; International Food Information Council, Washington; 2007.
2. VERSCHUREN, P.M.; Functional Foods – Scientific and Global Perspectives; *ILSI Europe Report Series*; Vol. 1, p. Brussels; 2002.
3. BELLISLE, F.; Functional foods in Europe – theme papers; *British Journal of Nutrition*; 1998, Vol. 80, p. 1–193.
4. DIPLOCK, A.T., AGGETT, P.J., ASHWELL, M. *et al.*; Scientific concepts of functional foods in Europe consensus document; *British Journal of Nutrition*; 1999, Vol. 81, no. 4, p. S1–S27.
5. Regulation (EC) No. 1924/2006 of the European Parliament and of the Council of on nutrition and health claims made on foods; 2006.
6. SOUTHON, S.; Model systems *in vitro* and *in vivo*, for predicting the bioavailability of lipid soluble components in food; Final Report FAIR CT97–3100; 2001.
7. PARADA, J., AGUILERA, J.M.; Food microstructure affects the bioavailability of several nutrients; *Journal of Food Science*; 2007, Vol. 72, no. 2, p. R21–R32.
8 Title 21 – Food and Drugs Chapter I – Food and Drug Administration, Department of Health and Human Services – Continued Part 320 – Bioavailability and Bioequivalence Requirements; 21CFR320; 2000.
9 Food Chemicals Codex, 6th edn; United States Pharmacopeia, Rockville, MD; 2008.
10. DRESSMAN, J.B., BERARDI, R.R., DERMENTZOGLOU, L.C. *et al.*; Upper gastrointestinal (GI) pH in young, healthy-men and women; *Pharmaceutical Research*; 1990, Vol. 7, no. 7, p. 756–761.
11. FALLINGBORG, J.; Intraluminal pH of the human gastro-intestinal tract; *Danish Medical Bulletin*; 1992, Vol. 46, no. 3, p. 183–196.
12. CHAHINIAN, H., SNABE, T., ATTIAS, C. *et al.*; How gastric lipase, an interfacial enzyme with a Ser-His-Asp catalytic triad, acts optimally at acidic pH; *Biochemistry*; 2006, Vol. 45, no. 3, p. 993–1001.
13. VERTZONI, M., DRESSMAN, J., BUTLER, J. *et al.*; Simulation of fasting gastric conditions and its importance for the *in vivo* dissolution of lipophilic compounds; *European Journal of Pharmaceutics and Biopharmaceutics*; 2005, Vol. 60, no. 3, p. 413–417.
14. KALANTZI, L., GOUMAS, K., KALIORAS, V. *et al.*; Characterization of the human upper gastrointestinal contents under conditions simulating bioavailability/bioequivalence studies; *Pharmaceutical Research*; 2006, Vol. 23, no. 1, p. 165–176.

15. JANTRATID, E., JANSSEN, N., REPPAS, C. *et al.*; Dissolution media simulating conditions in the proximal human gastro intestinal tract; an update; *Pharmaceutical Research*; 2008, Vol. 25, no. 7, p. 1663–1676.
16. ARMAND, M., BOREL, P., PASQUIER, B. *et al.*; Physicochemical characteristics of emulsions during fat digestion in human stomach and duodenum; *American Journal of Physiology – Gastrointestinal and Liver Physiology*; 1996, Vol. 34, no. 1, p. G172–G183.
17. STONE, B.G., ANSEL, H.J., PETERSON, F.J. *et al.*; Gallbladder emptying stimuli in obese and normal-weight subjects; *Hepatology*; 1992, Vol. 15, no. 5, p. 795–798.
18. FROEHLICH, F., GONVERS, J.J., FRIED, M.; Role of nutrient fat and cholescystokinin in regulation of gallbladder emptying in man; *Digestive Diseases and Sciences*; 1995, Vol. 40, no. 3, p. 529–533.
19. KOSSENA, G.A., CHARMAN, W.N., WILSON, C.G. *et al.*; Low dose lipid formulations: effects on gastric emptying and biliary secretion; *Pharmaceutical Research*; 2007, Vol. 24, no. 11, p. 2084–2096.
20. PRIEBE, M.G., WACHTERS-HAGEDOORN, R.E., STELLAARD, F. *et al.*; Oro-cecal transit time: influence of a subsequent meal; *European Journal of Clinical Investigation*; 2004, Vol. 34, no. 6, p. 417–421.
21. SCHILLER, C., FROHLICH, C.P., GIESSMANN, T. *et al.*; Intestinal fluid volumes and transit of dosage forms as assessed by magnetic resonance imaging; *Alimentary Pharmacology and Therapeutics*; 2005, Vol. 22, no. 10, p. 971–979.
22. PRIEBE, M.G., WACHTERS-HAGEDOORN, R.E., LANDMAN, K. *et al.*; Influence of a subsequent meal on the oro-cecal transit time of a solid test meal; *European Journal of Clinical Investigation*; 2006, Vol. 36, no. 2, p. 123–126.
23. HOAD, C.L., MARCIANI, L., FOLEY, S. *et al.*; Non-invasive quantification of small bowel water content by MRI: a validation study; *Physics in Medicine and Biology*; 2007, Vol. 52, no. 23, p. 6909–6922.
24. SARKER, S.A., DAVIDSSON, L., MAHMUD, H. *et al.*; *Helicobacter pylori* infection, iron absorption, and gastric acid secretion in Bangladeshi children; *American Journal of Clinical Nutrition*; 2004, Vol. 80, p. 149–153.
25. JOHNSON, K.C., SWINDELL, A.C.; Guidance in the setting of drug particle size specifications to minimize variability in absorption; *Pharmaceutical Research*; 1996, Vol. 13, no. 12, p. 1795–1798.
26. CLARYSSE, S., TACK, J., LAMMERT, F. *et al.*; Postprandial evolution in composition and characteristics of human duodenal fluids in different nutritional states; *Journal of Pharmaceutical Sciences*; 2009, Vol. 98, no. 3, p. 1177–1192.
27. RIGLER, M.W., HONKANEN, R.E., PATTON, J.S.; Visualization by freeze fracture, *in-vitro* and *in-vivo*, of the products of fat digestion; *Journal of Lipid Research*; 1986, Vol. 27, no. 8, p. 836–857.
28. STAGGERS, J.E., HERNELL, O., STAFFORD, R.J. *et al.*; Physical-chemical behavior of dietary and biliary lipids during intestinal digestion and absorption. 1. Phase-behavior and aggregation states of model lipid systems patterned after aqueous duodenal contents of healthy adult human-beings; *Biochemistry*; 1990, Vol. 29, no. 8, p. 2028–2040.
29. HERNELL, O., STAGGERS, J.E., CAREY, M.C.; Physical-chemical behavior of dietary and biliary lipids during intestinal digestion and absorption. 2. Phase-analysis and aggregation states of luminal lipids during duodenal fat digestion in healthy adult human-beings; *Biochemistry*; 1990, Vol. 29, no. 8, p. 2041–2056.
30. FENNEL EVANS, D., WENNERSTRÖM, H.; 4.4 Micellar solution play a key role in many industrial and biological processes; In: *The Colloidal Domain; Where Physics, Chemistry, Biology and Technology Meet*; VCH Publishers Inc., New York, 1999; p. 198–216.

31. PATTON, J.S., CAREY, M.C.; Watching fat digestion; *Science*; 1979, Vol. 204, no. 4389, p. 145–148.
32. KOSSENA, G.A., CHARMAN, W.N., BOYD, B.J. *et al.*; Probing drug solubilization patterns in the gastrointestinal tract after administration of lipid-based delivery systems: a phase diagram approach; *Journal of Pharmaceutical Sciences*; 2004, Vol. 93, no. 2, p. 332–348.
33. PERSSON, E.M., GUSTAFSSON, A.-S., CARLSSON, A.M. *et al.*; The effects of food on the dissolution of poorly soluble drugs in human and small intestinal fluids; *Pharmaceutical Research*; 2005, Vol. 22, no. 12, p. 2141–2151.
34. KAUKONEN, A.M., BOYD, B.J., CHARMAN, W.N. *et al.*; Drug solubilization behavior during *in vitro* digestion of suspension formulations of poorly water-soluble drugs in triglyceride lipids; *Pharmaceutical Research*; 2004, Vol. 21, no. 2, p. 254–260.
35. KAUKONEN, A.M., BOYD, B.J., PORTER, C.J.H. *et al.*; Drug solubilization behavior during *in vitro* digestion of simple triglyceride lipid solution formulations; *Pharmaceutical Research*; 2004, Vol. 21, no. 2, p. 245–253.
36. PORTER, C.J.H., POUTON, C.W., CUINE, J.F. *et al.*; Enhancing intestinal drug solubilisation using lipid-based delivery systems; *Advanced Drug Delivery Reviews*; 2008, Vol. 60, p. 673–691.
37. BARTHE, L., WOODLEY, J., HOUIN, G.; Gastrointestinal absorption of drugs: methods and studies; *Fundamental and Clinical Pharmacology*; 1999, Vol. 13, no. 2, p. 154–168.
38. HUSSAIN, N., JAITLEY, V., FLORENCE, A.T.; Recent advances in the understanding of uptake of microparticulates across the gastrointestinal lymphatics; *Advanced Drug Delivery Reviews*; 2001, Vol. 50, no. 1–2, p. 107–142.
39. LOMER, M.C.E., HUTCHINSON, C., VOLKERT, S. *et al.*; Dietary sources of inorganic microparticles and their intake in healthy subjects and patients with Crohn's disease; *British Journal of Nutrition*; 2004, Vol. 92, no. 6, p. 947–955.
40. DESAI, M.P., LABHASETWAR, V., AMIDON, G.L. *et al.*; Gastrointestinal uptake of biodegradable microparticles: effect of particle size; *Pharmaceutical Research*; 1996, Vol. 13, no. 12, p. 1838–1845.
41. ACOSTA, E.; Bioavailability of nanoparticles in nutrient and nutraceutical delivery; *Current Opinion in Colloid and Interface Science*; 2009, Vol. 14, no. 1, p. 3–15.
42. HEDREN, E., DIAZ, V., SVANBERG, U.; Estimation of carotenoid accessibility from carrots determined by an *in vitro* digestion method; *European Journal of Clinical Nutrition*; 2002, Vol. 56, no. 5, p. 425–430.
43. KANO, M., TAKAYANAGI, T., HARADA, K. *et al.*; Bioavailability of isoflavones after ingestion of soy beverages in healthy adults; *Journal of Nutrition*; 2006, Vol. 136, p. 2291–2296.
44. ULLMAN, U., METZNER, J., FRANK, TH. *et al.*; Safety, tolerability, and pharmacokinetics of single ascending doses of synthetic genistein (Bonistein™) in healthy volunteers; *Advances in Therapy*; 2005, Vol. 22, no. 1, p. 65–78.
45. DECROOS, K., EECKHAUT, E., POSSEMIERS, S. *et al.*; Administration of equol-producing bacteria alters the equol production status in the simulator of the gastrointestinal microbial ecosystem (SHIME); *Journal of Nutrition*; 2006, Vol. 136, p. 946–952.
46. WINIWARTER, S., BONHAM, N.M., AX, F. *et al.*; Correlation of human jejunal permeability (*in vivo*) of drugs with experimentally and theoretically derived parameters. A multivariate data analysis approach; *Journal of Medicinal Chemistry*; 1998, Vol. 41, no. 25, p. 4939–4949.
47. LENNERNAS, H.; Human intestinal permeability; *Journal of Pharmaceutical Sciences*; 1998, Vol. 87, no. 4, p. 403–410.

48. ANONYMOUS; US Department of Health and Human Services, Food and Drug Administration, Center for Drug Evaluation and Research (CDER); Guidance for Industry: waiver of *in vivo* bioavailability and bioequivalence studies for immediate-release solid oral dosage forms based on a biopharmaceutics classification system. Available from http://www.fda.gov/cder/guidance/3618fnl.pdf
49. MIRET, S., ABRAHAMSE, S.L., DE GROENE, E.M.; Comparison of *in vitro* models for the prediction of compound absorption across the human intestinal mucosa; *Journal of Biomolecular Screening*; 2004, Vol. 9, no. 7, p. 598–606.
50. CHARMAN, W.N.A., STELLA, V.J.; Estimating the maximal potential for intestinal lymphatic transport of lipophilic drug molecules; *International Journal of Pharmaceutics*; 1986, Vol. 34, no. 1–2, p. 175–178.
51. MANSBACH, C.M., GORELICK, F.; Development and physiological regulation of intestinal lipid absorption. II. Dietary lipid absorption, complex lipid synthesis, and the intracellular packaging and secretion of chylomicrons; *American Journal of Physiology – Gastrointestinal and Liver Physiology*; 2007, Vol. 293, no. 4, p. G645–G650.
52. LIPINSKI, C.A., LOMBARDO, F., DOMINY, B.W. *et al.*; Experimental and computational approaches to estimate solubility and permeability in drug discovery and development settings; *Advanced Drug Delivery Reviews*; 1997, Vol. 23, no. 1–3, p. 3–25.
53. VAN HET HOF, K.H., WEST, C.E., WESTSTRATE, J.A. *et al.*; Dietary factors that affect the bioavailability of carotenoids; *Journal of Nutrition*; 2000, Vol. 130, no. 3, p. 503.
54. LI, E., TSO, P.; Vitamin A uptake from foods; *Current Opinion in Lipidology*; 2003, Vol. 14, no. 3, p. 241–247.
55. ODEBERG, J.M., LIGNELL, A., PETTERSSON, A. *et al.*; Oral bioavailability of the antioxidant astaxanthin in humans is enhanced by incorporation of lipid based formulations; *European Journal of Pharmaceutical Sciences*; 2003, Vol. 19, no. 4, p. 299–304.
56. VERTZONI, M., FOTAKI, N., KOSTEWICZ, E. *et al.*; Dissolution media simulating the intraluminal composition of the small intestine: physiological issues and practical aspects; *Journal of Pharmacy and Pharmacology*; 2004, Vol. 56, no. 4, p. 453–462.
57 United States Pharmacopeia 31; General chapters: Physical Tests and Determinations; ⟨711⟩ Dissolution; In: USP31/NF26; 2009; p. 1578–1579.
58. MINEKUS, M., SMEETS-PEETERS, M.J.E., BERNALIER, A. *et al.*; A computer-controlled system to simulate conditions of the large intestine with peristaltic mixing, water absorption and absorption of fermentation products; *Applied Microbiology and Biotechnology*; 1999, Vol. 53, no. 1, p. 108–114.
59. KONG, F., SINGH, R.P.; A model stomach system to investigate disintegration kinetics of solid foods during gastric digestion; *Journal of Food Science*; 2008, Vol. 73, no. 5, p. E202–E210.
60. KONG, F., SINGH, R.P.; Disintegration of solid foods in human stomach; *Journal of Food Science*; 2008, Vol. 73, no. 5, p. R67–R79.
61. ALLEN, L., DE BENOIST, B., DARY, O., HURRELL, R.F.; Guidelines on food fortification with micronutrients; World Health Organization and Food and Agriculture Organization of the United Nations, Geneva; 2006.
62. LYNCH, S.; The precision of *in vitro* methods and algorithms for predicting the bioavailability of dietary iron; *International Journal for Vitamin and Nutrition Research*; 2005, Vol. 75, no. 6, p. 436–445.
63. LYNCH, S.; A comparison of methods for estimating the bioavailability of elemental iron food fortificants; *Faseb Journal*; 2006, Vol. 20, no. 4, p. A623.

64. VEBER, D.F., JOHNSON, S.R., CHENG, H.-Y. *et al.*; Molecular properties that influence the oral bioavailability of drug candidates; *Journal of Medicinal Chemistry*; 2002, Vol. 45, p. 2615–2623.
65. THOMAS, V.H., BHATTACHAR, S., HITCHINGHAM, L. *et al.*; The road map to oral bioavailability: an industrial perspective; *Expert Opinion on Drug Metabolism and Toxicology*; 2006, Vol. 2, no. 4, p. 591–608.
66. VAN DER PIJL, P.C., KIES, A.K., TEN HAVE, G.A. *et al.*; Pharmacokinetics of proline-rich tripeptides in the pig; *Peptides*; 2008, Vol. 29, no. 12, p. 2196–2202.
67. TAI, A., FUJINAMI, Y., MATSUMOTO, K. *et al.*; Bioavailability of a series of novel acylated ascorbic acid derivatives, 6-*O*-acyl-2-*O*-alpha-D-glucopyranosyl-L-ascorbic acids, as an ascorbic acid supplement in rats and guinea pigs; *Bioscience Biotechnology Biochemistry*; 2002, Vol. 66, no. 8, p. 1628–1634.
68. HUNT, J.N., SMITH, J.L., JIANG, C.L.; Effect of meal volume and energy density on the gastric emptying of carbohydrates; *Gastroenterology*; 1985, Vol. 89, no. 6, p. 1326–1330.
69. HUNT, J.N., STUBBS, D.F.; The volume and energy content of meals as determinants of gastric emptying; *Journal of Physiology*; 1975, Vol. 245, p. 209–225.
70. HUNT, J.N., KNOX, M.T.; A relation between the chain length of fatty acids and the slowing of gastric emptying; *Journal of Physiology*; 1968, Vol. 194, p. 327–336.
71. HUNT, J.N., CASH, R., NEWLAND, P.; Energy density of food, gastric emptying, and obesity; *Lancet*; 1975, Vol. 2, no. 7941, p. 905–906.
72. SIEGEL, J.A., URBAIN, J.L., ADLER, L.P. *et al.*; Biphasic nature of gastric-emptying; *Gut*; 1988, Vol. 29, no. 1, p. 85–89.
73. PAL, A., BRASSEUR, J.G., ABRAHAMSSON, B.; A stomach road or 'Magenstrasse' for gastric emptying; *Journal of Biomechanics*; 2007, Vol. 40, no. 6, p. 1202–1210.
74. MARCIANI, L., WICKHAM, M., SINGH, G. *et al.*; Enhancement of intragastric acid stability of a fat emulsion meal delays gastric emptying and increases cholecystokinin release and gallbladder contraction; *American Journal of Physiology – Gastrointestinal and Liver Physiology*; 2007, Vol. 292, no. 6, p. G1607–G1613.
75. BOREL, P.; Factors affecting intestinal absorption of highly lipophilic food microconstituents (fat-soluble vitamins, carotenoids and phytosterols); *Clinical Chemistry and Laboratory Medicine*; 2003, Vol. 41, no. 8, p. 979–994.
76. DOORNBOS, A.M.E., MEYNEN, E.M., DUCHATEAU, G.S.M.J.E. *et al.*; Intake occasion affects the serum cholesterol lowering of a plant sterol-enriched single-dose yoghurt drink in mildly hypercholesterolaemic subjects; *European Journal of Clinical Nutrition*; 2006, Vol. 60, no. 3, p. 325–333.
77. DEMONTY, I., RAS, R., VAN DER KNAAP, H.C.M. *et al.*; Continuous dose–response relationship of the LDL-cholesterol lowering effect of phytosterol intake: a meta-analysis of randomised controlled trials; *Journal of Nutrition*; 2008, vol. 139, p. 271–284.
78. MILLER, D.D., SCHRICKER, B.R., RASMUSSEN, R.R. *et al.*; An *in-vitro* method for estimation of iron availability from meals; *American Journal of Clinical Nutrition*; 1981, Vol. 34, no. 10, p. 2248–2256.
79. GUEGUEN, L., POINTILLART, A.; The bioavailability of dietary calcium; *Journal of the American College of Nutrition*; 2000, Vol. 19, no. 2, p. 119S–136S.
80. GRAF, B.A., MILBURY, P.E., BLUMBERG, J.B.; Flavonols, flavones, flavanones, and human health: epidemiological evidence; *Journal of Medicinal Food*; 2005, Vol. 8, no. 3, p. 281–290.
81. HU, M.; Commentary: Bioavailability of flavonoids and polyphenols: call to arms; *Molecular Pharmaceutics*; 2007, Vol. 4, no. 6, p. 803–806.
82. YANG, C.S., SANG, S., LAMBERT, J.D. *et al.*; Bioavailability issues in studying the health effects of plant polyphenolic compounds; *Molecular Nutrition and Food Research*; 2008, Vol. 52 Suppl 1, p. S139–S151.

83. PAPADOPOULOU, A., FRAZIER, R.A.; Characterization of protein–polyphenol interactions; *Trends in Food Science and Technology*; 2004, Vol. 15, no. 3–4, p. 186–190.
84. GREEN, R.J., MURPHY, A.S., SCHULZ, B. *et al.*; Common tea formulations modulate *in vitro* digestive recovery of green tea catechins; *Molecular Nutrition and Food Research*; 2007, Vol. 51, no. 9, p. 1152–1162.
85. LORENZ, M., JOCHMANN, N., VON KROSIGK, A. *et al.*; Addition of milk prevents vascular protective effects of tea; *European Heart Journal*; 2007, Vol. 28, no. 2, p. 219–223.

26

Coenzyme Q_{10}: functional benefits, dietary uptake and delivery mechanisms

I. Amar-Yuli, A. Aserin and N. Garti, The Hebrew University of Jerusalem, Israel

Abstract: Coenzyme Q_{10}, present in all cells and membranes, is essential for electron transport in the mitochondrial respiratory chain, antioxidant defence, and other functions of great importance for cellular metabolism. The essential advantages of CoQ_{10}, combined with its poor and slow absorption, generated the need to develop new technologies for delivery. Therefore, much effort has been expended to design delivery vehicles that can improve its aqueous solubility and overall bioavailability for oral and topical administration. This chapter summarizes the findings available today concerning CoQ_{10} chemical characteristics, human functionalities, its impact on human diseases, and new techniques developed to enhance its delivery.

Key words: coenzyme Q, coenzyme Q_{10}, mitochondrial respiratory chain, antioxidant, aging diseases.

26.1 Chemical characteristics and human functionality of coenzyme Q_{10}

Coenzyme Q_{10} (CoQ_{10}), the predominant human form of endogenous coenzyme Q, is synthesized in the mitochondrial inner membrane. The mitochondrial respiratory chain contains several coenzymes, including CoQ_1, CoQ_2, CoQ_4, CoQ_6, CoQ_7, CoQ_8, and CoQ_9, in addition to CoQ_{10}. It is known that CoQ_{10} is present in mammalian tissues, especially the heart, and CoQ_9 is found in rodents (i.e., mice and rats), while CoQ_6, CoQ_7, and CoQ_8 are found in yeast and bacteria (Warner 2000; Lekli *et al.* 2008). These coenzymes Q (CoQ) chemically differ from each other by the number of isoprene units in the tail; for example, CoQ_9 has nine units in contrast to the presence of ten units in CoQ_{10} (Fig. 26.1).

Coenzyme Q_{10} was originally isolated and characterized by Festenstein *et al.* in 1955; two years later it was established (Crane *et al.* 1957) as a

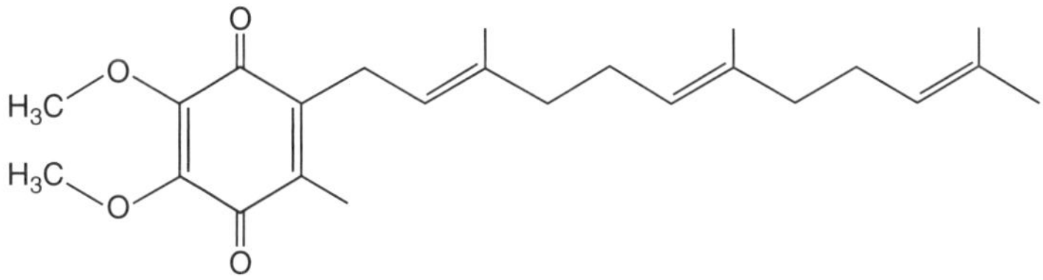

Fig. 26.1 The molecular structure of coenzyme Q_{10} (CoQ_{10}).

member of the mitochondrial respiratory chain. Moreover, CoQ_{10} was found to be an unusual lipid since its redox active benzoquinone ring is connected to a long isoprenoid side chain, requiring specific placement in a biological membrane (Fig. 26.1; Turunen *et al.* 2004). Its obligatory roles studied to date are wide-ranging: transporting electrons from complexes I and II to complex III in the mitochondrial electron transfer system; and depleting and reincorporating lipid into submitochondrial particles causing inactivation and reactivation of NADH and succinate dehydrogenase activities (Ernster *et al.* 1969) in the respiratory chain, participating in the protonmotive Q cycle, the cyclic electron transfer pathway through complex III involving ubisemiquinone. CoQ_{10} is now well known as an antioxidant molecule and involved in a number of aspects of cellular metabolism (Turunen *et al.* 2004).

This chapter summarizes the current structural knowledge on the CoQ_{10} human functionalities, its impact on human diseases, and the techniques that are available to enhance its bioavailability.

26.2 Functions of coenzyme Q_{10}

26.2.1 Participation as electron carrier in the mitochondrial respiratory chain

The inner mitochondrial membrane hosts the enzymes of the respiratory electron transport chain including five multiprotein enzyme complexes (I–V) and two electron carriers – coenzyme Q_{10} and cytochrome *c* (Fig. 26.2; Saraste 1999; Smeitink *et al.* 2001). The five complexes contain NADH:ubiquinone oxidoreductase (complex I), succinate:ubiquinone oxidoreductase (complex II, SQR), ubiquinone:cytochrome *c* oxidoreductase (complex III, cytochrome reductase, cytochrome *bc*1), cytochrome *c* oxidase (complex IV, cytochrome oxidase), and ATP synthase (complex V, F1F0-ATPase).

The main function of the system is the coordinated transport of electrons and protons, which leads to the production of ATP (Fig. 26.2). Generally, complexes I, III, and IV serve as proton pumps, using the energy of electron transfers for translocation of protons from the matrix to the cytosol of the mitochondrion, producing and sustaining an electrochemical gradient

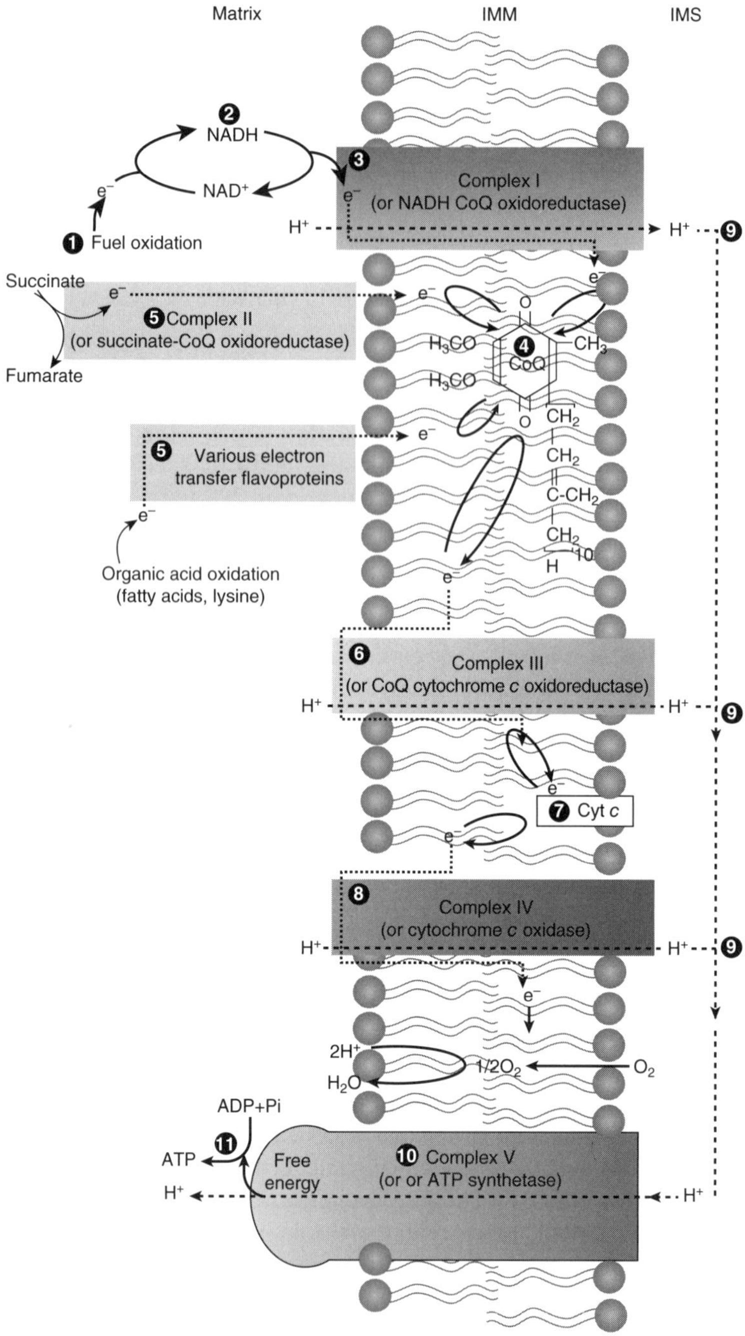

Fig. 26.2 The inner mitochondrial membrane containing the enzymes of the respiratory electron and proton transport chain that leads to the production of ATP, including five multiprotein enzyme complexes (I–V) and two electron carriers – coenzyme Q_{10} and cytochrome *c*. The number of subunits for each complex is indicated (CN, cyanide; FMN, flavin mononucleotide; mt, mitochondrial) (Smeitink *et al.* 2001).

across the inner membrane. Normally, complex V uses the free energy released from the flow of protons back across the membrane for producing ATP from ADP and inorganic phosphate. A steady state is achieved when the translocation of protons from the matrix into the intermembrane space is balanced by the utilization of the protons for ATP synthesis (Schultz and Chan 2001; Smeitink *et al.* 2001).

As seen in Fig. 26.2, electrons (e^-) from carbon oxidations (step 1 and dotted lines) are transferred via NADH (step 2) into complex I (step 3), which is embedded in the lipid bilayer of the inner mitochondrial membrane (IMM), then transported to coenzyme Q_{10} (step 4). Electrons from organic acid oxidations are transferred, via other flavin-containing enzyme complexes (step 5), directly to CoQ_{10}. CoQ_{10} delivers electrons via complex III (step 6) and cytochrome *c* (Cyt *c*) (step 7) to the final electron acceptor complex IV (step 8), where oxygen is reduced to water. The electrons lose free energy at each transfer step, and in complexes I, III, and IV, are coupled and utilized in the movement of H+ (step 9 and dashed lines) from the mitochondrial matrix to the intermembrane space (IMS). Finally, the proton gradient generated is used for the production of ATP by complex V (step 10) (Smeitink *et al.* 2001).

Part of the ATP is used for the mitochondrion's needs, but most of it is transported outside by the adenine nucleotide translocator and used for diverse cell functions (Saraste 1999).

26.2.2 Q-cycle mechanism of cytochrome bc_1

The Q-cycle mechanism for turnover of cytochrome bc_1, which was first proposed by Mitchell (1976), elucidated the phenomenon of oxidant-induced reduction (the reduction level of the *b* hemes in anaerobic, succinate-reduced mitochondria increased upon exposure of the mitochondria to dioxygen, particularly in the presence of the inhibitor antimycin) (Schultz and Chan 2001). The cycle, depicted in Fig. 26.3, takes advantage of the fact that ubiquinol is two-electron reductant but is oxidized in one-electron steps. The reaction cycle begins with ubiquinol binding to the P center of the enzyme. When the ubiquinol is oxidized, one electron is passed to the high-potential iron–sulfur cluster, which subsequently transfers the electron to cytochrome c_1, after which the electron is passed to ferricytochrome *c*. The second electron is transferred to heme b_L, then to heme b_H, where it is used to reduce a molecule of ubiquinone at the N site to its semiquinone form ($Q^\bullet$). The two protons released during the oxidation of the quinol molecule are released on the cytoplasmic side of the membrane. To complete the reaction cycle, a second molecule of ubiquinol is oxidized at the P center with the associated release of two protons to the cytoplasmic side of the membrane. Once more, one electron is transferred to the iron–sulfur protein, then to cytochrome c_1, and finally to a second molecule of ferricytochrome *c*. The second electron is transferred through hemes b_L and b_H

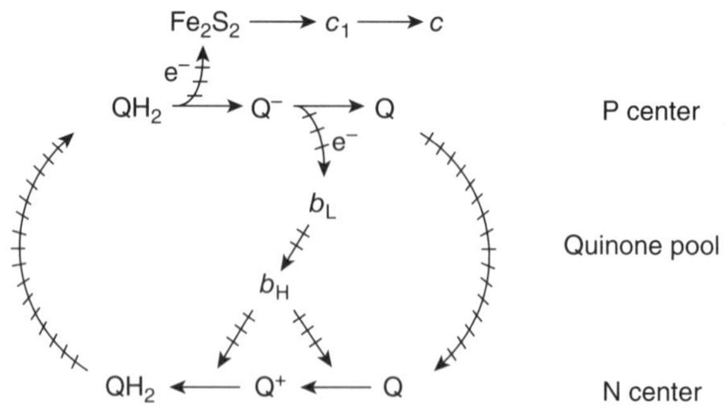

Fig. 26.3 Schematic diagram of the Q-cycle mechanism of cytochrome *bc*1. Thick arrows (→) denote substrate transformation or movement and thin, barbed arrows (⇸) denote electron transfer. Q: ubiquinone; $Q^•$: ubisemiquinone; QH_2: ubiquinol (Schultz and Chan 2001).

and used to promote the reduction of the semiquinone at the N center to ubiquinol, with the associated uptake of two protons from the matrix side of the membrane. Overall, four protons are released for every two molecules of ferricytochrome *c* reduced, giving a $2H^+/1e^-$ proton translocation stoichiometry (Schultz and Chan 2001).

The consequences of this cycle are: the branched electron transfer doubles the efficiency of proton translocation mediated by this enzyme. If the reaction catalyzed by this enzyme consisted solely of electron transfer from ubiquinol to cytochrome *c*, the reduction of one molecule of ferricytochrome *c* would be associated with the release of one proton, *not two as is observed*. Second, the electron transfer in the enzyme is under *kinetic control* rather than thermodynamic control that favors the transfer of both electrons from ubiquinol to ferricytochrome *c*, bypassing the *b* hemes altogether (Schultz and Chan 2001).

26.2.3 Antioxidant activity and generation of reactive oxygen species

Eighty percent of the normal mammalian oxygen consumption occurs in the mitochondria, of which 80% is coupled to ATP production (Papa 1996). Reactive oxygen species (ROS) account for 1–2% of the oxygen consumed by mitochondria, which is considered to be the major source of O_2^- and H_2O_2 production in the cell and known to depend on the state of respiration (Skulachev 1998). When the mitochondrial membrane potential is high and the ADP levels are low, the production of ROS is high. Alternatively, when the membrane potential is low, the ADP concentration is high, and the production of ROS is low. It is well known that the free radicals formed in the cell are able to damage lipids, proteins, and DNA, a concept known as oxidative stress. For example, lipid peroxidation, the most studied process, is initiated by abstraction of a hydrogen atom from a methylene group of a polyunsaturated fatty acid (PUFA). The results of lipid peroxidation are carbon-centered free radicals, peroxyl radicals, lipid hydroperoxide, alkoxyl radicals, and degradation to hydrocarbons, alcohols, ethers, epoxides, and aldehydes. The formed aldehydes are relatively long-lived, they can diffuse longer distances, and since they can also react with macromolecules, they further contribute to the damage caused by lipid peroxidation.

The reduced form of CoQ_{10} ($CoQH_2$) is a nonenzymatic antioxidant agent, among other molecules such as vitamins C and E, carotenoids, glutathione, α-lipoic acid, and flavonoids, which can prevent the formation of or remove ROS (Turunen *et al.* 2004). Antioxidant enzymes include superoxide dismutase and various peroxidases such as glutathione peroxidase, catalase, thioredoxin reductase, and peroxiredoxin (Wood *et al.* 2003).

It is well established that $CoQH_2$ is able to prevent lipid peroxidation in most subcellular membranes (Ernster and Dallner 1995). The $CoQH_2$ is oxidized during lipid peroxidation, yet it is efficiently regenerated by the respiratory chain and is normally reserved in a highly reduced state. It was suggested that $CoQH_2$ affects the initiation process and prevents the formation of lipid peroxyl radicals ($LOO^{\bullet}$), while vitamin E acts by quenching these radicals (Fig. 26.4; Ernster and Forsmark-Andree 1993). Apparently,

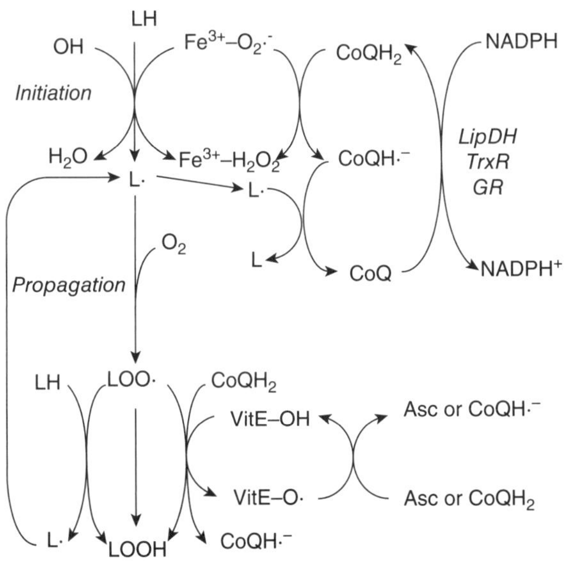

Fig. 26.4 Sites of action of CoQ_{10}, vitamin E, and ascorbate on lipid peroxidation. Asc – ascorbate; Asc^- – ascorbyl radical; $CoQH_2$ – reduced coenzyme Q; $CoQH^-$ – semiubiquinone; $Fe^3+O_2^-$ – perferryl radical; GR – glutathione reductase; L – carbon-centered fatty acid radical; LH – polyunsaturated fatty acid; LipDH – lipoamide dehydrogenase; LOO – lipid peroxyl radical; LOOH – lipid hydroperoxide; OH – hydroxyl radical; VitE-O – α-tocopheroxyl radical; VitE-OH – vitamin E (α-tocopherol); TrxR – thioredoxin reductase (Bentinger *et al.* 2007).

$CoQH_2$ reduces the initiating perferryl radical with the formation of ubisemiquinone and H_2O_2, and regenerates vitamin E from the α-tocopheroxyl radical (Fig. 26.4). Its lipid solubility, efficient continuous regeneration and involvement, both in the initiation and propagation steps of lipid peroxidation, elucidate why CoQ, even more than vitamin E, is considered a highly efficient antioxidant against radicals produced in biological membranes (Turunen *et al.* 2004; Bentinger *et al.* 2007).

Although the reduced form of coenzyme Q, ubiquinol, was generally considered to be the antioxidant, a patent in 1993 stated that the oxidized ubiquinone form had a significant antioxidation effect in food as well as cosmetic and pharmaceutical products, particularly those that were rich in PUFA (Bracco *et al.* 1993). This was in agreement with the observation that the main form of coenzyme Q present in postmortem light and dark muscles of mackerel was the oxidized form, ubiquinone (Petillo *et al.* 1998). The percentage of reduced coenzyme Q (ubiquinol) in mackerel light muscle was only 12.8% and in dark muscle it was 8.6% (per gram of lipid basis) (Petillo *et al.* 1998). Petillo *et al.* (1998) suggested that coenzyme Q may function as a prooxidant in mackerel dark muscle by producing some reactive oxygen species that escape the mitochondrial chain.

Petillo and Hultin (2008) aimed to determine whether the oxidized form of coenzyme Q, ubiquinone, was capable of acting as an antioxidant. Hence, its impact on the rate of oxidation of both methyl linoleate and methyl linolenate when exposed to a soluble free radical generator, 2,2′-azobis (2,4-dimethylvaleronitrile – AMVN), was tested. The results of the methyl linoleate and methyl linolenate experiments are presented in Fig. 26.5(a) and (b), respectively. The authors found that oxidized coenzyme Q, ubiquinone-10, functioned as an antioxidant at both 1:100 and 1:1000 (ubiquinone-10:substrate) ratios (Petillo and Hultin 2008). Some differences were noted between the substrates, methyl linoleate and methyl linolenate. A minor autoxidation, i.e., without AMVN, of methyl linoleate was detected (Fig. 26.5a). At a ratio of 1:100 (ubiquinone-10:methyl linoleate), ubiquinone-10 reduced the rate of oxidation to as low as that of autoxidation. However, the effectiveness of the antioxidant at a 1:1000 ratio was less pronounced, yet noticeable, compared with a sample without the antioxidant.

The autoxidation rate of methyl linolenate was six times greater than that of methyl linoleate based on the slopes of the linear regression curves for the two substrates. Additionally, the rate of AMVN-initiated oxidation without ubiquinone for methyl linolenate was approximately twice that for methyl linoleate (on the basis of initial slopes of the quadratic curves from the regression equations). Overall, ubiquinone-10 was an effective inhibitor at ratios of both 1:100 and 1:1000 with methyl linolenate. Petillo and Hultin (2008) could conclude that ubiquinone-10 was more effective as an antioxidant with fatty acids containing more than two double bonds.

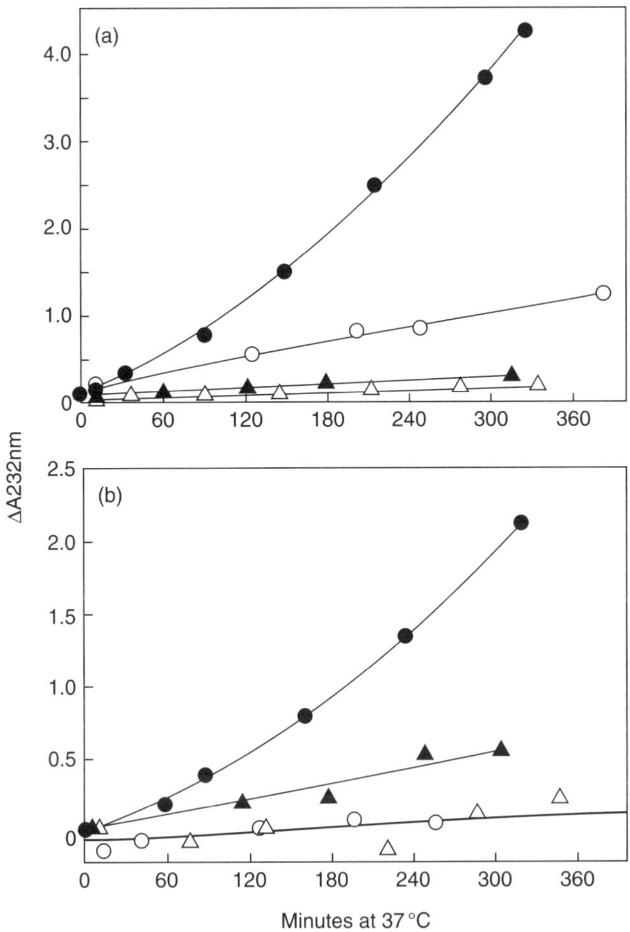

Fig. 26.5 Formation of conjugated dienes from (a) methyl linoleate (○); methyl linoleate, and AMVN (●); methyl linoleate, AMVN, and ubiquinone-10 (100:10:1, Δ); and methyl linoleate, AMVN and ubiquinone-10 (1000:100:1, ▲); (b) methyl linolenate (○); methyl linolenate and AMVN (●); methyl linolenate, AMVN and ubiquinone-10 (100:10:1, Δ); and methyl linolenate, AMVN and ubiquinone-10 (1000:100:1, ▲) in hexane at 37°C (Petillo and Hultin 2008).

Since ubiquinone-10 cannot donate hydrogen to free radicals, its antioxidant activity requires another mechanism to be involved. Ubiquinone was assumed to function as a free radical scavenger. A free radical scavenger, although not as efficient an antioxidant as a H donor (e.g., ubiquinol), can react with free radicals and lower their activation energy. In addition, free radical scavengers are known to interact with other antioxidants and provide mutual sparing. For example, astaxanthin and canthaxanthin were reported to be as effective as α-tocopherol as a radical-trapping antioxidant

(Palozza and Krinsky 1992a); synergistic action between β-carotene and α-tocopherol was also demonstrated (Palozza and Krinsky 1992b).

It was surmised by Petillo and Hultin (2008) and Cabrini *et al.* (1986) that the antioxidant behavior of ubiquinone might be due to its ability to (1) scavenge singlet oxygen and (2) structurally affect the lipid bilayer, thereby inhibiting hydroperoxide decomposition by metal-catalyzed reactions that promote spontaneous lipid peroxidation.

Other research comparing the antioxidant activity among carotenoids revealed that the oxo group at the 4 (4′) position and not the hydroxyl group at the 3 (3′) position of astaxanthin made this carotenoid more effective than β-carotene (Terao 1989). Ubiquinone-10 also has an oxo group at the 4-position; yet, unlike β-carotene, it does not possess a highly conjugated side chain, although it has approximately the same number of double bonds as β-carotene, astaxanthin, or canthaxanthin. Since its relatively long side chain is considered to be more flexible, the investigators believe it may facilitate reversible reduction of the quinone groups and then conversion to chromenol via cyclization with an isoprene unit (Petillo and Hultin 2008).

Another possibility raised by Petillo and Hultin involves the physical interaction between ubiquinone and the methylated fatty acid due to van der Waals forces that interfere with the formation of the conjugated diene. In addition, physical interaction between ubiquinone and AMVN could prevent the production of initiating radicals by AMVN. In either case, ubiquinone may interfere with the acceptance of a radical by the methylated fatty acid or the production of a radical by AMVN in an indirect way (Petillo and Hultin 2008).

26.3 Distribution of coenzyme Q

26.3.1 Tissues

CoQ is present in all tissues and cells (in human and rat) in variable quantities (Table 26.1). As mentioned above, the main species in human tissues is CoQ_{10}, which ranges from 8 μg/g in lung to 114 μg/g in heart. CoQ_9 was also found in the human body, yet in much smaller amounts, 2–7% in all human tissues. In rat the main species is CoQ_9, which varies from 17 μg/g in lung to 202 μg/g in heart (Åberg *et al.* 1992). In most rat tissues 10–20% of the total CoQ has 10 isoprene units, with the exception of brain, spleen, and intestines, where 30–40% of the total is CoQ_{10}.

The CoQ quantity, type, and extent of reduction *in vivo* can be estimated by employing rapid extraction, partition, and direct injection of the extract into high-performance liquid chromatography (HPLC) (Table 26.1; Åberg *et al.* 1992). The level of the CoQ reduced state was found to be very high, more in human than in rat, with the exception of lung and brain. The concentration of CoQ varies greatly not only among different organs, but also among various cells and regions of the same organ.

Table 26.1 Coenzyme Q_9 and Q_{10} quantities, type, and extent of reduction in human and rat tissues (Åberg *et al.* 1992)

	Rat			Human		
	CoQ_9	CoQ_{10}	% Reduced	CoQ_9	CoQ_{10}	% Reduced
Heart	202	17	22	3	114	47
Kidney	124	22	42	3	67	73
Liver	131	21	87	2	55	95
Muscle	43	3	40	1	40	60
Brain	37	19	27	1	13	23
Pancreas	37	3	62	2	33	100
Spleen	23	9	18	1	25	87
Lung	17	2	12	1	8	24
Thyroidea	44	7	45	1	25	68
Testis	32	5	49	1	11	78
Intestine	51	19	67	1	12	93
Colon	48	8	52	1	11	83
Venricle	56	5	52		12	59

26.3.2 Intracellular distribution

All organelles of the liver contain different types of mevalonate pathway lipids (Table 26.2; Turunen *et al.* 2004). It should be noted that the mevalonate pathway comprises the reactions beginning with acetyl-coenzyme A and ending with farnesyl pyrophosphate, the substrate for the biosynthesis of CoQ_{10}, cholesterol, dolicol, and isoprenylated proteins (Grünler *et al.* 1994). The largest quantities of CoQ_{10} are found in the outer and inner mitochondrial membranes, on protein basis lysosomes, and Golgi vesicles. Dolichol concentration is enriched in lysosomes and Golgi vesicles, while cholesterol exhibits a gradient character: rough microsomes→smooth microsomes→lysosomes→Golgi vesicles→plasma membranes. Golgi vesicles are the most enriched with α-tocopherol (α-T).

Mostly, there is one chain length of CoQ_{10} that is dominant, compared with dolichol, which is distributed in tissues as a family of polyisoprenoids with six to seven members (Grünler *et al.* 1994). It was proposed that the heterogeneity of CoQ_{10} is required for functional specializations, such as for mitochondrial respiration and for antioxidative action (Matsura *et al.* 1991). However, based on extracted beef heart submitochondrial particles, it was claimed that the efficiency of coenzyme Q as a respiratory chain redox carrier or as an antioxidant agent was not influenced by the length of the isoprenoid side chain, with either Q_9 or Q_{10} (Lenaz 1998).

In spite of these facts, there are cases where the type of CoQ species is important. Activation of uncoupling proteins and regulation of the mitochondrial permeability transition pore revealed selective requirements. It was observed that mumps virus infection of dorsal ganglion cells, which

Table 26.2 Coenzyme Q, dolichol, cholesterol, and α-tocopherol in subcellular organelles of rat liver (Turunen *et al.* 2004)

Organelle	CoQ	Dol + Dol-P (mg/mg protein)	Cholesterol	α-Tocopherol
Nuclear envelope	0.2	0.2	37.5	0.01
Mitochondria	1.4	0.09	2.3	0.04
Outer membranes	2.2	0.25	30	0.06
Inner membranes	1.9	0.009	5.0	0.04
Microsomes	0.2	0.4	28	0.07
Rough microsomes	0.2	0.5	16	0.04
Smooth microsomes	0.3	0.3	31	0.09
Lysosomes	1.9	4.7	38	0.18
Lysosmal membranes	0.4	0.6	6.1	
Golgi vesicles	2.6	1.7	71	0.48
Peroxisomes	0.3	0.8	6.4	0.02
Plasma membranes	0.7	0.8	128	0.008

contain both CoQ_9 and CoQ_{10}, led to a decrease of the coenzyme quantities and resulted in neuronal degeneration (Edlund *et al.* 1994). It was demonstrated by the authors that the cells could be rescued solely by the addition of CoQ_{10}, not by addition of CoQ_9 (Edlund *et al.* 1994).

26.3.3 Intramembranous localization

Lipids of the mevalonate pathway have distinct intramembranous locations that lead to a significant impact on membrane properties. The hydrophobic tails of the lipids, such as the polyisoprenoid chains of CoQ_{10}, dolichol, and dolichyl phosphate (dolichol-P), incorporate in the hydrophobic region, between the double layers of phospholipid fatty acids (Fig. 26.6; Lenaz *et al.* 1992). The active groups, the benzoquinone ring of CoQ_{10} and the phosphorylated α-isoprene of dolichol-P, locate adjacent to the phospholipid fatty acid polar area, on the outer or inner surface of the membrane, and were shown to be dependent on the functional requirement. Additionally, the hydrophobic tails of these three lipids are known to adopt a coiled assembly in the 'available phospholipid fatty acid space' (Fig. 26.6), thereby destabilizing the membranes and resulting in increased fluidity and permeability. In contrast, the shorter yet bulkier molecule, cholesterol, is distributed between the fatty acids solely on one side of the lipid (as seen in Fig. 26.6), and thus leads to decreased fluidity and permeability (Lenaz *et al.* 1992).

This lipid arrangement has two major consequences: (1) to achieve optimal function each membrane has to incorporate (solubilize) the appropriate lipid, while the level of solubilization is dependent on the type of structural assembly of the membrane; and (2) if the membrane lacks an

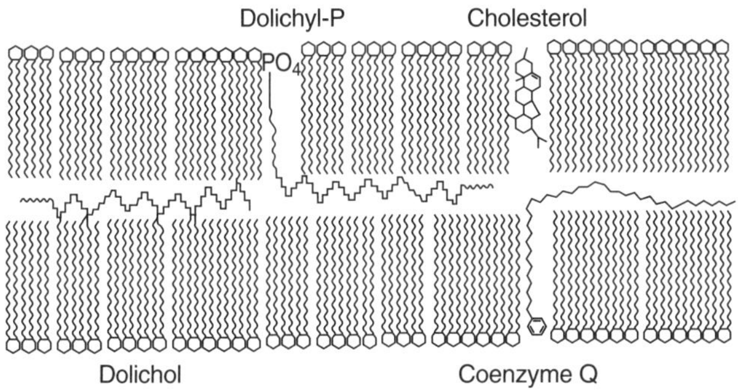

Fig. 26.6 Intramembranous distribution of mevalonate pathway lipids (Turunen *et al.* 2004).

Table 26.3 Mevalonate pathway lipids in human heart and pancreas during aging (Kalen *et al.* 1989)

Organ	Age (years)	Coenzyme Q	Dolichol (% of 2-day-old human)	Dolichyl-P	Cholesterol	Phospholipids
Heart	20	300	132	400	59	82
	80	129	605	2364	82	109
Pancreas	20	128	5450	176	50	140
	80	71	17502	500	68	181

isoprenoid, it will be deficient in fluidity – the outcome of isoprenoid presence. In this case an uptake from exogenous sources can be considered up to a limit level, while continuous uptake can result in further distribution in non-membranous locations. For example, lysosomes exhibited CoQ_{10} and dolichol content that exceeds the content of other membranes several-fold.

26.4 Aging

During aging, the lipid compositions are modified and known to have significant impact on the membranes' physicochemical structure, mevalonate pathway lipids, and function of the integral enzymes and their metabolic processes (Kalen *et al.* 1989). The pathway lipid content in human heart and pancreas during aging, comparing newborns (2 days old) to 20- and 80-year-old persons is shown in Table 26.3 (Kalen *et al.* 1989). In the first 20 years of life, in both heart and pancreas, the CoQ_{10} level is increased; however, up to the age of 80 years it decreases and in some organs it may be lower than at birth. Conversely, dolichol and dolichyl-P, in both heart

Table 26.4 Mevalonate pathway lipids in various pathological conditions (Turunen *et al.* 2004)

	(% of control)			
	CoQ	Dolichol	Dolichyl-P	Cholesterol
Noduli, rat liver	196	671	175	148
Noduli				
Mitochondria	104	116		
Microsomes	693	474		
Lysosomes	261	84		106
Cancer, rat liver	76	105	204	190
Cancer, human liver	40	889	94	212
Cardiomyopathy, human heart	40–80			
Alzheimer's disease, human brain	130	56	172	102
Prion disease, mice brain	250	67	158	103
Niemann–Pick type C disease, mouse liver	65	95	267	1100
Diabetes, type 2, rat liver	140			
Diabetes, type 2, rat testis, mitochondria. Mevinolin treatment of rat	125			
Heart	82	72	60	104
Muscle	83	75	68	92
Liver	89	134	91	85

and pancreas, increase significantly during the whole life. It is still questionable to what extent these modifications represent an actual deficiency in the membrane structure or are attributable to a change in cellular organization. Furthermore, in adult tissues CoQ_{10} is found mostly in its reduced form, but the degree of reduction in aged tissue has not yet been determined.

26.5 Diseases – coenzyme Q_{10} content dependence

Various diseases, in particular the most studied cardiomyopathies and degenerative muscle diseases, exhibit a decrease in CoQ_{10} content (Table 26.4; Manzoli *et al.* 1990). There is evidence that heart function can be improved upon administration of CoQ_{10} (Manzoli *et al.* 1990). CoQ_{10} is known to reach the heart via the blood, but is taken up only to a limited extent. Other mechanisms that do not require its entrance into the cell appear to exist, either of signaling type or by production of mediators.

During the first stage of the disease there is increased oxidative stress, which has been suggested to induce a response, resulting in cell self-protection by raising the concentrations of antioxidants (Dröge 2002). Similarly, in the noduli, the levels of dolichol and dolichyl-P are elevated. Upon disease progression, cancer develops and in humans, the quantity of CoQ_{10} decreases to only 40% of pre-disease levels, while the cholesterol level doubles in fully developed cancerous liver. In biopsy samples from human heart, a significant decrease of CoQ_{10} content in cardiomyopathy was found and was directly associated with the severity of the disease (Turunen *et al.* 2004).

It was suggested that CoQ_{10} levels are also modified in neurodegenerative diseases such as Huntington, Parkinson, and amyotrophic lateral sclerosis (Shults *et al.* 1997). In both experimental models and human patients, positive effects have been observed after supplementation (Beal and Matthews 1997). It is now generally accepted that increased production of free radicals is an important feature during the development of these diseases, and it is not surprising that cellular protection is induced to counteract these radicals; thus the CoQ_{10} concentrations are increased (Contestabile 2001). It should be noted that, in Alzheimer disease in humans, the level of dolichol decreases, dolichyl-P increases, and cholesterol is unchanged (Söderberg *et al.* 1992).

The importance of CoQ_{10} in living organisms, in general, is highlighted by the number of reports describing the genetic disorders in which CoQ_{10} synthesis was impaired. Lowered CoQ_{10} content in organs resulted in serious metabolic disturbances; however, its supplementation can re-establish mitochondrial and other functions.

26.6 Coenzyme Q_{10} dietary uptake

CoQ_{10} is taken up from the intestine into the circulation at a low rate; only about 2–4% can be recovered (Zhang *et al.* 1995). The mechanism of its uptake has not been clarified, but since it is found in the various lipoproteins, redistribution in the circulation is assumed. In the case of α-tocopherol, the liver possesses a specific binding protein that delivers it back to the circulation via very low density lipoprotein (VLDL) for further transport to various organs (Yoshida *et al.* 1992). The limited available information may imply that VLDL synthesized in the endoplasmic reticulum (ER)–Golgi system contains only *de novo* synthesized CoQ_{10} in a quantity that is required for antioxidant protection but not for redistribution to tissues (Elmberger *et al.* 1989). In liver, spleen, adrenals, ovaries, arterial endothelium, blood monocytes, and lymphocytes from rat, CoQ_{10} was found to be taken up from the circulation, while its uptake by heart, pancreas, pituitary gland, testis, and thymus was very limited. No uptake was observed in kidney, muscle, brain, thyroid gland, and blood polynuclear cells.

The uptake mechanism of CoQ_{10} from the blood into tissues is not yet clarified. Similar to cholesterol and α-tocopherol, LDL receptor was considered one of the mediators based on the fact that organs such as adrenals and ovaries are rich in this receptor (Turunen *et al.* 2004).

26.7 Coenzyme Q_{10} delivery techniques

The development of formulations for oral administration of the poorly and slowly absorbed CoQ_{10} (via foods and supplements from the gastrointestinal tract) is a complicated task. Hsu *et al.* (2003) concluded that the absorption of CoQ_{10} mainly occurs at the intestinal lymphatic tissues (the Peyer's patches). The epithelial cell layer overlying the Peyer's patches contains specialized M cells that facilitate transcytotic transport across the intestines. Small particles in the intestinal lumen localize to the apical side of M cells and can be internalized by the M cells through transcytosis.

Moreover, according to Desai *et al.* (1996), there is an exclusion phenomenon in the gastrointestinal mucosal tissue that is particle size-dependent; 100 nm size particles demonstrate significantly improved tissue uptake compared to larger particles. In general, particles less than 500 nm were found to be able to cross the M cells and the mesentery on the surface of gastrointestinal mucosa, successfully delivering a drug (Hussain *et al.* 2001). Consequently, the size of the carrier particles can potentially influence the internalization via the M cells.

CoQ_{10} is also known to have limited solubility in lipids, insolubility in water, oxidative instability, precipitation susceptibility, and to be of high molecular weight (863 Da) (Ankola *et al.* 2007; Bhagavan and Chopra 2007; Prosek *et al.* 2008). Therefore, much effort was devoted to designing new technologies and delivery vehicles to increase the aqueous solubility of CoQ_{10} and thus its loading in the vehicles, enhancing its chemical and physical stability, and improving its bioavailability. CoQ_{10} products currently available on the market include powder-based compressed tablets, chewable tablets, powder-filled hard-shell capsules, and softgels containing an oil suspension (presence of fats for promoting improved absorption of CoQ_{10}).

Miles *et al.* (2002) evaluated the pharmacokinetic properties of three solubilized formulations of CoQ_{10} compared with a powder-filled hard shell capsule formulation. The three solubilized products included a CoQ_{10} formulation as a syrup (LiQ10®), a softgel formulation (Q-Gel®), and a softgel formulation containing CoQ_{10} in its reduced form as ubiquinol (Q-Nol®). The three solubilized formulations were found to be much greater than the powder-filled capsules in terms of both increase (fold) and increase per 100 mg (Table 26.5; Miles *et al.* 2002). The solubilized ubiquinol, Q-Nol®, was found to be the best of the three solubilized formulations.

Schulz *et al.* (2006) examined an additional CoQ_{10} supplement (Solu™ Q_{10}) on 54 volunteers over 14 days. This formulation, consisting of Polysorb-

Table 26.5 Plasma CoQ_{10} response to ingestion of a single low/moderate dose of CoQ_{10} in adults using solubilized and powder-based formulations (Miles *et al.* 2002)

Formulation	Plasma CoQ_{10} (μmol/L)		Increase (fold)	Increase per 100 mg
	Baseline	C_{max}		
Solubilized (syrup)[a]	0.602	1.795	2.982	0.663
Solubilized (softgel caps)[b]	0.602	1.795	2.982	0.663
Solubilized (ubiquinol caps)[c]	0.602	2.073	3.444	0.817
Powder (caps)	0.602	0.741	1.231	0.077

[a] LiQ10®.
[b] Q-Gel®.
[c] Q-Nol®.

ate 80 and medium chain triglycerides, was found to be superior to oily dispersions and crystalline CoQ_{10} in overall bioavailability. Prosek *et al.* (2008) reported on preparation of a water-soluble CoQ_{10} in the form of a water-soluble paste, based on molecular encapsulation of CoQ_{10} into the β-cyclodextrin's lipophilic cavity. This formulation expressed enhanced bioavailability in beagle dogs compared with commercially available oil-based form of CoQ_{10}.

For an additional increase in oral bioavailability, micro- and nanoparticle-based techniques were utilized to encapsulate CoQ_{10}. For example, Kommuru *et al.* (2001) showed that microparticles containing polyglycolyzed glycerides resulted in a two-fold increase in CoQ_{10} bioavailability compared with the powder formulation.

Garti *et al.* (to be published) examined a liquid nano-sized structure based on Tween 60 and loaded with 150 mg of CoQ_{10} in comparison to a CoQ_{10} supplement available in the market (as bioavailable softgels) on eight volunteers, over 14 days. The liquid nano-sized formulations showed higher levels of CoQ_{10} in the blood, by 40%, than the CoQ_{10} that is available in the market (Fig. 26.7). It should be noted that, upon uptake of the CoQ_{10} liquid nano-sized structures, greater quantities of CoQ_{10} and higher levels of oxidized CoQ_{10} were found in the bloodstream of humans and also higher levels of vitamin E were detected in the blood even after 14 days, compared with the market available CoQ_{10}. These outcomes demonstrate greater bioavailability of the entrapped CoQ_{10} in addition to its high release levels. More surprising and encouraging was the fact that the levels of vitamin E were found to be high, since it is known that lipophilic drugs compete with CoQ_{10} and vitamin E, resulting in a reduction of the vitamin E levels in the blood. These new formulations suggest that the CoQ_{10} is adsorbed by an alternative pathway that leaves the solubilized vitamin E levels in the

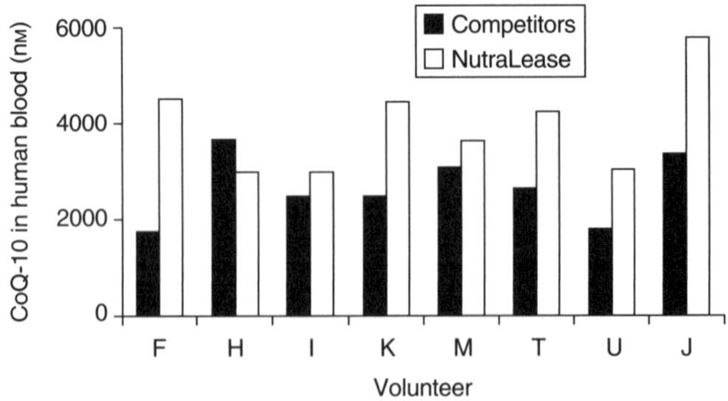

Fig. 26.7 CoQ_{10} levels in human blood of liquid nano-sized formulations (Tween 60-based) and the market available CoQ_{10} (Garti *et al.*, to be published).

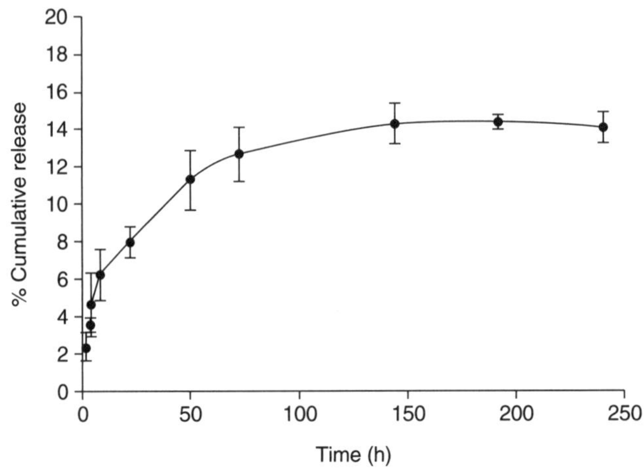

Fig. 26.8 *In vitro* release profile of CoQ_{10} from nanoparticles. The experiment was performed in 5% Tween 80 solution at 37°C (Hsu *et al.* 2003).

bile-salt micelles unaffected and, as a result, their levels are even higher than those of the control.

Hsu *et al.* (2003) reported on emulsifying wax-based nanoparticles (50–100 nm) for incorporation of CoQ_{10}. These carriers were prepared by cooling warm microemulsion precursors composed of emulsifying wax, CoQ_{10}, and Brij 78 and/or Tween 20, which was accompanied by lyophilization of the nanoparticles. Release profile in the *in vitro* study, including an initial rapid release followed by a slow release, which is characteristic for nanoparticle systems in general, was obtained (Fig. 26.8). A rapid release was monitored over the first 9 hours, during which over 7% of the CoQ_{10} was released. In contrast, after 9 hours, the release of CoQ_{10} from the nanoparticles slowed and eventually, after 72 hours, a total of 12% CoQ_{10} had been released. As discussed by the authors, in oral administration the slowly released CoQ_{10} may be passively partitioned into the gastrointestinal tract tissues resulting in improved bioavailability.

Recently, biodegradable poly(lactide-co-glycolide) (PLGA) nanoparticles have attracted considerable scientific attention due to their clinical biocompatibility, and possible uses in oral, intramuscular, and intravenous therapies. Such nanoparticles are able to solubilize hydrophobic drugs, flow through capillaries, and protect the guest molecules from enzymatic degradation. In addition, they are adjustable for receptor targeting and can be internalized by cells for cytoplasmic drug delivery (Sahoo *et al.* 2002). Ankola *et al.* (2007) prepared nanoparticulate formulations based on PLGA by an emulsion technique using the quaternary ammonium salt didodecyldimethylammonium bromide (DMAB) as a stabilizer. The intestinal uptake of CoQ_{10} as a suspension in carboxymethylcellulose (CMC), a commercial formulation, and the developed nanoparticulate formulation, was examined in rats and found to be 45%, 75%, and 79%, respectively. Moreover, the nanoparticles were tested for therapeutic potential in renal hypertensive animals, and revealed enhanced efficacy at a 60% lowered dose compared with a CoQ_{10} suspension, and also a greater efficiency than the commercial formulation at an equal dose.

The major drawback of the described systems is the use of surfactants as stabilizing agents to avoid nanoparticle aggregation. Surfactants are not always desirable in this type of formulation due to their problematic biocompatibility and irreversible incorporation in the nanoparticles that can affect the drug release (Sahoo *et al.* 2002). To overcome these disadvantages, a nanoprecipitation technique was utilized by Nehillla *et al.* (2008) to formulate CoQ_{10}-loaded nanoparticles with biodegradable PLGA, without using a surfactant. In this method, a water-miscible organic solvent (such as acetone or acetonitrile) containing the dissolved polymer and drug molecules was injected into an aqueous medium. As a result, nanoparticles were spontaneously precipitated, the organic solvent was evaporated, and the nanoparticle suspension was filtered. The obtained nanoparticles contained 7% drug with a total encapsulation yield of 65%. As shown in the atomic force microscopy (AFM) image (Fig. 26.9), these nanoparticles display spherical, non-aggregated morphology and diameter sizes less than 200 nm.

The obtained systems also demonstrated promising release properties of CoQ_{10} (Fig. 26.10). As mentioned above, typical drug release profiles from nanoparticles containing surfactant normally exhibit a short 'burst' (1–2 days) followed by slower, yet nearly 100%, drug release (Budhian *et al.* 2005). Two main deviations from the common release profiles were noted: (1) the 'burst' period was longer (~2 weeks), indicating more sustained drug release behaviour in these nanoparticles. As discussed by the authors, weeks-long drug release is preferable to a typical short and substantial 'burst' lasting hours; (2) CoQ_{10} remained encapsulated for as long as two

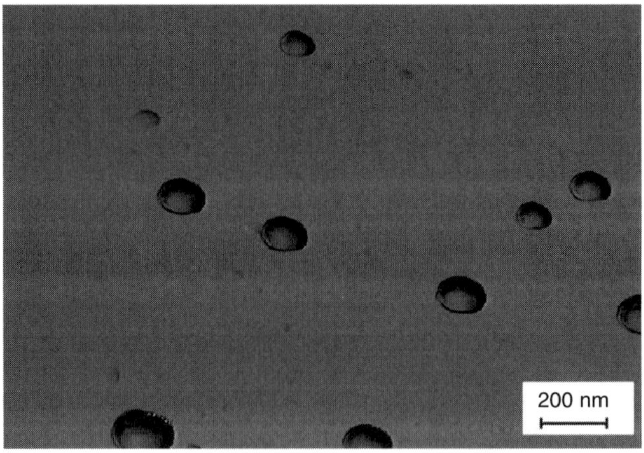

Fig. 26.9 Representative phase AFM image showed that surfactant-free CoQ_{10}-loaded PLGA nanoparticles maintained the spherical, non-aggregated, sub-200 nm diameter characteristics (Nehilla *et al.* 2008).

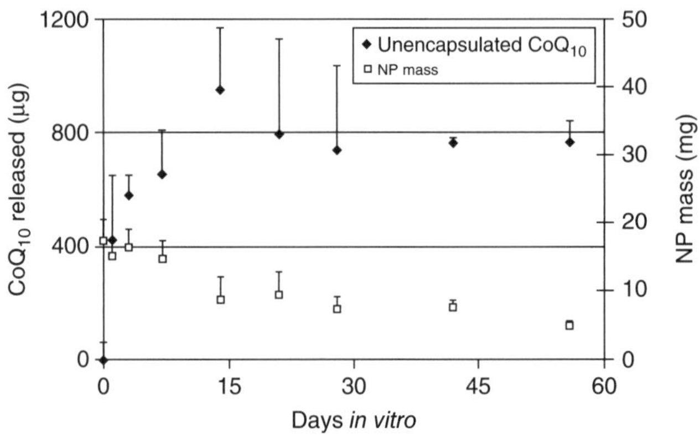

Fig. 26.10 Total CoQ_{10} release into phosphate buffered saline (PBS) and CoQ_{10}-loaded nanoparticle (NP) mass followed for 2 months (Nehilla *et al.* 2008).

months. Moreover, strong hydrophobic interactions between the polymer and CoQ_{10} were found, thereby preventing 100% drug release.

Liposomes are considered to be effective nano-sized drug delivery vehicles, since they can accumulate in regions of myocardial infarction, leading to enhanced permeability and retention (EPR) (Maeda 2001). Liposomes containing monoclonal antibodies specifically recognizing chemically damaged cells may also plug and seal the damaged myocyte membranes and protect cells against ischemic and reperfusion injury. Verma *et al.* (2007) presented *in vivo* data that revealed a significant cardio-protective effect of CoQ_{10}-loaded liposomes in rabbits subjected to a 30 min coronary artery occlusion. The investigators found that these nano-sized vehicles (177 ± 26 nm), loaded with CoQ_{10} successfully protected the myocardium from ischemia/reperfusion damage. This was achieved by decreasing the size of the irreversibly damaged zone in rabbits with an acute experimental myocardial infarction. Thus, it was shown that these liposomes can perform as an effective exogenous source of CoQ_{10} and protect damaged hearts suffering from reduced CoQ_{10} supply during an ischemic attack.

Combined administration of CoQ_{10} and vitamin E ('NanoSolve' formulations) was tested on 24 volunteers by Wajda *et al.* (2007). Upon administration of 'NanoSolve' formulations, the bioavailability of CoQ_{10} was found to increase five-fold and that of vitamin E was enhanced 10-fold, both compared with the pure substances.

Utilizing CoQ_{10} in topical delivery, in addition to the oral delivery, developed into an important issue. Hoppe *et al.* (1999) established that CoQ_{10} is able to act as an antioxidant against both hydrogen peroxide and UVA in cultured epidermal keratinocytes and UVA in dermal fibroblasts. Moreover, the investigators demonstrated a significant reduction in oxidation *in vivo* using ultra-weak photon emission.

Nanoparticle-based technique was also applied in topical delivery. Nanostructured lipid carriers (NLC) are widely used in cosmetic dermal products (Müller *et al.* 2007). NLC have greater loading capacity due to the decreased degree of organization of the lipid matrix, compared with solid lipid nanoparticles (SLN) (Fig. 26.11). By decreasing the internal order of these structures, important advantages in release properties can be provided. The drug molecules, accommodated between lipid layers, are not expelled from the carrier, implying that the drug release is controlled and its chemical stability is improved. NLC loaded with CoQ_{10} and composed of cetyl palmitate with various amounts of caprylic/capric triacylglycerols (as liquid lipid) were prepared by Teeranachaideekul *et al.* (2007). A scanning electron microscopy (SEM) image of CoQ_{10}-loaded NLC is shown in Fig. 26.12. The particles revealed an anisometric shape with a size of approximately 200 nm, with some agglomeration of individualized particles, possessing 100% of entrapment efficiency. The NLC were compared with

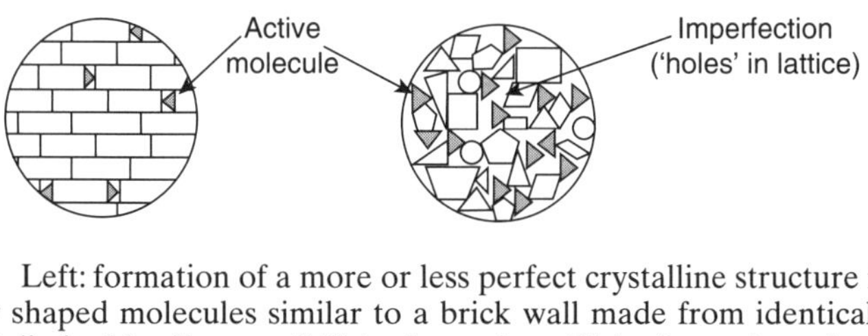

Fig. 26.11 Left: formation of a more or less perfect crystalline structure in SLN by identically shaped molecules similar to a brick wall made from identically shaped bricks with limited loading possibilities for actives. Right: formation of a crystalline particle matrix with many imperfections, while the increased number of imperfections leads to an increased loading capacity (Müller *et al.* 2007).

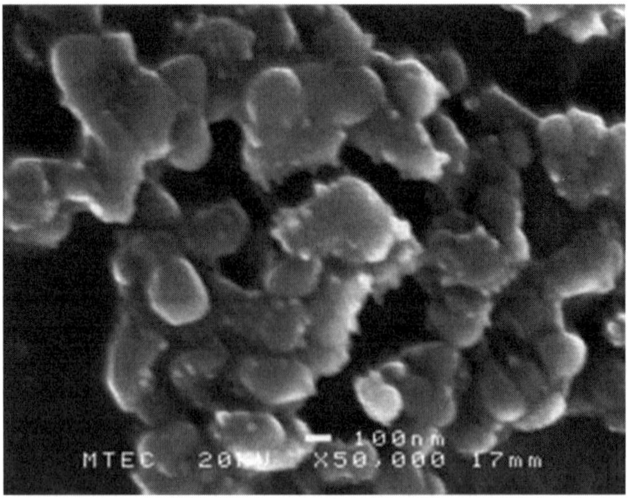

Fig. 26.12 SEM image of CoQ_{10}-loaded NLC (Teeranachaideekul *et al.* 2007).

nanoemulsions composed solely of liquid lipid. Using Franz diffusion cells, the authors showed that CoQ_{10}-loaded NLC exhibited a biphasic release pattern compared with CoQ_{10}-loaded nanoemulsions, which demonstrated almost constant release. The NLC release patterns were characterized by an initial fast release followed by a prolonged release, which was dependent on the oil content.

Use of CoQ_{10} was also found to be useful in intraocular administration. Nucci *et al.* (2007) revealed that intraocular delivery of CoQ_{10} minimized glutamate increase and provided neuroprotection, suggesting that oxidative stress might be implicated in the mechanisms of retinal ganglion cell (RGC) death. Using an established animal model of retinal ischemia/reperfusion, the authors discovered that synaptic glutamate increased at 130 min starting from reperfusion and delayed apoptosis in the RGC layer (at 24 h). Eye protection by CoQ_{10} was also shown by Brancato *et al.* (2002). Treatment of rabbit eyes before excimer laser photorefractive keratectomy (PRK) with CoQ_{10} and vitamin E lowered the number of apoptotic events. Moreover, vitamin E, which itself has less antiapoptotic activity than ubiquinone Q_{10}, when applied simultaneously, significantly enhanced the antiapoptotic properties of ubiquinone Q_{10} both *in vivo* and *in vitro*.

26.8 Summary

Coenzyme Q_{10} is a promising agent for treatment of mitochondrial disorders, cardiomyopathies, and degenerative muscle and neurological diseases such as Parkinson, Huntington, Alzheimer. Although it is known to be synthesized in the body, during aging its level is gradually decreased, and in some cases may be even lower than at birth. CoQ_{10} products currently available on the market include powder-based compressed tablets, chewable tablets, powder-filled hard-shell capsules, and softgels containing an oil suspension.

New technologies and delivery vehicles are presented to overcome its poor and slow absorption. It was shown that the beneficial properties of CoQ_{10} can be utilized for topical and oral administration by enhancing its aqueous solubility, and chemical and physical stability, and using nanoparticles as delivery vehicles, thereby improving its bioavailability. It was demonstrated that the size of the carrier particles can influence internalization via the M cells, thereby affecting the bioavailability of the entrapped molecule. Accordingly, the bioavailability of CoQ_{10} was tested in various carriers starting from powders, oil suspensions, emulsions, microemulsions, and micro- and nanoparticles (with or without surfactant). The advantages and disadvantages of the examined carriers were discussed.

26.9 References

ÅBERG F, APPELKVIST EL, DALLNER G and ERNSTER L (1992), 'Distribution and redox state of ubiquinones in rat and human tissues', *Arch Biochem Biophys*, **295**, 230–234.

ANKOLA DD, WISWANAD B, BIHARDWAY V, RAMARAO P and KUMAR MNVR (2007), 'Development of potent oral nanoparticulate formulation of coenzyme Q_{10} for treatment of hypertension: can the simple nutritional supplements be used as first line therapeutic agents for prophylaxis/therapy?', *Eur J Pharm Biopharm*, **67**, 361–369.

BEAL MF and MATTHEWS RF (1997), 'Coenzyme Q10 in the central nervous system and its potential usefulness in the treatment of neurodegenerative diseases', *Mol Aspects Med*, **18**, 169–179.

BENTINGER M, BRISMAR K and DALLNER G (2007), 'The antioxidant role of coenzyme Q', *Mitochondrion*, **7S**, S41–S50.

BHAGAVAN HN and CHOPRA RK (2007), 'Plasma coenzyme Q_{10} response to oral ingestion of coenzyme Q_{10} formulations', *Mitochondrion*, **7S**, S78–S88.

BRACCO U, LÖLIGER J and SAUCY F (1993), 'Protection of a food, cosmetic or pharmaceutical product against oxidation', US Patent No. 5,258,179.

BRANCATO R, FIORE T, PAPUCCI L, SCHIAVONE N, FORMIGLI L, ORLANDINI SZ, GOBBI PG, CARONES F, DONNINI M, LAPUCCI A and CAPACCIOLI S (2002), 'Concomitant effect of topical ubiquinone Q_{10} and vitamin E to prevent keratocyte apoptosis after excimer laser photoablation in rabbits', *J Refract Surg*, **18**, 135–139.

BUDHIAN A, SIEGEL SJ and WINEY KI (2005), 'Production of haloperidol-loaded PLGA nanoparticles for extended controlled drug release of haloperidol', *J Microencapsul*, **22**, 773–785.

CABRINI L, PASQUALI P, TADOLINI B, SECHI AM and LANDI L (1986), 'Antioxidant behavior of ubiquinone and β-carotene incorporated in model membranes', *Free Radic Res*, **2**, 85–92.

CONTESTABILE A (2001), 'Oxidative stress in neurodegeneration: mechanisms and therapeutic perspectives', *Curr Top Med Chem*, **1**, 553–568.

CRANE FL, HATEFI Y, LESTER RL and WIDMER C (1957), 'Isolation of a quinine from beef heart mitochondria', *Biochim Biophys Acta*, **25**, 220–221.

DESAI MP, LABHASETWAR V, AMIDON GL and LEVY RJ (1996), 'Gastrointestinal uptake of biodegradable microparticles: effect of particle size', *Pharm Res*, **13**, 1838–1845.

DRÖGE W (2002), 'Free radicals in the physiological control of cell function', *Physiol Rev*, **82**, 47–95.

EDLUND C, HOLMBERG K, DALLNER G, NORRBY E and KRISTENSSON K (1994), Ubiquinone-10 protects neurons from virus-induced degeneration, *J Neurochem*, **63**, 634–639.

ELMBERGER FG, KALEN A, BRUNK UT and DALLNER G (1989), 'Discharge of newly-synthesized dolichol and ubiquinone with lipoproteins to rat liver perfusate and to the bile', *Lipids*, **24**, 919–930.

ERNSTER L and DALLNER G (1995), 'Biochemical, physiological and medical aspects of ubiquinone function', *Biochim Biophys Acta*, **1271**, 195–204.

ERNSTER L and FORSMARK-ANDREE P (1993), 'Ubiquinol: an endogenous antioxidant in aerobic organisms', *Clin Investig*, **71**, 60–65.

ERNSTER L, LEE IY, NORLING B and PERSSON B (1969), 'Studies with ubiquinone-depleted submitochondrial particles. Essentiality of ubiquinone for the interaction of succinate dehydrogenase, NADH dehydrogenase, and cytochrome *b*', *Eur J Biochem*, **9**, 299–310.

FESTENSTEIN GN, HEATON FW, LOWE JS and MORTON RA (1955), 'A constituent of the unsaponifiable portion of animal tissue lipids (λ_{max} 272mμ)', *Biochem J*, **59**, 558–566.

GARTI N, SHARABI H and ASERIN A (to be published), Ubiquinone solubilized in microemulsion'.

GRÜNLER J, ERICSSON J and DALLNER G (1994), 'Branch-point reactions in the biosynthesis of cholesterol, dolichol, ubiquinone and prenylated proteins', *Biochim Biophys Acta*, **1212**, 259–277.

HOPPE U, BERGEMANN J, DIEMBECK W, ENNEN J, GOHLA S, HARRIS I, JACOB J, KIELHOLZ J, MEI W, POLLET D, SCHACHTSCHABEL D, SAUERMANN G, SCHREINER V, STÄB F and STECKEL F (1999), 'Coenzyme Q_{10}, a cutaneous antioxidant and energizer', *BioFactors*, **9**, 371–378.

HSU C-H, CUI Z, MUMPER RJ and JAY M (2003), 'Preparation and characterization of novel coenzyme Q_{10} nanoparticles engineered from microemulsion precursors', *Pharm Sci Tech*, **4**, 1–12.

HUSSAIN N, JAITLEY V and FLORENCE AT (2001), 'Recent advances in the understanding of uptake of microparticulates across the gastrointestinal lymphatics', *Adv Drug Del Rel*, **50**, 107–142.

KALEN A, APPELKVIST EL and DALLNER G (1989), 'Age-related changes in the lipid compositions of rat and human tissues', *Lipids*, **24**, 579–584.

KOMMURU TR, GURLEY B, KHAN MA and REDDY IK (2001), 'Self-emulsifying drug delivery systems (SEDDS) of coenzyme Q_{10}: formulation development and bioavailability assessment', *Int J Pharm*, **212**, 233–246.

LEKLI I, DAS S, DAS S, MUKHERJEE S, BAK I, JUHASZ B, BAGCHI D, TRIMURTULU G, KRISHNARAJU AV, SENGUPTA K, TOSAKI A and DAS DK (2008), 'Coenzyme Q_9 provides cardioprotection after converting into coenzyme Q_{10}', *J Agric Food Chem*, **56**, 5331–5337.

LENAZ G (1998), 'Quinone specificity of complex I', *Biochim Biophys Acta*, **1364**, 207–221.

LENAZ G, SAMORI B, FATO R, BATTINO M, PARENTI CASTELLI G and DOMINI I (1992), 'Localization and preferred orientations of ubiquinone homologs in model bilayers', *Biochem Cell Biol*, **70**, 504–514.

MAEDA H (2001), 'The enhanced permeability and retention (EPR) effect in tumor vasculature: the key role of tumor-selective macromolecular drug targeting', *Adv Enzyme Regul*, **41**, 189–207.

MANZOLI U, ROSSI E, LITTARRU GP, FRUSTACI A, LIPPA S, ORADEI A and AURELI V (1990), 'Coenzyme Q_{10} in dilated cardiomyopathy', *Int J Tissue React*, **12**, 173–178.

MATSURA T, YAMADA K and KAWASAKI T (1991), 'Changes in the content and intracellular distribution of coenzyme Q homologs in rabbit liver during growth', *Biochim Biophys Acta*, **1083**, 277–282.

MILES MV, HORN P, MILES L, TANG P, STEELE P and DEGRAUW T (2002), 'Bioequivalence of coenzyme Q_{10} from over-the-counter supplements', *Nutr Res*, **22**, 919–929.

MITCHELL P (1976), 'Possible molecular mechanisms of the protonmotive function of cytochrome systems', *J Theor Biol*, **62**, 327–367.

MÜLLER RH, PETERSEN RD, HOMMOSS A and PARDEIKE J (2007), 'Nanostructured lipid carriers (NLC) in cosmetic dermal products', *Adv Drug Deliv Rev*, **59**, 522–530.

NEHILLA BJ, BERGKVIST M, POPAT KC and DESAI TA (2008), 'Purified and surfactant-free coenzyme Q_{10}-loaded biodegradable nanoparticles', *Int J Pharm*, **348**, 107–114.

NUCCI C, TARTAGLIONE R, CERULLI A, MANCINO R, SPANÒ A, CAVALIERE F, ROMBOLÀ L, BAGETTA G, CORASANITI MT and MORRONE LA (2007), 'Retinal damage caused by high intraocular pressure-induced transient ischemia is prevented by coenzyme Q_{10} in rat', *Int Rev Neurobiol*, **82**, 397–406.

PALOZZA P and KRINSKY NI (1992a), 'Astaxanthin and canthaxanthin are potent antioxidants in a membrane model', *Arch Biochem Biophys*, **297**, 291–295.

PALOZZA P and KRINSKY NI (1992b), 'β-carotene and α-tocopherol are synergistic antioxidants', *Arch Biochem Biophys*, **297**, 184–187.

PAPA S (1996), 'Mitochondrial oxidative phosphorylation changes in the life span. Molecular aspects and physiopathological implications', *Biochim Biophys Acta*, **1276**, 87–105.

PETILLO D and HULTIN HO (2008), 'Ubiquinone-10 as an antioxidant', *J Food Biochem*, **32**, 173–181.

PETILLO D, HULTIN HO, KRZYNOWEK J and AUTIO WR (1998), 'Kinetics of antioxidant loss in mackerel light and dark muscle', *J Agric Food Chem*, **46**, 4128–4137.

PROSEK M, BUTINAR J, LUKANC B, MILIVOJEVIC FIR M, MILIVOJEVIC L, KRIZMAN M and SMIDOVNIK A (2008), 'Bioavailability of water-soluble CoQ_{10} in beagle dogs', *J Pharm Biomed Analysis*, **47**, 918–922.

SAHOO SK, PANYAM J, PRABHA S and LABHASETWAR V (2002), 'Residual polyvinyl alcohol associated with poly (D,L-lactide-*co*-glycolide) nanoparticles affects their physical properties and cellular uptake', *J Control Release*, **82**, 105–114.

SARASTE M (1999), 'Oxidative phosphorylation at the fin de siècle', *Science*, **283**, 1488–1493.

SCHULTZ BE and CHAN SI (2001), 'Structures and proton-pumping strategies of mitochondrial respiratory enzymes', *Annu Rev Biophys Biomol Struct*, **30**, 23–65.

SCHULZ C, OBERMÜLLER-JEVIC UC, HASSELLWANDER O, BERNHARDT J and BIESALSKI HK (2006), 'Comparison of the relative bioavailability of different coenzyme Q_{10} formulations with a novel solubilizate (Solu™ Q10)', *Int J Food Sci Nutr*, **57**, 546–555.

SHULTS CW, HAAS RH, PASSOV D and BEAL MF (1997), 'Coenzyme Q_{10} levels correlate with the activities of complexes I and II/III in mitochondria from parkinsonian and nonparkinsonian subjects, *Ann Neurol*, **42**, 261–264.

SKULACHEV VP (1998), 'Uncoupling: new approaches to an old problem of bioenergetics', *Biochim Biophys Acta*, **1363**, 100–124.

SMEITINK J, VAN DEN HEUVEL L and DIMAURO S (2001), 'The genetics and pathology of oxidative phosphorylation', *Nature Rev*, **2**, 342–352.

SÖDERBERG M, EDLUND C, ALAFUZOFF I, KRISTENSSON K and DALLNER G (1992), 'Lipid composition in different regions of the brain in Alzheimer's disease/senile dementia of Alzheimer's type', *J Neurochem*, **59**, 1646–1653.

TEERANACHAIDEEKUL V, SOUTO EB, JUNYAPRASERT VB and MÜLLER RH (2007), 'Cetyl palmitate-based NLC for topical delivery of coenzyme Q_{10} – development, physicochemical characterization and *in vitro* release studies', *Eur J Pharm Biopharm*, **67**, 141–148.

TERAO J (1989), 'Antioxidant activity of β-carotene-related carotenoids in solution', *Lipids*, **24**, 659–661.

TURUNEN M, OLSSONC J and DALLNER G (2004), 'Metabolism and function of coenzyme Q', *Biochim Biophys Acta*, **1660**, 171–199.

VERMA DD, HARTNER WC, THAKKAR V, LEVECHENKO TS and TORCHILIN VP (2007), 'Protective effect of coenzyme Q10-loaded liposomes on the myocardium in rabbits with an acute experimental myocardial infarction', *Pharm Res*, **24**, 2131–2137.

WAJDA R, ZIRKEL J and SCHAFFER T (2007), 'Increase of bioavailability of coenzyme Q_{10} and vitamin E', *J Med Food*, **10**, 731–734.

WARNER MG (2000), 'Complementary and alternative therapies for hypertension', *Complementary Health Prac Rev*, **6**, 11–19.

WOOD ZA, POOLE LB and KARPLUS PA (2003), 'Peroxiredoxin evolution and the regulation of hydrogen peroxide signaling', *Science*, **300**, 650–653.

YOSHIDA H, YUSIN M, REN I, KUHLENKAMP J, HIRANO T, STOLZ A and KAPLOWITZ N (1992), 'Identification, purification, and immunochemical characterization of a tocopherol-binding protein in rat liver cytosol', *J Lipid Res*, **33**, 343–350.

ZHANG Y, ÅBERG F, APPELKVIST EL, DALLNER G and ERNSTER L (1995), 'Uptake of dietary coenzyme Q supplement is limited in rats', *J Nutr*, **125**, 446–453.

Index